ENVIRONMENTAL MEDICINE

ENVIRONMENTAL MEDICINE

Stuart M. Brooks, M.D.
Professor and Chairman
Department of Environmental and Occupational Health
College of Public Health;
Director
Occupational and Environmental Medicine Residency Program
College of Medicine
University of South Florida
Tampa, Florida

Michael Gochfeld, M.D., Ph.D.
Director
Occupational and Environmental Medicine Residency
Program
Occupational Health Division
Environmental and Occupational Health Sciences Institute
Robert Wood Johnson Medical School
Rutgers University
Piscataway, New Jersey

Jessica Herzstein, M.D., MPH
Assistant Clinical Professor of Medicine
Temple University School of Medicine
Philadelphia, Pennsylvania;
Director
Center for Occupational and Environmental Health
Abington Memorial Hospital
Abington, Pennsylvania

Richard J. Jackson, M.D., MPH
Director
National Center for Environmental Health
Centers for Disease Control and Prevention
Atlanta, Georgia

Marc B. Schenker, M.D.
Professor and Chief
Divisions of Occupational and Environmental Medicine
and Epidemiology
University of California, Davis
Davis, California

with 163 illustrations

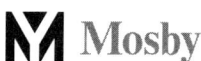

St. Louis Baltimore Boston Carlsbad Chicago Naples New York Philadelphia Portland
London Madrid Mexico City Singapore Sydney Tokyo Toronto Wiesbaden

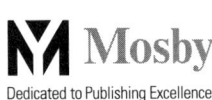

Mosby
Dedicated to Publishing Excellence

A Times Mirror
Company

Editor: Laura DeYoung
Editorial Assistant: Alicia E. Moten
Project Manager: Linda McKinley
Editing and Production: University Graphics Production Services
Manufacturing Supervisor: Karen Lewis

Copyright © 1995 Mosby–Year Book, Inc.

All rights reserved. No part of this publication may be reproduced, stored in a retrieval system, or transmitted, in any form or by any means, electronic, mechanical, photocopying, recording, or otherwise, without prior written permission from the publisher.

Permission to photocopy or reproduce solely for internal or personal use is permitted for libraries or other users registered with the Copyright Clearance Center, provided that the base fee of $4.00 per chapter plus $.10 per page is paid directly to the Copyright Clearance Center, 27 Congress Street, Salem, MA 01970. This consent does not extend to other kinds of copying, such as copying for general distribution, for advertising or promotional purposes, for creating new collected works, or for resale.

Printed in the United States of America
Composition by University Graphics, Inc.
Printing/binding by Maple-Vail Book Mfg. Group

Mosby–Year Book, Inc.
11830 Westline Industrial Drive
St. Louis, Missouri 63146

Library of Congress Cataloging in Publication Data

Environmental medicine / Stuart M. Brooks . . . [et al.].
     p. cm.
    Includes bibliographical references and index.
    ISBN 0-8016-6469-1
    1. Environmental health.   2. Environmentally induced diseases.
 I. Brooks, Stuart M.
    [DNLM: 1. Environmental Health.   2. Environmental Pollution—
adverse effects.   3. Environmental Pollution—prevention & control.
    4. Environmental Pollutants—toxicity.   WA 30 E63887 1995]
    RA565.E52   1995
    616.9′8—dc20
    DNLM/DLC
    for Library of Congress   94-42249
                                                CIP

94 95 96 97 98 / 9 8 7 6 5 4 3 2 1

We wish to dedicate this book to the primary care providers, physician specialists, nurses, and health professionals who seek more knowledge of the environmental medical problems they manage. We hope this book fulfills your needs and that it becomes a useful tool for translating complex environmental information into sound advice for you and your patients.

ACKNOWLEDGMENTS

I would like to thank Ms. Lynette Benson. Her organization and editorial assistance were important in bringing this book together. I must also mention the invaluable assistance furnished by the staff of Mosby. I especially want to acknowledge Mr. James Shanahan, who helped initiate this book, and Ms. Laura DeYoung, who was instrumental in bringing the project to completion.

On a more personal note I wish to say to my wife, Dena, and my son Cameron, I thank you for your continued support and encouragement. To my daughters, Cheri, Amy, and Melissa, I value your curiosity and views on environmental issues.

Stuart M. Brooks, M.D.

To my wife, Joanna Burger, our children, Deborah and David Gochfeld, and my parents, Anne and Alex Gochfeld—and all who strive for a healthier environment.

Michael Gochfeld, M.D., Ph.D.

I wish to acknowledge the two people who had the greatest impact on my career in occupational medicine: Drs. Donald Whorton and Mark R. Cullen. They first showed me the broad public health impact of this field when I was searching for a specialty within medicine, and the latter has been a source of knowledge and inspiration in this dynamic field.

It must be said that the editor, Laura DeYoung, had an enduring commitment to this book, which helped the editors and contributors overcome challenges and meet deadlines. Finally, I would like to dedicate the book to my family, who with patience and understanding witnessed the many weekends this project absorbed.

Jessica Herzstein, M.D., MPH

I wish to thank my wife, Heath, for her years of support, encouragement, and tolerance of my work, and my children, Yael, Phoebe, and Hilary, for being constant sources of joy, inspiration, and pride. I am grateful to Dr. Frank Speizer for his critical guidance and the development of my career, and Dr. Joseph Silva, Jr., for his steadfast support at U.C., Davis.

Marc Schenker, M.D.

I would like to acknowledge and give thanks to my colleagues at the California Department of Health Services and the California Environmental Protection Agency.

Richard Jackson, M.D., MPH

CONTRIBUTORS

Christine Abarca, B.A.
Research Associate
College of Medicine
University of South Florida
Tampa, Florida

Henry L. Abrons, M.D.
Associate Professor
Department of Pulmonary and Critical Medicine
West Virginia University
Morgantown, West Virginia

Khalid Ali, M.D.
Resident
Department of Internal Medicine
Baptist Medical Center
Montgomery, Alabama

Ilene B. Anderson, Pharm. D.
Assistant Clinical Professor of Pharmacy
University of California, San Francisco;
Poison Information Specialist
San Francisco Bay Area Regional Poison Control Center
San Francisco General Hospital
San Francisco, California

Daniel E. Banks, M.D.
Associate Professor
Department of Pulmonary and Critical Care Medicine
West Virginia University
Morgantown, West Virginia

C. Stuart Baxter, M.D.
Staff
Department of Environmental Health
University of Cincinnati Medical Center
Cincinnati, Ohio

Cynthia Bearer, M.D.
Assistant Professor of Pediatrics
Rainbow Babies and Childrens Hospital
Cleveland, Ohio

Lynette Benson, Ph.D.
Fellow—Medical Anthropology
ASTDR
Atlanta, Georgia

Jan Beyea, Ph.D.
Vice President and Chief
National Audubon Society
New York, New York

Sue Binder, M.D.
Chief
Lead Poisoning Prevention Branch
Centers for Disease Control and Prevention
Atlanta, Georgia

Eddy Bresnitz, M.D.
Professor and Chairman
Department of Community and Preventive Medicine
Medical College of Pennsylvania and Hahnemann University
School of Medicine
Philadelphia, Pennsylvania

Stuart M. Brooks, M.D.
Professor and Chairman
Department of Environmental and Occupational Health
College of Public Health;
Director
Occupational and Environmental Medicine Residency Program
College of Medicine
University of Florida
Tampa, Florida

Joseph P. Brown, Ph.D.
Acting Chief
Water Toxicology Unit
Pesticide and Environmental Toxicology Section
University of California
Berkeley, California

CONTRIBUTORS

Patricia A. Buffler, Ph.D., MPH
Professor
Epidemiology
School of Public Health
University of California
Berkeley, California

Lois Bullock, M.D.
Department of Environmental and Community Medicine
UMDMJ/Robert Wood Johnson Medical School
Rutgers University
Piscataway, New Jersey

Joanna Burger, Ph.D.
Professor of Biology;
Director
Graduate Program in Ecology and Evolution
Department of Biological Sciences
Rutgers University
Piscataway, New Jersey

Peter Casten, Jr., M.D.
Staff
Ochsner Clinic
Department of Occupational Medicine
New Orleans, Louisiana

Jim Cook, Ph.D.
Staff Scientist
National Audubon Society
Scully Science Center
Islip, New York

James Craner, M.D., MPH
Principal
Tahoe Associates in Occupational and Environmental Medicine
Carson City, Nevada

Mark R. Cullen, M.D.
Director
Occupational and Environmental Medicine Program
Yale University School of Medicine
New Haven, Connecticut

Francis N. Duke-Dobos, M.D.
Adjunct Professor
College of Public Health
University of South Florida
Tampa, Florida

Edward A. Emmett, M.D.
National Institute of Occupational Health and Safety
Worksafe Australia
Sydney, Australia

Enrique Fernandez-Caldas, Ph.D.
Associate Professor
Division of Allergy and Clinical Immunology
Department of Internal Medicine
University of South Florida
Tampa, Florida

Nancy Fiedler, M.D.
Associate Professor
Occupational Health Division
Environmental and Occupational Health Sciences Institute
UMDMJ/Robert Wood Johnson Medical School
Rutgers University
Piscataway, New Jersey

Lora E. Fleming, M.D.
Assistant Professor
Department of Epidemiology and Public Health
University of Miami School of Medicine
Miami, FLorida

Roger W. Fox, M.D.
Associate Professor
Department of Internal Medicine
University of South Florida
Tampa, Florida

Arthur Frank, M.D.
Professor and Chairman
Department of Preventive Medicine and Environmental Health
University of Kentucky College of Medicine
Lexington, Kentucky

David J. Garling, M.D., Ph.D.
Fellow
Occupational and Environmental Medicine
University of Cincinnati College of Medicine
Cincinnati, Ohio

Michael Gochfeld, M.D., Ph.D.
Director
Occupational and Environmental Medicine Residency Program
Occupational Health Division
Environmental and Occupational Health Sciences Institute
UMDMJ/Robert Wood Johnson Medical School
Rutgers University
Piscataway, New Jersey

David F. Goldsmith, Ph.D.
Senior Research Assistant
Western Consortium for Public Health
Berkeley, California

Jeanette Gomez, M.D.
Graduate School of Public Health
University of Pittsburgh
Pittsburgh, Pennsylvania

Yehia Y. Hammad, Sc.D.
Professor
Department of Occupational and Environmental Health
College of Public Health
University of South Florida
Tampa, Florida

Robert Harrison, M.D.
Staff
Air Toxicology and Epidemiology Section
University of California
Berkeley, California

David T. Harvey, M.D.
Chief Resident
Dermatology
Division of Dermatology and Cutaneous Surgery
College of Medicine
University of South Florida
Tampa, Florida

Edward B. Hayes, M.D.
Director
Year 2000 Project
Division of Disease Control
Augusta, Maine

Jessica Herzstein, M.D., MPH
Assistant Clinical Professor of Medicine
Temple University School of Medicine
Philadelphia, Pennsylvania;
Director
Center for Occupational and Environmental Health
Abington Memorial Hospital
Abington, Pennsylvania

Daniel J. Hogan, M.D., F.R.C.P.
Professor of Dermatology
Division of Dermatology and Cutaneous Surgery
College of Medicine
University of South Florida
Tampa, Florida

Patricia H. Hiatt, M.D.
Private Practice
Elkgrove, California

Richard J. Jackson, M.D., MPH
Director
National Center for Environmental Health
Centers for Disease Control and Prevention
Atlanta, Georgia

Susan Kim, Pharm.D.
Assistant Clinical Professor
School of Pharmacy
University of California, San Francisco;
Poison Information Specialist
San Francisco Bay Area Regional Poison Control Center
San Francisco General Hospital
San Francisco, California

Judith B. Klotz, M.D.
Program Manager
New Jersey Department of Health
Trenton, New Jersey

Jeffrey D. Laskin, M.D., Ph.D.
Professor
Occupational Medicine
Occupational Health Division
Environmental and Occupational Health Sciences Institute
UMDNJ/Robert Wood Johnson Medical School
Rutgers University
Piscataway, New Jersey

Douglas H. Linz, M.D., M.S.
Director
Occupational Medicine Residency Project
Center of Occupational Health
Holmes Hospital—Tate Wing
Cincinnati, Ohio

Michael Lipsett, M.D., MPH
Staff
Air Toxicology and Epidemiology Section
University of California
Berkeley, California

Katherine Loftfield, M.D.
Staff
Ochsner Clinic
New Orleans, Louisiana

Max R. Lum, Ph.D.
Health Education Program
ASTDR
Cincinnati, Ohio

Clement A. Maccia, M.D.
Private Practice
Cranford, New Jersey

Yogesh Manocha, M.Sc.
College of Public Health
University of South Florida
Tampa, Florida

Joyce Martin, J.D.
Private Practice
Indianapolis, Indiana

Todd McCune, M.D.
Staff
Ochsner Clinic
New Orleans, Louisiana

Donald R. Mattison, M.D.
Staff
Graduate School of Public Health
University of Pittsburgh
Pittsburgh, Pennsylvania

Tim Molon, M.D.
Staff
Department of Occupational Medicine
Ochsner Clinic
New Orleans, Louisiana

Kent R. Olson, M.D.
HIRAB CAL-EPA
Berkeley, California

Thomas R. Parker, M.Sc.
Toxicologist
State of California
Office of Environmental Hazard Assessment
Sacramento, California

David Parkinson, M.D.
Private Practice
Middle Island, New York

Susan Pollack, M.D.
Assistant Professor
Departments of Pediatrics and Preventive Medicine
University of Kentucky
Lexington, Kentucky

Leon Prockop, M.D.
Department of Medicine
College of Medicine
University of South Florida
Tampa, Florida

Lee A. Reed, M.D.
Associate Professor
Department of Pulmonary and Critical Care Medicine
West Virginia University
Morgantown, West Virginia

Karen M. Reiser, M.D.
Staff
Department of Medicine
School of Medicine
University of California, Davis
Davis, California

Ira S. Richards, M.D.
Staff
Department of Environmental and Occupational Health
College of Public Health
University of South Florida
Tampa, Florida

Mark G. Robson, Ph.D.
Executive Director
Occupational Health Division
Environmental and Occupational Health Sciences Institute
UMDMJ/Robert Wood Johnson Medical School
Rutgers University
Piscataway, New Jersey

Linda Rosenstock, M.D.
Director
NIOSH
Hubert H. Humphrey Building
Washington, D.C.

Jonathan M. Samet, M.D.
Professor and Chairman
Department of Epidemiology
School of Hygiene and Public Health
The Johns Hopkins University
Baltimore, Maryland

Marc B. Schenker, M.D.
Professor and Chief
Divisions of Occupational and Environmental Medicine and Epidemiology
ITEH
University of California, Davis
Davis, California

Steven M. Schrader, Ph.D.
Chief
Functional Toxicology Section
NIOSH
Cincinnati, Ohio

Paul A. Schulte
Chief
Screening and Notification Section
UWSB, DSHEFS
Cincinnati, Ohio

Randy L. Schuler, Ph.D.
Private Practice
Trenton, New Jersey

Stuart L. Shalat, M.D.
Assistant Professor
Department of Epidemiology and Public Health
University of Miami School of Medicine
Miami, Florida

Robert Snyder, Ph.D.
Chairman and Director
Joint Graduate Program, Toxicology
Rutgers University
Piscataway, New Jersey

Yuen T. So, M.D.
Staff
Department of Neurology
University of California General Hospital, San Francisco
San Francisco, California

Virginia H. Sublet, Ph.D.
Health Education Program
ASTDR
Cincinnati, Ohio

Doug Swift, M.D.
Chairman
Occupational Medicine
Department of Occupational Medicine
Ochsner Clinic
New Orleans, Louisiana

Andor Szentivanyi, M.D.
Staff
Department of Medicine
College of Medicine
University of South Florida
Tampa, Florida

Dennis D. Tolsma, M.D.
Senior Advisor for Prevention
NIOSH
Centers for Disease Control and Prevention
Atlanta, Georgia

Iris G. Udasin, M.D.
Clinical Associate Professor
UMDNJ/Robert Wood Johnson Medical School
Rutgers University
Piscataway, New Jersey

Mark J. Utell, M.D.
Director
Pulmonary/Critical Care Unit
Department of Medicine
University of Rochester
Rochester, New York

Timothy Varney, P.G.
Vice President
Environmental Risk Management
Lakeland, Florida

Gary Walker, M.S.
Deputy Director
Assistant Professor
College of Public Health
University of South Florida
Tampa, Florida

Daniel Wartenberg, M.D., Ph.D.
Associate Professor
Department of Environmental and Community Medicine
UMDMJ/Robert Wood Johnson Medical School
Rutgers University
Piscataway, New Jersey

Donald E. Wasserman, MSEE, MBA
Private Practice
Cincinnati, Ohio

Contents

PART I PRINCIPLES IN ENVIRONMENTAL MEDICINE

1 **Overview of Environmental Medicine,** 3
Michael Gochfeld

2 **Types and Sources of Environmental Hazards,** 9
Stuart M. Brooks, Lynette Benson, Michael Gochfeld

3 **Risk Assessment Applied to Environmental Medicine,** 30
David F. Goldsmith

4 **Principles of Exposure Assessment,** 37
Yehia Y. Hammad, Yogesh Manocha

5 **Uses of Epidemiology in Environmental Medicine,** 46
Patricia A. Buffler

PART II BASIC SCIENCE OF ENVIRONMENTAL MEDICINE: MECHANICS AND PRINCIPLES

6 **Principles of Toxicology,** 65
Michael Gochfeld

7 **Carcinogenesis,** 78
C. Stuart Baxter

8 **Assessment of Male Reproductive Function,** 95
Steven M. Schrader

9 **Female Reproductive System,** 101
Jeannette Gomez, Donald R. Mattison

10 **Developmental Toxicology,** 115
Cynthia Bearer

11 **Toxicology of Selected Neurotoxic Agents,** 129
Douglas H. Linz, David J. Garling

12 **Environmental Immunotoxicology,** 139
Andor Szentivanyi, Khalid Ali, Christine Abarca, Leon Prockop, Stuart M. Brooks

13 **The Immunology of Cancer,** 156
Andor Szentivanyi, Khalid Ali, Christine Abarca, Leon Prockop, Stuart M. Brooks

14 **Respiratory Toxicology,** 166
Ira S. Richards, Stuart M. Brooks

15 **Dermal Toxicology,** 182
Edward A. Emmett

16 **Neurobehavioral Toxicity and Testing,** 189
Nancy Fiedler, Joanna Burger, Michael Gochfeld

17 **Bone Marrow Toxicology,** 201
Robert Snyder

PART III   CLINICAL ENVIRONMENTAL MEDICINE

18 **Clinical Approach and Establishing a Diagnosis of an Environmental Medical Disorder,** 217
Mark R. Cullen, Linda Rosenstock, Stuart M. Brooks

19 **The Environmental History,** 232
Arthur Frank

TOPICS IN CLINICAL SYSTEMS

20 **The Eyes and Vision,** 240
Peter Casten Jr., Katherine Loftfield

21 **Disorders of the Ear and Hearing,** 250
Doug Swift, Tim Molon

22 **Common Environmental Dermatoses,** 263
David T. Harvey, Daniel J. Hogan

23 **Disorders of the Upper and Lower Respiratory Tract,** 282
Henry L. Abrons, Daniel E. Banks, Lee A. Reed

24 **Gastrointestinal Tract and Liver,** 298
Todd McCune, Stuart M. Brooks

25 **Kidney and Urinary Tract,** 311
David Parkinson, Stuart M. Brooks

26 **Nervous System,** 318
Yuen T. So

27 **Disorder of the Immunologic System** 326
Clement A. Maccia, Andor Szentivanyi, Khalid Ali, Christine Abarca, Stuart M. Brooks

PART IV SUSCEPTIBLE POPULATIONS AND SPECIAL PATIENT GROUPS

28 General Principles of Susceptibility, 351
Karen M. Reiser

29 Preexisting Conditions and the Elderly, 361
Jessica Herzstein

30 Multiple Chemical Sensitivity: Controversies in Clinical Diagnosis and Management, 368
Robert Harrison

UNIQUE ISSUES AS THEY RELATE TO CHILDREN

31 The Hazards of Pesticides to Children, 377
Richard J. Jackson

32 The Hazards of Lead to Children, 383
Edward B. Hayes

33 The Hazards of Air Pollution to Children, 390
Michael Lipsett

34 Poisoning Due to Household Products, 398
Ilene B. Anderson, Susan Kim

35 Work-Related Injuries and Exposures in Children and Adolescents, 408
Susan Pollack

36 Environmental Health in Minority Communities, 412
Lynette Benson

PART V SPECIFIC ENVIRONMENTAL EXPOSURE SOURCES

AIR POLLUTION

37 Indoor Air Pollution, 419
Enrique Fernandez-Caldas, Roger W. Fox, Ira S. Richards, Timothy C. Varney, Stuart M. Brooks

38 Asbestos Exposure in Buildings, 438
Michael Gochfeld

39 Man-Made Mineral Fibers, 455
Stuart M. Brooks

40 Air Pollution in the Outdoor Environment, 462
Mark J. Utell, Jonathan M. Samet

41 Fire and Pyrolysis Products, 470
Michael Gochfeld

42 Water Pollution, 479
Joseph P. Brown, Richard J. Jackson

43 **Food: Its Quality and Role as a Pathway of Exposure,** 488
James Craner

44 **Natural Carcinogens and Anticarcinogens in the Diet,** 512
Randy L. Schuler, Jeffrey D. Laskin

45 **Soil: Sources, Dynamics, and Routes of Exposure,** 515
Michael Gochfeld

PHYSICAL AGENTS

46 **Ionizing Radiation,** 524
Joanna Burger

47 **Radon,** 534
Judith B. Klotz

48 **Nonionizing Radiation,** 542
Joanna Burger, Michael Gochfeld

49 **Electromagnetic Fields,** 554
Daniel Wartenberg

50 **Vibration,** 557
Donald E. Wasserman

51 **Heat Stress,** 563
Francis N. Dukes-Dobos

52 **High-Altitude and Aerospace Medicine,** 576
Lois Bullock

53 **Chemical Agents,** 592
Michael Gochfeld

54 **Biologic Agents,** 615
Iris G. Udasin

WASTE

55 **Health Implications of Solid Waste Management,** 623
Michael Gochfeld

56 **Community Exposure to Hazardous Waste,** 635
Michael Gochfeld

57 **Assessment and Remediation of Hazardous Waste Sites,** 647
Michael Gochfeld, Joanna Burger

58 **Environmental and Human Health Perspectives on Municipal Composting,** 654
Jim Cook, Jan Beyea

59 **Reuse of Sludge,** 657
Mark G. Robson

60 Incinerator Waste Exposures, 660
Eddy Bresnitz

PART VI PREVENTIVE APPROACHES IN ENVIRONMENTAL MEDICINE

61 Global Aspects of Environmental Health, 669
Joanna Burger, Michael Gochfeld

62 Environmental Health Surveillance, 692
Lora E. Fleming, Jessica Herzstein, Stuart L. Shalat

63 Biomarkers, 698
Paul A. Schulte

64 Hazardous Materials Emergency Medical Response, 705
Patricia H. Hiatt, Kent R. Olson

65 Chemical Disaster Preparedness, 722
Thomas R. Parker

66 Helping Patients Adopt Healthful Life-Style Choices, 729
Dennis D. Tolsma, Jessica Herzstein

67 Health Risk Communication, 737
Virginia H. Sublet, Max R. Lum

APPENDIXES

A Environmental Legislation, 743
Gary Walker, Joyce Martin

B Poison Control Centers, 752
Patricia Hiatt, Kent R. Olson, Virginia H. Sublet,

C Good Information About Hazardous Substances, 755
Virginia H. Sublet

Part I

PRINCIPLES IN ENVIRONMENTAL MEDICINE

Chapter 1

OVERVIEW OF ENVIRONMENTAL MEDICINE

Michael Gochfeld

Focus of environmental medicine and relationship with other disciplines
Approach to environmental medicine
Boundaries of environmental medicine
Environmental medicine versus occupational medicine
The discipline of environmental medicine
Environmental physicians and the environment
Environment and cancer
Physician as risk communicator
Conclusion

Physicians in many types of practice, including primary care[11] and public health, are increasingly confronted by patients with signs, symptoms, or concerns that they attribute to one or more chemical, physical, or biologic agents in their home, community, or workplace. For example, questions arise concerning radon exposure, hazards of electromagnetic fields, and the neurodevelopmental consequences of early childhood lead exposure. Evaluating and managing such patients and identifying, quantifying, and preventing their exposure is the domain of environmental medicine.[17]

An important purpose of this book is to furnish a comprehensive resource of scientific information on environmental health, "the study of effects upon human beings of external physical, chemical, and biologic factors in the general environment."[6] This is a book for health professionals who must face these issues and especially for the practitioner who takes care of patients on a regular basis. A national study conducted by the Institute of Medicine showed that most environmental and occupational medical services are provided by primary care practitioners.[11] It is anticipated that by providing this resource, practitioners and other health professionals can effectively manage patients who are ill and communicate to healthy citizens who are concerned about the risks from various environmental exposures. There is a need for an approach to deal with the very important and unique features of environmental medicine.

FOCUS OF ENVIRONMENTAL MEDICINE AND RELATIONSHIP WITH OTHER DISCIPLINES

Environmental medicine centers on the interface between the person and the environment. Most diseases arise when the body is exposed to some agent or stressor in the environment, and the assessment of exposure assumes the utmost importance as the pivotal feature of environmental medicine.

The diseases one encounters in environmental medicine, for example, contact dermatitis, obstructive lung disease, nephritis, neuropathy, various cancers, and anxiety, are essentially the same diseases that confront colleagues in other fields of medicine and public health. It is the emphasis on the evaluation, documentation, modification, and prevention of an environmental exposure that gives environmental medicine its cohesiveness.

Environmental medicine is closely related to other medical and nonmedical disciplines, as shown in Fig. 1-1. Several disciplines focus on the environment: ecology, environmental science, environmental health, and environmental medicine. Fig. 1-2 expands on this theme, showing further relationships with other medical disciplines such as preventive medicine, community medicine, and occupational medicine.

4   PRINCIPLES IN ENVIRONMENTAL MEDICINE

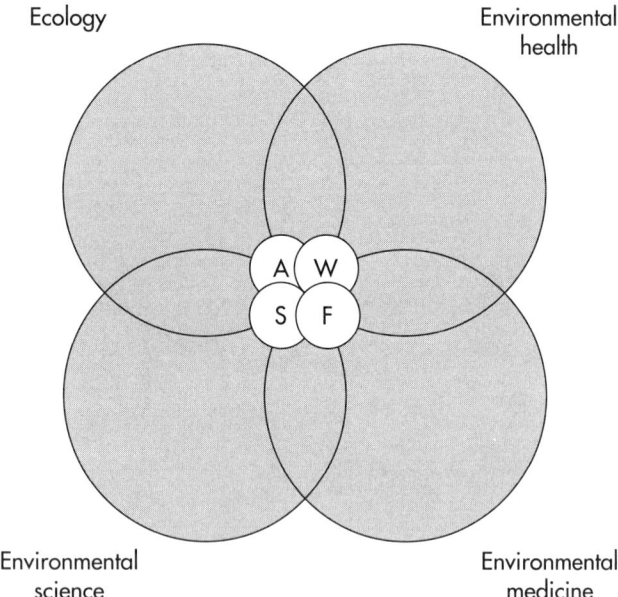

Fig. 1-1. Venn diagram showing relationships among four disciplines, all of which have some focus on the four major environmental media: A = Air, W = Water, S = Soil, F = Food. Ecology is primarily a basic science discipline with a heavy theoretical emphasis as well as an applied emphasis on conservation biology. Environmental science focuses more on the physical or abiotic components of the environment, air, water, and soil. Environmental health is a public health domain, partly overlapping environmental science but carrying it into the sphere of human health, and environmental medicine broadly overlaps environmental health and environmental science and serves as their clinical arm. (With permission of Environmental and Occupational Health Sciences Institute.)

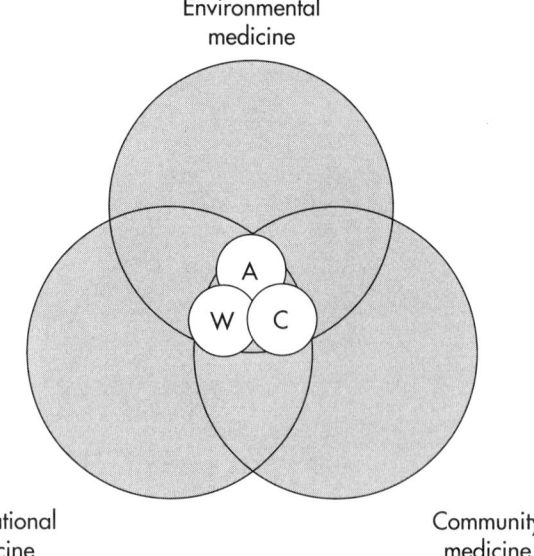

Fig. 1-2. Venn diagram showing relationships among three branches of medicine and their relationships to the three major human environments: A = Abode or Home, C = Community (including schools, shopping areas, recreational areas), W = Workplaces. There is a broad overlap between environmental medicine and occupational medicine. Both overlap community medicine, and all three are part of preventive medicine, although as often practiced some aspects of occupational medicine do not seem to be preventive in nature. Various permutations of the four disciplines are represented in academic departments in about two thirds of American medical schools. The void in the remaining one third of schools is disheartening. (With permission of Environmental and Occupational Health Sciences Institute.)

Ecology, environmental science, environmental health, and environmental medicine all deal with the four environmental media: air, water, soil, and food. Ecology, emerging mainly in the early twentieth century, is the basic and theoretical study of the relationships between living organisms (including humans) and their environment.[14] Environmental health emerged mainly after World War I as a public health endeavor studying the control of environmental factors harmful to human health, initially with a heavy emphasis on sanitation and control of communicable disease.[16] Environmental science, arising mainly after 1960, focuses mainly on the physical environmental media, particularly with regard to pollutants in air, water, and soil. Environmental medicine, arising mainly after 1975, can be viewed as the preventive medicine *and* clinical arm of environmental health, closely related to the above disciplines,[10] focusing on how pollutants in the environmental media enter the body and cause harm. A generic exposure matrix is shown in Table 1-1, and the relationships between contaminated media and routes of exposure are elaborated in Chapter 2 (Types and Sources of Environmental Hazards).

Although historically environmental health was heavily involved in studying and controlling infectious diseases, modern environmental medicine specialists are inclined to relinquish much of the area of infectious disease to other disciplines and to focus mainly on chemical and physical hazards in the environment.

Not only do the various disciplines overlap, but the media interdigitate as well. Airborne pollutants can be deposited on soil, water, and food. Waterborne pollutants can volatilize into the air, can contaminate soil, and may be taken up by plants, thereby entering the food chain. Soil-borne contaminants can enter the air when dust is created, can be carried into surface and groundwater, and can be taken up by plants. Food-borne contaminants contribute less to the other media, although microbial degradation of foods, potential foods, or food wastes can contribute to soil and water pollution.

The fact that there are overlaps among the disciplines is obvious. Pesticides provide an example. Pesticide residues in a community's soil can be a concern of all of these disciplines, albeit in somewhat different ways. Ecologists may focus on how pesticides alter the structure and function of ecosystems by eliminating one or more sensitive species. Environmental scientists may focus on how pesticides move through soil and how they are degraded. Environmental health may focus on the number of people exposed to pes-

Table 1-1. The generic media x route matrix for exposure assessment

Environmental medium	Routes of exposure		
	Ingestion	Inhalation	Dermal
Air	Particulates TSP	++++ PM-10	Variable Vapors Liquids
Soil	Children (100 mg/day)	Re-entrained dust	Muds
Water	++++	Showers Aerosols	Liquids
Food	++++	0	0

Modified from Gochfeld M: *A matrix of routes and media of exposure for risk assessment scenarios,* Piscataway, NJ, 1991, Environmental and Occupational Health Sciences Institute.

ticides. Finally, the practitioner interested in environmental medicine will focus on how individuals or a community are exposed and how exposure can be recognized and prevented.

APPROACH TO ENVIRONMENTAL MEDICINE

For the primary care practitioner, environmental medicine involves the familiar approach of individually evaluating and treating patients who report either an exposure or an illness implicating hazardous substances in the home, community, or workplace environment. Occupational medicine, the specialty involving the health of workers and workplaces, can be considered in part a special form of environmental medicine practice, but the emphasis of this book will be on the nonoccupational environment and the medical issues and disorders associated with exposures in the home, playground, school, highway, mall, and community at large.

In the final analysis no single health professional can address all aspects of environmental medicine such as documenting exposures or recognizing and preventing disease. Our hypothetical community with pesticide contamination in the soil will require an environmental scientist to measure contaminant levels in soil and basements, an environmental health professional to characterize the population at risk, and an environmental medicine practitioner to perform clinical evaluations of people.

BOUNDARIES OF ENVIRONMENTAL MEDICINE

Throughout the book *Enviromental Medicine: Concepts and Practice,* we will use the term *enviromental health* to denote the broader public health province, while the tasks of *environmental medicine* will refer to the responsibilities of the physician or public health specialist who provides assessment and/or management of the individual patient or community.

Confusion may arise regarding the term *environmental medicine* because a group of clinicians, often identified as "clinical ecologists," have called their field "environmental medicine" (they have developed a Board of Environmental Medicine, which, however, is not under the American Board of Medical Specialties). They focus attention mainly on patients who appear to be unusually responsive to very low levels of chemicals, and some of their therapeutic approaches are controversial and not adequately validated. Environmental medicine in the context of this book covers a much broader domain built on scientifically documented principles. However, the basic tenet that clinical ecologists voiced as early as the 1960s,[15] that illness can arise from hitherto unexpected interactions between human susceptibility and environmental hazards, is basic to environmental medicine by any definition.

While Fig. 1-1 examines the relationships of the environmental disciplines to the environmental media, Fig. 1-2 examines the relationships of several branches of medicine to the major human habitats or environments: the home, the community (including schools, shopping areas, places of recreation), and the workplace. The overlaps between the environments are shown in Fig. 1-1. A school may be a community environment for the children, but a work environment for the teachers and other staff. The home may be contaminated by chemicals brought home on the clothes of factory workers and may be the workplace of homemakers and other domestic workers.

ENVIRONMENTAL MEDICINE VERSUS OCCUPATIONAL MEDICINE

Occupational medicine became prominent mainly after 1930 and is concerned with the recognition and prevention of diseases related to the work environment. The tools of the specialty, epidemiology, toxicology, and public health and clinical expertise, are shared with environmental medicine.[6] Community medicine (arising mainly after 1960) shares many of the concerns of environmental health and environmental medicine but has more of a social science emphasis and is more likely to be concerned with health economics and the health infrastructure. Environmental medicine clearly overlaps occupational medicine when the workplace environment is the source of exposure. Environmental medicine somewhat less clearly overlaps community medicine when the community is the focus of exposure. Thus people who identify their specialty as community medicine may have only modest interest when a community being studied has chromium-contaminated soil, while most (though not all) occupational physicians would claim an interest in chromium contamination in the workplaces they encounter.

Although many occupational physicians have focused narrowly on their discipline and have tended to ignore diseases arising from other environments, there has been an increasing recognition that the agents of concern for the workplace (for example, pesticides, heavy metals, noise) are often the same agents that are of concern in the community.[7,9] In 1989 the directors of occupational medicine residency training programs responded to this recognition by agreeing to rename their training programs "occupational and environmental medicine." In 1991 the American College of Occupational Medicine followed suit by renaming itself the American College of Occupational and Environmental Medicine.[1] The American Board of Preventive Medicine considered renaming the subspecialty of occupational medicine but decided against it because its other subspecialties, public health/preventive medicine and aerospace medicine, are also heavily focused on environmental medicine.

Most classes of agents pose the greatest threat in occupational settings where the concentrations or amount of exposure is the greatest and the duration of contact and hence the opportunity to absorb hazardous materials is also the greatest. Moreover, because of their reliance on their income, workers usually do not feel free to walk away from hazardous conditions, particularly those that do not immediately cause adverse effects.

However, increasingly, people have realized that some of the vague and minor discomforts they experience in life may be due to hazardous exposures encountered in their home and community. While this is readily apparent to those who suffer the severe, acute, and time-limited symptoms of hay fever, it is often much less apparent to those who are exposed to vapors emitted by new building materials, household pesticides, and tobacco smoke, although certainly in the last case the risk of significant disease from secondhand smoke in the home is now well documented.

The challenge facing environmental medicine lies not only in the evaluation and management of patients with these exposures, but in research into the contribution of long-term low-level exposure to many environmental agents. Where such exposures are found to cause disease in many people or in a small proportion of unusually susceptible individuals, steps—analogous to those employed by industrial hygiene—must be taken to measure and control the exposures and to ultimately eliminate the hazards. Where exposures do not appear to cause disease, this should be documented as well. In either case a balanced and unbiased perspective, clear educational efforts, and sound public health policies are necessary goals.

THE DISCIPLINE OF ENVIRONMENTAL MEDICINE

Environmental medicine is a broad discipline. Historically clinicians have been trained in the importance of environmental factors as causes or influences of disease. The environment includes all agents outside of the body, including infectious organisms, toxins, and food. The intrinsic factors include the genetic makeup of the host as well as its underlying state of health and history of past illnesses. Disease results from an interplay of these factors when the host defenses are overcome by the agent.

Rosenau[16] defines the domain of preventive medicine in two parts: "... namely, that which deals with the person (hygiene) and that which deals with the environment (sanitation) ... in its relation to health and disease includ(ing) ... discussion of food, water, air, soil, disposal of waste, vital statistics, diseases of occupation, industrial hygiene, school hygiene, disinfection, quarantine, isolation and other topics of sanitary importance, as well as subjects of interest to health officers."

ENVIRONMENTAL PHYSICIANS AND THE ENVIRONMENT

Apparent in all these views of environmental health and environmental medicine is the emphasis on human health rather than environmental quality. The biodiversity and the survival of snail darters or whooping cranes, which capture the attention of conservationists, is not likely to be found in the literature on environmental health or environmental medicine. However, the factors responsible for the decline of some species, such as pollution by chlorinated hydrocarbon pesticides and the health status of fish-eating birds, may have human health significance. Environmental health may use biomonitoring of indicator species to provide early warning of some human health hazards. However, until recently even the major federal agencies responsible for research and protection of the environment (U.S. Environmental Protection Agency [USEPA] and National Institute of Environmental Health Sciences [NIEHS]) have focused almost exclusively on health rather than environmental quality.

The tide is changing, as we shall see. Ecological risk assessment is becoming an important aspect of environmental risk assessment,[2,13] but the distinction between environmental health (human) and ecological health (everything else) remains strong. Environmental medicine plays two major roles in environmental health. It provides the diagnosis and treatment of health complaints attributable to the environment, and it contributes to a much broader understanding of the unity of human health with environmental quality. It provides the basis for understanding what we must do in the next decade and century to ensure that environmental quality will be sufficient to sustain life as we know it.

Sadly, the recognition that this may very well not be the case has come from disciplines (meteorology, evolutionary biology, ecology) lying largely outside the health domain. Moreover, clinicians trained to be skeptical of new and loud claims have not been the first to recognize the importance of environmental impacts, both local and global, on human health.

A specific example is New Jersey, where year after year through the 1980s the public proclaimed environmental health and quality as the number one public policy issue (Eagleton Star Ledger Polls), yet practicing physicians infrequently recognize an environmental basis for their patients' fears or symptoms. Of course, this may be due to the fact that in some cases a patient's fears or concerns are unfounded, but to assert this the clinician bears the responsibility of adequately evaluating the patient—through history, physical examination, appropriate tests, and where necessary through consultation or referral. An environmental basis for disease should not be a diagnosis of exclusion.

ENVIRONMENT AND CANCER

Some of the naturally occurring and artificial substances encountered in air, soil, water, and food are known to cause cancer (see Chapter 25). Some substances can be shown to cause cancer in animals; others cause mutations in in vitro tests such as the Salmonella reversion test or Ames Assay. A few are actually linked to cancer in humans through epidemiologic studies. At present only about 40 to 50 compounds are known to be human carcinogens; an equal number are probable human carcinogens, but many others are listed as possible human carcinogens, based upon their carcinogenicity in animals.[12] It is equally important, however, to note that most chemicals do not have carcinogenic properties.

Frequently one reads that 75% of cancers are environmental in origin. This estimate can be traced to a World Health Organization Expert Committee on the Prevention of Cancer,[18] which actually said that 75% of cancers were preventable. This estimate, of course, refers to all environmental factors, including diet and smoking. The National Institute for Occupational Safety and Health estimated that as many as 20% of cancers might be related to occupation.[3] Two British epidemiologists challenged this view, arguing that no more than 4% were related to work and that the main environmental factor responsible for cancer was smoking (30% of cancers).[5] The truth is somewhere in between, as Davis[4] has proclaimed, relating some of the increases in cancer rates to changing environmental exposures. Recent research has suggested that even breast cancer may have a nondietary environmental component—Wolff et al.[18] reported excess breast cancer cases related to chlorinated hydrocarbon pesticide residues in tissue.

PHYSICIAN AS RISK COMMUNICATOR

Physicians play a unique role in communicating information about risks to patients. Opportunities for risk communication may be missed if the patient does not ask specific questions. However, it is not always easy to answer a patient's specific questions regarding the risks of developing disease or the urgency of eliminating a hazard from their lives.

Very often patients have unbalanced fears. They may worry about pesticide residues in their food while continuing to eat an otherwise unhealthy diet (see Chapter 25) or continuing to smoke. They may worry about the siting of an incinerator in their community while neglecting to test their homes for radon. The clinical interview offers the chance to put these risks into perspective.

Practitioners must be clear that estimates of risks fre-

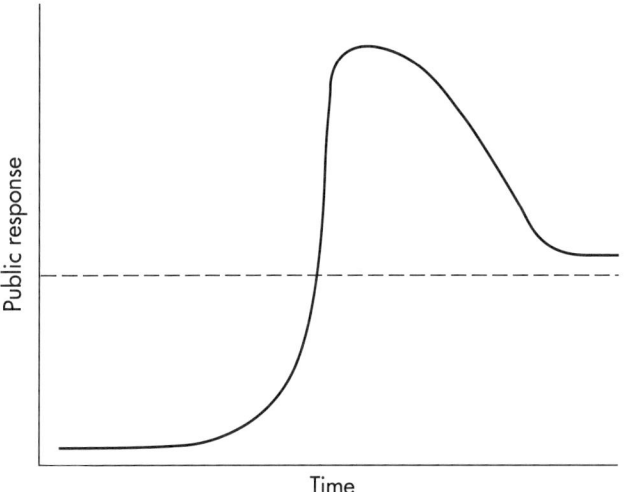

Fig. 1-3. This exemplifies the history over a period of years of a hypothetical environmental hazard. At first the public seems unaware or ignores it; hence zero response. Then the hazard potential is recognized and there may be a profound reaction of alarm. Thereafter the true hazard potential (*dashed line*) comes into focus, and the public response becomes (hopefully) more appropriate. This pattern describes societal response to hazards as diverse as nuclear power, asbestos, electromagnetic fields, and pesticide residues in food, although there often remains a gap between response and reality. (With permission of Environmental and Occupational Health Sciences Institute.)

quently change as we discover more about the health aspects of an environmental subject. The practitioner is an appropriate person to convey this information, perhaps using words such as "based on current understanding or knowledge." Fig. 1-3 exemplifies the history of a hypothetical hazard. At first society ignores it or takes it for granted; then the hazard potential is recognized and there may be a profound reaction of alarm, following which the true magnitude of the hazard may be recognized. This pattern describes societal response to hazards as diverse as nuclear power, asbestos, electromagnetic fields, and pesticide residues in food.

CONCLUSION

Environmental medicine, the clinical arm of environmental health, involves the diagnosis and prevention of illness caused or influenced by external agents (particularly chemical and physical agents) in a person's environment. It is a very important preventive discipline. Once an environmental disease has occurred, its treatment is often within the domain of internal medicine, but its recognition and prevention is the essence of environmental medical practice. Once hazards have been recognized, control and reduction of exposure should follow swiftly.

The closing of a century and a millennium is a perfect foil for writing about almost any topic. Most biomedical science developed in the past century, and most of what we know about the environment that we share with all manner of organisms has been learned this century as well. Predicting society's needs for the twenty-first century is no longer a quest for writers of science fiction. It is safe to say that we will need clinicians who are well versed in ecology and environmentalists who understand exposure and health. Both will play an important role in educating the public as well as public policy makers, preparing them for the difficult and costly decisions that we will face in the next century.

Clinicians should understand that people generally tend to underestimate risks that are large but voluntary (for example, smoking or riding in a car) and to overestimate risks that are much smaller, but involuntary (pesticide residues in food, electromagnetic waves). Usually, neither alarm nor complacency is warranted.

REFERENCES

1. American College of Occupational and Environmental Medicine: Scope of occupational and environmental health programs and practice. Committee on Occupational Medical Practice, *J Occup Med* 33:436-440, 1991.
2. Bartell SM, Gardner RH, O'Neill RV: *Ecological risk estimation,* Boca Raton, Fla, 1992, Lewis.
3. Bridbord K, Decoufle P, Fraumeni JF et al: *Estimates of the fraction of cancer in the United States related to occupational factors,* Rockville, Md, 1978, National Institute for Occupational Safety and Health.
4. Davis DL, Hoel D, Fox J et al: International trends in cancer mortality in France, West Germany, Italy, Japan, England and Wales, and the United States, *Ann New York Acad Sci* 609:5-48, 1992.
5. Doll R, Peto R: *The causes of cancer,* New York, 1981, Oxford University Press.
6. Ducatman AM: Occupational physicians and environmental medicine, *J Occup Med* 35:251-259, 1993.
7. Ducatman AM, Chase KH, Farid I et al: What is environmental medicine? *J Occup Med* 32:130-132, 1990.
8. Gochfeld M: *A matrix of routes and media of exposure for risk assessment scenarios,* Piscataway, NJ, 1991, Environmental and Occupational Health Sciences Institute.
9. Gochfeld M, Becker C: Taking poetic license with occupational and environmental medicine, *J Occup Med* 32:1108-1109, 1990.
10. Goldstein BD, Gochfeld M: Role of the physician in environmental medicine, *Med Clin North Am Environ Med* 74:245-262, 1990.
11. Institute of Medicine (Goldstein BD, Chair): *Role of the primary care physician in occupational and environmental medicine,* Washington, DC, 1988, National Academy Press.
12. International Agency for Research on Cancer: *Evaluation of the carcinogenic risk of chemicals to humans,* Lyon, France, 1982, IARC Monographs.
13. National Research Council: *Issues in risk assessment,* Washington, DC, 1993, National Academy Press.
14. Odum EP: *Fundamentals of ecology,* Philadelphia, 1953, WB Saunders.
15. Randolph TG: *Human ecology and susceptibility to the chemical environment,* Springfield, Ill, 1962, Charles C Thomas.
16. Rosenau MJ: *Preventive medicine and hygiene,* ed 3, New York, 1918, D Appleton.
17. Upton AC, editor: Environmental medicine, *Med Clin North Am* 74:235-540, 1990.
18. Wolff MS, Tonio PE, Lee EW et al: Blood levels of organochlorine residues and risk of breast cancer, *J Natl Cancer Inst* 85:648-652, 1993.
19. World Health Organization: Cancer prevention, *WHO Chronicle* 323-327, 1964.

Chapter 2

TYPES AND SOURCES OF ENVIRONMENTAL HAZARDS

Stuart M. Brooks
Lynette Benson
Michael Gochfeld

Introduction and scope
   "Dysfunctional" society
   Global crisis
   What can be done?
Hazards in the environment
   Environmental catastrophes
   How chemicals enter the environment
Causative agents and causality
   The three environments
   Environmental hazards
   The media of environmental hazards
Interaction between hazardous exposures and humans
   Important exposure characteristics
   Routes and pathways: "total human exposure"
   Relationship of magnitude, duration, and frequency
   Multifactorial etiology and lack of specificity
   Host susceptibility
   Latency
   Complexity of environmental pathogenesis
Cellular responses to human exposures
   Cellular stress responses
   Cellular stress proteins and toxicity
Health outcomes from environmental hazards
Recognition of human hazardous exposures
   Measurements of actual exposures
   Estimating exposures using mathematical models
   Use of environmental exposures databases
   Sentinel event strategies
   Geographic information system
   Biologic markers
Examples of exposures in air
   Outdoor air pollution
   Indoor air pollution
Examples of exposures in water
   Dumping of nuclear waste
   Oil spills
Examples of exposures in land and soil
   Solid waste and garbage
   Hazardous waste sites
   Extraction of ores and abandoned mines
   Nuclear wastes
Examples of exposures in other categories

INTRODUCTION AND SCOPE
"Dysfunctional" society

Modern Western society has been described as "environmentally dysfunctional."[1,2] This description refers to a prevalent attitude of many individuals who deny responsibility for future environmental consequences of their present-day actions. Such disregard may lead to a collision between the world's civilizations and its ecologic systems. The combination of a human population explosion and a scientific and technical revolution that enhances the human ability to manipulate nature may lead to a bleak future for Earth and its inhabitants.

Global crisis

Human activity has radically altered close to 50% of the Earth's ice-free land surface and has significantly modified much of the remaining area. About 40% of all photosynthetic energy has been appropriated for human use. The burning of fossil fuels and the destruction of forests have altered the global flow of energy within the biosphere, possibly contributing to a global warming trend. Pollution, hunting, and destruction of natural habitat have resulted in a critical reduction in the many plants and animals, as well as in the number of species (biodiversity).

Global population is expected to reach 10 billion by the year 2050.[37] It took hundreds of thousands of years for *Homo sapiens* to reach a population of around 5 billion, and now that population is expected to double in a little more than 50 years. Computerized simulations of the Earth's ecosystems predict that the Earth's capacity to sustain continued population growth may be reached within the next century.[28] These models cannot yet predict conclusively what the result of continued human activities resulting in an "overshoot" of the carrying capacity of the biosphere might be, although a permanently impoverished environment and substantial reductions in the current material standard of living are hypothesized. Formerly ubiquitous and inexpensive resources, such as water, agricultural land, and wood for fuel and construction, are increasingly inadequate to meet the growing demand. The unprecedented population increase drives efforts to increase the Earth's productivity, fueling an increase in the use of chemicals in agriculture and increased consumption of limited petroleum resources. In actuality, no one really knows the capacity of our biosphere to sustain human expansion, but the implications of continuing unrestrained growth are frightening.

What can be done?

Physicians and public health professionals play a unique role in communicating information about environmental health risks to patients and their communities. In fact, it may be said that there is no one who has greater responsibility for dealing with important environmental health issues than the medical practitioner and public health specialist. These professionals have the training to recognize environmental health hazards. As they have been for centuries, those with medical training must lead the search for remedies to those health threats created by social, political, and economic conditions. Practicing physicians and other health professionals, because of their concern with preventive and curative health issues, are uniquely placed to take a leading role in addressing the environmental crisis and developing "treatments" for it. The words of Vice President Al Gore, in his book *Earth in the Balance,* support the crucial role of physicians and other health professionals interested in environmental medicine: "We accept our responsibility to help make known to the millions we serve and teach, the nature and consequences of the environmental crisis, and what is required to overcome it."[12]

HAZARDS IN THE ENVIRONMENT
Environmental catastrophes

In the latter half of this century numerous public tragedies have increased awareness of environmental issues and potential health effects of chemical releases into the environment. Media coverage has enormous influence on public perceptions and attitudes about environmental catastrophes. Dioxins in Times Beach, Missouri; a hazardous waste site in Love Canal, New York; a nuclear energy leak at Three Mile Island, Pennsylvania; contaminated drinking water in Woburn, Massachusetts; and an accidental release of methyl isocyanate in Bhopal, India, were well-described environmental episodes brought to the public's attention by the media. While providing a forum for the exchange of information, such media coverage also heightens public perceptions of the adverse consequences of environmental contamination and lowers public confidence in the effectiveness of government response to such incidents.[1] As dramatic as these incidents were, an even greater and more enigmatic threat may be the repeated, low-level exposures to untested chemical compounds ubiquitous in the human environment, at home, at school, at work, and even at play.

How chemicals enter the environment

Six ways in which hazardous substances may enter the environment are illustrated in Fig. 2-1. There may be *direct exposure to the source of contamination,* as when a hazard is introduced either inadvertently or intentionally into the environment as a consumer product (such as pesticides, cigarettes, or lead in paint).[3] Toxic emissions from transportation, smokestacks, and incinerators; discharge of untreated sewage and chemicals into convenient lakes, rivers, and streams; and contamination of soil by leaking containers or from chemical application may result in *direct discharge into air, water, or soil. Inadequate landfills* may fail to prevent escape of pollutants from hazardous chemical or radioactive waste or from "sanitary" waste. Through processes of runoff or leaching, these contaminants may find their way into drinking water or the food chain, with humans as the ultimate consumers. There are also many reports of illegal dumping of hazardous substances into the environment by unscrupulous consumers, ranging from an individual dumping used oil in the backyard, to the mass dumping of toxic substances resulting in such episodes as the contamination of Times Beach with dioxins. Hazardous pollutants may be released into the environment due to *environmental catastrophic events,* including accidental releases of large quantities of extremely virulent toxins (such as the release of a cloud of methyl isocyanate in Bhopal or the nuclear accident in Chernobyl). Finally, there are *ecologic catastrophic events* that have serious consequences for human health. Frequently, several of these factors may be combined, proportionately increasing risks to human health.

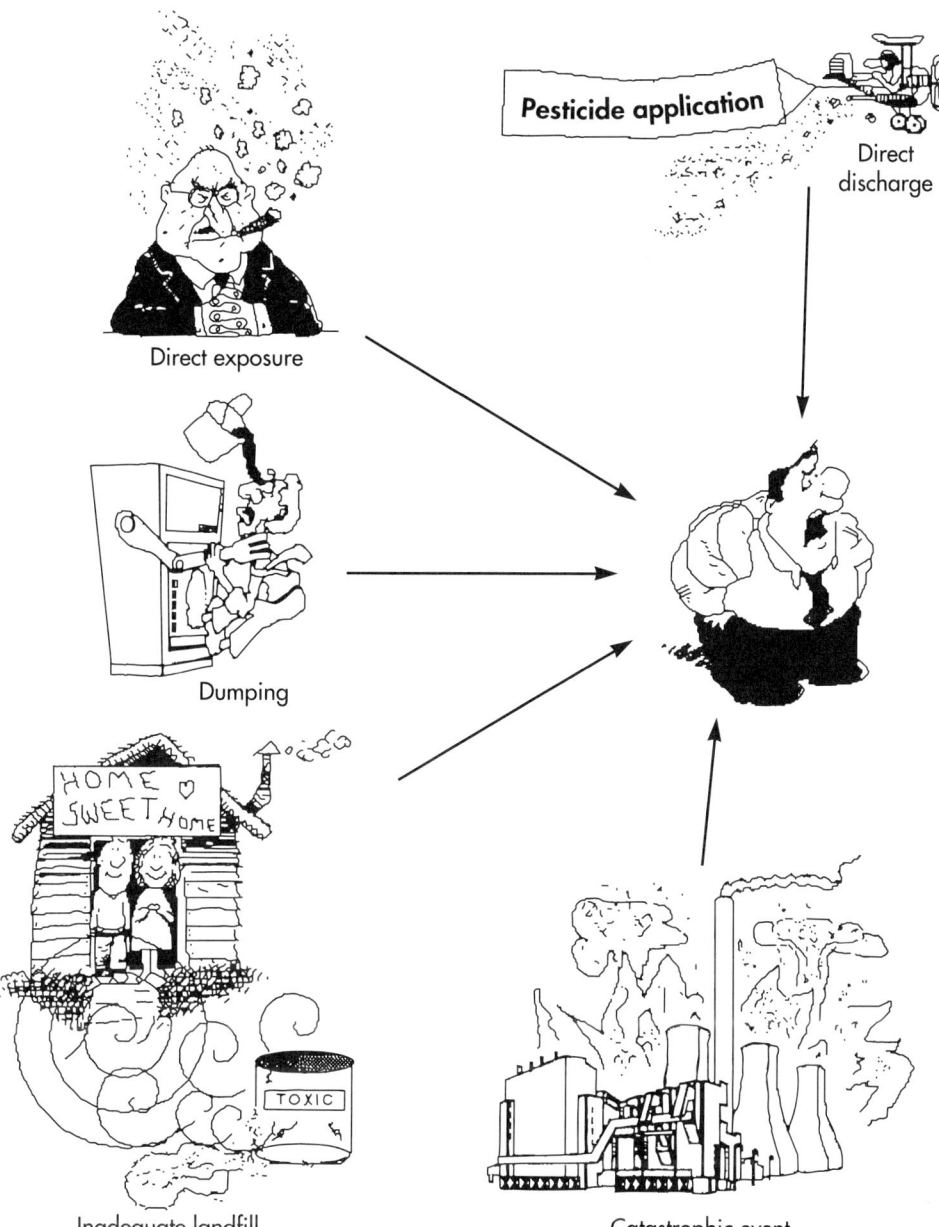

Fig. 2-1. Ways in which hazardous substances may enter the environment and be conveyed to humans. *Direct exposure to the source* occurs when a hazard is introduced either inadvertently or intentionally into the environment as a consumer product (e.g., lead in paint) or personal factor (e.g., environmental tobacco smoke). Examples of a *direct discharge into air, water, or soil* are toxic air emissions from transportation sources, smokestacks, and incinerators; discharge of untreated sewage and chemicals into convenient rivers and streams, and contamination of soil by leaking containers or from application of chemicals (e.g., pesticide application). *Inadequate landfills* occur when landfills, designed for disposal of waste (either ''hazardous''—chemical/nuclear or ''sanitary'') and engineered to prevent escape of pollutants, become deficient and result in runoff, leaching, or travel through the food chain. *Dumping* is the illegal release of environmental hazards into the environment. Additionally, hazardous pollutants may be released into the environment after *environmental catastrophic events,* such as accidental releases (e.g., Bhopal situation and release of methyl isocyanate or Chernobyl disaster). There are also *ecologic catastrophic* events that lead to human health consequences, such as volcanoes, floods, famine, and hurricanes (not shown). (From Blumenthal D: Perspective on environmental health. In Blumenthal D, ed: *Introduction to environmental health,* New York, 1985, Springer Publishing Company.)

CAUSATIVE AGENTS AND CAUSALITY
The three environments

Individuals divide their time among three major environments: the *home,* the *workplace,* and the *community at large.* Each environment has its own characteristic "toxic profile" (see Table 2-1), although exposures to a given agent often occur in more than one environment, increasing the complexity of estimating exposure. Different controls must be implemented to reduce toxic exposures in each type of environment. Contaminants in the home rely on individual knowledge of the situation and willingness and/or ability to remedy it. In the workplace, reduction of toxic exposures is dependent on the cooperation of a corporate structure and is often complicated by economic factors and conflicting objectives of workers and management. Individuals most at risk in the workplace tend to be those with the least control over their working environment. Remedies for toxic exposures in the community at large, although they may be initiated by individuals or corporations, are often the province of government agencies, which may be hampered by a bureaucratic structure that limits their ability to respond quickly to prevent or defend the community from acute or chronic environmental health threats.

Table 2-1. Classification of environmental hazards

Relative importance in various settings

Agents	Home	Community	Workplace
Chemical			
Heavy metals	+++	++	++++
Pesticides	++	++	++++
Solvents	++	+	++++
Chlorinated HC	+	+	++++
Polyaromatics	++	+++	+++
Physical			
Ionizing radiation	0	++	+++
Nonionizing radiation	++?	++?	+++
Noise	+	++	++++
Vibration	0	0	+++
Temperature	+	++	+++
Biologic			
Bacteria	+++	++++	+++
Viruses	++	++++	+++
Fungi	+	+++	+
Allergens	++++	++++	+++
Psychosocial			
Personal	+++	+	+++
Family	++++	+	+++
Co-workers	+++	+	++++
Trauma			
General	++++	++++	++++
Cumulative	+	0	++++

The intensity of the exposure is designated by plus signs reflecting none or minimal (0/+) to great (+++/++++).

Environmental hazards

The term *environmental hazard* refers to a wide array of diverse environmental phenomena that have the potential to cause adverse health effects. At present there are at least 26 groups of chemicals known to be human carcinogens, over 600 known rodent carcinogens, over 2000 known teratogens, and more than 50,000 chemicals or chemical compounds with no scientific study of toxicity.[22] Over 1400 active ingredients are formulated into more than 45,000 pesticide products. More than 6 billion tons of toxic waste with diverse chemical compositions are produced each year. Of the 5 to 6 million chemicals with a known molecular structure, 60,000 of which are currently in use in agricultural, manufacturing, or medical applications, only about 1% have been tested for toxicity. The problem of assessing toxicity is complicated by the fact that approximately 6000 new chemicals are synthesized each week. The fact that humans are virtually never exposed to a single chemical at a time adds to the complexity of predicting adverse health effects of chemical exposure, given our extremely limited knowledge about the interactions among chemicals occurring in infinite combinations.

Table 2-1 classifies the major *environmental hazards* and their relative importance in various environmental settings. *Chemical agents* are responsible for a majority of environmental toxic reactions; *physical agents* include ionizing and nonionizing radiation, vibration, temperature, and noise; *biologic agents* include infectious and allergic disorders; *psychosocial factors* are an important consideration for environmental medicine, especially at work and in the home; and *trauma,* or mechanical factors, includes cumulative or repetitive trauma, such as carpal tunnel syndrome, which may be more important in the workplace, and trauma induced by recreational activities or accidents in the home.

The media of environmental hazards

Air, earth, water, and food are the major environmental media or vectors through which exposures to hazardous environmental agents may occur. Additionally, fire, in the form of incineration, has emerged as a major and somewhat controversial issue in environmental medicine. Assessment of individual exposures includes an examination of actual and potential exposures to hazardous agents through food; water used for drinking, cooking, or washing; air; and soil. While soil is often overlooked as a route of exposure, in some cases such an oversight may result in a critical underestimate of actual exposure. Home gardeners may be exposed dermally or through inhalation to contaminants in soil, dust, or clay. Although most plants have limited pollutant uptake, such a possibility should not be overlooked where home-grown fruits and vegetables are an important input to diet. Perhaps most critical, soil contamination can affect children who play

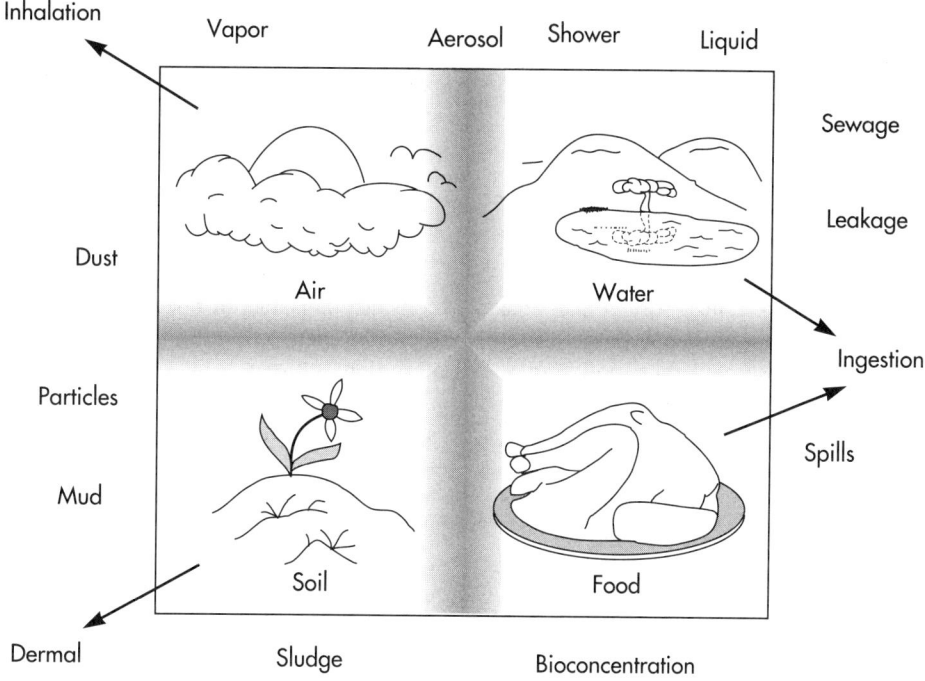

Fig. 2-2. Examples of the numerous exposure pathways for airborne and waterborne pollutants, as well as for pollutants deposited in food and soil. The medium of exposure may take various forms as it enters the body by inhalation, ingestion, or dermal absorption. There is considerable overlap among the various environments, media, and ways pollutants enter the body.

in the yard and then transfer contaminants from dirty hands to eyes, nose, or mouth.

There is considerable interaction among environmental contaminants, their media or vectors, and routes of exposure. This interaction reflects the complexity of ecologic processes in the environment. Fig. 2-2 presents an exposure matrix that demonstrates the relationship among the four environmental media and the three routes of exposure (inhalation, dermal, and ingestion). The parenteral environment has not been included, although it is important in many regards (for example, HIV, needle sticks, blood transfusions, and infected cuts and abrasions).

INTERACTION BETWEEN HAZARDOUS EXPOSURES AND HUMANS
Important exposure characteristics

There are four characteristics critical to exposure assessment: (1) route (inhalation, ingestion, dermal), (2) magnitude (concentration or dose), (3) duration (minutes, hours, days, lifetime), and (4) frequency (daily, weekly, monthly, seasonally).[36] The assessment of an environmental medical disorder requires an awareness of many other important factors, including multifactorial etiology, lack of specificity, host susceptibility, and latency.[41]

Routes and pathways: "total human exposure"

All of the environmental media are possible sources of chemical contamination, and each medium should be considered in an assessment of environmental exposure to toxic agents. Humans have access to environmental toxicants by eating contaminated food, drinking contaminated water, and breathing contaminated air.[1] Hazardous pollutants may also enter the human body through the skin or through a combination of these routes.[21] Rarely are humans exposed to a single pollutant along a single route. Lead exposure may result from exposure to lead in drinking water and food (ingestion), indoor and outdoor air (inhalation), house dust (inhalation and dermal), and paint and soil (dermal and ingestion). Although all sources contribute to blood levels and dose,[36] different routes of exposure may result in diverse clinical manifestations. The inhalation of mercury fumes results in very different pathology than its ingestion or percutaneous absorption. Just as all environmental media must be considered as possible sources of exposure, all routes of administration must also be considered in a clinical assessment of environmental exposure. The realization that many human exposures to a diverse array of toxicants occur through a wide range of environmental pathways and by different routes allows a better appreciation of the concept of "total human exposure." Fig. 2-2 illustrates the concept of multiple human exposure pathways for environmental pollutants. By examining all of the various pathways and routes, practitioners and other health professionals can construct a "human exposure topology" for each pollutant and estimate total human exposure.[23,27]

Relationship of magnitude, duration, and frequency

The concept of "dose" in environmental medicine is a function of the amount of the toxicant absorbed and time factors, including the duration and frequency of exposure. There may be a single, large exposure over a period of minutes or hours; intermittent, brief, but regularly or sporadically repeated exposures over a period of months or years; continuous or chronic exposure; or an infinite number of permutations of dose or concentration, duration, and frequency. At lower concentrations, repeated or continued exposure is usually necessary for the development of a clinical response, but this relationship is less clear for carcinogens. A toxicant may be present in very low, perhaps minute, concentrations, but depending on duration and frequency of exposure, physical and chemical characteristics of the substance, and biologic factors in the host, even a very small concentration of a highly toxic substance can cause a significant clinical response.

Multifactorial etiology and lack of specificity

The genesis of an environmental disorder should not be considered in isolation but examined by considering not only the toxic agent in question and pertinent information on the hazardous substance, but other factors that may modify the outcome. Factors that vary from one individual to another and may impact on pathogenesis include age, sex, nutritional status, life-style, preexisting health problems, and exposure to other toxicants. Any or all of these factors may combine with a single exposure to a toxic substance to produce unexpected health effects. It is also important to emphasize that unlike many other clinical conditions, there is often a lack

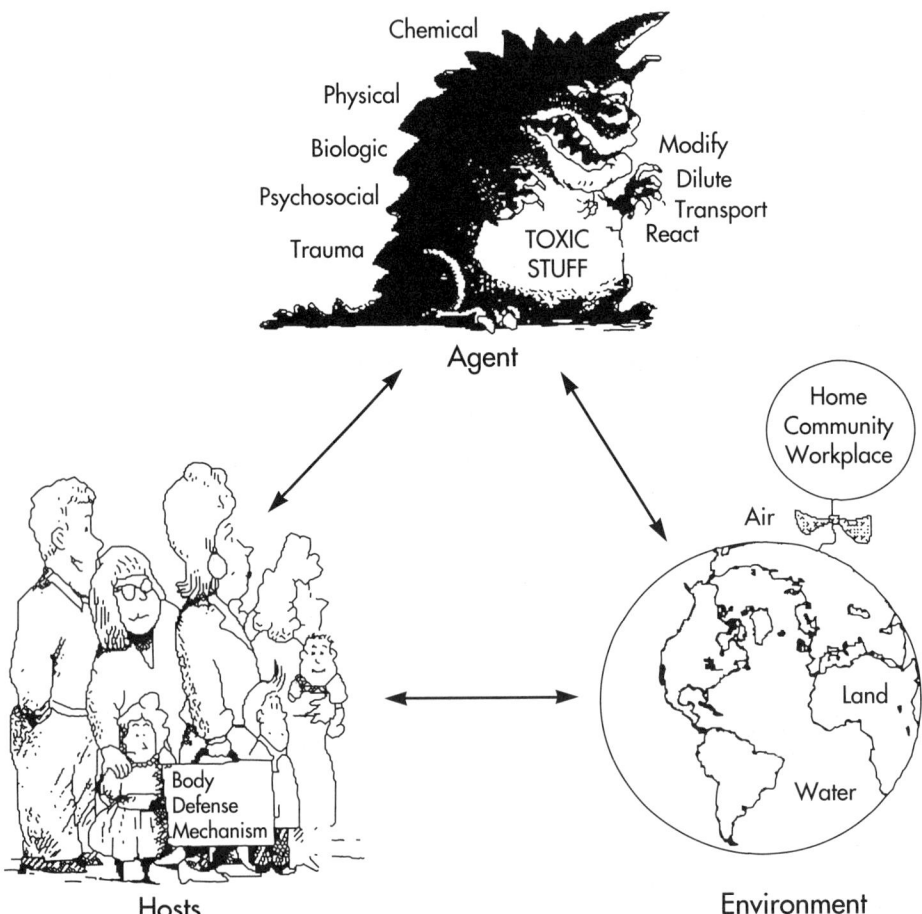

Fig. 2-3. The interaction that occurs among the three "key players" of environmental medicine. There is a continuous and dynamic interaction between the environment and hazardous agents, with the ultimate environmental modification of the agent occurring before it is presented to humans. Host defense mechanisms, susceptibility, and various human responses are influential in how humans respond to the hazardous agent.

of specificity in environmentally induced illness. It rarely occurs with any unique clinical presentation and evolves in a manner similar to other common medical disorders. It is only when the disease pattern and the circumstances of its appearance are viewed in a holistic context that toxic pathogenesis can be identified.

The type and magnitude of an individual's response to an environmental toxicant depend on a number of factors besides dose, duration, and frequency of exposure; chemical properties of the agent; and host factors. The observed clinical effect is directly related to what is actually delivered internally. The response of an organism to a toxic challenge is a reflection of response at the cellular level.

Host susceptibility

Such important factors as age, race, gender, intercurrent disease, genetic makeup, nutritional status, physiologic capacity, exposure history, and emotional state can all influence an individual's susceptibility, and thus response, to environmental pollutants. Differences in these factors are responsible for variations in response to a given exposure. The effectiveness of an individual's defense mechanisms

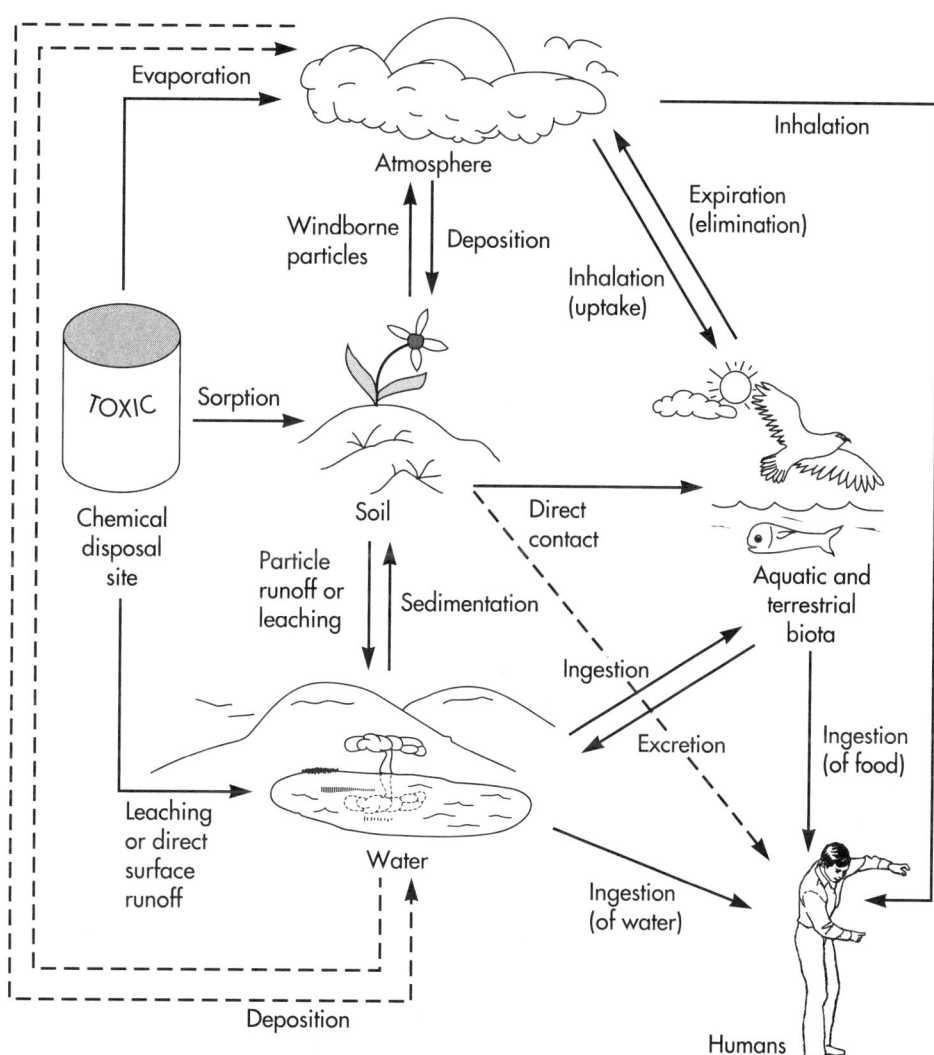

Fig. 2-4. The numerous and complex physical and biologic routes of exposure from disposal site. A chemical may be diluted, diffused, or concentrated by physical or biologic processes. It may be widely transported by air or water, or with solid particles and biologic life or undergo vaporization, sublimation, diffusion, and/or leaching. Pollutants in water can be chemically modified by reactions with other chemicals. Weather transports substances to different locales or media. Plants and animals may bioconcentrate the chemical to such a degree that it becomes hazardous to humans who may ingest the plant or animal. The most prominent route of exposure is through contaminated drinking water and usually ground water drawn from wells. (Modified from Grisham J: *Health aspects of the disposal of water chemicals,* New York, 1986, Pergamon Press.)

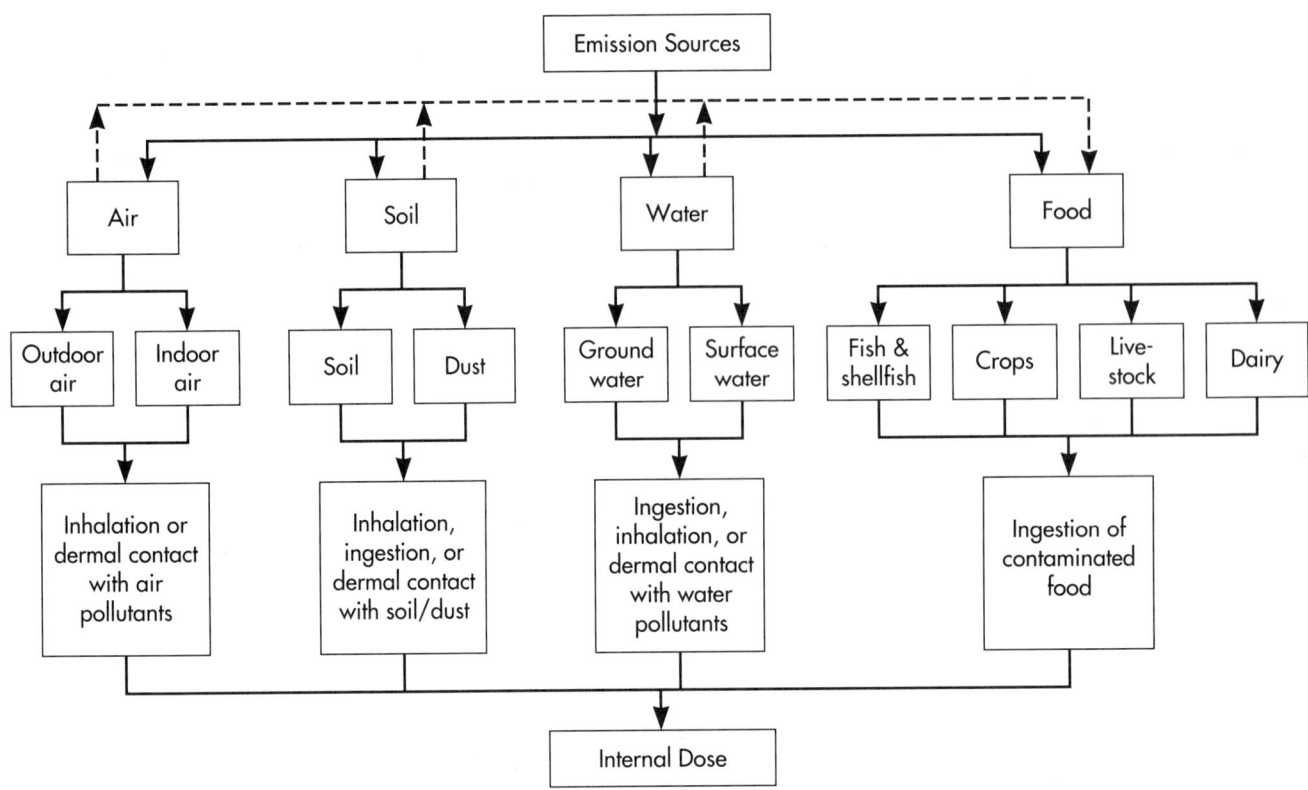

Fig. 2-5. Examples of multiple exposure pathways for airborne and waterborne pollutants from an emission source. Multiple pathways can contribute to an exposure and a dose for a single pollutant. Many human exposures occur through a wide range of environmental pathways and by different routes, allowing for an appreciation of the concept of "total human exposure." (Adapted from Sexton K et al: Estimating human exposures to environmental pollutants: availability and utility of existing databases, *Arch Environ Health* 47:398, 1992.)

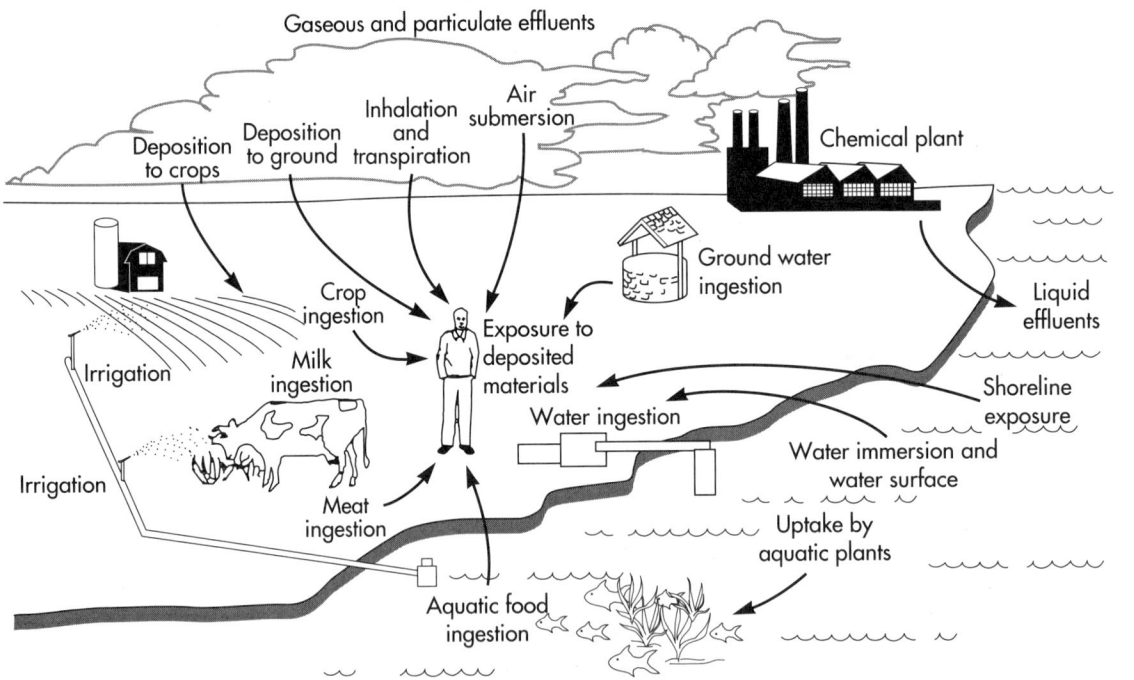

Fig. 2-6. Multiple exposure pathways for airborne and waterborne pollutants emitted from a hypothetical chemical plant. Not only is there human exposure and effects but there are ecologic consequences as well. (From Tarcher A: Principles and scope of environmental medicine. In Tarcher A, ed: *Principles and practice of environmental medicine,* New York, 1992, Plenum Medical Book Company, pp 3-18.)

will play a critical role in determining clinical manifestations and outcome of a hazardous exposure. Persons having "poor" or nonadaptive body defenses might develop overt and progressive disease, while individuals with strong defenses that allow them to adapt to the exposure may be asymptomatic or suffer only a mild clinical response. Of course, such factors as exposure dose and duration, and whether the exposure is high-level, repeated, low-level, or chronic, are also critical.

Latency

The concept of latency, that a disease agent may initiate pathogenesis that does not manifest overt disease for many years or even decades, requires a comprehensive assessment of the patient's exposure history and general health over a lifetime. Many environmental pathogens, especially carcinogens, exhibit long periods of latency. Thus even more so than other types of medical practitioners, the environmental health practitioner must view the patient's health status holistically, as a composite of the patient's total life experience.

Complexity of environmental pathogenesis

Environmental pathogenesis is the result of complex, dynamic interaction among the environment, the host, and the hazardous agent, often involving modification of the agent between the time it is released into the environment and its introduction to the human host. Such modifications may come about as a result of meteorologic conditions; interaction with other chemicals in the atmosphere; the influence of physical factors, such as sunlight, humidity, or biotransformation or other biologic processes within insect/animal vectors; or in the hosts themselves. Host defense mechanisms, cultural and biologic; host susceptibility; and societal responses affect how the individual human responds to the hazardous agent. In reality, host-agent-environment interactions are so complex that no definitive understanding of all that takes place is possible at this time. Fig. 2-3 graphically illustrates the multidimensional interactions among these three "key players" in environmental medicine. Each player contributes to the clinical manifestation of exposure and its final outcome.

The complexity of interactions among hazardous agents, the environment (including nonhuman life forms), and humans is so great that untoward or unexpected human outcomes, both "good" and "bad," can result from a chemical release into the environment. Thus careful analysis of all aspects of an environmental exposure is necessary in predicting outcome and developing a prognosis. Any exposure, small or large, can have unexpected consequences, and a judgment of whether an exposure is "safe" or "dangerous" should not be based on the face value of the chemical or magnitude alone. Fig. 2-4 provides an example of how hazardous substances originating from a disposal site can represent numerous and complex physical and biologic routes of exposure.[16] A chemical initially may be modified by the environment before it enters the human. The toxic agent can be carried by air or water or with solid particles or other forms of biologic life; transformed by chemical or biochemical reactions; and diluted, diffused, or concentrated by physical or biologic processes. It may undergo vaporization, sublimation, diffusion, or leaching. Pollutants being carried by air or water may be chemically modified by reactions with other chemicals (for example, reaction of chlorines and haloethers in treated water). Weather cycles may transport substances to different locales or through different media than those in which they were released. Wind, for example, may blow particulates across the land, runoff may carry them into the water, and evaporation may return them to the air, where they may be carried for hundreds of miles before returning to Earth as rainfall. Plants and animals may accumulate small doses of a chemical agent and bioconcentrate them to the degree at which they become a human hazard.

Once a hazardous substance is released into the environment, it may be transported and transformed in a variety of complex ways.[21] After modification by the environment and entering numerous media, the hazardous agent can be inhaled, ingested, or absorbed through the skin. Fig. 2-5 illustrates the multiple exposure pathways for airborne and waterborne pollutants emitted from an emission source, the various media entered, and the possible multiple exposure routes resulting in a final internal dose of a pollutant. The complexity of the situation is even greater considering the plethora of other sources, including motor vehicles, industrial waste, agricultural runoff, and consumer products, which release literally thousands of hazardous pollutants. This concept is shown in Fig. 2-6, which depicts multiple exposure pathways presented by the environmental contamination of air, soil, and water occurring from a chemical plant. Not only are there human exposure and health effects, but there are ecologic consequences as well that are beyond the scope of this text.

CELLULAR RESPONSES TO HUMAN EXPOSURES
Cellular stress responses

It has been known for many years that immediately after a sudden increase in temperature, all cells (from the simplest bacterium to the most complicated and sophisticated nerve cell) increase production of a certain class of molecules that buffer them from harm.[47] When the phenomenon was first observed some 30 years ago, it was designated as a "heat shock response," but subsequent investigations have realized that the same response occurs in cells after a variety of different environmental stimuli. Because there are so many different stimuli that elicit the same cellular defense response, it is now commonly referred to as the "stress response" and the expressed molecules as "stress proteins." Some conditions that induce the expression of stress proteins include heat shock, heavy metals, metabolic poisons that inhibit energy metabolism, viral infections, oxidant injury, ischemia, and inflammation. Stress proteins participate in a number of essential cellular functions, including the pathways by which cellular proteins are synthesized and assembled and regulation of growth and differentiation. Several pathways for folding and distributing proteins within cells are managed by stress proteins. There is evidence to suggest that stress proteins may be important, if not essential, for the ability of cells to recover from a metabolic insult. Increased levels of the proteins after a cellular injury from a toxic chemical seem to act as molecular chaperones that facilitate the synthesis and assembly of new reparative proteins.[47] Cells that produce high levels of stress proteins seem more able to survive ischemic damage, and stress proteins may also be influential for certain immunologic responses.

Stress proteins have been implicated in dioxin-induced injury. It has been reported that the aryl hydrocarbon (Ah) receptor, which is detectable in many tissues and organs, binds to many environmental pollutants such as polycyclic aromatic hydrocarbons, heterocyclic amines, and polychlorinated aromatic compounds (including dioxin, dibenzofurans, and biphenyls) and is responsible for mediating the carcinogenic effect of these agents. The components of the Ah receptor, a soluble protein complex, include a ligand-binding subunit of about 95 kD as well as a 90 kD unit which is a stress-induced protein.[19]

Cellular stress proteins and toxicity

Cellular stress protein responses may find future use in discerning the toxicity of a chemical agent. For example, recombinant-DNA techniques have allowed development of cultured cell lines of "stress receptor" cells that appear to have the potential for use as screening tools for screening biologic hazards.[47] In such cells, DNA sequences that control the activities of the stress protein genes are linked to a receptor gene that encodes an enzyme (such as b-galactosidase). When these cells experience environmental stress and produce more stress proteins, they also make the receptor enzyme, which can be detected easily by various laboratory assays. Thus by using such reporter cells, investigators can easily determine the extent of the stress response induced by a specific chemical agent. It may also be possible to use this technique as a biologic monitor. For example, genetic breeding has provided transgenic worms in which a reporter gene for b-galactosidase is under the control of the promoter for a stress protein.[47] When these worms are exposed to various pollutants, they express the reporter enzyme and turn blue. This phenomenon thus provides the potential for using these genetically altered reporter worms for monitoring a wide variety of pollutants, possibly in a specific locale.

HEALTH OUTCOMES FROM ENVIRONMENTAL HAZARDS

The EPA identifies seven categories of human health effects from hazardous exposures (Table 2-2)[38,44]: (1) carci-

Table 2-2. Outcomes from environmental hazards

Outcome	Example
Human health	
Carcinogenicity	Benzene
Heritable genetic and chromosomal mutation	Ionizing radiation
Developmental toxicity	1,3-Butadiene
Reproductive toxicity	Lead
Acute toxicity	Phosgene or mustard gas
Chronic toxicity	Carbon tetrachloride
Neurotoxicity	Mercury
Ecologic	
Environmental toxicity	Cadmium or aluminum
Persistence	1,1,1-Trichloroethane
Bioaccumulation	Chlordane

nogenicity—can cause cancer in humans and/or laboratory animals (benzene); (2) heritable genetic and chromosomal mutations—can cause mutations in genes and chromosomes that will be passed to the next generation (ionizing radiation); (3) developmental toxicity—can cause birth defects or miscarriages (1,3-butadiene); (4) reproductive toxicity—can damage the ability of men or women to reproduce (lead); (5) acute toxicity—can cause death from even short-term exposures, either through the lungs, the mouth, or the skin (phosgene or mustard gas); (6) chronic toxicity—can cause long-term damage other than cancer, such as liver, kidney, or lung damage (carbon tetrachloride); and (7) neurotoxicity—can harm the nervous system by affecting the brain, spinal cord, or nerves (mercury). The EPA also designates three ecologic effects of concern: (1) environmental toxicity—can harm wildlife and vegetation when released to water, soil, or air (cadmium or aluminum); (2) persistence—does not break down easily, thus persisting and accumulating in portions of the environment such as soil, sediment, and groundwater (1,1,1-trichloroethane); (3) bioaccumulation—can enter the bodies of plants and is not easily expelled, thus accumulating over time through repeated exposure (chlordane).

RECOGNITION OF HUMAN HAZARDOUS EXPOSURES

There are a number of ways of recognizing environmental exposure situations (box). The following discussion will explore some of the more accessible approaches.

Measurements of actual exposures

The only way to accurately determine to what extent persons come in contact with a specific environmental hazardous pollutant is to actually measure the exposure. There are at least three ways to accomplish this task: (1) use of microenvironmental samplers (for example, passive samplers in residences or offices that measure integrated concentrations

> **Recognition of human hazardous exposures**
>
> Measure of actual exposures
> Mathematical models
> Environmental exposures databases
> Sentinel event strategies
> Geographic information system
> Biologic markers

of airborne lead); (2) use of personal monitors (for example, active monitors worn by volunteers that measure real-time concentrations of airborne lead); or (3) use of biologic measurements in human tissues (for example, determining blood-lead concentration).[36]

Estimating exposures using mathematical models

Because obtaining individual exposure data on large numbers of persons in the United States is not possible, an alternative approach has been developed. Mathematical abstractions of physical reality are used to create "models" based on mathematical analyses of smaller numbers of measurements. The data are then extrapolated to fit the larger population. Three types of models typically used in exposure assessment include: (1) concentration models, which estimate the concentration of a pollutant in a particular environmental medium; (2) contact models, which estimate the exposure or the contact between pollution and persons; and (3) dose models, which estimate the internal or delivered dose, or the amount of pollutant that enters the body and that is finally deposited in specific human tissues and fluids.[36]

Use of environmental exposures databases

Human health effects have formed the basis of many epidemiologic investigations concerning hazardous agents in the environment. One promising approach to hazard assessment focuses on the use of exposure parameters. There are existing data systems that contain a substantial amount of information relevant to exposure estimation.[26,43] The highest priority for investigation would be directed at those locales where there is documentation of a significant number of persons having an elevated exposure to a pollutant that is very toxic and can cause harm at a low exposure dose.

Unfortunately, current exposure databases are geared more for regulatory use than for public health and human surveillance purposes. There are difficulties relying on exposure information using the current databases. There are inconsistencies in the data, and accessing and understanding their contents is often difficult. The databases fail to include information on important human exposures, such as tobacco smoke and allergens. There are differences in the frequency of data collection, and many databases do not represent national samples but are regional in scope and thus do not represent other geographic areas or populations. Temporal relationships of data collection may vary and databases are heterogeneous. Modification of the existing databases to accommodate much-needed human exposure information seems quite important and of a high priority. Goals for improving exposure information through use of databases have been entertained.[13]

There are currently a great number of available databases. In a recent inventory 67 reliable databases that met important criteria were identified.[36] About 54 contained pollutant concentration measurements in several media; 11 were emission inventories that document pollutant releases into air, water, and soil; and 13 contained biologic information from human tissues. Only 5 reported production and usage information; 10 elicited microenvironmental measurements; and 7 contained personal measurements. The database inventory contained the spectrum of exposure estimators, including production volumes (amounts produced in the United States annually); emission inventory (estimates or measurements of amounts of a chemical released into the environment annually); concentrations in the environment (air, water, soil, food); concentrations in the microenvironments (residences); personal exposure measurements (use of small portable monitors carried by individuals for 12 to 24 hours, which enables documentation of particle exposures); and concentrations in human tissues (blood and adipose tissue).[36]

An example of how database information can be effectively utilized is shown in the reporting of the EPA in Region IV, examining databases using the Toxic Chemical Release Inventory (TRI).[38,44] In 1989 there were almost 1 billion pounds of total releases and another 200 million in transfers.

Sentinel event strategies

For the practicing physician, the concept of sentinel events is important. Sentinel event strategies follow the philosophy that some events are particularly suggestive of occupational or environmental hazards and their occurrence suggests alterations that are known or suspected about a specific hazardous substance.[2] There may well be a need to have a system in place for monitoring communities around hazardous point sources so that one case of an unusual health event will be noticed or so that a pattern of unusual health events will be detected. Identifying clusters of disease events may uncover a hazardous substance point source that was not previously recognized. The emergence of exposure registries has allowed attempts at using available data to detect evidence of increased disease risk. Selective surveillance for certain health events can be productive because the events tend to be rare and thus their causation may also be more simple to study (box).

Because sentinel events include the occurrences of single cases of disease, they are amenable to preventive strategies.[32] Some examples of sentinel events that, when recognized by the practicing physician, could lead to preventive interventions include cervical cancer deaths (Pap smears), death dur-

Examples of sentinel health events and conditions

Health events

Liver cancer in nonsmoker and nondrinker
Glioblastoma
Amelanotic melanoma
Pediatric solid tumors
Genitourinary cancers in children
Exotic lymphoma cell type
Exotic leukemias in uncharacteristic age group
Bladder cancer in nonsmoker
Lung cancer in nonsmoker
Midline or septal birth defects

Health conditions

Unusual allergies
Unusual neurologic symptoms
Idiopathic hematuria
Persistent, unresolved rashes
Persistent, idiopathic nasopharyngitis
Extreme liver enzyme dysfunction in nonsmoker
Extreme renal function values in nonsmoker

Adapted from Aldrich TE, Leaverton PE: Sentinel event strategies in environmental health, *Annu Rev Publ Health* 14:205, 1993.

ing childbirth (natality care), and oral cancer in a person less than 30 years of age (smokeless tobacco).[2] Another approach is to examine localized clustering of rare events. Rare health events can be informative when they occur in a small aggregate or in unusual populations. Such examples might be pediatric osteogenic sarcoma within a single residential subdivision located near a nuclear waste disposal site.

Viewing incidence patterns on a population scale and not necessarily on a cause-and-effect level is another component of sentinel event strategy. Changes in the "logical" pattern of disease may reflect an underlying hazard. For example, noting a change in the distribution of bladder cancer to a greater frequency in younger individuals may reflect chemical contamination of a water supply. The strategy of searching for an increased occurrence along a spectrum of biologic effects provides an innovative approach. For example, the biologic spectrum leading to cancer may be reflected by other adverse health events that have a related etiology but whose occurrence precedes the cancer. Congenital anomalies (birth defects) are a logical consideration for this example. There might be a finding of a small cluster of rare cancers, which has marginal statistical significance, but a concordant increase in birth defects can provide additional evidence for a "problem" and need for further environmental investigations. There may be sentinel species, perhaps analogous to the canary in the mine. Animals who have an accelerated life span compared to humans may manifest adverse disease from an undetected hazardous chemical more quickly than humans. An example of this situation occurred in the Hunan province of China, where a community with high esophageal cancer rates was noted to share a higher prevalence of gullet cancer among local poultry.[25] The practice of eating strongly pickled vegetables was identified as the causal association; a similar pattern among chickens had been the result of shared food.

Geographic information system

The EPA has a relatively new tool, known as the EPA Geographic Information System (GIS), which can integrate diverse multimedia (air, water, soil) data, geographic features, census information, information about ecologic regions, and chemical toxicity information into a common database with spatial characteristics.[38,44] This approach provides an initial step in defining the geographic distribution of environmental releases of the TRI chemical releases and displays potential exposure zones. The chemical release data used in the study was provided through a new federal law, Section 313 of the Emergency Planning and Community Right-to-Know Act (EPCRA) of the Superfund Amendments and Reauthorization Act of 1986 (Public Law 99-499). The act is also known as Title III of the Superfund Amendments and Reauthorization Act (SARA). Under Section 313 certain businesses must submit annual reports to the EPA and the state in which they operate for certain specified toxic chemicals manufactured, processed, or used at the facility. In fact, the facilities must account for the total aggregate releases to the environment for each chemical listed under Section 313 for the calendar year. These aggregate data are referred to as the Toxic Chemical Release Inventory (TRI). There are over 300 chemicals and 20 chemical categories on the Section 313 list. The box lists some of the EPA priority chemicals. Fig. 2-7 shows the 25 top-ranking TRI facilities in the southeastern portion of the United States (Region IV) according to the facility-reported emissions (according to the 1980 census). Fig. 2-8 depicts the 25 top-ranking TRI facilities in the southeastern portion of the United States (Region IV) according to the facility-reported emissions information presumed to provide information on carcinogens in these locales.

There have been several investigations using these new surveillance tools. Williams and associates[49] used geographic analysis and three-dimensional mapping to show potential adverse health effects on newborn infants of contaminated air pollutants from incineration. Analyses of clusters of diseases have utilized algorithms coupled with population density equalized maps (i.e., cartograms).[35] Spatial clustering of diseases around geographic formations such as rivers and hazardous waste sites has been evaluated using proximity analysis.[20] Spatial autocorrelation has been used to analyze large-scale data and allows the examination of distributional characteristics of disease.[45,46] Investigations of spatial patterns and geographic comparisons of rates of disease across county regions in states can be accomplished by using mapping procedures.[24]

EPA priority chemicals

Priority 1 chemicals

Aldrin	Benzene
Benzo(a)pyrene	Beryllium
Chloroform	Chrysene
Dibenzo(a,h)anthracene	Di(2-ethylhexyl)phthalate
Lead	Nickel
Polychlorinated biphenyls	Vinyl chloride
	Benzo(a)anthracene
Arsenic	Cadmium
Benzo(b)fluoranthene	1,4-Dichlorobenzene
Cyanide	Methylene chloride
Heptachlor	2,3,7,8-Tetrachlorodibenzo-p-dioxin
N-Nitrosodiphenylamine	
Tetrachloroethylene	Trichloroethylene

Priority 2 chemicals

Benzidine	1,1,2-Trichloroethane
Carbon tetrachloride	Bis(chloromethyl)ether
3,3-Dichlorobenzidine	Chloroethane
2,4 and 2,6-Dinitrotoluene	1,1-Dichloroethane
	Isophorone
N-Nitrosodimethylamine	Pentachlorophenol
Selenium	Toluene
Zinc	Bis(2-chloroethyl)ether
Chlordane	p,p-DDT, DDE, DDD
1,2-Dichloroethane	Hexachlorocyclohexane
Mercury	N-nitrosodi-n-propylamine
Phenol	1,1,2,2-Tetrachloroethane

Priority 3 chemicals

Acrolein	Ammonia
Bromoform	Chloromethane
Creosote	1,2-Diphenylhydrazine
cis-, trans-, 1,2-Dichloroethene	Ethylbenzene
	Radium
Plutonium	Silver
Radon	Toxaphene
Thorium	Uranium
1,1,1-Trichloroethane	Asbestos
Acrylonitrile	Copper
Chlorobenzene	1,1-Dichloroethane
Di-n-butylphthalate	Ethylene oxide
Endrine/endrin aldehyde	Total xylenes
Polycyclic aromatic hydrocarbon	Naphthalene/2-methylnaphthalene
2,4,6-Trichlorophenol	

Priority 4 chemicals

Aluminum	Barium
Boron	1,3-Butadiene
Carbon disulfide	Creosols
1,2-Dibromethane	1,3-Dichloropropene
Fluorides	Manganese
Methyl parathion	Nitrophenol
Styrene	Tin
Vanadium	Antimony
2,3-Benzofuran	Bromomethane
2-Butanone	Cobalt
Dibromochloropropane	2,4-Dichlorophenol
Endosulfan	2-Hexanone
Methyl mercaptan	Thallium
1,2,3-Trichloropropane	Vinyl acetate

In order to illustrate how various databases can be used to study disease states known to be associated with environmental pollution, a specific example can be used. Felber[28] used sentinel events strategies by examining the prevalence of specific groups of cancers and congenital malformations through descriptive statistics, graphic plots, and mapping techniques for the state of Florida. The sources of data used in the investigation were the Florida Cancer Data System (which contained 226,000 cases of cancer over the period 1981 to 1985) and the Congenital Disease Surveillance Project (which contained 11,849 cases of congenital malformations). Significant correlations were noted for bone cancers and total birth defects, brain cancers and central nervous system defects, brain cancers and eye malformations, total cancers and certain cardiovascular defects, liver cancer and genitourinary defects, urogenital cancers and musculoskeletal defects, and kidney cancers and genitourinary defects. Several counties were identified as having a high risk for a number of classes of cancers or malformations.

The mapping systems have tremendous value for future hypothesis-generating investigations. For example, it might be productive to match maps of health outcome rates, such as cancer rate in a county,[28] with maps of the EPA's TRI facility's reporting of certain types of emissions. If there is a match between a carcinogen emission region and a county with a high cancer rate, then more definitive, hypothesis-testing epidemiologic methodology, such as a case control investigation, is warranted. Thus by using both sentinel event strategies to define health outcomes for mapping (for example, liver cancer in nonsmokers/nondrinkers) and emission mapping for the specific type of chemical (such as a carcinogen), high-priority efforts can focus attention on a potentially hazardous area and initiate corrective measures.

Biologic markers

Biologic markers in the context of environmental health are indicators of events in biologic systems or samples. Once an exposure has occurred, a continuum of biologic events can be detected. These events may serve as markers of the initial exposure, administered dose, biologically effective

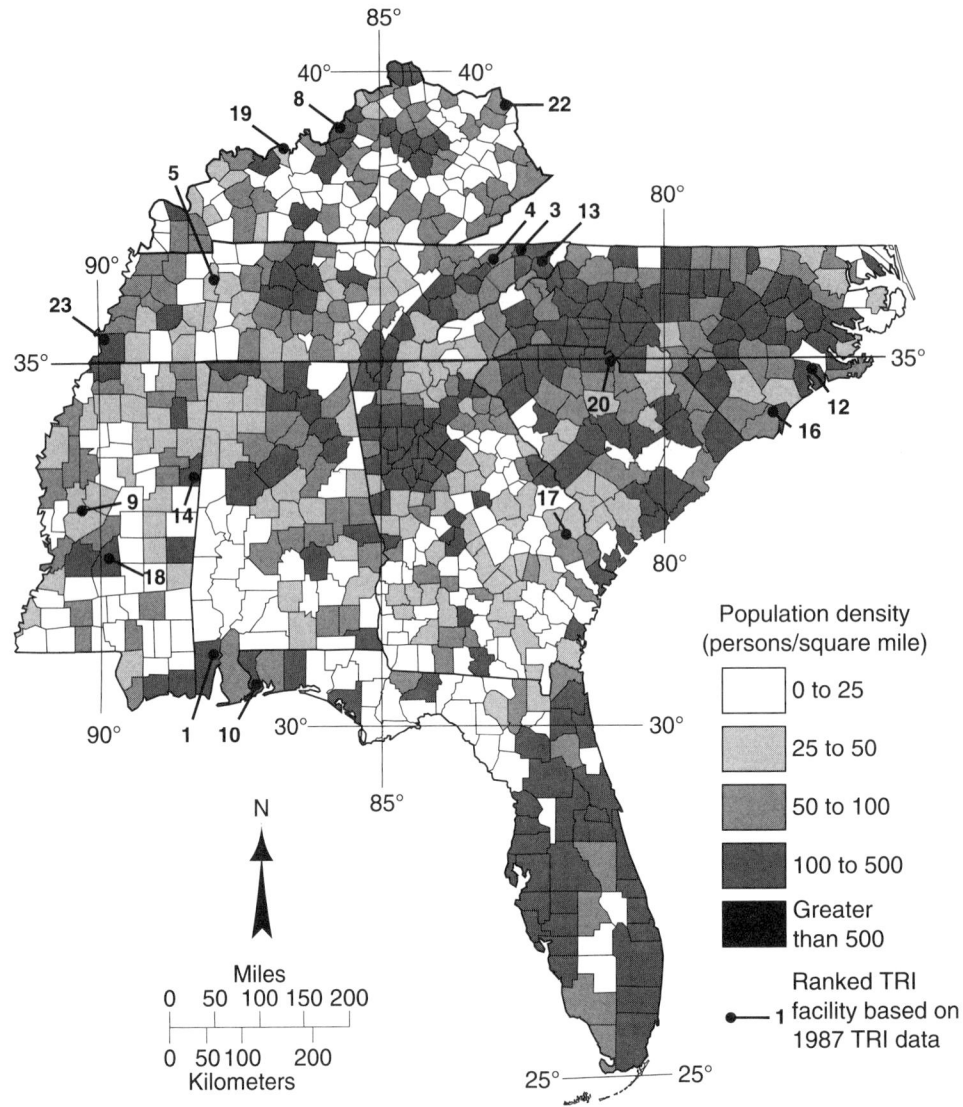

Fig. 2-7. The 25 top-ranking TRI facilities in the southeastern United States (Region IV). Data present rating according to the facility-reported emissions to surrounding populations according to the 1980 census. (From Stockwell J et al: *Risk Analysis* 13:155, 1993.)

dose, and altered structure or function with no ensuing pathologic effect or potential or actual health impairment.[39] Thus the biologic markers can represent a marker of effect (such as blood glucose), a marker of susceptibility (such as the presence of atopy), or a marker of exposure. The last can be defined as exogenous substances or metabolites of them or the product of an interaction between a hazardous agent and some target molecule or cell that is measured in a compartment within the body.[39]

EXAMPLES OF EXPOSURES IN AIR
Outdoor air pollution (see Chapter 37)

Outdoor air pollution may occur either in community or regional contexts or be confined to a specific area. Concentrations of air pollutants may be higher near a heavily traveled road or an industry producing noxious fumes and toxic gases. Although there are both natural and synthetic sources, natural sources are usually not a health concern and require no protective measures.

The six most widespread air pollutants in the outdoor environment include particulate matter (diameter <10 μm), sulfur dioxide, nitrogen dioxide, carbon monoxide, photochemical oxidants such as ozone, and lead. During 1991 a total of 514 counties and 20 cities were designated as nonattainment areas, representing an estimated 164 million persons.[7] Persons residing in nonattainment counties included 63% (about 31 million) of preadolescent children (<13 years), 60% (approximately 19 million) of persons aged >65 years, and about 64% (approximately 9 million) of persons with chronic obstructive pulmonary disease; there were also

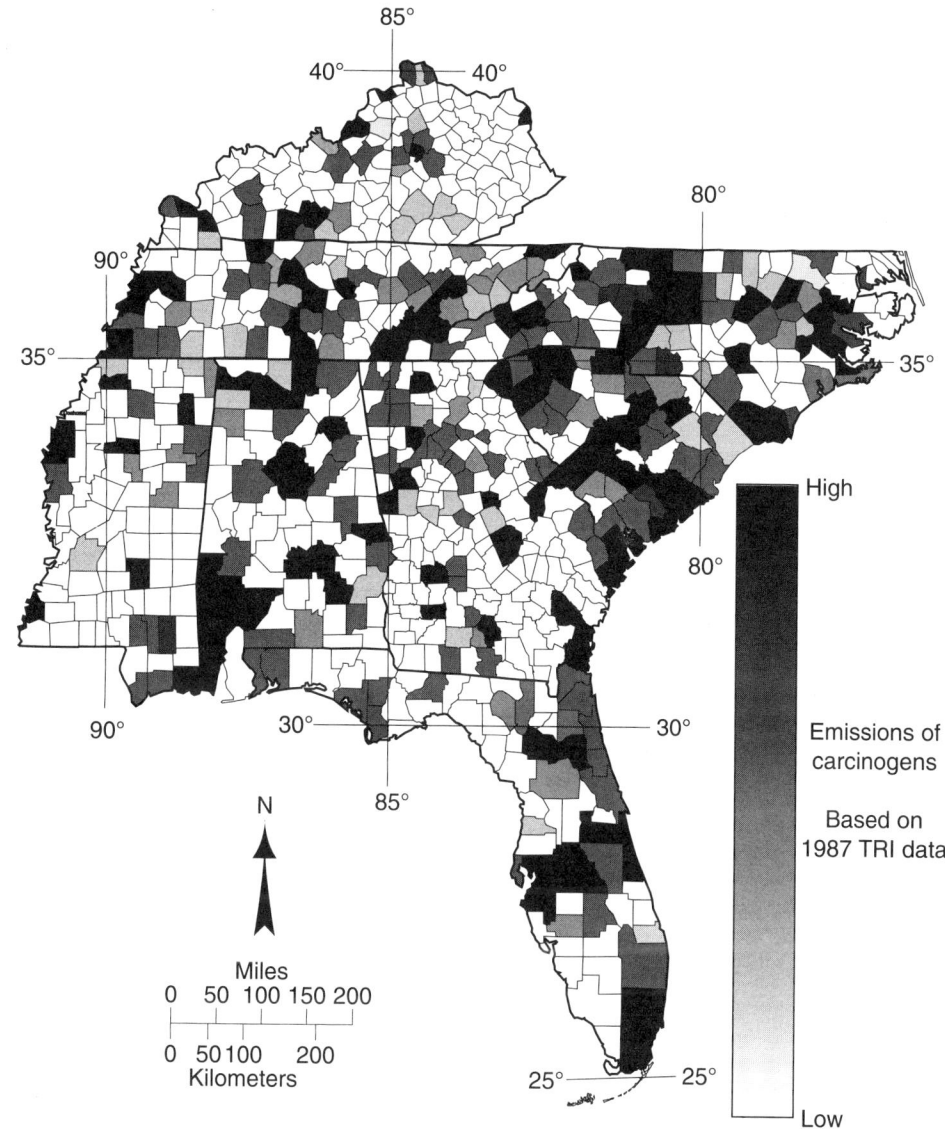

Fig. 2-8. The emissions in locales of the 25 top-ranking TRI facilities in the southeastern United States (Region IV) according to the facility-reported emissions presumed to be carcinogens. (From Stockwell J et al: *Risk Analysis* 13:155, 1993.)

some 4.3 million adults with asthma, 2.2 million children with asthma, and 3.5 million persons with coronary heart disease. About 1.6 million were estimated to be pregnant women.[7]

Photochemical air pollution contains virtually all oxidant gases and acidic aerosols and is especially severe during the summer, in urban areas, and in nearby suburbs downwind of an urban center. Photochemical air pollution contains oxides of nitrogen, carbon monoxide, nonmethane hydrocarbons, ozone, nitric acid, peroxyacetyl nitrate (PAN), acidic sulfates (such as sulfuric acid), salts, aldehydes, and organic particulates. The major source of photochemical air pollution is transportation, which accounts for 64% of the components of photochemical smog. Highway vehicles alone contribute 32% of nitrogen oxides, 29% of hydrocarbons, and 72% of the carbon monoxide emissions. The energy industry is responsible for about 10.6% of the nitrogen oxide emissions, and industrial processes release close to 11% of the hydrocarbons. Industrial processes and forest fires each contribute nearly 5.5% of annual carbon monoxide emissions in the United States.

Ozone (O_3), a powerful oxidizing agent and strong irritant formed from molecular oxygen (O_2) and oxygen free radicals (O^-), typically rises during the summer months, when higher temperatures and increased sunlight combine with static atmospheric conditions. Solar radiation breaks oxygen molecules into free radicals in the stratosphere and divides NO_2 into NO and free radicals in the lower atmosphere.

These free radicals then combine with atmospheric oxygen to create ozone. Other naturally occurring or synthetic pollutants, such as aldehydes and unsaturated hydrocarbons, may also be broken down by sunlight to form organic free radicals. Free radicals produced by these other pollutants may oxidize readily with NO, leaving little NO to react with ozone and allowing ozone to build up in the atmosphere. Ozone levels in and near urban centers may frequently exceed National Ambient Air Quality Standards (NAAQS) for several hours during the day and may often exceed the 8-hour daily NAAQS standard. High concentrations of ozone may be produced and persist for up to 3 weeks during a single episode.

Oxides of nitrogen include nitrogen oxide, nitrous oxide, and nitrogen dioxide; they also lead to evolution of nitrous and nitric acids and nitrite and nitrate salts. Oxides of nitrogen, in combination with sunlight, may also promote the formation of ozone. Nitrous oxide is a natural component of the atmosphere and is not usually significant as a factor in air pollution or as a health hazard in the quantities in which it is naturally present in the atmosphere. The primary pollutant, NO, is oxidized by atmospheric oxygen to produce NO_2, an irritating dark brown gas that helps to give photochemical smog its characteristic brown color. Nitrogen dioxide is considerably more toxic than NO and is more important in the formation of other toxic nitrogenous byproducts and ozone. Effects of NO_2 are similar to those of ozone but require exposure to higher ambient concentrations. As with carbon monoxide, individuals whose respiratory system is already compromised by illness may have a much lower tolerance for oxides of nitrogen.

Carbon monoxide is produced during the burning of carbon-based fuels when combustion is incomplete, resulting in the release of gaseous hydrocarbons and carbon particles.

A type of air pollution that has significant health effects is sulfur dioxide and associated sulfates. While this type of pollution has been significantly reduced in the United States, it is common in parts of the industrialized world that depend on high-sulfur coal as their primary combustion fuel source. In the United States, the energy industry is still the largest contributor to sulfur oxide levels in the air, accounting for 80% of emissions. Chemicals produced in this type of pollution that have significant health impacts include sulfur dioxide, sulfuric and sulfonic acid, neutralized sulfate salts, and carbon and carbon monoxide.[23]

Unlike photochemical smog, sulfurous smog episodes are more common in the winter, possibly due to the higher demand for heat and to atmospheric inversions associated with fog formation and higher levels of primary pollutants, such as SO_2 and soot, in the atmosphere. Liquid droplet chemistry speeds up the oxidation of SO_2 to sulfuric acid in the presence of fog and possibly a transition element, such as manganese, vanadium, or iron. While potentially very irritating at high concentrations, at ambient levels sulfate salts, sulfuric acid, and other acid aerosols may be neutralized by ammonia naturally present in the respiratory tract.

Particulates in the air may include such contaminants as asbestos, fiberglass, silica, cotton and other fibers, dusts, and heavy metals and particulates released by fires, volcanoes, and fly ash from waste incineration. Also included are the products of incomplete combustion from transportation, energy, and other industry sources.

The hazardous waste incineration industry experienced explosive growth in the 1980s as a result of two hazardous waste laws. The 1980 Superfund law legislated the cleanup of chemical dumps; the 1976 Resource Conservation and Recovery Act was intended to manage waste disposal more carefully. The effect of both laws was to make millions of tons of hazardous chemical wastes more valuable as a commodity that could be burned by charging up to a $1000 per ton.[33] In 1993 there were 184 hazardous waste incinerators in the United States.[33] About 20 are commercial incinerators, while 164 plants burn hazardous wastes as fuel in cement kilns, boilers, and industrial furnaces; 3 to 4 million tons, or about 1%, of all hazardous wastes are incinerated. Some 600,000 tons are burned in the 20 commercial hazardous waste incinerators, and perhaps 1 million are incinerated at a fee in 29 cement and other types of industrial kilns around the country. The rest is burned on a noncommercial basis in 135 boilers and industrial furnaces operated by chemical companies, refiners, and other generators of hazardous waste. Major criticisms are the lack of trained personnel at the facilities housing kilns and boilers to carefully monitor the waste entering the furnaces, the failure of furnaces to comply with federal air pollution requirements, and the failure to carefully analyze wastes before burning to determine what they contain.[33]

Emissions from hazardous waste incineration include polychlorinated dioxins and furans, two of the most potentially toxic chemicals that are extremely persistent in the environment. Other contaminants are known or suspected carcinogens, such as arsenic, cadmium, chromium, chlorinated dioxins and dibenzofurans, formaldehyde, polychlorinated biphenyls (PCBs), and polycyclic aromatic hydrocarbons. In addition, incinerator emissions include heavy metals (including mercury and lead), beryllium, carbon monoxide, chlorobenzenes and chlorophenols, hydrogen chloride, and nitrogen oxides.[14] Mercury pollution in Florida has been implicated in the contamination of fish and aquatic organisms. It has been estimated that about 15% of the total environmental mercury contamination comes from garbage incineration, 14% from medical waste incineration, 11% from paint application, 11% from fossil fuel burning, and 6% from fluorescent and other light bulbs, batteries, wiring, switches, and other electrical apparatus.[17] Other types of domestic burning, such as open leaf burning, are of concern as there are reports that such burning may affect asthmatic individuals and cause acute reductions in lung function.[9]

Emissions from incineration include dioxins, which may attach to particulate forms and be deposited in residential communities' soil or drinking water. The term *dioxin* is commonly used to refer to two families of chemicals that, taken together, comprise 210 closely related but unique compounds. These compounds are categorized as either polychlorodibenzo-p-dioxins ("dioxins") or polychlorodibenzofurans ("furans"). These compounds are extremely toxic to animal species and believed to be very toxic to humans. They are also produced during metal recovery, waste incineration, wood preservation, paper pulp bleaching, and chemical manufacturing. Each industrial process produces a different "fingerprint" pattern of dioxins and furan compounds that allows the chemicals to be traced back to their sources.[11] The amount of dioxins emitted from incinerators varies as much as 1000-fold, depending upon the sophistication of the technology used to burn the waste.[11] Table 2-3 lists various environmental sources of dioxins and furans.[11]

One approach to reducing the toxic pollutants associated with the burning of waste through incineration is limiting the development of new incineration sites and restricting the capacity of the current hazardous waste incineration facilities to burn more than a specified amount of chemical by-products a year.[33]

Other chemical substances that are significant air pollutants and have potentially hazardous effects on human health include mercury and lead compounds, cyanates, vinyl chloride, and organic pesticides. These tend to be distributed locally, near mines or industries that manufacture such substances or use them in the production process. Trace elements of such toxic substances as arsenic, beryllium, cadmium, chromium, mercury, lead, and nickel may also be present in the atmosphere. Appreciable airborne concentrations of volatile organic chemicals may exist at hazardous waste sites during cleanup operations.[42]

Indoor air pollution (see Chapter 37)

Chemical components of nonindustrial indoor air pollution include volatile organic chemicals (VOCs), formaldehyde, various pesticides, lead, carbon monoxide, carbon dioxide, nitrogen dioxide, sulfur dioxide, and polycyclic aromatic hydrocarbons. Several of these are present in environmental tobacco smoke, which has recently been receiving more attention as a source of toxic indoor air pollution. Tobacco smoke itself may be responsible for many adverse health effects, including carcinogenesis, and may aggravate existing cardiopulmonary disease or react synergistically with other chemical exposures.

VOCs include benzene from tobacco smoke and perchlorethylene from dry-cleaned clothing, rugs, and draperies; paints; and stored chemicals. Such common household items as pesticides, wood preservatives, cleaners, solvents, and polishes may contain and release VOCs. Formaldehyde is a common VOC contaminant of indoor air, as it is released from building materials, treated carpets and other textiles, and many synthetic surfaces found in homes and offices.

Odorants are another common type of indoor air pollutant. These chemicals are found in perfumes and room and body deodorants and are ubiquitous in household cleaning and personal care products. Chemicals found in odorants include organic compounds, such as nonane, decane, undecane, ethylheptane, pinene, and limonene. Substituted aromatics such as paradichlorobenzene have become one of the leading VOCs in indoor air.[5] A 1988 study by the U.S. House Subcommittee on Business Opportunities and NIOSH found 314 chemicals used in the fragrance industry that were known to be mutagens, 218 that caused reproductive problems, 778 that caused acute toxic reactions, 146 that were tumor-causing, and 376 that caused eye and skin irritations. Other chemical contaminants that may be present in fragrances include toluene, methyl ethyl ketone, and benzoine.

Organic solvents are an important component of indoor air pollution in many industrial contexts. This category of contaminants includes kerosene, acetone, and naphthas.

Biologic agents include bacteria, viruses, fungi, pollen, dust mites and other insects, and animal dander and matter that can travel in particulate form and be inhaled, ingested, or obtained through parenteral or dermal routes. Many are found within the inside environment, especially the home, but some occur outdoors. Excessive growth of bacteria and

Table 2-3. Sources of dioxins and furans

Process	Predominant dioxin/furan	Dioxin carrier
Chemical manufacture		
2,4,5-T	TCDD	Herbicide
Pentachlorophenol	Higher Cl dioxins	Pesticides
Other chlorophenols	Various	Pesticides
PCBs	Furans	Capacitor fluid
Incineration		
Industrial	Furans	Stack emissions, fly ash
Biomedical		
Garbage		
Wood preservation		
Pentachlorophenol	Higher Cl dioxins	Preserved wood
Paper pulp bleaching		
	TCDD, TCDF	Diapers, tea bags, milk cartons, coffee filters
Metal recovery		
Copper	Furans	Stack emissions, fly ash
Silver		
Nonpoint sources		
Automobiles	Furans	Exhaust fumes, smoke
Fires		
Wood stoves		

Cl, chlorinated; TCDD, tetrachlorodibenzodioxin; TCDF, tetrachlorodibenzofuran fungi occur in improperly maintained air ducts, air conditioners, humidifiers, dehumidifiers, air-cleaning filters, carpets, and poorly ventilated indoor spaces where moisture collects (bathroom, kitchen, laundry room, and basement). Viruses are spread by human contact. Dust mites and other insects reside in sofas, stuffed chairs, carpets, and bedding.

EXAMPLES OF EXPOSURES IN WATER

Chemical contamination of drinking water represents a major environmental medical problem. Chapter 24 explores this subject in more detail. The following examples may lead to serious consequences in the future.

Dumping of nuclear waste

The dumping of highly radioactive wastes at sea has been banned worldwide for more than 30 years and thus by global consensus has been ruled off limits because of the tremendous toxicity for human and oceanic life. Unfortunately, information has come to light indicating that the Soviet Union had repeatedly broken international rules and dumped vast amounts of highly radioactive waste into the ocean.[4] Such spent fuel includes contamination with cesium-137 and other highly toxic isotopes. Ten years ago the ban was extended to include all other forms of nuclear waste, including uranium mill tailings. It was reported that the Russians dumped some 2.5 million curies of radioactive wastes, including 18 nuclear reactors from submarines and an icebreaker; 16 were dumped into the Kara Sea and near major northern fisheries, while 2 were deposited into the Sea of Japan. In comparison, it has been estimated that the accident at Chernobyl nuclear power plant released 50 million curies of radiation, but most of that was in short-lived isotopes like iodine-131 that disappear in a few months. The sea-dumped radioactive wastes have half-lives of decades.

Oil spills

It has been estimated that in the United States alone oil spills represent a significant environmental contamination. Every day there is an oil spill somewhere in the nation, often due to leaky pipes that may be as old as 50 years. Many of the country's 700,000 underground oil storage tanks have leaked oil, contaminating soil and water. It has been estimated that about 44 million gallons of petroleum have leaked from oil refineries since the early 1980s. There have been major oil spills at sea or near ports, causing tremendous ecologic harm and potential human health effects.

EXAMPLES OF EXPOSURES IN LAND AND SOIL
Solid waste and garbage

Solid waste may pose a lesser potential threat to human health than air or water pollution, but it represents a major public concern. Chapters 56 to 58 deals with the issue of hazardous wastes and Chapter 45 explores the area of soil and contaminated sites. Municipal solid waste, generated by houses and offices, makes up about 10% of the total solid waste generated; household waste accounts for about only 4% of the total.[40] Typical trash in the United States contains about 5% textiles, rubber, leather, and wood; 8% metals; 8% plastics; 10% glass; 31% paper; 25% vegetables; and 13% others.[40] In lower- and middle-income countries, trash contains 47% to 60% vegetables.

Several companies are developing systems to transform garbage into slag.[10] The system utilizes a new generation of highly efficient plasma arc torches that pass a strong electric current through rarefied gas, ionizing it and producing a flame hotter than fire with temperatures up to 8000° C. Such intense heat with oxygen deprivation results in matter not burning but rather dissociating in a process of pyrolysis. The toxic hydrocarbons break down into simple gases, metals melt and disperse, and soil solidifies. This "plasma pyrolysis" may lead to the ultimate solution to municipal solid waste disposal.

Hazardous waste sites

The number of toxic chemical waste disposal sites in the United States is estimated to be more than 30,000.[42] Over the past four decades more than 750 million tons of chemicals have been deposited in these sites.[15] In May 1988 there were 29,997 sites listed by EPA as containing potentially hazardous materials. The nearly 1000 sites placed on the National Priorities List are distributed throughout the country, but four states contain 60 sites and New Jersey had at least 100. Many of the sites were landfills operated by local, state, or federal agencies and were used intentionally for hazardous waste disposal by permits or solicited dumping; some were used unintentionally either by accident or through lack of regulatory control. Some were associated with military facilities. Many were developed in conjunction with industrial operations producing hazardous wastes. The many sites include open waste heaps, filled pits, landfills, tanks, piles of drums, lagoons, pools, ponds, and sediments in water bodies contaminated by direct discharge.[42] Sites were located on hills and slopes, valleys, and drainage areas, with every type of disposal and with every imaginable route and degree of dispersion of contaminants to the various routes of dispersion. They are generally in the form of liquids, solids, and sludges. While chemical analyses have revealed about 400 different substances at the sites, the most common substances detected are halogenated hydrocarbons (for example, trichloroethylene, chloroform, PCBs, tetrachloro- and dichloroethanes, methylene chloride), aromatic hydrocarbons (for example, toluene, benzene, phenol, ethylbenzene, xylene), and metals (for example, lead, zinc, cadmium, arsenic, chromium, copper, mercury).

Contamination of water supply from leaking chemicals at hazardous waste sites has been relatively frequent, especially the release of heavy metals and organic solvents.[6,15] The state of Florida can be used as an example; the state's geologic structure increases the chances of chemical leaching.[31] There are 12,659 miles of streams and rivers in Florida and more than 7700 lakes, which when combined total 2.1 million acres of surface area.[18] In Florida the majority of designated hazardous waste sites are near densely populated areas, such as Miami, Tampa, and Jacksonville. The existence of large aquifer systems may distribute hazardous pollutants large distances and affect large numbers of inhabitants.

Extraction of ores and abandoned mines

Large-scale extraction of metals presents hazardous waste management problems. It has been estimated that by the year 2000 mining will have directly disturbed approximately 240,000 km of the Earth's surface, an area equivalent to about the size of Oregon.[29] Fig. 2-9 depicts types of contamination that might result from a large-scale metal extraction operation, including contamination of drinking water.[29]

Abandoned mines often represent sites of toxic mine wastes. The abandoned mines and waste include residues from mineral-processing plants and hard rock minerals. When it rains or snows, the water mixes with the remaining materials and forms acidic solutions that, by estimates, pollute some 10,000 miles of streams in the western United States.[34]

Nuclear wastes

Each year 120 million nuclear medicine procedures are performed in the United States.[48] Principle sources of low-level radioactive waste (LLRW) that are shipped for disposal include nuclear fuel cycles (nuclear power plants, fuel fabricators and processors, and research and development), industrial sources (manufacturing, mining research), institutional sources (hospitals, clinics), and government sites.[48] In 1986 about 3% of the volume and 0.06% of the activity of all LLRW received at commercial disposal facilities were from institutional sources.

The federal government disposes of high-level radioactive waste, like that from nuclear weapons production or spent fuel from nuclear plants, but each state is responsible for its own low-level waste. The disposal of this low-level radioactive waste is reaching a crisis state because public opposition and political conflict have impeded carrying out laws intended to make this type of waste disposal more equitable for the states with dump sites.[30] Under the law the three states that have been accepting and burying radioactive waste can exclude any waste generated outside their own region. Nevada planned to discontinue its site while Wash-

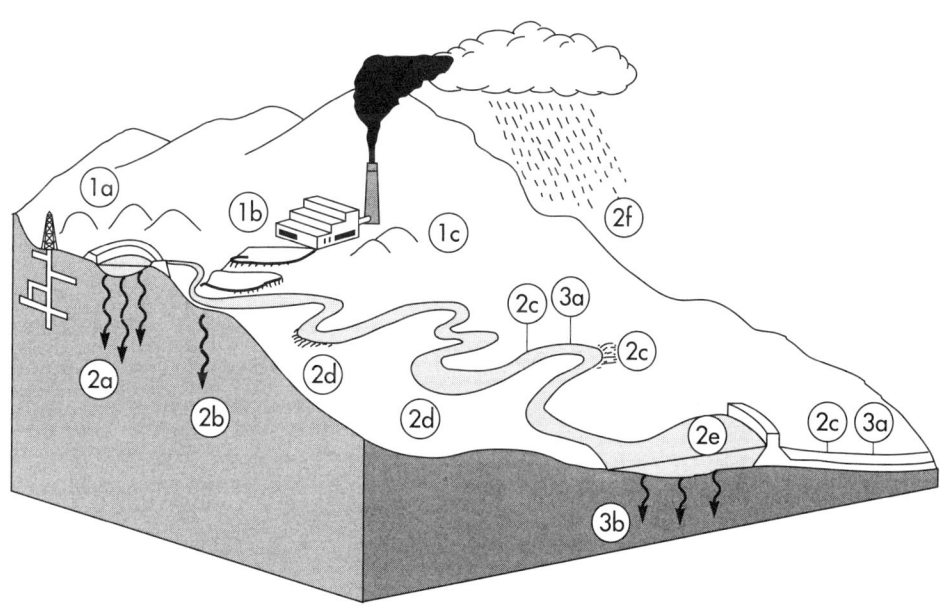

Primary	Secondary		Tertiary
1a. Waste rock	2a. Ground water at open pits	2d. Flood plain sediment/soil	3a. River sediment reworked from flood plain
1b. Tailings	2b. Ground water beneath ponds	2e. Reservoir sediment	3b. Ground water from contaminated reservoir sediment
1c. Slag	2c. Sediment in river channels	2f. Soils from air pollution	

Fig. 2-9. Types of contamination that might result from a large-scale metal extraction operation. (From Moore J, Luoma S: Hazardous wastes from large-scale metal extraction: a case study, *Environ Sci Technol* 24:1278, 1990.)

ington State planned to limit its intake from other regions. Consequently, only one dump, in Barnwell, South Carolina, plans to stay open for the rest of the country but will be closed to many outsiders by 1994 and shut down by 1996. After this time, with so much public opposition, it is unclear where the nation will store the thousands of cubic feet of low-level radioactive waste it generates. This will put hospitals, pharmaceutical companies, and electric utilities at a great loss to find a source for their radioactive wastes.

EXAMPLES OF EXPOSURES IN OTHER CATEGORIES

The category of physical agents includes such environmental hazards as ionizing and nonionizing radiation, electric and magnetic fields, noise, temperature extremes, and factors leading to traumatic injuries and accidents. The health consequences of exposure to these agents are diverse and, in some cases, still controversial.

Trauma and accidents are the fourth leading cause of death in the United States and the first for children and young adults.[3] This category includes all types of accidents, including vehicular and household, and violent injury and death, including suicide and homicide. Automobile accidents are the largest cause of accidental death in the country. Concern about suicide and homicide has been rising sharply over the past 20 years, as an epidemic of random violence seems to be sweeping our nation, particularly in urban areas. This has been attributed to poverty, the breakdown of the family, increasing stress, and the influence of the media, to give but a few examples. In fact, all of these factors are probably involved as our environment grows increasingly complex and confusing. Much of the fear and anxiety experienced by people in our nation may be attributable to a feeling of loss of control over the environment in which we live and work. Accidents in the home and workplace may be related to the greater sophistication of our technology, much of which we use without really understanding the way it works or the hazards it may present.

REFERENCES

1. Aldrich T, Griffith J: Public awareness, federal policy, and environmental epidemiology. In Aldrich T, Griffith J, eds: *Environmental epidemiology and risk assessment,* New York, 1993, Van Nostrand Reinhold.
2. Aldrich T, Leaverton P: Sentinel event strategies in environmental health, *Ann Rev Publ Health* 14:205, 1993.
3. Blumenthal D: Prospective on environmental health. In Blumenthal D, ed: *Introduction to environmental health,* New York, 1985, Springer.
4. Broad W: Russians describe extensive dumping of nuclear waste, *New York Times* April 27:A1, 1993.
5. Cone J, Shusterman D: Health effects of indoor odorants, *Environ Health Prospectives* 95:53, 1991.
6. Dix H: *Environmental pollution,* New York, 1981, J Wiley.
7. Editor: Populations at risk from air pollution, *MMWR Report* 42:301, 1993.
8. Felber E: *Childhood cancers and congenital malformations in the state of Florida: an ecologic study [MSPH],* College of Public Health, University of South Florida, 1993.
9. From L, Bergen L, Humlie R: The effects of open leaf burning on spirometric measurements in asthma, *Chest* 101:1236, 1992.
10. Gibbs W: Garbage in, gravel out, *Sci Am* May:130, 1993.
11. Goldman L et al: Dioxins in California: a widespread problem, California Department of Health Services, 1991.
12. Gore A: *Earth in the balance,* New York, 1992, Penguin.
13. Graham J et al: Role of exposure databases in risk assessment, *Arch Environ Health* 47:408, 1992.
14. Greenpeace: Municiple solid waste incinerators, Greenpeace Action, 1990.
15. Griffith J et al: Cancer mortality in U.S. counties with hazardous waste sites and ground water pollution, *Arch Environ Health* 44:69, 1989.
16. Grisham J: *Health aspects of the disposal of water chemicals,* New York, 1986, Pergamon Press.
17. Gunter B: Study details sources of toxic mercury, *Tampa Tribune* 25:1, 1992.
18. Hand J, Tauxe V, Friedman M: Water quality assessment for the state of Florida, Department of Environmental Regulation, 1988.
19. Hoffman E et al: Cloning of a factor required for activity of the Ah (dioxin) receptor, *Science* 252:954, 1991.
20. Knox E, Lancashire R: *Epidemiology of congenital malformations,* London, 1990, HMSO.
21. Koren H: Environment and humans. In Koren H, ed: *Handbook of environmental health and safety: principles and practices,* Chelsea, Mich, 1991, Lewis.
22. Lave L, Ennever F: Toxic substances control in the 1990s: are we poisoning ourselves with low-level exposures? *Ann Rev Public Health* 11:69, 1990.
23. Lioy P: Total human exposure assessment, *Environ Sci Technol* 24:938, 1990.
24. Mahoney M et al: Population density and cancer mortality differentials in New York State, 1978-1982, *Int J Epidemiol* 19:483, 1990.
25. Mason T, Hays HM: Disease among animals as sentinels of environmental exposures. In Leaverton P, Masse L, Simches S, eds: *Environmental epidemiology,* New York, 1982, Praeger.
26. Matanoski G et al: Role of exposure databases in epidemiology, *Arch Environ Health* 47:439, 1992.
27. McKone T: Human exposure to chemicals from multiple media and through multiple pathways: research overview and comments, *J Risk Anal* 11:5, 1991.
28. Meadows D, Meadows D, Randers J: *Beyond the limits: confronting global collapse, envisioning a sustainable future.* Post Mills, Vt, 1992, Chelsea Green.
29. Moore J, Luoma S: Hazardous wastes from large-scale metal extraction: a case study, *Environ Sci Technol* 24:1278, 1990.
30. Reinhold R: States, failing to cooperate, face a nuclear-waste crisis, *New York Times* Dec 28:A1, 1992.
31. Ritter D: *Process geomorphology,* Dubuque, Ia, 1986, William C. Brown.
32. Rutstein D et al: Sentinel health events (occupational): a basis for physician recognition and public health surveillance, *Am J Public Health* 39:1054, 1984.
33. Schneider K: Administration to freeze growth of hazardous waste incinerators, *New York Times* May 18:A1, 1993.
34. Schneider K: New approach to old peril: abandoned mines in west, *New York Times* April 27:A1, 1993.
35. Selvin S et al: Transformation of maps to investigate clusters of disease, *Social Science and Medicine* 26:215, 1988.
36. Sexton K et al: Estimating human exposures to environmental pollutants: availability and utility of existing databases, *Arch Environ Health* 47:398, 1992.
37. Stevens W: Humanity confronts its handiwork: an altered planet, *New York Times* May 5:B5, 1992.
38. Stockwell JR et al: The U.S. EPA geographic information system for mapping environmental release of toxic chemical release inventory (TRI) chemicals, *J Risk Anal* 13:155, 1993.

39. Subcommittee on Pulmonary Toxicology, Committee on Biologic Markers, National Research Council: *Biologic markers in pulmonary toxicology,* Washington, DC, 1989, National Academy Press.
40. Survey: waste and the environment, *Economist* May 29:1-19, 1993.
41. Tarcher A: Principles and scope of environmental medicine. In Tarcher A, ed: *Principles and practice of environmental medicine,* New York, 1992, Plenum.
42. Upton A, Kneip T, Toniolo P: Public health aspects of toxic chemical disposal sites, *Annu Rev Public Health* 10:1, 1989.
43. U.S. Environmental Protection Agency NCFHS and the Agency for Toxic Substances and Disease Registry: Inventory of exposure-related data systems sponsored by federal agencies, 1992.
44. U.S. Environmental Protection Agency RI: Categories of released chemicals reported to the toxic release inventory, 1993.
45. Walter S: The analysis of regional patterns of health data. I. Distributional considerations, *Am J Epidemiol* 36:730, 1992.
46. Walter S: The analysis of regional patterns of health data. II. The power to detect environmental effects, *Am J Epidemiol* 136:742, 1992.
47. Welch W: How cells respond to stress, *Sci Am* 56, 1993.
48. Wilkerson A et al: Low-level radioactive waste from U.S. biomedical and academic institutions: policies, strategies, and solutions, *Annu Rev Public Health* 10:299, 1989.
49. Williams F, Lawson A, Lloyd O: Low sex ratios of births in areas at risk from air pollution from incinerators, such as shown by geographical analysis and 3-dimensional mapping, *Int J Epidemiol* 21:311, 1992.

Chapter 3

RISK ASSESSMENT APPLIED TO ENVIRONMENTAL MEDICINE

David F. Goldsmith

Risk assessment process
    Hazard identification from review of the medical and toxicology literature
    Dose-response assessment
    Exposure assessment
    Risk determination
Assumptions used in risk assessment
Risk assessment for crystalline silica
    Background
    Assumptions for extrapolation from animals to humans
    Extrapolation methods
    Results of risk assessment
    Assessing human risk assessment
Guidelines for practitioners of environmental medicine

Risk assessment is a means of quantifying the probability that exposure to hazardous materials will damage the health of individuals in a population. Similar methods are being developed to enable risk assessors to estimate ecologic impacts on the health of environments, such as wetlands and coastal fisheries, but the focus in this chapter is on the health of human communities. For environmental health practitioners risk assessment is the yardstick by which agencies such as the U.S. Environmental Protection Agency (EPA) judge whether to take regulatory action, which is referred to as *risk management*. This chapter describes the risk assessment process used to evaluate chemicals causing cancer and those producing health effects other than cancer. With use of exposure to crystalline silica dust as an example, the risk estimation process is examined, and there is a discussion of how environmental health practitioners can play a greater role in risk-assessment activities.

RISK ASSESSMENT PROCESS

In 1983 the National Academy of Sciences (NAS) provided the EPA and other regulatory agencies with a framework for applying and standardizing health risk policies.[20] The NAS panel defined the terms and procedures that are now used when risk assessment is undertaken for individual chemicals or chemical processes. The EPA has elaborated on these recommendations to develop nomenclature to encompass the risk assessment process. For environmental health evaluations under the Superfund law, the EPA undertakes remedial investigation and feasibility studies to arrive at a determination by EPA managers of the degree of clean-up or control options.[26] With the exception of the regulations for pesticide chemicals, similar methods are used by federal and nonfederal agencies in evaluating the hazards from environmental chemicals.

After some determination that there is a likely environmental health hazard, a baseline risk assessment is begun. This assessment includes four interrelated steps: (1) hazard identification and data evaluation, (2) toxicity assessment focusing on dose-response findings, (3) exposure determination, and (4) risk characterization, including uncertainty analysis. Fig. 3-1 lists the steps in risk assessment (highlighted in bold) and the contributions of the attendant disciplines to each step. The flow of information into and out of the steps in the risk assessment process are interactive, as are the events between steps in the process. When new data emerge about environmental hazards—such as findings of carcinogenicity for a chemical previously thought to affect only the nervous system—the risk assessment equation is reconfigured to determine what is necessary to protect public health. A more stringent environmental lead standard is an example of a chemical exposure that has undergone recon-

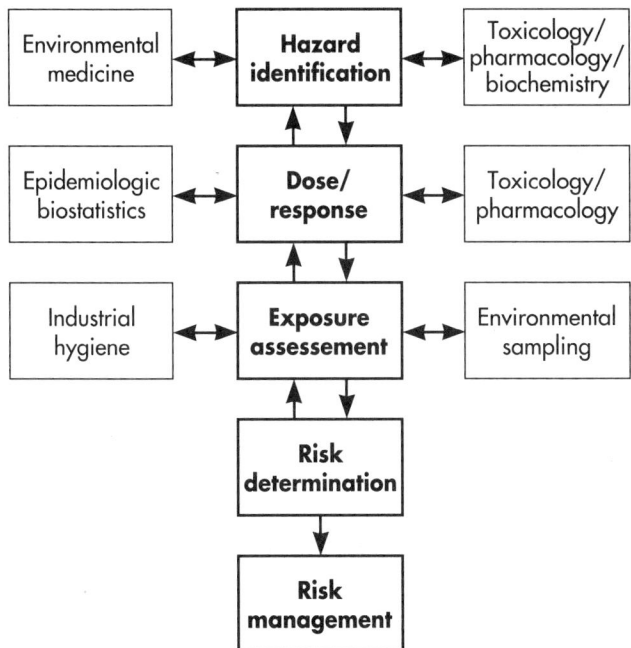

Fig. 3-1. Steps in risk assessment.

sideration as new findings of lead's ability to cause learning deficits at levels previously thought to be safe have emerged; however, when regulatory agencies conduct risk assessments, they do not consider the risk management impacts of their risk evaluations. That is, in theory, enforcement, or risk management, is separate from measurement of risk for a chemical or an environmental contamination.

Hazard identification from review of the medical and toxicology literature

Risk assessment begins with a review of the medical and toxicology literature to determine whether there is evidence of acute or chronic health effects related to use of or exposure to the chemical of concern. For many industrial chemicals or chemical wastes, there may be few or no human data; thus there is a great deal of reliance on animal toxicity and pharmacology findings, including structural-activity research from biochemistry. When evidence of human health effects appears in the environmental medicine literature, it may consist of case reports or epidemiologic studies with low statistical power. Useful places to begin this review include medical and toxicology texts on occupational and environmental health hazards.[6,17,23] For chemicals thought to cause cancer, the International Agency for Research on Cancer (IARC) provides a thorough review of the world's literature.[16] The Agency for Toxic Substances and Disease Registry, in Atlanta, Georgia, is a source for information on health effects from toxic chemical hazards, and many of its review documents are found in health science libraries. The EPA also provides access to an on-line database, Integrated Risk Information Service, that provides reviews of chemicals for the initial determination of hazard. The National Institute for Occupational Safety and Health has a toll-free telephone number, 1-800-35NIOSH, for occupational and medical toxicology information.

In the evaluation of data on health effects, it is appropriate to ascertain the medium from which the findings arose. Thus, if there is concern about a solvent's health effects, it is important to recognize where workers or residents contact the chemical. (Measurement of the material in the environment is described later.) Because human contact can occur through air, water, soil, and plants, toxic findings of effects on soil nematodes may be of limited relevance for human exposure experience. Solvent liquids may produce neurologic effects different from those caused by solvent vapors; thus temperature, air pressure, and prevailing winds must be considered. Experimental routes of exposure need to be examined for relevance; therefore a solvent-saturated pellet implanted into the bladder lumens of mice may be inappropriate for judging the solvent's risk for miscarriage in women exposed through drinking water.

The purpose of conducting the hazard identification is to determine the type of toxic health effect (usually divided into cancer or noncancer endpoints), acute or chronic conditions, the degree of toxicity of the chemical, and the appropriateness of the media in which the effects and exposure are found. If the chemical has toxic properties by inhalation, can it be assumed that the same findings will be obtained when risk assessment is undertaken of contamination of an Indian fisheries preserve? Alternatively, if a chemical has been studied with gavage methods in mice, these experimental findings are highly relevant for a pathway that includes ingestion by children.

Dose-response assessment

The next step in the risk assessment process is dose-response determination, which has some similarities and some differences in extrapolation for neoplastic health effects or for noncancer effects. Assuming that there are no usable epidemiologic findings of adverse human health effects, the process for cancer extrapolation involves three crucial assumptions: that high-dose findings can be extrapolated to low or ambient doses, that dose-response gradients observed in experimental studies can be extrapolated to humans, and that extrapolations from high to low doses follow a no-threshold model at low doses. The EPA and other regulatory agencies use the upper 95% confidence limit (UCL) of the linearized multistage model at 1 mg/m^3 to predict the excess lifetime risk from these extrapolations.[14] Other biostatistical models (such as Weibull or probit) produce different-shaped slope lines at low doses, but the linearized multistage model is used because it is the most health conservative when the slopes are compared. The ultimate goal in the dose-response assessment is to derive the cancer potency slope, which is usually presented at the unit cancer risk, that is, the probability of excess cancer risk from lifetime exposure to 1 mg/m^3. When there are positive epidemiologic findings (usually from occupational health studies), it is feasible to extrapolate these results to determine ambient cancer risks. However, the assumptions are fewer because epidemiologic findings pertain to the species of interest, humans. There is still a need to extrapolate from healthy workers to members of the general population, including sensitive groups such as children, the elderly, and those with preexisting medical conditions.

For noncancer health endpoints (such as respiratory, reproductive, or nervous system effects), the examination of dose-response extrapolations follows a different process.[26] Dose-response data for either humans or experimental animals are sought to determine thresholds, that is, the lifetime dose at which no findings were detected or the lowest dose at which findings were detected. The dose at which no findings are observed is called the no-observed-adverse-effect level (NOAEL), and the dose at which the lowest findings were detected is referred to as the lowest-observed-adverse-effect level (LOAEL). Once these levels are derived, they are divided by safety factors, referred to as uncertainty factors (UFs) or modifying factors (MFs), to determine the reference dose (RfD) or reference concentration (RfC) for airborne toxins. UFs of 10 are used when the following apply: protection of sensitive subpopulations (such as children, the elderly, and fetuses); extrapolation from animals to humans; a NOAEL is derived from a subchronic study (rather than a lifetime chronic study); and a LOAEL, rather than an NOAEL, is used. MFs range from 1 to 10 and reflect uncertainties in the entire database judged to exist by agency environmental scientists. The default value is 1. The equation for a noncancer RfD is

$$RfD = NOAEL \text{ or } LOAEL/(UF_1 \times UF_2 \ldots \times MF)$$

The RfD is also defined as the ambient dose of a noncancer toxin for which no health effects are likely.[26]

Exposure assessment

The next step in the risk assessment is to obtain an estimate of chemical concentration in the environment and potential for human exposure. This step is usually undertaken by industrial or environmental hygienists. For regulatory agencies, environmental consultants are often used to measure levels of toxins in the air, water, soil, plants, animals, and exposed humans. Once the exposure is determined by dermal, inhalation, or ingestion route of entry, the assessment is presented in milligrams per kilogram per day. Some standard assumptions are used, such as that an average adult human weighs 70 kg, breathes 20 or 23 m^3 of air per day, drinks 2 L water per day, lives an average of 9 years in one residence, and has a life span of 70 years. Other assumptions for risk assessment (such as a toddler's ingestion of soil and food intakes) are available from the EPA Superfund *Human Health Evaluation Manual.*[26]

Exposure data can be derived from three extant sources ordered by level of uncertainty: biologic monitoring of the community at risk for toxics in human tissues (such as blood lead monitoring or samples of hair or fat tissues for specific chemicals or metabolites); ambient monitoring of plants, air, and water for indicator pollutants (such as pesticide residues, longitudinal air pollutants, or coliform counts from drinking water supplies); or pollutant models based on transport of substances in or between air, water, or soil. Because the concern for developing risk assessments is to protect the general population or the public health, two things need to be kept in mind: there must be an exposed human receptor for risk assessment to be undertaken, and data on humans (even if derived from workers rather than from the general population) are preferable to approximations of human exposure via modeling. When potential human exposure data are obtained, it is feasible to proceed to the next step in risk assessment: risk determination.

Risk determination

To estimate the risk from a particular environmental exposure to a carcinogen, environmental concentrations derived from the exposure assessment are multiplied by the unit cancer probability, and the product becomes lifetime excess risk. For most regulatory agencies, if the cancer risk exceeds acceptable levels (usually predetermined to be 10^{-6} or one excess cancer in 1,000,000 persons), regulatory action is justified. The risk assessment can be used to guide or develop risk-management strategies. Thus if exposure to a certain amount of pollutant leads to a 10^{-4} cancer risk, cleanup (risk management) is needed to control exposure so that no excess cases (above the acceptable risk level) arise from the remaining exposure to the chemical in the environment. The lifetime risk level, a unitless measure, also can be presented by multiplying the cancer risk by the population at risk to estimate the excess cancer cases.

For noncancer health effects, risk characterization is simpler. Once the RfC is calculated, it is simply a matter of comparing the average pollutant concentration level from the exposure assessment with the RfC or RfD. If the exposure is less than the RfC, no regulatory action is needed; if the exposure level exceeds the RfC, then control or cleanup is needed so that exposure is equal or less than the RfC (RfD).

ASSUMPTIONS USED IN RISK ASSESSMENT

In addition to the assumptions used in determining dose and exposure, environmental medicine practitioners must be aware that other assumptions go into risk assessments. The first is that there is an assumption of worst-case scenarios when the risk assessment calculations are made. This assumption is made to protect public health, because as a society we would rather overprotect than permit potential overexposure to a known health hazard for any population or group. Seen in this context, there is a philosophy of calculations permitting sizable margins of error so that when risk management is undertaken, the possibility of false-negative results regarding exposure and subsequent illness is reduced. The no-threshold assumption for carcinogens is based on empirical epidemiology findings of elevated cancer risks among both light smokers and survivors with low-level exposures to radiation after atomic bomb blasts in Japan. A final assumption is that risk assessment is undertaken without regard to beneficial properties of the chemical or the costs of cleanup. By way of contrast, under the Federal Insecticide, Fungicide, and Rodenticide Act, risk assessment must weigh the benefits to growers of pesticide chemicals before determinations of risk management options are made, whereas other enabling federal (and state) legislation does not require any benefit assessment before risk management occurs.

RISK ASSESSMENT FOR CRYSTALLINE SILICA

Silica is a useful example for environmental medicine practitioners to consider, because silica exposure is widespread, it has both cancerous and noncancerous health effects, and animal and human data support its classification as a toxic substance. As with other airborne respiratory hazards, such as arsenic, asbestos, coke oven emissions, and radon, cancer risks have been assessed for ambient environmental exposures to quartz particulate. This process requires extrapolation of the risks, using the cancer potency slope or the geometric means of several slope lines according to an established method such as that recommended by a regulatory agency.[2,25,26] Cancer risk assessment for quartz was an outgrowth of two separate determinations of the carcinogenicity of silica by IARC[15] and the Science Advisory Board for California's Proposition 65.[22] IARC reviewed the evidence for carcinogenicity of silica and concluded that there was sufficient evidence for carcinogenicity in laboratory animals and limited evidence for carcinogenicity in humans and therefore that silica was a probable human carcinogen.[15,16] The Science Advisory Board also reviewed the animal and human evidence and judged that airborne, respirable silica was a carcinogen known to the state of California.[22] Because it was determined that silica was a carcinogen, a risk assessment extrapolation was required under California's air toxins law, AB2588.[2] This section describes the cancer risk assessment extrapolations used in California.

Background

The first findings demonstrating that quartz produced tumors were reported by Wagner and colleagues,[27] who showed that intrapleurally injected silica dusts produced histiocytic lymphomas in several strains of rats. Since 1983, silica (using the trade names Min-U-Sil and DQ12) has been shown to be a pulmonary carcinogen in four lifetime rat studies using both intratracheal injection and inhalation methods.[4,10,13,19] Because the studies by Holland et al,[13] Dagle et al,[4] and Muhle et al[19] used inhalation methods to expose the animals to silica (similar to the route of exposure in humans), their findings were used in the three extant risk-assessment extrapolations.[1,2,8] There have also been two epidemiologic studies of California diatomaceous earth workers and white South African gold miners exposed to inhaled silica dust showing dose-response gradients for lung cancer.[3,11] The cancer risk assessment for the human and animal data are presented herein.

Assumptions for extrapolation from animals to humans

For all three risk assessment extrapolations, some standard assumptions were used. First, the lifetime silica dust exposure in the experimental studies was converted from milligrams per cubic meter to milligrams per kilogram/day. Thus it is assumed that adult female rats' body weight (BW) is 0.207 kg and male rats' BW is 0.342 kg. The daily air intake of a rat (Ira) is assumed to be $0.8 \times BW^{0.8206}$.[25] The fraction of silica aerosol deposited (DF) in the lung is 23%, based on research done by Newton and Pfledderer.[21] Thus the animal dose (AD) is obtained by multiplying the Ira by the silica dust concentration (Sdc), by the hours exposed per day (Hexp), by days exposed per week (Dexp), by days exposed per exposure period (Mexp), by the respirable fraction (Rspf), by DF, and dividing this numerator by the rodent BW.

$$AD = (Ira \times Scd \times Hexp \times Dexp \times Mexp \times Rspf \times DF)/BW$$

Thus to obtain the AD (in milligrams per kilogram per day) for female F344 rats in the study by Dagle et al,[4] the calculation is as follows:

$$[0.8 \times 0.207 \text{ kg}^{0.8206} \times 51.6 \text{ mg/m}^3 \times 6 \text{ hr/24 hr} \times 5 \text{ days/7 days/wk} \times 494/730 \times 100\% \times 0.23]/0.207 \text{ kg} = 1.52 \text{ mg/kg/day}$$

To obtain the human equivalent dose (HED) from the animal dose,[25,26] we assume an average human weight (avgBW) of 70 kg and apply a surface area correction factor (SACf), which equals $(avgBW/BW)^{1/3}$. Thus

$$HED = AD/SACf$$

Continuing the example of Dagle et al,[4] SACF = $(70 \text{ kg}/0.207 \text{ kg})^{1/3}$ = 6.97 and HED = (1.52 mg/kg/day)/6.97 = 0.22 mg/kg/day.

Last, we assume a human inhalation rate of 20 m³ air/day and a 70-year lifetime exposure for those living where ambient silica levels are the greatest.[25,26]

Extrapolation methods

To conduct a cancer risk assessment, the linearized multistage model, developed by Crump and colleagues in the form of the GLOBAL 86 program,[14] was used to estimate the cancer potency slope for silica. This model has been used by the EPA and the California Department of Health Services for previous cancer health risk assessments. The model uses the animal tumor incidence data to compute maximum likelihood estimates (MLE) and UCLs, which are also referred to as the q1*. The UCL is regarded as the upper limit of the estimated risk, and because of the nonthreshold assumption regarding carcinogens, the MLE and UCL are linear at low doses. Furthermore, UCL provides greater protection for public health than does use of less conservative approaches such as the use of the Occupational Safety and Health Administration permissible exposure limit, which is 0.1 mg/m^3 for silica in occupational settings to protect against silicosis.[5] The q1* results were converted from milligrams per kilogram per day to micrograms per cubic meter by first multiplying the q1* value by 20 m^3 of air per day, multiplying that product by 10^{-3} mg/µg, and dividing the whole product by 70 kg, the average weight of an adult.

By using the methods presented above, we can assess the unit risk for this example. The cancer potency slope (q1*) from the study by Dagle et al[4] of female rat tumors, in micrograms per cubic meter per day for an adult who is a lifetime resident in a high-silica location is as follows[8]:

Unit cancer risk = (q1*) × (20 m^3/day) × (10^{-3} mg/µg)/70 kg
0.36 × 20 × 0.001/70 = 1.0 × 10^{-4} (µg/m^3)$^{-1}$

Another way of describing this information is that the adult lifetime excess cancer risk from inhalation of 1 µg/m^3 of silica, based on the study by Dagle et al[4] of female rats, is 1 in 10,000.

Results of risk assessment

To find the individual cancer risk from lifetime exposure to the silica levels, the unit cancer risk factor is multiplied by the measured silica concentration, or

Individual lifetime cancer risk =
silica exposure × unit cancer risk (q1*)

The cancer potency (or unit risk factor) estimated by Goldsmith et al[9] ranged from 2.3 × 10^{-5} (based on data from males in the study by Dagle et al[4]) to 6.0 × 10^{-3} (based on data from females in the study by Muhle et al[9]) for a (1-µg/m^3)$^{-1}$ lifetime air exposure to silica dust. These findings are similar to those estimated by California's Office of Health Evaluation and Assessment,[2] which range from 2.9 × 10^{-4} (µg/m^3)$^{-1}$ (without correction for surface area differences between rodents and humans) to 4.4 × 10^{-5} (µg/m^3)$^{-1}$ (with surface area correction). Brantner and Klein[1] also conducted a cancer risk assessment for silica exposure based on the same three animal studies. They derived a single q1* for quartz of 3.55 × 10^{-5} (µg/m^3)$^{-1}$, using some variations in methods from those used by Goldsmith et al.[9] Another way to interpret these findings is that if lifetime exposure to quartz is 1 µg/m^3, the cancer risk is greater than 1 in 100,000 and a Proposition 65 warning about cancer risk is required to be posted by the source of the emissions.

As seen from Fig. 3-2, the findings from Muhle et al[19] have the greatest cancer potency slope with the lowest dose and the results from Dagle et al[4] show the shallowest slope with the greatest dose. The latter result may be a function of high dose levels—51.6 mg/m^3—used in the study by Dagle et al.[4] (This level of exposure may exceed the maximum tolerated dose for rats.) Goldsmith et al[9] excluded these high dose levels, and a clear dose-related gradient emerged for the remaining animal data, suggesting that although these separate studies show that silica is a carcinogen in rodents, overall there appears to be a dose-related gradient except at high doses. This latter finding is consistent with the view that the animals receiving the high-dose silica levels exceeded the maximum tolerated dose and thus their results should not be included in the risk assessment calculation.[25]

Epidemiologic findings among white South African gold miners[11] and among diatomaceous earth workers[3] demonstrated dose-response lung cancer findings for quartz exposure. Ruble and Goldsmith[24] developed cancer potency slope estimations from the epidemiologic dose-response findings by modifying the silica exposure data to fit the Global 86 model. The cancer slope factors ranged from 6.8 × 10^{-7} to 1.85 × 10^{-5} for lifetime exposure to 1 (µg/m^3)$^{-1}$ silica dust.[9,24] Because of large uncertainties in the extrapolation to humans of animal data, more rational risk assessments are achieved with use of data from silica-exposed workers than from reliance on laboratory findings. Cancer potency estimation from silica-exposed workers produces a more shallow slope than that with extrapolations from rats and thus enables risk managers to develop recommendations consistent with a rational assessment of the risk.[9]

Silica's ability to cause silicosis, a chronic pulmonary disease characterized by shortness of breath, bloody sputum production, and cough and confirmed by biopsy or chest

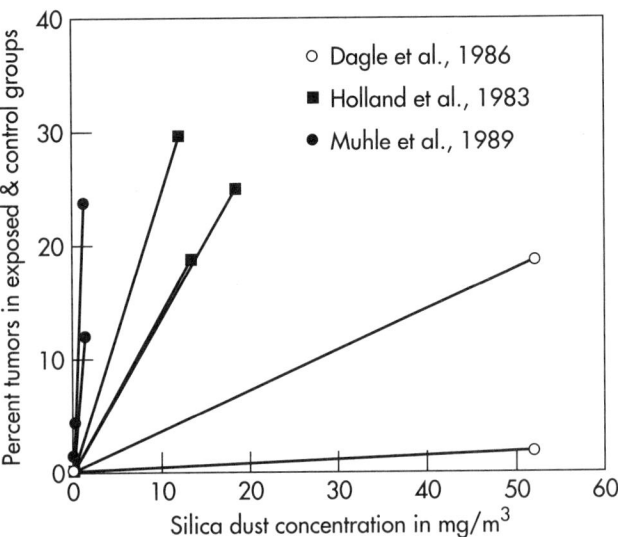

Fig. 3-2. Tumor rate by "crude" silica dust concentration.

radiographs, is not disputed.[17,23] The noncancer risk extrapolation focused on the risk of silicosis among workers exposed to quartz dust over a working life. Gift and Faust[7] have reviewed the silicosis epidemiology literature to determine the acceptability of studies for calculation of a RfC for silica. The NOAEL values were very close—between 0.05 mg/m^3 and 0.3 mg/m^3—and the RfCs range from 0.03 μg/m^3 to 2.06 μg/m^3. Taking the lowest RfC and applying it to the cancer risk values reported earlier means that lifetime exposure to 0.03 μg/m^3 would not result in an excess risk beyond acceptable levels based on human extrapolation but may result in excess cancer using the animal methods.

Assessing human risk assessment

The extrapolation procedure for risk assessment for crystalline silica seems straightforward and compelling as a means to protect public health; however, objections have been raised to extrapolation from animal studies,[12] because all studies with positive results were not done with use of the same protocol and because these studies were not initiated to evaluate the cancer hazards from silica. There is the possibility that costly emission controls that do little to reduce public lung cancer risk may be required. Goldsmith et al[9] have raised the issue of whether using animal data is appropriate when there are high-quality epidemiologic data on workers and on silicotics[3,8,11,18] demonstrating dose-response findings. Seen in this context, extrapolations from human findings must be seriously considered for risk assessment purposes. The reasons for adopting this approach are that these data reflect the species for which the risk assessment is directed—humans—and that the lung cancer risks were found at measured exposures. The last reason is that these findings represent risks in the realm of human exposures and biologic process whereas there have been no demonstrated respiratory cancer risks from ambient silica exposures. There needs to be more research on cancer risk-assessment procedures, an activity that may lead to extrapolations that are more rationally based on epidemiologic findings.

GUIDELINES FOR PRACTITIONERS OF ENVIRONMENTAL MEDICINE

Environmental health professionals can and should provide training to other practitioners and to their patients in the recognition and management of environmentally caused illnesses. This delivery of training also can provide credible and reassuring information to the public and to concerned patients. In this way, environmental health professionals can become leaders in guiding and interpreting risk assessments of hazardous materials.

Environmental health professionals should contact the EPA's Offices of Toxic Substances and Pesticide Programs in Washington, D.C., to make known their clinical findings and their views on environmental health hazards. The state agency or department that regulates pesticides and other hazardous materials also should be contacted. Professional involvement is the only way in which new findings in environmental medicine can be incorporated into the risk assessments that will be required for newly recognized insults to health.

Environmental health professionals must develop outreach programs in safety and prevention in collaboration with poison control centers, industry groups, worker organizations, and the environmental activist community. This professional outreach must include a working knowledge of the principles of environmental risk assessment.

REFERENCES

1. Brantner JH, Klein AK: Carcinogenic risk assessment for silica. Presented at the Society of Toxicology Meeting, Dallas, Tex, February 25–March 1, 1991.
2. California Air Pollution Control Officers Association: AB 2588 Risk Assessment Committee of the California Air Pollution Control Officers Association: Air Toxics "Hot Spots" Program, Risk Assessment Guidelines, January 1, 1991.
3. Checkoway H et al: Mortality among workers in the diatomaceous earth industry, *Br J Ind Med* 50:586, 1993.
4. Dagle GE et al: Chronic inhalation exposure of rats to quartz. In Goldsmith DF et al, eds: *Silica, silicosis, and cancer: controversy in occupational medicine,* New York, 1986, Praeger.
5. Department of Labor: Occupational Safety and Health Administration, 29 CFR Part 1910, Air Contaminants: final rule, *Federal Register* 54:2521, 1989.
6. Doull J et al: *Toxicology: an applied science,* New York, 1987, Houghton-Mifflin.
7. Gift J, Faust R: EPA's reference concentration (RfC) methodology and its potential application to silica dust, *J Exposure Anal Environ Epidemiol* (in press).
8. Goldsmith DF: Silica exposure and pulmonary cancer. In Samet JM, ed: *Epidemiology of lung cancer,* New York, 1994, Marcel Dekker.
9. Goldsmith DF, Ruble RP, Klein C: Comparative cancer potency for silica: human and animal extrapolations. Presented at the 2nd International Symposium on Silica, Silicosis and Cancer, San Francisco, October 28-30, 1993, *Scan J Work Environ Health* (in press).
10. Groth DH et al: Lung tumors in rats treated with quartz and other minerals by intratracheal instillation. In Goldsmith DF, et al, eds: *Silica, silicosis, and cancer: controversy in occupational medicine,* New York, 1986, Praeger.
11. Hnizdo E, Sluis-Cremer GK: Silica exposures, silicosis, and lung cancer: a mortality study of South African gold miners, *Br J Ind Med* 48:53, 1991.
12. Holland LM: Crystalline silica and lung cancer: a review of recent experimental evidence, *Regul Toxicol Pharmacol* 12:224, 1990.
13. Holland LM et al: Pulmonary effects of shale dusts in experimental animals. In Wagner WL et al, eds: *Health issues related to metal and nonmetal mining,* Boston, 1983, Butterworths.
14. Howe RB, Crump KS, Van Landingham C: *GLOBAL86: a computer program to extrapolate quantal animal toxicity data to low doses,* Ruston, La, 1986, K.S. Crump and Company.
15. International Agency for Research on Cancer: *Evaluation of the carcinogenic risk to silica and some silicates,* monograph no 43, Lyon, France, 1987, The Agency.
16. International Agency for Research on Cancer: *Summary of evaluation of the carcinogenic risk to chemicals and industrial processes,* monograph no 46, Lyon, France, 1988, The Agency.
17. Levy N, Wegman D: *Theory and practice of occupational medicine,* ed 2, Philadelphia, 1990, WB Saunders.

18. *Mortality from cancer among Ontario gold miners 1955-1977, Appendix C of Industrial Disease Standards Panel Report to the Workers' Compensation Board on the Ontario Gold Mining Industry,* Toronto, Ontario Ministry of Labour.
19. Muhle H et al: Lung tumor induction upon long-term low-level inhalation of crystalline silica, *Am J Ind Med* 15:343, 1989.
20. National Academy of Sciences: *Risk assessment and regulation of hazardous chemicals,* Washington, DC, 1983, National Academy of Sciences Press.
21. Newton PE, Pfledderer C: Measurement of the deposition and clearance of inhaled radiolabeled particles from rat lungs, *J Appl Toxicol* 6:113, 1986.
22. Proposition 65: Hearings of the Scientific Advisory Board for Proposition 65, State of California Safe Drinking Water and Toxic Enforcement Act of 1986: chemicals known to the State (of California) to cause cancer or reproductive toxicity, Davis, Calif, September 15, 1988.
23. Rom W: *Occupational and environmental medicine,* ed 2, Baltimore, 1992, Williams & Wilkins.
24. Ruble R, Goldsmith DF: A technique for estimation of silica cancer potency from occupational epidemiology studies. Presented at the 2nd International Symposium on Silica, Silicosis and Cancer, San Francisco, October 28-30, 1993.
25. US Environmental Protection Agency: Guidelines for carcinogen risk assessment, *Federal Register* 51:33992, 1986.
26. US Environmental Protection Agency: *Risk assessment guidance for Superfund: human health evaluation manual,* Part A, Solid Waste and Emergency Response (OS-230), 9285 701A, Washington, DC, 1989.
27. Wagner MMF et al: Silica induced malignant histiocytic lymphoma: incidence linked with strain of rat and type of silica, *Br J Cancer* 41:908, 1980.

Chapter 4

PRINCIPLES OF EXPOSURE ASSESSMENT

Yehia Y. Hammad
Yogesh Manocha

Exposure assessment
Routes of exposure
    Inhalation exposure
    Dermal exposure
    Ingestion exposure
    Eye exposure
    Parenteral exposure
Principles of exposure assessment
    Selection of agents to be measured
    Selection of an attribute of the agent to be measured
    Use of markers and surrogates of exposure
    Use of biologic markers
Technical terms and units
    Air ventilation
    Airborne contaminants
    Waterborne contaminants
Assessment of airborne exposure
    Aerosol sampling
    Sampling of gases and vapors
Assessment of waterborne exposure
Exposure limits
    Occupational standards
    Community standards

EXPOSURE ASSESSMENT

Exposure is an event or series of events in which a person (or population) comes in contact with a biologic, chemical, or physical agent. Assessment of this exposure is an important endeavor that is required as a first step in many applications, including compliance with legal standards, disease diagnosis and treatment, risk assessment and management, and occupational and environmental epidemiology. The underlying assumption is that there is a causal relationship between the amount of exposure to an agent and the extent of observed health effect. The concept of dose is used as a descriptor of the administered quantity of the agent. Thus the dose is the physiologically (and pathologically) significant characteristic of exposure. The National Research Council has defined the dose as the amount of the contaminant that is absorbed or deposited in the body of an exposed organism over a period of time. The dose can be portioned into these components: internal dose and biologically effective dose. The internal dose is the amount of a contaminant that is absorbed into the body over a given time, and the biologically effective dose is the amount of contaminant or its metabolites that has interacted with a target site over a given period so as to alter a physiologic function. A third complaint is the dose reaching the target tissue, whether or not it produces a biologic effect.[17] It should be noted that absorption includes any process in which the agent crosses body surfaces or membranes and reaches the bloodstream. Generally, the concentration of a chemical in an environmental medium is evaluated for calculations of the dose; however, in cases of exposure to physical agents, particulates, and fibers, attributes other than simple concentration, such as particle surface area, fiber length and diameter, and ultraviolet radiation at a given wavelength, are measured. The administered quantity can be further defined in several terms, including amount of agent per unit body weight, amount of agent per body surface area, and amount of agent per region of the lung per minute. In summary, exposure assessment is the measurement or estimation of the magnitude, frequency, duration, and route of exposure as well as a description of the size and nature of the exposed populations.

ROUTES OF EXPOSURE

The route of exposure affects the extent of absorption and therefore the absorbed dose. The main sites of absorption are the lungs, the skin, and gastrointestinal tract.

Inhalation exposure

Inhalation is the most important route of entry of many biologic and chemical agents into the body. Inhalation exposure per event is estimated based on the duration of each event, the inhalation rate of the exposed individual during the event, and the concentration of contaminant in the inspired air. Inhalation exposure occurs from breathing ambient air (community air pollution), indoor air (indoor air pollution), and contaminated air in the work environment. Airborne contaminants can be present in the gaseous phase (gases and vapors), liquid phase (droplets), and solid phase (particulates and fibers). Uptake of gases and vapors depends on concentration and relative solubilities of the agent in water and lipids, and deposition of particulates in the respiratory tract depends on size, shape, and density of the material. Host factors influencing uptake of gases and particulates include age, weight, sex, race, disease state, and respiratory rate.

Dermal exposure

Dermal exposure is determined by the concentration of hazardous substance in a contaminated medium that is contacted, the extent of contact, and the duration of such contact. Factors influencing dermal absorption of chemicals include molecular weight of the compound, its solubility in lipids, presence of other compounds that might facilitate passage of a chemical through skin, and the permeability of the skin. Dermal exposure takes place during swimming or bathing in contaminated water, skin contact with the soil, and various industrial operations.

Ingestion exposure

Exposures due to ingestion of contaminated food (drink) can be estimated as the product of contaminant concentration in the consumed food or drink and the amount of food or drink consumed per day. Daily ingestion exposure estimates are calculated in the same manner, regardless of the type of ingested food. In adults, ingestion exposure is mainly due to consumption of contaminated food and drinks, but in children, contaminated soil should also be taken into consideration. Children consume between 50 and 100 mg soil per day, but this amount may exceed 1000 mg in children with pica.

Eye exposure

Eye exposure results from accidental contact of the eyes with biologic, chemical, and physical agents. The eyes are very sensitive to these insults and can be affected by exposure to a minute amount of an agent. For example, the cornea must remain transparent; hence irritants causing scarring, a normal process of the body with little adverse effect in other organs, can destroy the function of the eye. Consequently, a small amount of an acid with no effects elsewhere in the body can cause blindness. Another example is cornpicker's pupil, which is mydriasis caused by operating machinery in cornfields containing jimson weed (Datura stramonium), from which hyoscyamine and related substances reach the eye to cause dilation of the pupils.[19] The significant effects on the eyes of the minute amounts of irritants present in food, such as those released from onions and capsaicin, the hot extract of pepper, are well known. On the other hand, there is a dearth of information on chemicals that can be absorbed through the eyes in amounts enough to induce systemic poisoning without causing damage to the eye itself. Examples include fluoroacetate, which caused convulsions and death without affecting the eyes of rabbits, and p-phenylenediamine, a major ingredient in Lash Lure (before regulation of chemicals used in cosmetics), which has been reported to cause a fatality after application to the eyelids.[19] It should be noted that many physical agents, such as ultraviolet radiation, also have direct effects on the eye.[30]

Parenteral exposure

Parenteral exposure is usually encountered in two scenarios: bites and stings by animals and occupational exposure among health professionals and veterinarians from cuts and pricks by sharp instruments such as needles contaminated with blood pathogens. Nosocomial infections with human immunodeficiency virus (HIV) among health professionals is well documented. In 1988 the Centers for Disease Control reported 26 cases of HIV infections in health care workers who had parenteral, nonintact skin, or mucous membrane exposures to HIV.[6]

Obviously, age, sex, race, and activity influence the average inhalation rate, the rate of food and water intake, the body area subject to dermal exposure, and the types of food consumed, all of which can affect the level of exposure actually experienced. It is also essential that assessment of exposure include all possible routes of entry of the agent into the body for all environmental media, that is, air, food, water, and soil.

PRINCIPLES OF EXPOSURE ASSESSMENT

Exposures are generally classified into two major categories: acute and chronic exposures. Acute exposure is usually associated with exposure to a single dose over a short period. Acute exposures can involve a single chemical or multiple chemicals, and the health effects associated with the exposure become apparent very quickly. Acute exposures generally last less than 24 hours. Long-term exposure, on the other hand, involves receiving a dose at frequencies over a longer period, which may range from hours or days to months or years. Health effects after long-term exposure are a function of the route of exposure and accumulation and metabolism of the chemical. Long-term exposures are usually of longer duration and low-level concentration. Exposures may be multiple and uneven, and the overall biologic response can be influenced by other environmental exposures, which may act synergistically or antagonistically.[23]

Selection of agents to be measured

Environmental and occupational epidemiologic investigations performed to develop dose-response relationships have improved significantly during the past four decades because of advances in the fields of biostatistics, epidemiology, industrial hygiene, and medicine. Earlier epidemiologic studies focused attention on measurement of disease outcomes, and little attention was paid to assessment of exposure. In these studies, duration of employment and questionnaires administered to study participants about their exposure were used instead of actual evaluation of environmental exposures. Other times, study participants were sorted into exposure categories that were based solely on their job titles. These practices resulted in inadequate descriptions of exposure and in many cases erroneous assignment of exposure categories.

Current studies require the participation of industrial hygienists or environmental engineers. These environmental scientists are trained not only to recognize the health effects of the various agents that may be present in the environment but also to measure the various attributes of the agent that are associated with the particular health effect under investigation. They are able to collect the right background and field information to answer the typical questions of what, where, how, and whose exposure to measure. The collected information is subsequently used to identify and quantify the exposure of each study participant and to develop uniform exposure categories that cover a range adequate for meaningful distinction among groups.

The National Research Council has established a hierarchy of exposure data that can be used in the development of sampling strategy.[17] In this scheme, seven categories are included, of which direct personal monitoring represents the best approximation to actual exposure. Other categories in the hierarchy are considered to be indirect measurements and are subdivided into information derived from quantification of concentration of the agent in the microenvironment (area or ambient measurement) and information that does not use quantitative estimates of exposure but rather surrogates of exposure, such as site of residence. The categories in the hierarchy are presented in Table 4-1.

It should be noted that often environmental conditions in which the airborne concentration of the agent is very low may arise. Reliance on personal sampling schemes would be self-defeating because of the very small volume of air that can be collected with battery-operated personal sampling pumps. This small volume results in the collection of a very minute amount of the contaminant that is below the limit of detection of the analytic procedure. Under these conditions, area samplers capable of collecting large volumes of air samples are used. The partial loss of information due to collection of samples by area samplers is compensated for by the large volume of air samples and the large amounts that can be collected of the agent, adequate for subsequent physical and chemical analysis. This change from personal to area samples represents a shift from category 1 to category 2 in Table 4-1.

Table 4-1. Hierarchy of exposure data or surrogates

Types of data	Approximation to actual exposure
1. Quantified personal measurement	Best
2. Quantified area or ambient measurements of the vicinity of residence or other sites of activity	
3. Quantified surrogates of exposure (such as estimates of drinking water use)	
4. Distance from site and duration of residence	
5. Distance or duration of residence	
6. Residence or employment in a geographic area in reasonable proximity to the site where exposure can be assumed	
7. Residence or employment in defined geographic area (such as a county) of the site	Poorest

Selection of an attribute of the agent to be measured

Perhaps no other category of toxic substances exhibits the degree of interdependence of physical characteristics and toxicity as aerosols. Some of the important properties of aerosols include shape, size, surface area, density, and chemical composition of the parent material. These factors affect site of deposition in the lung, interaction with lung tissue, solubility in lung fluids, and durability as well as persistence in lung tissue. A case in point is mineral fibers in general and asbestos fibers in particular. Stanton and Wrench[22] showed that fiber toxicity is related to fiber length and diameter, whereby long (more than 10 μm) and thin (less than 0.5 μm) fibers are the most toxic. The mineral type of asbestos affects not only the shape and size of fibers but also their durability in lung tissue and consequently fibrogenic and carcinogenic potential.[28] Another example is silica dust, the fibrogenicity of which is related to whether the dust is in amorphous or crystalline form, the type of crystalline structure, and particle size.[2] Thus, in the case of asbestos, the attributes of interest that should be taken into consideration are asbestos type and concentration of fibers in the various length and diameter categories. For silica dust, it is essential to measure the concentration of the fine fraction of the dust known as *respirable dust* (the dust fraction deposited in the nonciliated part of the lung, that is, the gas-exchange compartment); to know whether it is amorphous or crystalline; and, in the case of the latter, to determine the exact crystalline form, that is, quartz, cristobalite, or tridymite.

Evaluation of exposures to gases and vapors is relatively simple in comparison to sampling of particulates. Because the gas or vapor is present in molecular form, we have only one degree of freedom, that is, determination of the concentration or the number of molecules per unit volume. Some gases or vapors exist in more than one form, or isomer (that is, the compound exists in two or more forms that are identical with respect to percentage composition but differ as to the position of the atoms within the molecule). If the chemical and toxic potentials of the isomers are different, the exposure to each isomer should be determined.

For example, toluene diisocyanate (TDI) is a chemical with two isomers 2, 4-TDI and 2, 6-TDI. When the isomeric composition of airborne TDI was measured in the polyurethane foam industry, it was found that there is a large increase in the amount of airborne 2, 6-TDI relative to 2, 4-TDI as compared with the starting material. The magnitude of increase depended on the stage of production.[21] This finding is consistent with the lower reactivity of 2, 6-TDI, although it has often been assumed that the industrial environment consists primarily of the 2, 4 isomer or a mixture of the 2, 4 and 2, 6 isomers in the same ratio as that of the starting material. The significance of these findings becomes apparent in light of the fact that both the Occupational Safety and Health Administration (OSHA) permissible exposure limit (PEL) and American Conference of Government Industrial Hygienists' (ACGIH) threshold limit value (TLV) are for 2, 4-TDI only.[2] Further, the dose-response relationships that these standards are based on were developed with use of air-sampling methods that underestimated total TDI exposure because of the lower reactivity of 2, 6-TDI.[20]

Use of markers and surrogates of exposure

Markers and surrogates of exposure are new names applied to practices that have been used extensively in the past by many investigators. These practices are undergoing a process of redefinition in terms of applicability and use. In 1938 Dreessen and his colleagues[7] described asbestos exposure among 541 employees in asbestos textile plants in terms of total number of airborne particles, because at that time there was no known method for measuring airborne asbestos. Thus the total concentration of all types of airborne particulates was used as a surrogate for asbestos exposure. More recent epidemiologic investigations of the health effects of asbestos had to consider that part of the information on historic exposure was described in terms of total particles and available contemporary information was presented in terms of airborne asbestos fibers. To solve this problem, studies to estimate the relationship between total concentration of airborne particulates and airborne asbestos fibers were done.[9]

Another use of markers and surrogates is to describe exposure to complex mixtures in which either the active and causative agent has not been identified or an inordinate number of agents may be present at the same time. An example of the first case is cotton dust,[4] and typical examples of the second are diesel exhaust and cigarette smoke, in which more than 3800 compounds have been identified.[15] Markers are used to describe relative levels of exposure to a complex mixture when the underlying assumption is that if exposure to a mixture is related to the health effects, there should be a parallel correlation between exposure to the marker and exposure to the mixture. Markers of cigarette smoke include respirable particulates, carbon monoxide, and nicotine.

Use of biologic markers

Biologic markers are biologic materials obtained from humans exposed to contaminated media (see Chapter 63). A marker can be either an exogenous substance that indicates exposure, such as a heavy metal; a biochemical change that would indicate potential health effects; or variation in a vital body function, such as metabolism, that would be associated with exposure. Biologic markers constitute one of the most important and rapidly evolving areas in assessment of exposure. The National Research Council has described three types of biomarkers: markers of exposure, markers of effects, and markers of susceptibility.[17] In a recent monograph by Hulka et al,[10] *Biological Markers in Epidemiology,* the authors classified the types of biomarkers as internal dose markers, biologically effective dose markers, biologic response markers, markers of subclinical disease, and susceptibility markers. On the other hand, biologic markers are associated with a very wide margin of variability. The factors influencing this variability include individual variability, interactive effects of exposure, diet, and diurnal variation. Therefore, investigators should be aware of the possible misuse of these markers. For example, exhaled alcohol concentration is a good marker of alcohol concentration in the blood. It is used, however, by law-enforcement agencies as a test for neurotoxicity or intoxication that impairs driving ability. Obviously, different individuals with identical internal doses of alcohol vary widely in terms of effects on driving ability.[10]

An important development in the field of biologic markers is the publication of 37 biologic exposure indices by ACGIH.[2] Because of the advantages of breath analysis, which include immediate results, assessment of exposures by all routes, its noninvasive nature, and acceptability by workers, the ACGIH is also considering the publication of biologic exposure indices for volatile compounds.

TECHNICAL TERMS AND UNITS

In this section some of the important technical terms and units encountered during assessment of exposure are introduced and discussed. They are related to expression of air ventilation in buildings as well as expression of concentration of contaminants in air, food, and water.

Air ventilation

Cubic feet per minute (CFM) of outdoor air. The CFM is the unit of air flow usually specified in American

Society of Heating, Refrigerating and Air Conditioning Engineers (ASHRAE) standards.[5] It is the total quantity of outside air delivered to the building.

CFM of outdoor air per square foot. The CFM of outdoor air per square foot is another way of specifying ventilation rate of outdoor air. It is expressed in terms of the net habitable area, not the gross area of the building. This unit is also used in the ASHRAE standard.[5]

Air changes per hour. Air changes per hour is the conventional way of expressing the total actual dilution ventilation rate of a specific space. It is equal to the ventilation air flow rate in CFM divided by the volume of ventilated space in cubic feet; however, it can also be used to express air changes per hour of outdoor air.

Airborne contaminants

Concentration of gases and vapors. A gas is a substance that is in the gaseous phase at normal temperature and pressure (NTP). On the other hand, a vapor is the gaseous phase of a material that is usually a solid or a liquid at NTP. The concentration can be expressed as parts of contaminants per million parts of air by volume (ppm) or in terms of weight of contaminant (in milligrams) per unit volume of air (in cubic meters), that is, milligrams per cubic meter.

Concentration of particles. Concentration of particles is usually expressed in weight of dust (milligrams or micrograms) per unit volume of air, that is, milligrams or micrograms per cubic meter. Under some circumstances the concentration of dust that can be tolerated is very low, such as expression of concentration of particles in clean rooms used in electronics and the space industry or the case of asbestos fibers in indoor air. Under these conditions, concentration is expressed in terms of number of particles or fibers per milliliter of air, for example fibers per milliliter in the case of asbestos.

Waterborne contaminants

Although water that can be consumed without concern for adverse health effects is referred to as *potable water*, the term does not mean that it has to taste good. On the other hand, palatable water may taste good but is not necessarily safe. Community water systems are designed to provide water that is both potable and palatable. Different substances and contaminants that may be present in water are classified as follows.

Suspended, colloidal, and dissolved solids. Suspended solids are solids large enough to settle out of water. They can be removed by sedimentation or filtration. Dissolved solids are those that are in solution; that is, they are homogeneously dispersed in the water. They can be removed from water by extraction, precipitation, or distillation. Colloidal solids are in a size that ranges between suspended and dissolved solids. They are harder to remove from water but can be removed by filtration through small-pore filters and by centrifugation. Suspended and colloidal solids, including clay silt, organic material, and plankton, cause turbidity in water. The unit of measure is turbidity units (TU).

Color. Color in water can be due to the presence of dissolved or colloidal solids. Excessive amounts of algae and other microorganisms also affects color.

Taste and odor. Taste and odor in water can be caused by dissolved gases and inorganic and organic compounds. Consumers expect water to be odor- and taste-free.

Expression of concentration. The expression of concentration of various dissolved substances such as chlorides, fluorides, and sulfates is usually presented in milligrams of solids per liter of water. Because the density of water is equal to unity and because the dissolved salts at the concentrations encountered in surface water do not significantly affect water density, it can be shown that the concentration in milligrams per liter is numerically equal to the concentration expressed in parts of the contaminant per million parts of water on a weight basis. It should be noted that this is not true in the case of air.

ASSESSMENT OF AIRBORNE EXPOSURE

During sampling, a sufficient amount of the contaminant must be collected to perform subsequent qualitative and quantitative analytical procedures. The amount collected is proportional to the airborne concentration, sampling flow rate, and duration of sampling. Sampling can be performed to obtain either area or personal samples. The selection of the sampling method depends primarily on the airborne contaminant, the purpose of the survey, and subsequent sample analysis.

Before any sampling program is undertaken, it must be ascertained whether a particular situation is covered by statutory requirements of a federal, state, or local regulatory agency. If the situation is regulated, the decision to diverge from the official regulatory agency procedure is a major one, because the individual then carries the burden of proving the equivalency of the selected unofficial method. Sampling and analytic techniques are described in adequate details in several publications by the Environmental Protection Agency (EPA)[6] and the National Institute for Occupational Safety and Health (NIOSH).[14] Comprehensive descriptions of air sampling equipment and analytic methods available at the present time are presented in several recent publications.*

Aerosol sampling

Samples of particles may be collected by a variety of techniques, including filtration, electrostatic precipitation, and impaction. Particle collection can be obtained with or without size separation. Collection without size separation is used to obtain total suspended particulate matter for subsequent gravimetric, chemical, or physical analysis. Collection with size segregation is used to determine the particle

---

*References 1, 11, 12, 14, 18, 27.

size distribution of airborne particles or a specific fraction of the dust cloud, such as the inspirable particulate mass, thoracic particulate mass, and respirable particulate mass fraction.[3]

Sampling of gases and vapors

Sampling of gases and vapors can be conducted to obtain grab, intermittent, or continuous samples. Each sampling procedure provides data representing a range of averaging times. Grab samples can be collected with gas-sampling bags, evacuated bottles, gas syringes, and gas-detector tubes. Intermittent samples can be obtained by absorption of the gases in liquid media contained in bubblers and impingers or absorption of gases on solid media such as charcoal and silica gel.

A new technique that is becoming very popular is passive dosimetry, such as badges (analogous to radiation badges). Gases and vapors are allowed to diffuse into the collection medium of the dosimeter; therefore, the use of an air-moving device or an air pump is not needed. Another category is the direct reading instruments or meters used extensively in field evaluations. Generally, they can be operated intermittently or in a continuous mode and provide real-time sampling and readout. These instruments are based on some physical or physicochemical property of the gas or vapor. They include ultraviolet/visible photometry, infrared analysis, chemiluminescence, combustion, electrical conductivity, electrochemical analysis, coulometry, flame ionization, gas chromatography, and photoionization.[8,18] A major disadvantage of these types of instruments is their high cost.

ASSESSMENT OF WATERBORNE EXPOSURE

The water environment is composed of two interrelated phases: groundwater and surface water. Because of their close interrelationship, the complete assessment of impact involves consideration of both groundwater and surface water. Groundwater contamination is often harmful, and the source is sometimes very difficult to locate. Groundwater is contaminated mainly from septic tanks, injection wells, and leachates from waste disposal. The most frightening aspect of groundwater pollution is that by the time the problem is discovered, it is generally too late to do anything about it.[16]

The public health hazards posed by surface water pollution depend on many factors, including the ultimate use of water. A surface water pollution source generally is located above ground, which often leads to recognition of the presence of a problem before serious health or environmental effects are observed.

Physical, chemical, and biologic characteristics of water should be taken into consideration in assessment of waterborne exposure. Physical properties of water include turbidity, color, temperature, sediment, and floating solids. Chemical pollution of the water environment is mainly due to dissolved solids, phosphate, pesticides, petrochemicals, heavy metals, and other toxic substances. Biologic characteristics of water include bacteria, viruses, parasites, fungi, and other organisms. Adults usually drink about 2 L of water per day.

EXPOSURE LIMITS

A national consensus of safe working standards and regulatory standards has been developed by a variety of national organizations and governmental agencies. These standards, together with exposure assessment, are used to render judgments regarding the safety of environmental conditions. Therefore, the most useful information is obtained from quantitative data that can be related to the threshold exposure that may result in a health effect. A threshold is defined as the relationship of the lowest detectable level of a biologic or toxic response of the host to a specific concentration or dose of an agent, below which no toxic effect occurs. The following discussion focuses on several important types of standards for safe exposure.

Occupational standards

ACGIH threshold limit values. The ACGIH has established the TLV as guidelines for the control of health hazards in the work environment. TLVs are established on the basis of unconsciousness, irritation, or other forms of toxicity. TLVs are presented in two ways: time-weighted average concentrations and short-term exposure limits of airborne chemicals that would be acceptable for an 8-hour day, 40 hours per week, to which nearly all workers may be repeatedly exposed, day after day, for a working lifetime without suffering any adverse health effects.[2] Each year the ACGIH updates and publishes a list of TLVs and biologic exposure indices.[3]

OSHA permissible exposure limits. The 1970 Occupational Safety and Health Act established two new governmental organizations: OSHA, which is the policing and enforcing arm of the act, and NIOSH, which represents the research arm of the act. OSHA publishes health standards known as *PELs* and short-term exposure limits based on recommendations by NIOSH. They are conceptually similar to TLVs but differ in some specific allowable concentrations because of the time-consuming process required for the establishment of each new standard. As a result, PELs established by OSHA are not always the same as TLVs published by ACGIH. Traditionally, many of the ACGIH limits have been more conservative than those established by OSHA, because of flexibility in the process of establishing and updating the TLVs. The PELs are enforceable standards under the Occupational Safety and Health Act.[25]

NIOSH recommended exposure limits. NIOSH develops and periodically revises recommendations for limits of exposure to hazardous substances or conditions in the workplace. These recommended exposure limits (RELs) are published and transmitted to OSHA for use in promulgating the PELs.[13]

Another category established by NIOSH is that representing conditions that are immediately dangerous to life or health (IDLH). An IDLH condition means an atmospheric concentration of any toxic, corrosive, or asphyxiant substance that poses an immediate threat to life or would interfere with an individual's ability to escape from a dangerous atmosphere. In other words, IDLH can be defined as a concentration representing the maximal level of a pollutant from which an individual could escape within 30 minutes without escape-impairing symptoms or irreversible health effects. IDLH conditions most generally arise in emergency situations, thus making essential training for situations in which emergencies may arise. NIOSH's other responsibilities include development of methods for assessment of exposure, training of personnel in the field of occupational health, and, finally, publishing of information on occupational hazard assessments and special hazard evaluations and reviews.

Oxygen deficiency. The normal oxygen content of the air at sea level is 21%. Oxygen deficiency is defined as any concentration below 19.5%. A decrease in oxygen concentration to 16% can result in mental impairment, and the decrease of oxygen concentration below 16% can result in unconsciousness and death. Monitoring of the oxygen concentration in ambient air is required before entry into a confined space or unknown area. Because the pressure of oxygen also depends on air pressure (760 mm Hg at sea level), different criteria are used at high altitudes. (See Chapter 52.)

Community standards

Community air pollution. Although air-pollution abatement standards were enacted in many American cities, such as Chicago, as early as 1881, significant regulations at the federal level were promulgated only during the last three decades. This change was a result of social interest and national reaction to the rapid deterioration of environmental quality on all fronts, that is, air, water, and soil. As a result, the National Air Pollution Control Administration was dissolved and air pollution control functions, together with other environmental control responsibilities, were transferred to the EPA, an independent federal agency created by an executive order of the president.

National ambient air quality standards. Development of air-quality standards for ambient air assumes that some level of contamination is permissible but low enough so that it does not cause significant adverse health effects. Under the 1967 Air Quality Act and subsequent amendments of the Clean Air Act in 1970, 1977, and 1990, the federal government was charged with the responsibility of developing uniform National Ambient Air Quality Standards (NAAQS). These standards included primary standards to protect the health of the public and secondary standards to protect public welfare. The Air Quality Act also specified that promulgation of NAAQS must be preceded by the publication of Air Quality Criteria. These criteria are issued in document form and summarize all relevant scientific information on the health and welfare of individual pollutants so that air-quality standards are supported by good scientific evidence. NAAQS are not instantaneous standards but refer to average exposure over a period of hours to a year. NAAQS, averaging times, and recommended measurement methods are presented in Table 4-2.[24]

Indoor air pollution. The enforcement of OSHA's safety and health standards in the work environment is pos-

Table 4-2. National ambient air quality standards*

Pollutant	Averaging time	Primary standard	Secondary standard	Measurement method
Carbon monoxide	8 hr	10 mg/m^3 (9 ppm)	Same	Nondispersive infrared spectroscopy
	1 hr	40 mg/m^3 (35 ppm)	Same	
Nitrogen dioxide	Annual average	100 μg/m^3 (0.05 ppm)	Same	Colorimetry using Saltzman method or equivalent
Sulfur dioxide	Annual average	80 μg/m^3 (0.03 ppm)	Same	Pararosaniline method or equivalent
	24 hr	365 μg/m^3 (0.14 ppm)		
	3 hr		1300 μg/m^3 (0.5 ppm)	
Particulate matter	Annual arithmetic mean	50 μg/m^3	50 μg/m^3	Size-selective samplers
	24 hr	150 μg/m^3	50 μg/m^3	
Hydrocarbons (corrected for methane)	3 hr (6-9 AM)	160 μg/m^3 (0.24 ppm)	Same	Flame ionization detector using gas chromatography
Ozone	1 hr	235 μg/m^3 (0.12 ppm)	Same	Chemiluminescent method or equivalent
Lead	3-month average	1.5 μg/m^3	Same	Atomic absorption

*Standards other than those based on the annual average are not to be exceeded more than once a year.

sible because of the clear-cut relationship between the industrial processes and the resulting concentrations of airborne contaminants. Moreover, the exposed population is composed of healthy adults who are to some extent willing to accept the risks associated with the limited exposure for 8 hours per day, provided that levels are below the OSHA PEL. Unfortunately, such is not the case with indoor air-quality problems that occur at home and in offices, schools, and public buildings from indoor and outdoor sources. The exposed population covers the entire health spectrum, including infants, the infirm, pregnant women, and the elderly. In addition, persons with allergies or diseases of the heart and lungs are more susceptible to these problems. Hence, the development and enforcement of comprehensive indoor air-quality standards are virtually impossible. The OSHA PEL, ACGIH TLV, and NIOSH REL are derived for the industrial setting and should not be used as evaluation criteria for indoor air quality. Thus the only standards that seem to be applicable at the present time are those published by ASHRAE,[5] derived from recommendations by the World Health Organization.[29]

Building owners and managers concerned about the possibility of existence of indoor air-quality problems in their property may consult the *Guide for Building Owners and Facility Managers* published by the EPA.[26]

Soil and food contamination. It is difficult to identify all routes of exposure in any given case. Soil ingestion may be important for some small children, but it is unusual for soil to be ingested directly by adults. The Food and Drug Administration (FDA) Market Basket Survey consists of samples of groceries that include 234 different food items sampled four times each year in three cities in each of four regions. Comparisons are made between the measured residues and acceptable daily intakes (ADIs) established for individual contaminants. ADIs are established by the FDA as estimates of the daily amount of a chemical that can be safely ingested without substantially increasing an individual's lifetime risk of illness from that chemical.

Water contamination. Contamination of water bodies supplying drinking water to the general public led to laws initially passed by state legislatures and later by Congress, such as the Federal Water Pollution Control Act of 1948, that required intervention by the U.S. Public Health Service and subsequently by the EPA to ensure the safety of the nation's water supply. The National Safe Drinking Water Act of 1974 is designed to achieve uniform safety and quality of drinking water by identifying contaminants and establishing maximal acceptable levels for the contaminants. The major provisions of the act establish primary regulations for protection of public health and secondary regulations that are related to taste, odor, and appearance of drinking water. National revised primary drinking-water regulations—maximum contaminant levels and secondary maximum contaminant levels published by EPA in 1992—are presented in Tables 4-3 and 4-4, respectively.

Table 4-3. National primary drinking water regulations, U.S. EPA, 1992

Constituent	Maximum contaminant level
Arsenic	0.05 mg/L
Barium	2 mg/L
Cadmium	0.005 mg/L
Chromium	0.1 mg/L
Fluoride	4 mg/L
Lead	0.05 mg/L
Mercury	0.002 mg/L
Nitrate as N	10 mg/L
Nitrite as N	1 mg/L
Total nitrate and nitrite	10 mg/L
Selenium	0.05 mg/L
Asbestos	7,000,000 fibers/L (longer than 10 µm)
Vinyl chloride	0.002 mg/L
Benzene	0.005 mg/L
Carbon tetrachloride	0.005 mg/L
Trichloroethylene	0.005 mg/L
Ethylbenzene	0.7 mg/L
Monochlorobenzene	0.1 mg/L
Styrene	0.1 mg/L
Tetrachloroethylene	0.005 mg/L
Toluene	1 mg/L
1,2-Dichloroethane	0.005 mg/L
Para-Dichlorobenzene	0.075 mg/L
1,1-Dichloroethylene	0.007 mg/L
1,1,1-Trichloroethane	0.2 mg/L
1,2-Dichloropropane	0.005 mg/L
O-Dichlorobenzene	0.6 mg/L

Table 4-4. National secondary drinking-water regulations, U.S. EPA, 1992

Constituent	Maximum contaminant level
Aluminum	0.2 mg/L
Chloride	250 mg/L
Color	15 color units
Copper	1.0 mg/L
Corrosivity	Noncorrosive
Fluoride	2.0 mg/L
Foaming agents	0.5 mg/L
Iron	0.3 mg/L
Manganese	0.05 mg/L
Odor	3 threshold odor number
pH	6.5-8.5
Silver	0.1 mg/L
Sulfate	250 mg/L
Total dissolved solids	500 mg/L
Zinc	5 mg/L

REFERENCES

1. American Conference of Government Industrial Hygienists: *Air sampling instruments for evaluation of atmospheric contaminants,* ed 7, Cincinnati, Ohio, 1989, The Conference.
2. American Conference of Government Industrial Hygienists: *Documentation of TLVs and BEIs,* ed 6, Cincinnati, Ohio, 1991, The Conference.
3. American Conference of Government Industrial Hygienists: *1993-1994 TLVs for chemical substances and physical agents and biological exposure indices,* Cincinnati, Ohio, 1993, The Conference.
4. Ainsworth KA, Neumann RE: Chemotoxins in cotton dust: possible etiologic agents in byssinosis, *Am Rev Respir Dis* 124:280, 1981.
5. American Society of Heating, Refrigerating and Air Conditioning Engineers: *Standard 2-89: ventilation for acceptable indoor air quality,* Atlanta, Ga, 1990.
6. Centers for Disease Control: Update: acquired immunodeficiency syndrome and human immunodeficiency virus infection among health-care workers, *MMWR* 37:229, 1988.
7. Dreessen WC et al: A study of asbestosis in the asbestos textile industry, *Public Health Bulletin* No 241, 1938.
8. Hammad YY, Corn M, Dharmarajan V: Environmental characterization. In Weill H, Turner-Warwick M, eds: *Occupational lung diseases: research approaches and methods,* New York, 1981, Marcel Dekker.
9. Hammad YY, Diem JE, Weill H: Evaluation of dust exposure in asbestos cement manufacturing operations, *Am Ind Hyg Assoc J* 40:490, 1979.
10. Hulka BS, Wilcosky TC, Griffith JD: *Biological markers in epidemiology,* New York, 1990, Oxford University Press.
11. Lodge JP, ed: *Methods of air sampling and analysis,* ed 3, Chelsea, Mich, 1989, Lewis.
12. Maslansky CJ, Maslansky SP: *Air monitoring instrumentation,* New York, 1993, Van Nostrand Reinhold.
13. National Institute for Occupational Safety and Health: *Guide to chemical hazards,* DHHS (NIOSH) Pub No 85-114, 1989, US Department of Health and Human Services, CDC.
14. National Institute for Occupational Safety and Health: *Manual of analytical methods,* ed 4, Washington, DC, 1990, US Government Printing Office.
15. National Research Council: *Environmental tobacco smoke: measuring exposures and assessing health effects,* Washington, DC, 1986, National Academy of Sciences.
16. National Research Council: *Environmental epidemiology, public health, and hazardous waste sites,* Washington, DC, 1991, National Academy of Sciences.
17. National Research Council: *Human exposure assessment of airborne pollutants: advances and opportunities,* Washington, DC, 1991, National Academy of Sciences.
18. Ness SA: *Air monitoring for toxic exposure,* New York, 1991, Van Nostrand Reinhold.
19. Potts AM: Toxic response of the eye. In Ambdor MO, Doull J, Klaassen CD, eds: *Casarett and Doull's toxicology: the basic science of poisons,* ed 4, New York, 1991, McGraw-Hill.
20. Rando RJ, Hammad YY: Modified Marcali method for the determination of total toluenediisocyanate in air, *Am Ind Hyg Assoc J* 46:206, 1985.
21. Rando RJ, Abdel-Kader H, Hammad YY: Isomeric composition of airborne TDI in the polyurethane foam industry, *Am Ind Hyg Assoc J* 45:199, 1984.
22. Stanton MD, Wrench C: Mechanisms of mesothelioma induction with asbestos and fibrous glass, *J Natl Cancer Inst* 48:797, 1972.
23. Sullivan JB, Darcy J, Van Ert M: Evaluation of hazardous environments. In Sullivan JB, Krieger GR, eds: *Hazardous materials toxicology: clinical principles of environmental health,* Baltimore, 1992, Williams & Wilkins.
24. US Code of Federal Regulations, 40 CFR, part 50, Washington, DC, 1989, Government Printing Office.
25. US Department of Labor, Occupational Safety and Health Administration: *OSHA safety and health standards,* 29 CFR 1910, no 1910.1000, 1993.
26. US Environmental Protection Agency, Office of Air and Radiation, Office of Atmospheric and Indoor Air Programs, Indoor Air Division: *Building air quality: a guide for building owners and facility managers,* 1991.
27. US Environmental Protection Agency: *Environmental Response Team (ERT) and Response Engineering and Analytical Contract (REAC) standard operating procedures, air sampling and monitoring guidance documents,* 1992.
28. Weill H et al: Differences in lung effects resulting from chrysotile and crocidolite exposure. In Walton WH, editor: *Inhaled particles IV,* New York, 1977, Pergamon Press.
29. World Health Organization: *Indoor air quality research, report on a WHO meeting,* Stockholm, World Health Organization, Regional Office for Europe, Copenhagen, August 27-31, 1984.
30. Wilkening GM: Nonionizing radiation. In Clayton GD, Clayton FE, eds: *Patty's industrial hygiene and toxicology,* ed 4, vol 1, part B, New York, 1991, Wiley.

Chapter 5

USES OF EPIDEMIOLOGY IN ENVIRONMENTAL MEDICINE

Patricia A. Buffler

Epidemiologic studies
    Disease incidence and prevalence
    Cross-sectional or prevalence studies
    Longitudinal studies: cohort studies
    Longitudinal studies: case-control studies
    Proportional mortality studies
    Cluster studies and case series
Sources and validity of data
    Data sources
    Federal agencies
Comparability and bias
    Bias
Statistics: risk estimates
    Risk measures from a cohort study
    Standardized mortality/morbidity ratios
    Analytic role of confounders
    Attributable risk measures
    Confidence intervals
Statistics: type II error and power
Causal inference
    Judging positive associations
Summary

Any work which seeks to elucidate the cause of disease, the mechanism of disease, the cure of disease, or the prevention of disease must begin and end with observations on man whatever the intermediate steps may be.
                                            G.W. PICKERING
                                   Opportunity and Universities
                                          Lancet 2:895-898, 1952

EPIDEMIOLOGIC STUDIES

Epidemiology is generally defined as the study of the distribution of disease in human populations and the determinants of that distribution. Characteristics of people and their environment may be examined for possible causal associations with the occurrence of human disease.

Because epidemiology draws its conclusions from observations of the natural distribution of disease, it possesses both unique strengths and limitations. Since humans are the subjects of study, epidemiology avoids the problem of extrapolating from animal experiments in which both the exposure conditions and the appropriateness of the animal model are often questioned. As Hill[16] noted, there are no grounds for antagonism between experiment and observation. In public health they will—or should—constantly benefit from each other. Observation in the field suggests experiments that need to be done; the experiments lead back to more and better-defined observations. Observational researchers may have to be more patient than the experimenter, awaiting the occurrence of the natural chain of events they desire to study; they may have to be more imaginative, sensing the correlations that lie below the surface of their observations; and, importantly, they may have to be more logical and less dogmatic, avoiding the fallacy of *post hoc ergo propter hoc,* the mistaking of correlation for causation.[16]

Epidemiologic research generally provides less conclusive findings than experimental studies. The inability of epidemiologic research to offer direct proof of a cause-and-effect relationship results from its observational methods. In a laboratory investigation of a suspected harmful agent, it is assumed that the animals under study differ only on the basis of their exposure regimen. Any ensuing differences that are found between exposed and nonexposed animals can then reasonably be attributed to the exposure itself. Since obvious ethical and practical prohibitions on experimentation with humans exist, data must be collected on the "natural" occurrence of the disease and agent under study in human populations.

Human exposure to an agent is not a random phenomenon occurring among members of a homogeneous population. Exposed and nonexposed groups will differ in terms of age, residence, occupation, gender, and many other factors. Some of these variables are known to influence disease occurrence and can be accounted for in the design or analysis of a study. Other factors associated with both the disease and the exposure may not be known to the investigator and therefore cannot be accounted for. Such potentially "confounding" factors may lead to an incorrect interpretation of the relationship between the agent and the disease under study.

Other examples of design problems that can alter or bias observational studies include uncertainties in determining the actual exposure status of individuals, variations in disease definitions and diagnoses in different geographic areas or in different hospitals, loss of study subjects who leave the area, unwillingness of subjects to participate, and inaccuracies in frequently used data sources such as death certificates and clinical records. Practical solutions to many of these problems have been developed by epidemiologists, although frequently these sources of bias are not adequately addressed.

Although each epidemiologic investigation poses its own unique problems and solutions, the overall approach of a study generally follows one of several basic study designs. The choice of a study design will depend on many factors such as time and cost limitations, frequency of the disease(s) to be studied, frequency of the exposure, intended use of the information, and availability of required data.[2] Several commonly used designs are described below, along with a brief consideration of their particular advantages and limitations.

Disease incidence and prevalence

A fundamental division of epidemiologic research separates studies according to whether the investigation is done longitudinally or cross-sectionally. Longitudinal studies focus on a process over time to investigate changes, whereas cross-sectional reports focus on describing a state of phenomenon at a fixed or indefinite time.

Longitudinal studies can be of two types depending upon whether the subjects were selected on the basis of input or output variables. Input variables refer to presumed determinants of disease, and sampling on this basis produces studies commonly known as *cohort studies*. Sampling on the basis of output variables focuses on the status of subjects after treatment or follow-up and leads to case-control studies.

The terms *incidence* and *prevalence* will be used in the following descriptions of epidemiologic study designs. These two commonly used measures of disease occurrence have distinctly different meanings in epidemiology. In a population-based study, the prevalence of disease is the proportion of individuals in a population with the disease at a given time. For example, the number of persons with lung cancer in a population of 100,000 on December 31, 1990, might be 30. The prevalence of lung cancer in this population at this time is 30/100,000 or .0003. This figure would include *all* persons with lung cancer on December 31, regardless of whether the person has had the disease for 1 day or 3 years. Prevalence is dimensionless; that is, it has no units.

In contrast to prevalence, incidence is a measure of the new cases of disease occurring in a population in a given time interval. If 15 of the 30 persons with lung cancer in the previous example were first diagnosed in 1990, the incidence of lung cancer in this population would be 15 per 100,000 *per year* (also written 15/100,000/yr or 15 per 100,000 person-years). The dimension of time is the defining characteristic of incidence, making this measure of disease occurrence a rate. The term *rate* always implies that the measurement of disease or death in a population is related to a specified period of time. Thus although some scientists refer to prevalence as prevalence rate, the expression is a misnomer.

Cross-sectional or prevalence studies

Cross-sectional studies examine factors of interest in a defined population at a particular time. The study group may represent a random sample of a community working at a particular occupation or a sample chosen on the basis of some environmental variable. Through a questionnaire, physical examination, and/or other means, the presence or absence of the disease(s) in question is determined for each individual, along with other characteristics or exposures of interest (for example, age, whether the person smokes, exercise level, and proximity to industrial emissions).

Some of the advantages of cross-sectional studies include the following:
- They can generally be performed relatively quickly and inexpensively.
- They provide valuable descriptive information on the existing patterns of disease occurrence and exposure.
- They can examine a variety of factors and diseases simultaneously.

The major limitations include the following:
- The "snapshot" approach may not allow one to determine whether exposure actually preceded development of the disease.
- Diseases that generally have a longer duration are more likely to be detected than diseases with the same incidence rate but with a shorter duration. Thus an association between an exposure and a disease of short duration may be missed.
- Individuals who survive longer with a disease are more likely to be found than those with shorter survival times. Therefore the cases with short survival will not be available for study and the remaining cases may not be typical of all cases and a potential association be-

tween exposure and disease may be masked or exaggerated.

Longitudinal studies: cohort studies

Cohort studies typically start with the selection of groups of disease-free individuals on the basis of some exposure variable. Exposed and nonexposed individuals are then followed up to determine subsequent development of disease. There are two types of cohort or follow-up studies: prospective (or concurrent) and retrospective (or nonconcurrent or historical). These two types differ as to when exposure and disease occur in relation to the onset of the study.

Prospective (concurrent) cohort studies. Prospective cohort studies are most similar to the classic laboratory study. These studies first identify a group of persons (cohort) who are currently free of disease but whose members differ in terms of exposure to the agent under study. For example, the cohort may be a specified group of reproductive-age women, and the exposure variable may be the use of contaminated drinking water. The cohort is then "followed up" at some future time to determine the occurrence of adverse birth outcomes in the cohort. How soon follow-up begins or the length of time it must be conducted depends on the disease outcome(s) of interest and their characteristics (such as induction or latency periods). Incidence rates can then be compared for exposed and nonexposed groups. These rates, which must be adjusted for differences in age and other characteristics of the study subjects, are typically expressed as a ratio or "relative risk" for the exposed group.

The advantages of prospective cohort studies are significant:
- They allow the direct determination of incidence among exposed and nonexposed groups. This permits calculation of the increased disease risk (relative risk) associated with the exposure. They also permit calculation of the "attributable risk," which is that portion of the incidence of a particular disease that is due to a specific cause.
- They may yield more extensive and more reliable data on exposure levels, as well as on confounding factors (such as cigarette smoking).
- Many different disease outcomes can be investigated in a single study.
- Relatively rare exposures (or occupations) can be investigated.

Prospective cohort studies also have a number of limitations:
- They often require many years of follow-up, since many diseases have long latencies.
- A very large cohort and/or a long follow-up period would be required to investigate relatively rare diseases, including most cancers.
- Substantial effort and expense are necessary to follow a large number of people over a long period of time.

Longitudinal studies: retrospective (historical or nonconcurrent) cohort studies. Retrospective cohort studies differ in that both the exposure and the follow-up period have occurred prior to the onset of the study. These studies use data from existing records such as occupational records, professional registries, and death certificates to identify the cohort and conduct the follow-up. Studies of occupational groups are most often conducted using this approach. As with prospective studies, a disease-free cohort is first defined on the basis of exposure status. For example, the cohort may be defined as all the members of a particular occupation or all employees at Company X as of some specified time in the past. The subsequent occurrence of disease in the cohort (up to the time of the study) is then ascertained, generally by using death certificates. To reduce costs, an unexposed cohort is often not identified for comparison; instead, the mortality experience of the exposed group is usually compared to that experienced by the general population in the state, region, or country from which the study population was derived.

The advantages of retrospective cohort studies include the following:
- Much less time and less cost is required to complete the study compared to a prospective study, since the disease outcome has already occurred.
- These studies are widely used in occupational settings, where personnel records, industrial hygiene data, and other records can be used to both construct the cohort and establish some measures of estimated exposure.

The limitations of retrospective cohort studies include the following:
- Past exposures cannot be defined as precisely as current exposures. For example, it may be difficult or impossible to estimate exposures to workers that occurred 40 years ago if no industrial hygiene data are available and work practices have changed over time.
- Little information may be available on confounding factors, such as smoking history.
- It may be difficult to select a suitable population to which the cohort can be compared. Frequently, the study results will differ depending on whether national, regional, or local disease rates are used as the comparison. The problem of a suitable comparison population is avoided in large cohort studies in which internal comparisons can be made; that is, a particular category of exposed workers within the cohort can be compared to the complete cohort or the remaining unexposed workers within the cohort.

Some cohort studies involve both prospective and retrospective components. For example, a cohort may be defined through personnel and other records as everyone who worked at Company X at least 1 month between 1945 and 1985. The mortality experience of this population as of 1986 (the time the study is undertaken) can then be determined using state and national mortality records. Additional follow-up of this cohort might then be conducted in 1990 or 1995, for example.

Longitudinal studies: case-control studies

This is a common study design used in epidemiology. As outlined previously, cohort studies first identify the exposure status of nondiseased individuals, then determine the subsequent incidence of disease in the cohort. In contrast, case-control studies begin by first identifying individuals who have developed the disease under study (cases) and individuals without the disease (controls). Cases can be selected through hospitals, disease registries, health maintenance organizations, physicians' practices, or even death certificates. Controls may be selected from individuals who are "patients" at the same hospital as the cases or who live in the same neighborhood as the cases or from other sources. An attempt is then made to compare the previous exposure experience of the cases with that of the control subjects. Certain factors that can influence disease rates (such as age, race, sex) are taken into account in the design or analysis of these studies.

Case-control studies offer several advantages:
- They are generally much faster and less expensive to undertake than prospective cohort studies.
- Sample sizes can be much smaller than cohort studies, particularly in the case of relatively uncommon diseases. Whereas a cohort size of tens or hundreds of thousands might be required to demonstrate some cancer risk, several hundred or even fewer subjects in a case-control study might be sufficient to reveal the risk. For very rare diseases, the only practicable study design is a case-control study.
- A variety of previous exposure variables can be (and usually are) examined in a single study.

Case-control studies have a number of limitations as well:
- The cases selected for inclusion in the study may not actually be representative of all those who develop the disease. For example, the selected cases may represent only those individuals who entered particular hospitals, and these cases may differ from nonhospitalized cases.
- It is often difficult to select an appropriate control group that is sufficiently comparable to the cases as well as representative of the general population from which the cases arise. Comparability and representativeness are both important yet sometimes mutually exclusive goals in selecting controls. In some studies, two different control groups have been utilized (for example, hospital controls and neighborhood or population controls). Many of the controversies in epidemiology arise from case-control studies in which the appropriateness of the controls is questioned.
- It is difficult or impossible to ascertain accurately exposures that have occurred in the past.
- These studies are inefficient for studying rare exposures.

Proportional mortality studies

This study design is frequently used in exploratory or "hypothesis-generating" investigations, usually in occupational settings. The entire study is most often based only on death certificate information: age, sex, race, cause of death, residence, and in most states, usual industry and occupation. A proportional mortality study is conducted when only the deaths among the exposed group can be ascertained, but the structure of the population from which deaths came is unknown.

In a proportional mortality study, the proportion of deaths from a specified cause relative to all deaths among the exposed group is compared with the corresponding proportion in the nonexposed group or a general population. This comparison is done independently of any relationship to the incidence *rate* of the disease in the exposed and unexposed groups; that is, only *numerator* data are used to make the comparison. For example, a researcher might wish to investigate the hypothesis that exposure to electric and magnetic fields (EMF) is related to leukemia occurrence. Assuming that the job title "power lineman" is an adequate surrogate for exposure to job-related electric and magnetic fields, the researcher could plan a study to find out whether leukemia mortality in these workers was elevated in 1970 to 1979. A relatively quick way to do this would be to identify all power linemen (from death certificates) who died in that time interval, determine what proportion died of leukemia, and compare that proportion with the proportion of deaths due to leukemia among individuals of similar age and sex in the general population. The quotient of the proportion in all power linemen divided by the proportion in the general population is called the *proportional mortality ratio (PMR)*.

A similar type of study might also be done using incidence data from a disease registry such as a regional cancer registry. Such a study is referred to as a *proportional incidence study,* and a proportional incidence ratio (PIR) shows the observed-to-expected ratio of cases. The population of this type of study consists of those with cancers newly identified in a specified time period, and the study data are derived from the registry medical records. As with the mortality data, the proportions of cancers of different types can be compared among different groups.

PMR studies have the following advantages:
- They can be conducted very quickly and inexpensively, especially if the relevant data are already computerized (as they often are).
- Many different exposures and causes of death (or types of cancer) can be examined simultaneously.
- They can provide many useful leads for possible relationships between disease and environmental exposure that can be investigated further using more powerful study methods.

PMR studies also have some severe limitations:
- Unlike a cohort study, no information is collected on the population "at risk," only on those already de-

ceased. Therefore, no disease rates can be calculated. An elevation in the PMR may be due either to an increase in mortality from the cause of concern or to a reduction in mortality from another cause. For example, a PMR for leukemia may be elevated in one group because they are actually at an increased risk of leukemia or because they have a lower risk of some other common disease such as heart disease.

- Information on confounding factors (such as smoking) is usually not available.
- Accuracy and completeness of information obtained from death certificates or medical records is variable (see below).
- Study results can sometimes differ quite significantly when compared with results of more definitive studies such as cohort studies, especially if the overall mortality rates differ substantially among the groups (occupations) being compared.

Cluster studies and case series

A "cluster" of disease (for example, leukemia) is generally considered to be an unusually high number of cases appearing in the same setting (such as neighborhood, town, workplace) over a limited period of time. Considerable attention has been given to the study of disease clusters, particularly cancer clusters, and a number of statistical methods have been developed to analyze them. Nevertheless, no noninfectious agent has ever been consistently implicated in causation of any type of cancer by analyses of cancer clusters, except in the occupational setting where a subset of the employee population may have been exposed to high concentrations of a toxic material and the cases are of the same type of cancer.[32]

Cancer clustering in the nonoccupational setting is generally thought to be the result of random (nonuniform) distribution of disease cases in a population. Thus even when a significant elevation of a disease is noted for a specified time and place, it is very likely a statistical artifact and not the result of exposure of the cases to an agent in their environment. For example, three new cases of leukemia might occur in a community of 4000 persons in a 5-year period, and this incidence might be significantly elevated relative to the incidence in a comparison population for the same time period ($p = 0.04$). But such a cluster might not be unusual. The calculations used to determine the statistical significance of the increased incidence of leukemia imply that if there are 1000 communities of 4000 persons in the country, 20 or 40 communities throughout the country (depending on the type of statistical test used) might have an elevated incidence of leukemia because of random statistical variation alone. Thus such a cluster, while "statistically significant," would not be that rare. It is also unlikely that similar environmental agents, leukemia subtypes, or age or gender distributions of the cases would be found in these 20 or 40 communities.

It is possible that a cluster of cancer cases may be related to the presence of an environmental carcinogen. The fact that no such relationship has been established through cluster analysis may be due partly to the fact that cancer clusters generally consist of so few cases that it is not possible to rigorously test hypotheses relating environmental carcinogens to cancer risk. Thus the size of the population being studied in most settings is generally insufficient to yield statistically significant results.[32]

SOURCES AND VALIDITY OF DATA

In any scientific study, careful attention must be given to the validity and reliability of the data. Unfortunately, all data collection methods involve some degree of inaccuracy and variability. These data quality problems are addressed in scientific studies by such means as full descriptions of data collection techniques, calculation of likely or potential measurement errors, validation procedures, and replication of measurements.

Because of the wide variety of epidemiologic data sources, professionals outside the field may find it difficult to judge the validity, utility, reliability, and limitations of these data. Data on exposure of study subjects, for example, may range from direct measurements of chemicals or their metabolites within the body to the relatively imprecise information on a decedent's exposure history taken from interviews with next of kin.

The following discussion briefly describes the major sources and limitations of epidemiologic data, with particular emphasis on the determination of exposure and disease status. The overall consequences of data inaccuracies are also briefly considered.

Data sources

Population data. Census data are collected by the U.S. Department of Commerce, Bureau of the Census, every 10 years and provide age, race, and sex-specific counts for persons living in the various geographic subdivisions of the United States, plus certain additional demographic, socioeconomic, and household characteristics for those individuals. Census information is collected, analyzed, and presented for the country as a whole and for progressively smaller subdivisions such as states, counties, cities, and census tracts within cities. These published data supply the "denominator" (population at risk) for most commonly reported disease morbidity and mortality rates.

One of the major limitations of census data is that a count taken once every 10 years will not provide the up-to-date information necessary to accurately describe a growing (or shrinking), highly mobile population. This problem is, to a degree, offset by the Current Population Survey (CPS), conducted by the Bureau of the Census, which consists of monthly sample assessments of about 50,000 homes. There are many areas in the country, however, in which the population does not behave as expected and in which population projections are significantly in error by the end of the decade.

Such errors in the denominator (population at risk) of a rate calculation also can cause the rate to be significantly in error. For example, if population growth has been higher than expected, morbidity or mortality rates may appear artificially elevated for that area.

Environmental measurements. A variety of environmental measurements may be used to provide data on exposure levels either in the community or in the workplace. Data are sometimes available for specific industries from industrial hygiene surveys. These environmental measurements, coupled with detailed work histories (usually available from personnel records), are frequently used to establish exposure categories for individuals. Environmental levels can also be measured as part of the study.

The use of environmental measurements can involve several potential problems.[22] Complete data may not be available on past exposure, particularly if it occurred many years ago as is often the case in occupational studies. Even when data are available on past or current exposures, the measurement errors associated with a particular sampling method must be considered.

Another problem with environmental measurements is their relevance to personal exposure levels. Different individuals who live in the same community or work at the same job may experience quite different exposures to the same agent. More relevant personal exposure measurements may be obtained by the use of personal dosimeters, such as radiation film badges. However, even these "personal" measurements are not always an accurate indication of the biologically absorbed dose of an agent. In recent years, considerable attention has been given to identifying markers of exposure in individuals at the molecular or genetic level.

Thus environmental measurements of an exposure are an indirect index of personal exposures. Personal dosimetry provides a more direct measure of exposure, but even here, some degree of error may occur in classifying an individual's exposure. Fortunately, misclassification of a comparatively small proportion of individuals, if it is nondifferential, does not invalidate a study.

Exposure can best be determined if some biologic marker of exposure can be identified or if the agent (or an appropriate metabolite) can be measured in the individual. For example, the presence of antibodies to the hepatitis B virus in the blood can serve as a biologic marker of exposure to that virus. Lead levels in serum or in teeth can give a measure of either short-term or chronic exposure to lead, respectively.

State or local health departments. Nearly all states have some form of infectious and chronic disease reporting laws requiring physicians, hospitals, and/or schools to report cases of specific diseases that are considered to be of significant public health importance to that state or to the Centers for Disease Control (CDC) in Atlanta, Georgia. A number of states also have some form of occupational disease reporting law and/or surveillance activities. However, the reporting of such disease cases to state and local health departments is often neglected by many health professionals, and the reported cases for some diseases may represent a small proportion of the actual cases occurring in that state.

Federal agencies

Federal agencies, such as the U.S. Public Health Service Center for Disease Control and Prevention (CDC) or the National Center for Health Statistics (NCHS), maintain active and/or passive surveillance on a wide variety of infectious and chronic diseases and health status parameters for populations in the various geographic areas of the United States.

Medical records. Hospital or clinical records are a frequent source of information for identification or confirmation of study subjects. These records can also provide information about a person's age, sex, race, address, and additional relevant medical data.

The information contained in medical records is highly variable in accessibility, accuracy, and completeness. Access to medical records, even for scientific research, has been restricted due to privacy and legal concerns in many situations. Another practical problem involves the many judgments that must be made in reviewing and abstracting the data from medical records. Also important in many cases is the considerable variation in the definition and diagnosis of certain diseases. While some diseases can be routinely diagnosed with a higher degree of certainty (acute leukemia), others are not readily or consistently diagnosed (Alzheimer's disease). Diagnostic criteria can vary according to the physician, the hospital, and the geographic region.

Both diagnostic acumen and criteria for a particular disease can vary significantly over time. One common procedure for achieving some degree of standardization is to identify and code diseases according to the diagnostic classifications found in the International Classification of Diseases (ICD). Since major revisions of the ICD occur about every 10 years, it is important to specify which revision is followed (the ninth revision of the ICD was published in 1978, the tenth in 1990). When medical records are utilized in a study, diagnostic criteria should be explicitly established at the study outset, and these criteria should be clearly reported.

Although hospital medical records or hospital disease indexes occasionally provide valuable sources of disease morbidity data, information based upon hospital admissions is likely to contain significant biases. Many diseases require no medical intervention or the individuals are treated by physicians on an outpatient basis. Consequently, these cases will not appear routinely in incidence or prevalence data derived from hospital records. Additionally, many selective factors may influence any hospital admission. Therefore, the population base associated with particular hospitals or with all the hospitals in a given area may be undefined or poorly defined. Finally, hospital-generated disease statistics are often difficult to collect, in part because of the lack of computerized retrieval systems.

Sources and limitations of mortality data. The most routinely collected and commonly used source of data for surveillance of disease has been mortality data from death certificates. These data are readily accessible and inexpensive to use. Since death certificates are required by law in the United States and many other countries as well, very nearly all deaths in these countries are reported to the authorities and death certificates are filed. Finally, mortality data have been collected, tabulated, and published annually for many decades and for many different countries of the world, so both temporal and geographic disease trends may be studied. Few other databases exist that allow such comparisons.

There are a number of limitations associated with the use of mortality data for epidemiologic studies or as an indicator of disease frequency. Some of these limitations involve biases in mortality reporting that are dependent on the particular disease. For example, the mortality rates for diseases that have high case fatality rates, such as lung or liver cancer, are more likely to accurately represent the status for that disease than the mortality rates for a disease that less often results in death, such as diabetes mellitus. In addition, those diseases that are easily diagnosed may be overrepresented on the death certificates relative to diseases for which the diagnosis is more complex.

The cause of death may be inaccurately reported on the death certificate for a number of reasons, including unfamiliarity of the physician with the past medical history of the case. Causes of death that bear some social stigma, such as suicide, sexually transmitted diseases, or abortion-related deaths, may be significantly underreported on death certificates. Failure to perform an autopsy may result in not determining the true underlying cause of death. Revisions in the International Classification of Diseases (ICD) may result in changes in the way diseases are grouped together, which may in turn lead to apparent sudden changes in the mortality rate for a particular cause of death. Occasionally, the cause of death is recorded correctly but is then miscoded on the certificate. Sometimes a diagnostic "label" is used more heavily in one locale than in another. Furthermore, diagnostic "fads" may occur that result in the disproportionate assignment of death to a few particular disease codes.

Variations in the quality of medical care over time or from place to place may cause deceptive differences in mortality rates. For example, improvements in diagnostic procedures for a certain disease may result in an apparent increase in the mortality for that disease when it is only the ratio of diagnosed cases to undiagnosed cases that has changed.

Finally, elderly people may have several active disease processes at the time of death, and an accurate selection of the underlying cause of death may not be possible or feasible. For this last reason more and more authorities are recommending the use of multiple-cause coding for death certificates.[20]

Death certificate data are used frequently in epidemiologic studies not only to ascertain the cause of death, but also to identify the decedent's occupation (a possible indicator of occupational exposures) and certain other demographic data (such as age at death, date of death, sex). Several studies have shown that death certificate data vary considerably in accuracy and reliability. Certain causes of death are more accurately or more reliably reported on death certificates than are other causes. This variability is due to factors such as uncertain diagnostic criteria for some diseases, the presence of multiple diseases, whether the death occurred in a hospital, and whether an autopsy was performed.

Occupational data from death certificates have even greater variability. Death certificates generally list the decedent's "usual occupation," as reported by family members or other persons. Just as there is no routine confirmation of cause of death (by autopsy), there is no verification of occupational information provided by respondents. Studies show that certain occupations are systematically over- or underrepresented. For individuals with a multiple-job history, the most recent occupation may be listed rather than the usual occupation. Thus except for a decedent who held a single, well-defined occupation and for whom this information is accurately entered on the death certificate, the occupation shown on the death certificate may represent an incomplete and inaccurate characterization of a person's actual occupational history.

In conclusion, mortality data can, without question, assist epidemiologists in understanding fundamental disease trends and relationships and to help generate hypotheses about risk factors and etiologic agents. However, because of the potential problems with accuracy, caution should be used in the interpretation of the results of any mortality data analysis. Such findings should be considered preliminary, suggesting further exploration through more definitive methods.

Disease registries. In some areas disease registries have been established for the surveillance of diseases that are of major concern to public health. Cancer is one such disease entity. In 1972 the National Cancer Institute (NCI) established the Surveillance, Epidemiology, and End Results (SEER) Program, which consists of a number of population-based cancer registries located in different geographic areas across the United States. These SEER cancer registries systematically collect demographic, diagnostic, treatment, survival, and follow-up information on all patients in the geographic area who are newly diagnosed as having any of the various forms of cancer.

The term *population-based,* as used above, means that the registry has attempted to enroll every case of cancer that occurred among the residents of a particular geographic area such as a city, county, region, or state. When all (or very nearly all) cases from the geographic area have been ascertained and the "population at risk" is the total population of that area, it is possible to calculate a cancer incidence rate. This is in contrast to a "hospital-based" cancer registry, which may have enrolled every case of cancer that was diagnosed in (or admitted to) a particular hospital but which has insufficient information about the "population at risk." Thus cancer incidence rates cannot be determined.

Disease registries, particularly those for cancer, are becoming a widely used resource for epidemiologic studies of environmental exposures. The approximately 45 population-based cancer registries in the United States collect data on cancer cases in prescribed geographic areas. Some collect additional data on treatment and follow-up. These systems can be used to identify unusual clusters of cancer cases associated with exposures to particular environmental agents, to study occupational hazards, to assess the magnitude of and trends in cancer rates, to identify cases for case-control studies, and to facilitate the ascertainment of cancer among members of a study cohort.

Despite the obvious usefulness of registries, the completeness, timeliness, and accuracy of registry data can vary substantially from one registry to another, and these issues can be factors of concern in epidemiologic studies. In addition, limitations on access to personal identities may reduce the utility of these data for epidemiologic studies requiring follow-up or record linkage.

Special disease surveys or epidemiologic studies. Routinely collected data on illness from hospitals, registries, and other sources do not yield a complete picture of the illness and disability of a defined region. More comprehensive data for monitoring the health status of a region are provided by sample surveys, known as *morbidity surveys.* Such surveys may consist of a single, cross-sectional examination or longitudinal studies in which respondents are revisited periodically. Although the most ambitious of these surveys in the United States, the National Health Interview Survey (NHIS), collects data on all diseases, specific diseases and conditions may be studied in special surveys. In the United States, the NCI has conducted cancer surveys that have yielded basic data on the incidence of cancer by primary site, histologic type, and stage of disease at time of diagnosis.

Data on personal factors, exposures, and even disease status are often obtained from in-person or telephone interviews of study subjects or their relatives. The validity and reliability of these data are affected by many factors such as the training and experience of the interviewer(s), the length of the interview, and recency of the events questioned. In short, the quality of data obtained by interview depends on how carefully the interview protocol is designed and administered, as well as on the type of information being sought. Information obtained by interview is frequently confirmed by other data sources (such as medical records) to improve its validity.

Mailed questionnaires provide another source of data on demographic factors, exposures, and health status. As with interviews, the quality of questionnaire data is influenced by many factors, including questionnaire length, specific wording of questions, types of questions, motivation of the study subjects, and the perceived importance of the study. Questionnaire data are also frequently confirmed (validated) by other data sources such as medical records.

Misclassification. As indicated in the previous discussion, the data sources used by epidemiologists are each characterized by potential inaccuracies. These inaccuracies are usually well recognized by epidemiologists, and efforts are made to limit and/or quantify the extent and type of data errors. Inevitably, however, some error remains and must be examined in terms of its impact on overall study validity.

Epidemiologic studies usually involve the comparison of large groups of subjects, often hundreds or thousands of individuals. Study subjects are generally classified according to whether or not they are exposed to the agent in question, as well as according to their disease status. An error in assessing an individual's degree of exposure may affect the relative ranking in the exposed group but will not necessarily remove the person from the "exposed" category. Even if an occasional individual is completely misclassified on exposure status, the overall findings are not necessarily invalidated. As long as the exposed *group* has, on average, a significantly higher exposure level than the nonexposed group, a comparison can still be made and a correct conclusion reached, although the precise exposure-response effect will be somewhat in error. In general, occasional and random misclassification is likely to reduce the strength of but not eliminate or reverse a significant association between exposure and disease. Frequent or systematic misclassification, on the other hand, can obscure or even change the direction of an association or create an association where none exists.

Sound epidemiologic research strives to identify, assess, and reduce the inevitable inaccuracies in data collection. It is particularly important that frequent or systematic errors be recognized. This is accomplished through the usual scientific means of providing detailed descriptions of data sources, observing rigorous methodologic standards, and confirming the accuracy of the data whenever possible.

COMPARABILITY AND BIAS

A serious threat to the validity of any epidemiologic study is the possibility that the selection of study subjects or data collected are biased. In epidemiology, "bias" does not imply a prejudice or prejudgment on the part of the study investigators. Rather, "bias" generally refers to systematic or nonrandom errors, that is, errors due to factors other than sampling variability that prevent the true value of a disease rate or exposure status from being obtained. The introduction of bias renders study groups noncomparable in some important way that will distort study findings.

To understand how a study can become biased, it is useful to recall the degree to which the laboratory scientists strive to achieve comparability between exposed and unexposed animals in their experiments. This is accomplished by such means as using a single strain of test organism, random assignment of each study animal to an exposure group, maintaining uniform environmental and dietary conditions during the course of the study, and using a consistent protocol for examination. The examination for disease outcomes is performed with the investigator "blinded" to the subject's previous exposure history. Failure to achieve any of these major comparability elements can bias a study, and its conclusions must be regarded cautiously.

In epidemiologic research, using observational methods, an equivalent degree of comparability as that achieved in an experimental study cannot be achieved. The goal of the epidemiologist is to select from an existing population of exposed and nonexposed groups that are fundamentally comparable and from which equivalent data can be obtained. It is important to recognize that bias can be introduced in numerous ways, some of which cannot be known or controlled by the investigator. The following discussion provides examples of major types of biases that can occur in epidemiologic studies.

Biases

Bias can occur in virtually every aspect of epidemiologic research. However, the following examples illustrate only those biases that can arise (1) in the process used to specify or select study participants (selection bias), (2) in the process of collecting data on study participants (observation or information bias), and (3) due to the existence of factors that are associated with both the exposure and the disease (confounding bias). Some types of bias can only occur in a particular study design, while others must be considered as a possibility with any design.

Nonresponse bias. Some portion of those who are selected or identified as study subjects cannot or will not participate in the study. Bias can occur when this group of nonrespondents differs systematically from respondents with respect to exposure or disease status. For example, nonrespondents may have more serious health problems. To minimize this bias, considerable effort must be expended to achieve a high participation rate (90% or better) or at least to obtain a sample of nonrespondents to determine whether or how they may differ with regard to the risk of disease or exposure status.

Lost-to-follow-up-bias. A similar type of bias can occur when study participants are "lost to follow-up" in cohort studies. Those who are "lost" may differ in their disease status, thus removing from the study individuals with more serious health problems. Significant efforts must be made in cohort studies to minimize the proportion of individuals who cannot be located.

Detection bias. This bias refers to the situation in which a disease (such as a brain tumor) is more frequently diagnosed and ascertained in a particular population (such as an occupational group) than in the general population. This may result from better access to medical care or better diagnostic services. If the general population rates are used as a basis for comparison, it will appear that members of the particular population are at increased risk of the disease. In reality, they are at increased risk only of being diagnosed with the disease. Widespread publicity about some agent may prompt exposed persons to seek medical examination, again increasing the possibility of detection among members of that group.

Healthy worker effect. Overall the working population is healthier than the general population. Less healthy people are less likely to become or remain employed; thus employment serves as a selective factor. In occupational studies therefore a clear possibility of bias arises if the general population is used as the basis for obtaining expected disease rates as is often done in retrospective cohort studies. The use of general population rates can create the false appearance that employment in an industry actually affords protection against mortality or suggest that there is no excess mortality. This effect is more evident for some diseases than others. For example, in contrast to some chronic diseases, it does not appear that overall cancer mortality is typically lower than expected in occupational cohorts when compared with the general population. Cardiovascular disease on the other hand is typically found to be lower in an occupational cohort than would be expected based on general population rates.[26]

Incidence-prevalence bias. Newly diagnosed ("incident") cases of disease may differ in certain characteristics from all existing ("prevalent") cases of the disease. Studies that use prevalent cases are more likely to include longer duration cases and exclude both rapidly fatal and readily cured cases. Consequently, prevalence studies are more likely to yield information relating to disease duration rather than disease development.

Observation and measurement bias. Numerous biases involve noncomparable data or data collection procedures. For example, exposure data obtained from interviews will not be comparable to data obtained from environmental measurements.

Observation bias can also arise when interviews are used to obtain health outcome data. If the interviewer knows a subject's disease status as well as the hypothesis under study, the interviewer may subconsciously probe harder concerning past exposures. Furthermore, a subject who has been advised of a study's purpose may attempt to provide responses that are perceived as "favorable" or "helpful" to the interviewer. Thus, when possible, interviews are frequently conducted in a "double-blind" fashion where neither the interviewer nor the subject is aware of the specific hypothesis under investigation.

In follow-up studies, disease diagnosis may be influenced by the physician's knowledge of a subject's exposure history. This bias, which applies mainly to cohort studies, will tend to increase the association between exposure and disease.

Recall bias. A person who has developed a particular disease may be better motivated and better able to recall previous exposures compared with control subjects. The mother of a child born with a malformation may recall more completely (or perhaps exaggerate) exposures experienced during pregnancy compared with the mother of a healthy child. This is a serious potential bias in case-control studies.

Misclassification bias. This does not refer to random misclassification of some small proportion of the study population but to systematic misclassification of disease or exposure status. This could happen if, for example, the job title "electrician" is used to identify subjects occupationally exposed to electric and magnetic fields (EMF) and a large portion of these electricians work only on dead circuits, where EMF exposure is low. On the contrary, some other workers, who are identified as "nonelectricians," might be exposed to EMF.

Berksonian bias. This bias, first described by Berkson in 1946, can arise when controls are selected from hospitals (usually the same hospitals from which the cases have been selected). Hospitalized controls are generally not representative of the overall population with respect to certain characteristics, such as smoking, alcohol, or coffee consumption. In order to detect and prevent Berksonian bias, multiple controls are suggested. Therefore, some case-control studies have used both hospital and neighborhood controls at the same time to detect this bias.

Confounding bias. Confounding bias occurs when there is a third variable that is not of interest to the study but is related to the exposure and is a cause of the disease under study. A study of lung cancer, for example, will find a significant association between alcohol consumption and the development of lung cancer. In such a study smoking would be considered a confounding variable since it is associated both with alcohol consumption and lung cancer. If the effect of smoking is removed in the study (by design strategies such as matching or analytic techniques such as stratification or adjustment), the association between drinking and lung cancer might not remain.

Most epidemiologic studies attempt to control at least several well-established confounding variables such as age, sex, race, and socioeconomic class. Other variables may be examined in a particular study; however, not all potentially confounding variables can be examined. Thus some degree of confounding bias is probably present in all data.

Conclusions. Given the difficulty in recognizing and controlling all potential sources of bias, no study should be considered completely free of bias. For example, rarely does a study attain 100% follow-up of subjects. Critics can always attribute study findings to some form of bias since there are indeed so many potential sources. However, in practice, it is difficult to actually demonstrate that some bias may fully explain or even materially affect the findings of a study. Strict adherence to established procedures and standards can reduce many, but not all, possibilities for bias. In many well-reported studies, the authors frequently discuss the possible sources of bias in their study and attempt to show, through logic and/or data, that their findings are not likely to be due to some bias. But there still remains the possibility that some unknown bias is operating.

STATISTICS: RISK ESTIMATES

The following discussion addresses how rates and ratios are used to provide estimates of risk, with emphasis on the measures of risk derived from two major study designs: the cohort study and the case-control study.

Risk measures from a cohort study

A cohort study is similar to an experimental study in terms of the time sequence of events. A study group (cohort) of healthy people is identified and each individual is then classified according to whether exposed or not exposed to the agent under study. At some later point in time, which may be many years later, the cohort is rechecked (the "follow-up") to identify those study participants who may have developed disease. Two risk measures from cohort studies will be described: the relative risk and the standardized mortality ratio.

Relative risk. From the follow-up data, an actual disease rate can be tabulated separately for both the exposed and nonexposed groups. Depending on the specific disease in question, the rate may be either a morbidity or a mortality rate. As an example, consider that the exposure under study is cigarette smoking and the disease in question is lung cancer. Data from an actual study showed that the lung cancer mortality rate for a particular age group of nonsmokers was 19 deaths per 100,000 per year. In contrast, the rate for smokers in this same age group was approximately 190 per 100,000 per year.

These rates can be compared in several ways such that a quantified expression of risk can be obtained. The most common measure of risk in this type of study is the relative risk (RR). The RR indicates the increased (or decreased) degree of risk of disease among the exposed compared to the nonexposed. It provides a measure of the causative importance of the exposure under study. A RR with a value of one (1.0) indicates no association between the exposure and the disease.

The RR is calculated as follows:

$$\text{RR} = \frac{\text{Rate in the exposed}}{\text{Rate in the unexposed}}$$

For smokers and lung cancer, the RR is

$$\text{RR} = \frac{190/100,000/\text{year}}{19/100,000/\text{year}} = \frac{190}{19} = 10$$

This indicates that smokers of a particular age group have 10 times the risk of dying from lung cancer compared with nonsmokers of the same age group.

Confidence limits can (and should) be computed for RR to determine the precision of the risk estimate. Confidence limits are the range of the risk estimate that takes into account sample size and variability. A very wide confidence interval indicates an imprecise risk estimate. If the range of the estimate does not include 1.0, it is recognized as being consistent with statistical significance.

Standardized mortality/morbidity ratios

Standardized mortality ratios (SMRs) are used for adjusting mortality rates in order to compare health outcomes between populations that may have different distributions of important variables such as age, sex, or race. Indirect standardization (adjustment) involves applying mortality rates from some selected reference population, adjusted for age and possibly other factors, to the study population. This procedure generates the number of deaths that would be "expected" if the study population had experienced the same disease incidence as the reference population. Then a common way to compare this expected number with the actual observed number is to compute the SMR. This is done by dividing the observed number of deaths by the expected number and then multiplying the quotient by 100 to eliminate decimals:

$$\text{SMR} = \frac{\text{Observed deaths}}{\text{Expected deaths}} \times 100$$

An SMR of 100 means that the expected and observed deaths are essentially equal in number, and no excess risk is evident. An SMR of 120 means that there were 20% more deaths than expected, while an SMR of 80 would mean that the observed deaths were only 80% of the deaths expected based on the reference population. SMRs are used frequently in occupational studies.

In a typical occupational mortality study, the investigator has collected extensive information on who has worked in the industry, when, for how long, in what jobs, and if deceased, the cause of death. Thus, both numerator data (deaths) and denominator data (person-years or persons at risk) are collected, and an actual mortality rate for each disease can be determined. This serves as the basis for the observed number of deaths.

A similar ratio can be calculated using morbidity data. For example, a standardized incidence ratio (SIR) can be determined using only incident cases.

Proportional mortality ratio. An entirely different ratio, which appears frequently and almost exclusively in occupational studies, is the *proportional mortality ratio* (PMR). As previously described, proportional mortality expresses the proportion of all deaths that are due to one cause. For example, of those who worked in a particular industry, 20% of the deaths may have been due to cancer, whereas heart disease may have accounted for 35% of the deaths.

In a PMR study the data are often obtained completely from death certificates. Consequently, the investigator only has data on people who have already died. Recall that death certificates also list the usual occupation and other personal data such as age, race, and sex. The investigator does not (and perhaps cannot) obtain denominator data, that is, the total person-years or persons at risk (most of whom may even still be living). Thus a mortality rate cannot be determined; all that can be done is to compare, for example, the proportion of all deaths that were due to leukemia in one occupation with the proportion of deaths due to leukemia in another (reference) group.

Although the PMR and SMR superficially appear similar, they are quite different and are derived from different types of data. Because they are both used widely in occupational epidemiology, the distinctions are underscored here.

Risk measures from a case-control study. In a contrast to cohort studies, which determine subsequent disease rates between exposed and nonexposed people, case-control studies first identify diseased and nondiseased persons, then ascertain their previous exposure history. This approach does not permit determination of actual disease rates. Thus an RR cannot be determined. One can, however, compare "exposure ratios" between diseased and nondiseased groups. Under certain conditions these exposure ratios can be used to estimate the RR by calculating an odds ratio.

To illustrate the odds ratio calculation, it is first useful to categorize case-control study data in a 2 × 2 table according to disease and exposure status:

		EXPOSURE STATUS	
		Exposed	Unexposed
DISEASE STATUS	Cases	a	c
	Controls	b	d

The letters *a, b, c,* and *d* represent the number of study subjects who fall into the four categories. Omitting its derivation, the odds ratio (OR) is then calculated as

$$\text{OR} = \frac{a \times d}{b \times c}$$

As an example, consider the following data obtained from a case-control study:

		EXPOSURE STATUS		
		Exposed	Unexposed	Totals
DISEASE STATUS	Cases	85	15	100
	Controls	40	60	100

The OR is then calculated as

$$\text{OR} = \frac{85 \times 60}{15 \times 40} = 8.5$$

The OR will be a reasonable estimate of the RR if the disease in question is relatively rare (e.g., cancer), the exposure is relatively common, and, of course, there are no serious study biases.

The OR is interpreted exactly the same as the RR. If equal to one (1.0), it suggests no association between the exposure and disease. If greater than one, it indicates a positive association, and if less than one a negative association or a protective effect. As with RRs, confidence limits can be computed to determine the precision of the OR and whether the OR is significantly different from a value of one.

In some case-control studies, the controls are individually "matched" to the cases during the selection process. For each case identified, a systematic approach is used to select a control who is in the same age bracket, of the same sex and race, and so forth. This matching process avoids having to adjust for these variables later in the analysis. When this type of matching is used in a study, the OR is calculated differently than above.

Analytic control of confounders

In practice, analysis and interpretation of epidemiologic studies involves much more than a single 2 × 2 table. As previously described, epidemiologic studies involve examination of many different variables in addition to the exposure and disease under study since there are other factors that may be related to the risk of exposure and/or the disease being investigated. The challenge then is to tease out the effect of the exposure of interest in the presence of these other factors or covariates. If confounding variables are not controlled for in the design of a study, they must be controlled for in the analysis. Two approaches for the analytic control of covariates or confounding are stratification and mathematical modeling.

Stratification. If the number of variables to be controlled is not too large and the range of values for these variables is not too wide, stratification provides a simple and powerful analytic technique. In stratification the investigator looks at the relationship between exposure and disease among subsets of the study population that have been categorized according to the level of some other covariate. In a study of breast cancer, for example, it may be found that a late age at first birth has a positive association with breast cancer and that low parity also has a positive association. The investigation may suspect that age at first birth and parity are themselves related and that one is a confounder. Instead of a single 2 × 2 table, the investigator might construct a series of 2 × 2 tables showing the association of breast cancer and age at first birth for different parity levels (e.g., one child, two children, and three or more children). In other words, the investigator "stratifies" on the covariate parity. The investigator might also look at breast cancer and parity, stratifying on age at first birth (for example, under 30 years and 30 years and older). The investigator would then find that the late age at first birth shows an increased risk ratio regardless of parity level. Stratifying on age at first birth, the investigator would find that parity is no longer associated with breast cancer risk. Stratifying has thus eliminated the confounding of parity and age at first birth by examining each variable separately.

Where several 2 × 2 tables and risk ratios are constructed in an analysis, a summary OR can still be calculated. The usual technique for calculating a summary OR is the Mantel-Haenszel procedure.[24] This summary OR can be thought of as a weighted average of the individual ORs from the separate 2 × 2 tables. Actual techniques for calculating the summary OR and its confidence limits can be found in basic epidemiology or biostatistics texts.[36,8]

Mathematical modeling. Until relatively recently stratification was the main approach to analysis in epidemiologic research. The limitation, however, is that if more than a few variables are controlled for at one time, too few subjects fall into each stratum, and the resulting risk estimates become unreliable. In this situation the addition or deletion of even one subject in a stratum could change the risk estimate dramatically. Mathematical modeling overcomes this limitation. Many different mathematical models are available today, some of which are available on personal computers. The most commonly used model is logistic regression. Although developed originally for use with cohort studies, logistic regression is commonly employed in case-control studies. Discussion of the assumptions, use, and limitations of logistic regression and other models can be found in most recent epidemiology and statistics texts.[3,35]

Attributable risk measures

Simple attributable risk. Disease rates can also be compared in another fashion: by looking at the absolute difference in the rates between exposed and nonexposed groups. This measure is referred to as a *simple attributable risk*. The simple attributable risk is used to quantify the risk of disease in the exposed group that can be attributed to the exposure. Using the smoking data presented above,

$$\text{Rate difference} = (190/100{,}000/\text{year}) - (19/100{,}000/\text{year})$$
$$= 171/100{,}000/\text{year}$$

For this age group the excess lung cancer rate among smokers attributable to smoking is 171/100,000/year. Expressed as a percentage (171/190 × 100%), it would be said that 90% of lung cancer among smokers can be attributed to the fact they smoked, and 90% of lung cancer among smokers could be eliminated if they did not smoke.

Population attributable risk. Another more useful measure of attributable risk is referred to as the *population attributable risk*. It provides a useful measure of the proportion of disease that can be explained by the exposure under study. The population attributable risk has important public health implications since it provides an estimate of the potential impact of a preventive program. For example, if a population attributable risk of a disease is 40% for a specific factor, it is implied that 40% of the disease in the population can be attributed to the factor. It is further implied that eradication of that factor should result in the eventual elimination of 40% of the disease.

Although a number of methods have been proposed for calculating the population attributable risk (PAR), the most useful ("Levin's attributable risk") is as follows:

$$\text{PAR} = \frac{P(R-1)}{P(R-1)+1}$$

where P = the proportion of the population exposed to the factor and R = the relative risk (or OR if derived from a case-control study).

As an example, assume that 40% of the population is exposed to some agent (this is approximately the proportion of smokers in the United States) in which the RR (or OR) has been determined to be 10. Then:

$$\text{PAR} = \frac{0.40(10-1)}{0.40(10-1)+1} \times 100\% = 78\%$$

Thus by eliminating this particular exposure, 78% of the disease could potentially be eliminated.

Calculation of p value. There are a number of procedures for calculating p values depending on whether one is considering, for example, the difference between the means of a continuous variable (e.g., age, years of employment) or a categorical variable, such as the difference between the proportions of those in each group who have some characteristic (for example, residence near high-current distribution lines). These formulae and their applications can be found in great detail in any statistics text.[2] One common example is provided.

Consider a case-control study investigating whether the proportion of those with a specific exposure differs significantly between the case group and the control group. The common statistical method for comparing proportions (or percentages) is the X^2 (chi-square) test. To apply the X^2 test, it is helpful to arrange the data in the form of a 2 × 2 table. To demonstrate this, assume that the study involved 100 cases and 125 controls, where 35 of the cases were exposed to the agent, while 25 of the controls were exposed.

The table would then be constructed as follows:

	Cases	Controls	Totals
Exposed	35	25	60
Not exposed	65	100	165
Totals	100	125	225

The X^2 test statistic is defined as

$$X^2 = \sum \frac{(O-E)^2}{E}$$

where O = observed number of cases and E = expected number of cases, and the summation is over all cells of the table. Often, a correction for continuity is made by subtracting 0.5 from OE as shown below:

$$X^2 = \sum \frac{(O-E-0.5)^2}{E}$$

To calculate the X^2 statistic, the "expected" number for each cell in the table must be found. This is done by assuming that there is no association between exposure and disease and making use of the marginal totals in the table. The expected value can then be calculated with the following equation:

$$E = \frac{(\text{Row total}) \times (\text{Column total})}{\text{Grand total}}$$

To illustrate, consider the upper-left cell of the 2 × 2 table shown previously. The row table is 60, the column total is 100, and the grand total is 225. Thus the expected number of exposed cases is

$$E = (60 \times 100)/225 = 26.7$$

This calculation can be applied to each of the other cells of the table to obtain the other expected values. The expected (E) numbers thus obtained are shown in parentheses below:

	Cases	Controls	Totals
Exposed	35 (26.7)	25 (33.3)	60
Not exposed	65 (73.3)	100 (91.7)	165
Totals	100	125	225

Using the simple formula for X^2 gives: $X^2 = 6.39$. Using the corrected formula gives a X^2 value of 5.65.

Once this statistic has been calculated, the investigator can then refer to a table of the X^2 distribution, found in most statistics texts (Fienberg, 1980). These tables show the probability of obtaining a given X^2 statistic (the larger the value, the lower its probability or p-value). In this case, with a simple 2 × 2 table with one degree of freedom, our corrected X^2, whose value is 5.65, yields a p-value of approximately 0.0175.

Confidence intervals

A second, but related approach for assessing the significance of epidemiologic results is the use of confidence intervals. The principle of confidence intervals is very straightforward. A certain degree of variability occurs in sample data. The amount of this variability depends on such factors as the sample size, the inherent subject-to-subject variability in a measured characteristic, and/or the prevalence of a characteristic. Therefore the observed value of some characteristic of the sample (e.g., means, risk ratio) is only an estimate of the "true" value. More confidence, however, can be placed in some estimates than in others; that is, estimates may range from a "ballpark figure" to a very precise and narrow range of values.

One way to express the precision of a sample estimate is to calculate boundaries between which the true value is most likely to fall. These upper and lower limits, which bracket the estimated value, are referred to as the *confidence interval*. This is the range of values from the lower confidence limit to the upper confidence limit. Confidence intervals are very useful in showing the precision of sample estimates. The larger the confidence interval, the less precise the estimate.

In epidemiologic studies confidence limits are frequently calculated for risk ratios. A major purpose is to determine whether the interval around an estimate of the RR includes unity (1.0). Recall that an RR of a given value "x" is interpreted as meaning that subjects with the exposure are "x" times more likely to have the disease than those without the exposure. If the disease and the exposure are not associated with each other, the risk will be unity. Values less than 1.0 indicate a negative association (protective effects), while values greater than 1.0 indicate a positive association. If the confidence interval for an RR includes the value of 1.0, no association is considered to exist between the exposure and the disease.

As an example, consider the following data from a case-control study:

	Cases	Controls	Totals
Exposed	35	25	60
Not exposed	65	100	165
Totals	100	125	225

In a case-control study the OR quantifies the strength of the association as an approximation of the RR. In this example it is calculated as follows:

$$OR = \frac{35 \times 100}{25 \times 6} = 2.2$$

Thus the *point estimate* of the RR is 2.2.

The calculation of confidence limits will then show the precision of this estimate. Commonly, 95% confidence limits are used. This means that there will be a 95% chance that the true risk will be contained in the interval. The first step of the procedure is the calculation of the variance and the standard error of the risk ratio. For the above data a number of different formulas can be used. The standard error is then used in calculating the lower (LL) and upper (UL) confidence limits. In practice some of the simpler formulas provide results quite similar to the more complex formulas. A complete description of these calculations can be found in any standard epidemiology textbook.[15a]

In this example the variance for the natural logarithm (ln) of the OR will be calculated as the sum of the reciprocals of the cells in the 2 × 2 table.

$$\text{Variance of ln OR} = \frac{1}{a} + \frac{1}{b} + \frac{1}{c} + \frac{1}{d}$$
$$= \frac{1}{35} + \frac{1}{25} + \frac{1}{65} + \frac{1}{100}$$
$$= 0.09396$$
$$\text{Standard Error (SE)} = \sqrt{\text{variance}} = \sqrt{0.09396} = 0.3065$$

The logarithm of the lower and upper 95% confidence limits is then:

$$\ln LL = \ln OR - (1.96 \times SE) = 0.1877$$
$$\ln UL = \ln OR + (1.96 \times SE) = 1.3892$$

Converting from natural logs of these exponential values to obtain the actual lower and upper limits can easily be done on most scientific calculators:

$$LL = e^{0.1877} = 1.21$$
$$UL = e^{1.3892} = 4.01$$

Thus the 95% confidence interval for the OR is 1.2-4.0. This interval shows several things. One is that the observed OR (2.2) is not a highly precise estimate. The actual risk could range from a very weak 1.2 to a moderately high 4.0. All we know is that there is a 95% chance that the real risk ratio falls within this interval.

Another important aspect of this interval is that it does not include one (1.0). This is expected since the test for statistical significance (X^2 test) had already revealed that an association exists between the exposure and disease.

Many epidemiologists believe that a confidence interval conveys more information than a significance test because it indicates the lowest and highest likely true RR. It also reveals something about the precision of an estimate. An extremely wide confidence interval, whether or not it includes an RR of 1.0, suggests caution in interpreting the results of a study.

STATISTICS: TYPE II ERROR AND POWER

The discussion in the previous section considered techniques to avoid a mistaken conclusion regarding the presence of an association (type I error). Less frequently discussed is another type of error that may be equally important, that is, type II error. This is the chance of producing a conclusion of no association when one actually does exist. Just as chance can operate to produce an apparent association when none actually exists, chance can also obscure a difference that does exist. Failing to detect a true association is referred to as a *type II error*. The possible combinations of correct and incorrect conclusions are:

Study Conclusion vs. True Relationship

True relationship	Study conclusion	
	Association	No association
Association	Correct	Type II error
No association	Type I error	Correct

A relationship exists between type I and type II errors in that the more closely one guards against a type I error, the more likely a type II error will occur. In other words, the greater the difference required for a conclusion of a real association, the greater the chance that a real association will not be detected.

The probability that a real association will be detected in a study is referred to as the *power of the study*. It is determined by subtracting the probability of a type II error, expressed as β (beta), from 1.0. Although not commonly discussed in study reports because it is a design consideration, the power of a study to detect a particular level of risk is extremely important both in the planning of a study and in the evaluation of "negative" studies. Most recent epidemiologic and statistical texts provide detailed discussions of power and type II errors for various types of studies. Rather than review these methods for calculating power or sample size, this section will briefly outline the major factors that determine power and then show one example.

Four factors affect the probability of a type II error and therefore the power. The first is the level of confidence used to reduce the chance of a type I error. If one demands an extremely high level of confidence, that is, a very small p-value, a greater chance exists that a true association will not be recognized.

Another factor that affects the power of a case-control study is the prevalence of the exposure among the controls. Power is reduced where the exposure is either very rare or very common among the controls. In a cohort or cross-sectional study, power depends mainly on the "expected" number of diseased cases in the unexposed population, which is in turn related to sample size. (Sample size is discussed below.)

Obviously a study has a greater probability (power) to detect large RRs (or large differences in means or proportions) than small risks. A particular study may have a 90% chance of detecting an RR of 3, but less than a 25% chance of detecting a risk of 1.5. Another factor that affects the power of a study is the sample size of the study—the number of cases and controls in a case-control study, or the number of people and period of follow-up (person-years) in a cohort study. Obviously, the larger the study, the greater its power to detect a particular level of risk. Sample size is also quite important in type I errors. By increasing sample size, an investigator can simultaneously reduce the chance of both types of error. Because of the relationship of sample size to the probability of these errors and because sample size is one of the conditions that is under some control of the investigator, considerable emphasis is placed on sample size in the design of studies.

Unfortunately, sample size questions cannot be answered without consideration of many of the factors discussed above. For example, an appropriate sample size will depend on how small a difference (or how small a relative risk) the investigator wants to be able to detect, the desired confidence level (p value) to be used in significance testing, the power desired to detect a given difference or risk, and the expected prevalence of the exposure in the general population.

In many situations, sample size may not be readily under the control of the investigator. In an historical cohort study, for example, the sample size may be fixed by the number of individuals employed and the years of follow-up. In a case-control study, sample size may be determined by the number of new cases diagnosed over a set period of time at a hospital or through a disease registry. Time and costs are always practical constraints. Power calculations can be important in these situations by showing, for example, the power of a proposed study or a completed study to detect specified levels of risk.

To illustrate some of these interrelationships, the following example is taken from an actual study proposal. The proposed project is a case-control study to examine the possible association between leukemia and residential exposure to magnetic fields. Based on the population of a study area, expected cooperation rates, leukemia rates, and other factors, the investigators estimated that they would be able to compare 175 leukemia cases with 175 controls. Significance testing would be done at the 95% confidence level ($p < 0.05$). The investigators then determined the minimum detectable RRs (or ORs) that could be detected 80% of the time, that is, power = 0.80. Since reliable data on the prevalence of magnetic field exposure (however defined) in the general population were not available, several estimates were evaluated based on the findings of an earlier study.

The following estimated minimum detectable risks correspond to exposure prevalence in this study:

Prevalence of exposure	0.10	0.15	0.20	0.25	0.30
Minimum of detectable risk (RR)	2.41	2.15	2.02	1.95	1.90

Thus, depending on sample size, the exposure prevalence estimates, and use of the 95% confidence level for significance testing, an 80% chance exists that this study would detect an RR as low as 1.9 to 2.4. If the true risk were higher than 2.0, the power would be higher than 0.80. However, if the true risk were actually small (e.g., 1.5), the power would be much less than 0.80.

If an investigator considered it important to detect a risk of 1.5 with high probability, the study size would have to be increased. If the number of cases could not be further increased due to cost or availability, sample size and power could be increased by increasing the number of controls. For each case, 2, 3, or even 4 controls might be selected. Little further improvement in efficiency, however, would be gained beyond a ratio of 4 to 1, controls to cases.

The above calculations could have been determined for a power of 0.70 or 0.90 or any other desired level. Conversely, one could have been selected various relative risks (e.g., 1.5, 2.0, 5.0, 10.0) and then determined the power to detect that risk.

An understanding of the relationships among power, sample size, significance tests, and so on, is quite important to both the design and the evaluation of epidemiologic research. If a proposed study design requires a higher power to detect a certain magnitude risk that is considered important, then a larger sample size is needed. Of course, the power of a study should always be taken into account in evaluating a report of negative findings, that is, was the study sufficiently powerful to give the reader confidence that the author's claim of a negative study is valid?[4]

CAUSAL INFERENCE

In laboratory research a well-designed experiment that results in a statistically significant effect (i.e., one not due to chance variation) is usually interpreted as demonstrating a cause-and-effect relationship. The existence of a cause-and-effect relationship cannot be so readily inferred from observational epidemiologic studies. The epidemiologist, at best, can show that some association or relationship exists between an exposure (e.g., chemical, radiation) and a physiological or health-related effect (e.g., blood chemistry, disease, death). Typically, the epidemiologist further attempts to demonstrate that the association is unlikely to be due to chance and is not due to some third (confounding) variable.

Judging positive associations

Scientific "proof" of a cause-and-effect relationship cannot be established by an observational study. However, as a practical matter, explicit or implicit judgments of causality are frequently derived from such studies and strongly influence public health policy. Therefore, it is important to consider epidemiologic findings from a variety of perspectives such that a reasonable assessment can be made.[16] Epidemiologists have not established specific rules for determining when a positive association should be considered consistent with a cause-and-effect relationship. Different experts stress different factors in evaluating associations, and not all agree that certain items are particularly useful.[17,15] However, certain guidelines arise frequently in discussions of causal relationships, and these are discussed briefly here.

Perhaps the most widely quoted guidelines for evaluating an empirical association to determine whether it is causal are the nine aspects offered by Hill.[17] These are as follows:
- Strength of the association
- Consistency of the association
- Specificity of the association
- Temporality of the association
- Biologic gradient observed
- Biologic plausibility of the association
- Coherence
- Experimental or intervention effect
- Analogy

Hill regarded these nine different perspectives as useful in studying associations before concluding that a given association was causal, irrespective of statistical significance. These were not intended as "hard-and-fast rules" of evidence nor "criteria" that must be satisfied before accepting cause and effect. In his words[17]:

> None of my nine viewpoints can bring indisputable evidence for or against the cause-and-effect hypothesis and none can be required as a sine qua non. What they can do, with greater or less strength, is to help us to make up our minds of the fundamental question—is there any other way of explaining the set of facts before us; is there any other answer equally, or more likely than cause and effect?

No formal tests of significance can answer these questions. Such tests can, and should remind us of the effects that the play of chance can create, and they will instruct us in the likely magnitude of those effects. Beyond that, they contribute nothing to the proof of our hypothesis.

SUMMARY

Epidemiology is the simplest and most direct method of studying the causes of disease in human populations. Many significant contributions to environmental health and environmental medicine have been made by studies that have demanded nothing more than an ability to count, to think logically, and to have an imaginative idea. The rapid accumulation of knowledge that characterizes the past two to three decades, however, has made it more difficult for individuals working alone to make effective contributions. Epidemiologic research is becoming increasingly a matter of teamwork, not only because of the large number of people that may need to be studied and the large amount of data that have to be collected and analyzed, but also because of the need to bring together a number of disciplines for the design and conduct of the study. But even as epidemiologic research is becoming more complex, the core of the subject remains essentially simple, and a good epidemiologic study should be capable of description in such a way that all who are interested in the cause of disease can follow the argument and decide for themselves on the validity of the conclusions.[6]

REFERENCES

1. Altman DG et al: Statistical guidelines for contributors to medical journals, *Br Med J* 286:1489, 1983.
2. Bailar JC III, Mosteller F: *Medical uses of statistics,* ed 2, Boston, 1992, NEJM Books.
3. Breslow NE, Day NE: *Statistical methods in cancer research,* vol 1, *The analysis of case-control studies,* IARC Scientific Publication 32, New York, 1980, Oxford University Press.
4. Buffler PA: The evaluation of negative epidemiological studies: the importance of all available evidence in the risk characterization, *Regul Toxicol Pharmacol* 9:34, 1989.
5. Cole P: The evolving case-control study, *J Chron Dis* 32:15, 1979.
6. Doll R: Foreword. In Hennekens, CH, Buring JE: *Epidemiology in medicine,* Boston, 1987, Little, Brown.
7. Feinstein AR, Horwitz RI: Double standards, scientific methods, and epidemiologic research, *N Engl J Med* 307:1611, 1982.
8. Fleiss JL: *Statistical methods for rates and proportions,* ed 2, New York, 1981, J Wiley.
9. Fletcher RH, Fletcher SW, Wagner EH: *Clinical epidemiology—the essentials,* ed 2, Baltimore, 1988, Williams & Wilkins.
10. Friedman GD: *Primer of epidemiology,* ed 2, New York, 1980, McGraw-Hill.
11. Gladen B, Rogan WJ: Misclassification and the design of experimental studies, *Am J Epidemiol* 109:607, 1979.
12. Glasser JH: The quality and utility of death certificate data (editorial), *Am J Public Health* 71:231, 1981.
13. Goldsmith JR: *Environmental epidemiology: epidemiological investigation of community environmental health problems,* Boca Raton, Fla, 1986, CRC Press.

14. Greenberg RS, Kleinbaum DG: Mathematical modeling strategies for the analysis of epidemiologic research, *Annu Rev Public Health* 6:223, 1985.
15. Greenland S, ed: *Evolution of epidemiologic ideas: annotated readings on concepts and methods,* Chestnut Hill, Mass, 1987, ERI.
15a. Hennekens CH, Buring JE: *Epidemiology in medicine,* Boston, 1987, Little, Brown.
16. Hill AB: Observation and experiment, *N Engl J Med* 248:995, 1953.
17. Hill AB: The environment and disease: association or causation? *Proc R Soc Med* 58:295, 1965.
18. Horwitz RI, Feinstein AR: Metholodogic standards and contradictory results in case-control research, *Am J Med* 66:556, 1979.
19. Ibrahim MA: *The case-control study: consensus and controversy,* Oxford, 1979, Pergamon Press.
20. Kelsey JL, Thompson WD, Evans AS: *Methods in observational epidemiology,* New York, 1986, Oxford University Press.
21. Last JM, ed: *A dictionary of epidemiology,* ed 2, New York, 1988, Oxford University Press.
22. Lioy P: Assessing total human exposure to contaminants: a multidisciplinary approach, *Environmental Science Technology* 24:938, 1990.
23. MacMahon B, Pugh TF: *Epidemiology: principles and methods,* Boston, 1970, Little, Brown.
24. Mantel N, Haenszel W: Statistical aspects of the analysis of data from retrospective studies of disease, *J Nat Cancer Inst* 22:719, 1959.
25. Mausner JS, Kramer S: *Mausner and Bohn epidemiology—an introductory text,* Philadelphia, 1985, WB Saunders.
26. McMichael AJ: Standardized mortality ratios and the healthy worker effect: scratching beneath the surface, *J Occup Med* 18:165, 1976.
27. Monson RR: *Occupational epidemiology,* ed 2, Boca Raton, Fla, 1990, CRC Press.
28. Percy C, Stanek E, Gloeckler L: Accuracy of cancer death certificates and its effect on cancer mortality statistics, *Am J Public Health* 71:242, 1981.
29. Public Utility Commission of Texas, Electro-Magnetic Health Effects Committee (P.A. Buffler, Chair): Health effects of exposure to powerline-frequency electric and magnetic fields, appendix B, *Fundamentals of epidemiology,* pp. B1-22, 1992.
30. Rose G: Sick individuals and sick populations, *Int J Epidemiol* 14:32, 1985.
31. Rothman KJ: *Modern epidemiology,* Boston, 1986, Little, Brown.
32. Rothman KJ: A sobering start for the Cluster Busters' Conference: keynote presentation, *Am J Epidemiol* 132:S6, 1990.
33. Sackett DL: Bias in analytic research, *J Chron Dis* 32:51, 1979.
34. Schlesselman JJ: Sample size requirements in cohort and case-control studies of disease, *Am J Epidemiol* 99:381, 1974.
35. Schlesselman JJ: *Case-control studies: design, conduct, analysis,* New York, 1982, Oxford University Press.
36. Snedecor GW, Cochran WG: *Statistical methods,* ed 8, Ames, Iowa, 1989, Iowa State University.
37. Steenland K, Beaumont J: The accuracy of occupation and industry data on death certificates, *J Occup Med* 26:288, 1984.
38. Walker AM: Reporting the results of epidemiologic studies, *Am J Public Health* 76:556, 1986.

Part II

BASIC SCIENCE OF ENVIRONMENTAL MEDICINE: MECHANICS AND PRINCIPLES

Chapter 6

PRINCIPLES OF TOXICOLOGY

Michael Gochfeld

Historical information
What does the practitioner need to know?
Definitions
Classification or taxonomy of toxic agents
Temporal features of exposure and toxicity
Chemicals in the environment
    Environmental toxicology
    Biologic amplification
Pharmaceuticals and abused substances
Exposure and effect: the clinician's role
    Step 1
    Step 2
    Step 3
    Step 4
Special issues
Factors affecting toxicity
    Toxicokinetics
Metabolic activation versus detoxification
Excretion
What is the dose-response curve?
Thresholds
The no threshold dilemma
Latency
Chemical interactions: synergism and antagonism
Reversibility
Susceptibility
Mechanisms of toxicity
    Receptors and ligands
    Metabolic poisons
    Macromolecular binding
    Subcellular poisons
    Cellular poisons
    Immunotoxins
    Sensitizers
    Neuroendocrine poisons
    Mutagens
    Reproductive toxins
    Teratogens
Microsomal enzyme induction
Oxidative stress
Carcinogenesis: initiation and promotion

Assessing the significance of a toxic effect
    Hormesis
The significance of toxicity testing
Animal welfare and animal rights

Physicians in many types of practices are increasingly confronted by patients with signs, symptoms, or concerns that they attribute to one or more chemical, physical, or biologic agents in their home or community. Environmental medicine is concerned with the interface between the body and the environment, and the assessment of an exposure assumes importance as a major feature of environmental medicine. In fact, it is the unique focus on the evaluation of exposures that gives environmental medicine its cohesiveness. Once hazards have been properly assessed, procedures for control and reduction of exposure can follow.

Physicians play a unique role in communicating information about risks to patients. Opportunities for risk communication may be missed if the physician does not ask specific questions. The physicians must be able to anticipate patients' concerns, as well as react to specific questions. However, it is not always easy to answer patients' specific questions regarding the risks of developing disease or the urgency of eliminating a hazard from their lives. Very often patients have unbalanced fears. They may worry about pesticide residues in their food while continuing to eat an otherwise unhealthy diet or while continuing to smoke. They may worry about the siting of an incinerator in their community while neglecting to test their homes for radon. The clinical interview offers the chance of putting these risks into perspective. Clinicians must be clear that estimates of risks change, and they should be conveyed to the patients with words such as "based on current understanding or knowledge." In order to be able to explain the significance of an exposure to a patient, some basic understanding of how chemicals can injure a patient is necessary. Therefore, this chapter will deal with the principles of *toxicology,* the study of the harmful effects of chemicals, including drugs, on living organisms.[7,19] This chapter reviews some of the basic principles of toxicology that govern how foreign substances, also known as *xenobiotics,* cause harm. Information on specific groups of toxic chemicals will be found elsewhere in this book (see Part V, Specific Environmental Exposure Sources). This chapter will focus on toxic properties in general, how chemicals enter and move through the body, and the kinds of pathophysiologic damage to target organs that become manifest as disease.

HISTORICAL INFORMATION

Historians such as Oser[27] trace the history of toxicology back to Paracelsus (1493-1541), who seems to be the first physician to have pointed out a basic principle of toxicology: the *dose-response relationship.* Paracelsus indicated that one substance might be harmless at a low dose, therapeutic at an intermediate dose, and toxic at a high dose. Gallo and Doull[11] trace the history back more than two millennia but identify modern toxicology as arising in the nineteenth century. However, for most of the present century toxicology evolved hand in hand with pharmacology, as the study of the unwanted side effects of pharmaceuticals. There is also clinical toxicology, which deals mainly with the treatment of acute intoxications from pharmaceuticals. More recently the latter has come to include acute reactions to all xenobiotics.

Beginning in the 1970s the toxic effects of unwanted chemicals in the environment assumed a greater role in the field of toxicology. Today toxicologists work at various levels, including the molecular, cellular, organ system, whole person, and community or ecosystem. There are many branches of toxicology: descriptive, mechanistic, regulatory, forensic, environmental, and clinical.[19] Many toxicologists are involved in research on the effects of chemicals developed for pharmaceuticals and pesticides and may be involved in the registration of new substances with the Food and Drug Administration (FDA) or the Environmental Protection Agency (EPA). However, when the Food and Drug Act was first enacted in 1906 it was probably more attributable to Upton Sinclair's *The Jungle*[30] than to the exhortations of toxicologists.

WHAT DOES THE PRACTITIONER NEED TO KNOW

To fully evaluate how a chemical causes its effect, it is useful to have as much information as possible in the following areas:

1. The concentration of agent in an environmental medium or matrix
2. Exposure, dose, and route of entry into the body
3. Internal distribution, metabolism, excretion
4. Dose reaching target organ
5. Biochemical and physiologic effects on the target
6. Clinical manifestations

Chapter 2 considers how chemicals occur in air, water, soil, and food and describes how chemicals can enter the body by inhalation, ingestion, or through the skin. Once a substance has actually entered the body it may be absorbed into the circulation (depending on its bioavailability), and once absorbed it gets distributed to various parts of the body via the bloodstream. The xenobiotic may bind to carrier molecules in the blood or may enter organs where it undergoes intermediary metabolism, which may involve metabolic activation (or deactivation). In some tissues the xenobiotic or its metabolite may be stored for long periods of time (for example, PCBs in fat, lead in bone). Some of the material entering the body is eliminated directly without any absorption. Some of the absorbed chemical (or its metabolites) can be excreted by various routes, and this option is open even after a substance has been stored in an inactive tissue or depot for a long time period.[13] Fig. 6-1 presents these concepts diagrammatically.

By examining Fig. 6-1 more carefully, it becomes apparent that the uptake, distribution, metabolism, and excretion of a xenobiotic can be influenced at different steps and stages by endogenous and exogenous factors. This premise is better illustrated by the box, which depicts the factors that influ-

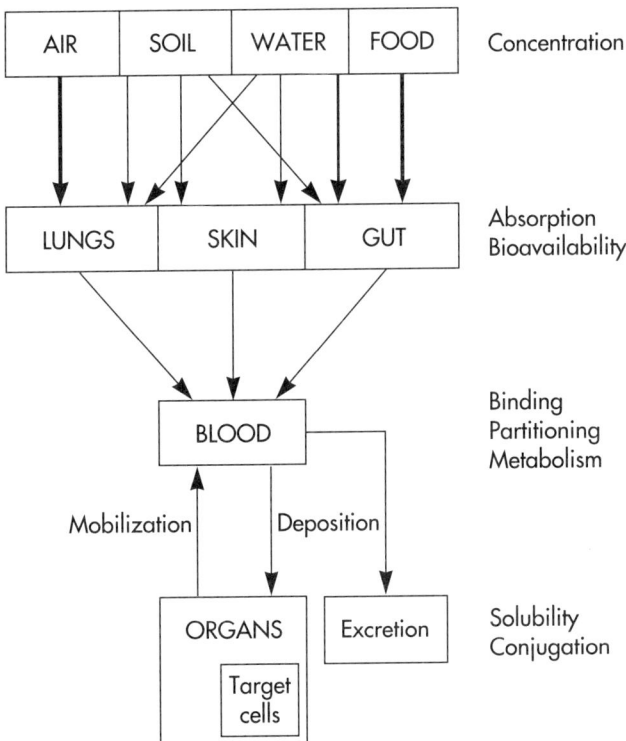

Fig. 6-1. A multicompartment model of toxicant distribution showing the relationship among uptake, metabolism, distribution, storage, and excretion. (Modified from Gochfeld M: Principles of toxicology. In Last JM, Wallace RB, eds: *Maxcy-Rosenau-Last's public health and preventive medicine,* Norwalk, Conn. 1992, Appleton & Lange.

> **Factors that modify toxicity in experimental animals or humans**
>
> *Host*
> Genetic factors
>   Species
>   Strain
>   Age
>   Gender
> Historical factors
>   Infectious/immunologic history
>   Behavioral stress history
>   Toxicant exposure history
> Activity level/fitness
> Nutritional status
>
> *Environment*
> Temperature
> Light (cycle, intensity, spectral distribution)
> Air (flow rate, humidity)
>
> *Toxicant*
> Matrix/bioavailability
> Physical form
> Chemical form

Modified from Gochfeld M: Principles of toxicology. In Last JM, Wallace RB, eds: *Public health and preventive medicine,* Norwalk, Conn, 1992, Appleton & Lange.

ence the uptake and toxicity of a material and the susceptibility of the host to handle the xenobiotic normally. Uptake varies by route of exposure and bioavailability. A given chemical may be readily absorbed from the lungs but may not be absorbed through the skin or intestinal tract.

Chapter 3 focuses on risk assessment and estimation, which is a critical process for determining the human toxicologic significance of a xenobiotic exposure. This chapter discusses the important contribution of toxicologic data to environmental risk assessment. The data can be used by regulatory agencies to assess chemical hazards, prioritize hazardous waste site cleanups, establish governmental policies, and set levels of allowable exposure. There is a lively controversy over how much reliance should be placed on toxicologic studies for influencing decisions.[8,36]

DEFINITIONS

It is best to provide some definitions to gain a better understanding of toxicology terminology.

Xenobiotic: A substance foreign to the body. Xenobiotics include all nonnaturally occurring chemicals and most pharmaceutical agents.

Toxin: Usually refers to a naturally occurring poisonous substance, for example, snake venoms.

Toxicant: Refers to a foreign or nonnatural poisonous substance and includes synthetic chemicals and pharmaceutical agents.

Toxicity: The intrinsic ability of a substance to harm living things. Even seemingly innocuous substances such as sodium chloride (where a dose of 0.9% is isotonic and therapeutic) can be toxic at high doses, whereas aflatoxin B1 or botulinum toxin are toxic at levels well below a part per trillion.

Potency: Used to compare two toxic agents with respect to the dosages capable of inducing harm (see x axis of dose-response curves).

Efficacy: Used to compare two toxic agents with respect to the amount of harm each can produce. Efficacy is compared on the y axis of the dose-response curve.

Selective toxicity: The property of producing one kind of harm or harming one kind of organism while not harming others.

Susceptibility: The ability of a living thing to be harmed by an agent. Gender, age, and genetics are important influences as well as one's state of health (for example, physical fitness, nutrition, immune status) and history of prior exposure.

Bioavailability: The ability of a substance that enters the body to be liberated from its environmental matrix (water, tissue, soil) and to enter the circulation.

Intermediary metabolism: The metabolic change(s) a chemical undergoes in various organs, particularly the liver. A xenobiotic can be rendered either less harmful (detoxification) or more harmful (metabolic activation).

Mechanism of action: How a xenobiotic harms the molecular, cellular, biochemical, or physiologic integrity of an organism. This includes formation of DNA adducts, metabolic poisons, cellular or intracellular membrane alteration, and others.

Threshold: The lowest dose at which some measurable effect occurs. For any xenobiotic that produces multiple effects, the threshold for each effect may differ. For example, for a neurotoxic chemical that produces dizziness, convulsion, coma, and death, the thresholds for these effects vary from relatively low for dizziness to high for fatality.

Toxic effect: Damage to an organism measured in terms of a loss, reduction, or change of function reported as a symptom or detected as a sign. Effects considered adverse in one individual may be desirable or therapeutic in another.

Structure activity relationship (SAR): Substances with similar structures tend to exert similar effects. Thus short-chain chlorinated alkanes (such as chloroform, trichloroethylene, trichloroethane) all tend to be CNS depressants. However, in some cases slight molecular alterations can strongly influence toxicity (for instance adding a methyl group to benzene removes its leukemogenic properties).

Octanol/water partitioning: The ratio of a substance's solubility in octanol to its solubility in water. This defines its relative lipophilic or hydrophilic properties, which in turn influence absorption, toxicity, and storage.

Depot: A tissue in which a chemical is stored for a long time. In some cases such as lead in bone or PCBs in fat, the depot is not a primary target organ. In other cases such as cadmium in the kidney, the depot is also a primary target.

CLASSIFICATION OR TAXONOMY OF TOXIC AGENTS

It is customary to divide the toxicologic hazards or external stressors that potentially can harm the body into broad categories such as physical (noise, temperature, radiation), biologic (infectious, immunologic), chemical, and psychosocial stressors. Generally, toxicologists focus on chemicals, both synthetic and of natural origin. There are interactions among classes of stressors. Thus radiation, infection, or psychologic stress may modify the effects of toxic chemicals, and vice versa; there is increasing attention to the effects of two or more chemicals administered together where synergistic or antagonistic effects may occur.

There are more than 75,000 named chemicals, many of which are used in commerce. Of these, probably only about 2000 are widely used and only about 200 are commonly encountered in environmental medicine practice. Therefore, if practitioners were knowledgeable in the details of these 200 chemicals, they could address more than 95% of patient concerns. Although learning about 200 chemicals may seem daunting, the principles of toxicologic knowledge are no different from understanding infectious organisms or pharmaceuticals. Just as one organizes infectious disease knowledge by virus, rickettsia, gram negative, gram positive, and so on, or drugs by mode of action, one can learn about classes of chemicals. How chemicals move through the environment how readily they are absorbed, how they undergo metabolism, distribution, and excretion and how they exert their toxic effects are strongly influenced by their chemical structure.[12] One of the basic structural features is the relative solubility in water versus organic solvents. This is usually defined by the octanol/water partitioning coefficient or ratio. This text emphasizes other aspects of chemical exposures, and Chapter 30 deals with the major features of many of the commonly encountered chemicals and provides information on obtaining further data when needed.

TEMPORAL FEATURES OF EXPOSURE AND TOXICITY

The terms *acute* and *chronic* can refer either to conditions of exposure or to the resultant health effects. A single "acute" exposure to a toxic chemical may be sufficient to induce health effects that in turn may be acute (followed by recovery), subacute, or chronic. Long-term or chronic exposure may be followed by no adverse health effects (if the dose is low), by acute effects (which may occur when a sufficient dose is accumulated), or by chronic effects. In addition to having a long duration, chronic effects are more likely to be irreversible. Fig. 6-2 illustrates these principles.

In animal toxicologic studies acute toxicity can be defined

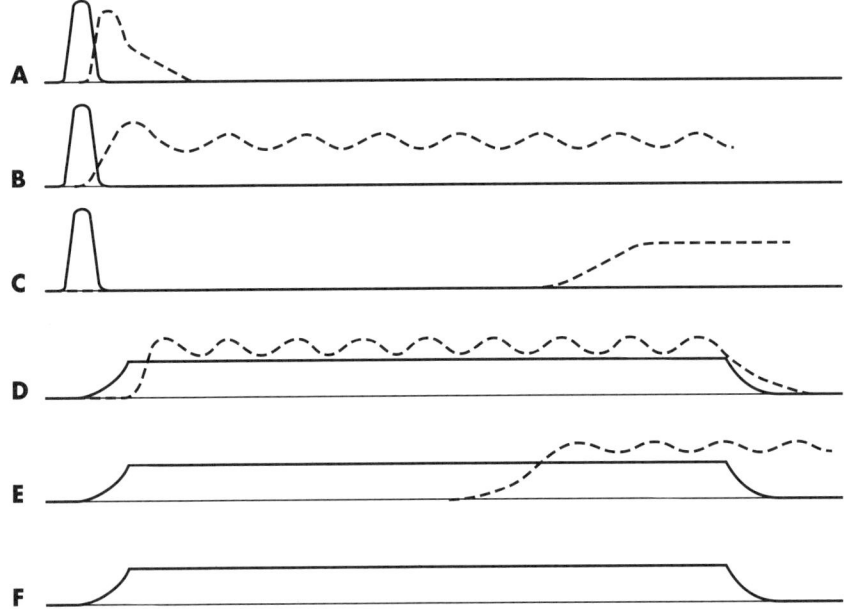

Fig. 6-2. Temporal relationships between exposure and effect. Curves *a, b,* and *c* show responses to a single acute, high-level exposure: *a,* an acute self-limited effect; *b,* an acute and persistent effect; *c,* a long-delayed effect after an acute exposure. Curves *d, e,* and *f* show response to a chronic, lower-level exposure: *d,* a chronic condition arising shortly after onset of exposure, and probably idiosyncratic; *e,* a chronic condition beginning after a long period of cumulative exposure; *f,* no appreciable response. *Solid lines* = exposure; *dashed lines* = effects. (Courtesy Environmental and Occupational Health Sciences Institute.)

Table 6-1. Relationship between exposure duration and dose in producing health effects

Dose	Duration of exposure	
	Brief	Long
Low	Usually innocuous	Household exposures
		Some workplaces
		Difficult to study
		Often controversial
High	"Accidents": fires, spills, explosions	Occupational settings
	Usually acute effects	Usually easy to study
		Usually consensus

Courtesy Environmental and Occupational Health Sciences Institute.

Table 6-2. How bioamplification might work for a hypothetical lipophilic contaminant in a hypothetical food chain*

Trophic level	Average concentration
Water	1 ppb
Plankton	10 ppb
Minute crustacean	100 ppb
Minnows, baby fish	1000 ppb = 1 ppm
Small fish	10 ppm
Commercial size large fish	100 ppm
Human	?

Plankton swimming in water with a 1 ppm concentration would contain 10 ppm, the fish larvae 100 ppm, the small fish 1000 ppm, and the large fish 10,000 ppm.

*Assumes a concentration factor of 10 throughout. Courtesy Environmental and Occupational Health Sciences Institute.

as effects occurring within 24 hours of a dose; subchronic toxicity occurs after exposure lasting less than 10% of one's life span[6] and chronic exposure refers to dosing animals for more than 10% of their life span.[31] Table 6-1 examines relationships between *exposure* and *dose* in producing a toxic effect. Long-term, high-level exposures such as those that occur in workplace settings readily cause disease, and it is often easy to identify a causal relationship. Explosions, fires, and spills may produce very high-level exposures but for a short period. Most effects are acute and either fatal or self-limiting, but sometimes chronic disease (for example, asthma, reactive airways disease) may follow. Short-term, low-level exposures to many toxic chemicals are innocuous for most people.

An active area of investigation concerns the effect of long-term, low-level exposures such as those that occur in the home, yard, or community and in some workplaces. For many agents that accumulate in the body even low-level exposure may have a cumulative effect when the body has received a sufficient dose over time. For other agents the body may reach an equilibrium between intake and excretion, and if this level is below a threshold, there may be no adverse effects.

CHEMICALS IN THE ENVIRONMENT
Environmental toxicology

Environmental toxicology deals with consequences of exposure to contaminants in air, water, soil, and food (see Chapters 2 and 4) that are encountered in our home, community, and workplace environments. Other chapters in this book deal with chemicals and exposures in all of these media (see Part V). Some toxic elements occur naturally in some soils, but fortunately many of the elements that are present in high concentrations in most soils (for example, calcium, silicon, aluminum, and iron) are relatively nontoxic. This perhaps should not be surprising, since plants and animals evolved with their environment and presumably have had to develop tolerances to elements with which they came in daily contact. For example, in those areas of New Caledonia where the soil has high concentrations of nickel, one finds unique plants that are tolerant of this chemical. Similarly salt-tolerant plants (halophytes) abound in brackish coastal marshes.

Food may contain toxic chemicals from a variety of sources. Regulations governing pesticide application (for example, the minimum number of days between spraying and harvest) are designed to minimize residual pesticides in food (see Chapter 43). Some chemical residues may be on the surface while others may have been taken up into the plant tissue. These differences have significant implications when considering methods for removing residues.

Biologic amplification

Biologic amplification is a process by which a chemical present at infinitesimal concentrations in air or water may be increasingly concentrated as it moves along the food chain, until humans consuming meat or fish encounter relatively high concentrations. This depends on the property of chemicals to bioconcentrate in certain cell fractions (particularly lipids) or in certain organs (for example, the liver). Biologic amplification was first shown for lipophilic chemicals such as chlorinated hydrocarbons and organometals such as methyl mercury. These substances may be present in water or soil at the parts per billion level, which would normally be considered innocuous. When taken up by planktonic organisms, they tend to concentrate in the lipids of these organisms, and only a small fraction of the uptake is excreted. When the plankton are consumed by low-level predators such as fish larvae or shrimp, they too retain the lipophilic contaminant. These minute animals are then eaten by small fish, which are in turn eaten by larger ones, and the larger ones are ultimately consumed by humans.

Table 6-2 illustrates a hypothetical bioamplification pathway for several trophic levels of a food chain. Each organism in the food chain retains more of the compound than it excretes (is in positive balance). The table assumes a concentration factor (CF) of 10 for each trophic level. This example leaves the hapless human consuming a huge dose of the amplified toxic material. The term *bioamplification* as used here is synonymous with biomagnifacation. The more general term *bioaccumulation* can include bioamplification.

PHARMACEUTICALS AND ABUSED SUBSTANCES

Certain chemicals with potent biochemical and physiologic effects are deliberately introduced into the body in very high concentrations. By whatever route and whether legal or illicit, these chemicals are used because of their high level of bioactivity, which can be either beneficial (efficacy) or harmful (toxicity). Even at therapeutic doses there are often undesired side effects that are actually manifestations of toxicity. These may be idiosyncratic and uncommon responses, such as anaphylactic reactions to penicillin, or common effects, such as drowsiness from antihistamines. The two most commonly abused substances are alcohol and tobacco, both of which have significant acute and chronic toxic effects.

EXPOSURE AND EFFECT: THE CLINICIAN'S ROLE

Recently the highly sophisticated field of exposure assessment has emerged, combining chemical analysis, behavioral studies, and mathematical modeling to estimate the dose received by an individual.[20] The patient's medical history provides very important information regarding potential and actual exposures, although the clinician must constantly add new questions to the traditional history.

Step 1

The first level in understanding exposure is knowing whether or not there is or has been a contaminant in the patient's environment. The environmental history provides critical information on how much of the material is likely to enter a person's body. This approach is presented in detail in Chapters 18 and 19. In many cases the patient has actual documentation in the form of a water analysis or a known pesticide application. In other cases the presence of a contaminant is only inferred. These are distinctly different situations. If a toxic chemical is present, that constitutes *potential exposure*. To determine whether *actual exposure* has occurred one needs to know about the proximity of the individual to the offending agent (for example, are they immediately adjacent to a hazardous waste site), the duration of exposure, and information about their life-style (for example, do they eat fish from nearby streams or produce from a garden on contaminated soil).

Step 2

It is important to obtain a complete and detailed medical history, indicating health complaints and temporal relationships. The medical history for environmentally induced illnesses is no different than for other medical problems, and the same clinical tools are utilized. This step requires defining the target organ affected, the degree of impairment, and the identification of non–environmentally induced disorders.

Step 3

In some cases the practitioner can validate exposure by *biologic monitoring* or the procedure of measuring a substance or its metabolite in body tissue or fluids. From the environmental history and information on bioavailability (often difficult to obtain), one can estimate the actual uptake into the system. This allows one to qualitatively estimate doses to target organs.[20]

Step 4

The clinician's next task is to determine whether there is an adequate linkage between the exposure history and the reported health effects. In a typical situation a primary practitioner sees a symptomatic patient who has no clue that there is something in the environment causing the illness. It may require multiple visits, various tests, and the ruling out of many common maladies before an environmental cause is suspected. In other cases, a patient complains about an exposure and is worried about future effects, even though there is no apparent health effect at the time.

Exposure to a specific substance is modified by the substance itself and its bioavailability, whether it is in soluble or insoluble form, volatile or not, whether there is a vehicle or carrier that promotes absorption into the body (or conversely whether it is bound to a matrix from which it cannot be released), and by the host condition and behavior (whether the skin is intact, whether dietary substances promote or inhibit uptake, and whether the host is breathing rapidly; for example, a jogger on a crowded urban avenue).

Potential exposure is commonly measured by analyzing water, food, air samples, and various products for their concentration of particular substances. In other cases a patient may actually have a fact sheet or material safety data sheet that provides written information.

SPECIAL ISSUES

Bioavailability is the ability of a substance to be released from its matrix.[35] This varies from 100% for ingested ethanol to less than 10% for lead ingested by an adult, to nearly 0% for many substances that contact only the skin. Bioavailability varies not only with the chemical itself but with the matrix. Thus dioxin had high bioavailability in the sandy soil of Times Beach but much lower bioavailability in the oily, clayey, urban soil of Newark.[35] The likelihood that a plant will take up a contaminant from the soil is also a function of bioavailability.

Vanishing zero: A common clinical problem is the patient who voices concern about exposure to very low levels of highly toxic chemicals. The past two decades have seen dramatic advances in analytic instrumentation, such that we are now capable of measuring contaminants at the parts per quadrillion level. This improved ability to analyze vanishingly small quantities of an agent has been a great boon to environmental science but also requires explaining the concept of adequate dose and threshold to patients.[39] A water analysis that would formerly have been listed as "undetectable" or "zero" now comes back with a detectable concentration in nanograms per gram or less. This has been referred to as the *vanishing zero*.[15]

FACTORS AFFECTING TOXICITY
Toxicokinetics

Toxicokinetics is the study of the distribution and differential concentration of a xenobiotic and/or its metabolites throughout the body. How a chemical behaves can be measured by the various rate constants that exist for each metabolic process in different tissues under different circumstances and on different partitioning coefficients, binding properties, and so on that influence rates of delivery to various organs and thus excretion or deposition. Some reactions are competitive, such that the amount of material available for metabolism depends on the amount that has been sequestered in fat, bound to protein, or excreted in the urine.

Every substance that enters the body undergoes a combination of absorption, transport, metabolism, storage, and excretion. The physicochemical properties of the xenobiotic or its metabolites (for example, binding properties, solubility) influence whether it will be stored or excreted, and dynamic equilibria exist for all of these processes; one can refer to Fig. 6-1 for the various state changes that enter into the toxicokinetic history of a substance.

The perfusion rate of an organ influences the delivery of a chemical. The passage of a chemical across a membrane is proportional to the concentration gradient, the membrane surface area, and the permeability coefficient, which depends on the compound's relative lipophilia and the condition of the membrane. Excretion via exhaled breath, urine, feces, or sweat is in turn determined by the relative solubility of the compound and its delivery to the appropriate organ (lungs, kidney, intestine, skin). In general, compounds that are water soluble or appropriately conjugated are excreted via urine, while lipid-soluble compounds are secreted via the bile into the intestine.

METABOLIC ACTIVATION VERSUS DETOXIFICATION

An important feature of metabolism is its ability to both reduce and enhance toxicity of a chemical.[18] Many toxic chemicals (for example, benzene) cannot exert an effect until they are changed into an active metabolite (bioactivation), usually through an oxidative reaction that produces reactive intermediate compounds that can interfere with other metabolic reactions or "attack" membranes, organelles, or macromolecules.

Alternatively, a xenobiotic may be sequestered in an organ where it produces little effect. This is not a permanent event, for there is usually an equilibrium between the amount of chemicals in any tissue and blood, and under certain conditions a chemical may be released from its depot tissue (for example, during starvation fat is broken down, and toxic chemicals stored in fat are released into the circulation).

EXCRETION

The amount of a xenobiotic in the body depends not only on exposure but on excretion. Volatile compounds are excreted through the lungs. At any moment the concentration of volatiles in expired air depends on how much has just been inspired (but not absorbed) as well as how much is released to the lungs from the bloodstream. Measurement of volatiles in expired air is gaining increasing utility as a means of monitoring exposure.

Chemicals that are not water soluble can be conjugated to molecules that allow them to be excreted via the urine. Highly volatile short-chain hydrocarbons may be excreted via the lungs or metabolized in the liver into water-soluble polar compounds.

WHAT IS THE DOSE-RESPONSE CURVE?

The hallmark of toxicology is the dose-response curve,[14,17] which stated simply means that a high dose of a xenobiotic usually has a greater effect than a low dose. This concept can be better illustrated by examining Fig. 6-3. Note that the magnitude of the exposure (dose, concentration, duration of exposure, or some other indication of exposure) is indicated along the x axis and the magnitude of the effect (response, number of animals with an outcome, or some other index of outcome) is plotted on the y axis. A typical dose-response curve has a sigmoid shape and is presented as a cumulative percent response. The characteristic features of dose-response curves are shown in Fig. 6-3, which represents an ideal case, and minor modifications in the shape

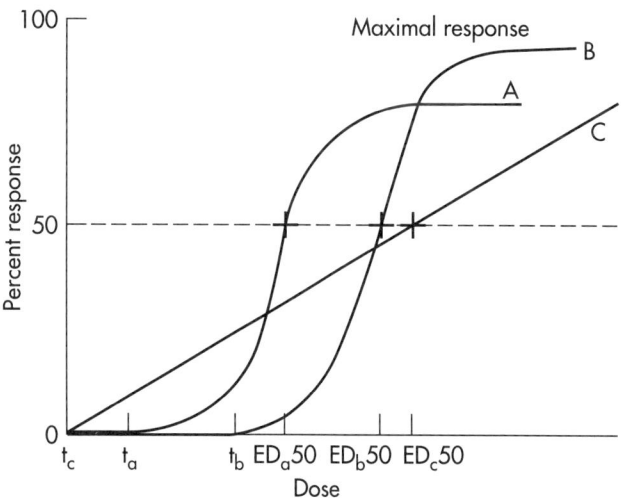

Fig. 6-3. The dose-response curve. *A* and *B* are typical sigmoid curves differing in potency and efficacy. *C* is a linear, no-threshold curve presumed to be characteristic of the causation of cancer by ionizing radiation. *B* has a higher threshold but also higher efficacy than *A*. Thresholds, indicated by 't', ED50s, and maximal responses, are indicated for curves *A*, *B*, and *C*. (Courtesy Environmental and Occupational Health Sciences Institute.)

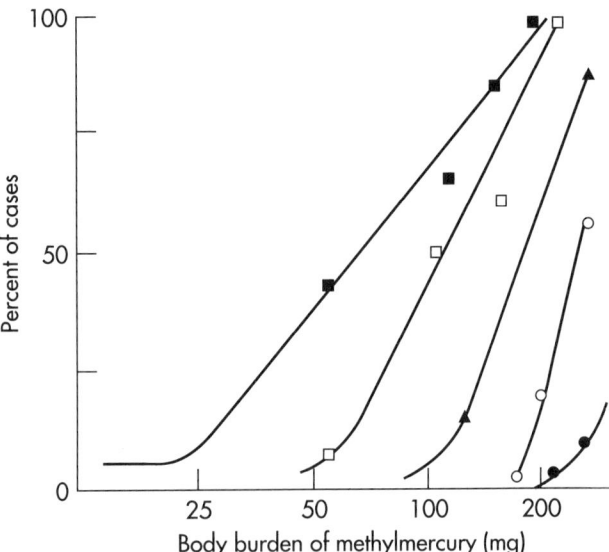

Fig. 6-4. Dose-response curves for different clinical manifestations of organomercury poisoning based on the epidemic in Iraq, showing the relative progression in thresholds from relatively minor sign of paresthesias to lethality, estimated at the time exposure ceased. Solid triangles = paresthesias, *open squares* = ataxia, *solid squares* = dysarthria; *open circles* = deafness; *solid circles* = death. (Modified from Takizawa Y: Epidemiology of mercury poisoning. In Nriagu J, ed: *The biogeochemistry of mercury in the environment,* Amsterdam, 1979, Elsevier-North Holland.)

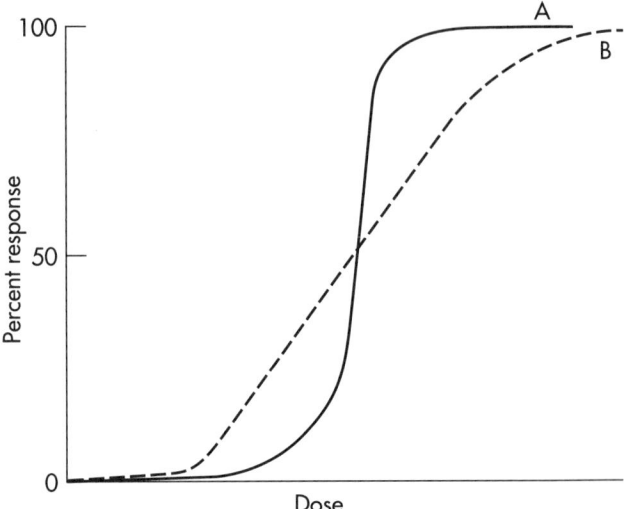

Fig. 6-5. Susceptibility curves, for *A* (*solid line*) an inbred laboratory animal showing very little variation in susceptibility and *B* (*dashed line*) for a highly variable human population. Both have similar ED50 and efficacy. (Courtesy Environmental and Occupational Health Sciences Institute.)

and slope of the curve may be noted in a "real-world" situation. Initially there is a flat portion where an increase in dose produces no effect (see curves A and B, Fig. 6-3). This is the subthreshold phase. The threshold is the lowest dose that produces an observable or measurable effect. Beyond that point the curve tends to rise steeply and enters a linear phase where the increase in response is proportional to the increase in dose. Eventually a maximal response is reached, and the curve flattens out. This usually means that all the exposed individuals or at least all the susceptible individuals have shown the effect.

Let us examine how a dose-response curve is developed. The first step in formulating dose-response curves is to identify the endpoints of concern. Fig. 6-4 illustrates a clinical example and represents a family of dose-response curves with different endpoints due to organomercury poisoning. The endpoints can vary from fatality to minor irritation and from objective (white blood count) to subjective (psychologic symptoms). In Fig. 6-4, the y axis shows the percent of cases with a specific response. Traditionally, in animal toxicology the y axis is the percent of animals showing a particular effect. Other endpoints commonly used in animal studies are the percent of animals developing tumors or the average number of tumors per animal. In the past the number of animals dying was commonly used as an endpoint; the dose that kills 50% of animals is referred to as the lethal dose 50% or LD50. Various chemicals can be ranked in terms of their LD50. This approach has been generally abandoned. However, for any quantitative effect one can estimate an ED50 (effective dose for 50% of animals) or an EC50 (an effective concentration in air or water). The ED50 and EC50 take into account that animals differ in their susceptibility to a toxic substance (Fig. 6-3). Notwithstanding, among the inbred animals customarily used in toxicology research, the genetic variability has been minimized. In humans the variation in susceptibility is much greater, as exemplified by the two dose-response curves shown in Fig. 6-5. The sigmoid-shaped solid line represents an inbred laboratory animal possessing very little susceptibility variability, while the dashed line exemplifies a highly variable human population. Both curves show similar ED50s and efficacy.

THRESHOLDS

Most physiologic and many pharmacologic actions have thresholds (see Fig. 6-3) that are levels of stimulus or dose below which there is no measurable response. Consequently, this type of dose-response curve is curvilinear in shape. Thresholds probably exist for most toxicologic exposures, allowing us to live normal lives even when exposed to numerous chemicals in water, food, and air at subthreshold levels. However, experience with ionizing radiation exposures indicates that even at very low doses there does not appear to be any detectable threshold below which there is no harm. A no threshold curve is one in which a threshold effect is not appreciated. Therefore, considering radiation exposures, there is no identifiable concentration of radiation below which a no response occurs. This type of dose-response curve is linear in nature and is illustrated in Fig. 6-3, *C.* Theoretically, in this instance one quantum of radiation may be sufficient to damage DNA. If in fact there is a threshold it must be so close to zero that it cannot be measured with the epidemiologic tools available today. The ability of ionizing radiation to cause cancer is therefore identified as a nonthreshold phenomenon, and this has led many scientists to view all cancer dose-response curves as having no threshold.[27]

THE NO THRESHOLD DILEMMA

Whether or not a threshold exists for any or all carcinogens has been the focus of controversy both in the scientific and legal arena. Governmental regulations have been challenged when based on a no threshold approach, yet theoretically at least, a single molecule may be the critical molecule that induces a cancer transformation in a cell.[8] Some scientists believe that there must be a threshold for cancer as there is for other toxicologic reactions. Others argue on theoretical grounds that since no threshold (below which no cancer risk exists) has been demonstrated, there must not be a threshold. Perhaps the largest group of scientists is undecided about the no threshold concept for carcinogens or believes that this may be true for some but not all carcinogens. A prudent approach adopted by regulatory agencies is to assume that there is no threshold until one has been documented. Thus the application of a no threshold approach to carcinogens can be viewed as a *policy decision* rather than a *scientific decision*.[8]

At the heart of this controversy is the Delaney Amendment to the Food, Drug, and Cosmetic Act, which states that a known carcinogen cannot be added to food at any concentration. This act was based on the presumption that there is no safe level (subthreshold) for a carcinogen. However, the Delaney Act does not restrict the sale of food that contains naturally occurring substances that may be carcinogens or pesticide residues, which are regulated separately.[25] It was implemented in 1958 when analytic methods were much less sensitive and when many substances that are now measurable would have been undetectable. Controversy over this clause continues.

LATENCY

A stimulus may produce an effect after a latency of milliseconds (nerve impulse inducing muscle contraction) or after decades (certain cancers). In the case of asbestos-induced mesothelioma, the latency may be on the order of 40 years. If the latency is very short, one can often identify a cause-and-effect relationship, but for chemicals with a long latency the cause-effect relationship is much more difficult to distinguish, and proof of its occurrence usually requires sophisticated epidemiologic approaches to recognize the adverse effect. On a clinical note, for diseases with long latency the patient may forget about exposures that occurred decades in the past. Latency itself may be plotted on the y axis of a dose-response curve. In certain studies the latent period, also called *time to tumor,* may vary with the dose of a carcinogen.

CHEMICAL INTERACTIONS: SYNERGISM AND ANTAGONISM

When two chemicals are administered together or when an individual is exposed to a mixtures of chemicals, there may be various interactions identified as follows: (1) independence or *additivity:* each substance produces its own effect in proportion to its dose; (2) *synergism:* the combined effect is greater than either substance would have produced alone; (3) *antagonism:* the combined effect is less than one would have expected from one or both chemicals administered alone; and (4) *potentiation* or *inhibition,* occurring when one agent that does not produce the effect in question increases or decreases the ability of a second agent to produce the effect. An example of synergism is workers exposure to asbestos fibers smoking cigarettes.[16] A worker with significant asbestos exposure has a risk about 5 times greater for developing lung cancer than a person without asbestos exposure. A cigarette smoker has about a tenfold greater relative risk for developing a lung cancer than a nonsmoker. A smoker exposed to asbestos does not have a 15 times greater risk for cancer (i.e., additive, whereby $5\times$ and $10\times = 15\times$) but rather a 50 times greater risk (i.e., synergistic, multiplicative, more than additive, whereby $5\times$ times $10\times = 50\times$).[16]

REVERSIBILITY

For the patient's welfare it is important to realize that many toxic events are reversible. The body has a tremendous potential for self-repair. If a substance inhibits a biochemical pathway, the inhibitory effect may subside as the substance is gradually eliminated from the body. In most organs, if a cell is killed, new cells are produced to take its place. Even damage to DNA molecules can be repaired, although human DNA repair capabilities decline with advancing age.

SUSCEPTIBILITY

Susceptibility is an essential ingredient of toxicology, and toxicologists are familiar with selecting experimental animals based on their susceptibility or resistance to a particular agent. Humans vary greatly in their susceptibility to chemical agents, partly due to genetic differences (for example, in constitutive or inducible enzymes) and partly due to their overall health status. Although some of the factors modifying susceptibility are well known, there is relatively little active research into human susceptibility. In experimental animals, species, strain, gender, and age influence susceptibility, and some strains are bred for enhanced susceptibility to certain diseases. Human susceptibility is discussed in greater detail in Part IV.

MECHANISMS OF TOXICITY

The following section provides a brief interpretation of common mechanisms of toxic action. More detailed explanations can be found in such resources as Casarett and Doull's textbook on toxicology.[19]

Receptors and ligands

Receptors are an important part of toxic interactions and may involve binding of a toxicant or ligand to a receptor site on a membrane, an enzyme, or some other macromolecules. Receptors are important components of normal cellular function and account for the specificity of many cell processes. Some toxic effects occur because a xenobiotic is able to bind to a hormone receptor or a neuroreceptor, thus interfering with the normal action of the endogenous chemical. For example, it has been shown that the very toxic chemical 2,3,7,8-TCDD (dioxin) binds to estrogen receptors.[12] In most cases this binding is reversible, but in some cases treatment is required to accelerate the reversibility. When a toxic chemical binds to a natural receptor, the complex is sometimes more stable than the normal agent-receptor complex; an example is the binding of carbon monoxide to hemoglobin.

Metabolic poisons

Metabolic poisons are substances that disrupt metabolic pathways, for example, by competitive inhibition. Some substances disrupt the tertiary structure of enzymes, interfering with their biologic activity.

Macromolecular binding

Macromolecular binding occurs when a xenobiotic binds with nucleic acids, proteins, or hemoglobin to form complexes (adducts) that interfere with the normal cellular function. The presence of DNA adducts may reflect genotoxic or carcinogenic properties, and the quest for these molecular markers of exposure is an important frontier in toxicologic research.

Subcellular poisons

Subcellular poisons act within cells, altering function or structural properties of organelles such as mitochondria or the endoplasmic reticulum. The mitochondria are a common target, and many chemicals disrupt intramitochondrial membranes and interfere with cellular energetics.

Cellular poisons

Cellular poisons cause cellular necrosis or membrane damage. Cell membranes are functional units as well as structural in nature. Xenobiotics may produce major consequences by virtue of interfering with membrane transport or membrane-bound functions. Many natural toxins, such as plant or snake venom hemolysins, act chiefly by lysing cells. Some chemicals act by increasing the fluidity of membranes through a process known as *lipid peroxidation*.[3]

Immunotoxins

Immunotoxins act on the immune system by either heightening or suppressing the immune response. Chemicals may affect gamma globulins; interfere with the production, function, or life span of the T and B lymphocytes; or have specific effects on antigens or antibodies. It is now possible to perform immunologic studies that quantify the subtypes of T cells and B cells. Although this is an active area of research, there have not been many applications to clinical environmetal medicine. Substances known to interfere with the immune system include polyhalogenated aromatic compounds (for example 2,3,7,8-TCDD), metals (e.g., lead and cadmium), pesticides, and even air pollutants, (for example, NO_2, SO_2, tobacco smoke). The chapter on immunotoxicology deals with this matter in more detail.

Sensitizers

Sensitizers act through the immune system and cause an immunologic response; there is recognition of a foreign agent and a heightened immunologic response to its subsequent introduction. Immune response occurs mainly in the skin and respiratory system. Sensitizers may be represented by either a hapten or a complete antigen. In a clinical vein, the syndrome of *multiple chemical sensitivity* is reported to reflect abnormal sensitivity of the immune system, but current scientific evidence documents no known immune mechanism.[9] This entity is discussed in greater detail in Chapter 13.

Neuroendocrine poisons

Neuroendocrine poisons have specific actions on components of the nervous and endocrine systems. The mechanisms of action of a neuroendocrine poison include interference with the active synthesis or release of a hormone or neurotransmitter; additionally, neuroendocrine poisons may competitively or destructively block hormone or neurotransmitter action. Some chemicals specifically interfere with excitable membrane function, for example, by altering the natural polarization, repolarization, or resistance to depolarization of a membrane.

Mutagens

Mutagens may alter the genetic material (are genotoxic), causing chromosomal damage, point mutations, sister chromatid exchanges, or functional defects in gene replication or cell division. Mutation is believed to be one of the events responsible for the initiation of cancer in many cases. A mutagenic effect refers to the event of a transmissible but hereditable change.

Reproductive toxins

Reproductive toxins can affect any of the processes ranging from gametogenesis, fertilization, implantation, embryogenesis, organogenesis, to birth. Major errors incompatible with life generally result in abortion, which can be viewed as a quality control procedure. Azoospermia in males has been attributed to the pesticide dibromochloropropane (DBCP).[38] In other reproductive situations gametes are formed but do not have normal structure or function. Once gametes are formed several factors may intervene to prevent the initiation of embryogenesis. There is concern that many synthetic chemicals, particularly those that bind to hormone receptors, may interfere with one or more of these steps. Many chemicals have been implicated in toxicity to the male reproductive system (including interfering with spermatogenesis, semen quality, erection, and libido). The list of chemicals affecting females includes heavy metals, anticancer drugs, insecticides, and various organic chemicals.[10] In order to predict the likelihood of future reproductive consequences, markers of reproductive toxicity have been investigated.[24,38]

Teratogens

Teratogens represent a subset of reproductive toxicants that interfere with the complex processes of developmental morphogenesis. Depending on the stage of embryogenesis and fetogenesis, they may affect different organ systems, leading to embryonic death, major structural birth defects, slowed maturation, or even postnatal effects such as learning difficulties.[26] Whereas exposure prior to implantation is often fatal, exposure in the first trimester during organogenesis is associated with major congenital anomalies. Exposure later in pregnancy retards fetal growth and may lead to fetal death or functional changes that interfere with birth or postnatal development. Recognizable birth defects occur spontaneously in approximately 3% of live births. Some of these are genetic or chromosomal in origin, but some are due to chemical exposures (including drugs taken by the mother). This 3% provides a background level that makes it difficult to identify slight increases in risk. Furthermore, the recognition that even relatively low levels of lead exposure in childhood are associated with slowed psychomotor development and impaired learning and school performance, as well as recognition of the fetal alcohol syndrome, has spawned an entire field of behavioral teratology as well as an aggressive assault on childhood lead poisoning.[1,26]

MICROSOMAL ENZYME INDUCTION

The body does not maintain a complete inventory of all the enzymes or antibodies that may be needed for every situation. However, when an exposure occurs, the appropriate enzymes or antibodies can be induced over a period as short as 12 to 24 hours, allowing the body to combat the insult. Constitutive enzymes are ones that remain present at approximately the same concentrations, whereas inducible enzymes are present at low levels and are increased by a specific exposure. Some enzyme systems are highly specific and act only on a single substrate; others are nonspecific and catalyze classes of reactions on a wide range of substrates. The cytochrome P-450 system is an inducible enzyme system that metabolizes a wide range of xenobiotics. The substrates vary in their potency and efficacy for inducing enzymes. Enzyme induction plays an important role in metabolizing xenobiotics, either enhancing their toxicity or reducing it. However, sometimes the most important consequence of the enzyme induction is the greatly accelerated metabolism of endogenous bioactive compounds.

OXIDATIVE STRESS

Oxygen is one of the most ubiquitous of poisons. Although it is essential to life, it also aids in the formation of destructive compounds referred to as *reactive oxygen species* that have been implicated in the pathogenesis of a variety of disease-causing processes including inflammation, aging, carcinogenesis, and toxicity.[29] Oxygen can receive an electron and form superoxide anion radical, which in turn forms hydrogen peroxide, which can react with electrons and hydrogen ion to form water and the highly reactive hydroxyl radical.

$$O\text{-}O + e^- \rightarrow O\text{-}O^{\cdot}$$
$$O\text{-}O^{\cdot} + e^- + 2H^+ \rightarrow H\text{-}O\text{-}O\text{-}H$$
$$H\text{-}O\text{-}O\text{-}H + e^- + H^+ \rightarrow H_2O + {}^{\cdot}OH$$

The OH radical can attach to macromolecules, leading to various effects. Since life has evolved in an oxygen-rich environment, organisms have evolved defense mechanisms[29] against the reactive oxygen species. Antioxidant vitamins A, C, and E; superoxide dismutase; and glutathione-dependent peroxidases are capable of scavenging free radicals. Many cells contain glutathione reductase, which reactivates the glutathione molecule, thereby promoting the scavenging. Free radicals exert damage on the molecular and membrane level and can form lipid peroxides with cell membranes, leading to cell damage and loss of function.

CARCINOGENESIS: INITIATION AND PROMOTION

The term *cancer* applies to a variety of diseases for which the uncontrolled proliferation of cells is a common denominator. Carcinogens can act either by initiating cancer, usually by interaction with DNA, or by promoting cancer in cells that have already been initiated. Cancer is currently viewed as a multistage process involving initiation and promotion. *Initiation* is the process by which the genetic material of the cell is altered, predisposing it to cancer.[37] All persons are regularly exposed to initiators throughout their lives, such as cosmic radiation. However, the early changes in DNA that might constitute initiation can be reversed by the body's normal DNA repair process; alternatively, DNA changes may lie dormant or inactive, perhaps controlled by immune mechanisms. *Promotion* is the process by which initiated cells are stimulated or allowed to become cancerous.[5] Carcinogenesis is presented in more detail in Chapter 7.

ASSESSING THE SIGNIFICANCE OF A TOXIC EFFECT

When is a toxic effect significant? When is a pathophysiologic change indicative of a disease process? The body is capable of adequately responding to various environmental challenges by evoking normal defense mechanisms (such as mucociliary clearance, inflammation). It is only when the body's defense mechanisms are overwhelmed that the environmental stressor exceeds the body's adaptive ability and disease is likely to arise. Some outcomes are not characterized as disease, but their significance is controversial or unknown. For example, is hyperplasia or hypertrophy a sign of a healthy physiologic adaptation or is it a pathologic process? An individual with hemolysis adequately compensated by reticulocytosis will show no sign of illness.[3] Does this natural biologic adaptation put an unacceptable and eventually unhealthful strain on the body? Is there a limit to the body's ability to compensate for stress? Is a certain level of stress beneficial? We currently do not know the answers to these questions.

Hormesis

Hormesis represents a reportedly beneficial effect by which a low-level exposure to a substance causes a beneficial effect while higher exposure causes disease.[22] It is a highly controversial topic, and will not be dealt with in detail in this chapter.

THE SIGNIFICANCE OF TOXICITY TESTING

Toxicologists employ a wide variety of systems and paradigms to test chemicals in order to predict their effects on human health or the environment. The factors affecting toxicity in humans (see box on p. 67) must be considered in designing the experiments. One must choose the appropriate animal model or in vitro test system. If using animals, the genetic strain, gender, and age of the animal must be selected appropriately. The dosage schedule, single or multiple, and acute subchronic or chronic, as well as appropriate dose levels must be chosen. The route of administration should be relevant to natural conditions of exposure. The experiment should last long enough to fully encompass any effects that have a long latency. And naturally appropriate controls must be selected. Quality assurance is essential to provide reliable data,[6,31] and laboratories should conform to the Good Laboratory Practices Standard.

ANIMAL WELFARE AND ANIMAL RIGHTS

Toxicologists have become increasingly attentive to the animal welfare/animal rights movements and in many cases are adopting in vitro testing. Animal welfare is clearly an important issue. Not only should experimental animals be spared unnecessary stress, discomfort, or pain, but stress may significantly interfere with the response of animals to the test conditions. The National Science Foundation and National Institutes of Health have recognized the importance of animal welfare not only from a humane perspective but because stressed animals may not provide an appropriate response in experimental situations. Increasingly, researchers have sought alternative models that do not require whole animals. At the same time animal research has been redesigned to use fewer animals and to minimize pain and stress. Accordingly, researchers using animals must take into account animal care guidelines, which stipulate the conditions under which animals must be kept and the availability of veterinary care. Research protocols must be reviewed by institutional animal care committees.

The conflict over animal welfare reaches its peak when primates are used. Primates are expensive to acquire and maintain, and most studies of primates can afford only a few animals, who often live under extremely stressed conditions. For example, highly social and mobile animals such as chimpanzees are confined individually in small cages. Chimpanzees are genetically very close to humans, but they are prohibitively expensive. On the other hand, monkeys are genetically more distant from humans, and there are dietary, social, and behavioral factors that interfere with extrapolation from monkeys to humans. The extensive use of monkeys for research during the 1940s, 50s, and 60s resulted in the virtual elimination of monkey populations in a number of countries, particularly Thailand. Many primate populations are threatened or endangered because of habitat destruction and commercial exploitation for food or research. Although basic research into primate biology continues to be of importance, particularly with regard to conservation of these species, research on primates is rarely justified in toxicology.

REFERENCES

1. Agency for Toxic Substances and Disease Registry (ATSDR): The nature and extent of lead poisoning in children in the United States: a report to Congress, US Dept HHS, Atlanta, 1988.
2. Amdur MO, Doull J, Klaassen CD: *Casarett and Doull's toxicology,* ed 4, New York, 1991, Macmillan.
3. Amoruso MA et al: Estimation of risk of glucose 6-phosphate dehydrogenase-deficient red cells to ozone and nitrogen dioxide, *J Occup Med* 28:473, 1986.
4. Amoruso MA, Witz G, Goldstein BD: Alteration of erythrocyte membrane fluidity by heavy metal cations, *Toxicol Industr Health* 3:135, 1987.
5. Armitage P: Multistage models of carcinogenesis, *Environ Health Perspect* 63:195, 1985.
6. Chan PK, O'Hara GP, Hayes AW: Principles and methods for acute and subchronic toxicity. In Hayes AW, ed: *Principles and methods of toxicology,* New York, 1982, Raven Press.
7. Christian MS et al: *Assessment of reproductive and teratogenic hazards,* Princeton, 1983, Princeton Scientific.
8. Cohrssen JJ, Covello VT: *Risk analysis: a guide to principles and methods for analyzing health and environmental risks,* Washington, DC, 1989, U.S. Council on Environmental Quality.
9. Cullen MR: The worker with multiple chemical sensitivites, *State-of-the-Art Reviews in Occup Medicine* 2:655, 1987.
10. Dixon RL, Hall JL: Reproductive toxicology. In Hayes AW, ed: *Principles and methods of toxicology,* New York, 1982, Raven Press.
11. Gallo M, Doull J: History and scope of toxicology. In Amdur MO et al, eds: *Casarett and Doull's toxicology,* New York, 1991, Macmillan.
12. Gallo MA et al: Interactive effects of estradiol and 2,3,7,8-tetrachlorodibenzo-p-dioxin on hepatic cytochrome P-50 and mouse uterus, *Toxicol Letters* 32:123, 1986.
13. Gibaldi M, Perrier D: *Pharmacokinetics,* New York, 1982, Marcel Dekker.
14. Gochfeld M: Principles of toxicology. In Last JM, Wallace RB, eds: *Maxcy-Rosenau-Last's public health and preventive medicine,* Norwalk, Conn, 1992, Appleton & Lange.
15. Gutherie FE, Perry JJ, eds: *Introduction to environmental toxicology,* New York, 1980, Elsevier.

16. Hammond EC, Selikoff IJ: Relation of cigarette-smoking to risk of death of asbestos-associated disease among insulation workers in the United States. In Bogovski, ed: *Biological effects of asbestos,* 1973, IARC.
17. Hayes AW: *Principles and methods of toxicology,* ed 2, New York, 1982, Raven Press.
18. Jakoby WB, Bend JR, Caldwell J, eds: *Metabolic basis of detoxication,* New York, 1982, Academic.
19. Klaassen CD, Eaton, DL: Principles of toxicology. In Amdur MO et al, eds: *Casarett and Doull's toxicology,* New York, 1991, Macmillan.
20. Lioy P: Total human exposure analysis: a multidisciplinary science for reducing human contact with contaminants, *Environ Sci Technol* 24:938, 1990.
21. Lowrance WW: *Of acceptable risk,* Los Altos, Calif, 1976, William Kaufmann.
22. Luckey TD, Venugopal B, Hutcheson D: Heavy metal toxicity, safety and hormology, *Environ Qual Safety* (suppl 1): 1975.
23. National Research Council: *Biologic markers in immunotoxicology,* Washington, DC, 1992, National Academy Press.
24. National Research Council: *Biologic markers in reproductive toxicology,* Washington, DC, 1989, National Academy Press.
25. National Research Council: *Regulating pesticides in food: the Delaney paradox,* Washington, DC, 1987, National Academy Press.
26. Needleman H et al: Deficits in psychologic and classroom performance of children with elevated dentine lead levels, *New Engl J Med* 300:689, 1979.
27. Oser BL: Toxicology then and now, *Regulatory Toxicol & Pharmacol* 7:427, 1987.
28. Ottoboni A: *The dose makes the poison,* Berkeley, Calif, 1984, Vincente Books.
29. Sies H: Oxidative stress: introductory remarks. In Sies H, ed: *Oxidative stress,* New York, 1985, Academic Press.
30. Sinclair U: *The jungle,* New York, 1946, Viking, (originally published 1905).
31. Stevens KP, Gallo MA: Practical considerations in the conduct of chronic toxicity studies. In Hayes AW, ed: *Principles and methods of toxicology,* New York, 1982, Raven Press.
32. Takizawa Y: Epidemiology of mercury poisoning. In Nriagu J, ed: *The biogeochemistry of mercury in the environment,* Amsterdam, 1979, Elsevier-North Holland.
33. Tallarida RJ, Jacob LS: *The dose-response relation in pharmacology,* New York, 1979, Springer-Verlag.
34. U.S. Department of Health, Education: *NIOSH pocket guide to chemical hazards,* Cincinnati, 1983, National Institute for Occupational Safety and Health.
35. Umbreit TH, Hesse EJ, Gallo MA: Bioavailability of dioxin in soil from a 2,4,5,-T manufacturing site, *Science* 232:497, 1986.
36. USEPA: Proposed guidelines for carcinogen risk assessment, *Federal Register* 49:46294, 1984.
37. USEPA: *Report of the EPA workshop on the development of risk assessment methodologies for tumor promotores,* Washington DC, 1987, Environmental Protection Agency EPA/600/9-87/013.
38. Whorton MD: Male reproductive hazards, *State-of-Art Reviews in Occup Med* 1:375, 1986.
39. Zweig G: The vanishing zero: the evolution of pesticide analyses, *Essays in Toxicology* 2:156, 1970.

Chapter 7

CARCINOGENESIS

C. Stuart Baxter

Definition and terminology of cancer
    Definition and characteristics of cancer
    Terminology of cancer and related tissue changes
    Tumor behavior and classification
    Classification of carcinogenic agents
Mechanisms of carcinogenesis
    Somatic mutation theory
    Aberrant differentiation theory
Animal modes
Presumptive human models
Implications for regulation
Mechanisms of initiation, tumor promotion, and progression
    Oncogenes and tumor-suppressor genes
Types of carcinogens
    Chemicals
    Oncogenic viruses
    Radiation
Etiology of environmental and occupational cancer
    Clues from epidemiology
    Identification of occupational carcinogens
    Experimental determination of carcinogenic activity and exposure
    Classification of potential human carcinogens
Factors modifying cancer susceptibility
    Host-dependent factors
    Cultural and dietary factors
    Agent-dependent factors
    Summary

Cancer continues to be a disease of high concern for many reasons, among which are the following:
- It is the second most common cause of death, and its very nature and conventional treatment procedures continue to instill disproportionate fear and misunderstanding.
- There is a widespread feeling that personal risk of cancer could be eliminated or minimized by individual action. This feeling does not allay feelings of anxiety stirred by cancer, because current knowledge of the complexity of carcinogenesis provides only tantalizing glimpses of appropriate actions to take.
- The general public has the impression, which has not been dispelled by continuing scientific disagreement, that the presence of a carcinogen in the diet or environment represents a significant hazard regardless of the concentration.

In the recent past considerable progress toward understanding mechanisms of carcinogenesis has been made. New approaches have also been developed for estimating cancer risk at low doses. There is still a great need to raise public awareness, however, from paranoia arising from each new discovery that a popular product, food, or beverage "contains known carcinogens" to some understanding of the relative risk involved from ingestion of the carcinogens at the concentrations involved. As understanding of the mechanisms of the cancer family of diseases continues to improve, personal strategies to reduce cancer risk will be placed on a surer scientific footing and improved treatment therapies will be developed.[20]

DEFINITION AND TERMINOLOGY OF CANCER

The induction of malignant neoplasms by a carcinogenic agent frequently involves a number of intervening alterations in cell morphology and tissue architecture. In addition, a number of abnormal growths of tissue are not associated with malignancy. Therefore it is necessary to clarify current nomenclature for abnormal tissue growth and accompanying tissue changes.

Definition and characteristics of cancer

A primary concept of the nature of cancer, which is increasingly supported by recent research findings, is tissue released from restraints that normally regulate growth to some degree. This is reflected in the cells of neoplasms' becoming increasingly refractory to the actions of growth factors and hormones as the malignancy of the tumor increases. The rate of growth of neoplasms never approaches that of embryonic tissue at its greatest and is in many instances slower than that of surrounding normal tissue; therefore rapid growth is not a *prima facie* characteristic of cancer. Embryonic and other normal tissue growth is under exquisite physiologic control; moreover, is limited with respect to size and boundary by surrounding tissues in the mature organism. Development of neoplasms, on the other hand, is associated with progressive liberation of tissues from external regulatory influence.

Terminology of cancer and related tissue changes

The most appropriate term describing the process that leads to the family of diseases described as cancer is *neoplasia* (new growth). Neoplasia indicates that the affected tissue is of a new type in comparison with that from which it arose. This concept is pivotal to carcinogenesis in relation to other toxic responses, in which the original tissue eventually returns to its normal state after termination of a nonlethal toxic insult. *Malignancy* is a term most aptly used to describe neoplasms expressing aggressive behavior, such as invasion of surrounding tissue and metastasis. In this respect *neoplasms* are to some investigators synonymous with *malignancies*, although theoretically some nonmalignant growths, such as benign tumors of aberrant tissue architecture that are suspected to be precursors of malignancies, could also be termed *neoplasms*. The term *tumor* is now accepted to be a very general term for an abnormal mass of tissue, with no implications for malignancy or otherwise.

A number of tissue alterations may be observed during the formation of neoplasms. Among those that have been most implicated in this process are the following, which are associated with increased tissue mass:

1. Hyperplasia: an increase in cell number
2. Hyperproliferation: an increase in cell growth rate
3. Hypertrophy: an increase in cell size

All of these changes have been observed to occur concurrently in the same tissue. Clear distinction among these alterations is necessary, however, because in some cases some responses are more closely associated with the neoplastic process than are others. Persistence of these changes also appears to be crucial.

There are further tissue changes involving changes in cell and tissue architecture:

1. Metaplasia: reversible replacement of one mature cell type by another
2. Dysplasia: a change in the arrangement and size of cells
3. Anaplasia: a change in relative organization of cells within the tissue (positional anaplasia) or subcellular organelles within the cell (cytologic anaplasia)

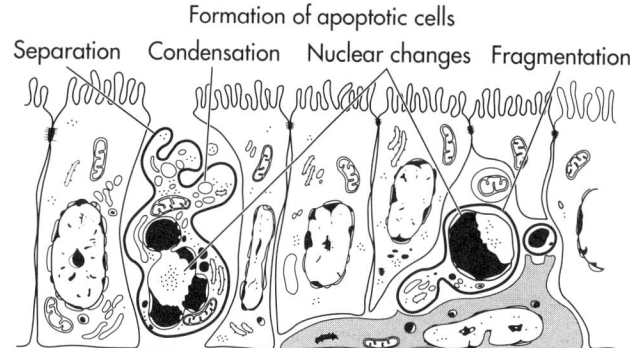
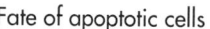
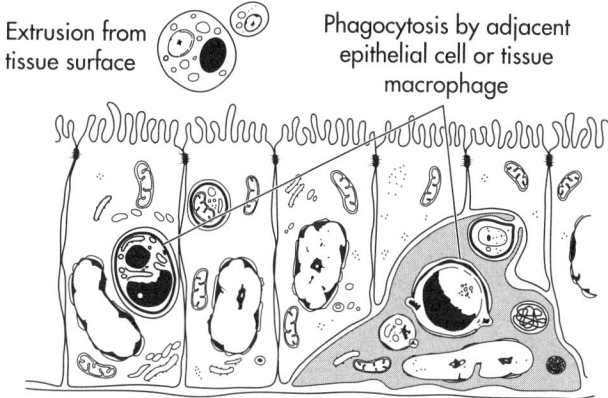

Fig. 7-1. Summary diagram of the morphologic events seen in apoptosis. (From Wyllie, AH: Cell death: a new classification separating apoptosis from necrosis. In Bowden ID, Lockshin RA, eds: *Cell death in biology and pathology*, London, 1981, Chapman and Hall.)

4. Apoptosis: programmed deletion of cells with nonrandom DNA fragmentation (Fig. 7-1)

None of these changes is specific to neoplasia, but they nevertheless have often been causally connected with the process.

Tumor behavior and classification

Exposure of organisms to carcinogens frequently results in the formation of tumors with a range of behavioral characteristics, although it has been most convenient to classify tumors into two major categories, benign and malignant. Medically these distinctions are important, but in experimental and regulatory areas they lead frequently to confusion. Debate continues on whether malignant tumors in some circumstances arise from benign counterparts. If treatment of experimental animals with an environmental contaminant leads to a significant increase in benign but not malignant tumors, controversy over whether the contaminant should be labeled carcinogenic therefore results. In this instance, histologic classification becomes crucial, and disagreement in pathologic interpretation is not uncommon. Some light is being shed on this debate, however, with increasing knowl-

Table 7-1. Characteristics of benign and malignant tumors

Benign	Malignant
Usually encapsulated	Nonencapsulated
Usually noninvasive	Invasive
Highly differentiated	Poorly differentiated
Few mitoses	Frequent mitoses
Normal growth	Often rapid growth
Rare anaplasia	Varying degrees of anaplasia
Nonmetastatic	Metastatic

edge of genetic changes present in benign and malignant tumors in the same tissue. If mutations associated with malignancy are already present in the cells of a benign tumor, that tumor may be suspected to be a precursor of a more malignant counterpart.

Despite current discussion, benign and malignant tumors continue to be classified according to several overall distinctions (Table 7-1).

Classification of carcinogenic agents

The term *carcinogen* for any compound or agent that causes malignant neoplasms actually has wider implications. Within this definition are included several types of agents whose properties may not always be identical. These include agents that induce a statistically significant increase in number of malignant and/or benign tumors in a treated group of animals in comparison with an untreated group; reduce the latency period for tumor appearance so that tumors appear much earlier, which in humans implies that carcinogens are agents that cause diagnosable tumors to arise within the expected lifespan; and induce tumors in tissues other than those observed in unexposed groups or different types of tumors.

Research in experimental animals has confirmed earlier pathologic findings in humans that cancer is a multistage process (Fig. 7-2). Most of the aforementioned concepts can therefore now be understood in light of findings that there are agents that can complete or accelerate one or more but not all of these stages.

MECHANISMS OF CARCINOGENESIS

Proposed mechanisms of carcinogenesis by chemicals and other agents center around two principal theories, the *somatic mutation theory* and the *aberrant differentiation theory,* although recent evidence suggests that these theories are different facets of one general theory or describe individual components of a *multistage* process.[2,30] These two theories reflect the two principal characteristics of neoplastic cells: heritability of the neoplastic phenotype (behavior) and aberrant control of cell growth and development.

Somatic mutation theory

A primary characteristic of cancer cells is the inheritance of phenotype (behavior); that is, cancer cells divide into other cancer cells. Because mutation is defined as a stable heritable change in phenotype and is synonymous with deoxyribonucleic acid (DNA) alteration, cancer has been postulated to arise as a result of mutation in normal cells. Many experimental findings support this theory, some of the most convincing of which are: certain normal cells can be neoplastically transformed by introducing tumor cell DNA or mutated normal genes into them; mutation and malignant transformation can occur concurrently in cells treated with agents that induce a specific alteration in their DNA; tissues that repair certain DNA lesions more efficiently have greater resistance to chemical carcinogens; oncogenic viruses induce mutations and rearrangements in the DNA of the cells they infect; and many carcinogenic chemicals and agents are mutagenic.

Aberrant differentiation theory

Despite the aforementioned evidence, there is still an argument that cancer rather rises as a *disease of differentiation.* Differentiation is the process whereby cells change in phenotype without changing in genetic composition, that is, mutation, and is intimately involved in the development of mature cells and tissues from stem and embryonic counterparts. This theory therefore does not require mutagenesis and is supported by findings that (1) under specific conditions, such as exposure to vitamin A analogues and growth hormones, leukemia and lymphoma cells of many types can be induced to change to mature leukocytes, which has led to a theory of oncology as blocked ontogeny, that is, cancer cells as immature cells restrained from differentiating into mature counterparts; (2) malignant tumors in experimental animals and humans are occasionally found to regress to tissues made up of normal cells; (3) some types of tumor cells, when implanted into pregnant animals, are able to generate viable embryos and normal intact adults, a finding that suggests that cancer cells have all the genetic information required for normal growth and development; (4) cell culture experiments suggest that the frequency at which chemicals induce cell mutation is much less than that at which they induce malignant transformation; (5) there are many carcinogens that are not mutagenic; and (6) not all mutagens are carcinogenic.

Much of the disagreement arising from these theories can be resolved by accepting that carcinogenesis is a multistage process. Pathologic findings in humans have suggested for a long time that such is the case, and there are now animal models for many tissues. In the best-characterized models, carcinogenesis may be divided into initiation, tumor-promotion, and tumor-progression stages[32] (Fig. 7-3). In some cases, especially when carcinogens are administered at a low dose rate, malignant tumors appear to arise directly, not from benign precursors (Fig. 7-4). Even in this case, there is evidence for processes equivalent to those that occur during promotion and progression, especially those that enable malignant cells to escape the controlling influences of normal neighbors. Although chemicals with initiating activity are generally identifiable in microbial assays on the basis of their

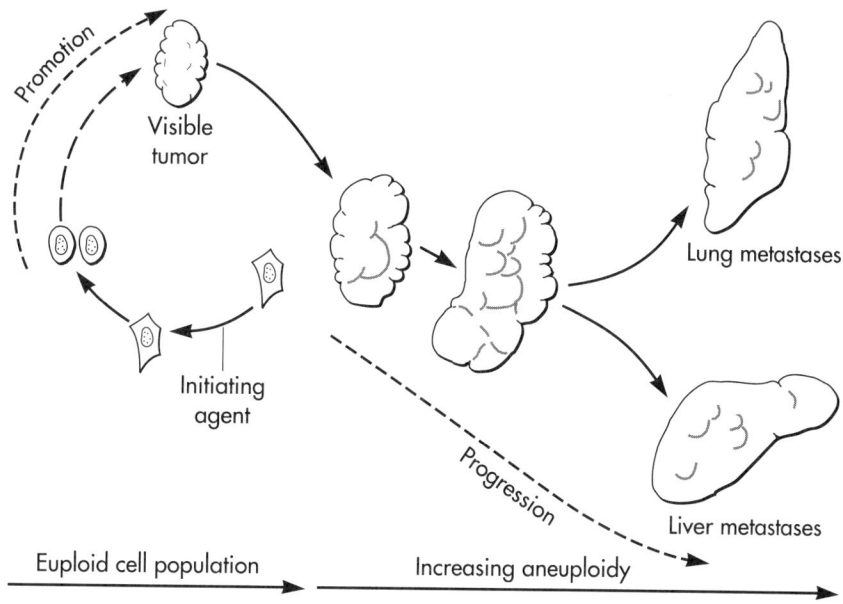

Fig. 7-2. The natural history of neoplasia, beginning with the initiated cell after application of an initiating agent (carcinogen) and subsequent promotion to a visible tumor, with progression of this neoplasm to malignancy. The relation to karyotype is presented as a generalization on the lower arrows. The reader should again be cautioned that not all neoplastic cells undergo this entire natural history. It is theoretically possible, although this has not yet been definitely shown, that some neoplasms, such as those induced in animals by radiation or high doses of chemical carcinogens, may enter this sequence in the stage of progression exhibiting aneuploidy and thus bypass the early euploid cell stage. (From Pitot HC: *Fundamentals of oncology,* ed 3, New York, 1986, Marcel Dekker.)

	Carcinogenesis	Initiation	Promotion	Progression
Normal cell	Adequate exposure to carcinogen ↓	Limited carcinogen exposure ↓		
Initiated cell			Continued carcinogen or tumor promoter ↓	
Benign tumor				Continued carcinogen or tumor progressor ↓
Malignant cell				
Malignant tumor				

Fig. 7-3. A summary of multistage carcinogenesis models.

mutagenic activity, less attention has been given to tumor-promoting agents or chemicals that accelerate the progression of tumors to malignancy and metastasis. Nevertheless these types of agents are a further important factor to be considered in assessment of the risk to populations exposed to environmental or occupational mixtures. Tumor-promoting agents are chemicals with little or no carcinogenic activity themselves but are nevertheless able to strongly potentiate the effects of carcinogens. With primary attention focused on testing chemicals for carcinogenic activity in microbes or animals singly, there has been relative little attention to assessing the activity of tumor-promoting agents or other type of cocarcinogens, even though some are consistent coconstituents with carcinogens in occupational mixtures such as petroleum products, coke oven emissions, and coal tar fractions. The same chemicals, for example, linear alkanes, are also found together with polycyclic aromatic hydrocarbon carcinogens in cigarette smoke. The potency of one of these chemicals was demonstrated by the finding that the minimum dose of the potent carcinogen benzo[*a*]pyrene required to produce skin cancer in mice could be lowered by a factor of 1000 if dissolved in *n*-dodecane, which is a cocarcinogen and tumor promoter.[8]

	Carcinogenesis
Normal cell	Sufficient exposure to carcinogen (low dose rate)
Malignant cell	
Malignant tumor	

Fig. 7-4. A summary of single-stage carcinogenesis.

ANIMAL MODELS

To date, multistage cancer models have been characterized in a range of tissues in several species. As illustrated in

Table 7-2. Animal models of two-stage tumorigenesis

Organ system	Initiator	Modifier (cocarcinogen-promoter)
Skin*	Polycyclic aromatics, cisplatin, ultraviolet light	Croton oil, phorbol esters, cigarette tar, aliphatic amphipaths, polycyclic aromatic hydrocarbons, mirex, wounds
Liver	2-Acetamidofluorene	Phenobarbital, PCBs, PBBs, TCDD
	Diethylnitrosamine	Acetylamidofluorene (mitoinhibition), hepatectomy
Esophagus	Diethylnitrosamine	Diet (marginal lipotrope)
	Methylphenylnitrosamine	Diet (zinc deficiency)
Colon	Dimethylhydrazine	Bile acids
Bladder	N-methyl-N-nitrosourea	Saccharin, cyclamate
Breast	Dimethylbenz[a]anthracene	Hormones
Stomach	N-methyl-N'-nitro-N-nitrosoguanidine	Surfactants
Lung*	Urethan	Butylated hydroxytoluene
Kidney	Nitrosamine	Lead acetate

PBB, Polybrominated biphenyl; *PCB*, polychlorinated biphenyl; *TCDD*, tetrachlorodibenzodioxin.
*Mouse; in other systems, rat.

Table 7-2, several agents of low carcinogenicity per se are promoting agents for the same tissue (saccharin, cyclamate, lead acetate). This is also true for physiologic agents suspected to play a role in cancer (bile acids, hormones, and zinc deficiency). In these cases the agents in question presumably promote spontaneously initiated cells. It has been estimated that lesions in DNA occur spontaneously at a very high rate because of damage caused by endogenous oxidative processes, error in replication, and natural instability. Although repair mechanisms to counteract such damage exist, they have seldom been found to be perfect.

PRESUMPTIVE HUMAN MODELS

Experiments demonstrating tumor-promoting activity for physiologic agents in animals supplement previous knowledge in humans. There is a long-standing association between bile-acid concentration and colon cancer, and hormone-dependent sites appear especially sensitive to malignancy. With regard to environmental exposure, a major role in tumor promotion has been proposed for cigarette smoking. For those who quit smoking, the risk of bronchogenic carcinoma essentially stays frozen at the time of quitting and may eventually decline with time. This scenario is consistent with cessation of exposure to tumor-promoting agents in the smoke, the degree of cancer risk being determined by the time of exposure to smoke carcinogens until the time of quitting.

IMPLICATIONS FOR REGULATION

Recognition of tumor-promoting and cocarcinogenic activity therefore has important ramifications for regulatory aspects of carcinogenesis. These include that the dose of a carcinogen estimated to present negligible or acceptable risk to a population of a stated size may need to be revised to a considerably smaller value if exposure occurs concurrently with a cocarcinogen or tumor-promoting agent; agents with weak carcinogenic activity may be potent tumor-promoting agents; examples that tests in experimental animals suggest minimal carcinogenicity but significant tumor-promoting activity in the same tissue are saccharin (bladder) and polychlorinated biphenyls (liver); and whereas it is debatable whether thresholds exists for carcinogens and initiators, they apparently exist for tumor-promoting agents.

MECHANISMS OF INITIATION, TUMOR PROMOTION, AND PROGRESSION

Mutations are now widely believed to be essential in the *initiation* and *progression* stages of carcinogenesis, and changes in normal patterns of growth regulation and differentiation are important in the *tumor-promotion* stage. Genes that have undergone mutation in tumors, moreover, are those that code for proteins involved in growth regulation.[1] All cells undergo mutation and hence initiation spontaneously; therefore many nonmutagenic carcinogens may induce neoplasms by promotion mechanisms. It is also known that mutations may be *silent*—that is, without immediate consequence—but later capable of activation. Cells may therefore show normal or malignant behavior, depending on whether a mutation is active or silent.

In the case of some types of carcinogenic agent, for example, transplanted films of inert materials and fibers such as asbestos, the mechanism of action is currently unclear.[10,12] Implantation of such materials does cause a chronic inflammatory response, although it is not believed to be completely responsible for it.

Oncogenes and tumor-suppressor genes

Two types of gene that recent research has strongly implicated in the process of carcinogenesis are *cellular protooncogenes* and *tumor-suppressor genes,* or *antioncogenes.* Cellular protooncogenes (abbreviated *c-oncs*) are normal cellular genes that are essential for regulation of cell growth and differentiation. The protein products of these genes include growth hormones or their specific cell-surface receptors, proteins that transmit growth signals across membranes, and factors that bind to DNA and regulate its processing.

Table 7-3. Tumor-suppressor genes and associated human cancers

Tumor-suppressor gene	Associated cancers
Retinoblastoma (Rb)	Retinoblastoma, osteosarcoma, breast cancer, SCLC
p53	Multiple; Li-Fraumeni syndrome
WT-1	Wilms' tumor of the kidney
NF-1	Neurofibromatosis
NF-2	Meningioma, neuroma, pheochromocytoma
DCC	Colon carcinoma
MCC	Adenomatous polyposis

DCC, Deleted in colon cancer; *MCC*, mutated in colon cancer; *NF*, neurofibromatosis; *SCLC*, small cell lung cancer.

Involvement of these genes in carcinogenesis is suggested by findings that they are closely similar to the genetic components (*v-oncs*) responsible for the cell-transforming abilities of oncogenic viruses. In many benign and malignant tumors *c-oncs* bear specific mutations, which can result in marked changes in properties of the corresponding protein products so as to reduce or corrupt their regulatory function. These findings have been very provocative in suggesting ways in which theories of mutation and altered growth regulation in the carcinogenic process may be unified. In other tumors there is a strong increase in expression (usage) of these genes, with higher cell levels of the corresponding ribonucleic acid and protein than in normal tissues.

Early studies on cancers with a high degree of inheritability, such as retinoblastoma and osteosarcoma, showed that in genetically predisposed individuals a portion of one chromosome had been deleted. In the retinoblastomas themselves, both chromosomes had suffered deletions. In individuals predisposed to retinoblastoma, one copy of chromosome 13 is therefore biochemically different from the other. These individuals are said to have a polymorphism at the retinoblastoma (Rb) gene locus.[17] Polymorphisms are detected by probing cell DNA with short lengths of DNA of complimentary sequence to the gene under study after digestion of cell DNA with specific enzymes termed *restriction endonucleases*. These enzymes cut DNA at a restricted number of sites and hence into fragments of specific sizes. Individuals who are predisposed to various types of cancer may therefore be identified on the basis of restriction fragment length polymorphisms in genes associated with these cancers. Since this finding, deletions in specific regions of various chromosomes have been reported in cancers from many sources. This finding therefore suggests that development of certain cancers requires loss of both active copies of genes that normally suppress malignant behavior. These genes are termed *tumor-suppressor genes*[36] (Table 7-3). The ability of these genes to suppress cancer development has been shown in malignant cells lacking both copies of the Rb gene. Reintroduction of active Rb genes into these cells results in the appearance of normal nonneoplastic cell behavior.

The normal cellular function of the Rb protein has recently been found to lie in control of cell division, where it forms complexes with important cell-cycle–regulating proteins termed *cyclins*. This finding again reinforces the idea

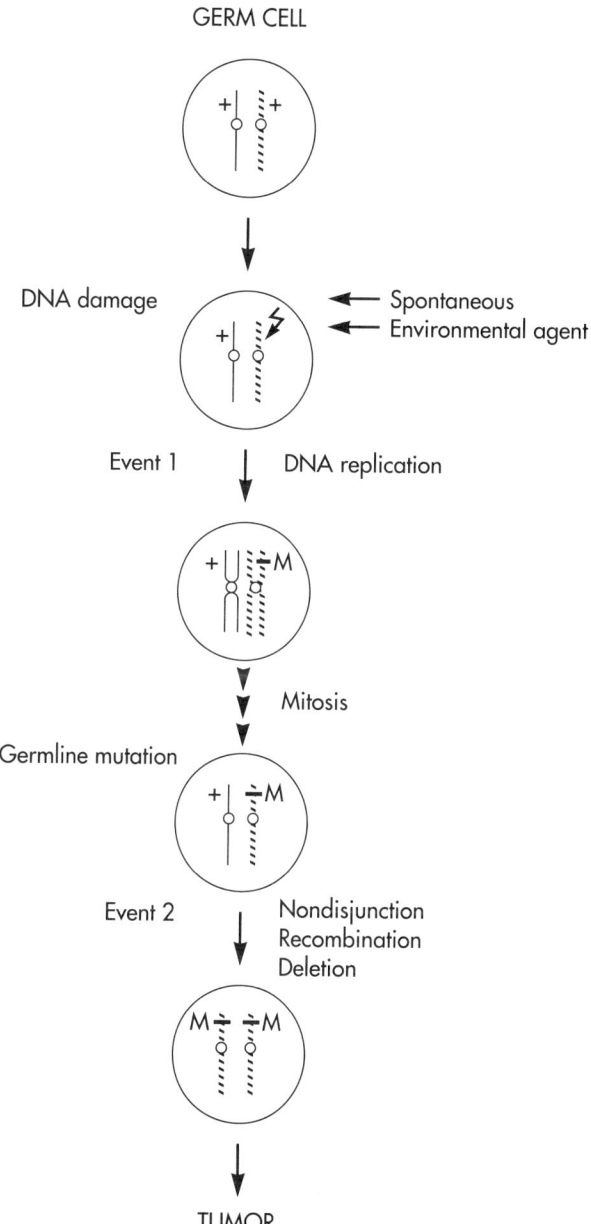

Fig. 7-5. Model for the involvement of recessive mutations in tumorigenesis. An initial mutation at a specific locus can be caused by a variety of agents (event 1). In hereditary cases this predisposing mutation is passed through the germline and is present in all cells of the progeny, whereas in sporadic cases this mutation occurs in a single somatic cell. In both instances a second somatic event eliminates the remaining wild-type allele, thereby unmasking the initial mutation and resulting in neoplastic transformation of the cell. (From Nordenskjold. In Klein G: *Tumor suppressor genes,* New York, 1990, Marcel Dekker, p 148.)

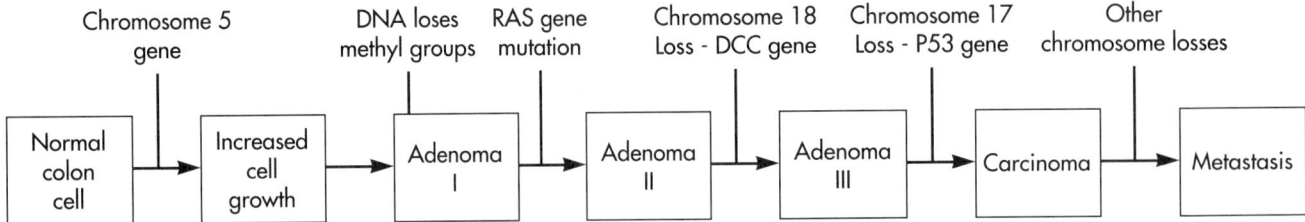

Fig. 7-6. Proposed multistage etiology of somes kinds of colon cancer. (From Marx J: Possible new colon cancer gene found, *Science* 251:1317, 1991.)

that cancer reflects a loss of normal growth regulation. The importance of normal Rb protein to mammals is demonstrated by the finding that mice in whom both genes are inactivated are unable to develop beyond the early fetal stage. Of additional relevance is that several types of oncogenic viruses, including adenoviruses and papillomaviruses, appear to act by producing proteins that bind to the protein products of tumor-suppressor genes, thereby rendering them unable to function correctly.

The discovery of tumor-suppressor genes has also provided an explanation for the existence of hereditary and nonhereditary forms of the same cancer (Fig. 7-5). As described earlier, the hereditary form of retinoblastoma involves inheritance of a deletion or inactivating mutation in one copy of chromosome 13. A deletion in the second copy of chromosome 13 then results in a tumor. Retinoblastoma may also result if both deletions in chromosomes 13 result after birth. In this case, termed *sporadic retinoblastoma,* the cancer is *unilateral* and tumors occur only in one eye, because the probability of two deletions in two cells, one in each retina, is very low. If one deletion is inherited, the cancer can be *bilateral,* because there is the same probability of a second deletion in each retina.

The induction of some tumors appears to involve changes in both protooncogenes and tumor-suppressor genes. A striking case is human colon cancer, in which a multistage process of this type is strongly indicated (Fig. 7-6).[15,25]

TYPES OF CARCINOGENS
Chemicals

The types of agent that induce cancer are very varied, and attempts to evolve a common mechanism for carcinogenesis by all carcinogens have therefore been very frustrating. Some clarity has recently been achieved, however, with the acceptance of the multistage models described earlier. These models have enabled carcinogenic agents to be divided to some extent into several categories:

1. Those that alter DNA qualitatively or quantitatively and hence act primarily as initiators. These agents *initiate* the sequence of events leading to cancer. Limited doses of most complete carcinogens can initiate the neoplastic process, but there are also other agents that are only initiators and cannot complete the carcinogenic process alone, even if animals are exposed to them repeatedly. *Initiation* is regarded to be an irreversible event, probably involving a mutation. Agents that alter DNA have also been termed *genotoxic carcinogens* and include organic compounds, which induce mutations directly; organic compounds, which alter DNA after activating metabolism; and metals and metal salts, which alter DNA and/or the fidelity of its replication. Examples of these types are given in Table 7-4.

2. Those that act by other mechanisms to corrupt growth control and act as tumor-promoting agents. These agents induce the formation of benign and malignant tumors in tissues that have previously been initiated by exposure to an initiating agent. The action of this kind of agent, in contrast to that of initiators, is reversible and is reflected in a requirement to apply this type of agent repeatedly. An important property of these agents is their ability to strongly reduce the time to appearance of tumors. Tumor-promoting agents are a type of *cocarcinogen,* an agent that potentiates the action of a carcinogen, but are specific in being active when administered following *initiators.* Cocarcinogens may act via diverse mechanisms, such as activation or inhibition of specific metabolic pathways and enhancement of absorption or tissue concentration, but do not induce cancer by themselves. Agents of this type have been termed *epigenetic carcinogens,* and examples are given in Table 7-5.

Table 7-4. Genotoxic carcinogens

Compound type	Example	Source
Aromatic hydrocarbon	Benzo[a]pyrene (soot, tar, fumes)	Fossil-fuel pyrolysis
Nitroarene	1-Nitropyrene	Diesel fumes
Aromatic amine	β-Naphthylamine	Dyestuff manufacture
Fungal contaminant	Aflatoxin B1	Contaminated cereals
Nitrosamine	Dimethylnitrosamine	Dietary amine and nitrite
Metals, salts	Nickel, chromates	Occupational exposure, smelting
Plant toxin	Cycasin	Cycads

Table 7-5. Epigenetic carcinogens

Type	Mechanism	Example
Tumor promoter	Selective cell growth stimulation, differentiation, inhibition; inflammation	Phorbol esters, alkanes, saccharin, lead ions, PCBs, TCDD, bile acids
Cytotoxin	Regenerative proliferation	Tetrachloroethylene
Burns, wounds	Release of growth factors	Kangri cancer
Growth promoters	Cell growth stimulation	Steroid, thyroid hormones
Inert materials	Unknown: inflammation?	Asbestos, plastic and metal films, gallstones
Immunosuppressants	Suppression of antitumor immunity	Azathioprine, human immunodeficiency virus type 1

3. Partial tumor-promoting agents. Experiments in animals have demonstrated that certain agents are able to complete only a part of the tumor-promotion process. These agents are nevertheless able to induce tumors in animals that have been initiated and treated with another noncarcinogenic agent. The recognition that cancer is a multistage process predicts that there are some agents whose action is specific to only one or a few of these stages.
4. Agents that enhance the progression of benign to malignant tumors (sometimes termed *progressors*). In some animal systems the efficiency of conversion of benign to malignant tumors can be strongly enhanced by genotoxic carcinogens (those that chemically modify DNA) or certain other agents, usually inflammatory, that are noncarcinogenic.

The aforementioned division into genotoxic and epigenetic carcinogens is readily seen to be somewhat artificial, because complete genotoxic carcinogens presumably have both initiating and tumor-promoting activities. Noninitiating nonmutagenic carcinogens in many cases have been found to induce inflammation and leukocyte activation, a response that results in the release of DNA-damaging species. Chronic inflammation associated with serious wounds or burns or with infection with certain viruses (for instance, hepatitis viruses B and C) has long been identified with cancer in humans.[5] In Himalayan tribesmen who carry charcoal pots for warmth, there is a predisposition to cancer of the abdomen (Kangri cancer), perhaps as a result of frequent burns in conjunction with tar.[5] Similarly, inherited disposition to chronic colitis and gastritis is recognized to result in predisposition to colon and gastric carcinoma, respectively. Gastritis associated with infection with the bacterium *Helicobacter pylori*[28] has recently been associated with gastric carcinoma. Wound healing and inflammation have recently been found to be mediated by peptides also released by carcinogens and tumor-promoting agents,[13] reviving an older theory that carcinogenesis represents a wound-healing process that fails to terminate appropriately.

The identification of protooncogene and tumor-suppressor gene involvement in neoplasias induced by agents of widely different types has also been highly enlightening in the classification of carcinogens. Many genotoxic carcinogens induce tumors whose cells bear mutations in cellular protooncogenes or loss of tumor-suppressor genes; however, both these types of genes code for proteins that are critically involved in control of cell growth. The common concept that binds the mechanisms of action of most if not all carcinogens therefore continues to be corruption of normal growth-control mechanisms.

Table 7-6. Viruses associated with human neoplasms

Virus	Cancer
Epstein-Barr virus	Burkitt's lymphoma
Human T-cell lymphotrophic virus I (HTLV-I)	T cell lymphoma
HTLV-II	Hairy cell leukemia
Hepatitis B and C viruses	Hepatocellular carcinoma
Human immunodeficiency virus type I	Kaposi's sarcoma
Human papillomaviruses	Genital papillomas and carcinoma

Oncogenic viruses

Although an association between various types of virus infection and human cancer has existed for a considerable time, it has been exceptionally difficult to establish a causal relationship.[35,40] Strong associations have been established between viruses and cancer in several instances, however.[35,40] Several of these associations are listed in Table 7-6.

In some cases, the etiology of the tumor involves interaction of the virus with a second agent, for example, the dietary carcinogen aflatoxin B1 with hepatitis B virus[5] and malarial infection with the Epstein-Barr virus.[19] There is widespread infection with viruses of this type in human populations that are not highly susceptible to the corresponding cancers. This finding therefore strongly suggests that other factors are able to disturb a normally innocuous relationship between human cells and oncogenic viruses. In experimental animals and cells in culture, strong interactions among viruses, chemical carcinogens, and tumor-promoting agents have been recorded. These findings therefore support the

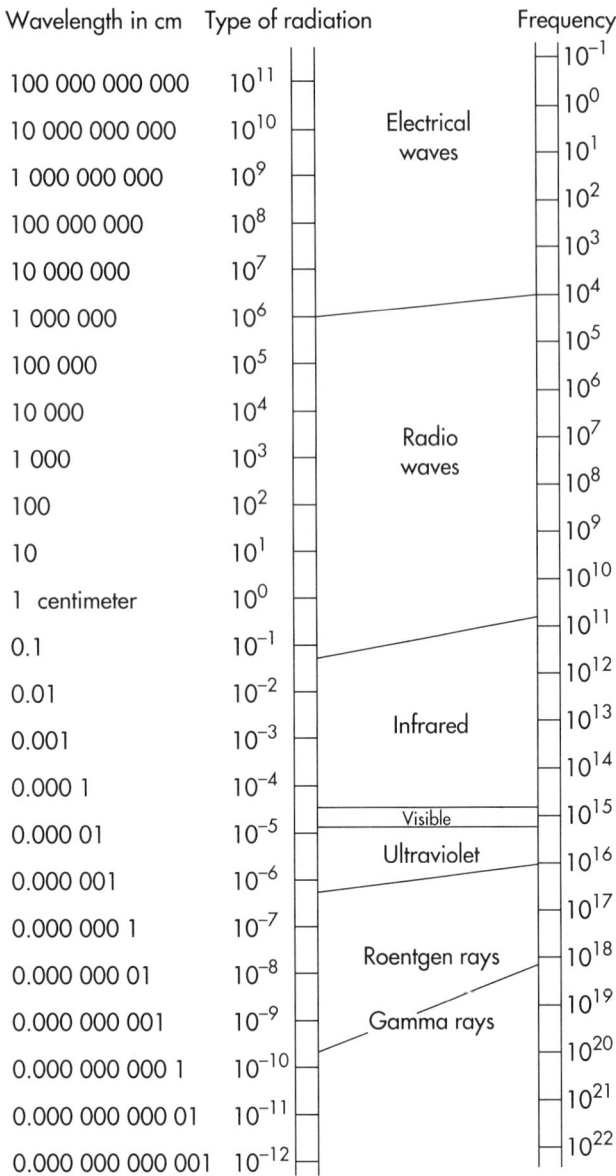

Fig. 7-7. The electromagnetic spectrum, showing the wavelength and frequency of the different classes of radiant energy.

idea that oncogenic viruses can be awoken from latency by other agents.

Oncogenic viruses are exceptionally efficient in their ability to transform sensitive cells malignantly, and studies on the mechanism by which they act have also been very informative on the overall mechanisms of carcinogenesis. The principal mechanisms by which viruses have been suggested to act are by producing proteins that are corrupted versions of cellular protooncogene proteins; causing protooncogenes to be overutilized, resulting in higher cellular levels of their protein products; and binding and inactivating the protein products of tumor-suppressor genes.

With current knowledge of the normal roles protooncogenes and tumor-suppressor genes play, corruption of normal cell growth controls therefore appears to be a major component of the mechanism of action of oncogenic viruses also.

Radiation

Ultraviolet radiation and other forms of higher frequency (Fig. 7-7) are well-characterized human carcinogens, although variations in lifestyle and methodology still complicate clear definition of dose-response relationships. Radiation of frequency lower than ultraviolet, including microwaves and high-frequency radio waves, also has been claimed by some to pose a carcinogenic risk, but there is considerable skepticism on this point. Currently, concern is primarily centered on issues relating to risk presented by low-dose diagnostic x-irradiation and on the relationship between ultraviolet irradiation and malignant melanoma, which is apparently increasing in incidence. The principal mechanism by which radiation induces cancer appears to involve DNA damage, although systemic effects, including immunosuppression, are involved in some cases. As with other types of carcinogens, there is continuing need to establish interactions between radiation and other factors such as diet.

ETIOLOGY OF ENVIRONMENTAL AND OCCUPATIONAL CANCER
Clues from epidemiology

The total cancer burden of each human being is made up of diverse components whose individual contributions will be different.[33] A number of years ago several eminent experimental cancer researchers announced their conclusion that cancer was an environmental disease and therefore its incidence could theoretically be dramatically reduced by appropriate avoidance of specific etiologic factors. This conclusion was derived after consideration of the recognized ways in which cancer could be induced, which are (1) iatrogenic, such as therapeutic administration of x-rays, diethylstilbestrol, and so on; (2) genetic predisposition, for example, in retinoblastoma and osteosarcoma; and (3) genetic predisposition with environmental insult, such as xeroderma pigmentosum and ataxia telangiectasia.

The aforementioned ways were estimated to account for no more than 15% of the total human cancer burden; therefore it was concluded that the remainder arose as a result of environmental exposure. Publication of this conclusion led to conviction of a large sector of the general public that the majority of cancers resulted from contamination of food and beverages with chemical additives and of air and drinking water with carcinogens released from industrial processes. It was later pointed out that environmental exposure includes dietary constituents and cultural components such as cigarette smoking although this was only partly successful in reducing public fears.[14] In recent years a vigorous debate has raged over the size of the risk associated with exposure to chemicals released as a result of industrial and agricultural processes. With the realization that a large number of common vegetables and other foodstuffs contain naturally oc-

Table 7-7. Change in mortality rate on migration from Japan to the United States*

Group	Stomach (M)	Colon (M)	Lung (M)	Breast (F)
Native Japanese	100	100	100	100
Japan-born Americans	72	374	306	166
U.S. whites	17	489	316	591

M, Males; *F*, females.
*Relative cancer mortality associated with stated tissue.

Table 7-8. Geographic hot spots and causes of esophageal cancer

High-incidence location	Suspected cause
United States	Heavy smoking and concentrated ethanol consumption
Pakistan	Consumption of very hot tea
Turkey	Natural promoters in food
Dutch West Indies	Natural promoters in tea
Sweden	Dietary deficiency
China	Dietary carcinogens and promoters

curring carcinogenic chemicals, which have presumably been synthesized to reduce depredation by animals, it has become apparent that elimination of exposure to carcinogenic agents may be impossible or at least impractical.

Evidence that a large component of human cancer results from dietary factors has come from studies on migrant populations. The results of these experiments show that populations migrating to a new geographic location undergo a shift in pattern of relative tissue susceptibility from that of the site of origin to that of the of the new one.[7] The best characterized of these studies involved Japanese who migrated to Hawaii or the western mainland of the United States. In Japan itself cancer susceptibility is characterized by a low incidence in the mammary gland and colon but a high incidence in the stomach, possibly as a result of frequent consumption of foods with high salt and fungal toxin content. In migrant Japanese, especially first-generation (Issei) or second-generation (Nissei), relative cancer susceptibility shifted toward that characteristic of American diets (Table 7-7). In this case, the incidences of colon and mammary gland cancer are high, probably as a result of high consumption of animal protein and saturated fat, and that of stomach cancer is low.[7] These findings therefore suggested that dietary rather than genetic differences are major determinants of cancer susceptibility in the general population.

In geographic terms there is a wide variation in cancer incidence at specific sites.[23] In different geographic hot spots for a particular tissue, different agents are responsible for cancer induction, leading to the suggestion that a common carcinogenic mechanism may be operating among these agents. A striking example of how cancer at the same site can result from exposure to different insults yet imply a common mechanism is provided by esophageal carcinoma. The suspected causes and areas of high incidence are shown in Table 7-8.

Although esophageal cancer appears to be induced by quite disparate agents among geographic hot spots, a common cause can be discerned, involving initial damage to the esophageal lining, which may result from the action of ethanol, very hot liquids, or dietary deficiencies. Neoplasia may be initiated in stem cells of the damaged esophageal epithelium by coadministered carcinogens as a result of increased permeability of outer cell layers. Tumor promotion and progression may then occur in response to naturally occurring tumor-promoting agents or as a result of the process of regenerative proliferation taking place after tissue injury.[28] Recent research findings indicate that tissue repair and tumor promotion appear to be mediated by similar peptide growth factors. In this respect it is interesting to note that skin wounding is a tumor-promoting stimulus.[13]

Identification of occupational carcinogens

Genetic factors and the complexity of personal dietary and cultural habits make it very difficult to identify specific chemical agents of significant carcinogenic risk for human beings. Although the same is true to some extent for exposure in the workplace, identification is considerably facilitated by the greater exposures involved. There are several instances in which carcinogen identification is least ambiguous.

When rare and agent-specific tumors are induced. Cases of hemangiosarcoma of the liver were reported to occur in workers exposed to high concentrations of vinyl chloride, a starting material in plastic manufacture. Although only a handful of cases were reported in any one situation, there was a tremendous increase in incidence in comparison with the general population, in whom this tumor is very rare. Furthermore, tumors of an identical type were induced by vinyl chloride in experimental rodents and thus provided a fingerprint for this carcinogen. A similar situation was provided with certain types of asbestos, which induced otherwise rare mesotheliomas of the pleural and peritoneal lining in exposed humans and laboratory rodents.

When tumor incidence is very high. There has been no ambiguity in assigning human carcinogenic potential to an industrial product in tragic cases in which a large fraction of the exposed population developed malignancies. In these cases, doubt was also removed by specificity of the neoplasm type and its reproducibility in a species of experimental animal. Examples of this type of agent are asbestos, inhaled during cleaning of cargo vessels, and exposure to dyestuff intermediates such as β-naphthylamine. In some situations the incidence of urinary bladder carcinoma in the exposed group was essentially 100%. Studies on aromatic amines such as β-naphthylamine have been instructive in pointing out the necessity of testing suspect human carcinogens in an appropriate animal species. In rodents these agents usually induce hepatic rather than bladder carcinoma, and these animals are therefore not an appropriate model for humans. Dogs, because of their more similar bladder physiology and aromatic amine metabolism, were found to model human exposure more closely.

Experimental determination of carcinogenic activity and exposure

Animal experiments. Other than the two categories discussed earlier, assignment of human cancer potential is very difficult and for regulatory purposes is supported in many cases by the results of animal experiments, which are inevitably controversial for several reasons, including the following:

1. The dose is customarily very high in order to achieve maximum sensitivity. Usually the maximum tolerated dose, the dose that results in mortality in 50% of the test group, is used.
2. The species of animal chosen may already have a high background cancer incidence or may be inbred. The basis for this choice is sensitivity and reproducibility.
3. The species may not be an appropriate model for humans with regard to the target tissue. β-Naphthylamine, for instance, induces liver carcinomas in rodents but bladder cancer in humans.
4. The exposure route may not be that by which humans are most commonly exposed, which is by inhalation or dermal exposure. Experimental animals are seldom exposed by these routes but generally through food or drinking water.
5. The size of the experimental groups in animal tests are relatively small because of economic factors.
6. Single agents are administered rather than the complex mixtures usually encountered in human experience.

Microbial and mammalian cell culture assays. In light of the expense of carrying out even limited animal experiments, for reasons including length of exposure, quality control, veterinary care, data collection, and pathologic evaluation, preliminary evaluation of carcinogenic potential in cultures of mammalian or microbial cells remains very common and necessary. In mammalian cells, chemicals are evaluated on the basis of their ability to induce mutation or foci of cells showing abnormal growth characteristics, including disoriented and three-dimensional growth (Fig. 7-8). Mutation assays are defended on the basis that many carcinogens are mutagenic. DNA is processed in basically similar ways in microbial and mammalian cells.

Cytogenetic assays. Exposure to carcinogenic agents frequently results in an increase in the number of *chromosome aberrations,* including breaks and translocations. More specific changes, such as *micronuclei* and *sister chromatid exchanges,* also are observed.[16] Micronuclei are formed during mitosis when chromosomes do not partition equally into the two daughter cells (Fig. 7-9). In the daughter cell con-

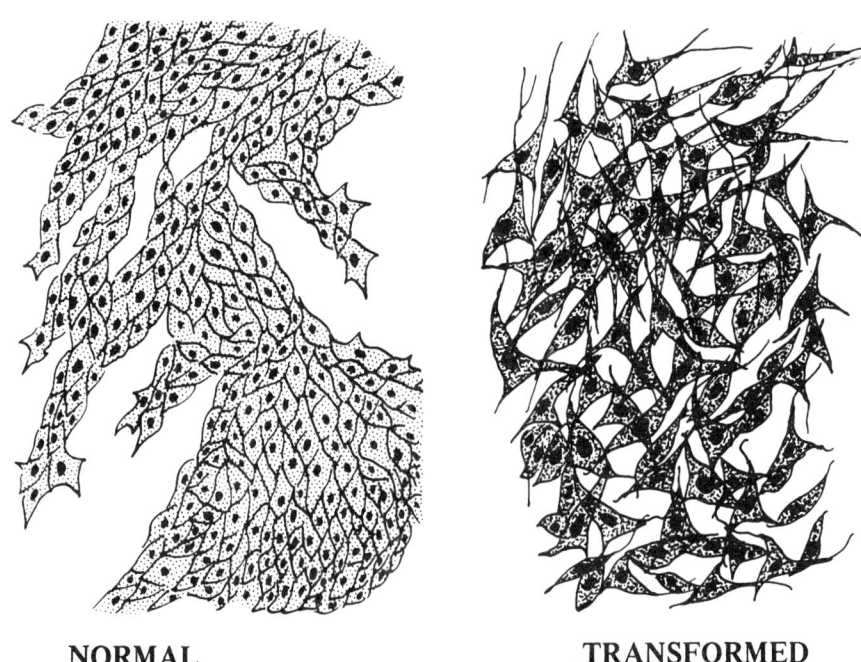

NORMAL   **TRANSFORMED**

Fig. 7-8. An artist's conception of the microscopic appearance of normal and transformed cells in culture. The single-cell layer of spindle cells is characteristic of normal cells, which ultimately exhibit contact inhibition of replication, whereas transformed cells exhibit cytologic anaplasia and ''piling up'' of one cell on another, with lack of contact inhibition of replication. (From Pitot HC: *Fundamentals of oncology,* ed 3, New York 1986, Marcel Dekker.)

taining the extra chromosome fragment, an additional small nucleus is formed. Sister chromatid exchanges involve extensive exchange of material between the two copies, or chromatids, of a chromosome (Fig. 7-10).

Chromosome smears can easily be prepared from blood leukocytes taken from consenting adults; therefore cytogenetic analysis can readily be applied to human populations. This method makes possible comparative studies between heavily exposed and unexposed groups in the same facility; however, the relevance of the measured endpoints is not clear. Chemicals that induce increases in chromosome alterations do so at much higher concentrations than do those that induce other types of mutation. In addition the changes induced are random, whereas in cancer cells, specific alterations are usually seen.

Biomonitoring. With the development of ultrasensitive assays it has become possible to monitor exposure of human populations to genotoxic carcinogens on the basis of their ability to produce DNA and protein adducts and induce excretion of molecules associated with their metabolism. Very low levels of DNA-carcinogen adducts (one adduct per 10^8 nucleotides) can be detected either by *immunoassay* using specific antibodies to the adducts[18] or by *phosporus 32 labeling*,[33] in which DNA is digested enzymatically and altered nucleotides are separated, radiolabeled, identified by chromatography, and measured by scintillation counting (Fig. 7-11).

Because erythrocytes in humans have a relatively long life span (120 days), hemoglobin-carcinogen adducts are also useful in measuring exposure to genotoxic carcinogens. Adduct levels are usually measured by release of the adduct by chemical methods, followed by an ultrasensitive analytical technique such as mass spectrometry. These methods have been successful in demonstrating elevated levels of adducts in the blood leukocytes or erythrocytes of selected industrial populations, such as coke oven operators. As a caveat it must be stated, however, that whereas they provide a

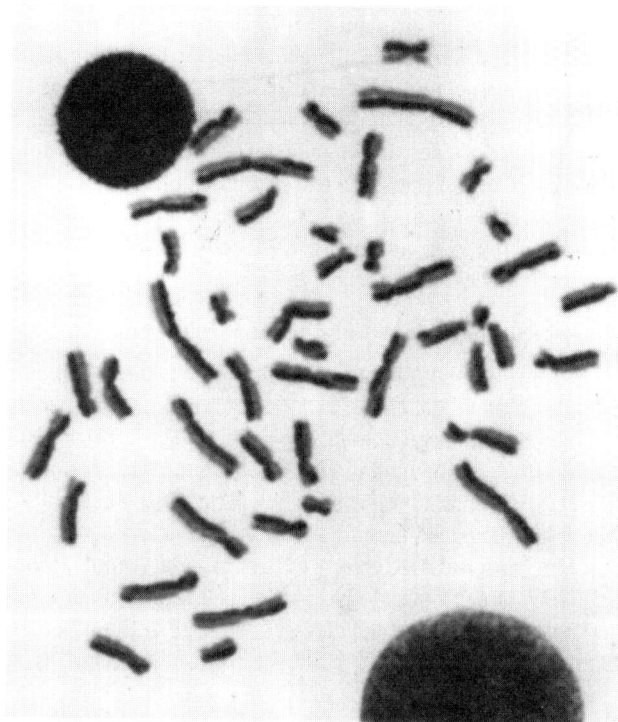

Fig. 7-10. Sister chromatid exchanges (SCEs) (denoted by arrow) in human chromosomes. In chromosomes with no SCEs, chromatids are uniformly stained dark or light. (Courtesy G.K. Livingston, Cincinnati, Ohio.)

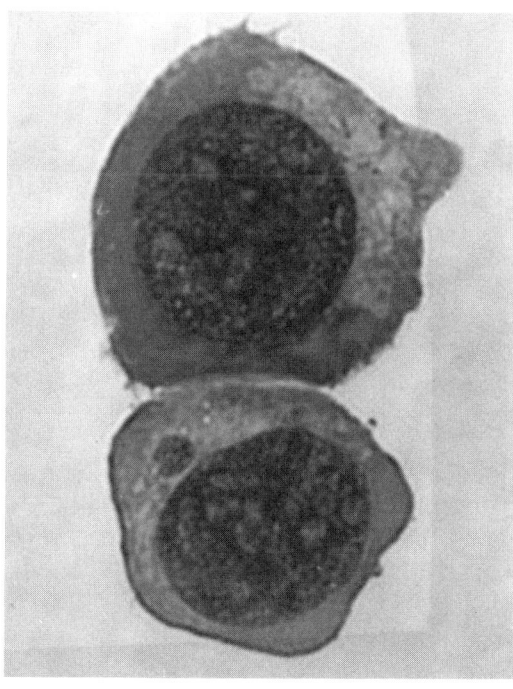

Fig. 7-9. Micronucleus formation in a nucleated cell. (Courtesy G.K. Livingston, Cincinnati, Ohio.)

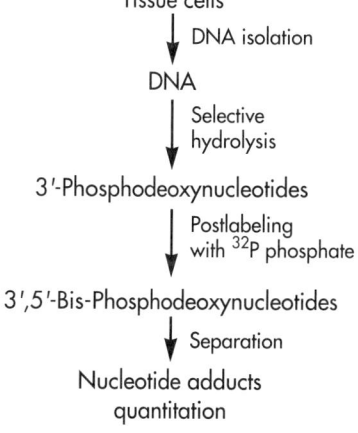

Fig. 7-11. Schematic of postlabeling method for quantitating DNA adducts.

measure of internal exposure, they do not provide a proven measure of risk.

Molecular epidemiology. With the advent of techniques for analysis of specific genes, the prospect of being able to associate cancer-related genetic alterations with exposure to specific agents has become more feasible. The polymerase chain reaction (PCR),[19] a technique by which it is possible to amplify the DNA contained in a tissue section or fragment and even from single cells (Fig. 7-12), has enabled any specific DNA sequence, such as that from an individual gene, to be obtained in a quantity sufficient for sequencing and other studies. Certain carcinogenic chemicals induce mutations at specific sites in cellular protooncogenes such as the *c-Ha-ras* protooncogene; therefore PCR can be applied to amplify these genes in human cells obtained in small numbers, such as blood leukocytes, exfoliated bladder cells, and alveolar cells obtained by lavage. Mutations can then be scored in the PCR-amplified DNA cells and, theoretically, related to specific carcinogen exposure.

Classification of potential human carcinogens

With use of both human epidemiologic and experimental animal testing data, classification of carcinogens, principally associated with occupational exposure, into categories of relative potential for human risk has been carried by various federal and international agencies. The most extensive of these are presented herein.

The National Toxicology Program. The Annual Report of the National Toxicology Program released its sixth report in 1991.[27] Known human carcinogens were defined as those substances for which the evidence from human studies indicates that there is a causal relationship between exposure to the substance and human cancer. Occupational exposures associated with a technologic process that are known to be carcinogenic are defined on a similar basis. Substances suspected or reasonably anticipated to be human carcinogens were defined as those for which there is a limited evidence of carcinogenicity in humans and/or sufficient evidence of carcinogenicity in experimental animals.

The International Agency for Research on Cancer (IARC) of the World Health Organization A somewhat different classification of industrial chemicals and processes has been compiled by the IARC.

A further potentially large group of potential human carcinogens are those occuring naturally in widely consumed foodstuffs as a result of either biosynthesis or the cooking process. Although potent dietary carcinogens such as aflatoxins have received a great deal of attention, there are many that have not. It has recently been reemphasized that exposure to certain dietary carcinogens may well exceed those to residual pesticides on the same foodstuff. The potential interaction between dietary and other types of carcinogens, such as occupational carcinogens and sunlight, has also been little explored. An example of this type of situation is the case of workers involved in the removal and replacement of asphalt roofing.

Factors Modifying Cancer Susceptibility

The many factors determining individual cancer risk can be divided into those derived from the genetic and physiologic profile of the individual, those dependent on environmental and cultural exposures, and those dependent on the

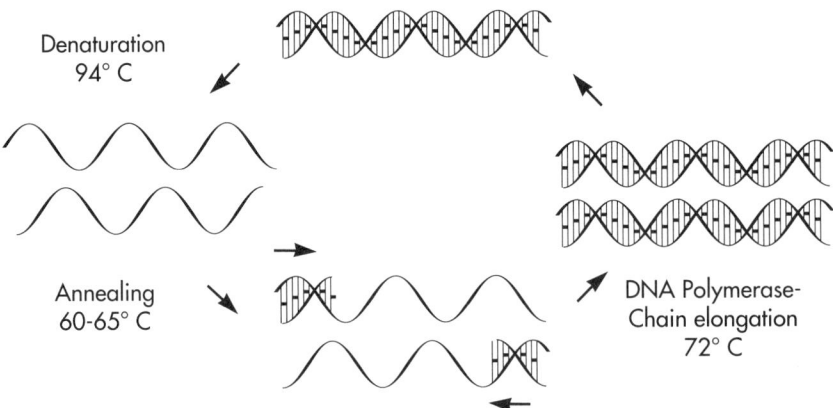

Fig. 7-12. Polymerase chain reaction. Unamplified target DNA is denatured by heating to 94° C. The solution, which also contains an excess of Taq polymerase, deoxyribonucleotides, and oligonucleotide primers, is then cooled to allow the primers to anneal to regions flanking the targeted sequence. The temperature of the solution is raised to 72° C, the temperature optimum of Taq polymerase. The enzyme catalyzes a chain elongation reaction from the primers in a $5' \rightarrow 3'$ direction. As this process is continued in each cycle, a DNA fragment (whose boundaries are defined by the 5' bases of each primer) increases 2^n where *n* is the number of PCR cycles. (From Cebula TA, Koch WH: In *New horizons in biological dosimetry,* New York, 1991, Wiley-Liss.)

nature of the agent to which the individual is exposed and the milieu in which the agent is contained at the time of exposure.

Host-dependent factors

Genetic profile. As described in the previous section, it has already been well established that there is considerable variation in susceptibility to cancer among races and individuals, as there are among species, strains within species, and individuals within strains. Genetic differences already mentioned that predispose to cancer are mutations in cellular protooncogenes and tumor-suppressor genes. There are also several other factors relating to the carcinogenic process that are subject to genetic variation.

Metabolism. Metabolism of carcinogenic agents to species that are more easily excreted or to others that react with crucial cellular nucleic acids and proteins to initiate cancer is a crucial aspect of carcinogenesis by many agents. Genetic variation in the activity of the enzymatic processes involved would therefore be expected to be a critical factor in cancer susceptibility.[23] The activity of these processes is frequently found to be subject to wide variation among species, which continues to befuddle attempts to extrapolate the results of animal tests to humans. Differences in drug sensitivity of individuals is already a major clinical concern to physicians, and individuals' susceptibility to carcinogenesis by a particular agent would also be expected to represent a balance of a number of metabolic factors. In all cases, enzymes that catalyze the conversion of carcinogens to both deactivated and activated species with respect to the carcinogenic process have been characterized.

A further aspect that has been shown to be important in regulating susceptibility to certain types of environmental carcinogen is the phenomenon of inducibility. After exposure to certain agents, the activity of the enzymes responsible for their metabolism is markedly increased or induced. The degree of inducibility is also under genetic control[23] and also appears to be correlated with cancer susceptibility. For the polycyclic aromatic hydrocarbons, which are ubiquitous components of pyrolysis products of fossil fuels and other organic materials, including tobacco, inducibility is genetically governed by the Ah locus. This locus controls inducibility of the aryl hydrocarbon hydroxylase (AHH) or cytochrome P-450 enzymes, and humans fall within clusters of low, intermediate, and high inducibility with respect to inducibility of these enzymes, which metabolize aromatic hydrocarbons to oxidized species implicated in their carcinogenicity. Previous studies have suggested that individual susceptibility to broncogenic carcinoma as a result of cigarette smoking is associated with low AHH inducibility and vice versa (Table 7-9).

Immunologic factors. The relationship between immune status and cancer susceptibility is complex and currently remains controversial; however, a number of observations suggest that a system of antitumor immunity is

Table 7-9. AHH inducibility in mitogen-stimulated lymphocytes from healthy individuals and bronchogenic carcinoma patients

	Number	Low AHH	Intermediate AHH	High AHH
Healthy individuals	230	42.2% (97)	46.9% (108)	10.9% (25)
Bronchogenic carcinoma patients	121	5.0% (6)	64.4% (78)	30.6% (37)

active in humans and can influence susceptibility to cancer. These observations include that cancer risk is highest in the very young and very old, the stages of life at which the immune system is least active; potent suppression of the immune system by drugs or human immunodeficiency viruses results in an elevated incidence of certain types of cancer; administration of carcinogens or tumor-promoting agents suppresses aspects of antitumor immunity; and carcinogens and tumor-promoting agents commonly induce inflammation and activation of leukocytes, responses that are immunologic in nature and that have frequently been associated with carcinogenesis.

The complexity of the immune system continues to make a relationship between itself and carcinogenesis controversial, and alternative explanations have been proposed to explain the aforementioned observations. Cancer risk may be high in the very young as a result of inheritance of deleted or inactivated tumor-suppressor genes, a situation found in retinoblastoma, for instance. In the inherited forms of these types of cancer, the disease occurs rapidly. In older individuals, exposure to carcinogens has occurred over a longer period and there has therefore been more opportunity for carcinogenic mutations to occur and also to be expressed. Recent research suggests that there is some increase in susceptibility to neoplasia in aging cells, however.

Factors relating to sex and endocrine balance. The established difference in tissue distribution of cancer susceptibility between males and females has long suggested that factors related to sex are potent determinants of cancer susceptibility. A proposal that these factors are based on differences in levels of endocrine hormones is basically suggested by the observation that the major sites of cancer in either sex are the tissues most susceptible to endocrine influence. In males these tissues are the colon and prostate, and in females they are the colon, endometrium, and mammary gland. High cancer susceptibility in these tissues presumably results from the abilities of endocrine peptides to induce cell proliferation and alter differentiation patterns. This proposal is further supported by the demonstrated carcinogenic potential of steroid hormones in experimental animals at large doses.[21] Estrogens are regarded as human carcinogens by the IARC.

Cultural and dietary factors

Smoking. Despite the expenditure of a large amount of effort to discourage it, smoking remains a significant cause of human cancer and in women has recently overtaken breast cancer as the leading cause of death outside heart disease. In addition to the cancer burden it itself imposes, smoking acts to strongly potentiate the carcinogenic action of other agents. In smoking workers exposed to asbestos, risk of bronchogenic carcinoma is increased synergistically in comparison with those who do not smoke and smokers not exposed to asbestos.[31] When compared with individuals who do not smoke, workers who smoke and are exposed to asbestos have a sixtyfold risk of cancer mortality. Smoking also acts synergistically in a similar way with radon daughters released in the uranium mining process.[3] In addition, the risk of cancer associated with exposure to rubber or fluorocarbon polymer fumes, chlorine, or carbon or cotton dust also is elevated by smoking. Although tar condensed from cigarette smoke contains a complex mixture of genotoxic carcinogens and cocarcinogens, epidemiologic studies on individuals who have quit smoking suggest that tumor promotion plays the major role in smoking-induced carcinogenesis.

Alcohol. Comparison of cause of death among those who consume large amounts of alcohol with those who imbibe moderately indicates that this agent contributes significantly to the total human cancer burden. Although alcohol itself has not been demonstrated to be a carcinogen in experimental animals, it has been found able to potentiate the carcinogenicity of other agents, including industrial chemicals. In humans there is good evidence to suggest that some types of alcoholic beverage are responsible for elevated cancer incidence. In combination with heavy tobacco smoking, excessive alcohol consumption has been especially associated with cancer of the upper digestive tract.[11] The extent of alcohol abuse is potentially serious in light of the possibility that alcohol increases cancer risk due to occupational chemical exposure.

Diet. The relationship between diet and cancer is of supreme interest to all who have a wide choice of diet, yet it is extremely complex.[39] The average Western diet contains a mixture of naturally occurring carcinogens, carcinogens produced by cooking, cocarcinogens, and anticarcinogens. Conflicting studies have suggested that the major dietary factor regulating cancer susceptibility is total caloric consumption, but others suggest it may be the fraction of calories that is consumed as saturated fat. Experimental studies indicate that the degree of caloric restriction required to reduce cancer incidence significantly in the general population would be unacceptably high and possibly physiologically hazardous. Beyond this, there is a general feeling that consumption of animal fats and protein should be minimized and that of fiber and fruits increased. Geographically there seems to be a good correlation between consumption of saturated fat and colon and breast cancer, which have therefore been termed *cancers of affluence*. In these studies it is difficult to divorce consumption of saturated fat from that of animal protein, because this major source of protein in the Western democracies, where colon and breast cancer is high, has a high fat content. Consumption of fish as an alternative source has been recommended, especially because animal experiments have suggested that fish oils contain unsaturated fatty acids of a type that reduces cancer susceptibility.

Although vegetables and other plant foodstuffs have been much expounded as alternatives to animal products, caution has been sounded in that plants have evolved against the pressure of animal predation and have developed a wide range of chemical defenses, including potent carcinogens.[3] Animals have concurrently developed defenses against these agents, moreover. With the possible exception of nonpoisonous fruit, in which animal consumption assists in the distribution of seeds, it should not be assumed that liberal consumption of plant products is free of risk and always beneficial. The consumption of plants as a source of fiber has also been widely popularized, although the ability of different types of fiber to reduce cancer risk has not been firmly established.

Cancer risk may also be reduced through the consumption of diets that contain sufficient levels of agents suggested by animal studies to antagonize the tumorigenic actions of carcinogens and tumor-promoting agents (Table 7-10). The added risk posed by chemicals added to food to retard spoilage has also been a cause for considerable public concern. It has been pointed out that the risk from these agents may be considerably less than that from naturally occuring carcinogens. In the case of nitrites added to fresh meat to maintain appearance, fear of risk due to added quantities of these agents has subsided somewhat since the realization that significant quantities are synthesized physiologically from urea and secreted into the saliva.

The complexity of the diet of any population will con-

Table 7-10. Dietary measures potentially capable of reducing or preventing cancer

Measure	Type of cancer
Dietary classes	
Increased fiber	Colon, rectum
Reduced fat	Breast, colon, rectum
Increased fruit	Stomach
Reduced nitrates	Stomach, esophagus (China)
Improved preservation of food	
Refrigeration	Stomach
Dietary constituents	
Vitamin A, β-carotene	Multiple sites
Vitamin C, E	
Vitamin B_2, B_6, B_{12}, folic acid	
Selenium	

tinue to make difficult identification of agents in that diet that affect cancer susceptibility positively or negatively. The interaction of specific dietary factors with other common components of the life-style of a particular population, such as smoking or alcohol consumption, or with specific occupational exposures therefore poses a continuing challenge to determination of the primary sources of the cancer burden in that population.

Agent-dependent factors

Structure-activity relationships. Within groups of chemicals of closely similar chemical structure, it is nevertheless very difficult to predict carcinogenicity or lack of it. A practical exception is nitrosamines; practically all chemicals of this class are carcinogenic. The tissue and species specificity of cancer depends markedly on the structure of a particular nitrosamine, however. Marked difference in activity among chemicals of closely similar structure also holds for tumor-promoting agents.

The complex mixture problem. Despite the certain knowledge that humans are exposed environmentally or occupationally to mixtures of carcinogens, relatively little attention is paid to the problem of interaction between two or more agents. The probable reason is the complexity of the problem, to which is added the possibility of frequent change in composition of the mixture. In a range of experiments using relatively high exposures, treatment with two carcinogens led to any of all the possible endpoints—inhibition, additivity, synergy, or no effect—with little predictability. It can be argued that at high doses a major factor will be saturation of one or more pathways of metabolism of one agent by another. At low doses, less interaction may therefore be observed. The dose of the mixture to which an individual is observed also is therefore a critical factor in assessing the potential effects of mixtures.

Anticarcinogenesis. Studies on multistage initiation/tumor-promotion/progression models of carcinogenesis have provided much evidence on the mechanisms underlying the different processes and concurrently identified many types of agent capable of inhibiting tumor promotion and carcinogenesis. These agents include those that inhibit cell division and hyperplasia; inhibit inflammation; maintain normal differentiation patterns; maintain cell-cell communication; enhance antitumor immunity; antagonize carcinogen- or tumor-promoter–induced alterations in the concentration of small growth regulatory molecules (cyclic nucleotides, polyamines, prostaglandins); and inhibit accumulation of reactive oxidants.

It is therefore apparent that many types of agents are capable of inhibiting the promotion and hence overall carcinogenesis processes. Many of the studies on which the aforementioned findings are based were carried out in a skin model with promoting agents to which humans would not normally be exposed. There is therefore great potential for studies on other agents and tissues, possibly leading to modification of diet and lifestyle to reduce cancer burden in human populations.

SUMMARY

Studies in both human populations and experimental animals continue to reinforce the concept that carcinogenesis resulting from environmental and occupational exposure is a multistage process. The agents currently described as carcinogens may affect any of these stages, with the overall result that at least one diagnosable tumor arises within the lifespan of the individual. The scope of the term *carcinogen* may therefore have to be expanded to include agents that affect stages other than those that involve genetic alterations. Currently, methods for at least initial identification of carcinogens are likewise based only on detection of their genetic effects; therefore, these methods may fail to identify many agents capable of significantly influencing human cancer risk. Studies on animal models of multistage carcinogenesis have also identified a wide range of agents with inhibitory activity toward various stages of carcinogenesis. For the future, several challenges can be raised regarding improvements in understanding of the factors that determine overall human cancer risk. These challenges include (1) determination of the interaction between occupational carcinogens and environmental factors such as viruses and ultraviolet radiation; (2) improvement of understanding of the relationship between diet and response to environmental and occupational carcinogens; (3) determination of the role that cocarcinogens and tumor-promoting and tumor-progressing agents play in environmental and occupational carcinogenesis; (4) identification of dietary factors that significantly and unambiguously reduce human cancer susceptibility; (5) improvement of the sensitivity and specificity of methods to measure human exposure to carcinogenic agents; and (6) identification of genetic factors that determine the relative sensitivity of different individuals to carcinogens and tumor-promoting agents.

REFERENCES

1. Aaronson S: Growth factors and cancer, *Science* 254:1147, 1991.
2. Ames BN: Carcinogenicity tests, *Science* 191:241, 1976 (letter).
3. Ames BN et al: Ranking possible carcinogenic hazards, *Science* 236:271, 1987.
4. Archer VE, Gillam JD, Wagoner JK: Respiratory disease mortality among uranium miners, *Ann NY Acad Sci* 271:280, 1976.
5. Beasley RP: Hepatitis B virus: the major etiology of hepatocellular carcinoma, *Cancer* 61:1942, 1988.
6. Becker FF, ed: *Cancer: a comprehensive treaties,* ed 2, vol 1, New York, 1982, Plenum.
7. Berg JW: World-wide variations in cancer incidence as clues to cancer origins. In Hiatt HH, Watson JD, Winsten JA, eds: *Origins of human cancer,* Cold Spring Harbor, NY, 1977, Cold Spring Harbor Laboratory.
8. Bingham E, Falk HL: Environmental carcinogens: the modifying effect of cocarcinogens on the threshold response, *Arch Environ Hlth* 19:779, 1969.
9. Birt DF: Update on the effects of vitamins A, C, and E and selenium on carcinogenesis, *Pro Soc Exp Biol Med* 183:311, 1986.

10. Bischoff F: Organic polymer biocompatibility and toxicology, *Clin Chem* 18:869, 1972.
11. Blot WJ et al: Smoking and drinking in relation to oral and pharyngeal cancer, *Cancer Res* 48:3282, 1988.
12. Brand KG et al: Etiological factors, stages, and the role of the foreign body in foreign body tumorigenesis: a review, *Cancer Res* 35:279, 1975.
13. Dolberg DS et al: Wounding and its role in RSV-mediated tumor formation, *Science* 230:676, 1985.
14. Doll R, Peto R: *The causes of cancer,* Oxford, England, 1981, Oxford University Press.
15. Fearon ER et al: Identification of a chromosome 18q gene that is altered in colorectal cancers, *Science* 247:49, 1990.
16. Fenech M: Optimisation of micronucleus assays for biological dosimetry. In Gledhill BL, Mauro F, ed: *New horizons in biological dosimetry: proceedings of the international symposium on trends in biological dosimetry,* New York, 1991, Wiley-Liss.
17. Hansen MF, Cavenee WK: Genetics of cancer predisposition, *Cancer Res* 47:5518, 1987.
18. Harris CC, et al: Detection of benzo(a)pyrene diol epoxide-DNA adducts in peripheral blood lymphocytes and antibodies to the adducts in serum from coke oven workers, *Pro Natl Acad Sci USA* 82:6672, 1985.
19. Harris CC: Molecular epidemiology of human cancer in the 1990s. In Gledhill BL, Mauro F, eds: *New horizons in biological dosimetry,* New York, 1991, Wiley-Liss.
20. Henderson BE, Ross RK, Pike MC: Toward the primary prevention of cancer, *Science* 254:1131, 1991.
21. Henderson BM, Ross R, Bernstein L: Estrogens as a cause of human cancer: the Richard and Linda Rosenthal foundation award lecture, *Cancer Res* 48:246, 1988.
22. Jacobs LR: Relationship between dietary fiber and cancer: metabolic, physiologic, and cellular mechanisms, *Proc Soc Exp Biol Med* 183:299, 1986.
23. Kouri RE, Schechtman LM, Nebert DW: Metabolism of chemical carcinogens. In Kouri RE, ed: *Genetic differences in chemical carcinogenesis,* Boca Raton, Fla, 1980, CRC Press.
24. Maclure KM, MacMahon B: An epidemiologic perspective of environmental carcinogenesis, *Epidemiol Rev* 2:19, 1980.
25. Marx J: Possible new colon cancer gene found, *Science* 251:1317, 1991.
26. Mueller GC, Gusberg SB, Stone A: Meeting report, the Mary Lasker conference on growth factors in hormone-related tumors, *Cancer Res* 51:4114, 1991.
27. National Toxicology Program: *Sixth annual report on carcinogens,* Washington, DC, 1991, Department of Health and Human Services.
28. Peterson WL: *Helicobacter pylori* and peptic ulcer disease, *N Engl J Med* 324:1043, 1991.
29. Preston-Martin S et al: Increased cell division as a cause of human cancer, *Cancer Res* 50:7415, 1990.
30. Rubin H: Carcinogenicity tests, *Science* 191:241, 1976 (letter). Ames BN, *ibid,* p 241, 1976.
31. Selikoff IJ, Seidman H, Hammond EC: Mortality effects of cigarette smoking among amosite asbestos factory workers, *J Natl Cancer Inst* 65:507, 1980.
32. Slaga TJ, ed: *Mechanisms of tumor promotion,* 4 vols, Boca Raton, Fla, 1983-1984, CRC Press.
33. Talaska G, Roh JH, Getek T: ^{32}P-postlabelling and mass spectrometric methods for Analysis Bulky, polyaromatic carcinogen-DNA adducts in humans, *J Chromatog* 580:293, 1992.
34. Tomatis L, ed: *Cancer: causes, occurrence and control,* Lyon, France, 1990, World Health Organization, International Agency for Research on Cancer, Scientific Publ 100.
35. Yu M-W et al: Association between hepatitis C virus antibodies and hepatocellular carcinoma in Taiwan, *Cancer Res* 51:5621, 1992.
36. Weinberg RA: Tumor suppressor genes, *Science* 254:1138, 1991.
37. World Health Organization, International Agency for Research on Cancer, 1987. IARC Monographs on the Evaluation of Carcinogenic Risks to Humans. Supplement 7: Overall Evaluations of Carcinogenicity: An Updating of *IARC Monographs* Volumes 1 to 42.
38. Wyllie AH: Cell death: a new classification separating apoptosis from necrosis. In Bowen ID, Lockshin RA, eds: *Cell death in biology and pathology,* London, 1981, Chapman and Hall.
39. Wynder EL: The dietary environment and cancer, *J Am Diet Assoc* 71:385, 1977.
40. zur Hausen H: Viruses in human cancers, *Science* 254:1167, 1991.

Chapter 8

ASSESSMENT OF MALE REPRODUCTIVE FUNCTION

Steven M. Schrader

Reproductive profile in human toxicology studies
Impact of toxic exposure
    Neuroendocrine system
    Testes
    Accessory sex glands
    Sexual function
    Summary

Environmental exposures have been shown to affect the male reproductive system.* Few human studies, however, have been conducted that evaluate environmental exposures.

There are four major indications that environmental exposures can be related to deficits in male reproductive function. First, approximately 15% of all couples are infertile,[1,60] with 10% to 20% of infertility of unknown etiology. Even when reduced male fertility is identified, the causes of the anomalies are often idiopathic.[59] Second, there are several reports that sperm numbers have declined over the last several decades as environmental exposures have increased.† Third, several occupational exposures to toxicants have been demonstrated to cause decreases in the reproductive potential of male workers.‡ Fourth, environmental contaminants that are toxic to other physiologic systems have been found in human seminal plasma.[3,78]

Because fertility is a couple event, it is very difficult to evaluate in independent fashion the effects of exposure to the man on fertility.[80,88] An assessment of human male fecundity, however, can be conducted. A complete assessment of male fecundity includes neuroendocrine measurements of blood samples and semen analysis, as well as medical and exposure histories.

REPRODUCTIVE PROFILE IN HUMAN TOXICOLOGY STUDIES

It is necessary to establish a male reproductive profile for assessing fecundity for both individuals and populations. The assessment profile described in this section is being used by the National Institute for Occupational Safety and Health (NIOSH) to assess populations that are or may be exposed to potential reproductive toxicants. If individual data (versus population comparisons) are to be used, it is appropriate to compare the results with the normal range of results from the laboratory conducting the analyses and not with previously published values from other sources. If a population-based study is being conducted, a concurrent comparable cohort must be used and the analyses should be blind to exposure status. A summary of assessments and specific methodologies follows, including identification of methodologies that are specific to individual or group comparisons.

Semen analyses provides a useful component in the development of the profile of male reproductive function. Exact instructions should be provided to each man to ensure that the semen sample is collected by masturbation after a set time of abstinence (usually 2 days). The semen sample should be delivered to the laboratory within 1 hour of the time of ejaculation. The men should be instructed to maintain the semen at room temperature to avoid any temperature

---
*References 16, 21, 45, 74, 85.
†References 9, 11, 33, 52, 56, 58.
‡References 61, 62, 71, 89, 90.

shock to the sperm cells. A videotape is available from NIOSH with these basic instructions.[12,24] At the time of collecting the semen sample, each subject should record the duration of abstinence, time of semen collection, and any information regarding spillage. A label attached to the collection jar facilitates the recording of this information.

Semen analyses can be conducted in two phases. The initial evaluation of the sample should be conducted when the sample arrives at the laboratory or field site. This evaluation consists of recording the temperature, turbidity, color, liquefaction time, volume, osmolality, and pH of the semen. Sperm counts, viability estimates, video recordings for motility assessments, preparation of slides for microscopic examination, and preservation of seminal plasma should also be conducted at this time. Morphologic and morphometric analyses of sperm on slides, as well as motility and velocity analyses of the sperm recorded on videotapes, may be conducted at a later time. The motility analyses may be performed manually or using a computer-assisted sperm analysis system (CASA). If CASA is used, several sperm motility variables can be measured. These variables provide information on the progression of sperm cells (curvilinear velocity, straight-line velocity, and linearity) and the sperm motility pattern (lateral head amplitude and beat cross frequency).

Sperm viability may be determined by two methods, eosin Y stain exclusion[19] and hypoosmotic swelling (HOS assay).[34] These techniques test for the structural and functional integrity of the cell membrane, respectively.[68] Sperm concentration and motility characteristics should be measured in a chamber at least 10 μm deep in order for the sperm to move freely in all dimensions.

Measurements of sperm motility and velocity should be conducted using a microscope stage maintained at 37° C. Results from 200 motile sperm per sample are desirable if one is interested in the distribution of velocity measurements,[67] but 50 motile sperm will suffice if means are to be compared among treatment groups.[72] If the videotapes are being used to calculate the percent motility one should avoid "hunting" for motile sperm. All fields examined or searched should be included in the calculations. Therefore, recording a certain number of arbitrary fields is advised. Some researchers have found it useful to record a consistent number of fields to determine sperm concentration and percent motility, followed by additional fields for velocity estimates. If a CASA system is being used for motility and velocity estimates, the number of sperm per field needs to be reduced to minimize cell collisions. Using a 10- to 20-μm-deep chamber, the sperm concentration should be less than 40 million/ml.[87] Diluents (including seminal plasma), however, alter sperm velocity up to a dilution of about 1:1.[13] The current recommendation is to dilute *all* samples 1 part semen in 1 part iso-osmotic buffer.[80] If this dilution does not reduce the sperm concentration below 40 million/ml, then an additional dilution in the same buffer should be performed on those samples to attain a concentration below 40 million/ml.

Sperm morphology analyses should be performed on air-dried, stained semen smears. During the past 30 years several schemes have been presented for the assessment of normal and abnormal sperm morphologies. Variation in sperm size and shape is not distinct but rather a continuum. This provides a challenge within and especially among laboratories to establish a repeatable system for morphological classification.[22,23,28,43] With recent advances of computerized image analyses, several methods of sperm morphometry have been introduced.* These morphometric analysis systems provide a more reproducible system of objective assessments for individual sperm head size and shape, as well as tail configuration. Comparisons of measurements between different analysis systems should be avoided. Sperm morphometry is now routinely used as part of the assessment of reproductive hazards to the male worker.[70]

IMPACT OF TOXIC EXPOSURE

Toxicants can affect the male reproductive system at one of several sites or at multiple sites. These sites and the assays associated with their respective functions are discussed individually. This does not imply that there exists an absolute one-to-one relationship between a particular measurement and the associated site of action. These sites include the neuroendocrine system, the testes, accessory sex glands, and sexual function.

Neuroendocrine system

The endocrine system, in concert with the nervous system, coordinates function of the various components of the reproductive axis. This system draws upon external (for example, sexual cues, temperature) and internal (for example, checks and balances between endocrine tissue function, metabolic status) inputs. The reproductive endocrine status of the male is best established by measuring the hormones in the circulation or in the urine. The hormones of interest are luteinizing hormone (LH), follicle stimulating hormone (FSH), testosterone, and prolactin.

Urinary testosterone levels may be assessed by measuring the parent compound, a metabolite, or hydrolysis of testosterone metabolites. When measuring steroid hormone metabolites in urine, consideration must be given to the potential that the exposure being studied may alter the metabolism of excreted metabolites. This is especially pertinent since most steroid metabolism occurs in the liver, which is a target of many toxicants. Lead, for example, was shown to reduce the amount of sulphated steroids that were excreted into the urine.[2]

FSH, LH, testosterone, and prolactin can all be evaluated in a population-based study by assessing the hormone levels in a single blood sample from each man.[73] If possible, samples should be collected about the same time of day to avoid circadian variations. In the study of an individual rather than a population, three blood samples should be collected 20

---

*References 15, 32, 35, 55, 65, 69, 85.

minutes apart or urinary assessment of testosterone metabolites and gonadotropins (FSH, LH) should be conducted.[77]

Testes

As noted previously, sperm count, sperm morphology, and sperm head morphometry all provide indices of the integrity of spermatogenesis and spermiogenesis. Thus the number of sperm in the ejaculate is directly correlated with the number of germ cells per gram of testis,[93] while abnormal morphology is probably a result of abnormal spermiogenesis. Azoospermia is the most severe observation, as it is often an indication that type A spermatogonia have been lost and recovery is unlikely. New methods that assess DNA stability and DNA adducts promise to provide information about spermatogenesis at the genetic level.

Genetic damage is difficult to detect in human sperm because most methods require induced replication, which cannot occur in haploid cells. Genetically damaged sperm may alter fertilization and lead to developmental anomalies or spontaneous abortions. Epidemiologic studies of large populations in some countries (for example, United Kingdom) have demonstrated increased frequency of spontaneous abortions in women whose husbands were working as motor vehicle mechanics[49] or had lead exposure.[42] Such studies indicate a need for methods to detect genetic damage in human sperm and to assess its significance. A growing research emphasis on germ cell genetics is beginning to unfold.[66]

Accessory sex glands

Seminal plasma is not essential for fertilization. This is demonstrated by the fact that artificial insemination with sperm collected from the epididymis results in conception. On the other hand, seminal plasma contributes importantly to the normal coitus-fertilization scenario. Seminal plasma serves as a vehicle for sperm transport, a buffer from the hostile acidic vaginal environment, and perhaps an initial energy source for the sperm. Cervical mucus minimizes passage of seminal plasma into the uterus. Some constituents of seminal plasma, however, are carried into the uterus to the site of fertilization by adhering to the sperm membrane.

The viability and motility of spermatozoa in seminal plasma is typically a reflection of seminal plasma quality. Alterations in sperm viability, as measured by stain exclusion, hypoosmotic swelling, or alterations in sperm motility parameters, would suggest an effect on the accessory sex glands producing seminal plasma.

Biochemical analysis of seminal plasma provides insights into the function of the accessory sex glands. Chemicals that are secreted primarily by each of the glands of this system are typically selected to serve as a marker for each respective gland. For example, the epididymis is represented by glycerylphosphorylcholine (GPC), the seminal vesicles by fructose, and the prostate gland by zinc. Note that this type of analysis provides only gross information on glandular function and little or no information on the other secretory constituents. Measuring semen pH and osmolality provide additional general information on the nature of seminal plasma.

Seminal plasma may be analyzed for the presence of a toxicant or its metabolite. Heavy metals have been detected in seminal plasma using atomic absorption spectrophotometry,[79] while halogenated hydrocarbons have been measured in seminal fluid by gas chromatography after extraction[45] or protein-limiting filtration.[92] It should be noted that the presence of an analyte in seminal plasma is not sufficient to indicate that this analyte is responsible for an observed effect, though it may be suggestive. A toxicant or its metabolite may act directly on accessory sex glands to alter the quality or quantity of their secretions. Alternatively, the toxicant may enter the seminal plasma[44] and thereby affect the sperm, be carried to the site of fertilization on the sperm membrane, and effect the ova or conceptus or be absorbed into the body of the female partner after intercourse.

Sexual function

Human sexual function refers to the integrated activities of the testes and secondary sex glands, the endocrine control systems, and the central-nervous-system-based behavioral and psychologic components of reproduction (libido). Erection, ejaculation, and orgasm are three distinct, independent, physiologic and psychodynamic events that normally occur in close temporal sequence in men. If detail on function or mechanisms are desired, several reviews and in-depth reports are available.[14,36,84]

Objective, unambiguous assessment of occupational-exposure-induced anomalies of sexual function is difficult. The practitioner usually must rely on the testimony and recall of the worker regarding his sexual function. This testimony often may be confounded by the bias of the individual to guard his ego or masculine image or to attribute a preexisting libido problem to exposures at work.

Burris and colleagues[10] recently reported application of a monitor for assessing erection at home. If substantiated, this may provide a convenient, nonclinical means by which to evaluate erectile function of exposed workers.

The assessment of ejaculate volume may provide information on the integrity of the emission phase of ejaculation. This is, of course, complicated by effects on the accessory sex glands' secretory capacity. Thus a semen sample of reduced volume but with a normal ratio of constituents (marker endogenous biochemicals) supports a diagnosis of an emission phase defect. This type of analysis must be considered in the context of population variation in such measures.

Effects of environmental exposures

Several occupational exposures have been shown to affect male fecundity. These include exposure to heavy metals such as lead,[38] pesticides (for example, dibromochloropropane)[90] ethylene dibromide,[71] and solvents (for example, glycol ethers[61,89]). Environmental (nonoccupational) effects

Table 8-1. Environmental effects on male reproduction selected references*

	Neuroendocrine	Testis	Accessory sex glands	Sexual function
Heat/climate		18, 39, 40 41, 53		
Stress	50, 81	26, 29, 81	26, 29, 81	50
Clothes		63, 75	63, 75	
Radiation†		48, 51, 54		
Pesticides‡	46	46	3, 46, 78	
Altitude	8	25		

*Number indicates reference number from references.
†Radiation data was collected from clinical treatment of cancer.
‡Most of the pesticide data is from occupational exposures.

Table 8-2. Life-style effects on male reproduction selected references*

	Neuroendocrine	Testis	Accessory sex glands	Sexual function
Alcohol	37, 31	37, 64	37	6, 57
Smoking	4	64, 82	30, 82	
Drug abuse	76	76	76	20
Exercise	5, 27	5 (?)	27 (?)	
Caffeine		47	7, 47	
Sauna		91		

*Number indicates reference number from references.
? Indicates a trend but not a significant difference.

on male fecundity have also been reported from a few studies. (Table 8-1). Environmental toxicant exposures rarely have been studied because of the difficulties associated with accurately characterizing populations and exposure levels. Occupationally exposed populations, on the contrary, tend to have higher and better defined exposure information.

Life-style practices may also have an negative effect on male fecundity (Table 8-2). Systemic illnesses,[24] infectious diseases,[24] alcohol, and many prescribed pharmaceuticals[17] have negative effects on male fecundity.

Summary

While environmental studies reveal that conditions and lifestyles do compromise male fecundity, very few studies have assessed the effects of environmental contamination. This reflects in large part the complexity of studying this problem. Occupational exposures are usually more discrete and better characterized, and therefore the studies are easier to conduct and interpret. Results from these studies may provide insight for those concerned with environmental hazards.

Each year several hundred new compounds are added to the 70,000 compounds and 4 million mixtures already in commercial use.[86] Little is known about the reproductive toxicity of these chemicals. The challenge to the physician and the toxicologist is to identify those that may be toxic and evaluate the potential effect they may have on human health.

REFERENCES

1. American Fertility Society: What you should know about infertility, *Contemp Obgyn* 15:101, 1980.
2. Apostoli P et al: Steroid hormone sulphation in lead workers, *Br J Indust Med* 46:204, 1989.
3. Arbjit K: Effect of environmental pollutants on human semen, *Environmental Contamination and Toxicology* 40:102, 1988.
4. Attia AM et al: Cigarette smoking and male reproduction, *Arch Androl* 23:45, 1989.
5. Ayers JWT et al: Anthropomorphic, hormonal and psychologic correlates of semen quality in endurance-trained male athletes, *Fert Steril* 43:917, 1985.
6. Bain CL, Guay AT: Reproducibility in monitoring nocturnal penile tumescence and rigidity, *J Urol* 148:811, 1992.
7. Beach CA, Bianchine JR, Gerber N: The excretion of caffeine in the semen of men: pharmacokinetics and comparison in the concentrations in blood and semen, *J Clin Pharmacol* 24:120, 1984.
8. Beall CM et al: Salivary testosterone concentration of Aymara men native to 3600m, *Annals of Human Biology* 19:67, 1992.
9. Bostofte E, Serup J, Rebbe H: Has the fertility of Danish men declined through the years in terms of semen quality? A comparison of semen qualities between 1952 and 1972, *Int J Fertil* 28:91, 1983.
10. Burris AS, Banks SM, Sherins RJ: Quantitative assessment of nocturnal penile tumescence and rigidity in normal men using a home monitor, *J Androl* 10:492, 1989.
11. Carlsen E et al: Evidence for decreasing quality of semen during past 50 years, *Br Med J* 305:609, 1992.
12. National Institute for Occupational Safety and Health: Collecting a semen sample, Cincinnati, 1986.
13. Davis RO et al: Effects of dilution with homologous seminal plasma (HSP) and phosphate-buffered saline (PBS) on computer-aided sperm analysis (CASA) measures of human seminal sperm motion, *Fertil Steril*, S65, 1989.
14. deGroat WC, Booth AM: Physiology of male sexual function, *Ann Intern Med* 92:329, 1980.
15. DeStefano F et al: Automated semen analysis in large epidemiologic studies, *J Androl* 8:24, 1987.
16. Dixon RL, Sherins RJ, Lee IP: Assessment of environmental factors affecting male fertility, *Environ Health Perspec* 30:53, 1979.
17. Drife JO: The effects of drugs on sperm, *Drugs* 33:610, 1987.
18. Effendy I, Krause WK: Environmental risk factors in the history of male patients of an infertility clinic, *Andrologia* 19:262, 1987.
19. Eliasson R, Treichl L: Supravital staining of human spermatozoa, *Fertil Steril* 22:134, 1971.
20. Fabro S: Drugs and male sexual function, *Reproductive Toxicology: A Medical Letter* 4:1985.
21. Fabro S: Reproductive toxicology: a medical letter on environmental hazards to reproduction, Editorial, *Reproduc Tox Center* 4:1985.
22. Fredricson B: Morphologic evaluation of spermatozoa in different laboratories, *Andrologia* 11:57, 1979.
23. Freund M: Standards for the rating of human sperm morphology, *Int J Fert* 11:97, 1966.
24. Gangi GR, Nagler HM: Clinical evaluation of the subfertile man, *Infertility and Reproductive Medicine Clinics of North America* 3:299, 1992.

25. Garciahjarles MA: Spermatogram and seminal biochemistry of high altitude natives and patients with chronic mountain sickness, *Archives de Biologia Y Medicina Experimentales,* 1989.
26. Giblin PT, Kmjajo MP: Effects of stress and characteristic adaptability on semen quality in healthy men, *Fert Ster* 49:127, 1988.
27. Grandi M, Celani MF: Effects of football on the pituitary-testicular axis (PTA)—differences between professional and non-professional soccer players, *Experimental and Clinical Endocrinology* 96:253, 1990.
28. Hanke LJ: Comparison of laboratories conducting sperm morphology, NIOSH Report TA78-28, Cincinnati, 1981.
29. KL Harrison VC, JH: Stress and semen quality in an in vitro fertilization program, *Fertil Steril* 48:633, 1987.
30. Holzki G, Gall H, Hermann J: Cigarette smoking and sperm quality, *Andrologia* 23:141, 1991.
31. Ida Y et al: Effects of acute and repeated alcohol ingestion on hypothalamic-pituitary-gonadal and hypothalamic-pituitary-adrenal functioning in normal males, *Drug and Alcohol Dependence* 31:57, 1992.
32. Jagoe JR, Washbrook NP, Hudson EA: Morphometry of spermatozoa using semiautomatic image analysis, *J Clin Path* 39:1347, 1986.
33. James WH: Secular trend in reported sperm count, *Andrologia* 12:381, 1980.
34. Jeyendran RS et al: Development of an assay to assess the functional integrity of the human sperm membrane and its relationship to other semen characteristics, *J Reprod Fert* 70:219, 1984.
35. Katz DF, Overstreet JW, Pelprey RJ: Integrated assessment of the motility, morphology, and morphometry of human spermatozoa, *Inserm* 103:97-100, 1981.
36. Krane RJ, Goldstein I, de Tejada IS: Impotence, *N Engl J Med* 321:1648, 1989.
37. Kucheria K, Saxen R, Mohan D: Semen analysis in alcohol dependence syndrome, *Andrologia* 17:558, 1985.
38. Lancranjan I et al: Reproductive ability of workmen occupationally exposed to lead, *Arch Environ Health* 30:396, 1975.
39. Levine R et al: Deterioration of semen quality during summer in New Orleans, *Fertil Steril* 49:900, 1988.
40. Levine RJ et al: Air-conditioned environments do not prevent deterioration of human semen quality during the summer, *Fertil Steril* 57:1075, 1992.
41. Levine RJ et al: Differences in the quality of semen in outdoor workers during summer and winter, *New Engl J Med* 323:12, 1990.
42. Lindbohm ML et al: Paternal occupational lead exposure and spontaneous abortion, *Scand J Work Environ Health* 17:95, 1991.
43. MacLeod J: Semen quality in 1000 men of known fertility and in 800 cases of infertile marriage, *Fert Steril* 2:115, 1951.
44. Mann T, Lutwak-Mann C: Passage of chemicals into human and animal semen: mechanisms and significance, *CRC Crit Rev Toxicol* 11:1, 1982.
45. Manseon JM, Simons R: Influence of environmental agents on male reproductive failure. In Hunt VR, ed: *Work and the health of women,* 1979.
46. Mattison DR et al: Reproductive toxicology of pesticides. In Baker, Wilkinson, editors: *Advances in modern environmental toxicology,* Princeton, 1990, Princeton Scientific Publishers.
47. Marshburn PB, Sloan CS, Hammond MG: Semen quality and association with coffee drinking, cigarette smoking, and ethanol consumption, *Fert Steril* 52:162, 1989.
48. Martin RH et al: An increased frequency of human sperm chromosomal abnormalities after radiotherapy, *Mutation Research* 174:219, 1986.
49. McDonald AD et al: Fathers' occupation and pregnancy outcome, *Br J Indust Med* 46:329, 1989.
50. McGrady AV: Effects of psychological stress on male reproduction: a review, *Arch of Androl* 13:1, 1984.
51. Meistrich ML, Samuels RC: Reduction in sperm levels after testicular irradiation of the mouse: a comparison with man, *Radiation Research* 102:138, 1985.
52. Menkveld R et al: Possible changes in male fertility over a 15-year period, *Arch Androl* 17:143, 1986.
53. Mieusset R et al: Association of scrotal hyperthermia with impaired spermatogenesis in infertile men, *Fertil Steril* 48:1006-1011, 1988.
54. Mikamo K, Kamiguchi Y, Tateno H: Spontaneous and in vitro radiation-induced chromosome aberrations in human spermatozoa-application of a new method, *Mutation and the Environment, Part B* 340:447, 1990.
55. Moruzzi JF et al: Quantification and classification of human sperm morphology by CAIA, *Fertil Steril* 50:142, 1988.
56. Nelson CKM, Bunge RG: Semen analysis: evidence for changing parameters of male fertility potential, *Fertil Steril* 26:503, 1974.
57. Nirenberg TD et al: The sexual relationship of male alcoholics and their female partners during periods of drinking and abstinence, *J Studies Alcohol* 51:565, 1990.
58. Osser O, Liedholm P, Ranstam J: Depressed semen quality: a study over two decades, *Arch Androl* 12:113, 1984.
59. Purvis K, Christiansen E: Male infertility—current concepts, *Ann Med* 24:259, 1992.
60. Rantala ML: Epidemiological and clinical studies on the etiology of infertility, academic dissertation, University of Helsinki, Finland, 1988.
61. Ratcliffe JM et al: Semen quality in workers exposed to 2-ethoxyethanol, *Brit J Ind Med* 46:399-406, 1989.
62. Rodamilans M et al: Lead toxicity on endocrine testicular function in an occupationally exposed population, *Human Toxicol* 7:125, 1988.
63. Sanger WG, Friman PC: Fit of underwear and male spermatogenesis—a pilot investigation, *Reproductive Toxicology* 4:229, 1992.
64. Savitz DA, Schwingl PJ, Keels MA: Influence of paternal age, smoking, and alcohol consumption on congenital anomalies, *Teratology* 44:429, 1991.
65. Schmassmann A et al: Quantification of human sperm morphology and motility by means of semi-automatic image analysis systems, *Microscopica Acta* 82:163, 1979.
66. Schrader SM: Data gaps and new methodologies in the assessment of male fecundity in occupational field studies, *Scand J Work Environ Health* 18 (Suppl 2):30, 1992.
67. Schrader SM et al: Laboratory methods for assessing human semen in epidemiologic studies: a consensus report, *Reprod Tox* 6:275, 1992.
68. Schrader SM et al: Sperm viability: a comparison of analytical methods, *Andrologia* 18:530, 1986.
69. Schrader SM et al: Morphometric analysis of human spermatozoa, *J Androl* 5:22, 1984.
70. Schrader SM et al: The use of new field methods of semen analysis in the study of occupational hazards to reproduction: the example of ethylene dibromide, *J Occup Med* 29:963, 1987.
71. Schrader SM, Turner TW, Ratcliffe JM: The effects of ethylene dibromide on semen quality: a comparison of short term and chronic exposure, *Reprod Toxicol* 2:191, 1988.
72. Schrader SM, Turner TW, Simon SD: Longitudinal study of semen quality of unexposed workers: sperm motility characteristics, *J Androl* 12:126, 1991.
73. Schrader SM et al: Measurement of male reproductive hormones for field studies, *JOM* (in press), 1993.
74. Sever LE, Hessol NA: Toxic effects of occupational and environmental chemicals on the testes. In Thomas JA ed: *Endocrine Toxicology,* New York, 1985, Raven Press.
75. Shafik A, Ibrahim IH, Elsayed EM: Effect of different types of textile fabric on spermatogenesis. I. Electrostatic potentials generated on surface of human scrotum by wearing different types of fabric, *Andrologia* 24:145, 1992.
76. Smith CG, Asch RH: Drug abuse and reproduction, *Fertil Steril* 48:355, 1987.
77. Sokol RZ: Endocrine evaluation in the assessment of male reproductive hazards, *Reprod Toxicology* 2:217, 1988.
78. Stachel B: Toxic environmental chemicals in human semen—analytical method and case studies, *Andrologia* 21:282, 1989.

79. Stachel B et al: Toxic environmental chemicals in human semen: analytical method and case studies, *Andrologia* 21:282, 1989.
80. Starr TB: Issues relating to surveillance of worker fertility, *Am J Ind Med* 9:579, 1986.
81. Steeno OP, Pangkahila A: Occupational influences on male fertility and sexuality, *Andrologia* 16:93, 1984.
82. Stillman RJ, Rosenberg MJ, Sachs BP: Smoking and reproduction, *Fertil Steril* 46:545, 1986.
83. Thomas JA: Reproductive hazards and environmental chemicals: a review, *Toxic Substance Journal* 2:318, 1981.
84. Thomas AJ Jr: Ejaculatory dysfunction, *Fertil Steril* 39:445, 1983.
85. Turner TW, Schrader SM, Simon SD: Sperm head morphometry as measured by three different computer systems, *J Androl* 9:45, 1988.
86. U.S. Environmental Protection Agency, Office of Toxic Substances: Chemical substance inventory, EPA publication 620-929/0027, 1985, supplement EPA publication 722-666, Washington, DC, 1990.
87. Vantman D et al: Computer-assisted semen analysis: evaluation of method and assessment of the influence of sperm concentration on linear velocity determination, *Fertil Steril* 49:510, 1988.
88. Welch LS, Plotkin E, Schrader S: Indirect fertility analysis in painters exposed to ethylene glycol ethers: sensitivity and specificity, *Am J Indust Med* 20:229, 1991.
89. Welch LS et al: Effects of exposure to ethylene glycol ethers on shipyard painters. I. Male reproduction, *Am J Ind Med* 14:509, 1988.
90. Whorton D et al: Infertility in male pesticide workers, *Lancet* 2:1259, 1977.
91. Brown-Woodman PDC et al: The effect of a single sauna exposure on spermatozoa, *Arch Androl* 12:9, 1984.
92. Zikarge A: Cross-sectional study of ethylene dibromide-induced alterations of seminal plasma biochemistry as a function of post-testicular toxicity with relationships to some indices of semen analysis and endocrine profile, dissertation to the University of Texas Health Science Center, Houston, Tex, 1986.
93. Zukerman Z et al: Quantitative analysis of the seminiferous epithelium in human testicular biopsies, and the relation of spermatogenesis to sperm density, *Fertil Steril* 30:448, 1978.

Chapter 9

FEMALE REPRODUCTIVE SYSTEM

Jeannette Gómez
Donald R. Mattison

Structure of the female reproductive system
    The hypothalamus and pituitary
    The ovary
    The fallopian tubes
    The uterus and cervix
    The vagina
Endocrine function
    The hypothalamic-pituitary relationship
    Hormones of the hypothalamus and the pituitary
    Hormones of the ovary
The menstrual cycle
Fertilization to implantation
Target sites for chemical injury in the female reproductive system
    The hypothalamus
    The pituitary
    The ovary
Mechanisms of action of reproductive toxicants
Direct-acting reproductive toxicants
Indirect-acting reproductive toxicants
Reproductive risk assessment
    Use of animal studies to define human reproductive risk
    Endpoints used in reproductive toxicity studies in animals
    Study design and statistical issues
Clinical evaluation
Conclusions

The female reproductive system is complex in both structure and function. These complexities, while necessary for normal function, also provide many sites at which female reproduction may be vulnerable to disruption by chemical, biologic, physical, or ergonomic stressors. The goal of this chapter is to review the structure and function of the female reproductive system up to implantation and use that framework to discuss sites of vulnerability to disruption by environmental factors. Early fetal development, teratology, fetal growth, and toxicity are covered in other sections of the book.

STRUCTURE OF THE FEMALE REPRODUCTIVE SYSTEM

The female reproductive system is controlled by components of the central nervous system (CNS), including the hypothalamus and pituitary.[31] It consists of the ovaries, the fallopian tubes, the uterus, and the vagina. The ovaries, the female gonads, are the source of oocytes and also synthesize and secrete estrogens and progestogens, the major female sex hormones. The fallopian tube transports oocytes and sperm to and from the uterus. The uterus is a pear-shaped muscular organ, the upper part of which communicates through the fallopian tubes to the abdominal cavity, while the lower part is contiguous through the narrow canal of the cervix with the vagina, which passes to the exterior.

THE HYPOTHALAMUS AND PITUITARY

The hypothalamus is located in the diencephalon, which sits on top of the brainstem and is surrounded by the cerebral hemispheres. The hypothalamus is the principal intermediary between the nervous and the endocrine systems, the two major control systems of the body.[62] The hypothalamus regulates the pituitary gland and produces two hormones of its own.

The pituitary lies deep in the cranial cavity within the sella turcica of the sphenoid. It is attached to the hypothalamus of the brain by a stalklike structure, the infundibulum.[62] The pituitary is divided structurally and functionally into anterior pituitary (adenohypophysis) and posterior (neurohypophysis) pituitary. The anterior pituitary has the microscopic structure of an endocrine gland, whereas the posterior pituitary has the structure of nervous tissue.

The anterior pituitary is under the influence of the hypothalamus by means of hormones released into a portal circulation, the hypophyseal portal system.[56] This hypophyseal portal system connects the blood supply of the hypothalamus with that of the anterior pituitary and is critical for the functioning of the pituitary. The hypophyseal portal system is composed of capillaries into which peptides and other neurotransmitters are secreted by cell bodies in the hypothalamus and are transported to the anterior pituitary.

The blood supply of the anterior pituitary and infundibulum originates principally from several superior hypophyseal arteries. These form a network or plexus of capillaries, the primary plexus. Regulating factors from the hypothalamus diffuse into the plexus, which drains into the hypophyseal portal vein. At the inferior portion of the infundibulum the veins form a secondary plexus in the anterior pituitary. From this plexus, hormones of the pituitary pass into the anterior hypophyseal veins for distribution. This transport system permits regulating factors to act on the anterior pituitary without circulating throughout the body.

The posterior pituitary does not synthesize hormones but contains the terminations of secretory neurons, called *neurosecretory cells,* which originate in the hypothalamus. The cell bodies of the neurons originate in the hypothalamus. Fibers project from the hypothalamus to form the hypothalamic-hypophyseal tract and terminate on blood capillaries in the posterior pituitary.

The blood supply to the posterior pituitary is from the inferior hypophyseal arteries, which form a plexus of capillaries called the *plexus of the infundibular process.* From this plexus, hormones stored in the posterior pituitary pass in the posterior hypophyseal veins for distribution.

The ovary

The ovary consists of three regions: the outer cortex, inner medulla, and hilum. The outer cortex, which is enveloped by the germinal epithelium, contains the follicles. These functional units of the ovary are present in different states of development or degeneration (atresia), and each generally contains a single oocyte. In addition to the oocyte, ovarian follicles have two other cellular components: granulosa cells that surround the oocyte and thecal cells that are separated from granulosa cells by a basement membrane. The inner medulla consists of stromal cells and cells with steroid-producing characteristics. The hilum serves as a point of entry of the nerves and blood vessels to the ovary. The major physiologic functions of the ovary are the periodic release of gametes (oocytes) and the production of the steroid hormones, estradiol and progesterone.[56]

Oocytes are formed prenatally in the female with no new formation after mid-gestation. At birth each ovary contains about 1 million oocytes, many of which undergo degeneration. By puberty this number will decrease to between 200,000 to 400,000. Of these, about 400 are destined to complete oogenesis and be ovulated. Any agent that damages oocytes will accelerate atresia and lead to reduced or absent fertility.[61]

Follicles begin to mature even before birth, but they do not mature or grow beyond the pre-antral state before puberty. At puberty, changes in the hypothalamus and pituitary result in a decreased resistance to the feedback inhibition by estrogens. As a result, follicle growth is further supported so that beginning at puberty follicles develop an antrum. Follicles develop throughout the life of the female until menopause, when the ovary is depleted of oocytes. Within the follicle the oocyte will mature and either be ovulated or undergo atresia. Growth of the follicle is accompanied by growth of granulosa cells, enlargement of the oocyte, and formation of an outermost connective-tissue layer, the theca, consisting of two layers, the theca interna and externa. The theca interna contains many blood capillaries.[7] The development of one or more follicles into a mature follicle is cyclic, occurring about once every 28 days. After ovulation, the ruptured follicle is transformed into a hormone-secreting glandular structure called the *corpus luteum.*[59]

The maintenance and growth of the follicle to maturity is brought about by follicle-stimulating hormone (FSH), which is secreted by the anterior pituitary. Another hormone, luteinizing hormone (LH), secreted by the anterior pituitary, works in conjunction whit FSH to stimulate maturing and antral follicles to secrete estrogens. The midcycle surge of LH causes a mature follicle to rupture and release the oocyte into the peritoneal cavity, which makes it available to be picked up and transported into the fallopian tubes.

The fallopian tubes

The fallopian tubes are anatomically separated into ampulla, isthmus, and infundibulum. The ampulla is the central region where fertilization takes place and in which the oocyte completes its second maturation division. The isthmus is nearest to the uterus, joining it at the uterotubal junction. The infundibulum is a funnel-shaped structure adjacent to the ovaries and is surrounded by finger-like projections (fimbriae) that are thought to play an important role in picking up the oocyte after it is released from the follicle.[19]

Once the oocyte has been released from the ovary, tubal fluids and cilia act together to transport the oocyte into the uterus and through the fallopian tube by a combination of peristalsis and the rhythmic beating of the cilia.[24] If fertilization occurs, the conceptus enters into the uterus within about 7 days of ovulation. An unfertilized oocyte disintegrates in either the tube or the endometrial cavity.[63]

The uterus and cervix

The uterus, a pear-shaped muscular organ located in the pelvis between the urinary bladder and rectum, functions in three reproductive processes: menstruation, pregnancy, and labor.[24] It consists of a fundus, a body (corpus uteri), and a neck (cervix uteri). The wall of the uterus consists of three layers: an inner endometrium, a middle myometrium, and an external peritoneal surface. The endometrium undergoes cyclic changes during the menstrual cycle that are governed by the interaction of hormones of the pituitary and ovary and is significantly modified in pregnancy. The myometrium, the bulky middle layer of the uterus composed of interlacing bundles of smooth muscle,[24] plays an active role during childbirth, contracting to expel the fetus through the cervix and birth canal.[19,24,64]

Once fertilization occurs the zygote enters the uterus, the zona pellucida is shed, and the conceptus attaches to and penetrates into the endometrium. Implantation most often occurs in the upper portion of the uterus, although other sites are possible. When fertilization does not occur, the endometrial lining is shed, in response to decreasing levels of ovarian hormones[8] resulting from the degeneration of the corpus luteum.

The vagina

The vagina lies between the bladder and rectum and is a muscular, tubular organ lined with mucous membrane extending from the cervix to the vestibule.[19,63] It is often called the *birth canal* because it serves as the passageway for delivery and for the menstrual flow to leave the body. Also, it receives the penis and semen during sexual intercourse.[19] At the opening of the vagina is a thin fold of vascularized mucous membrane, a developmental remnant of the urogenital sinus called the *hymen,* which forms a border around the orifice, partially closing it.

ENDOCRINE FUNCTION

The function of the endocrine system is communication and control between cells by means of hormones secreted into the blood. Endocrine organs are small and widely separated throughout the body. Some are mixed glands (both endocrine and exocrine in function); others are purely hormone producing.[62] Endocrine systems work together to maintain the body's functional status by releasing hormones, which are main regulators of metabolism, growth and development, reproduction, and many other body activities.[60]

After leaving the blood and entering target cells, hormones exert their effect by binding to a specific receptor. Hormone receptors are found on the cell membrane in the cytoplasm or nucleus of the cell and act with the hormone to perform important regulatory functions. Once hormone-receptor binding has occurred,[60] a series of changes occur, causing the cell to respond in a particular way. A cell that binds hormones with a specific receptor and responds in a defined way is called a *target cell* for that hormone.

The secretion of hormones is typically regulated by negative and positive feedback mechanisms. Negative feedback is the most common, in which rising levels of hormone 1 stimulate production of hormone 2, which in turn acts on the cells producing hormone 1 to inhibit further synthesis and/or release. For example, adrenocorticotropic hormone (ACTH) stimulates the release of glucocorticoids hormones by the adrenal cortex. Rising levels of the glucocorticoids inhibit ACTH release.[62] Positive feedback mechanisms, which are uncommon but of critical importance in female reproduction, act in the following way: hormone 2 stimulates the production of hormone 1 instead of diminishing it.[40] For example, rising levels of estrogen initially inhibit the release of LH. At concentrations above about 200 pgm/ml, however, the feedback mechanism changes and LH release is stimulated, producing the midcycle LH surge and ovulation.

The major endocrine components of the reproductive system are the hypothalamus, the pituitary, and the gonads, which are linked by inhibitory and stimulatory feedback mechanisms.[16] Gonadotropin-releasing hormone (GnRH), produced by the hypothalamus, is secreted in a pulsatile fashion and transported to the pituitary by the hypophyseal portal system. In the pituitary, GnRH stimulates the synthesis and secretion of the gonadotropins. FSH and LH are glycoprotein hormones composed of alpha and beta subunits.[16] These hormones are secreted into the bloodstream and distributed throughout the body, including the ovary, where they regulate and stimulate growth and development of the follicle. The gonads secrete a series of steroid hormones including progesterone (P), androstenedione (A), testosterone (T), estrone (E_1), and estradiol (E_2) in the female. The steroids produced in the largest quantities by the ovary are progesterone and estradiol.[16]

The hypothalamic-pituitary relationship

The anterior pituitary secretes several hormones, each of which stimulates the growth and secretion of hormones by other endocrine organs. Because the anterior pituitary exerts this control over other organs, it is sometimes referred to as the *master gland* of the body.[23,60] However, the pituitary does not act on its own because the release of its hormones is controlled (either stimulated or inhibited) by hormones produced by the hypothalamus.

Hormones of the hypothalamus and the pituitary

The hypothalamus, which is part of the nervous system, is also part of the endocrine system because it synthesizes two hormones, antidiuretic hormone (ADH) and oxytocin. In addition, the hypothalamus produces releasing and inhibiting factors that are transported by the portal system to the anterior pituitary, where they stimulate or inhibit the production and release of anterior pituitary hormones.

The hypothalamus also produces and releases the peptide hormone GnRH, which is secreted in a pulsatile manner about every 60 to 90 minutes. The pulsatile release of GnRH is subject to feedback from the ovarian sex steroids, estradiol and progesterone.

While the anterior pituitary secretes several major hormones, for the purposes of this chapter we will discuss only those involved in the reproductive cycle. The gonadotrope is a pituitary cell that is responsible for the synthesis, storage, and release of FSH and LH.[50] Both ovulation and spermatogenesis are controlled by FSH and LH, which promote follicular development and formation of sperm as well as stimulate estrogen and testosterone secretion.[40]

FSH stimulates follicular development. As follicles mature, they produce estrogen and prepare the oocyte for ovulation. LH acts with FSH to perform several functions, including stimulating folliculogenesis, stimulating follicle cells to secrete estrogens, and causing ovulation. Additionally, LH is thought to stimulate the formation of the corpus luteum in a ruptured follicle.[59]

Prolactin (PRL) is a protein hormone that promotes mammary growth and with other hormones the initiation and continuation of milk secretion.[21] Stimulation of mammary glands by PRL requires preparation by estrogens, progesterone, corticosteroids, growth hormone, thyroxine, and insulin. When the mammary glands have been primed by these hormones, PRL brings about milk secretion.[62]

The release of PRL is under the influence of both an inhibitory and an excitatory control system. During the menstrual cycle, prolactin inhibiting factor (PIF), a regulating factor from the hypothalamus, inhibits the release of PRL from the anterior pituitary. The secretion of PIF diminishes and PRL rises in the blood when the levels of estrogens and progesterone drop. However, this effect does not last long and as the menstrual cycle starts up again and the level of estrogens rises, PIF is again secreted and the level of PRL drops. PRL levels also rise during pregnancy and a regulating factor called *prolactin releasing factor (PRF)* stimulates PRL secretion after long periods of inhibition. PRL levels decline after delivery and rise again during breast feeding.

Hormones of the ovary

The second major function of the ovary is the secretion of estrogen and progesterone. Estrogens, primarily estradiol (E_2) and estrone (E_1), are produced by antral follicles and are responsible for development and maintenance of the female secondary sex characteristics (hair patterns, breast development, increased deposition of fat beneath the skin and particularly in the hips and breast) and the onset of the menstrual cycle. Estrogens prepare the uterus to receive a fertilized egg and assist in the maintenance of pregnancy and preparation of the breasts for lactation. The major source of progesterone is the corpus luteum, which develops from a ruptured mature follicle. The primary functions of progesterone are to induce secretory activity of endometrial glands and stimulate endometrial vascular development, thereby preparing the endometrium for implantation.[50]

THE MENSTRUAL CYCLE

The menstrual cycle is a sequence of events centered around ovulation, which prepares the female reproductive system, especially the uterus, to support implantation and pregnancy should fertilization occur. The hallmark of the menstrual cycle is the periodic discharge of blood and disintegrating endometrium following ovulation.[35] The principal events of the menstrual cycle are associated with the changes that occur in the endometrium, which are hormonally controlled by the ovary. Normal menstruation depends on the functional integrity of several endocrine sites: hypothalamus, anterior pituitary, and granulosa-theca cells of the ovary and endometrium. They are often referred to collectively as the *hypothalamic-pituitary-ovarian-uterine axis (HPOU-axis)*. Each cycle consists of three stages: menstrual, follicular, and luteal, with a typical menstrual cycle about 26 to 32 days long. Ovulation occurs midway through the cycle on day 14. The length of the cycle varies between 21 to 35 days, with the greatest variability occurring during the follicular phase.

The menstrual phase is caused by the sudden decrease in estrogen and progesterone and occurs over approximately the first 5 days of the cycle. During menstruation a group of primary follicles begins to grow and develop into secondary follicles. The secondary follicles secrete follicular fluid and produce estrogens, the dominant ovarian hormones during this phase. The production of estrogen stimulates the hypothalamus to secrete GnRH, which causes release of FSH, which in turn stimulates further ovarian follicle development.

The preovulatory or follicular phase is the part of the cycle with the greatest variation in duration. Increasing concentrations of estrogens secreted by the dominant follicle stimulate the growth of the endometrium. During this phase the dominant follicle matures to a large follicle that is ready for ovulation. Close to the time of ovulation, as a result of the change in feedback mechanism, LH is secreted in increasing amounts, and small amounts of progesterone may be produced by the graafian follicle a day or two before ovulation.

The process of ovulation sets in motion changes in the structure and function of the follicle: the basement membrane separating granulosa and thecal cells breaks down, blood vessels penetrate the degenerating basement membrane, and granulosa cells enlarge and form the corpus luteum.

The postovulatory or luteal phase is the most constant phase of 13 days' duration, lasting from days 15 to 28 in a 28-day cycle. Following ovulation LH stimulates the differentiation of granulosa cells into luteal cells. During this process granulosa cells change from small, compact cells that produce estrogen to large luteal cells that produce progesterone. The cells that form the corpus luteum consist of "luteinized" granulosa cells, as well as thecal cells, fibroblasts, and capillaries that invade the follicle following ovulation.[41] These changes in hormone secretion prepare the endometrium for implantation. During this phase the dominant ovarian hormone is progesterone, and FSH secretion gradually increases and LH secretion decreases.

If fertilization and implantation do not occur, the rising levels of progesterone and estrogen from the corpus luteum inhibit GnRH and LH secretion. As a result secretion of progesterone and estrogen decrease, the corpus luteum degenerates, and the menstrual cycle begins again. If fertilization and implantation do occur, corpus luteum function is maintained by human chorionic gonadotropin (hCG), a hormone produced by the placenta. As a result estrogen and progesterone continue to be secreted by the corpus luteum for about 8 to 10 weeks. After that time the placenta secretes the estrogen and progesterone needed to support pregnancy and breast development for lactation.[14]

Menopause is the cessation of menstrual cycles. It occurs because the ovaries are depleted of oocytes. Menopause generally occurs at about age 50 and is marked by diminished production of estrogen, bursts of GnRH release, sudden body-temperature fluctuations, and other longer-term changes.[39]

FERTILIZATION TO IMPLANTATION

Gametogenesis, release, and union of male and female germ cells are all preliminary events leading to a zygote.[61] Sperm cells deposited in the vagina must enter the cervix and move through the uterus and into the fallopian tube to meet the ovum.[59] Penetration of ovum by sperm and the merging of their respective DNA comprise the process of fertilization.[61] After fertilization cell division is initiated and continues during the next 3 or 4 days, forming a solid mass of cells called a *morula*. The cells of the morula continue to divide, and by the time the developing embryo reaches the uterus, it is a hollow ball called a *blastocyst*.[39,59]

Following fertilization, the developing embryo migrates through the fallopian tubes into the uterus. The blastocyst enters the uterus and implants in the endometrium approximately 7 days after ovulation. At this time the endometrium is in the preovulatory phase. Implantation enables the blastocyst to absorb nutrients from the glands and blood vessels of the endometrium for its subsequent growth and development.[63]

TARGET SITES FOR CHEMICAL INJURY IN THE FEMALE REPRODUCTIVE SYSTEM

As described in the preceding sections, normal reproductive function in the female requires intact structure and integration of HPOU-axis functions (Table 9-1). For example, disruption of hypothalamic or pituitary function by a xenobiotic may ultimately impair normal ovarian processes such as oogenesis, folliculogenesis, follicle function, ovulation, luteinization, and corpus luteum function. Clinically, disruption of the HPOU-axis may manifest as amenorrhea, menstrual irregularity, or reduced or absent fertility. The following section briefly reviews sites vulnerable to toxicity and basic mechanisms of action of reproductive toxicants.

Table 9-1. Target sites in the female reproduction system

Site	Process important for normal female reproduction	Process vulnerable to impairment by xenobiotics
Hypothalamus	Periodic GnRH release Synthesis of oxytocin/ADH	Synthesis and secretion of GnRH[1]
Pituitary	Synthesis, storage, and release of gonadotropins FSH, LH, and/or prolactin Steroid feedback mechanisms	Response to estrogen or progesterone Synthesis and release of FSH/LH Ovulation
Ovary	Synthesis and release of estrogen/progesterone Oocyte numbers Growth and development of oocyte Release of oocyte	Response to FSH/LH/PRL synthesis and release of estrogen or progesterone Folliculogenesis Ovulation Luteinization Corpus luteum function
Fallopian tubes	Final maturation of oocyte Pickup and transport of oocyte Site of fertilization Transport of conceptus into uterus	Tubal secretion Cilia function for transport of oocyte Fertilization of oocyte
Uterus	Site of implantation Placental growth Fetal development	Development of endometrium lining[2] Facilitation of sperm transportation Capacitation of the sperm Maintenance of pregnancy
Cervix	Retention and delivery of the fetus	Maintenance of pregnancy[3]
Vagina	Entrance for sperm Delivery of fetus	Collection of sperm

1. Interaction with endogenous hormones and neurotransmitters.
2. Delivery of chemicals to the very early embryo.
3. Physical barrier to infectious agents.

The hypothalamus

The hypothalamus has permissive control of the menstrual cycle through the pulsatile release of GnRH at a critical frequency and concentration. Deviations in the pattern of GnRH release can seriously alter normal pituitary secretion of the gonadotropins.[2,8,10] Experimental disruption of the hypothalamus or the communication pathways to the anterior pituitary results in gonadal atrophy and amenorrhea.[2,8,10]

A chemical might disrupt the reproductive function of the hypothalamus by altering the frequency or amplitude of GnRH pulses. The processes susceptible to chemical injury are those involved in the synthesis and secretion of GnRH, that is, transcription or translation, packaging or axonal transport, and secretory mechanisms. Altered frequency or amplitude of GnRH pulses could also result from disruptions in stimulatory or inhibitory pathways that regulate the release of GnRH. Catecholamine, dopamine, serotonin, GABA, and endorphins all have some potential for altering the release of GnRH. Therefore, xenobiotics that are agonists or antagonists of these compounds have the potential ability to modify GnRH release, thus interfering with communication with the pituitary.

The pituitary

FSH, LH, and PRL, secreted by the anterior pituitary, play a critical role in maintaining the ovarian cycle, and governing follicle recruitment and maturation, steroidogenesis, completion of ova maturation, ovulation, and luteinization. Precise control of the reproductive cycle is accomplished by the anterior pituitary in response to positive and negative feedback signals from the ovary. The appropriate release of FSH and LH during the cycle controls events of normal follicular development, and in their absence, amenorrhea and gonadal atrophy ensue.

Toxicant-induced alterations in the synthesis, storage, or secretion of gonadotropin would seriously disrupt reproductive capacity. Steroid receptor agonists and antagonists might initiate an inappropriate release of gonadotropin from the pituitary, thereby disrupting the ovarian cycle. Xenobiotics might also interfere with normal feedback dynamics of ovarian steroids or other ovarian factors. Chemicals that alter endocrine homeostasis would induce steroid-metabolizing enzymes, thus reducing steroid half-life and the circulating level of steroids at the pituitary.

The ovary

The follicle is responsible for maintaining the delicate hormonal environment necessary to support the growth and maturation of an oocyte during folliculogenesis. As a result there are a number of potential sites available for xenobiotic interaction. In addition, there are different follicle populations within the ovary, which allows for differential follicle toxicity. The patterns of infertility induced by a chemical agent may depend upon the follicle type affected. For example, toxicity to primordial follicles would not produce immediate signs of infertility but would ultimately lead to a shortened reproductive life span. On the other hand, toxicity to the antral or preovulatory follicles would result in an immediate loss of reproductive function.

The follicle has three basic components: (1) granulosa cells, (2) thecal cells, and (3) the oocyte, each with characteristics that may make it uniquely susceptible to chemical injury.

Granulosa cells. As a component of the follicle and as the supporting cell for oocytes, granulosa cells have several sites of vulnerability, including FSH and LH receptors and processes involved in steroid production and cell proliferation (Table 9-2). Chemicals that are gonadotropin antago-

Table 9-2. Granulosa cells as targets for chemical injury

Site of action	Mechanism of action	Outcome
FHS and LH receptors	Decreased receptor population	Decreased estradiol production
		Accumulation of androgens → atresia
	Competition for receptor	Inadequate luteinization
		Decreased progesterone production
	Uncoupling of receptor to secondary messenger	Luteal phase defects
Steroid production	Altered estrogen production:	Excessive follicular androgens → atresia
	Inhibition or depression of aromatase activity	
	Inadequate source of androgens	Decreased estrogen → altered follicle growth
	Altered progesterone production:	Decreased progesterone → inhibition of FSH surge
	Inhibition of enzymes responsible for biosynthesis of progesterone from cholesterol	Decreased progesterone → luteal phase defect
	Inadequate luteinization of granulosa cells	
Cell proliferation	General cytotoxicity	Follicular atresia
	Mitotic inhibitors	
	Reduced production of growth factors	

From Plowchalk DR, Mendows MJ, Mattison DR: Female reproductive toxicity. In Paul M, ed: *Occupational and environmental reproductive hazards: a guide for clinicians*, Baltimore, 1992, Williams & Wilkins.

nists, damage gonadotropin receptors, or uncouple the receptor from other molecules essential for action will clearly have an adverse effect on granulosa cell function. For example, a toxicant that is a gonadotropin antagonist and acts by blocking access to the receptor will impair FSH-stimulated estrogen synthesis during the follicular phase of the cycle.

Thecal cells. Thecal cells provide the androgen precursors for estrogens synthesized by the granulosa cells and are believed to be recruited from ovarian stroma cells during follicle formation and growth. Xenobiotics that impair cell proliferation, migration, and communication will alter thecal cell function (Table 9-3). In addition, alterations in thecal cell androgen production are expected to have a significant effect on follicle function. Excess production of androgens by thecal cells may lead to atresia, while impaired androgen production may lead to decreased estrogen synthesis by granulosa cells. At the present time, little is known about thecal cell vulnerability to xenobiotics.

Oocytes. Oocytes in both humans and experimental animals can be damaged or destroyed by xenobiotics. Sites of action for chemical injury include processes integral to oocyte maturation and meiotic cell division (Table 9-4). Ionizing radiation and alkylating agents have been shown to destroy oocytes in both humans and experimental animals.[3] Lead produces ovarian toxicity characterized by follicular atresia in rodents and nonhuman primates.[43,66,70] Other metals, including mercury and cadmium, have also been shown to produce ovarian damage that may be mediated through oocyte toxicity.[33]

MECHANISMS OF ACTION OF REPRODUCTIVE TOXICANTS

Reproductive toxicants can be classified as either direct or indirect acting based on their mechanism of action.[28]

Direct-acting reproductive toxicants

Direct-acting reproductive toxicants elicit their effects by virtue of their inherent chemical reactivity; or through structural similarity to endogenous compounds (Table 9-5).

Chemical reactivity. Compounds classified in this category are toxic due to their inherent chemical reactivity; that is, they react with and damage important cellular macromolecules or organelles, thereby disrupting processes essential for the structural and functional integrity of the reproductive system. For example, the electrophilic reactivity of alkylating agents allows them to interact with nucleophilic

Table 9-3. Thecal cells as targets for chemical injury

Site of action	Mechanism of action	Outcome
LH receptors	Decreased receptor population	Decreased androgen biosynthesis Insufficient substrate for granulosa cells Altered follicular growth
Steroid production	Inhibition of enzymes responsible for the biosynthesis of androgens from cholesterol	Altered androstenedione and testosterone levels Insufficient substrate for granulosa cells
Cell proliferation	Disrupted migration of stroma to form thecal cell layer General cytotoxicity Mitotic inhibitors Reduced production of growth factors	

From Plowchalk DR, Mendows MJ, Mattison DR: *Female reproductive toxicity.* In Paul M, ed: *Occupational and environmental reproductive hazards: a guide for clinicians,* Baltimore, 1992, Williams & Wilkins.

Table 9-4. Oocytes as targets for chemical injury

Site of action	Mechanism of action	Outcome
Oocyte maturation	Disrupted communication between oocyte and granulosa cells of the corona radiata	Loss of proper biochemical signals for maturation
	Interference with synthesis and secretion of the zona pellucida proteins	Abnormal sperm receptor content → nonviable ovum
	General cytotoxicity to cellular process	Oocyte death
	Damage to oocyte DNA	
Meiotic maturation	Disrupted communication with granulosa cells	Untimely meiotic divisions
	Interference with mechanisms that control germinal vesicle breakdown	

From Plowchalk DR, Mendows MJ, Mattison DR: *Female reproductive toxicity.* In Paul M, ed: *Occupational and in environmental reproductive hazards: a guide for clinicians,* Baltimore, 1992, Williams & Wilkins.

Table 9-5. Direct-acting reproductive toxicants

Compound	Clinical manifestation	Site	Mechanism	Ref
Chemical reactivity				
Alkylating agents	Altered menses	Ovary	Granulosa cell	3
	Amenorrhea	Uterus	Oocyte cytotoxicity	26
	Ovarian atrophy			47
	Decreased fertility			
	Premature menopause			
Lead	Abnormal menses	Hypothalamus	Decreased FSH	43,66,70
	Ovarian atrophy	Pituitary	Decreased progesterone	
	Decreased fertility	Ovary		
Mercury	Abnormal menses	Hypothalamus	Altered gonadotropin production and secretion	33
		Ovary	Follicle toxicity	
			Granulosa cell proliferation	
Cadmium	Follicular atresia	Ovary	Vascular toxicity	33
	Persistent diestrus	Pituitary	Granulosa cell	
		Hypothalamus	Cytotoxicity	
Structural similarity				
Oral contraceptives	Altered menses	Hypothalamus	Altered FSH, LH release	15
		Pituitary		
Azathioprine	Reduced follicle numbers	Ovary	Purine analog	49
		Oogenesis	Disruption of DNA/RNA synthesis	
Chlodecone	Impaired fertility	Hypothalamus	Estrogen agonist	5,18,20
DDT	Altered menses	Pituitary		
2,4-D	Infertility			
Lindane	Amenorrhea			
Toxaphene	Hypermenorrhea			

From Plowchalk DR, Mendows MJ, Mattison DR: *Female reproductive toxicity.* In Paul M, ed: *Occupational and environmental reproductive hazards: a guide for clinicians,* Baltimore, 1992, Williams & Wilkins.
These compounds are suggested to be direct-acting reproductive toxicants based primarily on toxicity testing in experimental animals.

sites of important cellular components (DNA, RNA, proteins/enzymes). A number of metals such as lead, mercury, and cadmium are also thought to be reproductive toxicants because of their chemical reactivity.[33]

Structural similarity. These compounds are toxicants as a result of similarity to biologically important molecules. They imitate the action of endogenous molecules or substitute for an endogenous compound in a metabolic pathway, or compete for the receptors of an endogenous compound. Moreover, they are capable of triggering inappropriate responses or blocking normal responses in the target cell or organ. These compounds are generally agonists or antagonists of endogenous hormones or neurotransmitters. One of the best examples of compounds that act via their structural similarity are the synthetic steroids found in oral contraceptives, which interfere with normal ovarian function by suppressing gonadotropin secretion. Other examples include polychlorinated biphenyls (PCB), polybrominated biphenyls (PBB), and organochlorine pesticides, many of which are estrogen agonists.[5,18,20]

Indirect-acting reproductive toxicants

Indirect-acting toxicants alter reproductive function either after metabolic activation to a reactive metabolite or by altering normal endocrine homeostasis (Table 9-6).

Metabolism. In the process of removing a xenobiotic from the body, normal detoxification pathways generate metabolites with a different structure, some of which may be more reactive than the parent compound. These metabolites may then produce reproductive toxicity by the mechanisms of direct-acting compounds. For example, cyclophosphamide is an indirect-acting reproductive toxicant in both the male and female, requiring metabolic activation by cytochrome P-450 monooxygenase enzymes before it can generate chemically reactive metabolites.[55] Some of these metabolites are responsible for several different types of female reproductive toxicity, including ovarian and uterine toxicity.[26,45,47] Similarly, polycyclic aromatic hydrocarbons (PAH) are also dependent on microsomal enzymes for their bioactivation to highly potent metabolites capable of destroying ovarian follicles.[58]

Endocrine homeostasis. This category includes compounds that alter the pattern of release or circulating levels of steroid hormones important in reproduction by affecting steroid production, secretion, or clearance. Altered circulating levels of steroids can disrupt the feedback loops of the HPOU-axis that control the normal reproductive cycle. Examples of these compounds include barbiturates, PAH, PCB, PBB, DDT, and other insecticides known to selectively induce enzyme systems.[1,5,18,20,69]

Table 9-6. Indirect-acting reproductive toxicants

Compound	Clinical manifestation	Site	Mechanism	Ref
Metabolic activation				
Cyclophosphamide	Amenorrhea	Ovary	Follicle destruction	26,45,47,55
	Premature ovarian failure	Uterus	Uterine toxicity	
	Impaired fertility			
Polycyclic aromatic hydrocarbons	Impaired fertility	Ovary	Follicle destruction	27,29,54,57,58
	Altered menses	Liver	Enzyme induction	
Cigarette smoke	Impaired fertility	Ovary	Follicle destruction	34
	Premature menopause		Impaired ovulation	
	Altered steroid clearance			
DDT metabolites	Metabolism	Liver	Enzyme induction	20
Disrupted homeostatis				
Halogenated hydrocarbons DDT, PCB, PBB	Abnormal menses	Hypothalamus	FSH	5,18,20,69
		Pituitary	LH	
		Liver	Enzyme induction	
Barbiturates	Increased steroid clearance	Liver	Enzyme induction	1

From Plowchalk DR, Mendows MJ, Mattison DR: *Female reproductive toxicity.* In Paul M, ed: *Occupational and environmental reproductive hazards: a guide for clinicians,* Baltimore, 1992, Williams & Wilkins.
These compounds are suggested to be indirect acting reproductive toxicants based primarily on toxicity testing in experimental animals.

REPRODUCTIVE RISK ASSESSMENT

Regulatory agencies have developed systematic scientific and administrative approaches to assess risks associated with chemical exposures.[38] The process begins with *hazard identification* followed by *hazard characterization, exposure assessment,* and *risk characterization.* If valid quantitative human data exist, they can be used for hazard identification and for determining an acceptable human exposure level.[30] However, risk assessment is typically based on findings from laboratory animal studies. This section reviews approaches to protecting human reproductive health using data from animal studies, emphasizing the evaluation of study quality and relevance to humans, and describes some commonly used methods for assessing reproductive effects in animals.

Use of animal studies to define human reproductive risk

When adequate human data are not available, animal studies must be used to protect human reproductive health. Unfortunately, the quality and quantity of animal data vary considerably, and data are often nonexistent or insufficient to evaluate the potential for reproductive toxicity of a given chemical. For example, it is estimated that only 34% of pesticides and inerts, 22% of cosmetics, 45% of drugs, and 20% of food additives have sufficient data for evaluation of reproductive toxicity.[37] A recent survey by the Organization for Economic Cooperation and Development found that sufficient data for determining reproductive hazard[6] existed for only 367 of 948 high-production-volume organic chemicals and 148 of 390 high-production-volume inorganic chemicals. Therefore, even for chemicals with high production volumes and likely human exposure, there may be little available data for assessing the potential risks to reproduction.

It is customary to conduct animal experiments at dosages exceeding estimated levels of human exposure to increase the likelihood that a weak toxicant will produce a detectable effect, to compensate for the relatively small numbers of animals used in the assay, and to ensure that a negative assay is meaningful. An important step in characterizing the dose-response relationship in these studies is to determine the "no-observed-adverse-effect level" (NOAEL), that is the highest dose level at which no adverse biologic effects occur. Depending upon the sensitivity of the endpoint monitored and the test species utilized, different NOAELs may be derived for the same chemical. Generally, if multiple endpoints suggest that the chemical is a reproductive toxicant, then the most sensitive one (the one that occurs at the lowest exposure level) should be used to establish the NOAEL. In defining the appropriate NOAEL the study selected should use an exposure route relevant to the human exposure whenever possible. If data from several species or strains are available, the most sensitive species should be used in determining the NOAEL, unless data from that species are not relevant to the human. A determination of relevance is based on the effect measured and the existence of comparable anatomic, physiologic, toxicologic, toxicokinetic, metabolic, and toxicodynamic processes for the effect in the test animal and in humans.

If sufficient data do not exist to determine the NOAEL for an endpoint, then the "lowest-observed-adverse-effect level" (LOAEL) should be used. Regardless of whether the NOAEL or the LOAEL is used, uncertainty or safety factors are typically applied to estimate an exposure level for humans at or below which there should be no adverse reproductive effects. This exposure level is often referred to as the reference dose or R_fD.[4] The total uncertainty factor usually ranges from 10 to 1000. Uncertainty factors of 10 each are applied (1) when the LOAEL must be used because a NOAEL was not established, (2) to account for differences between species, and (3) to provide an intraspecies adjustment for variable sensitivity among individuals. Additional adjustments may be made for inadequacy of the duration of the experiment, deficiencies in study design, or to account for special "sensitivity" of the human. Alternative approaches to the use of safety factors are being explored for both reproductive[30,36,42] and developmental toxicity.[9,13,48,65]

Endpoints used in reproductive toxicity studies in animals

Alterations in reproductive capacity measured in animals may be sufficient to classify an agent as a hazard to human reproduction (see box at right). Less conclusive results may indicate a potential hazard and suggest the need for further investigation.

Some chemicals cause reversible reproductive effects in the adult female. Exposures leading to effects in this category are likely to be of lower risk to human reproduction than those that cause permanent damage. However, exposure to a reversible reproductive toxicant may delay a desired pregnancy and result in a shifting of couples to a smaller completed family size. In other words, a temporary effect on fertility may permanently alter family size if that transient effect occurs during attempted reproduction.

Endpoints that are commonly evaluated in animal breeding studies and that may be most useful in identifying a potential human reproductive hazard are summarized in the box on p. 111. The first seven endpoints indicate the ability of animals to mate, conceive, or deliver live offspring and, as such, measure overall effects on female feundity. These endpoints should be considered collectively when evaluating study results. The survival indices measure pup survival from birth through postnatal day 21, expressed in increments over that time period. The body weights and growth of offspring are likely to be insufficient to definitively identify a reproductive hazard because of the myriad factors independent of test substance exposure that may affect these endpoints.

Biomarkers of female fecundity are listed in the box at right. Inhibition of ovulation or of implantation, delayed puberty, and early reproductive senescence[14,25] are the most compelling endpoints in defining a potential female reproductive hazard. The other endpoints listed are more difficult to interpret in terms of human reproductive risk. Recently, quantitative morphometric approaches have been developed to characterize the individual ovarian compartments affected by toxicants and the dynamic processes of ovarian toxicity.[44,46,68]

Study design and statistical issues

Several general principles guide the use of animal studies to assess potential human reproductive risk. In general, the relevance of animal studies to humans is based on (1) consistency among animal studies of patterns of exposure, ab-

---

Indices of female fecundity in laboratory animals

Estrous cycle disruption resulting in anovulation
Reduction in the number of ovarian follicles or oocytes
Altered uterine histology or function
Altered ovarian histology characterized by reduced corpora lutea or increased number of ovarian cysts
Altered concentration or temporal patterns of peptide or steroid hormones
Alterations in ovarian or uterine weight
Delayed puberty
Premature reproductive senescence

From Mattison DR et al: Criteria for identifying and listing substances known to cause reproductive toxicity under California's Proposition 65, *Reprod Toxicol* 4:163, 1990.

normal outcomes, and causal associations; (2) concordance of reproductive biology; and (3) evidence indicating biologic plausibility of mechanism of action. These factors must be consistent with human biologic principles.

In the interpretation of data from animal reproductive toxicology studies, the quality, design, conduct, and statistical analyses of the study must be taken into consideration; deficiencies in these factors may lead to the application of additional safety factors. The data used should be derived from studies of acceptable quality in mammalian species that are predictive of human responses. Animals should be exposed to the test compound by a route of administration relevant to the human route of exposure. Other routes may be relied upon by taking into consideration physiologic and toxicologic information. Also, exposures should be at the proper time and for the proper duration so as to maximize detection of an effect. In all cases, endpoints evaluated in animal reproduction studies should be predictive of adverse human reproductive outcomes (see boxes above and on p. 111).

For an agent to be identified as a reproductive hazard, adverse reproductive effects should occur at doses that do not cause significant systemic toxicity that could interfere with mating ability or frequency. When reproductive and systemic effects occur concomitantly, scientific judgment is needed to determine the probability of reproductive toxicity at lower doses.

Another important consideration is the power of the study, or the probability that the study demonstrates a true effect. Power is dependent on sample size, as well as on the background incidence and variability of the endpoint(s) examined. The apparent lack of an effect may be due to a true absence of activity or to the inability to identify an effect because of small sample size. Conversely, some statistically significant effects may arise by chance, especially if a large number of endpoints are analyzed. The use of appropriate historical control data and critical attention to toxicologic and reproductive biologic principles may prevent false assumptions in such cases.

Reproductive indices commonly used to assess female reproduction function in animal breeding studies

Female mating index $= \dfrac{\text{Number of females for which mating was confirmed} \times 100}{\text{Number of females used for mating}}$

Female fertility index $= \dfrac{\text{Number of females confirmed pregnant} \times 100}{\text{Number of females for which mating was confirmed}}$

Gestation index $= \dfrac{\text{Number of females delivering at least one live offspring} \times 100}{\text{Number of females confirmed pregnant}}$

Number of implantations per pregnant female

Number of pre- and postimplantation losses

Litter size at birth

Live birth index $= \dfrac{\text{Mean number of live offspring per litter} \times 100}{\text{Mean number of offspring per litter}}$

Survival indices $= \dfrac{\text{Number of live offspring on postnatal day 4} \times 100}{\text{Number of live offspring born}}$

$= \dfrac{\text{Number of live offspring on postnatal day 7} \times 100}{\text{Number of live offspring on postnatal day 4}}$

$= \dfrac{\text{Number of live offspring on postnatal day 14} \times 100}{\text{Number of live offspring on postnatal day 7}}$

$= \dfrac{\text{Number of live offspring on postnatal day 21} \times 100}{\text{Number of live offspring on postnatal day 14}}$

From Mattison DR et al: Criteria for identifying and listing substances known to cause reproductive toxicity under California's Proposition 65, *Repro Toxicol* 4:163, 1990.

The number of animals per dose group should be determined after consideration of a variety of factors, including the general toxicity of the substance being tested, which will affect the number of animals that survive to provide data and the expected variation of the reproductive endpoints being measured. The likely magnitude of the effect should also be considered, as well as the level of significance desired to establish a positive finding.

Reproductive toxicity studies often involve observations on animals from the same litter. Litter mates tend to respond more similarly to a test substance than animals from different litters.[22,67] This litter effect is taken into account by using the variation between litters rather than the variation within litters as the basis for statistical analysis.[12]

Data from replicate studies and multiple independent study types should be consistent and reinforcing. When data are discordant, sufficient additional evidence should be available to reconcile the differences. Confidence in a study outcome may be increased by the demonstration of a dose-response relationship. However, competing endpoints may obscure dose-response relationships in some cases.[52] Negative findings deserve special scrutiny regarding study design and conduct. In general, the highest dose used should produce systemic toxicity in the sexually mature animal. These studies must include sufficient numbers of animals to detect an adverse effect, appropriate dose levels and exposure routes, and appropriate statistical methods. Negative studies should also indicate the power to define an adverse effect or the confidence interval on the null hypothesis.

CLINICAL EVALUATION

A number of environmental exposures are known to produce adverse reproductive outcomes, including lead, ionizing radiation, cigarette smoking, infections, certain drugs and medications (estrogens, androgens, alkylating agents, anesthetic gases, anticonvulsants, and coumarin), and pesticides. To determine the etiology of reproductive disease it is essential that personal, medical, family, occupational, and reproductive history be taken into consideration.[39] Determining current and past medication taken is essential. The woman should be asked about types of occupational and environmental exposures. The exact date of her last menstrual period and the exact time sequence of any environmental exposure is important information to obtain. The period of organogenesis (18 to 55 days after fertilization) is a critical period for some reproductive hazards to produce their effects.

The anatomic evaluation should include physical examination of the external genitalia, vagina, and pelvis (Table 9-7). The major anatomical causes of subfertility or infertility in the female are structural abnormalities of the fallopian tubes and the uterus. Evaluation of the cervix, uterus, fal-

Table 9-7. Anatomic and functional techniques for evaluating female reproduction

Site	Test
External genitalia/vagina	Physical examination
Cervix	Physical examination
	Imaging techniques
	X-ray examination
	Magnetic resonance imaging (MRI)
	Ultrasound
Uterus	Physical examination
	Imaging techniques
	X-ray examination
	Magnetic resonance imaging (MRI)
	Ultrasound
	Hysterosalpingography
	Laparoscopy
Fallopian tubes	Hysterosalpingography
	Laparoscopy
Ovary	Ultrasound
	Laparoscopy
Hypothalamus	Response to GnRH agonist or antagonist challenge
	Indirect measure based on LH/FSH immunoassay
Pituitary	LH/FSH immunoassay
	Response to GnRH agonist or antagonist challenge
	Basal body temperature (BBT)
Pituitary gonadotropins	Immunoassay of serum for pattern of FSH/LH
Gonadal steroids	Measure of steroids (estrogen, pregnanediol, pregnanetriol) in 24-hr urine collection and/or serum with immunoassays
Estradiol	
Progesterone	
Human chorionic gonadotropin (hCG)	Immunologic assay
Ovary	LH
	Estrogen/progesterone
	Basal body temperature
	Endometrial assay
	Cervical mucus
Uterus	Regular bleeding (response to hormone changes)
	Endometrial biopsy
Cervix	Cervical mucus

lopian tubes, and ovary is generally not possible without imaging or invasive techniques.

After structural evaluation of the reproductive system has been completed, functional competence is assessed. The major functional abnormality associated with subfertility or infertility in the female is a result of disorders of ovulation. For that reason initial attention should be directed toward the evaluation of the ovary, pituitary, and hypothalamus.

An infertility examination addressing the presence of anovulation may require serial recording of basal body temperature, obtaining serum progesterone levels, and performing an endometrial biopsy during the luteal phase. Ovarian function may be assessed by measurements of serum or urinary estrogen, blood FSH, and LH. It may also be necessary to measure G_nRH.

If fetal abnormalities are suspected, prenatal evaluation of a fetus may require such techniques as ultrasound, radiography and more invasive fetoscopy, fetography, and aminography. There may be a need to analyze fetal tissue through amniocentesis, chorionic villus sampling, fetoscopy for fetal blood, or skin or liver specimens.

CONCLUSIONS

The female reproductive system is complex and requires precisely regulated local and circulating hormones for proper functioning. Multiple sites along the HPOU-axis are available for disruption of reproduction in the female. Unfortunately, few data are currently available addressing the actual vulnerability of human female reproduction to xenobiotics. When experiments have been conducted, impairment of reproduction or reproductive processes has been demonstrated for many chemicals. Careful attention to the design of animal experiments focusing on the vulnerable processes in female reproduction and broadening our knowledge of the impact of many chemicals on female reproductive function are essential for the development of public health strategies that protect reproductive health.

When attempting to characterize the potential hazard of a drug or chemical exposure on reproduction, it is necessary to evaluate a hierarchy of information. In a very few cases, sufficient human data are available to accomplish this task. In those instances it may be a relatively simple exercise to counsel the patient appropriately[30,32] or to define an exposure level that protects public health.

More often, it is necessary to rely on animal data. In general, animal studies correctly identify most human reproductive toxicants.[11,17] However, animal studies also identify many more chemicals as reproductive toxicants than have been confirmed in humans.[17,51,53] This may not be a problem from a public health perspective, as it is probably better to overestimate than underestimate risk to humans.

After the chemical has been identified as a potential hazard, it is necessary to characterize the dose-response relationship, as well as the site and mechanism of action. These steps are necessary to appropriately extrapolate the animal data to humans to estimate qualitatively or quantitatively the risk to reproduction. After hazard identification and hazard characterization have been completed, the next step is characterization of exposure. What was the concentration, duration, and relationship of the exposure to the critical milestones of reproduction? Chemicals that are reproductive toxicants may have biologic windows during which they produce adverse effects. Exposure outside of these windows may be associated with substantially smaller or no risk to the vulnerable reproductive process.

Unfortunately, there are often insufficient data even to characterize a chemical as a reproductive hazard. In these cases, proper clinical guidance is indeed difficult. In some cases, careful comparison of the structure of the chemical to that of known reproductive toxicants may be useful in estimating the potential for harm. Other factors that may be of value in determining whether the exposure or treatment carries risk include timing and duration of exposure and the presence or absence of systemic toxicity.

In the face of inadequate data, two different approaches may be useful in protecting public health. One approach assumes that the chemical is a potent reproductive and toxicant until proven otherwise and allows *no* human exposure. Another approach assumes that a stringent safety factor (at least 1000-fold) applied to the NOEL will protect human reproductive health. This method may be insufficient for some chemicals or sensitive subpopulations. It has been suggested that protection against cancer also prevents reproductive toxicity; unfortunately, this assertion does not seem to be correct.[13] For those chemicals to which large numbers of humans are exposed or where human exposure is to high concentrations, even more stringent safety factors may be necessary until adequate testing is available.

Consideration should be given to the redesign of many of the existing toxicologic testing protocols with reproductive endpoints specifically in mind. However, it will still be many years before the large number of untested chemicals receives any evaluation in a bioassay. Rapid and inexpensive alternative approaches are needed to screen chemicals for reproductive and developmental toxicity and to prioritize chemicals for the more expensive and time-consuming bioassays.

The structure and function of the female reproductive system and its vulnerability to damage by xenobiotics is complex and the concepts that underlie our understanding are changing. The references listed provide a more detailed introduction to the appropriate topics and the experimental literature that supports these concepts. In addition, the reader is also encouraged to perform a current literature review on any topic of importance to a patient or community before providing clinical advice.

REFERENCES

1. Aronson JK, Grahame-Smith DG: Clinical pharmacology: adverse drug interactions, *Br Med J* 6260: 282, 1981.
2. Baker TG: The control of oogenesis in mammals. In Migley AR, Sadler WA, eds: *Ovarian follicular development and function,* New York, 1979, Raven Press.
3. Barber HRK: The effect of cancer and its therapy upon fertility, *Int J Fertil* 26:250, 1981.
4. Barnes DG, Dourson M: Reference dose (RfD): description and use in health risk assessments, *Regul Toxicol Pharmacol* 8:471, 1988.
5. Bitman J, Cecil HC: Estrogenic activity of DDT analogs and polychlorinated biphenyls, *J Agric Food Chem* 18:1108, 1970.
6. Brydon JE et al: OECD's work on investigation of high production volume chemicals, report prepared for the Organization for Economic Cooperation and Development (OECD), May 2, 1990.
7. Davson H, Segal MB: Reproduction and lactation. In Davson H, Segal MB, eds. *Introduction to physiology, basic mechanisms,* vol 2, New York, 1975, Grune & Stratton.
8. diZerega GS, Hodgen GD: Folliculogenesis in the primate ovarian cycle, *Endocr Rev* 2:27, 1981.
9. Faustman EM et al: Characterization of a developmental toxicity dose-response model, *Environ Health Perspect* 79:229, 1989.
10. Fink G: Gonadotropin secretion and its control. In Knobil E, Neill JD, eds: *The physiology of reproduction,* New York, 1988, Raven Press.
11. Frankos VH: FDA perspectives on the use of teratology data for risk assessment, *Fundam Appl Toxicol* 5:615, 1985.
12. Gad SC, Weil CS: Statistics for toxicologists. In Hayes AW, ed: *Principles and methods of toxicology,* ed 2, New York, 1989. Raven Press.
13. Gaylor DW: Quantitative risk analysis for quantal reproductive and developmental effects, *Environ Health Perspect* 79:243, 1989.
14. Greep RO, ed: Recent progress in hormone research. Proceedings of the 1985 Laurentian hormone conference, vol 42, Orlando, Fla, 1986, Academic Press.
15. Harrington JM et al: Occupational hazards of formulating contraceptives: a survey of plant employees, *Arch Environ Health* 33:12, 1978.
16. Huff RW, Pauerstein CJ: *Human reproduction physiology and pathophysiology,* New York, 1979, Wiley.
17. Jelovsek FR, Mattison DR, Chen JJ: Prediction of risk for human developmental toxicity: how important are animal studies for hazard identification? *Obstet Gynecol* 74:624, 1989.
18. Kimbrough RD: The toxicity of polychlorinated polycyclic compounds and related chemicals, *Crit Rev Toxicol* 4:445, 1974.
19. Korach KS, Quarmby VE: Morphological, physiological, and biochemical aspects of female reproduction. In Dixon RL, ed: *Reproductive toxicology,* New York, 1985, Raven Press.
20. Kupfer D: Effects of pesticides and related compounds on steroid metabolism and function, *Crit Rev Toxicol* 44:83, 1975.
21. Lachelin GCL: The hypothalamus and the pituitary gland. In Coates D, ed: *Introduction to clinical reproductive endocrinology,* Oxford, Boston, 1991, Butterworth-Heinmann.
22. Mantel N: Some statistical viewpoints in the study of carcinogenesis. In Homburger F, ed: *Progress in experimental tumor research,* vol 11, New York, 1969, S Karger.
23. Marieb EN: Endocrine system. In Adams M, ed: *Essentials of human anatomy & physiology,* Redwood City, Calif. 1991, Benjamin/Cummings.
24. Marieb EN: The reproductive system. In Adams M, ed: *Essentials of human anatomy & physiology,* Redwood City, Calif, 1991, Benjamin/Cummings.
25. Mastroianni L Jr, Paulsen CA, eds: *Aging, reproduction, and the climacteric,* New York, 1986, Plenum Press.
26. Mattison DR, Plowchalk DR: Reproductive toxicity of cyclophosphamide in the C57BL/6N mouse. II. Effects on uterine structure and function, *Reproductive Toxicology* 6:423, 1992.
27. Mattison DR, Shiromizu K, Nightingale MS: Oocyte destruction by polycyclic aromatic hydrocarbons, *Am J Ind Med* 4:191, 1983.
28. Mattison DR, Thomford PJ: Mechanisms of action of reproductive toxicants. In Working P, ed: *Toxicology of the male and female reproductive systems,* New York, 1989, Hemisphere.
29. Mattison DR, Thorgeirsson SS: Ovarian aryl hydrocarbon hydroxylase activity and primordial oocyte toxicity of polycyclic aromatic hydrocarbons in mice, *Cancer Res* 39:3471, 1979.
30. Mattison DR: An overview on biological markers in reproductive and developmental toxicology: concepts, definitions and use in risk assessment, *Biomed Environ Sci* 4:8, 1991.
31. Mattison DR: Clinical manifestations of ovarian toxicity. In Dixon RL, ed: *Reproductive toxicology,* New York, 1985, Raven Press.
32. Mattison DR: Drug effects on the fetus. In Rayburn WF, Zuspan FP, eds: *Drugs therapy in obstetrics and gynecology,* St. Louis, 1992, Mosby.
33. Mattison DR: Ovarian toxicity: effects on sexual maturation, reproduction and menopause. In Clarkson TW, Nordberg GF, Sager PR, eds: *Reproductive and developmental toxicity of metals,* New York, 1983, Plenum Press.

34. Mattison DR: The effects of smoking on reproduction from gametogenesis to implantation, *Environ Res* 28:410, 1982.
35. Mattox JH: The menstrual cycle. In Wilson JR, ed: *Obstetrics and gynecology,* St Louis, 1991, Mosby-Year Book.
36. Meistrich ML: Calculations of the incidence of infertility in human populations from sperm measures using the two distribution model. In Liso AR, ed: *Sperm measures and reproductive success: Institute for Health Policy Analysis forum on science, health and Environmental Risk,* 1990.
37. National Research Council: *Toxicity testing: strategies to determine needs and priorities,* Washington, DC, 1984, National Academy Press.
38. National Research Council: *Risk assessment in the federal government: managing the process,* Washington, DC, 1983, National Academy Press.
39. Office of Technology Assessment: Principals of reproductive biology and development. In *Reproductive health hazards in the workplace,* Washington, DC, 1985, Government Printing Office.
40. Ojeda SR, Griffin JE: Organization of the endocrine system. In Ojeda SR, Griffin JE, ed: *Textbook of endocrine physiology,* New York, 1992, Oxford University Press.
41. Ojeda SR: Female reproductive system. In Griffen JE, Ojeda SR, eds: *Textbook of endocrine physiology,* New York, 1992, Oxford University Press.
42. Pease W, Vandenberg J, Hooper K: Comparing alternative approaches to establishing regulatory levels for reproductive toxicants: DBCP as a case study, *Environ Health Perspect,* 91:141, 1991.
43. Petrusz P et al: Lead poisoning and reproduction: effects on pituitary and serum gonadotropins in neonatal rats, *Environ Res* 19:383, 1979.
44. Plowchalk DR, Mattison DR: Ovarian morphometric changes following cyclophosphamide treatment. In Hirshfield AN, ed: *Growth factors and the ovary,* New York, 1989, Plenum Press.
45. Plowchalk DR, Mattison DR: Phosphoramide mustard is responsible for the ovarian toxicity of cyclophosphamide, *Toxicol Appl Pharmacol* 107:472, 1991.
46. Plowchalk DR, Mattison DR: Reproductive toxicity of cyclophosphamide in the C57BL/GN mouse. I. Effects on ovarian structure and function, *Reprod Toxicol* 6:411, 1992.
47. Plowchalk DR, Mattison DR: Reproductive toxicity of cyclophosphamide in the C57BL/6N mouse. I. Effects on uterine structure and function, *Reprod Toxicol* 6:423, 1992.
48. Rai K, Van Ryzin J: A dose-response model for teratological experiments involving quantal responses, *Biometrics* 41:1, 1985.
49. Reimers TJ et al: B1-generation effects of 6-mercaptopurine on reproduction in mice, *Biol Reprod* 22:367, 1980.
50. Sacks PC: The menstrual cycle. In Scialli AR, Zinaman MJ, eds: *Reproductive toxicology and infertility,* New York, 1993, McGraw-Hill.
51. Schardein JL: *Chemically induced birth defects,* New York, 1985, Marcel Dekker.
52. Selevan SG, Lemasters GK: The dose-response fallacy in human reproductive studies of toxic exposures, *J Occup Med* 29:451, 1987.
53. Shepard TH: *Catalog of teratogenic agents,* ed 5, Baltimore, 1989, John Hopkins University Press.
54. Shiromizu K, Mattison DR: The effect of intraovarian injection of benzo(a)pyrene on primordial oocyte number and ovarian aryl hydrocarbon [benzo(a)pyrene] hydroxylase activity, *Toxicol Appl Pharmacol* 76:18, 1984.
55. Shiromizu K, Thorgeirsson SS, Mattison DR: Effect of cyclophosphamide on oocyte and follicle number in Sprague-Dawley rats, C57BL/6N and DBA/2N mice, *Pediatr Pharmacol* 4:213, 1984.
56. Speroff L, Glass RH, Kase NG: *Clinical gynecologic endocrinology & infertility,* Baltimore, 1983, Williams & Wilkins.
57. Takizawa K et al: Experimental ovarian toxicity following intraovarian injection of benzo(a)pyrene or its metabolites in mice and rats. In Dixon RL, ed: *Reproductive toxicology,* New York, 1985, Raven Press.
58. Takizawa K et al: Murine strain differences in ovotoxicity following intraovarian injection with benzo(a)pyrene, (+)-(7R,8S)-oxide,(−)-(7R,8R)-dihydrodiol, or (+)-(7R,8S)-diol-(9S,10R)-epoxide-2, *Cancer Res* 44:2571, 1984.
59. Thiobodeau GA, Patton K: The reproductive systems. In Allen D, ed: *The human body in health and disease,* St Louis, Mo, 1992, Mosby–Year Book.
60. Thiobodeau GA, Patton K: The endocrine system. In Allen D, ed: *The human body in health and disease,* St Louis, Mo, 1992, Mosby–Year Book.
61. Thomas JA: Toxic responses of the reproductive system. In Amdur MO, Doull JD, Klaassen CD, eds: *Casarett and Doull's toxicology: the basic science of poisons,* New York, 1991, Pergamon Press.
62. Tortora GJ, Anagnostakos NP: The endocrine system. In Wilson C, Gensburg R, Gordon HD, eds: *Principles of anatomy and physiology,* New York, 1984, Harper & Row.
63. Tortora GJ, Anagnostakos NP: Development and inheritance. In Wilson C, Gensburg R, Gordon HD, eds: *Principles of anatomy and physiology,* New York, 1984, Harper & Row.
64. Tortora GJ, Anagnostakos NP: The reproductive system. In Wilson C, Gensburg R, Gordon HD, eds: *Principles of anatomy and physiology,* New York, 1984, Harper & Row.
65. Van Ryzin J: Risk assessment for fetal toxicity, *Toxicol Ind Health* 1:299, 1985.
66. Vermanda-VanEck GJ, Meigs JW: Changes in the ovary of the rhesus monkey after chronic lead intoxication, *Fertil Steril* 11:223, 1960.
67. Weil CS: Selection of a valid number of sampling units and a consideration of their combination in toxicological studies involving reproduction, teratogenesis or carcinogenesis, *Food Cosmet Toxicol* 8:177, 1970.
68. Weitzman GA et al: Morphometric assessment of the murine ovarian toxicity of 7,12-dimethylbenz(a)anthracene, *Reprod Toxicol* 6:137, 1992.
69. Welch RM et al: Effect of halogenated hydrocarbon insecticides on the metabolism and uterotropic action of estrogens in rats and mice, *Toxicol Appl Pharmacol* 19:234, 1971.
70. Wide M: Interference of lead with implantation in the mouse: effect of exogenous oestradiol and progesterone, *Teratology* 21:187, 1980.

Chapter 10

PEDIATRIC DEVELOPMENTAL TOXICOLOGY

Cynthia Bearer

Exposure
    Physical location
    Breathing zones
    Oxygen consumption
    Quantity and quality of food consumed
    Normal behavioral development
Absorption
    Transplacental route
    Percutaneous route
    Respiratory tract
    Gastrointestinal tract
Distribution
Metabolism
Excretion
Target organ susceptibility
Summary

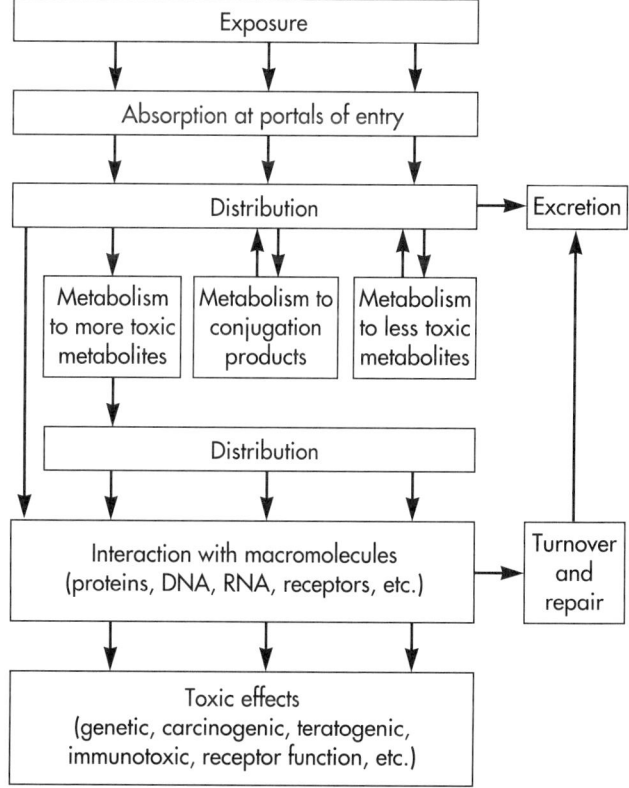

Fig. 10-1. Sequence of events following exposure of an individual to exogenous chemicals. Each of these processes is dependent on the developmental stage of the individual.[28] (From Hodgson E, Levi P, eds: *A textbook of modern toxicology*, New York, 1987, Appleton & Lange.)

Several factors alter an individual's risk for an environmentally related illness. They include genetic background, nutrition, age, lifestyle, and the like. These categories are not mutually exclusive but are influenced by each other. This chapter focuses on age as a susceptibility factor, specifically how exposure, absorption, metabolism, distribution, and target organ susceptibility change during development. Fig. 10-1 illustrates these processes.[28] Each of these processes is dependent on the stage of development of the individual. Developmental toxicology is the science of how these processes change throughout the growth and development of the individual. The changes in each of these processes are discussed individually with relevant clinical examples.

EXPOSURE

Exposure to an environmental agent is the first step in the sequence of environmentally related health effects. Exposures differ with developmental stage because children's environments are different from those of adults.

Consideration of exposures must examine the exposures of an individual over the course of a day. In general it is true that people may move through several environments during the course of a day—going on errands, going home, going to sleep—and such is also true for infants and children—going to school, going to day care, going to play (Fig. 10-2). What is needed is a sum total of all the exposures and/or some idea of the maximal exposure, but we are not usually able to put monitors on people and measure them. Usually our estimates of exposure are from retrospective estimates. Although the total exposure in a day may be the same for two individuals, the pattern of exposure may result in totally different health effects. For example, nitrates in well water may cause methemoglobinemia; however, if they are ingested at a rate at which the methemoglobin reductase can continue to keep the iron in hemoglobin in the reduced state, no health effect will occur, but if the dose exceeds the capacity of methemoglobin reductase, methemoglobinemia results[40] (Fig. 10-3). This is one mechanism that results in a threshold effect.

Exposures with profound health effects on an individual may occur at periods that frequently are not considered; for example, an exposure that happened to a woman prior to the conception of her child may have a profound effect on that child. For example, women who conceived after eating cooking oil contaminated with polychlorinated biphenyls (PCBs) gave birth to infants with yusho.[74] The mechanism responsible is thought to be storage of PCBs in adipose tissue during exposure that are then mobilized during preg-

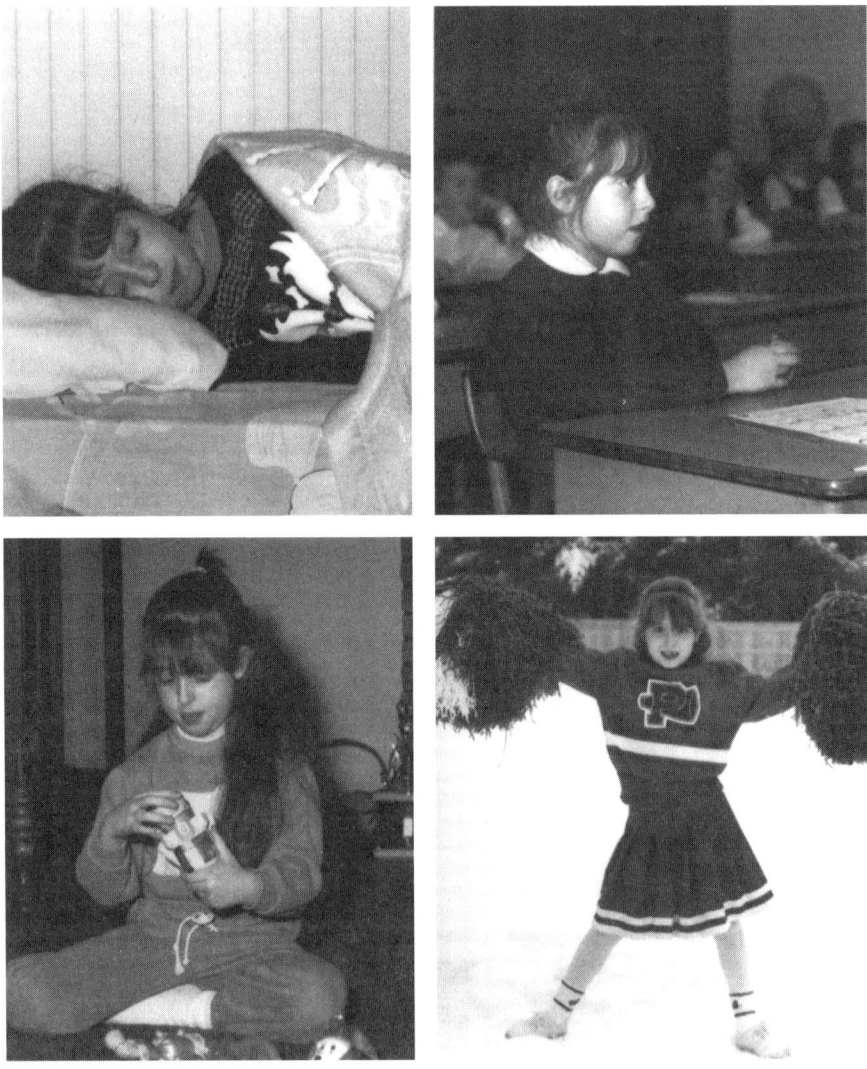

Fig. 10-2. A day in the life of a child. (Courtesy Joe Calderone and Kevin Mellott.)

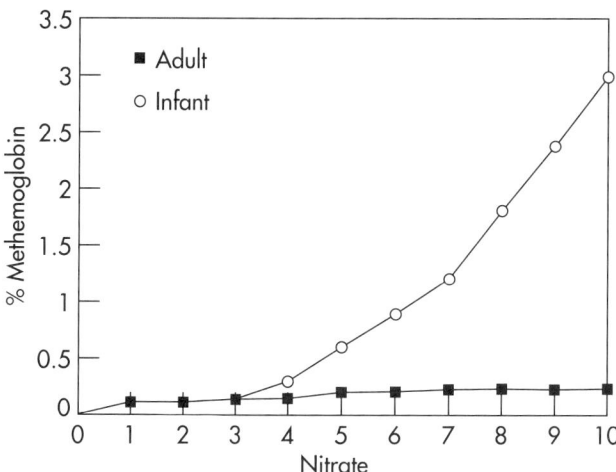

Fig. 10-3. Theoretical curve showing difference in adult versus infant erythrocytes to reduce methemoglobin. At low concentrations of an oxidant, nitrate, adult and infant erythrocytes are able to reduce methemoglobin. However, at higher levels of nitrate the infant's erythrocyte reducing capability is overwhelmed, resulting in accumulation of methemoglobin. This appears as a threshold effect.

nancy.[73,85] Another example is that of a woman who was inadequately treated for plumbism in childhood who gave birth to an infant with congenital lead poisoning.[65] Storage of the lead in bone with mobilization during pregnancy is the most logical explanation for this result[67] (Fig. 10-4).

Another exposure prior to conception that may result in effects on an individual is a preconception exposure that directly affects the ovum or sperm. The ovum, formed within the future mother during the fetal stage of her development, depends on the exposures to the grandmother and then to the mother (Fig. 10-5). The ovum, therefore, is a stage of development that sums all the exposures to the other stages of development. Studies have measured xenobiotics in follicular fluid, showing the potential for exposure.[75] Sperm, in contrast, are created only a few hours to days prior to conception. Thus the exposures to the sperm appear to depend on paternal exposure in the periconception period. There are few data about the influences of preconception paternal exposure on fetal development.

In most instances, exposures to the fetus depend on exposures to the mother; however, premature infants delivered after 24 weeks have very different exposures in the newborn intensive care unit (NICU), such as noise, light, compressed gases, intravenous solutions, and benzyl alcohol[8] (Fig. 10-6). Not only is the NICU a unique environment but these infants often remain in the same environment for months.

Exposures to newborns, infants, toddlers, school-aged children, and adolescents can be discussed with reference to changes in physical location, breathing zones, oxygen consumption, food consumption, types of foods consumed, and normal behavioral development.

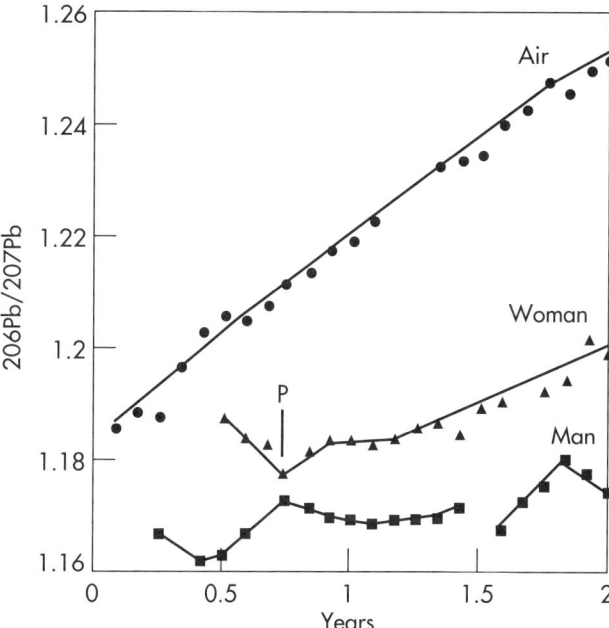

Fig. 10-4. Isotope ratio of lead in air and blood of a man and peripartum women in 1974 and 1975. P is the time of birth. The declining isotope ratio in the woman's blood before birth indicates a different source of lead than that of the man. Dietary lead was the same. The only different source of lead for the women is that coming from her bones during pregnancy.[41] (From Manton WI: Total contribution of airborne lead to blood lead, *Br J Ind Med* 42:168, 1985.)

Physical location

The physical location of children changes with development. The newborn is usually near the mother or held by the mother, so exposures are like those experienced by the mother. The newborn frequently spends more time in a single environment, such as a crib, for prolonged periods rather than in several different environments (Fig. 10-7). Infants and toddlers are frequently placed on the floor, carpet, or grass. Therefore, they have much more exposures to chemicals associated with these surfaces, such as formaldehyde and volatile organic chemicals off-gassing from synthetic carpet[5] and pesticide residues from flea bombs.[21]

Preambulatory children also may experience sustained exposure to noxious agents because they cannot remove themselves from their environment. An example is infants who are badly sunburned because of an inability to protect themselves. It has been shown that the risk of skin cancer is most closely related to the amount of sun damage the skin sustains during the first 18 years of life.[29]

School-aged children spend a significant amount of time at school, a physical environment very different from the home. Schools are frequently built on relatively undesirable land for economic reasons. These sites are frequently near

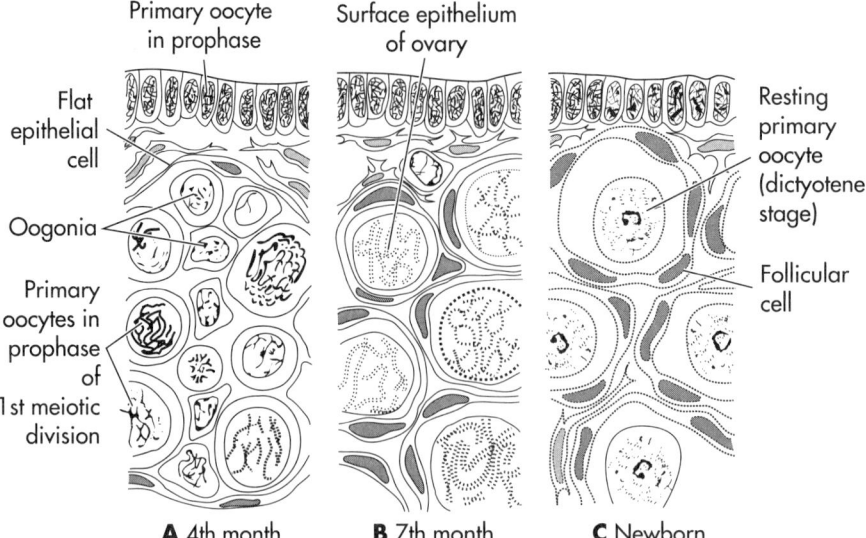

Fig. 10-5. Schematic representation of a segment of the ovary at different stages of development. **A,** At 4 months gestation. The oogonia are grouped in clusters in the cortical part of the ovary. Some show mitosis; others have already differentiated into primary oocytes and have entered the prophase of the first meiotic division. **B,** At 7 months gestation. Almost all the oogonia are transformed into primary oocytes in the prophase of the first meiotic division. **C,** At birth. Oogonia are absent. Each primary oocyte is surrounded by a single layer of follicular cells, thus forming the primordial follicle. The oocytes have entered the dictyotene stage, in which they remain until just before ovulation. Only then do they enter the metaphase of the first meiotic division.[35] (From Langman J: *Medical embryology,* Baltimore, 1975, Williams & Wilkins.)

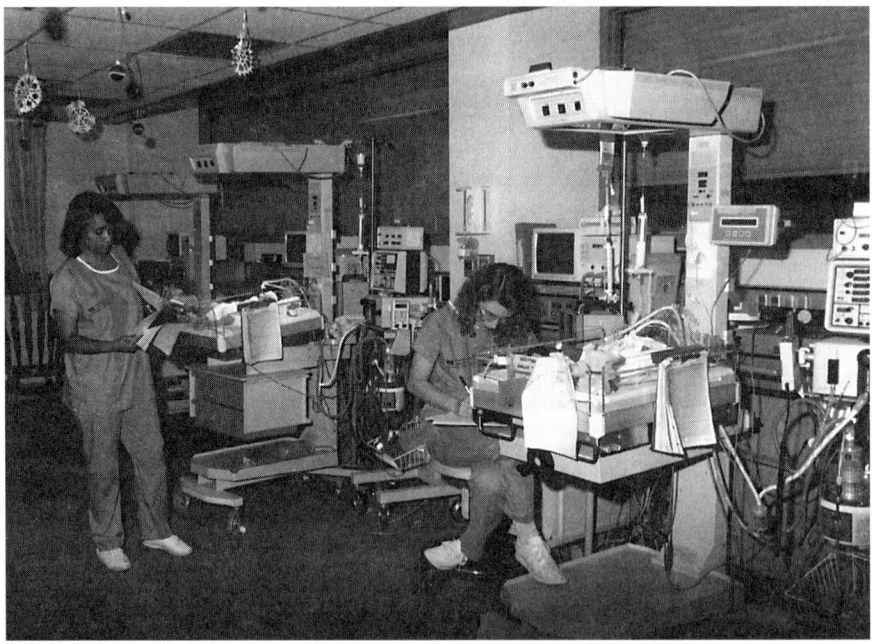

Fig. 10-6. A typical neonatal intensive care unit. (Courtesy Joe Calderone and Kevin Mellott.)

highways (and thus automobile emissions and lead), under power lines (and electromagnetic fields), or on old industrial sites (with benzene or arsenic). Schools made frequent use of asbestos as a building material[1] (Fig. 10-8).

Adolescents not only have a new school environment but begin to self-determine physical environments, often misjudging or ignoring the risks to themselves.[52] In addition, many adolescents have part-time jobs that place them in

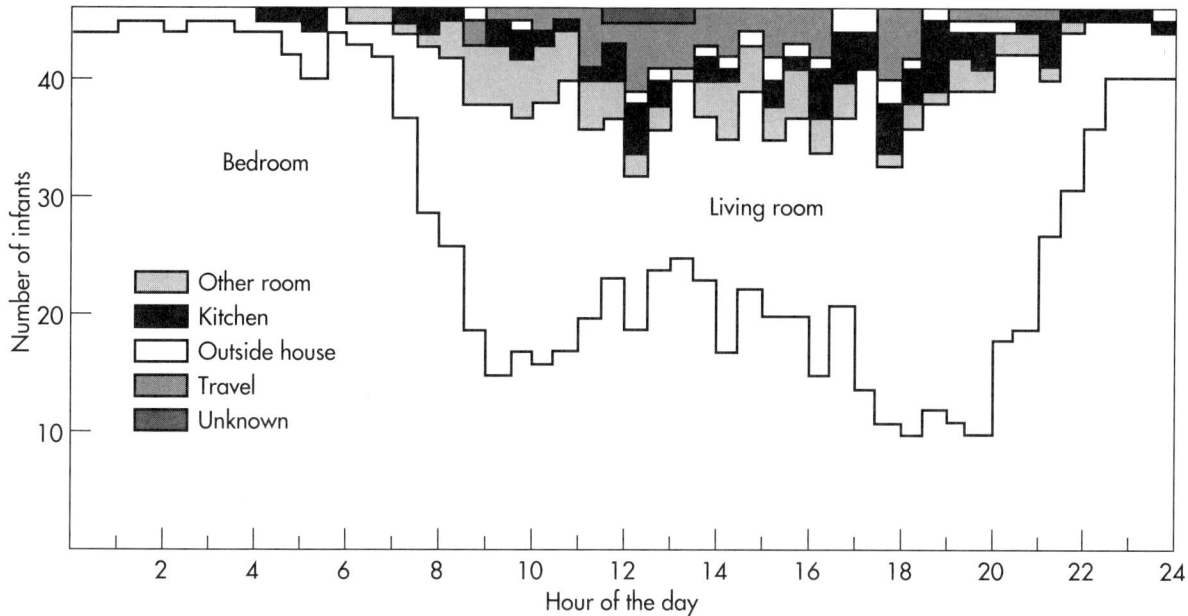

Fig. 10-7. Time location patterns for 46 infants.[78] (From US Department of Health and Human Services: *The health consequences of involuntary smoking; a report of the surgeon general*, USDHHS, PHS, CDC, DHHS Publication No. [CDC] 87-8398, 1986, p 144.)

ESTIMATED POPULATIONS AFFECTED BY
ASBESTOS IN SCHOOLS

- Affected School Districts: 5442 out of an estimated U.S. total of 15,854 (34%)
- Affected Public Schools: 11,588 out of an estimated U.S. total of 91,667 (12.6%)
- Affected Students: 2,992,347 out of an estimated U.S. total of 40.1 million students (7%)

Fig. 10-8. The national totals of estimates for the number of school districts, public schools, and students who may be affected by the U.S. EPA rule on identification and notification of asbestos containing materials in schools. (From US EPA, Office of Pesticides and Toxic Substances: *Asbestos containing materials in schools: economic impact analysis of identification & notification;* Proposed Rule, Section 6, Toxic Substances Control Act, Washington, DC, 1980, p 178.)

physical environments that may be hazardous because of occupational exposures.[56]

Breathing zones

The breathing zone of an adult is typically 4 to 6 feet above the floor; however, that of a child is closer to the floor and depends on the child's height and mobility. It is within these lower breathing zones that heavier chemicals such as methyl mercury and large respirable particulates settle[36] and radon accumulates.[7] This is a factor that may have accounted for the case of acrodynia in Michigan caused by latex house paint.[12]

Oxygen consumption

Because of their larger surface-to-volume ratio, children's metabolic rate is higher and hence their oxygen consumption is greater. Therefore, their exposure to any air pollutant is greater (Fig. 10-9). For example, if radon is present at 2 pCi/L, an adult with an average oxygen consumption rate of 3.5 ml/kg body weight per minute receives an exposure of 48 pCi/kg in 24 hours. In contrast, a 6-month-old child with an average oxygen consumption rate of 7 ml/kg body weight per minute receives an exposure of 96 pCi/kg in 24 hours, which is twice as much.[83]

Quantity and quality of food consumed

Just as children's oxygen requirement is higher as a function of their surface-to-volume ratio, so is their caloric requirement. Not only do children maintain homeostasis but they also grow. Therefore, the amount of food they consume per kilogram is higher than that consumed by an adult[6] (Fig. 10-10). Consider the amount of water consumed by an infant who receives formula reconstituted with boiled tap water. Average consumption is 6 oz/kg. In comparison, for the average male adult, this rate is equivalent to drinking 35 cans of soda per day (Fig. 10-11). Blood lead levels above 10 μg/dL have been found in infants with exposure to tap water in formula.[65] It has also been shown that the types of food that children consume differ from adults.[77] The diets of many

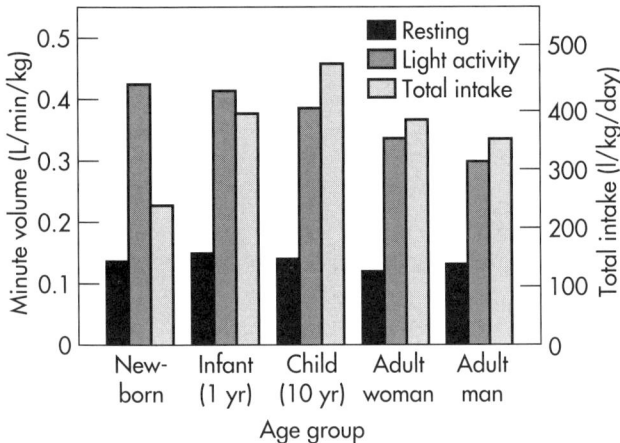

Fig. 10-9. Body-weight-adjusted air intake. (From Plunkett LM, Turnbull D, Rodricks JV: In Guzehan PS, Henry CJ, Olin SS, eds: *Similarities and differences between adults and children affecting exposure assessment*, Washington, DC, 1992, ILSI Press, p. 81.)

	Total intake (g/kg/day)	Metabolizable intake (per kg/day)	Cal (metabolizable)
Water		150-200 ml	
Protein/amino acid	3.5-4	3 g	14
Lipid	3.5-4.6	3-4 g	36
Carbohydrate	12-14	12-14 g	50
Total			100

Fig. 10-10. Daily water, macronutrient, and metabolizable energy requirement for the newborn.[71] (From Swyer PR, Heim T: Nutrition, body fluids, and acid base homeostasis. In Fanaroff AA, Martin RJ, eds: *Neonatal-perinatal medicine*, St Louis, 1987, Mosby, p 449.)

newborns are limited to breast milk, which has been documented to contain many environmental pollutants, including lead, PCBs, and dioxins.[24,51,58] Children's diets contain more milk products and more fruit and vegetables. When the level of exposure of children to daninozide (Alar) was calculated, using a child's daily consumption of apples and apple products, an unacceptable level of risk for cancer was found[86] (Fig. 10-12).

Normal behavioral development

A child's normal behavioral development also influences environmental exposures. Preambulatory infants are not able to remove themselves from a noxious environment, as mentioned earlier (Fig. 10-13). Normal children pass through a developmental stage of intense oral exploratory behavior. Most objects grasped are placed in the mouth. This behavior is a common source of lead poisoning in environments with high levels of lead dust.[14] It also places the child at risk in environments that have not taken the oral orientation of children into account. An example is arsenic- and creosote-treated wood in playgrounds. Children frequently place their mouths on this material in the course of normal play.[34] The ability to walk often places the child in unusual situations for play, such as used drums, mud puddles, and empty lots, environments in which adults spend little time and that have the potential for deleterious exposures. As children become adolescents, they gain more freedom from parental authority; however, they are at a stage of development in which physical strength and stamina are at a peak, yet they continue to acquire abstract thinking.[10] Therefore, they do not consider cause and effect, particularly delayed effects, in the same way as adults do. They often place themselves in situations with greater risk because of this lack of perception. An example is the higher incidence of farm injuries involving adolescents than in adults[32] (Fig. 10-14).

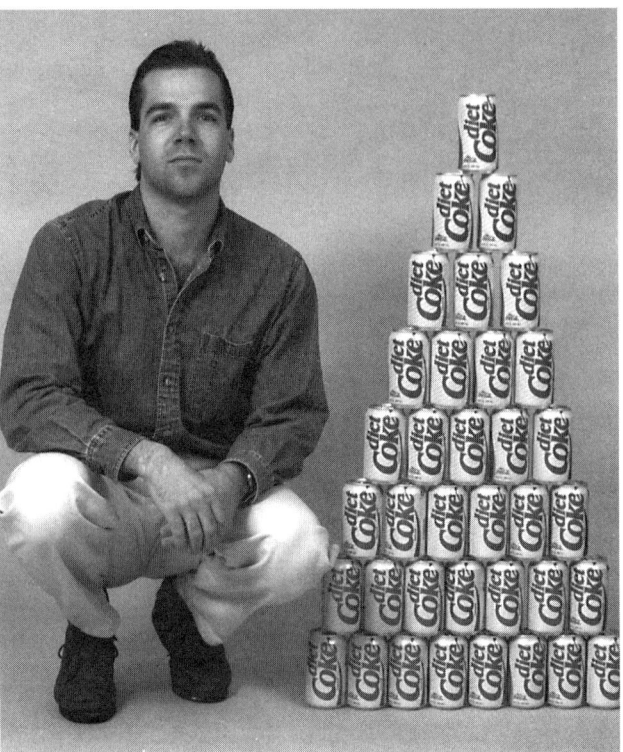

Fig. 10-11. An adult with 35 cans of soda. (Courtesy Joe Calderone and Kevin Mellott.)

ABSORPTION

Absorption generally occurs by four major pathways: the transplacental route, the percutaneous route, the respiratory tract, and the gastrointestinal tract. Each of these portals depends on the developmental stage of the child.

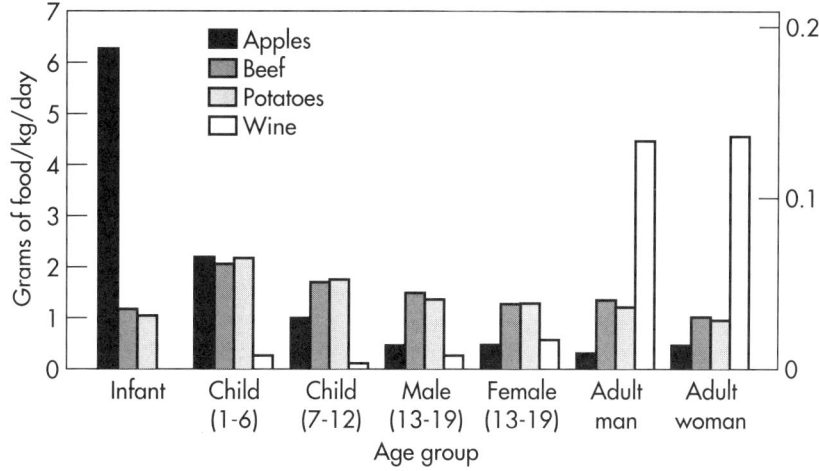

Fig. 10-12. Body-weight-adjusted food consumption. (From Plunkett LM, Turnbull D, Rodricks JV: In Guzehan PS, Henry CJ, Olin SS, eds: *Similarities and differences between children and adults: implications for risk assessment,* Washington, DC, 1992, ILSI Press, p. 81.)

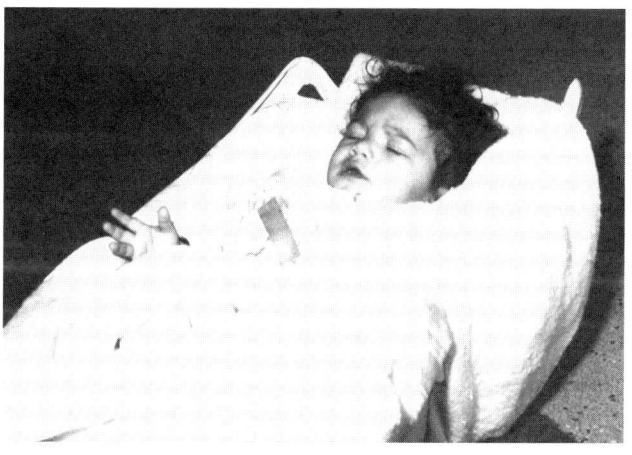

Fig. 10-13. A baby cannot move out of the sun. (Photo courtesy Joe Calderone and Kevin Mellott.)

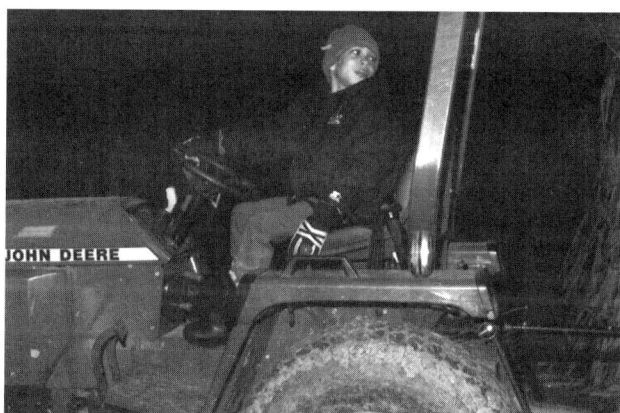

Fig. 10-14. A teenager driving a tractor. (Photo courtesy Joe Calderone and Kevin Mellott.)

Transplacental route

During the fetal stage, a major pathway of absorption is through the placenta. Until the late 1950s, the placenta was thought to protect the fetus from any maternal exposure; however, the experience with thalidomide drastically changed this paradigm.[50] It is now known that several classes of compounds readily cross the placenta. Compounds of low molecular weight cross the placenta readily. Carbon monoxide is a good example of this type of chemical. Because carbon monoxide has a higher affinity for fetal than for adult hemoglobin, the concentration of carboxyhemoglobin is higher in the fetus than in the mother.[81] Lipophilic compounds such as polycyclic aromatic hydrocarbons and ethanol also readily gain access to the fetal circulation. PCBs have been measured in equal concentration in fetal and maternal blood.[9] Fetal and maternal blood levels of ethanol are equal in pregnant ewes[16] (Fig. 10-15). The fetal liver does not express alcohol dehydrogenase until near term.[60] Therefore, most ethanol back-diffuses across the placenta and is metabolized by the mother. In addition, specific transport mechanisms in the placenta actively transport specific nutrients. Calcium is such a nutrient; an accretion of 100 to 140 mg/kg/day is required by the fetus in the third trimester.[70] Lead is transported via the calcium transporter. Fetal blood lead concentration is equivalent to maternal blood lead concentration.[22]

Percutaneous route

Transdermal pathways of absorption are particularly important for lipophilic compounds. The skin undergoes enormous changes with development that affect the properties of absorption.

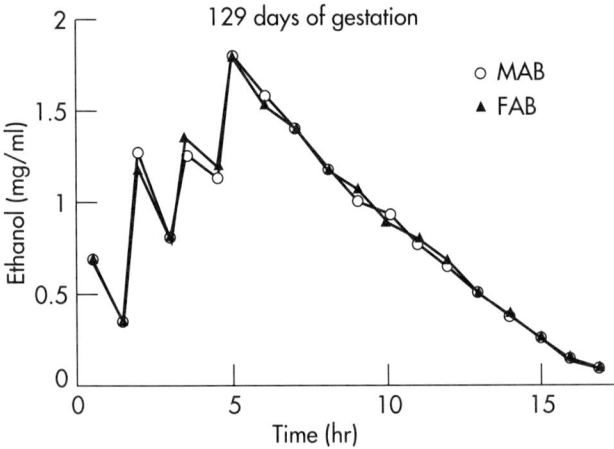

Fig. 10-15. Maternal arterial blood and fetal arterial blood ethanol concentration-time curve for maternal administration of four doses of 0.5 g ethanol/kg maternal body weight to the once conscious instrumented pregnant ewe at 129 days of gestation. Each ethanol dose was administered as a 0.5-hour maternal intravenous infusion with a 1-hour interval between each dose.[16] (From Clarke DW et al: Activity of alcohol dehydrogenase and aldehyde dehydrogenase in maternal liver, fetal liver and placenta of the near-term pregnant ewe, *Dev Pharmacol Ther* 12:35, 1989.)

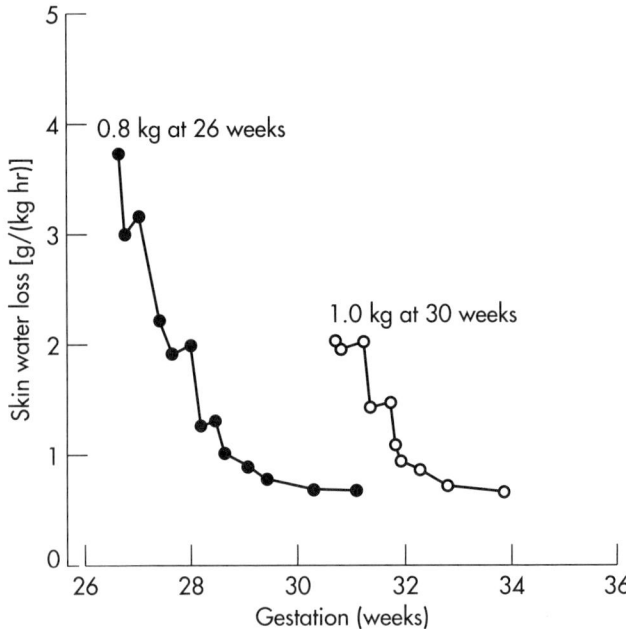

Fig. 10-16. Skin water loss falls rapidly in the first 2 weeks after birth as the skin becomes better keratinized. Enhanced skin maturation in response to premature delivery results in a 1-month-old baby born at 26 weeks gestation having a much more "waterproof" skin (and sweat glands that are more functionally mature) than a 1-week-old baby of 30 weeks gestation.[25] (From Hey E, Scopes JW: Thermoregulation in the newborn. In Avery GB, ed: *Neonatology*, Philadelphia, 1987, JB Lippincott, p 206.)

	Adult	Infant
Surface area	17,000 cm	2200 cm
Topical dose	100 mg	13 mg
Patient weight	70 kg	3.4 kg
Systemic dose	$\dfrac{100 \text{ mg} \times 0.2}{70 \text{ kg}}$	$\dfrac{13 \text{ mg} \times 0.2}{3.4 \text{ kg}}$
Actual dose	0.28 mg/kg	0.76 mg/kg

Fig. 10-17. Systemic availability in the newborn and adult following topical application. (From Plunkett LM, Turnbull D, Rodricks JV: In Guzelian PS, Henry CJ, Olin SS, eds: *Similarities and differences between children and adults: implications for risk assessment*, Washington, DC, 1992, ILSI Press.)

The dermis of a fetus is unkeratinized[11] and thus lacks one of the skin's major barriers. Although the presence of xenobiotics in amniotic fluid has been described,[80] the transdermal absorption of these compounds has not been studied. Keratinization occurs during the initial 3 to 5 days after birth and is independent of gestational age (Fig. 10-16). Therefore, the skin of a newborn remains particularly absorptive (Fig. 10-17). Several epidemics involving percutaneous absorption of xenobiotics, including hypothyroidism from iodine in povidone-iodine (Betadine) scrub solutions,[18] neurotoxicity from hexachlorophene baths,[66] and hyperbilirubinemia from a phenolic disinfectant,[84] have been reported. An additional factor in the transdermal absorption of these chemicals is the larger surface-to-volume ratio of newborns than that of older children and adults.

Respiratory tract

During prenatal life, the fetus makes breathing motions. Although the net flux of fluid is from the lungs out of the trachea into the amniotic fluid, some xenobiotics in amniotic fluid may come in contact with the respiratory epithelium. Studies of this pathway are limited. It has been noted that maternal smoking during pregnancy is associated with significant reductions in forced expiratory flow rates in the offspring.[23]

The surface absorptive properties of the lung probably do not change during development; however, from birth to adolescence, the lung continues to develop alveoli[26] (Fig. 10-18). A consequence of this development is an increasing surface absorptive area in the lung.

Gastrointestinal tract

The gastrointestinal tract undergoes numerous changes during development. The fetus actively swallows amniotic fluid.[43] Xenobiotics are known to be present in amniotic fluid, but prenatal absorption from the gastrointestinal tract is unknown.

After delivery, the gastric pH is relatively high and does not achieve adult levels of acidity until several months of

	30 weeks' gestation	Full term	Adult	Fold increase after birth
Lung volume	25 ml	150–200 ml	5 l	23
Lung weight	20–25 g	50 g	800 G	16
Alveolar no.	–	50 m	300 m	6
Surface area (SA)	0.3 m^2	3–4 m^2	75–100 m^2	23
SA kg		0.4 m^2	1 m^2	2.5
Alveolar diam.	32 μ	150 μ	300 μ	2
No. of airways	24	23–24	22–24	0
Tracheal length		26 mm	184 m	7
Main bronchi (L)		26 mm	254	10

Fig. 10-18. Changes in lung size with growth.[27] (From Hodson WA: Normal and abnormal structural development of the lung. In Fox RA, Polin WW, eds: *Fetal and neonatal physiology*, vol 1, Philadelphia, 1991, WB Saunders.)

age[42] (Fig. 10-19). The difference in pH markedly affects xenobiotic absorption from the stomach because it changes the ionization status of these chemicals.[15] In addition, under low levels of acidity, bacterial overgrowth in the small bowel and stomach may result. The absorption of nitrites formed by bacteria from ingestion of formula reconstituted with well water with nitrate contamination resulted in several cases of methemoglobinemia in Iowa.[19]

The small bowel is thought to express specific transport mechanisms in the newborn. In the newborn mouse and rat, maternal immunoglobulin M and immunoglobulin G present in colostrum are specifically transported across the small bowel and into the blood. Whether these mechanisms are present in humans has not been proved.[68] The bowel also responds to increased nutritional needs by increasing absorption of the particular nutrient. For example, growing children require more calcium than do adults for continued bone growth. Thus they absorb more calcium from intraluminal contents than adults; however, they also absorb more lead from the gastrointestinal tract than do adults because of this enhanced absorption. It is estimated that an adult absorbs 10% of ingested lead whereas a 1- to 2-year-old child absorbs 50% of ingested lead[61] (Fig. 10-20).

DISTRIBUTION

The tissue distribution of chemicals varies with the developmental stage of the child. For example, many drugs have higher apparent volumes of distribution in the newborn.[46] In animal models, it has been shown that lead is retained to a larger degree in the infant animal brain than in the adult brain.[45] Lead also accumulates more rapidly in children's bones, doubling between infancy and the late teen years.[4]

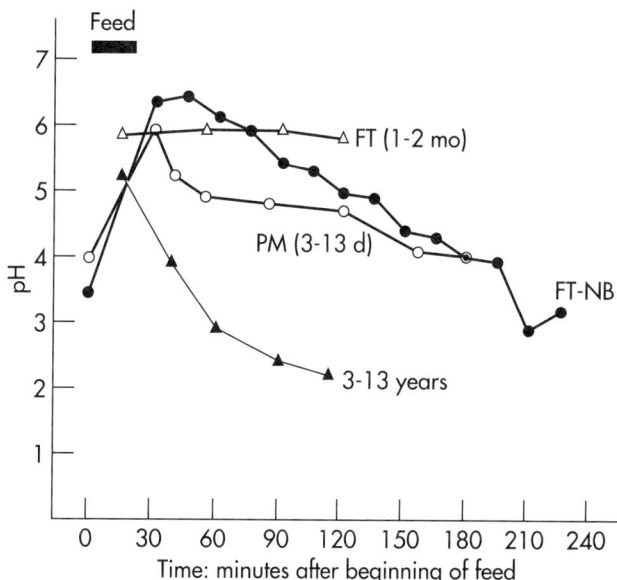

Fig. 10-19. Effect of feeding on pH values of the stomach contents of infants of different ages. (PM) 10 premature babies, 3 to 13 days old; (FT-NB) 25 full-term newborn infants; (FT) infants 1 to 2 months old; (3-13) equals children 3 to 13 years old.[33] (From Koldovsky O: Small and large intestine. In Fox RA, Polin WW, eds: *Fetal and neonatal physiology*, vol 1, Philadelphia, 1991, WB Saunders.)

Age, years	Average GI absorption rate (%)
0–1	42–53
1–2	42–53
2–3	30–40
3–4	30–40
4–5	30–40
5–6	30–40
6–7	18–24
Adult	7–15

Fig. 10-20. Differences in GI absorption of lead.[54] (From Plunkett LM, Turnbull D, Rodricks JV: In Guzehon PS, Henry CJ, Olin SS, eds: *Similarities and differences between children and adults: implications for risk assessment*, Washington, DC, 1992, ILSI Press.)

METABOLISM

Metabolism of chemicals may result in their activation or deactivation. These enzymes involved in the biotransformation of chemicals can be categorized into two groups, phase I and phase II enzymes. Phase I enzymes promote formation of a conjugable group, and phase II enzymes catalyze the conjugation of a more polar compound to the conjugable group such that the resulting conjugate is more polar and therefore more easily excreted. Not only does developmental stage determine the activity of these metabolic pathways but also the genetic polymorphisms of each locus determine the activity of each component enzyme. The family of glutathione S-transferase (GST), phase II enzymes, illustrates both of these points. The GSTs are a large and complex family of enzymes that share the catalytic activity of glutathione conjugation to a second substrate with a conjugable group.[53] They can be separated into four families of enzymes: alpha, mu, pi, and microsomal. The mu family is not present in 50% of individuals.[64] Smokers with lung cancer are more likely to lack the mu GSTs than are smokers without lung cancer.[63] Thus these individuals have a genetic susceptibility to carcinogenesis from cigarette smoke. The expression of the families of GST show a marked tissue specificity. GST pi is found only in placenta,[55,62] and the Yc isozyme of GST alpha is not expressed in brain, but the Yb3 isozyme of GST mu is expressed only in brain.[2,39] Developmental regulation is evident in that 50% of GST activity in fetal liver is GST pi, which is not expressed in adult liver.[82]

Developmental regulation is more complex in the P-450 cytochrome family. (For a complete review, see Nebert and Gonzalez' article.[47]) Clinically this knowledge is important for the pediatrician to prescribe medications accurately. Theophylline is metabolized by the P-450 cytochrome system. Initially, during the newborn period, the half-life of theophylline is prolonged, requiring twice-a-day dosing; however, P-450 cytochrome expression increases over the first few months of life, decreasing drug half-life and necessitating more frequent dosing (Fig. 10-21). If urinary metabolites of theophylline are examined during this period, a difference in the pattern of metabolites can be seen, denoting complex developmental stages in the expression and activity of the P-450 cytochromes.[46] The half-life of theophylline is again prolonged during adolescence, possibly as a consequence of competition with steroid hormones (Fig. 10-22).[38] Dosage must again be adjusted to avoid toxicity.

Another clinical example of developmental changes in metabolism is the case of acetaminophen. In the adult, especially the pregnant woman, high levels of acetaminophen may cause fatal hepatotoxicity; however, infants delivered to mothers with high acetaminophen levels also have elevated acetaminophen levels in blood but do not sustain liver damage. It is thought that the lack of the ability of the fetus to metabolize the acetaminophen protects the fetus from end organ damage.[57,59]

From these three examples, it can be concluded that biotransformation of xenobiotics is developmentally regulated and may either protect or harm the individual.

EXCRETION

Kidney function is also developmentally regulated. At birth, the glomerular filtration rate is a fraction of normal adult values. It gradually increases to adult values by approximately 1 year of age. The ability to concentrate urine is also developmentally regulated, concentration of urine being relatively poor in the newborn. By 16 months of age, renal function has reached adult capabilities.[31]

TARGET ORGAN SUSCEPTIBILITY

Children also are different from adults in that their organs are undergoing growth and differentiation. Both these processes may be affected by xenobiotics. The result of exposure to xenobiotics may differ between children and adults both in the degree of severity of effect and also in the nature of the effect. Because children's bodies are growing and developing, these processes may be disrupted as a result of environmental exposures, leading to uniquely different outcomes. Examples of such outcomes are prenatal and post-

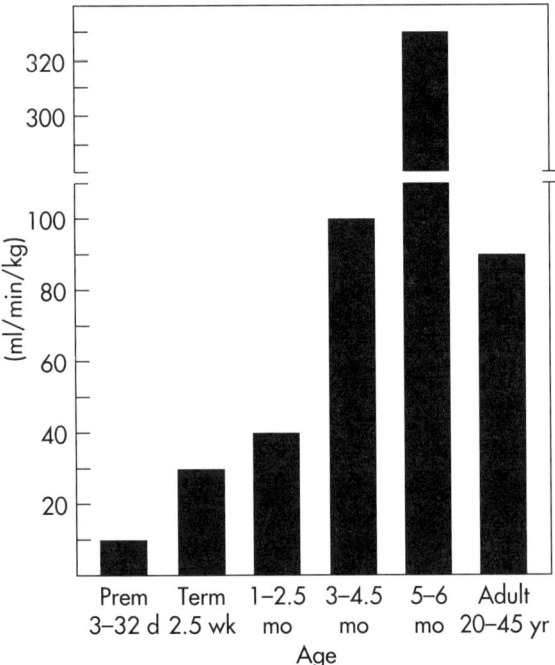

Fig. 10-21. Postnatal maturation of plasma caffeine clearance (ml/min/kg) in humans.[3] (From Aranda JW et al: Methyxanthine metabolism in the newborn infant. In Soyka LF, Redmond GP, eds: *Drug metabolism in the immature human,* New York, 1981, Raven Press.)

	Urinary excretion (% dose/24 hr)	Urinary conjugates (% of total)		Acetyl/Glycine
		Acetyl	Glycine	
Preterm newborn	61	45	31	1.5
Full-term newborn	68	39	43	0.9
Child (9–11 yr)	87	24	55	0.4

Fig. 10-22. Age dependence of acetylation and glycine conjugation of *p*-aminobenzoic acid in humans.[87] (From Zoltan G, Klaasen CD: Hepatic disposition of xenobiotics during prenatal and early postnatal development. In Fox RA, Polin WW, eds: *Fetal and neonatal physiology,* vol 1, Philadelphia, 1991, WB Saunders, p 1107.)

natal growth retardation, diminished intelligence quotient, precocious puberty, microcephaly, and diminished lung volumes.

Growth occurs by several mechanisms: auxetic, in which growth occurs by cells becoming larger; multiplicative, in which growth occurs by cells dividing; and accretionary, in which ground substance and nonliving structural components accumulate.[69] Multiplicative growth is believed to be complete at 6 months of gestation for those tissues not undergoing continual turnover, such as epithelia cells. All subsequent growth is accretionary or auxetic. Cells undergo two further processes to become the adult organism: differentiation and migration. Differentiation is the process by which cells take on their particular biochemical functions and lose the ability to divide. These events may be triggered by hormone-receptor interactions. Some environmental agents may mimic hormones and alter the differentiation of some tissues. Chlorinated insecticides are an example of this agent. Recent studies have shown effects on the reproductive system from exposure to kepone (Chlordecone).[76]

Cell migration is necessary for certain cells to reach their destination for function. Neurons, for example, originate in the germinal matrix, then migrate out along radial glia to a predestined location in one of the many layers of the brain[44] (Fig. 10-23). Xenobiotics may have a profound effect on this process, as shown in children with fetal alcohol syndrome. Prenatal exposure to ethanol may result in an interruption in this process severe enough to cause lissencephaly.[17]

Examples of organs with a prolonged period of postnatal development are the brain and the lungs. Myelination of the brain[26] and complete formation of alveoli[27] are not complete until adolescence. This protracted period of growth and development increases the vulnerability of these organs. For example, intracranial tumors are frequently treated with radiation therapy in adults, with uncomfortable but reversible side effects. However, in infants, radiation therapy is avoided because of its profound and permanent effects on the developing central nervous system.[20]

Another example of the unique vulnerability of children is the neurotoxic effect of lead. The current blood concentration of concern for children is 10 µg/dl.[13] This level is based on studies by numerous investigators[48] that children with blood lead concentrations above 10 µg/dl have measurable decreases in intelligence quotient. The occupational limit for adults is 60 µg/dl, at which no encephalopathy is noted but kidney function, fertility, and peripheral nerves may be impaired[61] (Fig. 10-24).

That the developing lung may also be compromised by

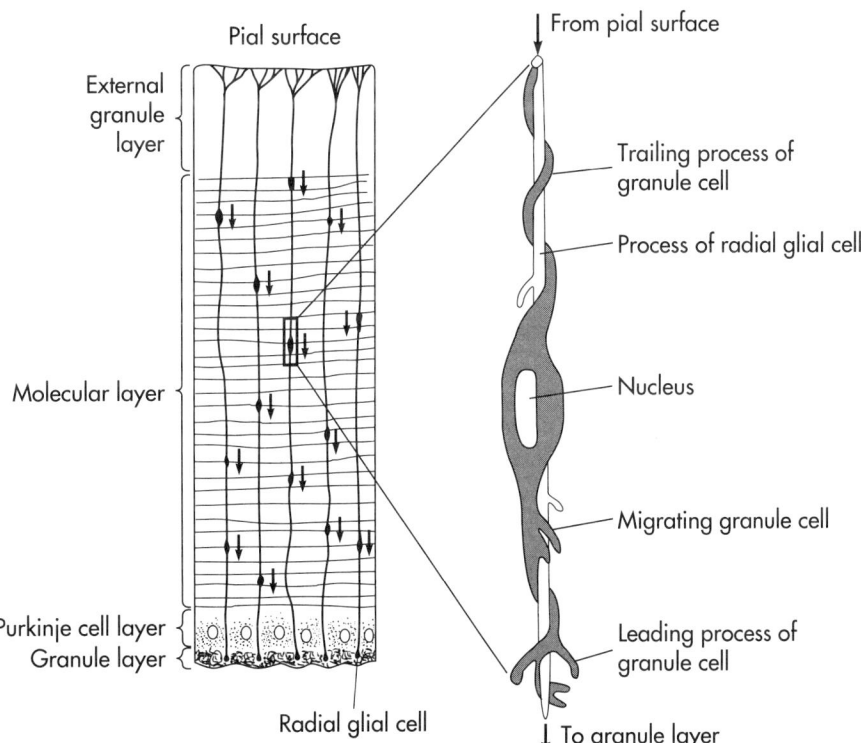

Fig. 10-23. Neurons use radial glial cell fibers as scaffolds for migration. Granule cells migrate through the molecular and Purkinje cell layers along processes of radial glial cells (Bergmann astrocytes), which extend from the granule layer to the pial surface. The cell bodies of the radial glial cells are located near the junction of the Purkinje and granule cell layers.[30] (From Jessell TM: Cell migration and axon guidance. In Kandel ER, Schwartz JH, Jessell TM, eds: *Principles of neural science,* New York, 1991, Appleton & Lange, p 91.)

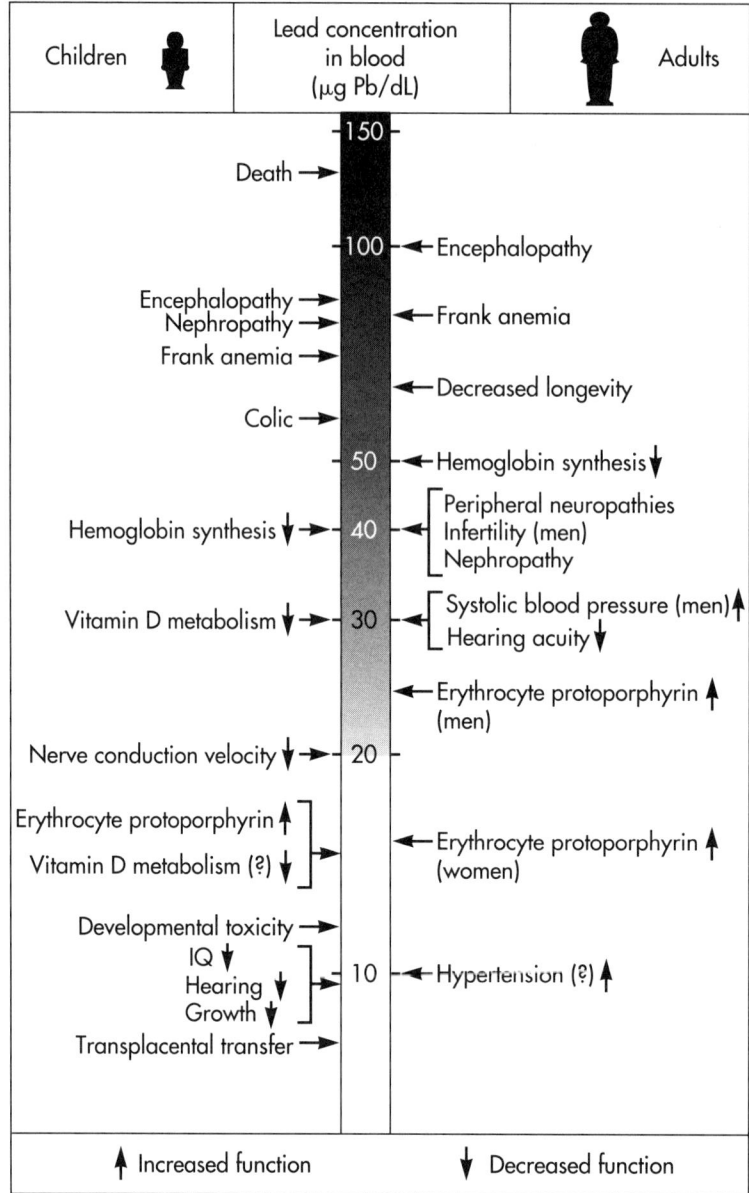

Fig. 10-24. Effects of inorganic lead on children and adults—lowest observable adverse effect levels.[61] (From Royce SE, ed: *Case studies in environmental medicine: lead toxicity.* Washington, DC, 1990, ATSDR, US Department of Health and Human Services.)

exposure to environmental agents is illustrated by studies of the effects of environmental tobacco smoke on children. It has been shown that the forced expiratory volumes in 1 second of children exposed to environmental tobacco smoke are measurably lower than those of children without exposure.[72]

Tissues undergoing proliferation and terminal differentiation are particularly susceptible to carcinogenesis.[37] This increased susceptibility is due to the shortened time period for deoxyribonucleic acid (DNA) repair and the multiple changes occurring within the DNA, such as interaction with growth factors and the switching on and off of genes. All are likely sites for interaction with chemicals that interrupt the sequence of events. A clinical example is the epidemic of scrotal cancer among the pubertal chimney sweeps of Victorian England.[49] Chimney sweeps were usually adolescents with developing secondary sexual characteristics. Occupational exposure to carcinogens such as soot was common, but the site of the tumor is uncommon outside this situation. Thus it can be hypothesized that the scrotum had increased susceptibility to the carcinogen while undergoing terminal differentiation.

SUMMARY

This chapter has attempted to outline the reasons why children cannot be considered simply as little adults in the area of environmental medicine or elsewhere in the practice of medicine. Their exposures are different, their pathways of absorption are different, their tissue distribution is different, their ability to biotransform and eliminate chemicals is different, and their bodies respond differently to environmental chemicals and radiation. Each of these differences depends on the developmental stage of the child; thus all children are not the same. Each of these differences must be taken into account when the health impacts of a particular exposure on the population are considered. Our data base with regard to pediatric environmental medicine is still incomplete.

What can the practitioner do? The roles of educator, investigator, and advocate are extremely important when children's environmental health is assessed. Prevention is the most important intervention in this field. Parents, children, teachers, community leaders, and policymakers need to be educated about the unique vulnerability of children to environmental pollution. Most environmentally caused diseases have been diagnosed by an alert clinician. Publication of case studies has allowed further description of environmentally mediated diseases. Finally, clinicians must be advocates for their patients. Most regulatory policies do not take the unique vulnerability of children into account when setting limits. To be an effective advocate a clinician must understand the basis for this unique vulnerability and all the factors that influence it.

REFERENCES

1. AAP Committee on Environmental Hazards: Asbestos exposure in schools, *Pediatrics* 79:301, 1987.
2. Abramovitz M, Listowsky I.: Selective expression of a unique glutathione S-transferase Y_{b3} gene in rat brain, *J Biol Chem* 262:7770, 1987.
3. Aranda JV et al: Methylxanthine metabolism in the newborn infant. In Soyka LF, Redmond GP, eds: *Drug metabolism in the immature human,* New York, 1981, Raven Press.
4. Barry PSI: A comparison of concentrations of lead in human tissues, *Br J Ind Med* 32:119, 1975.
5. Bernstein RS et al: Inhalation exposure to formaldehyde: an overview of its toxicology, epidemiology, monitoring, and control, *Am Ind Hyg Assoc J* 261:1183, 1984.
6. Biller JA, Yeager AM, eds: *The Harriet Lane handbook,* ed 9, Chicago, 1981, Year Book.
7. Blot WJ et al: Indoor radon and lung cancer in China, *J Natl Cancer Inst* 82:1025, 1990.
8. Brown AK, Glass L: Environmental hazards in the newborn nursery, *Pediatr Ann* 8:698, 1979.
9. Bush B, Snow JT, Koblintz R.: Polychlorinated biphenyl congeners, p,p'-DDE, and hexachlorobenzene in maternal and fetal cord blood from mothers in upstate New York, *Arch Environ Contam Toxicol* 13:517, 1984.
10. Campbell SF, ed: *Piaget sampler: an introduction to Jean Piaget through his own words,* Ann Arbor, 1976, Books on Demand.
11. Cartlidge PHT, Rutter N: Skin barrier function. In Polin RA, Fox WW, eds: *Fetal and neonatal physiology,* vol 1, Philadelphia, 1991, WB Saunders.
12. Centers for Disease Control: Mercury exposure from interior latex paint: Michigan, *MMWR* 39:125, 1990.
13. Centers for Disease Control: *Preventing lead poisoning in young children: a statement by the Centers for Disease Control,* Atlanta, 1991, Centers for Disease Control.
14. Chao J, Kikano GE: Lead poisoning in children, *Am Fam Physician* 47:113, 1993.
15. Chemtob S: Basic pharmacologic principles. In Polin RA, Fox WW, eds: *Fetal and neonatal physiology,* Philadelphia, 1991, WB Saunders.
16. Clarke DW et al: Activity of alcohol dehydrogenase and aldehyde dehydrogenase in maternal liver, fetal liver and placenta of the near-term pregnant ewe, *Dev Pharmacol Ther* 12:35, 1989.
17. Clarren SK et al: Brain malformations related to prenatal exposure to ethanol, *J Pediatr* 92:64, 1978.
18. Clemens PC, Neumann RS: The Wolff-Chaikoff effect: hypothyroidism due to iodine application, *Arch Dermatol* 125:705, 1989.
19. Comly HH: Cyanosis in infants caused by nitrates in well water, *JAMA* 129:112, 1945.
20. Duffner PK et al: Postoperative chemotherapy and delayed radiation in children less that three years of age with malignant brain tumors, *N Engl J Med* 328:1725, 1993.
21. Fenske RA et al: Potential exposure and health risks of infants following indoor residential pesticide applications, *Am J Public Health* 80:689, 1990.
22. Goyer RA: Transplacental transport of lead, *Environ Health Perspect* 89:101, 1990.
23. Hanrahan JP et al: The effect of maternal smoking during pregnancy on early infant lung function, *Am Rev Respir Dis* 145:1129, 1992.
24. Hayward DG et al: PCDD and PCDF in breast milk as correlated with fish consumption in California, *Chemosphere* p. 206, 1989.
25. Hey E, Scopes JW: Thermoregulation in the newborn. In Avery GB, ed: *Neonatology,* Philadelphia, 1987, JB Lippincott, p. 206.
26. Hoar RM, Monie IW: Comparative development of specific organ systems. In Kimmel CA, Buelke-Sam J, eds: *Developmental toxicology,* New York, 1981, Raven Press.
27. Hodgson E, Levi PE, eds: *A textbook of modern toxicology,* New York, 1987, Appleton & Lange.
28. Hodson WA: Normal and abnormal structural development of the lung. In Fox RA, Polin WW, eds: *Fetal and neonatal physiology,* vol 1, Philadelphia, 1991, WB Saunders.
29. Jackson RJ: Testimony to US House of Representatives Select Committee on Children, Youth and Families, 1990.
30. Jessell TM: Cell migration and axon guidance. In Kandel ER, Schwartz JH, Jessell TM, eds: *Principles of neural science,* New York, 1991, Appleton & Lange.
31. John EG, Guignard J-P: Development of renal excretion of drugs during ontogeny. In Polin RA, Fox WW, eds: *Fetal and neonatal physiology,* Philadelphia, 1991, WB Saunders.
32. Karlson T, Noren J: Farm tractor fatalities: the failure of voluntary safety standards, *Am J Public Health* 69:146, 1979.
33. Koldovsky O: Small and large intestine. In Polin RA, Fox WW, eds: *Fetal and neonatal physiology,* vol 1, Philadelphia, WB Saunders.
34. Kosnett M, ed: *Case studies in environmental medicine: arsenic toxicity,* Washington, DC, 1990, ATSDR, US Department of Health and Human Services.
35. Langman J: *Medical embryology,* Baltimore, 1975, Williams & Wilkins.
36. Leaderer BP: Assessing exposures to environmental tobacco smoke, *Risk Anal* 10:19, 1990.
37. Levi PE: Toxic action. In Hodgson E, Levi PE, eds: *A textbook of modern toxicology,* New York, 1987, Appleton & Lange.
38. Levitsky LL et al: Effect of growth hormone therapy in growth hormone–deficient children on cytochrome P-450–dependent 3-N-demethylation of caffeine as measured by the caffeine $^{13}CO_2$ breath test, *Dev Pharmacol Ther* 12:90, 1989.

39. Li N-Q et al: Expression of glutathione S-transferase in rat brains, *J Biol Chem* 261:7596, 1986.
40. Luykens JN: The legacy of well-water methemoglobinemia, *JAMA* 257:2793, 1987.
41. Manton WI: Total contribution of airborne lead to blood lead, *Br J Ind Med* 42:168, 1985.
42. Marino LR: Development of gastric secretory function. In Polin RA, Fox WW, eds: *Fetal and neonatal physiology,* vol 2, Philadelphia, 1991, WB Saunders.
43. Miller AJ: Deglutition, *Physiol Rev* 62:129, 1982.
44. Miller MW: Effects of prenatal exposure to ethanol on cell proliferation and neuronal migration. In Miller MW, ed: *Development of the central nervous system: effects of alcohol and opiates,* New York, 1992, Wiley-Liss.
45. Momcilovic B, Kostial K: Kinetics of lead retention and distribution in suckling and adult rats, *Environ Res* 8:214, 1974.
46. Nagourney BA, Aranda JV: Physiologic differences of clinical significance. In Polin RA, Fox WW, eds: *Fetal and neonatal physiology,* vol 1, Philadelphia, 1991, WB Saunders.
47. Nebert DW, Gonzalez FJ: P450 genes: structure, evolution, and regulation, *Annu Rev Biochem* 56:945, 1987.
48. Needleman HL, Bellinger D: Low-level lead exposure and the IQ of children: a meta-analysis of modern studies, *JAMA* 263:673, 1990.
49. Nethercott JR: Occupational skin disorders. In LaDou J, ed: *Occupational medicine,* San Mateo, Calif 1990, Appleton & Lange.
50. Newman CGH: The thalidomide syndrome: risks of exposure and spectrum of malformations, *Clin Perinatology* 13:555, 1986.
51. Ong CN et al: Concentrations of lead in maternal blood, cord blood, and breast milk, *Arch Dis Child* 60:756, 1985.
52. Perry CL, Silvis GL: Smoking prevention: behavioral prescriptions for the pediatrician, *Pediatrics* 79:790, 1987.
53. Pickett CB, Lu AYH: Glutathione S-transferases: gene structure, regulation, and biological function, *Annu Rev Biochem* 58:743, 1989.
54. Plunkett LM, Turnbull D, Rodricks JV: In Guzehan PS, Henry CJ, Olin SS, eds: *Similarities and differences between adults and children affecting exposure assessment,* Washington, DC, 1992, ILSI Press.
55. Polidoro G et al: Glutathione S-transferase activity in human placenta, *Biochem Pharmacol* 29:1677, 1980.
56. Pollack SH, Landrigan PH, Mallino DL: Child labor in 1990: prevalence and health hazards, *Annu Rev Public Health* 11:359, 1990.
57. Riggs BS et al: Acute acetaminophen overdose during pregnancy, *Obstet Gynecol* 74:247, 1989.
58. Rogan WJ et al: Polychlorinated biphenyls (PCB's) and dichlorodiphenyl dichlorethene (DDE) in human milk: effects of maternal factors and previous lactation, *Am J Public Health* 76:172, 1986.
59. Rosevear SK, Hope PL: Favourable neonatal outcome following maternal paracetamol overdose and severe fetal distress: case report, *Br J Obstet Gynaecol* 96:491, 1989.
60. Rout UK, Holmes RS: Postnatal development of mouse alcohol dehydrogenases: agarose isoelectric focusing analyses of the liver, kidney, stomach and ocular isozymes, *Biol Neonate* 59:93, 1991.
61. Royce SE, ed: *Case studies in environmental medicine: lead toxicity,* Washington, DC, 1990, ATSDR, US Department of Health and Human Services.
62. Schaffer J, Gallay O, Ladenstein R: Glutathione transferase from bovine placenta: preparation, biochemical characterization, crystallization, and preliminary crystallographic analysis of a neutral class Pi enzyme, *J Biol Chem* 263:17405, 1988.
63. Seidegard J et al: A glutathione transferase in human leukocytes as a marker for the susceptibility to lung cancer, *Carcinogenesis* (*Lond*) 7:751, 1986.
64. Seidegard J et al: Hereditary differences in the expression of the human glutathione transferase active on trans-stilbene oxide are due to a gene deletion, *Proc Natl Acad Sci USA* 85:7293, 1988.
65. Shannon MW, Graef JW: Lead intoxication in infancy, *Pediatrics* 89:87, 1992.
66. Shuman RM, Leech RW, Alvord EK: Neurotoxicity of hexachlorophene in the human. I. A clinicopathologic study of 248 children, *Pediatrics* 54:689, 1974.
67. Silbergeld EK: Lead in bone: implications for toxicology during pregnancy and lactation, *Environ Health Perspect* 91:63, 1991.
68. Simister ME, Mostov KE: An Fc receptor structurally related to MHC class I antigens, *Nature* 337:184, 1989.
69. Sinclair D: *Human growth after birth,* ed 5, Oxford, 1989, Oxford University Press.
70. Steichen JJ, Tsang RC: Osteopenia and rickets of prematurity. In Polin RA, Fox WW, eds: *Fetal and neonatal physiology,* vol 2, Philadelphia, 1991, WB Saunders.
71. Swyer PR, Heim T: Nutrition, body fluids, and acid base homeostasis. In Fanaroff AA, Martin RJ, eds: *Neonatal-perinatal medicine,* St Louis, 1987, Mosby.
72. Tager IB et al: Longitudinal study of the effects of maternal smoking on pulmonary function in children, *N Engl J Med* 309:699, 1983.
73. Taylor PR et al: Polychlorinated biphenyls: influence on birthweight and gestation, *Am J Public Health* 74:1153, 1984.
74. Tilson HA, Jacobson JL, Rogan WJ: Polychlorinated biphenyls and the developing nervous system: cross-species comparisons, *Neurotoxicol Teratol* 12:239, 1990.
75. Trapp M et al: Pollutants in human follicular fluid, *Fertil Steril* 42:146, 1984.
76. Uphouse L, Mason G, Hunter V: Persistent vaginal estrus and serum hormones after chlordecone (kepone) treatment of adult female rats, *Toxicol Appl Pharmacol* 72:177, 1984.
77. US Department of Agriculture: *Nationwide food consumption survey: continuing survey of food intakes by individuals, women 19-50 years and their children 1-5 years,* Washington, DC, 1985, Human Nutrition Information Service, CSFII.
78. US Department of Health and Human Services: *The health consequences of involuntary smoking: a report of the surgeon general,* USDHHS, PHS, CDC, DHHS Pub No (CDC) 87-8398, Washington, DC, 1986.
79. US Environmental Protection Agency, Office of Pesticides and Toxic Substances: *Asbestos containing materials in schools: economic impact analysis of identification & notification;* Proposed Rule, Section 6, Toxic Substances Control Act, Washington, DC, 1980.
80. Van Vunakis H, Longone JJ, Milunsky A: Nicotine and cotinine in the amniotic fluid of smokers in the second trimester of pregnancy, *Am J Obstet Gynecol* 120:64, 1974.
81. Visnjevac V, Mikov M: Smoking and carboxyhaemoglobin concentrations in mothers and their newborn infants, *Hum Toxicol* 5:175, 1986.
82. Warholm M et al: Glutathione S-transferases in human fetal liver, *Acta Chem Scand* B35:225, 1981.
83. World Health Organization: *Environmental health criteria 59: principles for evaluating health risks from chemicals during infancy and early childhood: the need for a special approach,* Geneva, 1986.
84. Wysowski DK et al: Epidemic neonatal hyperbilirubinemia and use of a phenolic disinfectant detergent, *Pediatrics* 61:165, 1978.
85. Yu M-L et al: In utero PCB/PCDF exposure: relation of developmental delay to dysmorphology and dose, *Neurotoxicol Teratol* 13:195, 1991.
86. Zeise L et al: Alar in fruit: limited regulatory action in the face of uncertain risks. In Garrick BJ, Gekler WC, eds: *The analysis, communication, and perception of risk,* New York, 1991, Plenum.
87. Zoltan G, Klaasen CD: Hepatic disposition of xenobiotics during prenatal and early postnatal development. In Polin RA, Fox WW, eds: *Fetal and neonatal physiology,* vol 1, Philadelphia, 1991, WB Saunders.

Chapter 11

TOXICOLOGY OF SELECTED NEUROTOXIC AGENTS

Douglas H. Linz
David J. Garling

Environmental neurotoxicants
Anatomy and physiology
Neuronal response to injury
Toxicology of selected neurotoxic chemicals
    Metals
    Organic solvents
    Pesticides
    Dioxins and related compounds
    Carbon monoxide
Summary

The nervous system has historically been a principal target organ for environmental toxicants, rivaled only by the lungs and skin. Widespread lead toxicity among Roman patricians from consumption of cider and spirits containing lead as a sweetener has been implicated in the downfall of the Roman Empire.[28] This use of lead continued to be prevalent throughout the Middle Ages.[29] Minamata disease,[78] due to consumption of methyl mercury–containing fish, and ginger jake paralysis,[73] caused by consumption of an alcoholic extract of Jamaican ginger adulterated by tri-*ortho*-cresyl phosphate (a nonpesticidal organophosphorous ester), are additional examples of devastating neurotoxic environmental illness. Other historical incidents of exposure to neurotoxicants include those of Yusho (Japan) and YuCheng (Taiwan) from eating foods cooked in polychlorinated biphenyl–contaminated rice oils.[39]

A number of excellent reviews are available on neurotoxicology* and neuropsychological or neurobehavioral toxicology.† Lippmann[46] has compiled a review of environmental toxicants, including a number of neurotoxicants and there are other resources available.[2,63] Anger and Johnson's[6] compendium of 750 neurotoxicants and their related industrial exposures, neurotoxic effects, and literature references is a source of information. A summary of neuropsychologic toxicology, including distinctions between laboratory and work-site research, a compilation of tests used in work-site research, and considerations in the selection of individual neuropsychologic tests and neurobehavioral test batteries for epidemiological research purposes, has been reported by Anger.[5] The clinical aspects of nervous system disorders are presented in Chapter 26.

Selected environmental neurotoxicants implicated as causing adverse human neurologic and neuropsychologic effects are highlighted in this chapter. The distinction between occupational and environmental sources is not always clear-cut. Exposures from occupations performed out of doors, such as forestry and farming, and from avocations and hobbies, for example, car painting, furniture refinishing, and gardening, are addressed.

ENVIRONMENTAL NEUROTOXICANTS

Lead, mercury, and arsenic are the neurotoxic metals of principal environmental concern. Residential lead exposure occurs from home remodeling and refinishing projects and flaking of leaded paints. Additional sources include bullet

---
*References 8, 10, 11, 33, 55, 64, 76.
†References 5, 7, 31, 32, 37, 67.

making, pottery glazing, stained-glass working, consuming foodstuffs from incompletely fired lead-glazed earthenware, and drinking water contaminated by leaching from lead pipes or lead-containing pipe solders. Industrial effluents containing lead, for example, from smelters, leaded gasoline exhaust, and pollution of homes through the clothing of lead workers, contribute to the environmental lead burden. Both mercury and arsenic have been identified in well water from mountainous regions with high indigenous concentrations of these metals. Sources of environmental mercury include gassing from the earth's crust, contamination from industrial operations, hazardous waste incineration, and accidental consumption of organomercurial-treated seed grain. Arsenic exposure occurs from a variety of metal smelters, arsenic-type pesticides, and certain glass and chemical manufacturers. Mercury of both natural and industrial origin is readily transformed into organomercurials by microorganisms and is bioaccumulated up the food chain.

Sources of volatile organic solvent exposure are numerous and include many home and commercial cleaning and degreasing products, paints, and lacquers. Among home businesses employing organic solvents are furniture dipping and refinishing, car painting, and printing. Typically, these operations are performed in poorly ventilated areas such as basements, attics, and garages. Airborne residential contamination occurs from dry-cleaning and painting operations, backflow of sewer gases, and leaks from underground gasoline and fuel-oil storage tanks.

Environmental pesticide sources include drift from nearby farm and forestry operations and use of home pesticide products, often overzealously or improperly diluted. Many products removed from the market in past years are still employed by homeowners, farmers, and small-business operators, with quantities taken from caches stockpiled in garages and basements.

Dioxin and related compounds have been introduced into the environment through releases from industrial sources, indiscriminate handling of contaminated wastes, and consumption of tainted foodstuffs.

Exhaust fumes from cars left running in attached garages and emissions from improperly functioning fireplaces, wood stoves, and furnaces remain disturbingly frequent sources of carbon monoxide intoxication.

ANATOMY AND PHYSIOLOGY

The range of human neurologic and neuropsychologic response to toxicant exposure is critically dependent on the anatomy and physiology of the nervous system. The uniquely elongated neuron is adapted to allow propagation of electrical potentials through transmembrane ion currents. The terminal axon houses neurotransmitter-containing microvesicles allowing synaptic transmission (Fig. 11-1). The discontinuous myelin envelope elaborated by oligodendrocytes and Schwann cells speeds conduction in larger neu-

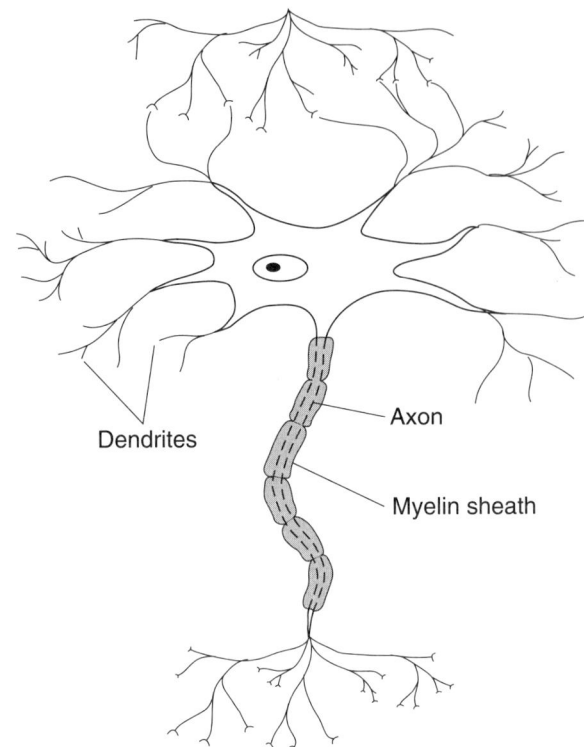

Fig. 11-1. Schematic representation of a neuronal cell with dendritic and axon extensions.

rons. Astrocytes provide a basic supportive role to neurons and contribute to the blood-brain barrier.[45]

Neurons, on the basis of immense cellular volume and length, require highly developed transport systems for delivery of nutrients, proteins, and cytoskeletal components.[8] The blood-brain and, in the case of the peripheral nervous system, blood-nerve barriers limit entry of nonlipophilic molecules from adjacent tissues via tight junctions between vascular endothelial cells. This defense is discontinuous at certain ganglions and at several locations within the central nervous system and is poorly developed in the fetus and young child, suggesting enhanced susceptibility to polar and water-soluble neurotoxicants. An area of recently intense investigation is the role of anatomic and physiologic neuroplasticity in learning and memory.[50] Expanding appreciation of the alteration in synaptic architecture, membrane receptors, neuronal interconnections, and amplitude and frequency of action potentials that occur in response to experience may provide a glimpse of the basis for higher cognitive functions.

NEURONAL RESPONSE TO INJURY

Neurotoxicants[74] may affect the neuron itself (mercury), the dendrites (monosodium glutamate), the axons (n-hexane, carbon disulfide, acrylamide), myelin (hexachlorophene, triethyl tin), and blood vessels (lead). Injury to the neuronal cell body may lead to degeneration of neuronal processes and cell death. The high metabolic state of neurons makes them more susceptible to depletion of high-energy compounds. Neurons do not regenerate. There is apparent functional improvement after injury, most likely reflecting recovery of neurons from nonfatal injuries, and some development of collateral branches from existing neurons, especially motor neurons. Structures in proximity to the ventricles, the autonomic ganglia, and the dorsal roots[74] have poorly developed blood-brain barriers and are particularly sensitive.

Axonal degeneration (distal axonopathy), producing both central and peripheral polyneuropathy, is the most common neurologic response to intoxication by chemicals of environmental significance (Fig. 11-2). Disruption of the axon at a site distant from the neuronal cell body initiates degeneration of the distal axon segment. Peripheral nerves are capable of regeneration over periods lasting weeks to months, whereas regeneration of central axons is limited, if it occurs at all.

TOXICOLOGY OF SELECTED NEUROTOXIC CHEMICALS

Table 11-1 lists major neurotoxicants of environmental medical significance. Important toxic metals include lead, mercury, and arsenic.

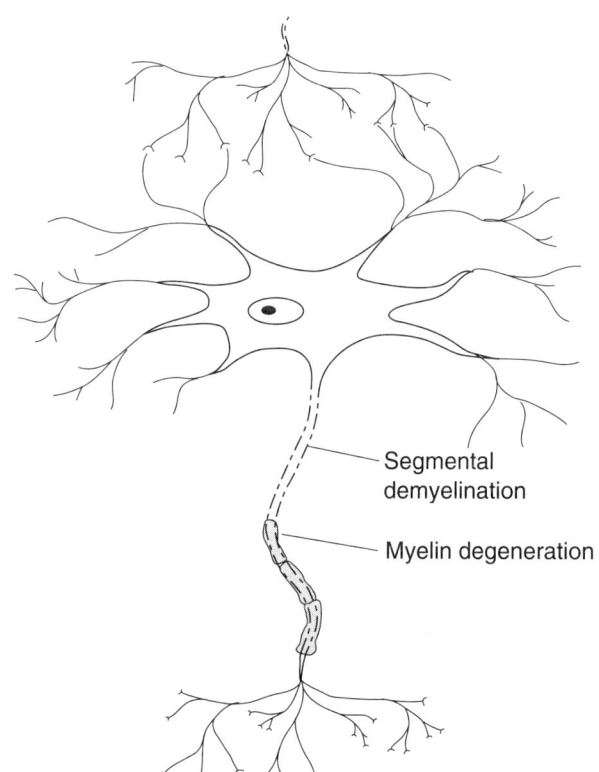

Fig. 11-2. A neuropathy may result from segmental demyelination or from myelin degeneration.

Metals
Lead

Lead's effects on human health and its neurotoxicology have been subjects of numerous publications.* The two principal exposure routes are the respiratory system, inhaled in dust and fumes, and the gastrointestinal system, especially ingestion of contaminated food. Respiratory retention of lead dust is a function of particle size. Alveolar absorption is generally rapid and complete. Gastrointestinal absorption is much lower, ranging from 10% to 15% in adults and approaching 40%[30] in children. The major target organs are the central and peripheral nervous systems, kidneys, and blood. Approximately 90% of the total body lead burden is in bone, with a mean half-life of 30 to 50 years, although the metabolically and toxicologically active lead pool may turn over considerably more rapidly.[48] This accounts in part for the persistence of lead toxicity after discontinuation of exposure and the relative lack of efficacy of chelation as treatment in individuals with markedly elevated total body lead burdens.

The important neurologic manifestations are a peripheral polyneuropathy, with motor neurons more vulnerable than sensory, and central nervous system effects, including short-term memory loss, new learning deficits, and reduction in psychomotor speed and dexterity. Depression, confusion, and anger are prominent emotional consequences.[31]

Lead's neurotoxic mechanisms are not completely understood.[14,70] Lead is directly toxic to blood vessels; causes distal axonopathy, predominantly in motor neurons; and damages peripheral myelin[23] via Schwann-cell degeneration. Because most of the systems implicated in lead's neurotoxicity are calcium dependent, alteration of calcium transport[48] may represent the basis for a unifying hypothesis. Lead inhibits cholinergic function by decreasing neurotransmission. It decreases dopamine uptake by synaptosomes; impairs the function of gamma-aminobutyric acid; binds to sulfhydryl groups, interfering with multiple enzyme systems; is a potent inhibitor of mitochondrial function; and may replace calcium in the activation of protein kinase C,[49] which mediates processes of cell differentiation and proliferation. δ-Aminolevulinic acid, generated through altered porphyrin metabolism, may itself be neurotoxic.[80] Altered tryptophan metabolism in the liver due to lead poisoning may cause elevated brain levels of tryptophan, serotonin, and 5-hydroxyindoleacetic acid.[71]

Mercury

The neurologic and neuropsychologic toxicity of mercury have been the subjects of numerous publications.† Elemental, monovalent (mercurous), and divalent (mercuric) inorganic salts and organic mercury compounds have distinctly different toxicologic effects.[30]

---
*References 6, 7, 14, 26, 30-32, 37, 41, 48, 68, 70.
†References 6, 7, 13, 17, 30-32, 37, 43, 57, 68.

Table 11-1. Common neurotoxicants

Metals	Solvents	Pesticides	Gases	Others
Lead	Xylene	Organophosphate	Carbon monoxide	Ethyl alcohol
Arsenic	Styrene	Organochlorine	Nitrous oxide	Hallucinogens
Mercury	Toluene	Methyl bromide	Hydrogen cyanide	Cocaine
Manganese	Carbon disulfide	Carbamates	Ethylene oxide	Marihuana
Thallium	Trichloroethylene		Methyl chloride	Mood alterers
Aluminum	Perchloroethylene			Tri-*ortho*-cresyl phosphate
Gold	Methylene chloride			Strychnine
Manganese	Acrylamide			Isoniazid
Triethy tin	*n*-Hexane			Dioxins
	Methyl alcohol			
	Ethylene oxide			
	Ethylene glycol			
	Methyl ethyl ketone			
	Benzene			
	1,1,1-Trichloroethane			
	Mixed solvents			
	Hexachlorophene			

Elemental mercury is absorbed through the lungs as a vapor, whereas inorganic mercury salts and organic mercury compounds are principally absorbed through the gastrointestinal tract. Absorption of elemental mercury is approximately 80% efficient after inhalation exposure, and 90% to 95% of methyl mercury is absorbed from the gastrointestinal tract. In distinct contrast, less than 0.01% of elemental mercury is absorbed from the gut. Biologic half-lives of mercury also vary as a function of its form and range from approximately 1.5 to 2.5 months.[13]

Manifestations of acute inhalation of high concentrations of mercury vapor include bronchitis and interstitial pneumonitis, because of its corrosive effects on lung tissue, as well as nervous system effects of tremor and excitability.[13] After chronic pulmonary exposure to elemental mercury, nervous system effects predominate, with early symptoms of "micro-mercurialism,"[30] which combines neurasthenic symptoms (headache, fatigue, dizziness, memory loss, depression) with three or more of a number of clinical findings: tremor, thyromegaly or increased thyroid uptake of radioiodine, tachycardia or pulse irregularity, gingivitis, dermatographism, hematologic changes, and elevated urine mercury levels. With increasing severity of intoxication, the classic triad of erethism (withdrawal, memory loss, excitability, and depression), tremor, and gingivitis emerges. A subacute, diffuse polyneuropathy also has been described.[68]

In contrast, the clinical picture after ingestion of inorganic mercury salts includes abdominal pain and diarrhea, with renal effects, including oliguria and proteinuria. Divalent (mercuric) compounds are more toxic than monovalent (mercurous) compounds. The lipid-soluble organomercurials pass rapidly through the blood-brain barrier, and clinical intoxication is characterized by circumoral and acral paresthesia, gait abnormality, dysarthria, dysphagia, spasticity, vision and hearing loss, tremor, and generalized weakness.[30]

Neuropsychologic effects combining behavioral and cognitive disturbances are the earliest effects associated with mercury exposure.[25] Among the deficits are visuospatial abnormalities, visual and short-term memory deficits, and delayed reaction times.[31]

Arsenic

The primary neurologic effect of arsenic is a peripheral neuropathy.* Arsenic, in both its inorganic and organic forms, may be trivalent or pentavalent. Common trivalent inorganic compounds are arsenic trioxide, sodium arsenite, and arsenic trichloride, and pentavalent forms include arsenic pentoxide, arsenic acid, and arsenates, including calcium and lead arsenate.[30]

The routes of exposure include inhalation of dust and ingestion of contaminated food. Arsenic is cleared predominantly through the kidneys, with a half-life ranging between approximately 10 hours for inorganic compounds and 30 hours for methylated arsenic.[30] Acute arsenic intoxication following ingestion is manifest by serious, at times hemorrhagic, gastroenteritis and shock.[44] Pathologic changes can be seen at autopsy in multiple organs. Chronic effects[44] include dermatitis, several varieties of skin cancer, hepatomegaly and cirrhosis, peripheral vascular occlusive disease (black foot disease), megaloblastic anemia, and respiratory effects, including nasal septal perforation and lung cancer.

Inorganic arsenic may cause a distal axonopathy[68] within weeks of a single high-dose exposure or more gradually after

---
*References 13, 30, 31, 44, 68.

long-term lower-level exposures. The single-exposure type begins as a sensory neuropathy with distal paresthesia and hypoesthesia, followed by motor involvement, generally first noticed in the lower extremities. The long-term–exposure type begins with constitutional symptoms of malaise, weakness, anorexia, and vomiting, followed by mucous membrane irritation, hyperkeratosis with hyperpigmentation, pitting edema, and Mee's lines, transverse white lines across the nails. A frank, predominantly sensory peripheral neuropathy, with numbness and painful burning, loss of position and vibratory sense, and, perhaps, mild weakness, develops as a final stage after chronic exposure.[68]

The mechanism of arsenic's neurotoxicity is incompletely known. Trivalent arsenic compounds are significantly more toxic than are pentavalent arsenicals or organic varieties, and this comparative toxicity may be at least partially based on the longer biologic half-life of trivalent arsenic. In addition, the cellular mechanisms are valence dependent. Trivalent arsenic binds to sulfhydryl groups and interferes with respiration and adenosine triphosphate production through disruption of the tricarboxylic acid cycle. Pentavalent arsenic compounds uncouple oxidative phosphorylation by substituting for inorganic phosphate.[13]

Organic solvents

The organic solvents, by virtue of their volatility and solubility, are in widespread use in commercial and industrial products. The same properties that contribute to their usefulness also helps explain their toxicity, tendency for absorption through the lungs and concentration in body fat and lipid-rich organs, including liver, kidneys, and the central and peripheral nervous systems.

Of the seemingly limitless number of solvents, only a relatively limited subset has particular importance in the field of environmental medicine. Primary among these are the solvent mixtures, often manufactured on the basis of boiling-point separation in petroleum distillation. Gasoline, kerosene, painter's naphtha, mineral spirits, petroleum, and other familiar names head the list. Of the pure products, toluene, ethyl benzene, and xylene are the alkyl benzene aromatics of greatest environmental concern. The principal halogenated alkanes and alkenes include trichloroethylene, trichloroethane (methyl chloroform), methylene chloride (dichloromethane), perchloroethylene (tetrachloroethylene), and methylchloroform. Lest we forget, ingested ethanol is clearly the most significant environmental neurotoxicant of them all. Many of the organic solvents of major toxicologic concern in the occupational setting, including carbon tetrachloride, benzene, carbon disulfide, styrene, *n*-hexane, methyl *n*-butyl ketone, and vinyl chloride, are not currently significant sources of environmental neurotoxicity.

Manifestations of organic solvent neurotoxicity can be clearly separated into acute, self-limited intoxication, with symptoms of headache, dizziness (both vertigo and light-headedness), feelings of drunkenness, disorientation, nausea, dysarthria, and ataxia; and a chronic psychoorganic syndrome also referred to as *chronic encephalopathy*.[9,19] After years characterized by recurrent episodes of acute intoxication at work, chronic symptoms, including short-term memory loss, depression, headache, dizziness, fatigue, loss of libido, irritability, distractibility, and social withdrawal, may emerge. Signs on clinical neurologic examination are limited to an accentuated postural tremor and, in severe cases, disturbances in immediate memory or recall after distraction.

Neuropsychologic abnormalities define both the acute and chronic syndromes.[33] Acute effects have been associated with impairments in attention, concentration, and reaction time.[4] Conversely, chronic effects include deficits in both auditory and visual memory, visuospatial functions, and psychomotor coordination. Intellectual functions tend to be relatively preserved but can be affected when the chronic encephalopathy is severe. Personality testing typically verifies the depression noted clinically.

Reviews of organic-solvent toxicology[3,9,19] are recommended for a more detailed description of the absorption, distribution, metabolism, clearance, and proposed toxic mechanism of individual solvents. The principal routes of exposure of the various individual solvents and solvent mixtures are closely related to their volatility, lipophilicity and the specific circumstances of their use. Organic solvents are efficiently absorbed across the alveolar membrane and quickly distributed throughout the body. Percutaneous absorption, although less avid, can be a major exposure route in individuals with prolonged or extensive cutaneous exposure or in the presence of underlying skin disease. Absorption through the gastrointestinal tract is the principal route of exposure of ethanol.

Organic solvents partition within body fat and fatty tissues, as a function of their lipid solubility and the local blood supply. The simpler molecules are cleared through the lungs and, to an extent, as metabolites or parent compounds through the urine. Several organic solvents are partially metabolized in the liver. The biologic half-life of organic solvents is predictably variable and agent specific. Persistence beyond 1 or 2 weeks is not typically seen.

It is likely that different neurotoxic mechanisms cause the acute narcotizing effects and the long-term effects of organic solvents. Acute narcotic manifestations have been associated with neuronal cell membrane changes, presumably related to the lipid solubility of solvents. Although the long-term central and peripheral nervous system effects have been speculatively linked to permanent alteration of neuronal structural proteins, these mechanisms remain unproven.

Pesticides

The third major category of environmental neurotoxicants consists of the pesticides, the major classes being the anticholinesterase and organochlorine insecticides.

Pyrethroid insecticides[24] have considerable potential environmental health importance because of their widespread use, including aerial spraying for mosquito control, and they are neurotoxic in their primary insecticidal action; generally, the potential for pyrethroid neurotoxicity has not been realized from environmental exposures. The only neurotoxic effects in humans have been self-limited burning and numbness after cutaneous exposure.

Anticholinesterase insecticides

The neurologic and neuropsychologic toxicology of anticholinesterase insecticides has been the subject of intense investigative interest.* Much of the neurotoxicity related to organophosphorous compounds has been associated with epidemics in which nonpesticidal forms adulterate foodstuffs, causing severe distal axonopathy. Ginger jake paralysis related to tri-*ortho*-cresyl phosphate[38] is one example. Both carbamate ester– and organophosphorous ester–type insecticides cause acute intoxication through interaction with acetylcholinesterase. Nicotinic and muscarinic symptoms include headache, nausea, dizziness, anxiety, restlessness, muscle twitching and weakness, tremor, incoordination, vomiting, abdominal cramping, and diarrhea. Bronchorrhea, rhinitis, tearing, salivation, and profuse diaphoresis contribute to a clinical picture of hypersecretion. Chest constriction, wheezing, and, at times, noncardiogenic pulmonary edema may occur. Pupillary constriction and bradycardia are important findings to monitor in the assessment of the course and efficacy of treatment.[52] A number of the organophosphorous compounds bind irreversibly to acetylcholinesterase, leading to prolonged intoxication; the carbamate esters bind reversibly to the reactive site and are associated with self-limited, although at times serious, intoxication.

Organic phosphorous esters[27] are absorbed slowly through the skin and efficiently absorbed through the lungs and gastrointestinal tract. Hundreds of heterogeneous chemicals are included within the class of organophosphorous compounds, and the different compounds' absorption, distribution, penetration into the central and peripheral nervous systems, neurotoxicity, metabolism, and clearance vary considerably. In general, persistence is minimal. The carbamate[12] insecticides are also a chemically diverse group. They too are absorbed through the skin, lungs, and gastrointestinal tract and are rapidly metabolized and cleared without bioaccumulation.

Certain organophosphorous esters, most having no pesticidal uses, are associated with organophosphate-induced delayed neurotoxicity (OPIDN). The carbamates have not been associated with polyneuropathy. The total number of reported cases of neuropathy caused by organophosphorous pesticides is less than 100.[27] The specific organophosphorous compounds implicated include triorthocresyl phosphate, mipafox, leptophos, diisopropylfluorophosphate, *O*-ethyl-*O*-4-nitrophenyl phenylphosphonothioate (EPN), merphos, and one of the trithiobutyl compounds 5,5,5-tributyl phosphorothioate (DEF).

The mechanism of the initiation of OPIDN is based on the permanent inhibition of neuropathy target esterase (NTE) in an ''aging'' process.[35] Induction of paralysis in adult hens correlates with inhibition of brain NTE and is the most reliable predictor of delayed neuropathy in humans. The experience with neurotoxicity testing in the hen has been summarized and tabulated.[20,27]

It is as yet unclear whether organophosphorous esters cause chronic central nervous system or neuropsychologic effects, although these are areas of current research interest.[66] Acute intoxication is characterized by cognitive and affective symptoms, and there have been reports of chronic neuropsychologic deficits after both acute poisoning and long-term exposure in agricultural and industrial workers.[31,32]

Organochlorine insecticides

The organochlorine insecticides[72] are a highly diverse group of agents. They fall into three chemical classes: the dichlorodiphenylethane-related compounds, the chlorinated cyclodienes, and the chlorinated cyclohexane and chlorinated benzene-related groups.[24] Individual insecticides vary widely in their toxicity and biopersistence. Nevertheless, some generalizations regarding their clinical effects, mechanisms of action, and significance as sources of medical illness in environmentally exposed human populations are possible.

Most of the organochlorine compounds have been removed from the market in the United States because of their long persistence in ecosystems, toxicity to fauna, and bioaccumulation up the food chain. Examples include 1,1,1-trichloro-2,2-*bis* (4-chlorophenyl) ethane (DDT), dieldrin, heptachlor, mirex, chlordecone, and chlordane. Many of these compounds, however, still are in widespread use in other countries and remain important to global environmental considerations.

The organochlorine insecticides tend to have low volatility and high lipid solubility and are slowly metabolized. They are chemically stable in the environment and slowly degraded. Organochlorine pesticides have largely been replaced by the organophosphorous ester compounds, and episodes of acute clinical intoxication are relatively rare.

In general, these compounds have an excitatory effect on central and peripheral nervous system functions. Early symptoms may include headache, nausea, vomiting, dizziness, hyperesthesia and paresthesia of the extremities and face, tremor, incoordination, and confusion.[52] With more severe intoxication, myoclonic jerking and generalized seizures, followed by coma and death, may occur. Sudden, high fever, at times delayed in onset, has been described, particularly with benzene hydrochloride.[72] Intoxication by the cy-

---
*References 1, 8, 11, 20, 21, 24, 27, 31, 32, 36, 37, 47, 69.

clodienes and toxaphene may present initially as status epilepticus without any of the premonitory symptoms noted previously, and seizures related to the cyclodienes (such as dieldrin, aldrin, and chlordane) may be highly resistant to pharmacologic intervention and may recur for days.[52] Neuropsychologic effects are likely, based on the clinical scenario of acute intoxication, but have not been documented. Nonneurologic effects, including hepatic and blood effects, occur with one or more compounds. Many of the compounds are carcinogenic in mice and other species, although human carcinogenicity is controversial. The toxicity of chlordecone (Kepone) has been well described in occupational groups,[15,77] with symptoms of ataxia, opsoclonus, headache, tremor, weight loss, impotence, and hepatosplenomegaly. Chlordecone is not a likely source of environmental intoxication, because it was banned prior to widespread distribution. All of the chlorinated hydrocarbon insecticides are absorbed percutaneously and via oral and respiratory routes. Absorption characteristics of the various chemicals, however, are extremely variable. DDT, for instance, is poorly absorbed through the skin. Low volatility predicts that inhalation is relatively unimportant except when these materials are aerosolized. All the representative agents in this group accumulate in fat, and their metabolism and biologic half-life are quite compound specific.[72]

The mechanisms of the neurotoxicity of chlorinated hydrocarbon insecticides are probably multiple and, again, are agent specific. All the compounds appear to affect Na^P-K^P ion currents across neuronal membranes and likely decrease the threshold for depolarization, resulting in repetitive neuronal discharge. DDT and its analogs inhibit Ca^{PP}-ATPase. Some compounds block the inhibitory action of gamma-aminobutyric acid–mediated neuronal uptake of chloride ions, also causing a state of uncontrolled excitation. There are additional effects on a variety of enzyme systems.[72]

Dioxins and related compounds

Evidence of neurotoxicity from environmental exposures to dioxin and related compounds is limited. A brief overview is provided here, because questions and concerns regarding these materials are so common in the practice of environmental medicine. Most concerns regarding potential chronic toxicity are directed at its potential carcinogenesis, immunotoxicity, and developmental and reproductive effects.

The toxicology of the halogenated aromatic hydrocarbons, including polychlorinated dibenzo-p-dioxins, polychlorinated biphenyls (PCBs), and the polychlorinated dibenzofurans (PCDFs), has been summarized.[42,57,65,68] The scientific literature linking environmental exposures to these materials with neurotoxicity is primarily limited to clinical evaluations of populations exposed to releases from industrial facilities or situations wherein these materials were introduced into food.

A chemical manufacturing plant in Seveso, Italy,[59] experienced a runaway reaction during the manufacture of 2,4,5-trichloroacetic acid, releasing large quantities of 2,3,7,8-tetrachlorodibenzo-p-dioxin (dioxin) into the environment. Among other effects, including chloracne and hepatomegaly, both peripheral and central nervous system findings were more common in individuals residing near the plant than in those living further away.[59] Abnormal results on nerve conduction studies did not correlate with the occurrence of chloracne, however.

Environmental intoxication from PCBs and the closely related and more toxic PCDFs and polychlorinated quaterphenyls (PCQs) has been responsible for severe multiorgan-system disease in populations in Japan (Yusho) and, 10 years later, in Taiwan (YuCheng). The source of the PCBs, PCDFs, and PCQs was traced to consumption of food cooked in contaminated rice oil. A clinical picture of sensory polyneuropathy,[18,53] including extremity numbness and abnormal results of nerve conduction velocity testing, have been described.

As yet, no epidemiologic evidence links environmental exposures to the halogenated aromatic hydrocarbons with neurotoxicity. Sport fishermen develop elevations in serum PCBs as high or higher than levels reported to occur in occupational groups; consumption of contaminated fish has not been implicated specifically as a cause of neurotoxic disease.

These materials[54] are principally absorbed through the gastrointestinal tract, although absorption through inhalation of contaminated aerosols and percutaneous absorption are possible, particularly when the compounds are suspended in a lipophilic vehicle. These agents are highly fat soluble and are stored in body fat pools and organs with relatively high lipid content, for example, bone marrow, brain, peripheral nerve, liver, and kidneys. Metabolism is, in general, limited and specific to the chemical structure. The presumed mechanism of action of these compounds is related to their common ability to induce hepatic cytochrome P-450 microsomal enzyme systems, especially aryl hydrocarbon hydroxylase, and alteration of the control of structural genes coding for several proteins.[54,60]

Carbon monoxide

Carbon monoxide as a source of environmental neurotoxicity, occurs not from outdoor but rather from indoor air pollution. Carbon monoxide is emitted from all sources of incomplete combustion of carbon-containing fuel, including fireplaces, gas and oil stoves, space heaters, ovens, faulty furnaces, and tobacco smoke.[40]

The clinical picture of carbon monoxide intoxication is well described,[22,75] with symptoms somewhat related to carboxyhemoglobin levels. At relatively low levels, headache is common; there is progression to giddiness, malaise, nausea and occasional emesis, weakness, and dyspnea occur as levels increase. Disturbances of alertness and consciousness are seen at carboxyhemoglobin levels above 40% to 45%.

There are two major issues regarding carbon monoxide and neurotoxicity. The first relates to evidence of behavioral effects at relatively low levels of carboxyhemoglobin, (that occur less than 10%), which may be from tobacco smoking and outdoor air pollution. Results of experimental studies at less than 5% are inconsistent, although some have shown impairment of time-interval discrimination at carboxyhemoglobin levels of 2.5%.[2] At a 5% carboxyhemoglobin level, rapid performance of complex dual tasks are impaired.[6] The human responses at various carboxyhemoglobin concentrations have been summarized.[56]

The second issue concerns the occurrence of delayed neuropsychiatric syndromes after acute high-level carbon monoxide intoxication, presumably due to delayed demyelination.[16,51,58,61] Although neuropsychologic testing was apparently not performed,[51] the clinical characteristics of 86 patients with carbon monoxide–induced delayed neurotoxicity suggests major impairments, with apathy, amnesia, disorientation, irritability, distractibility, and memory deficits. Neurologic findings may also include urinary or fecal incontinence, gait disturbance, mutism, masked facies, increased muscle tone, retropulsion, steppage gait, and a positive glabellar sign and grasp reflex.[51]

After inhalation, carbon monoxide passes rapidly through alveolar membranes and binds to hemoglobin with an affinity 240 times greater than oxygen. The biologic half-life varies with minute ventilation, cardiac output, and concentration of oxygen in ambient air, falling after 4 hours in room air; 60 to 90 minutes in 100% oxygen and decreased after less than 25 minutes in hyperbaric oxygen at 2 atm.[37]

Carbon monoxide causes hypoxia by competing with oxygen for binding sites on hemoglobin, reducing the oxyhemoglobin saturation. Peripheral utilization of oxygen is also impaired through a leftward shift of the oxyhemoglobin dissociation curve at high levels of carboxyhemoglobin. It increases the level of 2,3- diphosphoglycerate, further shifting the dissociation curve to the left. It also binds to cytochrome oxidase and cytochrome P-450 and impairs the diffusion of oxygen to mitochondria.[42] As a result, electron-transport processes, and therefore cellular energy production, are disrupted. The organs most sensitive to hypoxia are the nervous system and the heart, particularly if it occurs in a patient with coronary artery–occlusive disease.

SUMMARY

Neurotoxic disorders have long held a prominent place in the annals of environmental medicine. The clinical manifestations of a neurotoxic illness is closely linked to the normal anatomy and physiology of the nervous system and its pattern of responses to insult. The number of neurotoxicants causing disease from environmental exposures is relatively small. The toxicology of these agents remains incompletely understood. Research aimed at enhancing knowledge of normal neurologic and neuropsychologic function at the cellular and systemic levels will provide a fuller appreciation of neuronal function under stressed or diseased states.

REFERENCES

1. Abou-Donia MB, Lapadula DM: Mechanisms of organophosphorus ester-induced delayed neurotoxicity: type I and type II, *Annu Rev Pharmacol Toxicol* 30:405, 1990.
2. Amdur MO: Air pollutants. In Amdur MO, Doull J, Klaassen CD, eds: *Casarett and Doull's toxicology,* ed 4, New York, 1991, Pergamon.
3. Andrews LS, Snyder R: Toxic effects of solvents and vapors. In Amdur MO, Doull J, Klaassen CD, editors: *Casarett and Doull's toxicology,* ed 4, New York, 1991, Pergamon.
4. Anger WK: Worksite behavioral research: results, sensitive methods, test batteries and transition from laboratory data to human health, *Neurotoxicology* 11:629, 1990.
5. Anger WK: Assessment of neurotoxicity in humans. In Tilson HA, Mitchell CL, editors: *Neurotoxicology,* New York, 1992, Raven Press.
6. Anger WK, Johnson BL: Chemicals affect behavior. In O'Donoghue JL, ed: *Neurotoxicity of industrial chemicals,* vol 1, Boca Raton, Fla, 1985, CRC Press.
7. Anger WK, Johnson BL: Human behavioral neurotoxicology: workplace and community assessments. In Rom WN, ed: *Environmental and occupational medicine,* ed 2, Boston, 1992, Little, Brown.
8. Anthony DC, Graham DG: Toxic responses of the nervous system. In Amdur MO, Doull J, Klaassen CD, eds: *Casarett and Doull's toxicology,* ed 4, New York, 1991, Pergamon.
9. Baker EL: Organic solvent neurotoxicity, *Annu Rev Public Health* 9:223, 1988.
10. Baker EL: Neurologic disorders. In Rom WN, ed: *Environmental and occupational medicine,* ed 2, Boston, 1992, Little, Brown.
11. Baker EL, Feldman RG, French JG: Environmentally related disorders of the nervous system, *Med Clin North Am* 74:325, 1990.
12. Baron RL: Carbamate insecticides. In Hayes WJ, Laws ER, eds: *Handbook of pesticide toxicology,* vol 3, San Diego, 1991, Academic Press.
13. Bhamra RK, Costa M: Trace elements: aluminum, arsenic, cadmium, mercury and nickel. In Lippmann M, ed: *Environmental toxicants: human exposures and their health effects,* New York, 1992, Van Nostrand Reinhold.
14. Bressler JP, Goldstein GW: Mechanisms of lead neurotoxicity, *Biochem Pharmacol* 41:479, 1991.
15. Cannon SB et al: Epidemic Kepone poisoning in chemical workers, *Am J Epidemiol* 107:529, 1978.
16. Chang KH et al: Delayed encephalopathy after acute carbon monoxide intoxication: MR imaging features and distribution of cerebral white matter lesions, *Radiology* 184:117, 1992.
17. Chang LW: Mercury. In Spencer PS, Schaumburg HH, eds: *Experimental and clinical neurotoxicology,* Baltimore, 1980, Williams & Wilkins.
18. Chen RC et al: Polychlorinated biphenyl poisoning: correlation of sensory and motor nerve conduction, neurologic symptoms, and blood levels of polychlorinated biphenyls, quaterphenyls and dibenzofurans, *Environ Res* 37:340, 1985.
19. Cranmer JM, Goldberg L: Proceedings of a workshop on the neurobehavioral effects of solvents, *Neurotoxicology* 7:1, 1986.
20. Davis CS, Johnson MK, Richardson RJ: Organophosphorus compounds. In O'Donoghue JL, ed: *Neurotoxicity of industrial and commercial chemicals,* vol 2, Boca Raton, Fla, 1985, CRC Press.
21. De Bleecker J, Van Den Neucker K, Willems JL: Neurological aspects of organophosphate poisoning, *Clin Neurol Neurosurg* 94:93, 1992.
22. Dinman BD: The management of carbon monoxide intoxication, *J Occup Med* 16:662, 1974.

23. Duncan ID: Toxic myelinopathies. In O'Donoghue JL, ed: *Neurotoxicity of industrial and commercial chemicals,* vol 1, Boca Raton, Fla, 1985, CRC Press.
24. Ecobichon DJ: Toxic effects of pesticides. In Amdur MO, Doull J, Klaassen CD, eds: *Casarett and Doull's toxicology,* ed 4, New York, 1991, Pergamon.
25. Feldman RG: Neurological manifestations of mercury intoxication, *Acta Neurol Scand Suppl* 92:201, 1982.
26. Fischbein A: Occupational and environmental lead exposure. In Rom WN, ed: *Environmental and occupational medicine,* ed 2, Boston, 1992, Little, Brown.
27. Gallo MA, Lawryk NJ: Organic phosphorus pesticides. In Hayes WJ, Laws ER, eds: *Handbook of pesticide toxicology,* vol 2, San Diego, 1991, Academic Press.
28. Gilfillan SC: Lead poisoning and the fall of Rome, *J Occup Med* 7:53, 1962.
29. Gockel E: cited in Fischbein A: Occupational and environmental lead exposure. In Rom WN, ed: *Environmental and occupational medicine,* ed 2, Boston, 1992, Little, Brown.
30. Goyer RA: Toxic effects of metals. In Amdur MO, Doull J, Klaassen CD, eds: *Casarett and Doull's toxicology,* ed 4, New York, 1991, Pergamon.
31. Hartman DE: *Neuropsychological toxicology: identification and assessment of human neurotoxic syndromes,* New York, 1988, Pergamon.
32. Hartman DE, Hessl S, Tarcher AB: Neurobehavioral disorders. In Tarcher AB, ed: *Principles and practice of environmental medicine,* New York, 1992, Plenum.
33. Isaacson RL, Jensen KF, editors: *Vulnerable brain and environmental risks,* vol 2, New York, 1992, Plenum.
34. Jackson DL, Menges H: Accidental carbon monoxide poisoning, *JAMA* 243:772, 1980.
35. Johnson MK: Receptor or enzyme: the puzzle of NTE and organophosphate-induced delayed neuropathy, *Trends Pharmacol Sci* 8:174, 1987.
36. Johnson MK: Organophosphates and delayed neuropathy: is NTE alive and well? *Toxicol Appl Pharmacol* 102:385, 1990.
37. Kelley JP, Filley CM: Neurobehavioral toxicology. In Sullivan JB, Krieger GR, eds: *Hazardous materials toxicology: clinical principles of environmental health,* Baltimore, 1992, Williams & Wilkins.
38. Kidd JG, Langworthy OR: Paralysis following ingestion of Jamaica ginger extract adulterated with tri-ortho-cresyl phosphate, *Johns Hopkins Med J* 52:39, 1933.
39. Kimbrough RD: Human health effects of polychlorinated biphenyls (PCBs) and polybrominated biphenyls (PBBs), *Annu Rev Pharmacol Toxicol* 27:87, 1987.
40. Kleinman MT: Health effects of carbon monoxide. In Lippmann M, ed: *Environmental toxicants: human exposures and their health effects,* New York, 1992, Van Nostrand Reinhold.
41. Krigman MR, Bouldin TW, Mushak P: Lead. In Spencer PS, Schaumburg HH, eds: *Experimental and clinical neurotoxicology,* Baltimore, 1980, Williams & Wilkins.
42. Kurt TL: Chemical asphyxiants. In Rom WN, ed: *Environmental and occupational medicine,* ed 2, Boston, 1992, Little, Brown.
43. Kuznetsov DA: Minamata disease: what is a keystone of its molecular mechanism? A biochemical theory on the nature of methyl mercury neurotoxicity, *Int J Neurosci* 53:1, 1990.
44. Landrigan PJ: Arsenic. In Rom WN, ed: *Environmental and occupational medicine,* ed 2, Boston, 1992, Little, Brown.
45. Lewis AJ: Functions of supporting cells. In Lewis AJ, ed: *Mechanisms of neurologic disease,* Boston, 1976, Little, Brown.
46. Lippmann M, ed: *Environmental toxicants: human exposures and their health effects,* New York, 1992, Van Nostrand Reinhold.
47. Lotti M: The pathogenesis of organophosphate polyneuropathy, *Crit Rev Toxicol* 21:465, 1991.
48. Mahaffey KR, McKinney J, Reigert JR: Lead and compounds. In Lippmann M, ed: *Environmental toxicants: human exposures and their health effects,* New York, 1992, Van Nostrand Reinhold.
49. Markovac J, Goldstein GW: Picomolar concentrations of lead stimulate brain protein kinase C, *Nature* 334:71, 1988.
50. Milgram NW, MacLeod CM, Petit TL, eds: *Neuroplasticity, learning and memory,* New York, 1987, Alan R Liss.
51. Min SK: A brain syndrome associated with delayed neuropsychiatric sequelae following acute carbon monoxide intoxication, *Acta Psychiatr Scand* 73:80, 1986.
52. Morgan DP: *Recognition and management of pesticide poisonings,* ed 4, Pub No EPA-540/9-88-001, Washington, DC, 1989, US Environmental Protection Agency.
53. Murai Y, Kuroiwa Y: Peripheral neuropathy in chlorobiphenyls poisoning, *Neurology* 21:1173, 1971.
54. Nessel CS, Gallo MA: Dioxins and related compounds. In Lippmann M, ed: *Environmental toxicants: human exposures and their health effects,* New York, 1992, Van Nostrand Reinhold.
55. O'Donoghue JL, ed: *Neurotoxicity of industrial and commercial chemicals,* Boca Raton, Fla, 1985, CRC Press.
56. O'Donoghue JL: Carbon monoxide, inorganic nitrogenous compounds, and phosphorous. In O'Donoghue JL, ed: *Neurotoxicity of industrial and commercial chemicals,* vol 1, Boca Raton, Fla, 1985, CRC Press.
57. Parkinson DK: Mercury. In Rom WN, ed: *Environmental and occupational medicine,* ed 2, Boston, 1992, Little, Brown.
58. Plum F, Posner JB, Hain RF: Delayed neurological deterioration after anoxia, *Arch Intern Med* 110:56, 1962.
59. Pocchiari F, Silano V, Zampieri A: Human health effects from accidental release of tetrachlorodibenzo-p-dioxin (TCDD) at Seveso, Italy, *Ann NY Acad Sci* 320:311, 1979.
60. Poland A, Knutson JC: 2,3,7,8-Tetrachlorodibenzo-*p*-dioxin and related halogenated aromatic hydrocarbons: examination of the mechanism of toxicity, *Annu Rev Pharmacol Toxicol* 22:517, 1982.
61. Remick RA, Miles JE: Carbon monoxide poisoning: neurologic and psychiatric sequelae, *Can Med Assoc J* 117:654, 1977.
62. Rogan WJ, Gladen BC: Neurotoxicology of PCBs and related compounds, *Neurotoxicology* 13:27, 1992.
63. Rom WN, ed: *Environmental and occupational medicine,* ed 2, Boston, 1992, Little, Brown.
64. Rosenberg NL: Neurotoxicology, In Sullivan JB, Krieger GR, ed: *Hazardous materials toxicology: clinical principles of environmental health,* Baltimore, 1992, Williams & Wilkins.
65. Rosenman KD: Dioxin, polychlorinated biphenyls, and dibenzofurans. In Rom WN, ed: *Environmental and occupational medicine,* ed 2, Boston, 1992, Little, Brown.
66. Rosenstock L et al: Chronic neuropsychological sequelae of occupational exposure to organophosphate insecticides, *Am J Ind Med* 18:321, 1990.
67. Russell RW, Flattau PE, Pope AM, eds: *Behavioral measures of neurotoxicity,* Washington, DC, 1990, National Academy Press.
68. Schaumburg HH, Berger AR, Thomas PK: Occupational, biologic and environmental agents. In Schaumburg HH, Berger AR, Thomas PK, eds: *Disorders of peripheral nerves,* ed 2, Philadelphia, 1992, FA Davis.
69. Schenker MB, Albertson TE, Saiki CL: Pesticides. In Rom WN, ed: *Environmental and occupational medicine,* ed 2, Boston, 1992, Little, Brown.
70. Silbergeld EK: Mechanisms of lead neurotoxicity, or looking beyond the lamppost, *FASEB J* 6:3201, 1992.
71. Silbergeld EK, Hruska RE: Neurochemical investigation of low level lead exposure. In Needleman HL, ed: *Low level lead exposure,* New York, 1980, Raven Press.
72. Smith AG: Chlorinated hydrocarbon insecticides. In Hayes WJ, Laws ER, eds: *Handbook of pesticide toxicology,* vol 2, San Diego, 1991, Academic Press.

73. Smith MI, Lillie RD: The histopathology of triorthocresyl phosphate poisoning: the etiology of so-called ginger paralysis (third report), *Arch Neurol Psychiatry* 26:976, 1931.
74. Spencer PS, Arezzo J, Schaumburg HH: Chemicals causing disease of neurons and their processes. In O'Donoghue JL, ed: *Neurotoxicity of industrial and commercial chemicals,* vol 1, Boca Raton, Fla, 1985, CRC Press.
75. Stewart RD et al: Experimental human exposure to carbon monoxide, *Arch Environ Health* 21:154, 1970.
76. Taylor JR: Disorders of the nervous system. In Tarcher AB, ed: *Principles and practice of environmental medicine,* New York, 1992, Plenum.
77. Taylor JR et al: Chlordecone intoxication in man. I. Clinical observations, *Neurology* 28:626, 1978.
78. Tsubaki T, Irukayama K: *Minamata disease,* New York, 1977, Elsevier.
79. Urabe H, Koda H, Asahi M: Present state of Yusho patients, *Ann NY Acad Sci* 320:273, 1979.
80. Whetsell WO, Sassa S, Kappas K: Porphyrin-heme biosynthesis in organotypic cultures of mouse dorsal root ganglia, *J Clin Invest* 74:600, 1984.

Chapter 12

ENVIRONMENTAL IMMUNOTOXICOLOGY

Andor Szentivanyi
Khalid Ali
Christine Abarca
Leon Prockop
Stuart M. Brooks

Cellular and molecular foundations of immunity, immunologic inflammation, and hypersensitivity
    Chemical mediators of immunologic responses
    The immune response
    The effector molecules of immune response
    Effector molecule responses from antigen-antibody interactions
Pathotoxicologic mechanisms of immunologic and related diseases
    Immunotoxicology of acquired immunodeficiency syndrome
Environmental agents reported to cause immunologic alteration
    Immunodeficiency or immunosuppression
    Autoimmunity and immune enhancement
    Allergic or hypersensitivity reactions
    Immune system tumors

Immunotoxicology is a developmental component of immunopharmacology concerned with the study of toxicity of the immune system induced by environmental chemicals or drugs. The discussion that follows is organized in three major sections: the first section describes the cellular and molecular foundations of immunity, immunologic inflammation, and hypersensitivity; the second section describes the pathotoxicology of the altered immune responses; and the third section reviews the various categories of the most widely known agents which are toxic to the immune system.

CELLULAR AND MOLECULAR FOUNDATIONS OF IMMUNITY, IMMUNOLOGIC INFLAMMATION, AND HYPERSENSITIVITY[1-4]

Human life and development are marked by encounters with an infinite range of potentially injurious and destructive agents and stimuli. The various defense systems that establish and sustain homeostasis against injurious agents and stimuli involve elements that manage first encounters (the inflammatory response), and elements that utilize experience upon reencounters (the specific immune response). These systems, or defense functions, are anatomically interrelated and physiologically interdependent. Each is in continuous interplay with elements of the internal milieu of the host as well as with elements of the host's environment, and therefore closely linked with neurohumoral defense mechanisms.

Regardless of the purpose for which the inflammatory response is set in action, the first encounter is a more or less stereotyped reaction; for example, predictable cells are drawn into the injured area and proceed to engulf the foreign material by phagocytosis. Vascular occlusion, fibrin barriers, and other aspects of the inflammatory response serve to localize infection or other injury and initiate repair.

The immunologic system includes cells involved in immunity and immunologic inflammatory reactions (including reactions of hypersensitivity), the effector molecules stored or synthesized and released by these cells, the target cells on which these molecules act, the amplification systems (i.e., complement and kinin systems), and the biochemical controlling mechanisms that modulate the functioning of these various cell types, including their intracellular messenger systems (i.e., cyclic nucleotides).

The functions of the immune defense system are carried out by cells distributed throughout the body and include (1) free or circulating cells of the blood, lymph, and intravascular spaces; (2) similar type cells collected into units that allow for close interaction with lymph or circulating blood (lymph nodes, spleen, liver, and bone marrow); and (3) a source or control organ for the system (the thymus gland). Constant interchange of cells between the units provides for rapid dissemination of information to each unit. Therefore these systems are dynamic and change constantly in structure and functional capacity in response to stimuli. Defects in genetic endowment, injuries to cell lines, and factors that alter the rate or quality of accumulation of the memory store of immunologic experience alter the normal developmental patterns and result in clinical immunologic disorders.

Cells storing or synthesizing chemical mediators of immunologic inflammatory responses

Neutrophilic leukocytes (PMN)

Cytoplasmic granules include azurophil granules (lysosomal hydrolases—cationic proteins and myeloperoxidase—and antibacterial lysozyme); and specific granules (alkaline phosphatase, lysozyme, and lactoferrin). Preformed molecules include vascular permeability factors, kinins–complement-activating factor generating C5a, histamine releasers, and neutrophil inhibitory factor (NIF). Factors released on PMN activation are pyrogens and molecules with properties of SRS-A and ECF-A.

Basophilic leukocytes and mast cells

Contain histamine and ECF-A and a substance platelet activating factor (PAF) causing release of histamine and serotonin from platelets. SRS-A is not stored but elaborated during secretion of other mediators. Basophilic leukocytes and mast cells have an extraordinary binding affinity for IgE antibody.

Eosinophilic leukocytes

Facultative histamine carrier, possibly for detoxification and disposal of histamine. Contain peroxidase that catalyzes histamine, SRS-A, and PAF. Capable of synthesizing SRS-A-leukotrienes LTC4 and LTD4; kills antibody-coated parasites; may act synergistically with mast cells to destroy ticks.

Platelets

Interact with damaged endothelium and participate in hemostasis and coagulation and adhere to immune complexes; release mediators stored in granules. Serotonin and histamine contained by platelets; epinephrine, norepinephrine, serotonin, and/or histamine content is result of uptake from the plasma.

Thymic epithelial cells and Hassall's corpuscles

Collectively, represent a hormonal secretory cell system, enclosed in one organ that controls operation of immune responses. Thymic epithelial cells and Hassall's corpuscles secrete immunomodulatory hormones affecting terminal differentiation of T-lymphocytes.

Lymphocytes

T-cells (thymus-derived, or thymus-dependent lymphocytes) and B-cells (bone marrow–derived or bursal-equivalent cells, e.g., antibody-secreting plasma cells and precursors). T-lymphocytes functional subclasses are helper cells, suppressor cells, lymphokine-producing cells, and cytolytically active cells. Lymphokine-producing lymphocytes attract and activate macrophages. Cytolytically active T-cells or "killer" T-cells are induced during graft rejection and viral infections.

Monocytes

Arise in bone marrow, pass into blood for 24 to 36 hours, then enter tissues, where they persist for long periods of time. Precursors of tissue macrophages.

Macrophages

In connective tissue (histiocytes) and serous cavities (pleural and peritoneal macrophages); in "filter" organs on endothelial cells and reticulum fibers, they act as sentry networks of reticuloendothelial system (mononuclear phagocyte system). Found in liver (Kupffer cells), lung (alveolar macrophages), and spleen and lymph nodes (free and fixed macrophages). Phagocytes (monocytes and macrophages) ingest and kill bacteria; produce lysozyme, proteins of complement and fibrinolytic systems, and monokines. Program lymphocytes for antibody formation and containment and/or killing of intracellular parasites, viruses, protozoa, certain fungi, and mycobacteria.

Chemical mediators of immunologic responses[2,4,5,6]

The mediator-storing, synthesizing, and transporting cells (in mediators that have identified cell types) include (1) neutrophil leukocytes (SRS-A, ECF-A, enzymes, vascular permeability factors, kinin-generating substances, a complement-activating factor, histamine-releasers, and a neutrophil inhibitory factor—NIF); (2) basophilic leukocytes (histamine, SRS-A, ECF-A, NCF, and PAF); (3) murine basophilic leukocytes (histamine, SRS-A, ECF-A, PAF, and serotonin); (4) eosinophilic leukocytes (histamine, PAF, and possibly SRS-A); (5) mast cells (histamine, SRS-A, ECF-A, NCF, and PAF); (6) murine mast cells (histamine, SRS-A, ECF-A, PAF, NCF, and serotonin); (7) "chromaffin-positive" mast cells (dopamine in ruminants; in other mammals possibly norepinephrine); (8) enterochromaffin cells (serotonin); (9) chromaffin cells (catecholamines); (10) platelets (depending on species—histamine, serotonin, catecholamines, and prostaglandins); (11) neurosecretory cells (histamine, serotonin, catecholamines, acetylcholine, and prostaglandins); and (12) nerve cells (potentially all amine-mediators as well as prostaglandins and kinins). Details pertaining to the cells are shown in the box.

The immune response[3,7-10]

Overview. T-lymphocytes are the product of the lymphatic tissues. A negative-feedback loop is created by the reaction of antibodies and reactive T-lymphocytes with immunogen because the reaction results in neutralization or inactivation, which diminishes its input to the system. The pathway followed by the input signal, or immunogen, to the lymphatic tissues (central processing apparatus) is called the afferent limb; the pathway of the output signal of antibody and reactive T-lymphocytes from the lymphatic tissues is called the efferent limb.

Immunogens, antigens, and allergens. The term immunogen is currently the preferred name for a substance or material that will stimulate an immune response in a sensitive and immunocompetent host. An immunogen is considered a special class of antigen which is capable of immune stimulation. The immunogens that give rise to hypersensitivity through the specific stimulation of IgE antibody production are called *allergens*. Other types of antigens that are not considered allergens may exhibit reactivity with antibodies or sensitized lymphocytes but do not produce a stimulatory effect.

To be considered an immunogen, an antigen must elicit an immune response, which may be either antibody production or proliferation of specifically reactive T-lymphocytes. Each of the different populations of cells leading to production of antibody or sensitized lymphocytes reacts only with specific sites, called determinants, on the immunogens. The terms used to denote the structure of immunogenic determinants are *carrier-determinant* and *haptenic determinant*. Naturally occurring immunogens and antigens possess a variety of determinants, so the total immune response to an immunogen is quite varied and diverse. In the blood of a person that has developed an immune response, there are different populations of antibodies and sensitized T-lymphocytes, each reactive with a different individual antigenic determinant. This explains the considerable heterogeneity of an immune response to an immunogen and the great diversity of an immune response of similar immunogens in different animals.

Macromolecules increase in their effectiveness as immunogens depending on their size. Small macromolecules of molecular weights less than 6000 daltons usually do not behave as immunogens. Those ranging in size from 6000 to 30,000 daltons are often poor immunogens and require the use of adjuvants. Large macromolecules, especially those above molecular weights of 35,000 to 40,000 daltons, are usually good immunogens. In fact, some molecules can become immunogenic by being chemically linked or coupled to a larger macromolecule. The coupled molecule becomes the haptenic determinant, and the substrate macromolecule provides the carrier determinants.

Most immunogens require *processing,* a type of modification, before they are able to react effectively with the receptors on lymphocytes, which occurs in monocytes and histiocytes. Processing has a particular sequence of events which begins with phagocytosis of the antigen. The processed antigen then moves to the cell surface, where contact with recognition lymphocytes occurs. Processing of the antigen puts it in a form that is reactive with the lymphocyte receptors. Contact with the receptors then causes the activation sequence which leads to lymphocyte proliferation and differentiation.

Development and maturation of lymphoid tissues.[9,11-13] An immune response to a particular immunogen depends on genetically determined immunogen receptors in normally developed and functioning lymphocytes. Immature lymphocytes (in addition to erythrocytes, myelocytes, and megakaryocytes) are derived from primitive cells that accumulate in long bone. The primitive lymphocytes segregate into two major types: Primitive, or immature T-lymphocytes that have a high affinity for localization in the thymus; B-cells, or bursal-equivalent cells, that move from the stem cell foci to other areas in the bone marrow, and in the chicken, localize preferentially in a structure of the hind gut known as the *bursa of Fabricius.*

After localization in their respective tissues, the immature T- and B-lymphocytes undergo a period of maturation and differentiation. When they become mature cells, they enter the circulation and are disseminated throughout the body to populate the peripheral lymphatic tissues, which include the lymph nodes, lymphoepithelial tissues, spleen, and recirculating pool of lymphocytes in blood and lymphatic channels. By traversing postcapillary venules, the T- and B-lymphocytes can rapidly reenter the lymph nodes from the circulation and travel through the sinuses of the node, exiting along the medullary sinuses into draining lymphatic channels.

Then they enter subsequent lymph nodes in the chain and eventually return to the blood by draining through the thoracic duct.

Mature T- and B-lymphocytes have specific molecules on their cell membranes that recognize and bind to specific immunogenic determinants. These recognition molecules vary in T- and B-lymphocytes and in specificity among the individual lymphocytes. The specific individual determinant that binds to an individual lymphocyte's recognition molecules is usually quite different from its neighbor's. This high degree of selectivity and specificity represents an almost complete genetic (allelic) exclusion within each individual lymphocyte. Genes that determine the ability of recognition molecules to respond to various immunogens are contained within histocompatibility gene loci; in humans, they are designated by the abbreviation HLA (human leukocyte antigens). Immune response genes or IR genes are different regions along the genetic loci that determine an individual's immune response capabilities. Within IR genes are specific loci that code for the recognition of individual immunogenic determinants. Only one of these loci becomes a membrane receptor for each B- or T-lymphocyte.

Receptors on mature B-lymphocytes are identical to the particular immunoglobulin the cell will form after differentiating into a plasma cell. In B-lymphocytes that are not fully mature, there is an initial shift in the type of cell surface immunoglobulin receptor from IgM to IgD. The receptor continues changing until the lymphocytes reach final maturity; at this stage, the immunoglobulin receptor is identical to the type of receptor that the B-lymphocyte will secrete when stimulated. Although the membrane receptors on T-cells are not immunoglobulins, they do possess a high degree of specificity to their immunogens, and like B-cells, they also exhibit a wide range of receptor specificities from cell-to-cell. The T-cell receptor occurs in close physical association with the HLA on the cell surfaces.

B-cells and T-cells increase their numbers exponentially by a process called *clonal expansion*. The binding of antigen on a B-lymphocyte results in a phenomenon called *capping*, which results in movement of the antigen to one area on the cell membrane. After the movement, the B-cell undergoes blast transformation, an increased synthetic metabolic activity accompanied by cellular enlargement and an increase in nuclear size. Soon after blast transformation, the enlarged cells enter the mitotic cycle and divide, which leads to numerous identical, specific lymphocytes. T-cells undergo a similar increase in numbers as a consequence of immunogen stimulation.

As T- and B-lymphocytes increase in numbers following their first exposure to an immunogen, some of them differentiate into specialized effector cells, while others remain as memory cells that will respond to subsequent immunogen exposures. The B-lymphocytes that continue differentiation form plasma cells, which manufacture and secrete antibodies. T-cells however, differentiate into subclasses of reactive cells. They become either helper or suppressor cells, or antigen-reactive sensitized cells. In experimental studies, it has been shown that some animals fail to respond to a particular immunogen because of the effects of suppressor cells, while in other instances failure of response is due to lack of a T-helper cell effect. Some of the antigen-reactive cells can directly bind to antigens on tissue cells and cause death; T-lymphocytes that kill on direct contact with tissue are called *killer (K) T-lymphocytes.* Some antigen-reactive sensitized cells respond to antigen-binding by the production of soluble factors known as lymphokines, which promote cellular infiltration and other reactions in tissue.

Characteristics of the immune response.[14-16] After the entry of antigens into the tissues or circulation, nonspecific inflammatory and cellular reactions occur, leading to clearance, degradation, or sequestration of the antigens in the tissues. Phagocytic cells, especially polymorphonuclear leukocytes, tissue macrophages, and cells of the mononuclear phagocyte system, are the main participants in the phagocytic encounter with an immunogen. The majority of antigens may be effectively eliminated by the first encounter. (During this reaction the antigen becomes processed.)

The processed antigen is released to the surface of the phagocyte (macrophage) where contact with recognition lymphocytes occurs. Some processed antigen is also released into the circulation and may randomly interact with specific recognition lymphocytes either in the circulation or in the lymphatic tissues. Lymphocytes that react on this first exposure to immunogen follow the proliferative sequence of events and may differentiate further to give rise to a limited amount of antibody production, formation of specifically reactive T-cells, or production of abundant memory cells. The responding cell may be either T- or B-type or both, depending on the immunogen characteristics and recognition by virgin lymphocyte recognition.

The combination of events that occur on the lymphocyte's first encounter with antigen is described as the primary immune response, which usually requires a period of 4 to 7 days to fully develop after antigen exposure. The actual tissue sites where this cellular reaction will occur are determined by the location of antigen contact: T-cells traversing the tissues may encounter either native or processed immunogens at their site of entry; B-lymphocytes and other T-lymphocytes encounter antigens in regional lymph nodes after drainage from the site of entry. In the early phase, the lymph node (where the lymphocytes encounter antigens) appears hypercellular as a result of sinus plugging—engorgement of all lymph node sinuses within cells. As the engorgement of the cell declines in the paracortex, hyperplasia of the follicles appears in the cortical area. The lymph node becomes grossly enlarged and may become tender because of pressure and stretching on the surrounding tissues. After 5 to 7 days, plasma cells accompanied by immature cells that appear to be blast forms of plasma cells can be found in the medullary sinuses. Increases in antibody concentration can be detected in the draining lymph as well as in the peripheral circulation. The plasma cells remain in the sinuses and do not leave the node, secreting antibodies into the exiting lymph fluid. Similar cellular responses occur in the malpighian follicles of the spleen, where the lymphocytes are arranged in clusters.

The overall effect of a first exposure to an immunogen is an increase in the number of specific recognition lymphocytes, which raises the potential level of immune response to the immunogen when encountered at a later time. After the first exposure, an individual is *sensitized*—possesses a specific antibody to the initiating immunogen as well as a population of reactive T-lymphocytes. There are also increased numbers of recognition T- or B-lymphocytes (or both), depending on the nature of the primary reaction. Therefore the individual is in a condition of heightened responsiveness and will have a more significant reaction on subsequent exposure to the same or similar immunogen.

The secondary immune response, or *anamnestic response* (meaning "to recall" or "to recollect"), occurs in a sensitized individual. The biochemical and cellular changes parallel those of the primary response but occur more quickly and in much greater quantities. IgG is the major class of antibody in the secondary response, while IgM predominates in the primary response. The secondary immune response is reflected in the increase of peripheral lymphocytes and specific antibodies in circulation. These products of the immune response can be measured to provide pertinent clinical information regarding the immunocompetence and immunoresponsiveness of an individual.

Specifically reactive T-cells.[10,11,17-19] Several classes of specifically reactive T-cells have been described, but those most pertinent to this discussion are the regulatory T-cells (helper or suppressor cells) and effector T-cells. The effector T-cells are distinguished by their response to contact with antigens, which results in either synthesis and release of cytokines or cell death. Regulatory T-cells function by helping or suppressing the B-cell antibody response or T-cell effector response. Although the details of molecular and cellular regulation are not fully known, it has been shown that an important part of the regulatory activity is represented by soluble factors (i.e., cytokines) formed by helper and suppressor T-cells that are specifically reactive with antigen and closely associated with histocompatibility antigens of the cell membranes. It has been shown that some T-lymphocyte regulatory cells have receptors for an Fc structure of IgG and that others have receptors for the Fc of IgM. Those with Fc gamma (IgG) receptors appear to have a helper function; those with FcMu (IgM) have been associated with suppressor activity.

Effector T-cells are key participants in immunologic reactions known under varied labels, such as delayed hypersensitivity, cell-mediated immunity, tuberculin-type hypersensitivity, and cellular hypersensitivity. When an effector T-lymphocyte reacts with an antigen, the interaction triggers biochemical activities leading to cell division. Before division however, there is a secretory phase in which lymphokines are produced and secreted into local tissue from cytoplasm of activated lymphocytes. Lymphokines exhibit a wide range of biologic activities, but their principal activity causes monocyte/macrophage recruitment (chemotaxis) into tissue, followed by phagocytosis of the antigen and formation and release of digestive enzymes that destroy the antigen and produce tissue necrosis.

The other principal activity of T-cell effectors is killing cells. Cell death is a result of cytotoxic factors from T-lymphocytes called *killer T-cells* (NK cells). This occurs when the reactive antigen is part of (or closely linked to) a cell membrane which is in close association with histocompatibility antigens. The corresponding T-lymphocyte reacts with the specific surface antigen and therefore comes in close contact with the cell, inducing a biochemical sequence that causes death of the antigen-bearing cell.

Immunologic memory. Immunologic memory is generated during the primary immune response because (1) proliferation of antigen-triggered virgin lymphocytes creates a large number of memory lymphocytes through the process called clonal expansion, (2) memory cells have a much longer lifespan than virgin cells and recirculate between the blood and lymphoid organs, and (3) each memory cell able to respond more readily to antigen than each virgin cell.

Immunologic tolerance. Tolerance is induced by an antigen thus the immune system is inherently capable of responding to itself (but learns early in its development not to do so). Two general cellular mechanisms cause tolerance: clonal deletion, in which particular clones of T- or B-cells are eliminated or inactivated; and suppression, in which the clones are present but unresponsive because of excessive activity of T-suppressor cells. Either mechanism can cause tolerance of T-dependent antigens, but only deletion (or inactivation) of the appropriate B-cells can cause tolerance of T-independent antigens. This deletion of B-cells by antigen contact at a critical early stage in their differentiation into immunologically competent cells is called clonal abortion.

The effector molecules of immune responses

Immunoglobulins.[20,21] There are five classes of immunoglobulins, designated by the prefix Ig and a letter denoting the specific class (i.e., IgG, IgA, IgM, IgE, and IgD). The alphabetic class designation is derived from the Greek letters assigned to the larger polypeptide chains (known as heavy (H) chains) which make up part of each immunoglobulin. They are gamma (γ) (IgG), mu (μ) for (IgM), alpha (α) (IgA), epsilon (ε) (IgE), and delta (δ) (IgD).

Each molecule of IgG contains four polypeptide chains; two identical longer chains known as *heavy (H) chains* and two identical shorter chains called *light (L) chains*. They are held together in a three-dimensional configuration by interchain and intrachain disulfide bonds. Each of the polypeptide chains (heavy and light) have constant regions and a variable region. The constant regions of the heavy chains are the same for all molecules of a given immunoglobulin class of a single individual (isotypes). The constant regions of the light chains are the same for either of two light chain classes—kappa (κ) or lambda (λ)—in a given individual. The variable regions of both heavy and light chains differ among immunoglobulins in a single individual. These variable regions contribute to the structure of the antigen-binding site on the antibody molecule, and it appears that the variability is directly related to the specificity for antigen-binding.

The fragment antigen binding (Fab) portion of IgG contains the parts of heavy and light chains that form the two antigen-binding sites. The Fc portion of the molecule is composed of the two segments of each heavy chain, including the interchain disulfide bond.

The Fc portion of the immunoglobulin molecule is responsible for biologic activities (other than antigen-binding) including complement-fixing activity (exhibited by IgM and IgG), specific transfer across the placental barrier (IgG), specific attachment to the cell membranes of basophils and mast cells (IgE), and fixation to cell membrane receptors of lymphocytes, monocytes, and macrophages (IgG and IgE).

All immunoglobulins have basic structures similar to IgG and have similar physical and chemical characteristics. The immunoglobulins IgG, IgE, and IgD typically exhibit the four-chain, sedimentation coefficient of 7S, whereas IgA and IgM occur as polymers of the 7S units and are larger with higher sedimentation coefficients. IgA may occur as a monomer similar to the IgG basic unit but also occurs as a dimer and trimer with sedimentation coefficients ranging up to 13S. IgM normally occurs as a pentamer composed of five 7S units linked together by a disulfide glycopeptide chain known as the J chain, and has a high sedimentation coefficient of 19S. The J chain provides the link for IgA polymeric forms, and is synthesized by all plasma cells, even those that do not produce polymeric forms of immunoglobulin.

The class and specificity of immunoglobulins produced by plasma cells differ according to stimulating immunogens that selectively react with immunoglobulin receptors on particular virgin, or recognition, B-lymphocytes. The marked degree of diversity in immunoglobulin response is a result of the diverse recognition lymphocytes in a given individual. Antibodies are produced to the many different determinants of a single immunogen, which will usually be of different classes and subclasses as well as varying antigen reactivity. Because of this heterogeneity, there is a wide range of antibody reactivity in a given antiserum for different determinants. Some antibodies will have high affinities for some antigen determinants and bind strongly; others will have low affinities and will bind weakly. In general, larger immunogens with an abundance of heterogeneous determinants elicit an extremely heterogeneous antibody response, whereas more homogeneous responses result from immunogens of uniform composition.

In humans and other vertebrates, IgG predominates the relative concentration of immunoglobulins in the circulation, with average serum values in a human adult measuring approximately 1200 mg/dl; IgM values are about 124 mg/dl, IgA values are around 210 mg/dl, IgE values are between 40 and 100 ng/dl, and IgD is usually present in trace quantities. Normal levels of serum immunoglobulins generally indicate a normal state of immunocompetence and immunoresponsiveness.

Lymphokines, monokines, and cytokines.[22-26] Lymphokine and monokine activities have an essential role in communication between immunocompetent and accessory cells, and consequently, in the regulation of the immune system. In addition, many of these agents, such as lymphotoxins, growth inhibitory factors, interferons, and colony-stimulating factors, are produced by a wide variety of normal, damaged, or infected cells (fibroblasts, keratinocytes, Langerhans cells, tumor cells, etc). The discussion that follows is limited to a brief account of some of the best known of the regulatory molecules.

The interleukins. There are 15 major classes of interleukins, and each affects a variety of target cells. Details of the interleukins are provided in the box.

Transfer factor. Sensitized lymphocytes contain a substance known as transfer factor that is released by either disruption or stimulation of the cells with a specific antigen. Transfer factor (first described and named by Lawrence) earned its name from the fact that in humans it is possible to transfer delayed-type hypersensitivity (DH) to previously unreactive recipients. The transfers are made with extracts of sensitized cells obtained from skin test-positive donors. Transfer factor can specifically transfer DH without preparing the host to make antibody against the same antigen.

The lymphotoxins. In response to specific antigens or mitogens, sensitized human lymphocytes release an effector molecule or molecules (lymphotoxins—LT) that have cytotoxic effects on certain target cells. The physiochemical properties of human LT are heterogeneous, and there are at least three distinguishable molecular species—α-LT, β-LT, and γ-LT. A lymphocyte, activated by intimate contact with target cell membranes, is induced to synthesize LT, which binds to the target cell membrane where it affects target cell lysis. Disruption or physical dislodgment of the target cell membrane promotes the lymphocyte's release from the target cell and subsequent cessation of LT secretion.

Interferons. Interferons represent a group of vertebrate glycoproteins first described by Isaacs and Lindenmann as soluble factors interfering with viral multiplication. Their most recent classification, based on their antigenicities and molecular structures, defines the three antigenic types and numerous subtype interferons: (1) the antigenic type α, formerly called ''human leukocyte'' and ''lymphoblastoid''; (2) type β, fibroblast interferon; and (3) type γ, for the type II, immune, or T-type interferons.

Sequencing the genes of several of the interferons has shown that α-interferons are a heterogeneous group of pro-

Interleukins

Interleukin-1

Two different types (IL-1α and IL-1β); cellular sources are macrophages, T- and B-cells, NK cells, endothelial, glial, and epithelial cells. Both forms synthesized from 31,000 MW precursors, but biologically active forms have MW of 17,500; capacity to induce synthesis of colony-forming factors; contributes to activation and clonal expansion of T- and B-cells; contributes to inflammation by activating macrophages, fibroblasts, and endothelial cells; upregulates synthesis of β_2-adrenergic receptors on human pulmonary epithelial cells.

Interleukin-2

133 amino acid single protein that is variably glycosylated with a MW of 15,500; carbohydrates unnecessary for IL-2 activity in vitro; single gene for IL-2 on long arm of chromosome 4 at g26-28; T-lymphocytes and "large granular lymphocytes" are cell sources; principal effects are activation of T- and NK-cells.

Interleukin-3

MW of 28,000; produced by activated T-lymphocytes; has high degree of species specificity; viewed as colony-stimulating factor for most hematopoietic cell lines; promotes growth of early myeloid progenitor cells, and clonal expansion of basophils and mast cells; members of related effector molecules include T-cell stimulating factor, histamine-producing cell-stimulating factor, and mast cell growth factor.

Interleukin-4

Previously called *B-cell stimulatory factor (BSF-1)*; pleiotropic glycoprotein of 20,000 MW; has capacity to (1) costimulate anti-IgM activated B-cells, (2) induce Ia antigen on resting B-cells, (3) increase IgE and IgG_1 production, (4) enhance expression of low-affinity receptor for IgE ($FcER_1$) on B-cells—an effect inhibited by γ-interferon, (5) induce expression of class II HLA antigens on resting B-lymphocytes, and (6) promote IgE switch and mast cell growth; exerts regulatory effects on the macrophages, including induction of macrophage-mediated tumor cytotoxicity, Ia antigen expression, and increased Fc-dependent binding of IgG immune complexes to bone marrow-derived macrophages; Considered one of the "macrophage activating factors".

Interleukin-5

Previously called TRF/BCGF-II; derived from Th2 cells; primary molecule consists of single chain 112 or 113 amino acid polypeptide, heavily glycosylated; usually occurs as a 50,000 to 60,000 MW oligomer; cellular source is the Th_2 cell; principal effects are stimulation of B-cells, eosinophils, and promotion of IgA switch and eosinophilia; has precise molecular structure of eosinophil differentiation factor.

Interleukin-6

Formerly referred to as $interferon_2$ or BSF-2; glycoprotein of 184 amino acids with a MW of 25,000; produced by fibroblasts, T-cells, tumor cells, and macrophages; biological functions include (1) antiviral activity, (2) inhibition of fibroblast growth, (3) induction of growth myeloma cells and certain mouse-rat hybridomas; (4) production of acute-phase proteins as a hepatocyte-stimulating factor; (5) activation of hematopoietic stem cells as multi-CSF; (6) induction of cytotoxic T-cells as killer helper factors (7) NCF-like activity on PC 12 cells; (8) induction of B-cell differentiation for terminal maturation of activated B-cells into antibody producing cells, (9) paracrine growth factor for human B-cells activated by EBV.

Interleukin-7

MW of 25,000; product of stromal cells; a lymphocyte growth factor; generates pre-B and pre-T-cells.

Interleukin-8

Produced by macrophages; MW of 8800; chemoattractant of neutrophils and T-lymphocytes; regulates lymphocyte homing and neutrophil infiltration.

Interleukin-9

MW of 30,000 to 40,000; produced by activated T-lymphocytes; serves as a T-cell growth factor and a hematopoiesis stimulant; together with IL-2, increases fetal thymocyte proliferation and stimulates erythroid precursor cell proliferation.

Interleukin-10

MW of 18,000; primary cell sources are B- and Th_2 lymphocytes and thymocytes; shows homology with EBV proteins; function includes (1) inhibiting cytokine synthesis by Th_1 cells, (2) inducing proliferation of mature and immature thymocytes in presence of IL-2 and IL-4, (3) stimulating mast cells, when combined with IL-3 and/or IL-4 (4) exhibiting interference effect on antigen presentation.

Interleukin-11

MW of 23,000; effector molecule of bone marrow stromal cells; functions include (1) B-cell growth factor, (2) regulates stem cell cycle, (3) cofactor—hematopoiesis, (4) stimulates megakaryocyte colony-forming units, (5) enhances Ig synthesis in presence T-cells.

Interleukin-12

Previously called natural killer cell stimulatory factor (NKSF); is a heterodimer of p35-197aa and p40-306aa; produced by B-cells and macrophages; functions include (1) initiation of cell mediated immunity by induction of the differentiation of Th1 cells from uncommitted T-cells; (2) stimulation of the growth and functional activity of natural killer and T-cells.

Interleukin-13

MW of 10,000; derived from T-cells; functions include (1) induction of B-cell growth and differentiation; (2) inhibition of inflammatory cytokine production by monocytes/macrophages.

Interleukin-14

Previously called high molecular weight B-cell growth factor (HMW-BCGF); produced by T-cells and some malignant B-cells; functions include (1) induction of the proliferation of activated B-cells (but not resting B-cells); (2) inhibition of immunoglobulin secretion of mitogen-stimulated B-cells.

Interleukin-15

Chemical characterization and biological functions are under investigation at the time of this writing.

teins. Similar heterogeneities are expected to be found in ongoing investigations of β-and γ-interferons. The three types of interferons are not only antigenically distinct but are also distinct with respect to several other properties (e.g., molecular weights, stabilities, cross-species activities, and biologic activities).

Extensive work on γ- and β-interferons as purely antiviral agents has also revealed several nonantiviral activities, including inhibition of nonviral agents (bacteria, protozoans), cellular multiplication and inhibition, toxicity enhancement, increased or depressed cellular synthetic activities, and cell surface alterations. In addition, α- and β-interferons have become known for their immunomodulatory activity, such as enhancement of immunocytolysis (either cell-mediated or antibody-dependent), promotion of phagocytosis, macrophage activation, inhibition of delayed-type hypersensitivity and graft-versus-host reactions, and effects on humoral antibody production.

Overall, α-interferons appear to have much higher antitumor activity than the other types of interferon; specifically, a more potent influence on the antitumor activity of macrophages. α-Interferons immunomodulatory activities include both immunosuppressive and immunoenhancing properties. In a comparison between β- and α-interferons, the immunosuppressive activity of β-interferons produces effects on β-lymphocytes, and the immunoenhancing activity of α-interferon produces effects on T-lymphocytes.

Hematopoietic colony stimulating factors. Only the three most well-known factors that affect hematopoiesis will be mentioned here. Granulocyte colony stimulating factor (G-CSF; MW = 18,000-22,000) is a myeloid growth factor which generates neutrophils and is primarily produced by monocytes. Another factor that is also primarily produced by monocytes is the monocyte colony stimulating factor (M-CSF; MW = 18,000-26,000) which is a macrophage growth factor that generates macrophages. The best characterized agent is the granulocyte macrophage colony stimulating factor (GM-CSF; MW = 14,000-38,000), a glycoprotein produced by T-cells and endothelial cells that drives the formation of mixed colonies of granulocytes and macrophages from normal bone marrow. In contrast to other cytokines, the hematopoietic effects of GM-CSF are species specific. GM-CSF also participates in the activation of neutrophils, eosinophils, and macrophages, in addition to its effects on hematopoeisis.

Tumor necrosis factors (cachectin, TNF). TNF is a highly toxic, proinflammatory cytokine that acts both locally and systemically. TNF-α (MW = 17,000) also produces a wide range of other effects including activation of endothelial cells, granulocytes and macrophages; enhanced differentiation of myeloid cells; angiogenesis; and effects on growth and antibody secretion of B-cells. Another substance in this group, LT-TNF-β (MW = 25,000), is produced by T-lymphocytes and has essentially the same effects as the lymphotoxins.

Transforming growth factors (TGF-β). TGF-β (MW = 25,000) consists of two identical subunit chains joined covalently by disulfide bonds. Many cells, including activated T-cells, macrophages, platelets, bone and others, produce this agent. TGF-β has effects on several normal and neoplastic cells, such as T- and B-cells, platelets, and bone, resulting in fibroplasia, immunosuppression, wound healing, and bone remodeling. It may also potentiate an ongoing inflammatory process by its ability to attract and activate monocytes.

Histamine-releasing factors (HRFs). HRFs (MW = 12,000) induce a noncytotoxic histamine release from human basophils; they are nondialyzable and heat stable. Recently, factors similar to HRFs have been described which are derived from alveolar macrophages, platelets, endothelial cells, a macrophage cell line, and biological fluids, primarily in IgE-mediated, late-phase responses.

Thymosins and other thymic hormones. The thymus is responsible for the normal maturation of many different functional subclasses of T-lymphocytes (e.g., helper, suppressor, and cytotoxic effector cells). The thymus exerts its influence by releasing various effector molecules both within its own microenvironment and in distant target tissue sites (e.g., peripheral lymphoid tissues) via these effector molecules secreted into the blood. The thymus-derived effector molecules behave like hormones, and the thymus itself acts as an endocrine organ. These immunomodulatory hormones are produced by the medullary thymic epithelial cells and Hassall's corpuscles. The thymic products with immunomodulatory activity include thymosin fraction 5, thymopoietin I and II (TP), thymic humoral factor (THF), facteur thymique serique (FTS), and thymic Factor X (TFX).

Effector molecule responses from antigen-antibody interactions[4-7,16,27-31]

Individual components of immunologic or hypersensitive inflammatory responses are initiated by antigen-antibody interactions. If the interactions are on the surface of a basophil, mast cell, lymphocyte, or any of the other components of the spectrum of cells described earlier, they may trigger the release of effector molecules (mediators). Activation of the amplification systems (kinin or complement) by antigen-antibody interactions (or a secondary mechanism) also induces the generation of biologically active mediators. Both primary and secondary mediators induce pathophysiologic changes by mechanisms that include contraction of vascular and other smooth muscle, chemotaxis of inflammatory cells, and either activation or inhibition of secretion from inflammatory cells.

The chemical mediators of immunologic and hypersensitive inflammatory reactions include (1) amines, (2) peptides, (3) lipid substances, (4) Hageman factor pathway enzymes, (5) other enzymes (mast cell granules), and (6) proteoglycans. Collectively, the various groups of these effector molecules produce an increase in components of the anaphylactic and acute allergic inflammation including an increase in blood flow, capillary permeability, smooth muscle constriction, mucous gland secretion, and anticoagulation.

The amine category of chemical mediators consists of chemically defined amine mediators such as histamine, serotonin, catecholamines, and acetylcholine. The peptide category includes bradykinin, a nonpeptide whose amino acid sequence is His-Arg-Pro-Pro-Gly-Phe-Ser-Pro-Phe-Arg, and the eosinophil chemotactic factors of anaphylaxis (ECF-A).

The first established member of the lipid category is the slow-reacting substance of anaphylaxis (SRS-A), which consists of two leukotrienes that are cysteine-containing products of the lipoxygenase pathway of arachidonic acid metabolism. The first SRS-A is 5-hydroxy-6-S-glutathionyl-7, 9, 11,14-eicosatetraenoic acid (LTC_4), and the second SRS-A is 5-hydroxy-6-sulfidocysteinyl-glycine-7,9,11-14-eicosatetraenoic acid (LTD_4). A third biologically active leukotriene (LTE_4) can be formed by metabolic removal of glycine from LTD_4. Other important mediators in this group are the prostaglandins which are also derived from arachidonic acids but through the cyclooxygenase pathway. The prostaglandins are 20-carbon unsaturated carboxylic acids with a cyclopentane ring. Of the prostaglandins, the E_1, E_2, D_2, I_2, F_2, F_{2-} classes and thromboxane A_2 and B_2 have been proven as authentic mediators of hypersensitivity responses, although they are synthesized and released by a variety of nonimmunologic inflammatory and other stimuli. A final group of mediators in the lipid category are called *platelet activating factors (PAF)*. PAFs (1) are produced by basophils, mast cells, and neutrophils, (2) are released by immunologic and other stimuli, and (3) activate platelets to aggregate and release mediators. The structure of human PAF has not yet been defined, but rabbit PAF has been purified, and its structure has been identified as two closely related phospholipids (1-0-hexadecyl/octadecyl-2-acetyl-sn-glyceryl-3-phosphorylcholine).

The fourth category of mediators involves several high MW, Hageman factor pathway-associated proteolytic enzymes that were originally described as arginine esterases. There are at least three enzymatic activities associated with Hageman factor pathways in immunologic reactions: (1) kinin-generating (i.e., kallikrein-like)—the original kinin-generating activity associated with basophils is called BK-A, or basophil kallikrein of anaphylaxis; (2) prekallikrein-activating; and (3) Hageman factor-cleaving and Hageman factor-activating.

The fifth category of mediators includes a number of enzymes that are found in recast cell granules, such as chymotrypsin (rodents), trypsin (humans), superoxide dismutase, peroxidase, carboxypeptidase A, exoglycosidases, and arylsulfatases. These enzymes either contribute to the tissue destruction accompanying late-phase hypersensitivity reactions or participate in antiparasitic infection responses.

Finally, the last group of effector molecules is composed of the family of high MW proteoglycans, which are sulfated acid mucopolysaccharides that are preformed and stored in the granular storage sites of mast cells and other storage cells and are released by the antigen-antibody interaction.

Complement system. The complement system consists of a series of serum glycoproteins that possess many effector functions. There are two distinct pathways for complement activation, classical and alternative. Since both pathways utilize sequential activation reactions (i.e., the enzyme product of one step of a reaction catalyzes the next step), the amount of activated component can be markedly amplified in each succeeding step. The intermediate products of the complement pathway are involved in several biologic activities, including chemotaxis of cells, activation of cells for mediator release, and smooth muscle contraction. Activation of the entire complement sequence results in cell lysis.

Activation of the classical complement pathway by immune complexes results in the immunopathologic features of the Arthus phenomenon, serum sickness, and a variety of immune complex diseases. Conversely, the alternative pathway is not directly involved in atopic or nonatopic manifestations of immediate hypersensitivities, although there is some suggestive evidence that under certain circumstances histamine release may be activated by some complement components.

PATHOTOXICOLOGIC MECHANISMS OF IMMUNOLOGIC AND RELATED DISEASES[32-35]

The pathotoxicologic mechanisms of immunologic-related disorders may be classified into four categories: (1) immunodeficiency diseases which involve some, many, or all major components of the immune system including lymphocytes, phagocytic cells, and complement proteins (regardless of whether the disorder is genetically determined or acquired); (2) cancer; (3) autoimmunity and autoimmune reactions encountered in human disease; (4) immunologic tissue injuries. Overall, the immune system is the body's defense against various viral, bacterial, and certain other injurious stimuli and is manifested as (1) B-cell or antibody-mediated immunity, (2) T-cell or cell-mediated immunity, (3) phagocytic mechanisms, and (4) the complement system. Each of these networks can act independently or in conjunction with one or more of the others.

Immunodeficiency disorders may occur as a result of (1) antibody or B-cell deficiency diseases, (2) cellular or T-cell immunodeficiency diseases, (3) combined B- and T-cell immunodeficiency diseases, (4) diseases with phagocytic dysfunction, or (5) complement abnormalities and immune deficiency diseases. A classification of primary immunodeficiency disorders follows.

Secondary or acquired immune deficiency disorders occur as a result of infections, malignant conditions—especially those involving the lymphoid system[32], loss of proteins from the body, drug therapy, environmental and occupational chemical exposure, the aging process,

> **Classification of primary immunodeficiency disorders**
>
> *I. B-cell (antibody) immunodeficiency diseases*
>
> X-linked congenital hypogammaglobulinemia
> X-linked immunodeficiency of IgG and IgA with hyper IgM
> Common variable immunodeficiency
> Selective IgA deficiency
> Selective IgM deficiency
> Selective deficiency of IgG subclasses
>
> *II. T-cell (cellular) immunodeficiency diseases*
>
> Congenital thymic hypoplasia
> Chronic mucocutaneous candidiasis
>
> *III. Combined B-cell and T-cell immunodeficiency diseases*
>
> Severe combined immunodeficiency diseases
> Cellular and antibody immunodeficiency with abnormal immunoglobulin synthesis (Nezelof's syndrome)
> Wiskott-Aldrich syndrome (immunodeficiency with eczema and thrombocytopenia)
> Immunodeficiency with short-limbed dwarfism
> Immunodeficiency with enzyme deficiency
>   Adenosine diaminase deficiency
>   Nucleoside phosphorylase deficiency
>
> *IV. Phagocytic dysfunction*
>
> Chronic granulomatous disease
> Glucose-6-phosphate dehydrogenase deficiency
> Myeloperoxidase deficiency
> Chediak-Higashi syndrome
> Job's syndrome
> Tuftsin deficiency
>
> *V. Complement abnormalities and immunodeficiency diseases*
>
> C1q, C1r, C1 deficiency
> C2 deficiency
> C3 deficiency
> C5 dysfunction

> **Examples of secondary immunodeficiency syndromes**
>
> *I. T-cell (cellular) immunodeficiency*
>
> Malignant diseases such as Hodgkin's disease and chronic infections (e.g., leprosy, sarcoidosis)
> Aging
> Intestinal lymphangiectasis (obstruction of lymph flow)
>
> *II. B-cell (antibody) immunodeficiency*
>
> Lymphomas (decreased antibody synthesis)
> Nephrotic syndrome (increased loss and catabolism of immunoglobulins)
> Multiple myeloma, macroglobulinemia (increased abnormal and defective immunoglobulins and decreased synthesis of normal immunoglobulins and antibody)

and debilitating diseases. The consequences of acquired immunodeficiency can affect both humoral and cellular immunity; in many instances, both the T- and B-cell systems are suppressed to variable degrees.

Immunotoxicology of acquired immunodeficiency syndrome

AIDS is a highly lethal epidemic; it is an acquired immunodeficiency disorder of unclear immunotoxicologic basis that primarily affects the T-cell system. The disorder was first reported in homosexual males, but currently there are three groups of individuals who appear to be at the greatest risk for developing AIDS include: homosexual men, abusers of intravenous drugs who share needles and have no history of homosexuality, and hemophiliacs who have repeated blood-product transfusions. Patients with this syndrome present with life-threatening opportunistic infections, with Kaposi's sarcoma, or both. In addition, patients may present with non-Hodgkin's lymphoma or lymphoma of the brain.

The immunologic abnormalities found in AIDS are those of a severe and profound cellular immunodeficiency, which manifest as (1) an absence of delayed hypersensitivity, (2) an absolute lymphopenia caused by an absolute deficiency of helper T-cells ($CD4^+$ cells), (3) reversal of the usual ratio of phenotypic T-helper to T-suppressor blood cells, (4) depressed lymphocyte response to mitogens, and (5) impaired natural killer (NK) cell function in vitro. In contrast, hypergammaglobulinemia is common and antibody titers to a wide range of antigens are often very high; nevertheless, there is some evidence of a B-cell defect as well. Complement components are normal, but elevated interferon and thymosin levels are reported in most of these patients.

The etiologic agent for AIDS is human immunodeficiency virus (HIV), a retrovirus of *Lentiviridae* family, formerly known as human T-cell lymphotropic virus, or HTLV-III. The other members of this family are the feline and simian immunodeficiency viruses. There are two types of HIV; HIV1 causes AIDS worldwide, HIV2 causes AIDS or AIDS-like illnesses in Europe, West African nations, South America, and African Americans.

HIV infection results from an interaction between the viral envelope glycoprotein gp120 and the CD4 surface antigen of various target cells. CD4 antigen is primarily found on T-helper lymphocytes and is present on many different cell types in the body, including B-cells, phagocytic cells, tissue macrophages, and circulating monocytes. Emergence of HTLV as an etiologic agent also raises the possibility that infection with HIV also causes an immune complex-mediated thymic dysfunction. Indeed, the histopathologic changes formed in the thymus glands of patients with AIDS are consistent with an organ-specific immune complex attack on Hassall's corpuscles and thymic epithelial cells. In addition, HIV contains an internal structural protein (p19) that strongly cross-reacts with the epithelial cells of the thymus; some of the abnormal laboratory values found in AIDS patients reflect an autoimmune process. Often there are very large elevations in the immunoglobulins, especially polyclonal IgG and circulating immune complexes. There are significant changes in circulating T-lymphocytes in AIDS; their differentiation is thymus-dependent. Elevations of β_2-microglobulins and thymosin α_1 may reflect cellular death of lymphocytes and thymic epithelial cells, respectively. When normal thymus is incubated with serum from AIDS patients and then with FITC-goat antihuman globulin, the Hassall's corpuscles are fluorescent, a finding not found in normal sera or with sera from other autoimmune syndromes. These observations form the basis of the postulate that AIDS may represent an organ-specific immune complex attack by polyclonal immunoglobulins directed against the thymic epithelial cells and Hassall's corpuscles.[34]

ENVIRONMENTAL AGENTS REPORTED TO CAUSE IMMUNOLOGIC ALTERATION[37-39]

The immune system, with its diverse humoral and cellular components distributed throughout the body, is an easy target for many drugs, chemicals of indoor and outdoor air pollution, and chemicals from environmental and occupational sources. These agents act as immunotoxicants on the immune system by impairing host defenses. Environmental immunotoxicants may also exert indirect effects on the immune system by affecting other organs (e.g., liver, kidneys etc). The following discussion presents scientific information on specific environmental agents, gained mainly from animal and human in vitro experiments (there are few human epidemiologic investigations on the subject). The immunotoxicants' effects on the immune system will be classified into four categories: (1) immunodeficiency or immune suppression; (2) autoimmunity or immune enhancement; (3) allergy and hypersensitivity reactions; (4) tumors of the immune system.

Immunodeficiency or immunosuppression

Pesticides and insecticides.[40-43] There is no substantial evidence in humans which proves that occupational and environmental exposure to pesticides leads to clinically significant immunosuppression, and therefore to increased risk of infection or cancer. However, studies conducted in animals indicate that certain pesticides, when administered at high doses, may cause suppression of both cell-mediated and humoral immunity. The effects of 2-isopropoxyphenyl methylcarbamate (Unden) on the immune system of mice were investigated and shown to exert immunosuppressive effects (determined by the mice's plaque forming cells (PFC) and their humoral responses to sheep red blood cells); in some cases, stimulatory effects on spleen and lymph nodes were also observed. High doses of chlordane and hepatochlor modulated the immune responses in the peripheral blood mononuclear cells of rhesus monkeys by suppressing the lymphocytes' proliferation response to mitogenic stimuli and inhibiting the release of IL-2. Sublethal doses of the herbicide atrazine (Atrex) in female mice (1) caused transient suppression of the primary humoral IgM response to sheep erythrocytes and (2) caused a transient inhibition of a specific T-cell response to alloantigens in a mixed lymphocyte reaction. After 14 to 40 days of exposure, humoral and cellular responses reverted to normal; the effect did not seem to be dose related. High doses of cypermethrin caused significant leukopenia, a dose-dependent decrease in delayed-type hypersensitivity reaction, and a significant decrease in spleen weight when given orally to male albino rats. Low doses of this compound did not produce adverse effects on immunocompetence.

An investigation was conducted on the effects of human ingestion of an acetylcholine-esterase inhibitor (Aldicarb) from contaminated well water over a 1 to 5 year period. Data suggested that there was an increase in CD^{+8} T-lymphocytes. The investigators hypothesized that this alteration could predispose exposed individuals to immune deficient states because of their altered CD^{+4}/CD^{+8} ratios; however, there was no substantiation for this conclusion. A similar study on a human population exposed to technical chlordane reported various alterations of T- and B-lymphocyte function; some cases of B-cell dysfunctions involving reduced proliferative responses to pokeweed mitogen in mixed lymphocyte culture were noted.

Metals.[44-46] Exposure to chromium results in suppression of both T- and B-cell functions as documented by in vitro studies; chromium inhibited T-lymphocyte responses, and at higher concentrations, B-lymphocyte responses were also affected. High concentrations of chromium inhibit antigen-induced thymidine uptake in mixed lymphocyte cultures. Hexavalent chromate produces a concentration-dependent effect—it inhibits [^{3}H]-TdR incorporation by B-cells, as well as blastogenic transformation (i.e., the precondition of B lymphocytes for immunoglobulin synthesis in response to antigenic stimulation). In a study in which mice were fed nickel, the B-cells demonstrated significantly depressed IgG and IgM responses to antigenic stimulation. Depressed proliferative responses to mitogenic lipopolysaccharides were also noted in the same study, and a resulting hypothesis stated that dietary exposure to certain trace metals may induce alterations in immunity. Copper suppressed the delayed-type hypersensitivity response of sheep red blood cells orally administered to mice in a dose-duration relationship. The results of a study to evaluate the effects of lead acetate on the immune function of the red-tailed hawk suggest that chronic lead exposure depresses T-lymphocyte mitogenic responses, whereas humoral immunity is not affected.

Halogenated polyaromatic hydrocarbons.[44-46] Experimental data report findings of consistent immunosuppressive effects of the various halogenated polyaromatic hydrocarbons on humoral immunity; their effects on cell-mediated immunity are less clear. The halogenated aromatic hydrocarbons (HAHs) include 2,3,7,8-TCDD (tetrachlorodibenzo-p-dioxin); 2,3,4,7,8-pentachlorodibenzofuran (PeCDF); and 2,3,7,8-tetrachlorodibenzofuran) (TCDF). When the HAHs were tested using the Misshell-Dutton in vitro immunization model, there was a concentration-dependent immunosuppressive effect on the humoral immune responses to sheep red blood cells. An in vivo investigation in which mice were fed salmon contaminated with HAHs, demonstrated suppressed IgM, IgG, and IgA PFC responses to sheep red blood cells; no effects on T-lymphocyte responses to allogeneic tumor target cells was noted. Single low doses of TCDD injected subcutaneously into a primate *(Callithrix jacchus)*, were capable of causing a 20% reduction in CD^{4+} cells (helper-inducer) with a concomitant increase in the percentage of CD^{8+} cells (suppressor cells). The overall effects seem to manifest as suppression of both humoral and cell-mediated immunity. Dietary TCDD (25 ppt), given to rhesus monkeys and their offspring reduces the 1 year survival rate of the offspring to only 22%. The low survival rate may indicate that TCDD has a lethal immunosuppressive effect, but this conclusion is only conjectural.

Other physical and chemical agents.[47-50] Ozone (O_3); a component of photochemical smog and a common air pollutant, is suspected of enhancing the susceptibility to infections by compromising the host defense mechanisms. These conclusions are based on in vitro investigations[37] using human T- and B-lymphocyte culture exposed to O_3; B-cell production of IgG is suppressed, and suppressive mitogenic responses of T-cells to pokeweed mitogen—PWM and SAC (*Staphylococcus aureus* Cowan I). This study also reported decreased T-cell–dependent IgG production, resulting from alterations in T-cell production of B-cell regulatory cytokines (IL-2, IL-4, IL-6 and INF-α) after O_3 exposure. It has also been reported that a one hour pre-exposure to O_3(0.12 ppm) can enhance a sensitized atopic person's sensitivity to a grass allergen challenge. This could be a result of ozone altering bronchial mucosal permeability and allowing the antigen better access and penetration into the airways. The immunotoxic effects of benzene in drinking water when administered to male mice were characterized by involution of the thymic mass, suppression of both B- and T-cell proliferative responses to mitogens and alloantigens in mixed lymphocyte cultures. Benzene administration also resulted in suppressed lytic tumor activity in cytotoxic T-lymphocytes as revealed by 51Cr-release assay. Benzene also decreased the IL-2 secretion from Concanavalin A-stimulated mouse T-cells. Toluene, which frequently contaminates ground water with benzene, inhibited the immunotoxic effects of benzene in the same animal model at higher doses.

Mainstream tobacco smoke may also modify the immune response. Subchronic and chronic exposure of animals to environmental tobacco smoke induced immunosuppressive changes, which were characterized by decreased lymphocyte proliferative response to PHA (phytohemagglutinin) and LPS (lipopolysaccharide) mitogens; a reduction in airway-associated lymphoid tissue; and suppression of antibody production. When the smoke-exposed animals were challenged with metastasizing tumors or viruses, they exhibited a higher incidence of tumorigenic and infectious diseases, suggesting suppressive effects of tobacco smoke on immunity. (The effects of tobacco smoke exposure on animal immune processes are summarized in Table 12-1.) Generally, tobacco smoke exposure in humans alters their host defense mechanisms which leads to enhanced susceptibility to microbial infections.

Table 12-1. Immunologic Effects of Tobacco Smoke

Immunologic Parameters	Increase/Decrease
WBC count	↑
Cytotoxic/suppressor T-cell ratio	↑
Inducer/helper T-cell ratio	↓
Natural killer cell activity	↓
Serum IgA, IgG, and IgM levels	↓
Serum IgE levels	↑

Mice that are fed the organotin, tri-n-butyltin oxide (TBTO) and tri-n-butyltin chloride (TBTC) for 7 days, develop thymic gland changes characterized by thymic atrophy and lymphocytic depletion of the cortex. After 28 days, most of the thymic lesions have reverted to normal; at this stage, the thymus is markedly smaller in relation to body weight. Note: The immunotoxicity of TBTO seems greater than that of TBTC.

Ionizing radiation is known to affect immune function in humans. Epidemiological investigations of 455 pregnant and nonpregnant women living in the vicinity of the Chernobyl nuclear power plant for at least 13 months after the Chernobyl power plant accident demonstrated that the women had a suppressed humoral immunity; this finding was supported by a decrease in the production of immunoglobulins and decreased monocyte phagocytic activity. Frequent immune alterations resulting from ionizing radiation were also alleged in a study of cleanup workers of the Chernobyl power plant accident.

Autoimmunity and immune enhancement

The association between the development of autoimmune disorders or autoimmune-like illnesses and exposure to certain environmental chemicals is inconclusive and poorly understood. However, there is some evidence (based primarily on experimental animal studies) that autoimmune phenomena and immunostimulation may occur with a number of chemicals and metals.

Pesticides and insecticides.[51] Termiticide technical chlordane is suspected of causing immunologic changes, including the potential for autoimmune activation resulting from aberrations in peripheral T- and B-cell regulation; however, the conclusion is not well founded by epidemiologic investigations. Immune enhancement also include increased numbers of cortical thymocytes (CD1) in the circulation, decreased frequency of the suppressor-inducer phenotype CD45RA/T4, and elevated levels of both kappa and lambda light-chains. Furthermore, a mixed lymphocyte culture assay demonstrates reduced proliferative responses to mitogens, PHA, CON-A, PWM, and allogeneic lymphocytes. In addition, there was a case report of deildrin-induced autoimmune hemolytic anemia characterized by antidieldrin antibodies to red blood cells (Hamilton et al, 1979).

Metals.[52-56] In rodent species, mercury causes a lupus-like autoimmune syndrome with autoimmune glomerulonephritis. Autoimmunity in rodent species is generally caused by mercuric chloride ($HgCl_2$) in doses below the toxic levels in humans; it is also associated with increased IgE production. $HgCl_2$-induced autoimmunity seems to be a T-cell dependent phenomenon since athymic rats fail to develop autoimmune activity after $HgCl_2$ treatment. Normally, T-helper cells activate B-cells to produce antibodies. It has been suggested that $HgCl_2$-induced autoimmune reactions in rodents causes hyperstimulation of B-cells as a result of T-helper cell activation by $HgCl_2$. Mercury is known to cause renal damage in humans; there are reports of glomerulitis occurring in humans exposed to mercury and as an aftereffect of mercury poisoning. Workers occupationally inhaling inorganic mercury demonstrate B-lymphocyte overactivity with elevated plasma levels of IgA and IgM, suggesting immune enhancement.

When given to pregnant mice, cadmium affects the immune system development of their offspring. The postnatal immune system manifestations of prenatally exposed offspring are the following: enhanced spleen cell proliferative response to mitogenic and antigenic stimuli (concanavalin A, phytohemagglutinin and lipopolysaccharide); enhanced serum IgM antibody response to sheep red blood cells; enhanced activity of peritoneal macrophages (NBT, H2O2); and decreased delayed-type hypersensitivity to sheep red blood cells. The data suggest that prenatal exposure to cadmium may enhance the immune system's activity or enhance the body's susceptibility to autoimmune disorders in later life.

Zinc is a co-factor for several important enzymes and regulates many immune cell functions. Animals with induced zinc deficiencies show suppressed cell-mediated and humoral immunities and decreased phagocytic and complement activity; they are also more likely to get life-threatening infections. Administration of physiological concentrations of zinc to experimental animal models document the stimulatory effect of Zn on humoral and cell-mediated immunity; there is an apparent enhanced proliferative responses to different mitogens. High level exposure to zinc in environmental and occupational settings has not yet been fully explored. The high level oral administration of copper in the form of $CuSO_3$ to mice in drinking water (50 to 100 ppm) for 3 weeks induced a proliferative response to lipoprotein saccharide (LPS). It also induced autoantibodies directed to bromelin-treated mouse erythrocytes when administered acutely and chronically to mice in various doses. Inhalation of various nickel aerosols by mice caused immune system dysfunctions that were dose-dependent and influenced by the type of nickel salt administered. Inhalation of nickel oxide (NiO) and nickel subsulfide (Ni_3S_2) by mice caused an increase in antibody-forming cells (AFC) in lung-associated lymph nodes (LALN) and increased total numbers of LALNs (increase in LALN were also reported as a result of nickel sulfate hexahydrate ($NiSO_4$, $6H_2O$)); the same nickel compounds cause decreases in thymic weights and decreases in the number of AFCs in the thymus.

Human environmental exposures to asbestos reportedly result in an elevation in the number of antinuclear antibodies and elevated IgA, IgG and serum complement C3 levels. In the occupational setting, low level asbestos exposure, as demonstrated by x-ray findings of pleural plaques, is associated with increased levels of IgA, in addition antinuclear antibodies presence in some cases. In therapeutic human doses, *lithium carbonate* increased IgG and IgM production in experimental animals. Mitogenic doses of lithium carbonate enhance immune system activity by increasing the incorporation of ^3H-thymidine into peripheral blood mononuclear (PBM) cells. At concentrations greater than 1 mM, production of IL-2 is enhanced.

Polychlorinated biphenyls (PCB).[57-59] Epidemiologic investigations of Michigan farmers consuming dairy products contaminated with polybrominated biphenyls (PBB) disclosed high levels of serum IgA and IgG; lymphocyte cultures disclosed an increased production of IgG resulting from nonspecific activation of B-lymphocytes. Chronic exposure of female rhesus monkeys to Aroclor 1254-(PCB) revealed a dose-dependent increase in NK cell activity and increased thymosin alpha-1 and interferon levels.

Other physical and chemical agents.[39,60] A scleroderma-like syndrome was reported in workers occupationally exposed to quartz and vinyl chloride. Women with silicone breast implants were described as developed a connective tissue-like syndrome suggesting lupus erythematosus (SLE) and scleroderma-like illnesses. These conclusions have been challenged by some scientists. Persons chronically consuming the synthetic food color tartrazine are also reported to develop an SLE-like disease.

A number of pharmaceuticals induce autoimmune manifestations, including procainamide, penicillin, D-penicillamine, para-aminosalicylic acid, phenytoin, sulphasalazine, methyldopa, hydralazine, gold salts, reserpine, chlorpromazine, isoniazid, antithyroids, beta-blockers and quinidine. Human exposure to low-frequency electromagnetic fields caused in vivo alterations in immune function. In fact, evidence shows alterations of neuroendocrine and immune systems in many different animal species repeatedly exposed to magnetic fields. Static magnetic fields which were locally applied to the brains of rats exerted an in vivo, immunopotentiating effect on humoral and cell-mediated immune responses. The immunomodulating effects of a centrally applied magnetic field depends on the time of exposure and the region of brain exposed; the highest immunopotentiating effect is observed over the occipital region of the brain.

Allergic or hypersensitivity reactions

Allergens, whether high molecular (antigens) or low molecular agents (haptens) comprise a diverse group of substances that include biologically derived materials (plant and animal products), drugs, inorganic and organic chemicals.

Pesticides and insecticides.[39,61,62] Pesticides are reported to cause asthma, rhinitis, and allergic contact dermatitis. Repeated human exposures to 2,4-dichlorophenoxyacetic acid (2,4-D) caused new-onset asthma, rhinitis and anaphylaxis; there was however, the absence of specific IgE antibody formation against 2,4-D. Specific IgE antibodies to malathion and 2,4-D were detected after intraperitoneal injection of the chemical into mice. Patients with a preexisting atopic status may report exacerbation of allergic symptoms after the pesticide exposure. Allergic contact dermatitis may result from an exposure to organophosphates, fungicides, fumigants, and pyrethroid compounds. Dinitrochlorobenzene (DNCB) produces skin sensitization in humans at concentrations below 0.2%.

Malathion, naleb, maneb, captan, sodium chlorate, and benomyl are strong sensitizers for guinea pigs; whereas, sodium dichloropropionate is classified as a mild sensitizer. Patch testings for pesticide reactivity on various populations showed positive reactions primarily for thiophthalimides, captan, folpet, and difolatan.

Metals.[63-67] Few toxic effects are attributed to trivalent chromium, an essential trace element in humans and animals, even in large concentrations. Acute and chronic immunotoxicity is noted primarily for hexavalent chromium salts. Contact dermatitis, urticarial and eczematous skin reactions, and allergic asthma are consequences of repeated exposures to chromium via dermal, inhalation, and ingestion routes of entry. Workers engaged in platinum refining become sensitized to the halogenated platinum salts and develop specific IgE antibodies to these salts. Positive skin prick tests and serum RAST result from platinum salts conjugated with human serum albumin. Eczematoid skin lesions developed after exposure to nickel-containing compounds. Patch testing revealed that beryllium oxide elicits a delayed cutaneous hypersensitivity reaction. Other metals reported to cause hypersensitivity responses are mercury, copper, potassium dichromate, and medicinal use of gold salts.

Pharmaceuticals.[8,39] The most common allergic-type drug reactions are anaphylaxis, urticaria, contact dermatitis, serum sickness syndrome, and asthma. Metabolites of some drugs act as allergenic haptens and are capable of eliciting allergic reactions without binding to the carrier protein. Certain macromolecular proteins and drugs, such as sera, vaccines, and biologicals (insulin) are reported to induce allergic sensitization. Beta lactam antibiotics, such as penicillin and cephalosporins, are the most common drugs to cause allergic reactions. Penicillin induces both Type I and Type IV allergic reactions; Type I (anaphylaxis) may be life threatening. Other types of hypersensitivity reactions elicited by beta lactams are serum sickness, urticaria, allergic fever, rashes, allergic contact dermatitis, and hemolytic anemia. Patients with penicillin sensitivity, demonstrated IgE formation as a result of administration of penicilloyl-polylysine, penicillin, and penicilloic acid as measured by RAST and ELISA (Szentivanyi et al, 1987). The macrolide antibiotics (i.e., streptomycin and erythromycin) however, are less toxic antibiotics. Immediate hypersensitivity reactions to nonbetalactam drugs have also been noted. Farmers and pharmaceutical workers with occupational exposure to tylosin and spiramycin may develop chronic contact dermatitis, as well as occupational asthma; the diseases were documented by positive skin patch and bronchial provocation testing. When aspirin and other analgesics are ingested by sensitized persons, they may precipitate asthma attacks of a nonimmunologic basis, which are believed to be the result of inhibition of arachidonic cyclooxygenase pathways. Allergic reactions to morphine result from a nonspecific release of histamine from mast cells. Other drugs and products which produce allergic contact dermatitis after topical application include cosmetics, topical antibiotics, antihistamines, and local anesthetics; the various antigenic additives and antimicrobials incorporated into cosmetics include paraben esters, sorbic acid, phenolics, organic mercurials, quaternary ammonium compounds, and EDTA.

Other chemicals.[68-71] Trimellitic anhydride (TMA), used in plastics and epoxy resins, can elicit three different types of hypersensitivity syndromes: (1) an IgE-mediated hypersensitivity response (i.e., TMA-asthma); (2) specific IgG and IgM serum antibodies to TMA conjugated with human serum; (3) a more serious pulmonary hemorrhage with anemia; the latter is seen after exposure to TMA fumes. These patients are characterized by anemia, hemoptysis, dyspnea, pulmonary infiltrates, and restrictive lung disease. There are high titers of serum IgG, IgA, and IgM antibodies directed to TMA-protein complex and TMA-erythrocytes. In some workers, after TMA dust exposure for 4 to 12 hours a variant type illness developed with features of both asthma and hypersensitivity pneumonia, and has been referred to as hypersensitivity pneumonitis or TMA flu. Toluene diisocyanate (TDI) is used in upholstery, spray painting, wire coating, plastic, the rubber industry and in manufacturing polyurethane foam; exposed workers usually develop occupational asthma within the first three years of exposure (Brooks, 1993). Formaldehyde is a common contact allergen but an uncommon cause of asthma. It is present in cosmetics and personal care products, dishwashing liquids, water-based paints and photographic products.

Immune system tumors

Conditions that cause host immune suppression, secondary to immunotoxic effects of various environmental pollutants and immunosuppressive therapy, may increase the susceptibility of affected individuals to various malignancies. Chemical agents suspected of being human carcinogenics primarily include pesticides, insecticides, and some metals.

Pesticides and insecticides.[72,73] Patients with acute myeloid leukemia (AML) and occupational exposure to pesticides showed myelodysplasia of CD34 stem cells; cytogenetic studies revealed chromosomal aberrations involving chromosome 5 and/or 7. Recurring chromosomal changes in pesticide-exposed groups with non-Hodgkin's lymphoma (NHL) were total or partial monosomy 17p, structural aberrations involving the band 16q22, trisomy 11q, and band breaks in 6p23, 7p14, 11q13. Epidemiologic studies performed in an area having a high incidence of multiple myelomas identified phenoxyacetic acids and DDT as risk factors. Studies conducted in Sweden, Kansas, Nebraska, and Canada reported that frequent use of phenoxyacetic acid herbicides, particularly 2,4-dichlorophenoxyacetic acid, was associated with a 2- to 8-fold increase of NHL. Canine malignant lymphoma is also associated with 2,4-dichlorophenoxyacetic acid and other commercial lawn pesticides applied by dog owners. Triazine herbicides, organophosphate insecticides, fungicides, and fumigants also increased the risk of NHL. When analyzed in vitro, subthreshold doses of dimethoate and omethoate, two common organophosphorus insecticides, induced a dose-related increase in the frequency of sister-chromatid exchanges (SCEs) in human lymphocytes. Two other common pesticides, deltamethrin and benomyl, induced a modest increase in frequency of SCEs. A slightly elevated risk for NHL was identified by epidemiologic studies of farmers and agricultural exposures. An elevated risk was found for persons handling, mixing, or applying several types of pesticides including carbaryl, chlordane, dichloro-diphenyl-trichloroethane, diazinon, dichlorvos, lindane, malathion, nicotine, toxaphene, and herbicide 2,4-dichlorophenoxyacetic acid.

Metals.[74,75] Most metals having carcinogenic potential also affect immune function. Metals or metal salts rarely cause leukemias or lymphomas. Humans may be exposed to (VI) metals through contaminated drinking water; the pathogenesis of malignancies induced by chromium (VI) involves formation of DNA-protein crosslinks (DPC) in the target cells. Experimental data on rats suggest that DPC in isolated splenic lymphocytes are formed only when the cells are exposed to high doses of chromium in vitro. Oral exposure of chromium reportedly does not include measurable DNA-protein crosslinks because blood levels are too low. Cadmium exposure demonstrated a high frequency of chromosomal aberrations in cell culture studies of peripheral lymphocytes in individuals living in a cadmium-polluted area. It was suggested this situation might explain the higher incidence of malignancies among the affected exposed individuals.

Other physical and chemical agents.[76] The cultured peripheral lymphocytes of cotton-field workers exposed to different pesticides revealed chromosomal aberrations with gaps, breaks, dicentrics, exchanges, rings, and polyploidy. The frequency of total chromosomal aberrations increased significantly among male pesticide applications.

REFERENCES

1. Burnet M: *Cellular immunology,* Melbourne, 1969, University Press.
2. Karnovsky ML, Bolis L, eds: *Phagocytosis—past and future,* New York, 1982, Academic Press.
3. Dean JH, Adams DO: The effect of environmental agents on cells of the mononuclear phagocyte system. In Hadden JW, Szentivanyi A, eds: *The reticuloendothelial system: a complete treatise,* vol 8, New York, 1985, Plenum Press.
4. Movat HZ, ed: *Inflammation, immunity and hypersensitivity: cellular and molecular mechanisms,* ed 2, Hagerstown, Md, 1979, Harper and Row.
5. Kelsall MA, Crabb ED: *Lymphocytes and mast cells,* Baltimore, 1959, Williams and Wilkins.
6. Mahmound AAF, Austen KF, eds: *The eosinophil in health and disease,* New York, 1980, Grune and Stratton.
7. Plaut M, Lichtenstein LM: Cellular and chemical basis of the allergic inflammatory response: component parts and control mechanisms. In E Middleton Jr, CE Reed, E Ellis, eds: *Allergy: principles and practice,* ed 2, vol 1, St Louis, 1983, Mosby.
8. Parker CW, Samter M, eds: *Hypersensitivity to drugs,* vol 1, London, 1972, Pergamon Press.
9. Bach FH et al, eds: *T- and B-lymphocytes: recognition and function,* New York, 1979, Academic Press.
10. Khan A, Hill NO, eds: *Human lymphocytes: the biological immune response modifiers,* New York, 1982, Academic Press.
11. Bona CA: *Idiotypes and lymphocytes,* New York, 1981, Academic Press.
12. Fudenberg HH et al: *Basic immunogenetics,* New York, 1978, Oxford University Press.
13. Williams RC Jr, ed: *Lymphocytes and their interactions: recent observations,* New York, Kroc Foundation Series, no 4, 1975, Raven Press.
14. Barrett JF: Textbook of immunology, ed 4, St Louis, 1983, Mosby.
15. Szentivanyi A, Gillissen G, Friedman H, eds: *Antibiosis and host immunity,* New York, 1987, Plenum Press.
16. Unanue ER, Rosenthal AS, eds: *Macrophage regulation and immunity,* Proceedings of the Conference on the Regulatory Role of Macrophages in Immunity, New York, 1980, Academic Press.
17. Herberman RB: *NK cells and other natural effector cells,* New York, 1982, Academic Press.
18. Virella G, Patrick CC, Goust JM. In Virella G, Goust JM, Fundenberg HH, ed: *Introduction to medical immunology,* New York, 1990, Marcel Dekker.
19. Talmage DW: Allergy and immunology, *Annu Rev Med* 3:239-256, 1957.
20. Szentivanyi A, Maurer P, Janicki BW, eds: *Antibodies: structure, synthesis, function, and immunologic intervention in disease,* New York, 1987, Plenum Press.
21. Kindt TJ, Capra JD: *The antibody enigma,* New York, 1984, Plenum Press.
22. Hadden JW, Stewart WE III, eds: *The lymphokines: biochemistry and biological activity,* Clifton, NJ, 1981, Humana Press.

23. Mizel SB, ed: *Lymphokines in antibody and cytotoxic responses,* vol 6, *Lymphokines: a form for immunoregulatory cell products,* New York, 1982, Academic Press.
24. Pick E, ed: *Lymphokines,* vol 7, New York, 1982, Academic Press.
25. Merigan TC, Friedman RM, eds: *Interferons,* New York, 1982, Academic Press.
26. Stewart WE II: *The interferon system,* ed 2, Vienna, 1981, Springer-Verlag.
27. DeGaetano G, Garattini, S, eds: *Platelets: a multidisciplinary approach,* New York, 1978, Raven Press.
28. Fujii S, Moriya H, Suzuki T, eds: *Kinins—II: biochemistry, pathophysiology and clinical aspects.* New York, 1978, Plenum Press.
29. Fujii S, Moriya H, Suzuki T, eds: *Kinins—II: systemic proteases and cellular function,* New York, 1978, Plenum Press.
30. Haberland GL, Hamberg U, eds: *Current concepts in kinin research,* Oxford, 1979, Pergamon Press.
31. Szentivanyi A et al: The pharmacology of microbial modulation in the induction and expression of immune reactivities. I. The pharmacologically active effector molecules of immunologic inflammation, immunity, and hypersensitivity, *Immunopharmacology Rev* 1:159-272, 1990.
32. Cory JG, Szentivanyi A, eds: *Cancer biology and therapeutics,* New York, 1987, Plenum Press.
33. Dixon FJ, Fisher DW, eds: *The biology of immunologic disease,* Sunderland, Mass, 1983, Sinauer Associates.
34. Szentivanyi A, Friedman H, eds: *Viruses, immunity, and immunodeficiency,* New York, 1986, Plenum Press.
35. Szentivanyi A, Szentivanyi J: The pathophysiology of immunologic and related diseases. In Sodeman TM, Sodeman WA, eds: *Sodeman's pathologic physiology: mechanisms of disease,* Philadelphia, 1985, WB Saunders.
36. Selikoff IJ, Tierstein AS, Hirshman S: *Acquired immune deficiency syndrome,* New York, 1984, NY Academy of Sciences.
37. Dean JH, Cornacoff JB, Luster MI: Toxicity to the immune system: a review, *Immunopharmacology Rev* 1:377-408, 1990.
38. Virella G, Patrick CC, Goust JM. In Virella G, Goust JM, Fudenberg HH, eds: *Introduction to medical immunology,* New York, 1990, Marcel Dekker.
39. Kimber L, White JR. In Miller K, Turk J, Nicklen S, eds: *Principle and practice of immunotoxicology,* Oxford, 1992, Blackwell Scientific Publications.
40. Fournier M et al: Limited immunotoxic potential of technical formulation of the herbicide atrazine (AAtrex) in mice. *Toxicol Lett* 60(3):263-74, 1992.
41. Gieldanowski J, Kowalczyk-Bronisz S, Bubak B: Studies on affinity of pesticide Unden-2-isopropoxyphenyl N-methylcarbamate to immunological system, *Immunol Ther Exp* 39(1-2):85-97, 1991.
42. Chuang LF et al: Modulation by the insecticides heptachlor and chlordane of the cell-mediated immune proliferative responses of rhesus monkeys, *In Vivo* 6(1):29-32, 1992.
43. McConnachie PR, Zahalsky AC: Immune alterations in humans exposed to the termiticide technical chlordane, *Arch Environ Health* 47(4):295-301, 1992.
44. Cleland GB, McElroy PJ, Sonstegard RA: Immunomodulation in C57Bl/6 mice following consumption of halogenated aromatic hydrocarbon-contaminated coho salmon (Oncorhynchus kisutch) from Lake Ontario, *J Toxicol Environ Health* 27(4):477.
45. Davis D, Safe S: Halogenated aryl hydrocarbon-induced suppression of the in vitro plaque-forming cell response to sheep red blood cells is not dependent on the Ah receptor, *Immunopharmacol* 21(3):183-190, 1991.
46. Neubert R et al: Polyhalogenated dibenzo-p-dioxins and dibenzofurans and the immune system. 1. Effects on peripheral lymphocyte subpopulations of a non-human primate (Callithrix jacchus) after treatment with 2,3,7,8-tetrachlorodibenzo-para-dioxin (TCDD), *Arch Toxicol* 64(5):345-359, 1990.
47. Gardener DE: Effects of gases and airborne particles on lung infections. In McGrath J, Barnes CO, eds: *Air pollution,* New York, 1982, Academic Press.
48. Szentivanyi A, Filipp G, Legeza I: Investigations on tobacco sensitivity, *Acta Med Hung* 2:175, 1952.
49. Bressa G et al: Immunotoxicity of tri-n-butyltin oxide (TBTO) and tri-n-butyltin chloride (TBTC) in the rat, *J Appl Toxicol* 11(6):397-402, 1991.
50. Iakovlev NI et al: The immune status of nonpregnant and pregnant women living constantly under ionizing radiation exposure conditions, *Akush Ginekol (Mosk)* (11):42-5, 1991.
51. Blaylock BL et al: Cytotoxic T-lymphocyte and NK responses in mice treated prenatally with chlordane, *Toxicol Lett* 51(1):41-49, 1990.
52. Bencko V et al: Immunological profiles in workers occupationally exposed to inorganic mercury, *J Hyg Epidemiol Microbiol Immunol* 34(1):9-15, 1990.
53. Soukupova D, Dostal M, Piza J: Developmental toxicity of cadmium in mice. II. Immunotoxic effects. *Func Devel Morphol* 1(4):31-36, 1991.
54. Kruse-Jarres JD: The significance of zinc for humoral and cellular immunity, *Trace Elem Electrol Health Disease* 3(1):1-8, 1989.
55. Pocino M, Baute L, Malave I: Influence of the oral administration of excess copper on the immune response, *Fundam Appl Toxicol* 16(2):249-256, 1991.
56. Schiffer RB et al: The effects of exposure to dietary nickel and zinc upon humoral and cellular immunity in SJL mice, *J Neuroimmunol* 34(2-3):229-239, 1991.
57. Lipson S: Effects of PCBs on the growth and maturation of human peripheral blood lymphocytes, *Clin Immunol Immunopathol* 43:65-72, 1987.
58. Bekesi J et al: Immunotoxicology: environmental contamination by PBBs and immune dysfunction among residents of the state of Michigan, *Cancer Detect Prev Suppl* 1:29-37, 1987.
59. Tryphonas H et al: Effects of PCB (Aroclor 1254) on non-specific immune parameters in rhesus *(Macaca mulatta)* monkeys, *Int J Immunopharmacol* 11(2):199-206, 1989.
60. Jankovic BD et al: Magnetic fields, brain and immunity: effect on humoral and cell-mediated immune responses, *Int J Neurosci* 59(1-3)25-43, 1991.
61. Botham PA: Are pesticides immunotoxic? *Adverse Drug Reactions Acute Poisoning Rev* 9(2):91-101, 1990.
62. Peluso AM et al: Multiple sensitization due to bis-dithiocarbamate and thiophthalimide pesticides, *Contact Dermatitis* 25(5):327, 1991.
63. Dannaker CJ, White IR, Rycroft RJ: Long-term prognosis in occupational chromate allergy: an attempted 18-year follow-up study, *Contact Dermatitis* 21(1):59, 1989.
64. Decaestecker AM et al: Hypersensitivity to dichromate among asymptomatic workers in a chromate pigment factory, *Contact Dermatitis* 23(1):52-3, 1990.
65. Haley PJ et al: The immunotoxicity of three nickel compounds following 13-week inhalation exposure in the mouse, *Fundam Appl Toxicol* 15(3):476-487, 1990.
66. Kiec-Swierczynska M: Allergy to chromate, cobalt and nickel in Lodz 1977-1988, *Contact Dermatitis* 22(4):229-31, 1990.
67. Paustenbach DJ et al: Review of the allergic contact dermatitis hazard posed by chromium-contaminated soil: identifying a "safe" concentration, *J Toxicol Environ Health* 37(1):177-207, 1992.
68. Bousquet J, Michel FB: Allergy to formaldehyde and ethylene-oxide, *Clin Rev Allergy* 9(3-4):357-370, 1991.
69. Cronin E: Formaldehyde is a significant allergen in women with hand eczema, *Contact Dermatitis* 25(5):276-282, 1991.
70. Flyvholm MA, Menne T: Allergic contact dermatitis from formaldehyde: a case study focusing on sources of formaldehyde exposure, *Contact Dermatitis* 27(1):27-36, 1992.

71. Brooks SM: Occupational asthma. In Weiss EB, Stein M, eds: *Bronchial asthma: mechanisms and therapeutics,* ed 3, New York, 1993, Plenum Press.
72. Zahm SH, Blair A: Pesticides and non-Hodgkin's lymphoma, *Cancer Res* 52(suppl 19):5485-5488, 1992.
73. Dolara P et al: Sister-chromatid exchanges in human lymphocytes induced by dimethoate, omethoate, deltamethrin, benomyl and their mixture, *Mutat Res* 283(2):113, 1992.
74. Tang XM et al: Cytogenetic investigation in lymphocytes of people living in cadmium-polluted areas, *Mutat Res* 241(3):243-249, 1990.
75. Coogan TP et al: Differential DNA-protein crosslinking in lymphocytes and liver following chronic drinking water exposure of rats to potassium chromate, *Toxicol Appl Pharmacol* 109(1):60-72, 1991.
76. Rupa DS, Reddy PP, Reddi OS: Clastogenic effect of pesticides in peripheral lymphocytes of cotton-field workers, *Mutat Res* 261(3):177-180, 1991.

Chapter 13

THE IMMUNOLOGY OF CANCER

Andor Szentivanyi
Khalid Ali
Christine Abarca
Leon Prockop
Stuart M. Brooks

Tumor antigens
    Introduction
    Deletion of normal surface cell antigens
    Membrane alterations of tumor cells
    Tumor-specific antigens (TSA) and tumor-specific transplantation antigens (TSTA)
    Phase-specific fetal antigens associated with human tumors
The immune response to tumor
    Overview
    Lysis of tumor cells with activated T cells
    Lysis of tumor cells in the presence of antibody and complement
    Antibody-dependent cellular cytotoxicity (ADCC) of tumor cell
    Lysis of tumor cells by armed macrophages
Immune surveillance, immunodeficiency, and cancer
    Overview
Mechanisms of tumor escape and immunologic enhancement
    Afferent blockade
    Efferent blockade
    Central blockade
Immunologic evaluation and diagnosis of cancer
    Virus-induced or virus-associated antigens
    Fetal or embryonic antigens
    Tissue antigens
    Assays for tumor-associated antigens
    Tests for immune competence in immunodiagnosis of cancer
    Immune response to tumor-associated antigens
Immunotherapy
    Overview
    Active nonspecific immunotherapy
    Immunorestoration
    Active specific immunotherapy
    Adoptive immunotherapy
    Transfusion of normal T lymphocytes
    Transfusion of sensitized T lymphocytes
    Treatment with transfer factor
    Transfer of immune RNA
    Passive immunotherapy
    Local immunotherapy

At various points in the preceding chapter, we repeatedly referred to observations indicating an important relationship between some impairment of the immune status and the occurrence of cancer. It is appropriate therefore that in the sequential order of this chapter the immunology of cancer follows the presentation of diseases of immunodeficiency.

Cancer can be defined as a disease that can be triggered and influenced by a wide variety of factors such as viruses, genes, and chemical and physical agents. The factors involved in a particular tumor may be single or multiple. The objectives of tumor immunology are to explore the complex immunologic interrelationship between the host and the tumor and to manipulate this relationship for the purpose of diagnosis, prevention, and treatment of cancer.

TUMOR ANTIGENS*
Introduction

It is well established that the existence of specific antigens on tumors induced by chemical, physical, or viral agents may elicit an immunologic response in the host. Antigens associated with the tumor that can be qualitatively, quantitatively, or temporally different from normal cells are called *tumor-associated antigens* (TAA). Antigens that are able to induce an immune response or resistance to tumor growth in the autochthonous host have been called *tumor-specific transplantation antigens* (TSTA). The majority of the tumors, including those induced by chemical carcinogens and viruses as well as spontaneously arising tumors, carry antigens that elicit an immune response in the host.

During carcinogenesis there is often a retrogressive dedifferentiation, normally repressed in the mature normal cell, that leads to increased expression of the genetic information. This process leads to increased formation of fetal or embryonic components of the cell. With the advent of sensitive immunologic assay methods, there has been increasing evidence that extremely small amounts of fetal antigens may be present in normal adult persons. With development of a tumor, there is a reversion of the cell to the embryonic form, and the fetal antigens are formed in increasing amounts. Therefore the quantitative measurement of fetal antigens is useful—practically diagnostic—in the characterization of certain tumors that produce large quantities of these antigens. The embryonic or fetal antigens are more correctly referred to as *tumor-associated phase-specific antigens* (TAPSA) since such antigens are found in high concentration in fetal and tumor tissues and in very low concentration in normal adult tissues.

The tumor cells, when compared with their normal counterparts, may show the following features: (1) deletion of normal surface cell antigens, (2) membrane alteration with changes in composition and immunochemical reactivity, (3) formation of tumor-specific antigens (TSA), and (4) retrogressive dedifferentiation with formation of tumor-associated phase-specific antigens (TAPSA) or fetal antigens.

Deletion of normal surface cell antigens

An early loss of the blood group antigens A, B, and H has been shown in many human epithelial cancers such as squamous cell carcinoma of the cervix, head, and neck. Tests for the presence or absence of A, B, and H antigens on histologic sections of tumor have been used for early immunologic diagnosis of carcinoma. The exact mechanism leading to deletion of normal surface antigens in tumor cells is unknown. One postulated mechanism is that the cell surface may combine with the carcinogen to form a neoantigen leading to antibody production; the resulting autoantibody causes the deletion of the surface antigen.

Membrane alterations of tumor cells

When compared with their normal counterparts, the surface membranes of tumor cells demonstrate many physicochemical and immunochemical differences. Surface membrane changes in tumor cells definitely involve a difference in the distribution and density of normal membrane macromolecules. Tumor cells are more susceptible than normal cells to agglutination by plant agglutinins such as concanavalin A and wheat germ agglutinins. In addition, there are alterations in the lipid and glycoprotein composition of tumor cell membranes.

Tumor-specific antigens (TSA) and tumor-specific transplantation antigens (TSTA)

Tumors may be induced experimentally by chemical or physical agents and viruses. Individually distinct antigens are expressed in tumors induced by chemical or physical agents, so cross-immunization is rarely possible even in the presence of tumors of similar morphology induced by the same carcinogen. In contrast to the virus-induced tumor, each new tumor has unique properties of its own antigenic specificity. However, tumors induced by the same virus in different species may display identical tumor antigens that are related and specific for the virus-induced tumor. Individually specific neoantigens may be shown in several tumors of one host induced by the same carcinogen. The absence of immunologic cross-reactivity in certain tumor antigens induced by chemical carcinogens such as methylcholanthrene has been proved. The neoantigens of chemically induced tumors are best demonstrated by in vitro serologic techniques such as immunodiffusion and immunofluorescence.

There are two major categories of tumor-associated antigens in virus-induced neoplasms: (1) the virus-specific antigens and (2) the newly formed antigens that were not present in normal cells before neoplastic transformation. Virus-induced tumors have been shown to have individually specific antigens in addition to the common antigens coded by the virus. Antigens belonging in the second category may arise as a product of specific interaction of the viral genome with the host genome resulting in uncovering of normal or preexisting cell products such as fetal embryonic antigens.

Two categories of tumor antigens have been distinguished: (1) those that form part of the cell surface and (2) those that do not. Those that do not form a part of the cell surface are exemplified by certain virus-related antigens of the DNA viruses. They may be products of viral genes, although not incorporated into virus particles, and may continue to be produced within tumor cells that no longer release infectious virus. The group-specific antigens of RNA oncogenic viruses provide another example; in this case the antigens are components of the virus particle and are not

---
*References 2, 4, 9, 10, 13, 14, 17.

known to play any part in the rejection of tumor cells. The group-specific antigens are located intracellularly and elicit an immune response that can be demonstrated serologically. The antigens responsible for rejection reactions and relevant to immunotherapy are at the cell surface where they make the cell vulnerable to attack by humoral and cellular immune responses. These cell-surface antigens are called TSTA because the usual techniques for their demonstration involve transplantation of tumor cells from one host organism to another. There is a common belief that a distinction could be made between chemically induced tumors and virus-induced tumors since chemically induced tumors possess unique TSTA and virus-induced tumors share a TSTA common to all tumors. This difference is relative rather than absolute, and thus individually distinct TSTA may be a characteristic of tumors generally. This feature of individually distinct TSTA is often overlooked in virus-induced tumors with a virus-related cross-reacting antigen.

One of the best examples of the existence of a human tumor virus is the Epstein-Barr virus (EBV), which is a DNA virus. EBV is closely associated with infectious mononucleosis, Burkitt's lymphoma, and nasopharyngeal carcinoma, and it is believed to be the etiologic agent in infectious mononucleosis. However, the EBV genome has not been found in a variety of other lymphoproliferative diseases.

There is some indirect evidence that cervical carcinoma may result from herpes simplex virus type II infection. Preliminary studies for herpes simplex viral genome in cervical cancer biopsies with nucleic acid hybridization have produced both positive and negative results.

RNA tumor viruses have been demonstrated in association with mouse mammary carcinoma, mouse leukemia, and mammary carcinoma in rhesus monkeys. The hypothesis for the viral etiology of human breast cancer stems from the various studies of mouse mammary cancer. The evidence for etiologic association of an RNA tumor virus in human breast cancer is still incomplete. A recognizable virus has not been isolated from human breast cancer tissue, and the viruslike particles that have been isolated from human milk have not been shown to have biologic tumor-inducing activity.

There are experimental data to support the concept that RNA viruses may be involved in the pathogenesis of human leukemia. However, there is no convincing evidence that viral particles seen with the electron microscope are regularly present in leukemic cells. In addition, the viruslike particles have been noted in normal patients.

Phase-specific fetal antigens associated with human tumors

Trace amounts of fetal antigens and the probable regression of gene activity at a given phase in the adult differentiated call can be detected in normal adult tissue. Many of the fetal antigens that can be considered as phase-specific gene products appear in malignant tumors in larger amounts than in normal tissue. The tumor cells can arise from (1) a transformation of normal cells with a retrogressive dedifferentiation of phase-specific gene products, (2) undifferentiated cell populations that express significant amounts of the fetal phase-specific gene produced, or (3) undifferentiated cell populations that express significant amounts of the fetal phase-specific gene product.

Table 13-1 lists some of the more common fetal and placental antigens associated with human tumors. The fetal antigens that can be transported across the cell membranes are significant since immunologic tests for the quantitation of such antigens are useful as tumor markers. Alpha-fetoprotein (AFP) has a high binding affinity to estrogen and may play a role in hormonal regulation. There is some evidence that AFP has immunoregulatory properties with a suppressive effect on antibody synthesis. This phenomenon has been demonstrated in vitro to a T-cell–dependent antigen in both the primary and secondary antibody response. The exact physiologic role for most of the other fetal proteins is not well known. However, certain fetal proteins such as carcinoembryonic antigen (CEA) and AFP are tumor markers,

Table 13-1. Fetal and placental antigens associated with human tumors

Antigen	Fetal tissue of origin	Principal type of tumors
I. Fetal antigens		
1. Alpha-fetoprotein (AFP)	Liver	Hepatomas, teratomas
2. Carcinoembryonic antigen (CEA) and subspecies CEA-S	GI tract	GI tract and variety of other tumors
3. α_2H-ferroprotein	Liver	Leukemia, Hodgkin's disease
4. Fetal sulfoglycoprotein	GI tract	Stomach cancer
5. β-Oncofetal antigen	Fetal organs	All types of carcinoma
6. γ-Fetoprotein (γFP)	GI tract, spleen, thymus	Many different tumors
6. Pancreatic oncofetal antigen	Pancreas	Pancreatic tumors
II. Placental antigens		
1. Human chorionic gonadotropin (HCG)	Trophoblasts	Choriocarcinoma, teratocarcinoma
2. Placental alkaline phosphatase	Placenta	Various tumors

and assays for the antigens are useful to monitor the tumor growth as discussed subsequently.

THE IMMUNE RESPONSE TO TUMOR*
Overview

It is generally accepted that cell-mediated and humoral immune responses play a major role in host-tumor relationships. Histologic evidence of immune response to the tumor is indicated by infiltration of several types of mononuclear inflammatory cells, including lymphocytes and histiocytes, and increased cellularity of the regional lymph nodes. The host's ability to distinguish the tumor-associated antigens, as well as foreign antigens, and to respond to them forms the basis of the classic immunologic surveillance theory of host defense against neoplasia. Immune cells play a significant role in these host defense mechanisms against neoplasia.

The cell-mediated immune mechanisms play a significant role in tumor-rejection responses. The tumor-specific immune responses can be monitored in vitro by employing a cytotoxicity test that demonstrates the cytotoxic or cytostatic effects of sensitized lymphocytes by determining their capacity to inhibit the growth of tumor cells in culture. In vitro studies have shown that immunocompetent cells can destroy tumor cells. At least four distinct reactions against tumor cells have been described. They are discussed subsequently.

Lysis of tumor cells with activated T cells (Fig. 13-1, A)

The contact of a sensitized T lymphocyte with a target cell results in selective destruction and increased permeability of the plasma membrane of the target cells.

Lysis of tumor cells in the presence of antibody and complement (Fig. 13-1, B)

This is the classic reaction of lysis of cells with antibody and complement. The binding of complement components requires suitable aggregation of surface-bound immunoglobulin; such aggregation requires close apposition of several molecules of the membrane tumor antigens.

Antibody-dependent cellular cytotoxicity (ADCC) of tumor cell

ADCC is mediated by nonimmune and nonspecific effector cells that lack T-cell or B-cell markers. The effector cells

*References 2, 5-10, 14, 16.

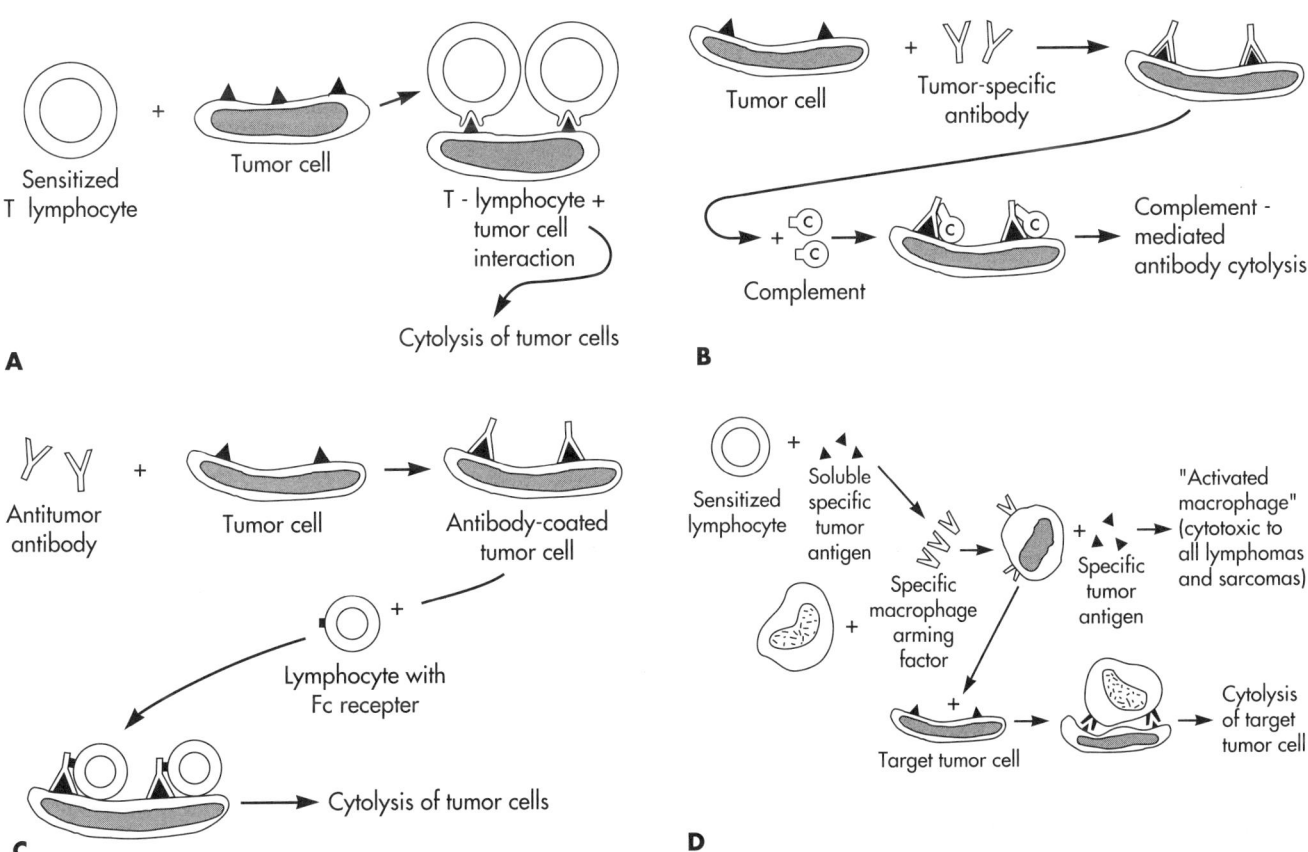

Figure 13-1. A, Lysis of tumor cells by activated T cells. **B,** Lysis of tumor cells by antibody and complement. **C,** Antibody-dependent cellular cytotoxicity of tumor cells. **D,** Lysis of tumor cells by macrophages and specific macrophage arming factor.

are called K or killer cells. They initiate lysis of the tumor cells bound with sensitizing antibody to specific tumor antigens. The cytotoxicity is mediated by nonimmune mononuclear cells attacking antibody-sensitized target cells through the Fc receptors (Fig. 13-1, *C*). Free immune complexes can inhibit the K-cell function, presumably by binding to the Fc receptors. There may be competition for these receptors between free immune complexes and target-bound antibodies. Very low dilutions of antiserum insufficient to induce complement-dependent lysis may still be effective in inducing ADCC. There is evidence to demonstrate that the effector cells are neither T cells nor the classic B cells.

Lysis of tumor cells by armed macrophages

Peritoneal macrophages can become specifically cytotoxic after incubation with either immune lymphoid cells or cell-free supernatant from cultures consisting of sensitized lymphocytes and specific macrophage arming factor (SMAF) (Fig. 13-1, *D*). The SMAF is believed to be smaller than the intact immunoglobulin and has a specific recognition site for the target cells. The type of lymphocyte involved in the generation of SMAF has not been definitely characterized. This phenomenon has been primarily demonstrated in experiments with mice.

IMMUNE SURVEILLANCE, IMMUNODEFICIENCY, AND CANCER[2,4,9,10-11,17]
Overview

Immune surveillance is the mechanism whereby the host mounts an immune response against antigens expressed by the tumor. By somatic mutation or other equivalent processes, the immune system is able to recognize and eliminate foreign patterns of antigens arising in the body. The concept of immune surveillance suggests that a mutant cell that is potentially responsible for neoplastic transformation develops neoantigens and elicits an immunologic host response. The immunologic response monitored against this antigen is sufficient so that a clone of immunocompetent cells can appear and eliminate the abnormal mutants.

It is generally accepted that some form of immune surveillance mechanism occurs continuously, but there is considerable controversy as to whether the surveillance mechanism requires immunologic rejection rather than elimination by nonimmunologic mechanisms. The evidence for an immune surveillance system is as follows: (1) after renal transplantation, patients taking immunosuppressive drugs develop an increased incidence of tumor; (2) stimulation of immune reactivity by specific immunization or nonspecific methods causes a decreased incidence of tumor after infection with certain oncogenic viruses; and (3) there is increased incidence of both lymphoreticular and solid tumors in patients with immunodeficiency diseases.

The increased incidence of cancer with old age has been cited as an example of the association of human malignancy with impaired immunologic status and thus as evidence supporting the concept of immunosurveillance. Observed exceptions to the increased incidence of cancer with old age are germ-cell tumors of the testes, which occur mostly in young men, and nodular sclerosing Hodgkin's disease, which is seen mostly in young women.

It is well established that the incidence of malignancy is greatly increased in patients with congenital immunodeficiency diseases in comparison with the general population. The incidence of cancer is roughly 10% for patients with Wiskott-Aldrich syndrome, common variable immunodeficiency, or ataxia telangiectasia, and it is about 5% for patients with Bruton-type agammaglobulinemia or severe combined immunodeficiency.

If the concept of immunosurveillance is valid, one would predict an excess of cancer in patients with impaired immunity secondary to other diseases. In patients with respiratory sarcoidosis and lepromatous leprosy, a depressed T-lymphocyte function has been demonstrated, although there is no evidence that leprosy is associated with increased risk of malignancy. However, the risk of developing cancer in patients with respiratory sarcoidosis was found to be greater than in the general population.

Recipients of renal transplants constitute the largest group of patients receiving immunosuppressive drugs over a prolonged period. Renal transplant patients showed an increased incidence of lymphoma 35 times that of the general population, and the tumors were mostly reticulum cell sarcomas. Risk of skin cancer was four times higher than normal, and the risk of other types of cancer was slightly higher than expected. It has been postulated that herpesvirus infection in a setting of prolonged antigenic stimulation may be responsible for the increased incidence of lymphoid malignancy and epithelial tumors of the skin, lip, and cervix in patients on immunosuppressive therapy. It is well known that the majority of transplant recipients showed evidence of infections with herpesvirus, especially cytomegalovirus. The evidence for herpesvirus etiology for other cancers is weaker than it is for the EBV and Burkitt's lymphoma; however serologic evidence points to the association of the EBV with nasopharyngeal carcinoma and herpes simplex type II with cervical carcinoma. It is of interest that cervical carcinoma is among the few nonlymphoid malignancies, occurring with greater frequency among transplant patients than in the general population.

The immune surveillance theory has been challenged with the observation that malignancies in individuals with immunodeficiency are usually in the lymphoreticular system. Perhaps the defect in immunity does not involve a failure of surveillance against neoplastic cells but that the disordered immune system in immunodeficient patients is unable to terminate the lymphoproliferative response to antigenic stimulation and the subsequent formation of lymphoreticular tumors.

In transplant patients the majority of the tumors (60%)

were reported to be of lymphoid origin, and the frequency was even higher in patients who were congenitally T-cell deficient. This is not consistent with the immune surveillance concept, which states that neoplastic cells should appear spontaneously in the body and be rejected by the immune system. There is no increased incidence of mammary carcinoma, a common tumor in immunodeficient patients. Skin, lip, and cervical cancers are the only epithelial tumors that show a slightly increased incidence in transplant patients. It is suspected that these epithelial tumors are of viral origin. Thus patients with defective T-cell systems are more susceptible to virus infections and virus-related tumors.

MECHANISMS OF TUMOR ESCAPE AND IMMUNOLOGIC ENHANCEMENT[2,9,10,16]

Numerous factors can facilitate the escape of tumor cells from the immune surveillance mechanism. Some of the important considerations are as follows:
1. Modulation of the cell-surface antigenic structure with alteration of the host immune response
2. Rapid turnover of antigenic cell-surface antigens with release of large amounts of free tumor-associated antigens and immune complexes
3. Production of tumor cell, specific antibody and host tissue enzymes that inactivate suppressor lymphoid cells
4. Rapid growth of the malignant cells with formation of a large tumor mass
5. Development of a varying tumor cell population that is less immunogenic to the host
6. Appearance of suppressor cells that dampen host immune response against the tumor cells
7. Immunosuppressive agents responsible for neoplastic transformation
8. Immuno deficiencies in the host

Many serum factors, including antigen-antibody complexes, antigens, and antibody capable of blocking the cytotoxic effect of sensitized cells, can provide important escape mechanisms. The nature of blocking serum factors and the mechanism of blocking have been only partially elucidated. Blocking may occur by binding of serum factors to antigens, thus preventing cellular recognition by specific lymphoid effector cells. The degree of blocking produced by immune complexes is critically related to their physical configuration. The most effective complexes are small and soluble because large complexes are readily removed from the circulation by the reticuloendothelial cells. Small complexes with a molecular weight of less than 1,000,000 are stable and are potent inhibitors of effector cells in antibody-dependent cytotoxicity.

Proposed mechanisms for the ability of serum factors to suppress host immune response against neoplastic cells have been categorized as afferent, central, or efferent inhibition, depending on which portion of the immune system is blocked.

Afferent blockade

Antibodies or antibody parts of immune complexes bind to antigenic determinants on the tumor and mask the antigenic sites, thus preventing recognition by the host immune cells.

Efferent blockade

The antigenic sites of the tumor are masked by antibody or immune complexes or both, preventing recognition and destruction of the tumor cells by immune effector cells. Soluble antigens and antigen-antibody complexes may bind to recognition sites of the immune effector cells and interfere with the ability of these cells to recognize the target tumor cells.

Central blockade

Tolerogenic soluble serum factors, suppressor cells, or both could induce a state of tolerance and prevent a tumor-destructive immune response.

The afferent blockade is an important mechanism for enhancing tumor growth in vivo. The effector mechanism is a plausible explanation for blocking in vitro with the use of hyperimmune antisera. Enhancement is often achieved with a single injection of antiserum, yet the binding of antibody to tumor cells is a transient phenomenon. The masking hypothesis is difficult to explain with the observation that very small quantities of antiserum are sufficient to induce enhancement. It seems more plausible that enhancement may be the result of an effector cell inhibition or central blockade.

IMMUNOLOGIC EVALUATION AND DIAGNOSIS OF CANCER[6,7,11,12,15]

There are several approaches to the immunodiagnosis of cancer, as shown in the box below. A popular approach is the detection of tumor-associated antigens. Several of the various assays may seem promising, although the usefulness, sensitivity, and specificity of most of them remain to be determined.

The tumor-associated antigens may be found in larger quantities in tumor cells than in normal cells. To be useful for immunodiagnosis, the tumor antigens should be common to a variety of tumors, at least of the same histologic type, and should appear and persist in circulation or in biologic fluids.

Immunodiagnosis of cancer

I. Detection of tumor-associated antigens on tumor cells and in plasma and biologic fluids
II. Immune competence of cancer patients
III. Immune response to tumor-associated antigens
   A. Humoral immunity
   B. Cell-mediated immunity

Common antigens in tumors have been identified and classified in the following categories:

Virus-induced or virus-associated antigens

Tumors induced by the same virus may share some of the same common tumor-associated antigens even when they differ in morphologic appearance.

Fetal or embryonic antigens

Such antigens are present on normal fetal cells and in a variety of tumors regardless of etiology.

Tissue antigens

Normal tissue antigens may be expressed in larger amounts in tumor cells, and some of these may be specific for the organ from which the tumor is derived.

Assays for tumor-associated antigens

Circulating antigens potentially useful for immunodiagnosis of cancer may be divided into categories of fetal antigens, hormones, and miscellaneous. A useful test would have the features of a high specificity with high sensitivity, with a definite quantitative difference from normal to benign cases. Currently, many of the tumor cell markers are useful for following patients known to have tumors, but they have not been proved useful for early detection of cancer patients prior to metastatic lesions.

The fetal and placental antigens suggested for possible diagnostic application are listed in Table 13-1. CEA is present in nonmalignant adult tissue and normal plasma. The use of serum CEA assays to differentiate between patients with tumors and patients with benign disease depends on relative concentrations of CEA in tumor tissue versus other nontumor tissues and the destruction of the barrier to leakage of CEA into the plasma. Many of the studies of patients with benign gastrointestinal disease and cancer patients with localized disease have demonstrated a large percentage of false positives, and many patients with localized GI cancer do not have elevated CEA values. More recently, a subspecies assay for CEA, called CEA-S, has been developed. The assay for CEA-S detected a higher proportion of patients with GI cancer and demonstrated a very low incidence of false-positive and false-negative results in noncancer patients. Currently, CEA and CEA-S assays are most useful in monitoring patients with cancer known to produce CEA substances to indicate prognosis.

Alpha-fetoprotein (AFP) has been found to be present in small amounts in normal serum. Serum AFP assays are useful in the differential diagnosis and serve to monitor patients with hepatoma, choriocarcinoma, and testicular tumors. More recently, serum and amniotic fluid AFP assays have been useful for the detection of neural tube defects of the fetus during pregnancy.

Investigations of the various other tumors associated with fetal antigens are currently under way; however, their practical usefulness has not been sufficiently documented.

Certain hormones have been reported to be useful as tumor markers. Human chorionic gonadotropin (HCG) and human placental lactogen (HPL) may be ectopically produced by a small proportion of tumors arising in areas outside the reproductive tract. HCG assays have been useful in monitoring choriocarcinoma and certain testicular tumors known to produce HCG. Pro-ACTH (adrenocortical trophic hormone) may be useful in the diagnosis of lung cancer, and a high percentage of patients with lung cancer have demonstrated elevated serum ACTH in preliminary studies.

Tests for immune competence in immunodiagnosis of cancer

There is a correlation between general immunocompetence and the level of specific tumor immunity with extent of disease and prognosis in patients in a wide variety of malignancies. The changes in levels of general immunocompetence and specific tumor immunity will parallel the changes in the clinical status of the patient with cancer. In almost every type of human cancer tested, patients who have a poor, depressed immune competence have a worse prognosis than patients demonstrating a normal immune system. Parameters of immune competence that can be assayed are outlined on page 163.

Immunocompetence declines markedly with advancing disease, and the patient becomes more immunodeficient. Progressive tumor growth with resulting immunodeficiency has been observed in Hodgkin's disease, leukemia, lymphomas, and a wide variety of solid epithelial tumors such as carcinomas of the breast, lung, colon, head, and neck. In Hodgkin's disease there is often a depressed cell-mediated immune reaction; in chronic lymphocytic leukemia humoral antibody response is impaired, whereas the cell-mediated immunity is slightly depressed. Cell-mediated immunity and inflammation may be markedly suppressed in various solid tumors, whereas the antibody response is only mildly impaired.

The depression of the immune competence of cancer patients may be useful diagnostically. In the normal or benign disease population decreased immune competence may have diagnostic implications. It has been demonstrated that immune functions that are impaired in cancer patients include delayed hypersensitivity responses, peripheral blood lymphocyte counts, lymphocyte blastogenic responses, T-lymphocyte levels, B-lymphocyte levels, serum immunoglobulin levels, complement levels, primary and secondary antibody responses, specific antitumor levels, in vivo delayed hypersensitivity to tumor antigens, and in vitro lymphocyte cytotoxicity to target cells.

Immune response and various nonimmunologic host defense mechanisms can be evaluated in cancer patients by a

> **Assays for immune competence in tumor patients**
>
> I. Cellular immunity
>   A. Skin tests for delayed hypersensitivity
>   1. Tests for previous sensitization with recall antigens (e.g., Candida, streptokinase-streptodornase, trichophytin, mumps)
>   2. Primary sensitization (e.g., dinitrochlorobenzene)
>   B. Quantitation for circulating T and B lympyocytes
>   1. E-rosette assay for T lymphocytes
>   2. Immunofluorescent assays for B lymphocytes
>   C. Lymphocyte function
>   1. Total WBC and total lymphocyte count
>   2. Response to mitogens, PHA, Con A, and pokeweed
>   3. Production of lymphokines
>   D. Macrophage function
> II. Humoral immunity
>   A. Quantitative immunoglobulins
>   B. Isoantibody levels (blood group isoagglutinins)
>   C. Serum complement level
>   D. Primary antibody response to typhoid, keyhold limpet hemocyanin
>   E. Secondary antibody response to antigens such as tetanus and diphtheria

variety of techniques. Cellular immunity can be evaluated in many ways: for example, the delayed hypersensitivity skin test, measurement of the lymphocyte blastogenic response to mitogens or antigens, and the production of migration inhibitory factor. Measurements as simple as lymphocyte and monocyte counts in the peripheral blood may be useful and may correlate with prognosis.

One can quantitate humoral immunity by measuring immunoglobulin levels, isoantibody titers, complement levels, primary antibody response to antigens (such as typhoid or keyhole limpet hemocyanin), and secondary response to antigens (such as tetanus and diphtheria).

Immune response to tumor-associated antigens

There have been several human studies involving immune response to specific tumor-associated antigens. The tests for delayed hypersensitivity reactions to extracts of tumors have been done in a manner similar to the tests for the common bacterial-fungal antigens. Routine hypersensitivity skin test reactions have been observed in patients with leukemia, colon cancer, breast carcinoma, carcinoma of the lung, and cancer of the cervix. Skin test reactivity to leukemia-associated antigens has been shown to correlate with the patient's clinical status. In general, delayed hypersensitivity skin tests to the the specific tumor-associated antigens correlate with the clinical state and are useful for monitoring response to therapy. Because of the possible hazard of inoculation of cancer antigen into patients who do not have cancer, the potential usefulness of such skin tests for cancer screening and diagnosis is limited.

Cell-mediated cytotoxicity assays may have a possible application in immunodiagnosis. The lymphocytes removed from patients with cancer can exhibit in vitro growth of the tumor cells or may demonstrate cytotoxic inhibition of the cultured tumor cells. Such assays are performed primarily in the larger diagnostic cancer centers, primarily on a clinical investigation basis.

Leukocyte migration inhibition assays have been performed with the use of patient cells reacted with the extract of the tumor tissue. Reactivity to common tumor-associated antigens has been observed by this method in patients with breast cancer, malignant melanoma, lymphoma, and leukemia. Furthermore, the leukocyte migration assay has been reported to show good correlation with delayed hypersensitivity skin test reactions.

Potential fruitful approaches that remain to be developed are useful tests for the detection of antibodies to tumor-associated antigens. Antibodies to common tumor antigens have been described in melanoma and osteosarcoma. The specificity of the reactions in melanoma and osteosarcoma must be studied further. This approach is very sensitive and can be useful for the early diagnosis of cancer.

IMMUNOTHERAPY[1,3,5,16]
Overview

There are many problems associated with current methods of immunotherapy. The human tumor antigens have not been well defined in terms of location (for example, cytoplasm or surface), immunogenicity, cross-reactivity with normal tissue antigens, and interaction with host immune surveillance systems. The approaches to enhance the normal immune system to combat and contain the growth of cancer have been (1) increasing cell-mediated immunity, (2) augmenting antibody-mediated immunity, and (3) stimulating the general immunocompetence with use of specific and nonspecific reagents.

There are seven major approaches to immunotherapy listed in Table 13-2.

Active nonspecific immunotherapy

This mode of therapy usually involves use of adjuvants such as BCG or *Corynebacterium parvum* to increase the general immunocompetence with augmentation of cell-mediated and humoral responses. These nonspecific adjuvant reagents may have one or more of the following immunologic effects: (1) increase in general immunocompetence, (2) augmentation of cell-mediated or humoral responses, (3) expansion of T-lymphocyte population and activation of the macrophages, or (4) enhancement of the reticuloendothelial system. This approach has been used in the therapy of many tumors such as melanoma, leukemia,

Table 13-2. Approaches to immunotherapy of cancer*

Approach	Mechanism of action
1. Active nonspecific	Increases general immunocompetence Activates macrophages
2. Immunorestorative	Restores immunocompetence
3. Active specific	Increases specific cell-mediated and humoral antitumor immunity
4. Adoptive	Transfers tumor immunity from immune cells
5. Passive	Transfers humoral tumor-specific antibodies, cytotoxic deblocking, opsonizing, antibody-dependent cellular cytotoxicity or drug- or isotope-transporting antibody
6. Local	Locally active macrophage kills tumor cells by bystander effect of delayed hypersensitivity; induces specific tumor immunity
7. Combination of above	

*From Hersh EM et al. Immunotherapy of cancer. In Becker FF, ed: *Cancer, a comprehensive treatise,* vol 6, New York, 1977, Plenum Press.

colon cancer, lung carcinoma, and breast carcinoma with variable degrees of success.

Immunorestoration

Certain agents such as levamisole and thymosin have been used to restore cell-mediated responsiveness. Levamisole is a chemical agent that probably acts through a cyclic nucleotide or prostaglandin system in lymphocytes and helps restore cell-mediated responsiveness in sensitized hosts.

In patients who are immunodeficient and immunosuppressed, the administration of thymic hormones has been shown to increase the percentage of peripheral circulating E-rosette T-cell types of lymphocytes. The possibility of thymic factors that can augment cell-mediated response of cancer patients has been shown to enhance in vitro cell function. Preliminary results have demonstrated some clinical improvement in tumor patients; however, further studies are needed to determine the true therapeutic benefits.

Active specific immunotherapy

This mode of therapy includes immunization with tumor cells or antigens. The tumor cells may be modified with virus or chemicals prior to immunization to enhance specific cell-mediated and humoral immunity in the host. Specific stimulation of immunity has been attempted by the following methods.

Unmodified cancer cells or cell surface antigens as immunogens. Allogeneic cancer cells as immunogens have been used in the immunotherapy of human leukemia. The human leukemia cells were irradiated to prevent cell division and injected periodically into recipients previously induced into remission of acute lymphocytic leukemia by chemotherapy. Concurrent with the tumor vaccine, BCG was administered. The immunotherapy with both irradiated allogeneic cells and BCG was synergistic, whereas either modality alone was ineffective.

Treatment of cancer cells with neuraminidase. This is based on the hypothesis that enzymatic removal of sialic acid residues from cancer cell membranes increases their immunogenicity and facilitates immunospecific rejection. The efficacy of this treatment has not been established.

Virus-modified cancer cells. Virus infections of cells may produce strongly immunogenic viral antigens on the cell surface that enhance the immunogenicity of weak tumor-specific antigens. The immune response is not directed to the virus alone because rejection of subsequent tumor challenge is tumor specific. These studies have been extended to humans with malignant disease on a limited basis. No therapeutic benefits have been noted in patients with osteogenic sarcoma given influenza virus-infected autologous or allogeneic tumor cells.

Chemically modified membranes on cancer cells. Chemicals can be coupled to tumor cell membranes and enhance the cell-mediated cytotoxicity in experimental animal tumor models. Most of the experimental work has been in animal models using substances such as 2,4-dinitrophenol. This approach is still in the early stages of clinical experimentation for treatment of human tumors.

Adoptive immunotherapy

This mode of therapy utilizes transfer of cells or cell products from a specifically immunocompetent donor to a tumor-bearing recipient. The therapy may involve transfer of T lymphocytes, transfer factor, or immune RNA extracted from sensitized lymphocytes.

Transfusion of normal T lymphocytes. Often in cancer patients the T lymphocytes are depressed primarily or secondarily and the therapeutic infusion of normal T cells will initiate or augment an antitumor response. One major obstacle of adoptive immunotherapy is the histocompatibility antigen difference. Without HLA matching, the donor cells will survive and a severe graft-versus-host reaction may occur in an immunosuppressed recipient.

Transfusion of sensitized T lymphocytes. The transfusion of allogeneic sensitized T lymphocytes in the form of leukocyte transfusion was one of the first methods used in immunotherapy of human cancer. The donors and recipients should be matched with respect to the ABO blood group and HLA antigens. This mode of therapy has been only partially successful in humans.

Treatment with transfer factor. Transfer factor has been used to activate the immune response in cancer patients and other immunodeficient diseases. The small molecular weight transfer factor derived from sensitized T lymphocytes can program recipient lymphocytes to develop certain aspects of specific cellular immunity such as T-cell–mediated cytotoxicity. Transfer factor therapy has been used in cases of human malignant melanomas resulting in prolongation of life span and an interval of time for clinical recurrence of the tumor.

Transfer of immune RNA. RNA is extracted from sensitized donor immune lymphocytes and injected into the recipient host. Experimental studies have shown that immunotherapy with immune RNA is more effective in inhibiting tumor growth if administered at a period when there is small tumor mass with growth in the early stages. This mode of therapy is not very effective when immune RNA is given to an animal with a well-established growing tumor. This approach in humans is still in the early stages of clinical investigation and the mechanism of action and beneficial effects have yet to be determined.

Passive immunotherapy

This refers to transfer of antitumor antibodies from an immune donor to a recipient host with tumor. The use of tumor-specific antibodies has been applied with some success in experimental animal models. However, studies of immunotherapy with antibodies in humans have not been adequately tested. Most of the reported human studies have not been very successful. There has been hesitation on the part of oncologists since it is possible to enhance the growth of the tumor by administration of tumor antibodies by blocking specific cell-mediated immunity. A better approach currently being used is to couple certain cytotoxic agents (for example, organic chemicals and radioactive substances) to specific antibodies and to employ such reagents to kill tumor cells selectively.

Local immunotherapy

This method refers to the injection of active nonspecific or adoptive immunotherapeutic reagents directly into the tumor in order to induce local killing and enhance specific tumor immunity of the general host immune system.

Combinations of the aforementioned modes of immunotherapy have been used with variable results. In general, one can summarize by stating that immunotherapy by itself has not been found to be very effective in most cases, although it has demonstrated some benefit when administered in conjunction with cancer chemotherapy.

REFERENCES

1. Burnet M: *Cellular immunology,* Victoria, Australia, 1969, Melbourne University Press.
2. Cochran AJ: *Man, cancer and immunity,* New York, 1978, Academic Press.
3. Corey JG, Szentivanyi A, editors: *Cancer biology and therapeutics,* New York, 1987, Plenum Press.
4. Friedman H, Klein TW, Szentivanyi A, editors: *Immunomodulation by bacteria and their products,* New York, 1981, Plenum Press.
5. Hadden JW, Szentivanyi A, editors: *The pharmacology of reticuloendothelial system,* New York, 1985, Plenum Press.
6. Hadden JW, Szentivanyi A, editors: *Immunopharmacology reviews,* vol 1, New York, 1990, Plenum Press.
7. Herberman RB, editor: *NK cells and other natural effector cells,* New York, 1982, Academic Press.
8. Herberman RB, Friedman H, editors: *The reticuloendothelial system: a comprehensive treatise,* vol 5, New York, 1983, Plenum Press.
9. Klein T, Specter S, Friedman H, Szentivanyi A, editors: *Biological response modifiers in human oncology and immunology,* New York, 1983, Plenum Press.
10. Oettgen HF: Immunologic aspects of cancer. In Dixon FJ, Fisher DW, editors: *The biology of immunologic disease,* Sunderland, Mass, 1983, Sinauer Associates.
11. Siegal FP: Cellular differentiation markers in lymphoproliferative disease. In Dixon FJ, Fisher DW, editors: *The biology of immunologic disease,* Sunderland, Mass, 1983, Sinauer Associates.
12. Sell S, editor: *Cancer markers: developmental and diagnostic significance,* Clifton, NJ, 1980, Humana Press.
13. Szentivanyi A, Szentivanyi J: Cellular and molecular foundations of immunity, immunologic inflammation and hypersensitivity: component parts and their relation to neurohumoral control mechanisms. In *Sodeman's pathologic physiology—mechanisms of disease,* Philadelphia, 1985, WB Saunders.
14. Szentivanyi A, Szentivanyi J: The pathophysiology of immunologic and related diseases. In Sodeman WA, editor: *Sodeman's pathologic physiology—mechanisms of disease,* Philadelphia, 1985, WB Saunders.
15. Trentin JJ, editor: *Cross reacting antigens and neoantigens (with implication for autoimmunity and cancer immunity),* 1967, Williams & Wilkins.
16. Waters H, editor: *The handbook of cancer immunology,* 9 vols, New York, 1978-1981, Garland STPM Press.
17. Yamamura Y, Kotani S, editors: Immunomodulation by microbial products and related synthetic compounds. Proceedings of an International Symposium, Osaka, Japan, July 27-29, 1981, Amsterdam, 1982, Excerpta Medica.

Chapter 14

RESPIRATORY TOXICOLOGY

Ira S. Richards
Stuart M. Brooks

Respiratory and environmental interface
    Unique features of the respiratory system
Anatomic features of the respiratory tract
Pulmonary defense mechanisms
    Clearance
    Biochemical mechanisms
    Bronchoconstriction
    Airway epithelium
    Olfaction
    Alveolar macrophages
    Immunologic mechanisms
Important environmental airborne pollutants
    Ozone
    Sulfur dioxide
    Oxides of nitrogen
    Aldehydes
Mechanisms of respiratory tract disease: failure of defense mechanisms
    Pulmonary fibrosis
    Bronchial asthma

The respiratory system is frequently the target for airborne environmental contaminants. For the average adult at rest, approximately 12 kg of air is inhaled each day. When this amount is compared with the average daily intake of water (2 kg) or food (1.5 kg), it becomes apparent that inhaled air is a major source for potential exposure to airborne environmental toxicants. In addition to being the target of toxicity, the respiratory system can be the principal route of exposure for neurotoxicants (for example, mercury, carbon disulfide, organic solvents); carcinogens (for example, benzo[A]pyrene, vinyl chloride, benzene); hepatotoxic agents (for example, carbon tetrachloride, bromobenzene); and other systemic toxicants.

Occasionally, situations in which the levels of environmental airborne chemical contaminants have increased to concentrations that were immediately hazardous to human health have developed. These rare instances have involved the accidental release of a specific chemical into the environment, as happened in Bhopal, India, in 1984, when approximately 40 tons of methyl isocyanate was discharged from a pesticide-manufacturing plant into the atmosphere. More than 2000 people died from this exposure, and many more became chronically ill after the incident. In a short-term episode of air pollution that occurred in London in 1952 as the result of a meteorologic inversion, approximately 4000 deaths were attributed to the smoke and sulfur dioxide (SO_2) that accumulated in the atmosphere over several days. On the worst day, the concentration of SO_2 was 1.34 ppm, and smoke was 4.5 mg/m^3.[3] The mortality and morbidity occurred principally among the elderly and those with pre-existing cardiopulmonary disease. Although such short-term and massive exposures are fortunately rare episodes, ambient levels of air pollution can contribute to the pathogenesis or exacerbation of disease, especially in urban populations. These diseases consist mainly of chronic bronchitis, pulmonary emphysema, and bronchial asthma; there is also the consideration of air pollution's contribution to the incidence of lung cancer.

Chemicals of biologic origin may be dispersed as a result of human activity and contribute to the aggravation of an existing disease state. For example, the processing of material from grain handling or milling and the release of dusts into the atmosphere may result in aeroallergenic contributions to the provocation of a bronchial asthmatic attack in susceptible individuals.

The exact relationship between long-term low levels of exposure to environmental airborne chemical pollutants and respiratory disease remains to be elucidated. Consider asthma as an example. The incidence and prevalence of asthma mortality and morbidity have been increasing in the United States since the 1980s. The greatest increases have been occurring in children and adolescents, especially in inner-city minority populations. Although the reasons for these increases are poorly understood, a possibly contributing factor to the development of asthma and other diseases of the respiratory system might be related, at least in part, to exposure to airborne environmental pollutants. Paradoxically, although the incidence and prevalence of asthma have been increasing over the past 2 decades, the quality of air with respect to ambient concentrations of the criteria pollutants (Table 14-1) has greatly improved.

There is concern about the health effects of other toxic air pollutants that were identified in the Clean Air Act Amendment of 1990. More than 180 air toxicants have been identified as hazardous in Title III of the Clean Air Act Amendment of 1990; however, the health effects of chronic respiratory exposure to most of these toxicants are virtually unknown. Because most information on the toxic effects of these and other chemicals of environmental concern is the result of research in laboratory animals, the practitioner and public health official must be mindful that it is difficult to extrapolate from controlled laboratory studies to the human situation. Often, even in comparison of data between laboratory species, different results are obtained. For example, benzo[A]prynene inhalation exposure was shown to produce nasal tumors in hamsters but not in rats. On the other hand, it produced pulmonary tumors in rats but not in hamsters.[114]

It becomes even more challenging to study chemical interactions such as synergism, potentiation, and antagonism. (See the section on principles of toxicology.) Although chemical exposures to individual toxicants under controlled laboratory conditions have provided useful toxicologic information, the implication of any particular chemical as a causative agent in the pathophysiology of an environmentally produced or exacerbated respiratory disease in humans may not be defensible.

Of further concern are underlying health-related factors that may influence the development or progression of disease. As an example, consider the relationship between air pollution, respiratory irritation, and the development of lung cancer. When benzo[A]pyrene was administered to rats with chronic irritation of the respiratory tract, as produced by SO_2 inhalation, there was a higher incidence of bronchogenic carcinoma.[70] In this case a preexisting condition produced by one chemical agent resulted in the greater likelihood for the development of disease produced by another chemical. On a broader scope, the question of whether respiratory irritation, as produced by physical, chemical, or biologic agents, represents a predisposing factor in the process of chemical carcinogenesis remains largely to be determined.

This chapter was written in the anticipation that it will provide the practitioner and public health professional with an overview of pulmonary toxicology as it relates to toxicant exposures of environmental concern. In some instances, when studies in different species of laboratory animals provide most of the information on a particular topic, several studies have been summarized so that interspecies variations would be omitted when comparisons between toxicants are made. The reader is referred to the appropriate references for more detailed and comprehensive discussions in those areas of particular interest.

RESPIRATORY AND ENVIRONMENTAL INTERFACE

The importance of the respiratory system lies well beyond that of maintenance of life through the exchange of gases. It also includes numerous essential nonrespiratory functions, such as the maintenance of an active immune system, metabolism of endogenous substances (for example, prosta-

Table 14-1. National ambient air quality standards

Pollutant	Sensitive population	Health effects	Averaging time	Primary standard
Ozone	None identified	Increased respiratory symptoms, reduced pulmonary function	1 hr	0.120 ppm
SO_2	Asthmatics	Increased respiratory symptoms, reduced pulmonary function	24 hr Annual	0.140 ppm 0.030 ppm
Nitrogen dioxide	Young children and asthmatics, individuals with preexisting respiratory disease	Increased pulmonary symptoms, reduced pulmonary function	Annual	0.053 ppm
Carbon monoxide	Individuals with heart disease	Aggravation of angina pectoris	8 hr 1 hr	9 ppm 35 ppm
Particles	Individuals with preexisting respiratory disease	Changes in mortality in sensitive populations; increase in respiratory symptoms, reduced pulmonary function	24 hr Annual	150 $\mu g/m^3$ 50 $\mu g/m^3$
Lead	Fetuses and young children	Neurobehavioral development, impaired heme synthesis	Quarterly	1.5 $\mu g/m^3$

glandins and angiotensin), and metabolism of environmental pollutants, including those of xenobiotic origin. All portions of the respiratory system, from the nose to the gas-exchange surfaces, have a role in the recognition, metabolism, detoxification, and elimination of airborne environmental pollutants. The human respiratory system consists of both conducting and respiratory portions. The structure of the system is complex. For a comprehensive discussion, the reader is referred to works by Murray[86] and Weibel.[114]

Unique features of the respiratory system

The surface of the respiratory system is composed of an extensive interface that is exposed to the external gaseous environment via the inhaled breath. Along with the exchange of gases, the inhaled air contains a variety of nonessential gases, vapors, aerosols, particulates, and so on, which may have the potential to produce local injury. In addition, depending on the chemical in question, the respiratory system can serve as a route for the systemic absorption of xenobiotics, as well as being the target of chemical toxicity. For example, inhaled nitrogen dioxide (NO_2) can produce pulmonary fibrosis without producing systemic toxicity. In this case, the lung serves as both the organ of exposure and the target of toxicity. Inhaled volatile organic compounds are absorbed systemically and can produce effects at the central nervous system level. Furthermore, the lungs may serve as the target organ of toxicity for chemicals that may enter the body from routes of exposure other than inhalation. For example, the herbicide paraquat produces pulmonary damage after its accidental (or intentional) ingestion. From a toxicologic perspective, then, the respiratory system is unique. In addition to direct exposure to airborne toxicants, all xenobiotics present in the cardiac output must first enter the pulmonary circulation before entering the systemic circulation. Consequently, it is easy to understand why the distribution of toxicants to other organs can be so rapid, producing systemic toxicity.

Despite the myriad of environmental chemicals capable of producing toxic injury to the respiratory system, the responses produced can be placed into one or more categories, including irritation and/or inflammation, bronchoconstriction (either nonimmunologically or immunologically mediated), edema, fibrosis, oncogenesis, and cellular death and necrosis. The degree of toxicity produced by an inhaled pollutant depends on several factors, including the concentration of the pollutant in the air, the duration of exposure, the level of physical activity of the individual who is exposed, and the physicochemical properties of the chemical (for example, solubility).

Depending on the chemical, any part of the respiratory system may be the target of toxicity. For example, chlorine and ammonia gas are capable of producing irritation and bronchoconstriction in the airways. Exposure to high concentrations of these gases can result in the inability to breathe deeply and rapidly enough to satisfy respiratory demands, resulting in the feeling of dyspnea. Because both gases are very water soluble, they are removed primarily in the upper airways, where they produce their effects.

ANATOMIC FEATURES OF THE RESPIRATORY TRACT

The respiratory system can be divided into three major divisions: the nasopharyngeal, tracheobronchial, and pulmonary regions). The nasopharyngeal region extends from the nares to the larynx and possesses a well-vascularized mucosa, which warms and humidifies inhaled air before it passes through the tracheobronchial tree. The nose is a complex organ that serves numerous functions, such as olfaction, metabolism, and the transport and conditioning of the inspired air. It contains a rich and complex blood-lymphatic system and innervations from the sympathetic and parasympathetic nervous systems and the olfactory nerves. The mucosal lining of the nose is complex and is divided into several major types of epithelia, including squamous, respiratory, transitional, and olfactory.

The tracheobronchial region (conducting portion) contains the trachea, bronchi, and bronchioles, which serve to conduct air between the nasopharynx and the gas-exchange surfaces of the lungs. This region contains approximately 23 generations of airways, which are composed of numerous reactive cellular components, including epithelial, nervous, secretory, and smooth muscle cells.[32] The epithelium of the airways is composed of at least eight types of cells and represents an important environmental interface that responds to toxic insult through several different mechanisms, including particulate clearance via the mucociliary escalator and metabolism of xenobiotics, that may, depending on the chemical, result in either their detoxification or their bioactivation. Clara cells are nonciliated cells in the epithelial lining of distal portions of the conducting airways.[17,93] They are located mainly in the central or proximal portion of the transition zone between the conducting airways and gas-exchange areas. The cells are cuboid to columnar and contain long, apical microvilli; extensive agranular endoplasmic reticulum; large mitochondria; and osmophilic granules. These cells can contain high levels of cytochrome P-450 monooxygenase isozymes and may represent important participants in the process of xenobiotic metabolism in the airways. In addition to xenobiotic metabolism, the Clara cells are believed to be a source of secretory material of the acellular bronchiolar linings. The conducting airways contain airway smooth muscle, which is regulated by both neural and cellular mediators, including those produced by the airways epithelia. Cholinergic enervation of the airways produces airway smooth muscle contraction, whereas adrenergic and nonadrenergic inhibitory mechanisms produce relaxation.

The pulmonary regions (respiratory portions) of the lungs are the sites at which gas exchange occurs and includes the respiratory bronchioles, alveolar ducts and sacs, alveoli, and other associated tissues, including capillaries and lymphatics. The basic unit of structure and function in the pulmonary region is the acinus, of which the human lung contains approximately 200,000. The alveolar surface area of the adult human lung is approximately 100 m² and provides a total surface area for exposure to environmental toxicants that is well over 50 times that of the skin. The luminal surface of the alveolar basement membrane is lined by the type I pneumocyte, which composes more than 90% of the alveolar surface area. These cells are characteristically thin to facilitate the exchanges of gases. The type II pneumocytes are cuboid and compose only 7% of the alveolar surface area, even though they are more numerous than the type I cells. These cells can develop into type I pneumocytes after pulmonary injury from inhaled toxicants.

The respiratory system has developed defense mechanisms to deal with environmental exposure to inhaled toxic materials. These mechanisms help reduce both local damage to the respiratory system and the absorption of toxicants into the systemic compartment. Alveolar macrophages are phagocytic cells that reside in the alveoli. They originate in the bone marrow and circulate in the blood stream as monocytes. On arrival at the lung interstitial tissue, they may or may not divide. Interstitial macrophages appear to become a distinct population of phagocytes that retain the capacity to undergo mitotic division. Macrophages that are destined to become pulmonary macrophages migrate into the air spaces of the alveoli. They are important in that they ingest inhaled particulates (Fig. 14-1) and represent the main mechanism of clearance in the pulmonary region of the respiratory system. Many environmental toxicants have been shown to influence the phagocytic behavior of these macrophages in laboratory animals. Some of these studies have been summarized (Table 14-2). Alveolar macrophages also are known to play a significant role in the repair process of oxidant injury to the alveolar epithelium by releasing factors that promote the growth of type II cells during injury repair.[43]

PULMONARY DEFENSE MECHANISMS
Clearance

A major component of pulmonary defense processes involves the physical removal of foreign material that contacts the epithelial interface, generically referred to as clearance mechanisms (Fig. 14-2). The clearance mechanisms of the respiratory system provide an important nonspecific mechanism for the removal of particulate material and dissolved chemicals and vary with the site of deposition.[106] Humans generally breathe through their mouths, which can cause greater deposition in the tracheobronchial tree, more-peripheral airways, and lung than with nasal breathing. Within the airways are submucosal glands and goblet cells, which secrete mucus, forming a serous-type fluid layer coating the epithelium. The mucus layer of the tracheobronchial region

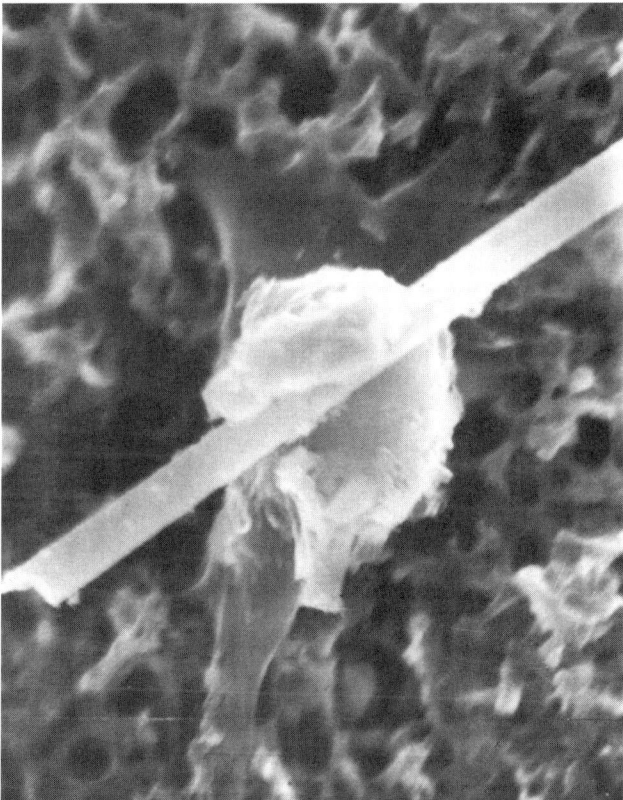

Fig. 14-1 Scanning electron photomicrograph of macrophage cells grown on culture with ceramic fibers (9600×).

Table 14-2. Effects of toxicants on phagocytic activity of alveolar macrophages in the rat

Toxicant	Exposure concentration	Exposure duration	Response	Reference
Ozone	0.8 ppm	20 days	+	31
	2.5 ppm	5 hr	−	47
	0.8 ppm	4 hr	−	89
Nitrogen dioxide	10, 25 ppm	24 hr	− at 25 ppm	62
Cadmium	1.5, 5.0 mg/m³	0.5 hr	+ at 1.5 mg/m³, − at 5 mg/m³	46

−, Depression of phagocytic activity; +, enhancement of phagocytic activity.

is biphasic, with an epiphase that floats on the surface of a less viscous layer below, the hypophase.[77] Mucus moves upward through the action of the coordinated beating of specialized mucosal ciliated cells. There are approximately 270 cilia per cell, each of which is approximately 6 mm long.[69] Macrophages containing ingested particles, in addition to free particles and dissolved gases and vapors in the mucus, are moved upward, where they can be swallowed or expectorated. Alterations in the efficiency of the clearance mechanisms can modify the ultimate disposition of inspired xenobiotics.

The mucociliary transport system is sensitive to a wide variety of environmental agents, including such irritants as ozone, cigarette smoke, and oxides of sulfur. This sensitivity has been well studied in laboratory animals (Table 14-3). Similar studies have been conducted with human subjects. Mucociliary clearance in humans can be determined with timed clearance after the inhalation of radiolabeled inert particles. In humans the mucus of the mucociliary escalator is normally cleared continuously from the airways at a rate of about 4 m per minute. Under normal conditions, clearance is relatively rapid and completed within a period of 1 to 2 days. Using sulfuric acid–radiolabeled aerosols, Leikauf et al.[73] demonstrated an increase in the clearance rate after a 1-hour exposure to the acid at a concentration of 100 mg/m^3 and a decrease of clearance after exposure to 1000 mg/m^3.

It is now well established that in humans, many types of airborne toxicants can alter the speed of mucus flow (Table 14-4) by altering cellular physiology or modifying the physical and chemical properties of mucus. Chronic exposure to smoke, for example, can result in prolonged impairment of the tracheobronchial clearance mechanism to inhaled particles.[105] These data and others from similar observations provide a plausible explanation linking exposure to certain types of airborne pollutants with development of chronic bronchitis.[75] As in the airways, the mucociliary apparatus of the nose plays an important role in protection of the respiratory tract from the toxic effects of inhaled particles. Cilia move the mucus of the nasal epithelium and tracheobronchial tree to the pharynx, where it is swallowed or expectorated.

In the pulmonary region, clearance occurs by phagocytosis and then removal via the mucociliary escalator, the blood capillaries, or lymphatic drainages. Clearance depends on the physiochemical properties of the particles. Soluble particles may dissolve and be absorbed into the pulmonary capillaries, and insoluble particles may move from the alveolar air sacs into the vascular system or lymphatic system.

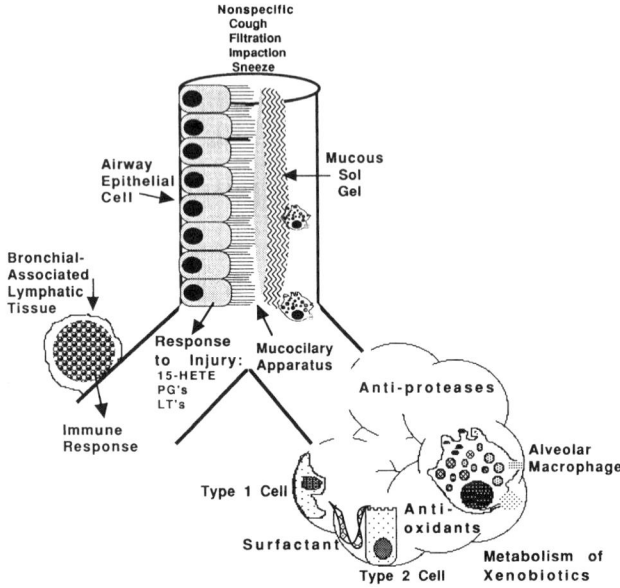

Fig. 14-2 Major pulmonary defense mechanisms include the mucociliary apparatus at the bronchial region and the alveolar macrophage at the respiratory level. There are also other defense processes operating, including antiproteases, antioxidants, and immunologic, metabolic, and cellular mechanisms.

Table 14-3. Effects of inhaled toxicants on respiratory clearance in the rat

Toxicant	Exposure concentration	Exposure duration	Response	Reference
Ozone	0.4-1 ppm	4 hr	+ at 0.8, 1 ppm	64
NO$_2$	3-24 ppm	7 hr/day, 5 days/wk, 2-3 wk	+ at low concentrations × time values; − at high concentrations × time values	40
Formaldehyde	20 ppm	4 hr	NE	76
SO$_2$	0.1-20 ppm	7 hr/day, 5 days/wk, 2-5 wk	+ at low concentrations × time values; − at high concentrations × time values	40
Sulfuric acid	3.6 mg/m^3 (1 μm)	4 hr	−	84
	3.6 mg/m^3	4 hr	NE	84
Chromium	0.2 mg/m^3	Continuous, 42 days	−	46
Diesel exhaust particles	0.2-4.1 mg/m^3	7 hr/day, 5 days/wk, 18 wk	− at 4.1 mg/m^3	51

NE, No effect; +, acceleration of clearance rate; −, reduction of clearance rate.

Macrophages are found to contain ingested particles within minutes after their inhalation, and by several hours inhaled particles are ultimately engulfed.

Biochemical mechanisms

Biochemical defense mechanisms in the respiratory system include, for example, the metabolism of xenobiotics, protective proteins, and antioxidant mechanisms. All portions of the respiratory tract from the nasal mucosa to the pulmonary alveolus contain enzymes capable of metabolic transformations of environmental xenobiotics, including potential carcinogens. Studies have included whole animals, perfused lungs, tissue explants, and cultured cells.[11] Many types of cells are active in pulmonary xenobiotic metabolism, including Clara cells, alveolar macrophages, epithelial cells, and pulmonary endothelial cells. Over the past few decades an increasing number of in vitro studies have used cell-culture systems to assess the effects of environmental toxicants on numerous aspects of cellular function. These studies have been well reviewed by Leikauf and Driscoll.[72]

Most data suggest that the pulmonary and nasal tissues have a greater metabolic capacity toward inspired environmental organic chemicals than do the conducting portions of the respiratory tract, such as the trachea and the bronchi,[34] although some cells, such as Clara cells in the bronchiolar region, may contain unusually high concentrations of certain enzymes. Because the mucosa is in direct line with air pollutants, it is susceptible to direct toxic damage. Let us use the nose as an example. The nose contains several types of epithelia, including the sensory or olfactory epithelium, the respiratory epithelium, and squamous epithelium. These tissues are frequently exposed to the highest levels of airborne toxicants of any tissue. Nasal metabolism plays a major role in the ultimate response of this organ to environmental xenobiotics.[6,10] The nasal cavity contains a wide range of enzymes capable of metabolic transformations, including cytochrome P-450,[76] 15-lipoxygenase,[59] epoxyhydrolase,[44] and glutathione S-transferase.[12,44]

Most information concerns the phase-I enzyme systems and, principally, cytochrome P-450 monooxygenase. Little information is available on phase-II transformations. Principal phase-I metabolizing enzymes in the respiratory system are cytochrome P-450 and flavin-containing monooxygenases. These systems cover a broad range of biologic transformations of inhaled organic toxicants, including aromatic and aliphatic hydroxylations, epoxidation, deamination, sulfoxidation, N-and O-dealkylations, and other biochemical transformations.[7,13,53] Enzyme systems are important in metabolizing compounds into more water-soluble ones, which can be more easily eliminated by the body. It is now clear, however, that the same enzyme systems that perform these xenobiotic transformations also can bioactivate compounds with relatively low toxicity into reactive metabolites capable of producing cellular injury, including the induction of cancer. These enzyme systems produce products less toxic than the inhaled compound; however, metabolic transformations may result in the bioactivation of the parent compound into a product more toxic than the parent compound. In general, when compared with hepatic cytochromes P-450, the nasal cytochromes P-450 are easily inhibited by common inhibitors of hepatic cytochrome P-450 but are relatively resistant to induction by xenobiotics.

That the nasal mucosa is important in xenobiotic metabolism is further supported by observations that show that antioxidants (such as ascorbate) are present.[68] The capacity of the nasal mucosa to transform xenobiotics metabolically may be responsible for both nasal protection and damage. For example, depletion of glutathione, an essential cosubstrate for formaldehyde dehydrogenase–mediated breakdown of formaldehyde, can result in increase in the covalent binding of formaldehyde with cellular deoxyribonucleic acid (DNA).[27] Research with laboratory animals strongly suggests that the activities of nasal enzymes are important links in the chain of events that lead to the production of nasal tumors.[1,18,22,33,34]

Other examples of biochemical protection in the respiratory system include protective proteins and antioxidant systems (Fig. 14-2). As an example, a major protective pro-

Table 14-4. Toxicant effects on mucociliary clearance in humans

Toxicant	Concentration	Duration of exposure	Region examined	Response	Reference
Ozone	0.2, 0.4 ppm	2 h (with exercise)	B	+	42
SO$_2$	1, 5, 25 ppm	6 h	N	−	4
	5 ppm	3 h	B	NE	111
	5 ppm	2 h (with exercise)	B	+	83
Carbon	50 mg/m^3	Few minutes	T, B	+	25
Sulfuric acid	0.1-10 mg/m^3	1 h	T, B	NE on T, + or − B (depending on concentration)	70
Cigarette smoke	2 cigarettes		T, B	+	49
	''Heavy'' smoking		T, B	−	49

B, Bronchial tree; *N*, nasal passages; *T*, trachea; *NE*, no effect; +, acceleration of clearance rate; −, reduction of clearance rate.

tein in the lung is alpha$_1$-antitrypsin. The primary source of this glycoprotein is the liver. Because of its low molecular weight, it diffuses freely to the alveolar surface, where it is found in concentrations similar to those in the serum. Because this molecule functions as an antiprotease, it serves a number of important functions in the normal physiology of the lung, including inhibition of plasmin, thrombin, and neutrophil elastase. Neutrophil elastase is a broad-spectrum protease capable of breaking down many of the extracellular matrix structural proteins. Exposure of the alveolar surface to oxidants, which may be contained in polluted air, can produce major alterations in the binding of alpha$_1$-antitrypsin and elastase. Antioxidant systems may further protect the respiratory system from chemical injury. The respiratory system is subjected to significant oxidant stress from direct environmental sources of oxidants (for example, NO$_2$, ozone, cigarette smoke) and endogenous oxidants released by respiratory cells in response to inhaled toxicants. Oxygen, which is essential for cellular respiration, also is involved in the generation of potentially toxic oxygen radicals. The respiratory system has developed sophisticated mechanisms for reducing oxidant stress, including enzyme systems such as superoxide dismutase, catalase, and other oxidant scavengers, including fat-soluble (such as vitamin E) and water-soluble (such as vitamin C) compounds. The topic of pulmonary antioxidant defense has been well reviewed by Heffner and Repine.[58]

The toxic effects of ozone, for example, have been ascribed to its reactive and oxidative capacities resulting in the generation of free radicals and consequent lung damage, which is due to the oxidation of unsaturated fatty acids and proteins in the membranes of pulmonary cells.[81] Biochemical studies conducted in rodents have shown that exposure to ozone stimulates the induction of the enzyme system glutathione peroxidase.[30] Induction of this enzyme system may be a mechanism protective against exposure to gases such as ozone or NO$_2$. Dietary vitamin E may serve as a protective agent during pulmonary exposure to ozone, because this vitamin serves as a scavenger for fatty-acid peroxides and may indirectly enhance the effectiveness of the glutathione peroxidase system.[93] Supplementation of rodent diet with vitamin E prior to the exposure to ozone resulted in elevated lung levels of glutathione peroxidase and other important enzyme systems (for example, glutathione reductase, glucose-6-phosphate dehydrogenase).

Bronchoconstriction

Exposure to airborne pollutants can change the responsiveness of the smooth muscle of the airways to normal endogenous bronchoconstrictor agents. This reduction may be particularly pronounced in individuals who are asthmatic. Acute inhalation of large concentrations of environmental chemicals such as NO$_2$ and ozone has been associated with an increase in nonspecific responsiveness of the smooth muscle of the airways.[15] Different mechanisms may be responsible for the bronchoconstriction produced in response to respired particulate matter and chemicals. For example, acute exposure to SO$_2$ for several minutes can result in bronchoconstriction (which may be significant and accompanied by wheezing in asthmatics) at concentrations as low as 0.4 ppm. The response is probably due to the activation of irritant nerve receptors and the release of acetylcholine through a vagal reflex mechanism and a histaminergically mediated mechanism involving the release of inflammatory mediators from resident airway cells. By reducing air flow to the lungs, bronchoconstriction is protective in that it provides an additional mechanism to limit pulmonary exposure to inhaled toxicants.

Airway epithelium

Damage to the epithelial lining of the airways from the inhalation of toxicants can initiate a cascading series of reactions that may ultimately produce an inflammatory response (Fig. 14-2). Airway epithelial cells have been shown to produce many types of inflammatory mediators (for example, arachidonic acid metabolites) that can promote alterations in vascular permeability and recruit inflammatory cells to the site of injury. In addition, damaged epithelial cells may not produce epithelium-derived relaxation factor or prostaglandin E$_2$, two important endogenous mediators that help maintain the normal tone of airway smooth muscle. The airway epithelium is thus an important component in the down-regulation of airway smooth muscle contractions. Respired environmental toxins may even produce nonimmunologically mediated bronchoconstriction, as was recently demonstrated by Richards et al.[98] with red tide toxins (brevetoxins). These environmental toxins produced depolarization of airway smooth muscle cells through the apparent activation of peripheral cholinergic nerves and the release of the transmitter acetylcholine.

Olfaction

The olfactory area is found in the roof of the nasal cavity and contains an epithelium composed of several types of cells, including the olfactory receptor cells, basal cells, and sustentacular (supporting) cells. The olfactory receptor cells are modified by bipolar neurons, each of which contains a cell body with a dendritic region extending to the surface of the epithelium and an axon extending into the lamina propria. The proximal portion of the cell contains the olfactory cilia, which are believed to play an important role in chemoreception and transduction. The unmyelinated axon of each bipolar receptor extends into the underlying lamina propria, where it joins with other axons to form bundles of olfactory nerve fibers that reach the olfactory bulbs of the brain by way of foramina in the cribriform plate of the ethmoid bone.

The mechanism of odor perception is not clearly understood. Olfactory receptors can respond to a wide range of odoriferous substances. From a toxicologic point of view, the olfactory system can be viewed as an important defense mechanism. Recognition of airborne odorants may result in appropriate adaptive behaviors, which can result in avoidance behavior to reduce further exposure. This is particularly significant because many noxious airborne pollutants have odor thresholds well below levels that can produce cellular injury.

Alveolar macrophages

Many of the alveolar macrophages, containing their engulfed particles, are transported to the mucociliary escalator, where they are removed from the respiratory system (see Fig. 14-2). Alveolar macrophages, unlike the polymorphonuclear leukocytes, adhere to the surface of the pulmonary epithelia and cannot metabolize effectively under conditions of hypoxia. It is unlikely that they would retain much of their function on removal from the humidified gas phase of the lungs and airways. Because the alveolar regions of the lung do not possess a mucociliary transport mechanism, particles deposited in these portions of the respiratory system are cleared at a much slower rate than that in the airways. This slower rate reflects the transport time of macrophages to more proximal portions of the respiratory system that contain ciliated epithelia. Most of the insoluble particles that deposit in the alveolar regions are phagocytized by macrophages that can migrate to the bronchoalveolar junctions to enter the mucociliary escalator for subsequent removal from the lung.[50] The macrophage plays a key role in the pathogenesis of pulmonary fibrosis. (See later discussion.)

Immunologic mechanisms

The lung is replete with immunologic capacity and rich in lymphatic tissue. This extensive immunologic capacity allows the lung to react more efficiently to foreign agents. A more extensive discussion of the immunologic system is presented in the immunotoxicology section.

IMPORTANT ENVIRONMENTAL AIRBORNE POLLUTANTS

Inhaled toxicants, such as carbon monoxide, oxides of sulfur, oxides of nitrogen, particulate matter, hydrocarbons, halogenated compounds, ketones, aldehydes, aromatic amines, and polycyclic aromatic hydrocarbons, are introduced into the respiratory system with inhaled air. Usually inhaled compounds are components of complex mixtures that occur in the environment either as vapors or adsorbed onto respirable particles. Virtually no information in available on potential human health risks associated with inhalation exposure to chemical mixtures. A discussion of the myriad chemicals of environmental concern is beyond the scope of this section. Instead, several well-studied agents have been selected as examples.

Ozone

Ozone occurs naturally in high concentrations in the upper atmosphere, where it functions to shield the earth's surface from the effects of ultraviolet radiation. Ozone also is an important component of urban air pollution, particularly during the summer, when oxides of nitrogen produced from the internal combustion of engines and hydrocarbons from these and other man-made sources react to form ozone.[54] These episodes often occur with elevations of levels of other airborne pollutants, such as sulfuric acid and nitric acid, which may potentiate the effects of ozone through multiple-chemical interaction as previously mentioned. Ozone is extremely irritating to the respiratory system, even in healthy individuals. The human respiratory system is the only organ known to be affected by inhalation of ozone at concentrations typically found in the environment. In urban environments, many individuals are commonly exposed to concentrations of ozone sufficient to produce reversible symptomatic and functional respiratory effects.[88] It has been demonstrated in exercising individuals that low-level ozone exposure over several hours produces reversible alterations in normal pulmonary function.[56,80] Short-term human respiratory exposure to ozone at concentrations that can occur during episodes of air pollution have been shown to produce rapid-onset chest tightness and discomfort on deep inspiration, more rapid shallow breathing during exercise, decreased maximal inspiratory capacity, increased specific airway resistance, increased mucociliary transport, airway hyperresponsiveness to methacholine challenge, and increased respiratory epithelial cell permeability.[28,41,56,64,67]

Because ozone is less soluble than are other irritant gases such as SO_2 and chlorine, it can penetrate more effectively through the tracheobronchial tree to the pulmonary regions of the respiratory system. At concentrations of ozone below 1 ppm, the more distal portions of the lung, including the terminal airways and the proximal alveolar regions, are affected.[8] Because it is a very powerful oxidizing agent and is highly reactive when in contact with cellular membranes, it produces disruptive changes that may be measured by alterations in pulmonary function, including increases in pulmonary permeability. For example, Kehrl et al.[64] have shown that human exposure to ozone at levels that produce significant alterations in pulmonary function produced a corresponding increase in lung permeability to technetium-labeled diethylenetriaminepentaacetic acid. Ozone exposures have also been shown to produce inflammation in the respiratory system. Devlin et al[36] studied nonsmoking males who were randomly exposed to either filtered air or air containing ozone (0.10 ppm or 0.08 ppm) during moderate exercise (40 L/min). Bronchoalveolar lavage (BAL) was performed 18 hours after a 6.6-hour exposure to ozone. Exposure to levels as low as 0.08 ppm was sufficient to initiate an inflammatory reaction in the lung as inferred from significant increases in neutrophils, protein, prostaglandin E_2, interleukin-6, lactate dehydrogenase, and α_1-antitrypsin.

Koren et al.[67] showed that in healthy, exercising human subjects exposed to ozone for several hours there was an eightfold increase in the number of polymorphonuclear leukocytes obtained by BAL. In addition, they observed a corresponding recovery of a number of inflammatory mediators, including prostaglandin E_2 and plasminogen activator. Generally, the peak inflammatory response occurs several hours after ozone exposure and appears not to correlate well with changes in airway function. Other studies have shown similar results and suggest that exposures below the National Ambient Air Quality Standard of 0.12 ppm may result in an inflammatory response suggestive of acute bronchiolitis.[104]

Zwick and coworkers[120] examined the lasting effects of high ozone concentrations (maximal levels of 0.188 ppm and above 0.06 ppm 45% of the time) under environmental conditions and discovered that long-term exposure to high ozone concentrations may lead to persistent bronchial hyperresponsiveness and subclinical effects on lymphocyte subpopulations in children. The low-concentration group had a maximal level of 0.095 ppm, but less than 0.5% of the time the level was 0.06 ppm). Even though the changes observed are of questionable clinical significance, the authors believed that they represent sensitive indicators for the assessment of the influence of air pollution.

Low ozone concentrations of 0.120 ppm for 1 hour at rest caused an increased sensitivity to the dose of inhaled allergen necessary to elicit an asthmatic response.[83] It was hypothesized that the short-term ozone exposure possibly could lead to a low-grade inflammatory response, with vasodilatation and thus greater absorption of allergen, although the exact mechanism could not be verified.

Sulfur dioxide

SO_2, one of the major environmental air pollutants, is produced by the combustion of such sulfur-containing fossil fuels as coal and oil. Major outdoor sources include power plants, smelters, and oil refineries. Indoor sources include kerosene space heaters. Commercially available kerosene can contain varying amounts of sulfur and under some conditions may produce indoor atmospheres containing as much as 5 ppm SO_2, which is approximately 30 times higher than the primary air quality standard for this irritant. The irritant effects of SO_2 are produced primarily in the upper airways. Individuals who are asthmatic are especially sensitive to the effects of SO_2.[107]

Some environmental chemicals such as SO_2 are capable of producing a nonimmunologically mediated airway smooth muscle contraction, which may involve both neural and nonneural mechanisms. Laboratory studies have shown that prior SO_2 exposure may greatly influence the response in immunologically sensitized animals during subsequent challenges with the sensitizing agent. For example, Riedel et al.[99] demonstrated that exposure to 0.16 to 4.3 ppm SO_2 in ovalbumin-sensitized guinea pigs for several hours per day over a period of 5 days resulted in the production of a greater degree of bronchoconstriction during a subsequent challenge with ovalbumin than in control animals exposed to air. This finding suggests that some airborne chemical pollutants that produce pulmonary effects via nonimmunologically mediated mechanisms may make certain individuals more susceptible to other chemicals that may produce effects through immunologic mechanisms.

Oxides of nitrogen

Oxides of nitrogen, such as NO_2, are produced by outdoor sources such as emissions from power plants, oil refineries, and automobile exhaust. Indoor sources include emissions from gas stoves and furnaces, kerosene space heaters, and cigarette smoke. NO_2, like ozone, produces effects at the level of the respiratory bronchioles and alveoli through peroxidation of cellular membranes. Large short-term exposures to ozone or oxides of nitrogen can produce pulmonary edema, and long-term exposures may result in the production of emphysema. Exposures to oxidants such as NO_2 may result in increases in the permeability of the alveolar epithelium, which may lead to the development of pulmonary edema. Clinically, this may be assessed by examination of BAL for increases in serum proteins (such as IgG and albumin), which may or may not appear after the exposure.[42,67] Studies in laboratory animals have shown that NO_2 exposure produces pathologic changes in the distal airways and proximal alveolar regions.[38,48] These effects were characterized by proliferation of type II epithelial cells and Clara cells and increases in bronchial epithelial permeability.

Aldehydes

Aldehydes of various types are formed during the photooxidation of hydrocarbons. The major aldehydes of interest are formaldehyde (which accounts for approximately 50% of total aldehydes) and acrolein (which accounts for approximately 5% of total aldehydes). These chemicals contribute to the eye irritation and odor that characterize photochemical smog. Formaldehyde, which is very soluble in water, is an irritant to the mucous membranes of the nose, upper respiratory tract, and eyes. It has an odor threshold of about 0.5 ppm, and at 4 to 5 ppm, it is intolerable to most individuals exposed. Formaldehyde may be present in indoor atmospheres as a result of the presence of urea-formaldehyde foam insulation and other sources (for example, cigarette smoke and particle board–constructed furniture). Because formaldehyde is used in both industry and consumer products, isolated laboratory reports of the ability of this chemical to produce cancer must be viewed with caution because epidemiologic studies have failed to show increased incidences of nasal cancer in exposed workers.

Acrolein is an unsaturated aldehyde that is more reactive

and irritating than formaldehyde and, at concentrations well below 1 ppm, can produce irritation to the eyes and mucous membranes of the respiratory tract. Because of the complex mixtures often present in polluted air, the effects on lung function could be reversible or irreversible. Irreversible loss of function could reflect the development of airway fibrosis, emphysema, or interstitial fibrosis. Acute but reversible loss of pulmonary function could occur secondary to bronchoconstriction, inflammation, or other mechanisms.

MECHANISMS OF RESPIRATORY TRACT DISEASE: FAILURE OF DEFENSE MECHANISMS

Several pathophysiologic pulmonary processes result from environmental exposures and lead to disease states, such as noncardiac pulmonary edema, inflammation (pneumonia), asthma, fibrosis, and cancer. Two common processes, fibrosis and asthma, are particularly pertinent because of the frequency of their occurrence and, more important in the context of this discussion, their demonstration of how the normal lung defense mechanisms may be overwhelmed or modified, leading to a disease state. Fig. 14-3 summarizes some of the more important defense processes. Nonspecific protective mechanisms, such as sneezing and coughing, may discharge particles or be a reaction to environmental agents' entering the upper respiratory tract. The mucociliary apparatus carries inhaled particles deposited on the bronchi upward toward the mouth to be swallowed or expectorated as sputum. It is believed that an initial step in the pathogenesis of asthma involves bronchial epithelial cell damage, which leads to a cascade of occurrences that eventuate as asthma. Bronchial-associated lymphatic tissue plays a role in the various allergic mechanisms that may be prominent in asthma. In the alveolar region, an activation and recruitment of alveolar macrophages seem important in the pathogenesis of pulmonary fibrosis. Other defense mechanisms influence other diseases processes, such as the relationship between the antiproteases and emphysema. The alveolar epithelial cells (type 1 and 2) have important defensive functions but when significantly overwhelmed by injury are unable to limit the extent of lung damage and thus the development of disease. Other important processes include the lung's ability to metabolize xenobiotics and the role of surfactant as a neutralizing factor for inhaled chemical pollutants. More detailed discussion of the lung's defense mechanisms can be obtained in specialized texts dealing with this topic.[32]

Pulmonary fibrosis

Investigations have recognized the key role of the alveolar macrophage in augmenting and suppressing fibroblast proliferation, a process that is central to the development of pulmonary fibrosis. Whether fibroblasts are stimulated or not seems to depend on the balance between secreted factors that increase fibroblast proliferation (growth factors) and factors that can inhibit fibroblast proliferation (Fig. 14-3). For example, supernatants of human alveolar macrophages obtained from BAL fluid that is stimulated with silica, contain large amounts of growth factor activity for human lung fibroblasts.[21] Prostaglandin E_2 seems to be an inhibitor of fibroblast proliferation; other arachidonate metabolites and, possibly, somatomedin-like growth factors also may be important in the balance.[111]

It has been suggested that one stimulus for the promotion of growth-factor secretion relates to a chemical-physical interaction between the fibrosis-producing agent (for example, silica) and the alveolar macrophage cellular surface, perhaps through the hydrogen donor ability of the silanol groups or a negative surface charge from the ionized silanol groups (SiO^-) on the quartz crystal surface. One hypothesis considers the role of spatial arrangement of oxygen atoms on the crystal structure in the formation of molecular contacts during crystal-cell interactions.[118] A similar mechanism can be used to explain how fibers may produce lung fibrosis. A fiber surface–cell interaction is an essential first step, but there are likely at least two separate interactions between the fiber and the cell surface.[23] The first is a charge-mediated effect that occurs with positively charged fibers, and the second is mediated by fibronectin, which first binds to the fiber. A serum factor may promote the interaction of the fibers with the cell membrane and vacuoles within the cell.[62]

Once the macrophage becomes activated and the process of phagocytosis begins, there is an expenditure of energy and a burst of mitochondrial respiration, with evolution of toxic free-radical oxygen metabolites, which exert an amplifying and modulating function on the inflammatory process.[57,115] Furthermore, when the macrophage is stimulated, a number of fibrogenic cytokines are released, including interleukin-1α, platelet-derived growth factor, basic fibroblast growth factor, transforming growth factor-β, and tumor necrosis factor-α (TNF). It has been suggested that there may be sustained local release of TNF, perhaps at higher levels than those of other potential fibrogens.[91]

Not only is the fiber surface important but the fiber dimensions are also critical; long fibers induce fibrosis, but short fibers do not. Additionally, clearance mechanisms may be influenced by fiber type. Chrysotile asbestos fibers are more actively translocated from the lung to other tissue than are amosite asbestos fibers.[112] Usually, asbestos fibers are retained in lung tissue for many years, and there is an enhanced ability of long fibers to cause fibrosis.[37] A length of about 10 μm is key in terms of leading to inflammation. The investigation of Adamson and Bowden[2] focused on the differences between alveolar macrophage responses to long and short asbestos fibers. Alveolar macrophages exposed to short asbestos fibers secrete a factor(s) that enhance DNA synthesis by fibroblasts in culture but do not produce fibrosis *in vivo*. Long fibers also secrete a growth factor, but at lower levels, which do not cause fibrosis. Alveolar macrophage secretion of a growth factor seems to be an amount-depen-

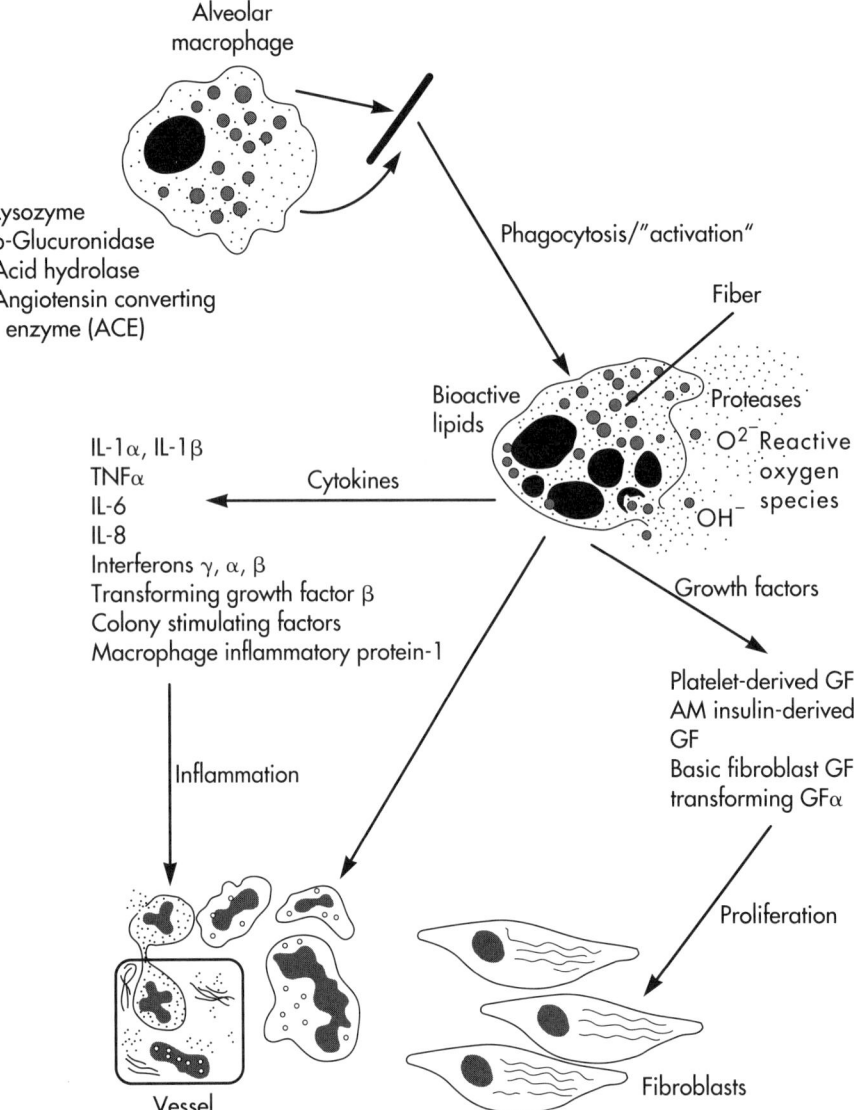

Fig. 14-3. Hypothetical mechanisms for pulmonary fibrosis.

dent response. Ingestion of the longer fibers is associated with a lower phagocytic rate than that with the shorter fibers and leads to a lower level of fibroblast growth-factor release. Thus the development of fibrosis seems dependent less on secretion of an alveolar macrophage growth factor than on fiber clearance from the lung. Long fibers are not cleared by alveolar macrophages. They penetrate the bronchiolar surface and are translocated to the peribronchiolar interstitium. It is in this critical location that activation of interstitial macrophages occurs and leads to pulmonary fibrosis. Macrophage-derived growth factor and fibronectin synergistically promote replication of fibroblasts, a prerequisite for fibrosis. Therefore, pulmonary fibrosis induced by long asbestos fibers may relate to growth factors secreted by interstitial rather than alveolar macrophages. This proposed mechanism is supported by the finding that the earliest pathologic changes of asbestosis occurs in the peribronchiolar interstitium. Subsequently, there is progression of the fibrosis, with promoting and protracting events such as hypoperfusion, mural and luminal edema, deposit of hyaline membranes, alveolar collapse, collapse induration, organization of exudates, and fibroplasia.[24] There may be exudate incorporation (septal and mural), collapse induration (obliterative and interseptal), and, possibly, intraluminal granulation tissue (luminal).

In addition to elaborating growth factors, the macrophages generate tissue-damaging free-oxygen radicals, with extracellular calcium playing an important role in the production of the superoxide anion. Chrysotile asbestos can open calcium channels on the macrophage surface, allowing extracellular calcium to enter the cell, which in turn serves to prolong superoxide anion production.[61] Inflammatory mediators released by alveolar macrophages include a neutrophil chemotactic factor.[55,101] Another potent inflammatory mediator secreted by activated alveolar macrophages is plasminogen activator (PA), a 50- to 55-kd neutral protease capable of converting the proenzyme plasminogen to plasmin.[26] Plasmin is a serine protease with a wide spectrum of potential substrates, including fibronectin, laminin, fibrinogen, and other glycoproteins, and can enhance macrophage-mediated elastin degradation. Because many of the substrates for plasmin are present in basement membranes and the extracellular matrix of normal alveolar structures and because PA activity has been shown to be increased in certain inflammatory lung disease, it has been suggested that alveolar macrophage–derived PA may be relevant to lung tissue destruction in asbestosis. Cantin et al.[26] hypothesize that lung inflammatory cell PA secretion is increased in the early stages of an asbestos-induced alveolitis and subsequently either decreases or is suppressed by the presence of fibrinolytic enzyme inhibitors in the more advanced stages of asbestosis. For PA to play a role in modulating the extracellular matrix of the lung, it is essential that the substrate plasminogen be present within the alveolar structures. Both plasminogen and PA activity are normally present in sufficient amounts within the lower respiratory tract to mediate the formation of plasmin. The increased PA activity in the asbestos-exposed lung may potentiate the conversion of alveolar plasminogen and mediate interstitial matrix alterations characteristic of asbestosis.

Animal models help identify the target cell on which inhaled asbestos fibers are deposited and the cells showing initial response by migration and phagocytosis.[19] The location of the early changes was at the bronchiolar-alveolar region, with activity noted in type II alveolar epithelial cells of the first alveolar duct bifurcation. Shoji and associates[110] demonstrated that bronchial epithelial cells produce fibronectin, which can act as a chemotactic factor for lung fibroblasts and perhaps plays some role in the regulation between bronchial epithelial cells and mesenchymal fibroblasts underlying the bronchial epithelial basement membrane. Different fibroblast populations may be operating, because Phipps et al.[92] delineated two populations of pulmonary fibroblasts based on the expression of Thy1 antigen, one population with the antigen (Thy1+) and the other without (Thy1−); morphologically, differences were noted and response to some lymphokines also varied. The Thy1− population may involve promotion of chronic inflammation and subsequent pulmonary fibrosis. The significance of lymphocytes in BAL in asbestos-exposed persons is not clear, nor is the role of immunologic mechanisms in the evolution of pulmonary fibrosis.[100,109]

The bisbenzylisoquinone alkaloids are agents investigated extensively by the Chinese, for antifibrotic potential. The data suggest a strong relationship between the antifibrotic potential of these alkaloids and their ability to bind to alveolar macrophages and inhibit particle-induced activation of these cells. In another study Jabbour et al.[60] demonstrated that constituents of surfactant extract can modify chrysotile bioactivity for alveolar macrophages. An example of how basic research can lead to possible clinical tools is an Italian study that examined serum aminoterminal propeptide of type II procollagen as an early marker of fibrosis in asbestos-exposed workers and found good correlations with asbestos dose and perhaps pulmonary function tests.[29]

Bronchial asthma

The mechanisms to explain how individuals become sensitized to environmental allergens is not fully understood. In the context of environmental asthma, exposure to chemicals in the environment is pertinent for an understanding of the pathogenesis. An important type is diisocyanate-induced asthma; toluene diisocyanate (TDI) asthma has been the most extensively studied. Airway epithelial cell damage and mucosal inflammation are important events in the pathogenesis of nonspecific airway hyperresponsiveness, a critical feature of asthma[102] (see Fig. 14-2). Patients with occupational asthma show pathologic changes of the bronchial mucosa that are similar to those in nonoccupational, environmental bronchial asthma. Thus the mechanisms of development for both occupational and nonoccupational asthma share similarities. There is infiltration of inflammatory cells (eosinophils, leukocytes, mast cells, and mononuclear cells, mainly of the CD45-positive type); evidence of bronchial epithelial damage; and thickening of subepithelial collagen. The mechanism of the thickening of the reticular basement membrane is not known but has been assumed to be due to an increase in collagen synthesis by myofibroblasts located in the lamina propria. Avoidance of exposure (that is, to TDI) may lead to a reversal of the reticular basement membrane thickening but not of the bronchial mucosal inflammatory cell infiltration, presence of specific airway sensitivity to the allergen, and nonspecific airway hyperresponsiveness to methacholine.[103]

The response of a subject with bronchial asthma due to an environmental allergen is associated with at least one of three different clinical airway manifestations. There may be an immediate response developing within 15 minutes; there may be a late asthmatic response, the development of which can begin 1 hour after an exposure but generally begins about 3 to 5 hours later; or there may a combination of both, a dual reaction. The late asthmatic response seems to be the type most directly associated with the presence of airway mucosal inflammation. The late asthmatic reaction seen in environmental asthma seems to be similar to occupational asthma and is associated with an increase in the numbers of suppressor-cytotoxic lymphocytes and eosinophils in peripheral blood; the immediate response is not so associated. Alterations of CD4-positive subsets of lymphocytes but not of CD8-positive subsets have been reported after allergen-induced asthma.[40] In contrast, TDI asthma is associated with an increase in CD8-positive cells. Whether this is an unique manifestation of TDI asthma needs to be established. The CD8 lymphocyte subset in humans is believed to be suppressor cells, possibly responding to leukotriene B_4 release during the asthmatic reaction.

Although human investigations help explain pathophysiologic manifestations of asthma, they do not really explain why some chemicals cause sensitization and others do not. One hypothesis is based on the premise that there should be a correlation between the ability of a chemical to react with proteins and its potential to induce respiratory tract sensitization.[116] A tri-amino acid peptide, L-lysl-L-tyrosol-L-lysine-2-formiate (LTL), was chosen because it showed the best separation on chromatography. Although there seemed to be a relatively good correlation between the ability of a chemical to cause allergic sensitization and its ability to react significantly with LTL, it did not occur in 100% of cases. The isocyanates and anhydrides were very reactive with LTL and are known to be potent allergic sensitizers. Other known sensitizers, such as ethylene oxide, platinum salt, and ethylenediamine, were not good reactors. Another approach to the understanding of chemical immunologic reactivity measured the capacity of topically applied trimellitic anhydride (TMA, a respiratory sensitizer with immunoglobulin E (IgE)–generation potential) and 2,4-dinitrochlorobenzene (DNCB, a potent cause of contact dermatitis) to stimulate IgE production and induce hapten-specific immunoglobulin G1, G2, and G2b (IgG1, IgG2, and IgG2b) antibodies.[35] Both TMA and DNCB elicited comparable lymph node cell proliferation, contact sensitization, and total IgG antihapten antibody responses in BALB/c-strain mice; however, the chemicals were shown to stimulate qualitatively different immune responses. There was a marked difference in their ability to stimulate IgE and in the isotype distribution of IgG antibodies. TMA preferentially elicited IgG2b, and TMA, but not DNCB, elicited IgE antibodies.

Although our understanding of allergic asthma due to sensitization has improved, it is only recently that investigators have realized that nonimmunologic mechanisms also are important in the pathogenesis of bronchial asthma. For example, persons exposed to high levels of irritating chemicals, which might occur after an environmental accident or large environmental-gas exposure, may develop the sudden onset of asthma. An example of this type of catastrophy is the Bhopal disaster. There appears to be more than one clinical type of environmentally induced reactive airways syndrome, but an important prototype is reactive airways dysfunction syndrome (RADS),[20] a condition that develops without a preceding latent period and occurs shortly after a brief high-level exposure to an irritant agent (usually gas or vapor) in the environment (always as an accident). The high-level exposure leads to sudden asthma development, with physiologic manifestations of persistent nonspecific airway hyperreactivity. In other words, the onset is abrupt, the exposure is massive, and atopy does not seem to be a necessary prerequisite. Bronchial biopsies show airway inflammation without eosinophilia.

There have been other reports of irritant-induced asthma that appear different from RADS.[45,113,114] There have been reports of RADS caused by an environmental accident, (three Philadelphia police officers exposed to toxic fumes from a roadside truck accident[96]); exposures in situations believed to be free of pollutants (a female computer operator exposed to a floor sealant[74]); exposure to TDI[78]; exposure to acetic acid[97]; exposure to SO_2[5]; after smoke inhalation[84]; after a spill of 100% glacial acetic acid[66]; after chlorine exposure in an atopic person[84]; and in a welder with concurrent metal-fume fever.[71]

The exact prevalence of morbidity after high-level irritant exposure is unknown. Blanc and coworkers[9] suggested that although symptomatic inhalation exposures due to irritants are frequently reported to poison centers, residual morbidity seems uncommon and does not relate to the degree of irritant exposure. Persistent complaints did not appear to be a simple function of the irritant exposure; it is more likely that host risk factors are the most important influencing parameter. A premorbid lung condition (such as asthma) and a history of cigarette smoking appear to be risk factors for persistent health complaints after an irritant exposure.

Environmental asthma and RADS exemplify the synergistic and complementary role played by immunologic and nonimmunologic processes. From the studies of RADS we learn that high levels of irritants can induce airway inflammation that may persist and be associated with an asthma-like condition with persistently hyperresponsive airways perhaps similar to adult-onset, intrinsic asthma. A similar condition can occur in individuals who have environmental asthma from a sensitizer and who have no further exposure to the offending allergen but continue to suffer asthma symptoms. What is not known is how these two divergent exposures lead to a similar clinical disorder. Investigations into the pathogenesis of environmental and occupational reactive airways disorders (allergic and nonallergic) provide a model for pulmonary medicine to study mechanisms of bronchial asthma in general, including the development of rational therapeutic and diagnostic approaches for treatment.

REFERENCES

1. Acteo A et al: Glutathione transferases in human nasal mucosa, *Arch Toxicol* 63: 427, 1989.
2. Adamson IY, Bowden DH: Pulmonary reaction to long and short asbestos fibers is independent of fibroblast growth factor production by alveolar macrophages, *Am J Pathol* 137:523, 1990.
3. Amdur MO: Air pollutants. In Amdur MO, Doull J, Klaassen CD, editors: *Cassaret and Doull's toxicology,* ed 4, New York, 1991, Pergamon Press.
4. Anderson I et al: Human response to controlled levels of sulfur dioxide, *Arch Environ Health* 28:31, 1974.
5. Axford A et al: Accidental exposure to isocyanate fumes in a group of firemen, *Br J Ind Med* 33:65, 1976.
6. Baron J et al: Sites of xenobiotic activation and detoxification within

the respiratory tract: implications for chemically induced toxicity, *Toxicol Appl Pharmacol* 93:493, 1988.
7. Baron J, Voigt JM: Localization, distribution, and induction of xenobiotic metabolizing enzymes and aryl hydrocarbon hydroxylase activity within the lung, *Pharmacol Ther* 47:419, 1990.
8. Barr BC et al: Distal airway remodeling in rats chronically exposed to ozone, *Am Rev Respir Dis* 137:924, 1988.
9. Blanc PD et al: Morbidity following acute irritant inhalation in a population-based study, *JAMA* 266:664, 1991.
10. Bogdanffy MS: Biotransformation enzymes in the rodent nasal mucosa: the value of a histochemical approach, *Environ Health Perspect* 85:177, 1990.
11. Bond JA: Contributions of the respiratory tract to the metabolic fate of inhaled organic chemicals. In Jerrity TR, Henry CJ, editors. *Principles of route-to-route extrapolation for risk assessment,* New York, 1990, Elsevier.
12. Bonnefoi M, Monticello TM, Morgan KT: Toxic and neoplastic responses in the nasal passages: future research needs, *Exp Lung Res* 17:853, 1991.
13. Boobis AR, Davies DS: Human cytochromes P-450, *Xenobiotica* 14:151, 1984.
14. Boulet L-P: Increase in airway responsiveness following acute exposure to respiratory irritants: reactive airways dysfunction syndrome or occupational asthma? *Chest* 94:476, 1988.
15. Boushey HA et al: Bronchial hyperreactivity: state of the art, *Am Rev Respir Dis* 121:389, 1980.
16. Brandtzaeg P: Immune functions of human nasal mucosa and tonsils in health and disease. In Bienenstock J, editor: *Immunology of the lung and upper respiratory tract,* New York, 1984, McGraw-Hill.
17. Breeze RG, Wheeldon EB: The cells of the pulmonary airways, *Am Rev Respir Dis* 116:705, 1977.
18. Brittebo EB et al: Metabolism of xenobiotics and steroid hormones in the nasal mucosa. In Barrow CS, editor: *Toxicology of the nasal passages,* New York, 1986, Hemisphere.
19. Brody AR, Overby LH: Incorporation of tritiated thymidine by epithelial and interstitial cells in bronchoalveolar regions of asbestos-exposed rats, *Am J Pathol* 134:133, 1989.
20. Brooks S, Weiss MA, Bernstein IL: Reactive airways dysfunction syndrome: persistent asthma syndrome after high-level irritant exposure, *Chest* 88:376, 1985.
21. Brown GP, Monick M, Hunninghake GW: Fibroblast proliferation induced by silica-exposed human alveolar macrophages, *Am Rev Respir Dis* 138:85, 1988.
22. Brown HR: Neoplastic and potentially preneoplastic changes in the upper respiratory tract of rats and mice, *Environ Health Persp* 85:291, 1990.
23. Brown RC et al: Factors affecting the interaction of asbestos fibers with mammalian cells, *Ann Occup Hyg* 35:25, 1991.
24. Burkhardt A: Pulmonary perspective: alveolitis and collapse in the pathogenesis of pulmonary fibrosis, *Am Rev Respir Dis* 140:513, 1989.
25. Camner P, Hellstrom PA, Phillipson K: Carbon dust and mucociliary transport, *Arch Environ Health* 26:294, 1973.
26. Cantin A, Allard C, Begin R: Increased alveolar plasminogen in early asbestosis, *Am Rev Respir Dis* 139:604, 1989.
27. Casanova M, Heck HD: Further studies of the metabolic incorporation and covalent binding of inhaled [3H] and [14] formaldehyde in Fischer-344 rats: effects of glutathione depletion, *Toxicol Appl Pharmacol* 89:105, 1987.
28. Castleman WL et al: Acute respiratory bronchiolitis: an ultrastructural and autoradiographic study of epithelial cell injury and renewal in rhesus monkeys exposed to ozone, *Am J Pathol* 98:811, 1980.
29. Cavalleri A et al: Evaluation of serum aminoterminal propeptide of type III procollagen as an early marker of active fibrotic process in asbestos-exposed workers, *Scand J Work Environ Health* 17:139, 1991.
30. Chow CK, Dillard CJ, Tappel AL: Glutathione peroxidase system and lysozyme in rats exposed to ozone or nitrogen dioxide, *Environ Res* 7:311, 1974.
31. Christman CA, Schwartz LW: Enhanced phagocytosis by alveolar macrophages induced by short-term ozone insult, *Environ Res* 28:241, 1982.
32. Crystal RG et al, editors: *The lung: scientific foundations,* New York, 1991, Raven.
33. Dahl AR: Activation of carcinogens and other xenobiotics by nasal cytochrome P-450. In Boobis AR et al, editors: *Microsomes and drug oxidations,* Philadelphia, 1985, Taylor & Francis.
34. Dahl AR, Hadley WH: Nasal cavity enzymes involved in xenobiotic metabolism: effects on the toxicity of inhalants, *Crit Rev Toxicol* 21:345, 1991.
35. Dearman RJ, Kimber I: Differential stimulation of immune function by respiratory and contact allergens, *Immunology* 72:563, 1991.
36. Devlin RB et al: Exposure of humans to ambient levels of ozone for 6.6 hours causes cellular and biochemical changes in the lung, *Am J Respir Cell Mol Biol* 4:72, 1991.
37. Donaldson K et al: Inflammation generating potential of long and short amosite asbestos samples, *Br J Ind Med* 46:271, 1989.
38. Evans MJ et al: Renewal of alveolar epithelium in the rat following exposure to NO_2, *Am J Pathol* 70:175, 1973.
39. Ferin J, Leach LJ: The effects of selected air pollutants on clearance of titanic oxide particles from the lungs of rats. In Walton WH, editor: *Inhaled particles,* vol 4, part 1, Oxford, 1977, Pergamon Press.
40. Finotto S et al: Increase in numbers of CD8 positive lymphocytes and eosinophils in peripheral blood of subjects with late asthmatic reactions induced by toluene diisocyanate, *Br J Ind Med* 48:116, 1991.
41. Foster WM, Costa DL, Langenback EG: Ozone exposure alters tracheobronchial mucociliary function in humans, *J Appl Physiol* 63:996, 1987.
42. Frampton MW et al: Effects of nitrogen dioxide exposure on bronchoalveolar lavage proteins in humans, *Am J Respir Cell Mol Biol* 1:499, 1989.
43. Gail DB, Lenfant DJM: Cells of the lung: biology and clinical implications, *Am Rev Respir Dis* 127:366, 1983.
44. Gervasi PG et al: Xenobiotic-metabolizing enzymes in human respiratory nasal mucosa, *Biochem Pharmacol* 41:177, 1991.
45. Gilbert R, Auchincloss J Jr: Reactive airways dysfunction syndrome presenting as a reversible restrictive defect, *Lung* 167:55, 1989.
46. Glaser U et al: Low level chromium (VI) inhalation effects on alveolar macrophages and immune functions in Wistar rats, *Arch Toxicol* 57:250, 1985.
47. Goldstein E et al: The effect of ozone on lysosomal enzymes of alveolar macrophages engaged in phagocytosis and killing of inhaled *Staphylococcus aureus, J Infect Dis* 138:299, 1978.
48. Gordon RE, Solano D, Kleinerman J: Tight junction alterations of respiratory epithelium following long term NO_2 exposure and recovery, *Exp Lung Res* 11:179, 1986.
49. Gordon T, Amdur MO: Responses of the respiratory system to toxic agents. In Amdur MO, Doull J, Klaassen CD, editors: *Cassaret and Doull's toxicology,* ed 4, New York, 1991, Pergamon Press.
50. Green GM: Alveolobronchiolar transport mechanisms, *Arch Intern Med* 131:109, 1973.
51. Greenspan BJ, Morrow PE: The effects of in vitro and aerosol exposures to cadmium on phagocytosis by rat pulmonary macrophages, *Fundam Appl Toxicol* 4:48, 1984.
52. Griffis LC et al: Clearance of diesel soot particles from rat lung after a subchronic diesel exhaust exposure, *Fundam Appl Toxicol* 3:99, 1983.
53. Guengerich FP: Purification and characterization of xenobiotic-metabolizing enzymes from lung tissue, *Pharmacol Ther* 45:299, 1990.
54. Haagen-Smit AJ: Chemistry and physiology of Los Angeles smog, *Ind Eng Chem* 44:1342, 1952.

55. Hayes AA et al: Neutrophil chemotactic release and neutrophil alveolitis in asbestos-exposed individuals, *Chest* 94:521, 1988.
56. Hazucha MJ, Bates DV, Bromberg PA: Mechanism of action of ozone on the human lung, *J Appl Physiol* 67:1535, 1989.
57. Hedenborg M, Klockars M: Quartz-dust-induced production of reactive oxygen metabolites by human granulocytes, *Lung* 167:23, 1989.
58. Heffner JE, Repine JE: Pulmonary strategies of anti-oxidant defense, *Am Rev Respir Dis* 140:531, 1989.
59. Henke D et al: Metabolism of aracidonic acid by human nasal and bronchial epithelial cells, *Arch Biochem Biophys* 267:426, 1988.
60. Jabbour A et al: Lung lining fluid modification of asbestos bioactivity for the alveolar macrophage, *Toxicol Appl Pharmacol* 110:283, 1991.
61. Kalla B et al: Role of extracellular calcium in chrysotile asbestos stimulation of alveolar macrophages, *Toxicol Appl Pharmacol* 104:130, 1990.
62. Kamp DW et al: Serum promotes asbestos-induced injury to human pulmonary epithelial cells, *J Lab Clin Med* 116:289, 1990.
63. Katz GV, Laskin S: Effect of irritant atmospheres on macrophage behavior. In Sander C et al, editors: *Pulmonary macrophage and epithelial cells*, Springfield, Va, 1977, NITS.
64. Kehrl HR et al: Ozone exposure increases respiratory epithelia permeability in humans, *Am Rev Respir Dis* 135:1124, 1987.
65. Kenoyer JL, Phalen RF, Davis JR: Particle clearance from the respiratory tract as a test of toxicity: effect of ozone on short and long term clearance, *Exp Lung Res* 2:111, 1981.
66. Kern D: An outbreak of reactive airways dysfunction syndrome following a spill of glacial acetic acid, *Am Rev Respir Dis* 144:1058, 1991.
67. Koren HS et al: Ozone-induced inflammation in the lower airways of human subjects, *Am Rev Respir Dis* 139:407, 1989.
68. Koren HS, Hatch GE, Graham DE: Nasal lavage as a tool in assessing acute inflammation in response to inhaled pollutants, *Toxicology* 60:15, 1990.
69. Krahl DE: Microstructure of the lung, *Arch Environ Health* 6:37, 1963.
70. Kuschner M: The causes of lung cancer, *Am Rev Respir Dis* 98:573, 1968.
71. Langley R: Fume fever and reactive airways dysfunction syndrome in a welder, *South Med J* 84:1034, 1991.
72. Leikauf G, Driscoll K: Cellular approaches in respiratory tract toxicology. In Gardner DE, Crapo JD, McClellan MO, editors: *Toxicology of the lung*, ed 2, New York, 1993, Raven Press.
73. Leikauf G et al: Effects of sulfuric acid aerosol on respiratory mechanics and mucociliary particle clearance in healthy non-smoking adults, *Am Ind Hyg Assoc J* 42:273, 1981.
74. Lerman S, Kipen H: Reactive airways dysfunction syndrome, *Am Fam Physician* 38:135, 1988.
75. Lippermann M: Background on health effects of acid aerosols, *Environ Health Perspect* 79:3, 1989.
76. Longo V et al: Metabolism of diethylnitrosamine by microsomes of human respiratory nasal mucosa and liver, *Biochem Pharmacol* 38:1867, 1989.
77. Lucas AM, Douglas LC: Principles underlying ciliary activity in the respiratory tract. II. A comparison of nasal clearance in man, monkey, and other mammals, *Arch Otolaryngol* 20:518, 1934.
78. Luo J-CJ, Nelsen K, Fischbein A: Persistent reactive airway dysfunction after exposure to toluene diisocyanate, *Br J Ind Med* 47:239, 1988.
79. Mannix RC et al: Effects of sulfur dioxide and formaldehyde on particle clearance in the rat, *J Toxicol Environ Health* 12:429, 1983.
80. McDonnell WF et al: Pulmonary effects of ozone during exercise: dose-response characteristics, *J Appl Physiol* 54:1345, 1983.
81. Menzel DB: Ozone: an overview of its toxicity in man and animals, *J Toxicol Environ Health* 13:183, 1984.
82. Moisan T: Prolonged asthma after smoke inhalation: a report of three cases and a review of previous reports, *J Occup Med* 33:458, 1991.
83. Molfino NA et al: Effect of low concentration of ozone on inhaled allergen responses in asthmatic subjects, *Lancet* 338:199, 1991.
84. Moore B, Sherman M: Chronic reactive airway disease following acute chlorine gas exposure in an asymptomatic atopic patient, *Chest* 100:855, 1991.
85. Morgan MS, Frank R: Uptake of pollutant gases by the respiratory system. In Brain JD, Proctor DF, Reid LM, editors: *Respiratory defense mechanisms*, New York, 1977, Marcel Dekker.
86. Murray JF: *The normal lung*, Philadelphia, 1986, WB Saunders.
87. Newhouse MT, Dolovich M, Obminski G: Effect of TLV levels of SO_2 and H_2SO_4 on bronchial clearance in exercising man, *Arch Environ Health* 33:24, 1978.
88. Office of Air Quality Planning and Standards, United States Environmental Protection Agency: National Air Quality and Emissions Trends Report: 1988. Pub No EPA-540/4-90-002, Washington, DC, 1990, US Government Printing Office.
89. Phalen RF et al: Effects of sulfate aerosols in combination with ozone on elimination of tracer particles by rats, *J Toxicol Environ Health* 6:797, 1980.
90. Phipps PD et al: Characterization of two major populations of lung fibroblasts: distinguishing morphology and discordant display of Thy 1 and class II MHC, *Am J Respir Cell Mol Biol* 1:65, 1989.
91. Piguet PF et al: Requirement of tumour necrosis factor for development of silica-induced pulmonary fibrosis, *Nature* 344:245, 1990.
92. Plopper CG: Comparative morphologic features of bronchiolar epithelial cells: the Clara cell, *Am Rev Respir Dis* 128:S37, 1983.
93. Plopper CG et al: Pulmonary alterations in rats exposed to 0.2 and 0.1 ppm ozone: a correlated morphological and biochemical study, *Arch Environ Health* 34:390, 1979.
94. Prasad SB et al: Effects of pollutant atmospheres on surface receptors of pulmonary macrophages, *J Toxicol Environ Health* 24:385, 1988.
95. Proctor DF: The mucociliary system. In Proctor DF, Andersen I, editors: *The nose, upper airway physiology and the atmospheric environment*, Amsterdam, 1982, Elsevier.
96. Promisloff R et al: Reactive airways dysfunction syndrome in three police officers following a roadside chemical spill, *Chest* 98:928, 1990.
97. Rajan K, Davies B: Reversible airways obstruction and interstitial pneumonitis due to acetic acid, *Br J Ind Med* 46:67, 1989.
98. Richards IS et al: Florida red-tide toxin (brevetoxins) produce depolarization of airway smooth muscle, *Toxicon* 28:1105, 1990.
99. Riedel F et al: Effects of SO_2 exposure on allergic sensitization in the guinea pig, *J Allergy Clin Immunol* 82:527, 1988.
100. Rom W et al: Lymphocyte-macrophage alveolitis in nonsmoking individuals occupationally exposed to asbestos, *Chest* 101:779, 1992.
101. Rom WN et al: Characterization of the lower respiratory tract inflammation of nonsmoking individuals with interstitial lung disease associated with chronic inhalation of inorganic dusts, *Am Rev Respir Dis* 136:1429, 1987.
102. Saetta M et al: Airway mucosal inflammation in occupational asthma induced by toluene diisocyanate, *Am Rev Respir Dis* 145:160, 1992.
103. Saetta M et al: Effect of cessation of exposure to toluene diisocyanate (TDI) on bronchial mucosa of subjects with TDI-induced asthma, *Am Rev Respir Dis* 145:169, 1992.
104. Schelegle ES, Siefkin AD, McDonald RJ: Time course of ozone-induced neutrophilia in normal humans, *Am Rev Respir Dis* 143:1353, 1991.
105. Schlesinger RB: Comparative deposition of inhaled aerosols in experimental animals and humans: a review, *J Toxicol Environ Health* 15:197, 1985.
106. Schlesinger RB: The interaction of inhaled toxicants with respiratory tract clearance, *Crit Rev Toxicol* 20:257, 1990.

107. Sheppard DA et al: Exercise increases sulfur dioxide–induced bronchoconstriction in asthmatic subjects, *Am Rev Respir Dis* 123:486, 1981.
108. Shoji S et al: Bronchial epithelial cells produce lung fibroblasts chemotactic factor: fibronectin, *Am J Respir Cell Mol Biol* 1:13, 1989.
109. Sprince N et al: T-cell alveolitis in lung lavage of asbestos-exposed subjects, *Am J Ind Med* 21:311, 1992.
110. St George JA et al: Cell populations and structure-function relationships of cells in the airways. In Gardner DE, Crapo JD, Massaro EJ, editors: *Toxicology of the lung,* New York, 1988, Raven Press.
111. Stiles AD, Moats-Staats BM: Production and action of insulin-like growth factor I/somatomedin C in primary cultures of fetal lung fibroblasts, *Am J Respir Cell Mol Biol* 1:21, 1989.
112. Suzuki Y, Kohyama N: Translocation of inhaled asbestos fibers from the lung to other tissues, *Am J Ind Med* 19:701, 1991.
113. Tarlo S, Broder I: Irritant-induced occupational asthma, *Chest* 96:297, 1989.
114. Thyssen J et al: Inhalation studies with benzo(a)pyrene in Syrian golden hamsters, *J Natl Cancer Inst* 66:575, 1981.
115. Wallaert B et al: Superoxide anion generation by alveolar inflammatory cells in simple pneumoconiosis and in progressive massive fibrosis of nonsmoking coal workers, *Am Rev Respir Dis* 141:129, 1990.
116. Wass U et al: An in vitro method for predicting sensitizing properties of inhaled chemicals, *Scand J Work Environ Health* 16:208, 1990.
117. Weibel AR: *The pathway for oxygen: structure and function in the mammalian respiratory system,* Cambridge, Mass, Harvard University Press.
118. Weissner JH et al: The effects of chemical modification of quartz surface on particulate-induced pulmonary inflammation and fibrosis in the mouse, *Am Rev Respir Dis* 141:111, 1990.
119. Wolff RK et al: Sulphur dioxide and tracheobronchial clearance in man, *Arch Environ Health* 30:521, 1975.
120. Zwick H et al: Effect of ozone on the respiratory health, allergic sensitization and cellular immune system in children, *Am Rev Respir Dis* 144:1075, 1991.

Chapter 15

DERMAL TOXICOLOGY

Edward A. Emmett

Structure and function of the skin
Percutaneous absorption
    Nature of the substance
    Properties and state of the skin
    Vehicle
    Experimental measurement of percutaneous absorption
Biotransformation in the skin
Photochemical transformation and photosensitivity
Excretion from the skin
Contact sensitivity-allergic contact dermatitis
    The mechanism of contact sensitivity
    Predictive testing

This chapter covers relevant toxicology related to the skin. It commences with a description of the structure and function of the skin, especially some characteristics of this layered organ that affect its responses. Because the first step in toxic responses of skin to applied substances is percutaneous absorption, this subject is covered in some detail. Percutaneous absorption also is increasingly recognized as a critical step in systemic toxicity of many xenobiotics.

Foreign substances in the skin may be altered in two major ways: biotransformation and photochemical conversion. Both are important determinants of toxicity. The role of the skin in excretion of some substances is described.

There are some unique features of immune reactions in the skin, particularly those associated with allergic contact dermatitis, one of the important types of occupational and environmental skin disease. Accordingly, the mechanism of allergic contact dermatitis is described.

STRUCTURE AND FUNCTION OF THE SKIN

An understanding of the structure and function of the skin provides a basis for understanding and anticipating the effects of hazardous agents.

The skin has three major layers of interest: the epidermis, a layer of surface epithelial tissue; the dermis, a layer of loose connective tissue; and the hypodermis, which lies under the dermis and is of variable thickness and composed of connective tissue and fat (Fig. 15-1).

The epidermis contains a number of cell types. In addition to the predominant keratinocytes, there are melanocytes, Langerhans' cells, and Merkel's cells. The epidermis is generally described as having a number of layers with different appearances resulting from the different behavior of the keratinocytes. The innermost, basal layer of the epidermis contains rapidly dividing, metabolically active keratinocytes. After their formation by cell division in the basal layer, keratinocytes move toward the surface of the skin, differentiate, and become less metabolically active as they undergo the process known as keratinization. The layer immediately above the basal layer is called the spinous, or prickle cell, layer because of the cells' appearance on light microscopy. Above the spinous layer is the granular cell layer, named because of the keratohyalin granules that contribute to the keratinization process. On the outer surface of the skin is the stratum corneum, or horny cell layer. This layer is of great importance to the toxicology of the skin because it constitutes the major barrier for the passage of water and most xenobiotics through the skin. The cells in the stratum corneum are dead, flattened, and cornified. They are the nonviable end product of the synthetic activity of the lower layers. In the process of keratinization, filaments of prekeratins formed in the lower layers are aggregated so that the cells fill with a network of keratin proteins embedded in a matrix containing mucus and lipids, and surrounded by a

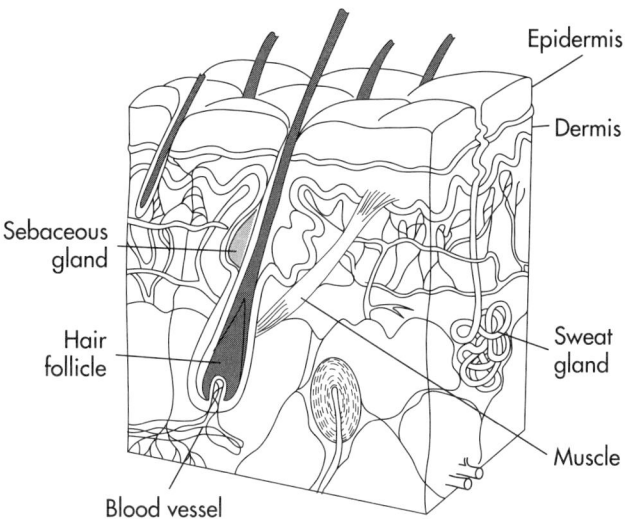

Fig. 15-1. Anatomical representation of a section of skin.

highly chemically resistant envelope. Between the cornified cells is an intercellular material containing ceramides that contributes to the barrier. The complex structure of the stratum corneum is responsible for the effective barrier function.[17]

The epidermis contains a constantly renewing cell population. Cornified material is lost from the surface, usually as an imperceptible fine scale. Usually the transit time from the basal layer through the viable epidermis and granular layer is approximately 14 days. It takes approximately another 15 days for the residual cell material to pass through the stratum corneum and be lost. The structure and composition of the epidermis and the turnover rates may be markedly altered in skin diseases, so the barrier characteristics may be quite different in abnormal skin.

A number of specifically differentiated skin structures are formed from epidermal cells, including the eccrine sweat glands, apocrine sweat glands, hair follicles, nails, and sebaceous glands. They are collectively referred to as the epidermal appendages.

The eccrine sweat glands produce sweat in response to thermal, nervous, or gustatory stimuli. The sweat ducts pass through the dermis and epidermis, and the sweat is produced by a secretory portion located just beneath the dermis in the hypodermis. Eccrine sweat glands are located over the entire body surface. Apocrine glands, in contrast, are found only in the axillae, genitalia, and nipples. They produce a clear secretion, the function of which has not been determined, that becomes odorous after bacterial decomposition.

The hair follicles also are located below the epidermis and contain some of the most metabolically active tissue in the body, with a rapid turnover rate. They are accordingly susceptible to toxic damage. Nails and hair contain keratin that is immunologically distinct from that of the stratum corneum and has a higher cystine content.

Sebaceous glands are composed of cells that fill with lipids, break down, and discharge an oily material called sebum onto the skin surface. They are associated with hair follicles on all skin areas except the palms, soles, and dorsa of the feet. They are particularly active and abundant on the scalp, forehead, and upper back. These glands are involved in the various forms of chemically induced acne.

The most important cells of the pigmentary system are the melanocytes, which are dendritic cells located in the lower epidermis. They synthesize melanin in a specialized organelle called the melanosome. Melanosomes are transferred to keratinocytes, where in whites they become aggregated, fused with lysosomes, and destroyed; however, both melanosomes and keratinocytes contain more melanin and remain discrete in the keratinocytes of dark-skinned races such as blacks and indigenous peoples of Australia and the South Pacific. Ultraviolet radiation stimulates increased production of melanin within the melanosomes, as well as increased melanosome transfer to keratinocytes, leading to darkening of the skin. Melanin functions as both an oxygen scavenger and a sunscreen. Its role, if any, in modifying chemical damage to the skin has not been fully determined, but it may function to remove mutagenic and carcinogenic oxygen radicals from the surrounding keratinocytes and Langerhans' cells.[18]

Another dendritic epidermal cell, the Langerhans' cell, is responsible for antigen recognition and presentation in the skin. The cells are necessary for the induction of allergic sensitization and have a variety of immunologic functions.[9] They normally have a relatively circumscribed distribution in squamous epithelial tissue (e.g., epidermis, cervix, gingiva) but occur occasionally in the dermis and some lymphoid tissue. Langerhans' cells are derived from bone marrow, where they exist in an immature form. They constitute roughly 5% to 10% of the epidermis and are located just above the basal layer in a network in which the cellular processes, if adjacent to Langerhans' cells, almost touch. These cells contain distinctive cytoplasmic inclusions that may be seen on electron microscopy and the function of which remains obscure.[1]

The dermis, the main constituent of which is loose connective tissue, poses much less of a barrier to water-soluble hazardous substances than does the epidermis. The dermis supplies flexibility and elasticity to the skin. Its major components are collagen, reticulin, elastic fibers, and ground substance. The ground substance provides a slow diffusion medium for constituent fluids. Fibroblast cells maintain the dermal components and have a major role in wound repair. Other cells, including macrophages, mast cells, and lymphocytes, contribute to dermal inflammatory, phagocytic, and immune reactions. The dermis has a substantial vascular supply, much greater than would be required for the metabolic activity of the skin, to contribute to temperature regulation through dilatation and constriction. The dermis also contains a plexus of lymphatic vessels and plentiful nerve endings.

Although the basic structure of the skin remains similar, there are substantial differences among body regions in the thickness of the epidermis, the distribution of the epidermal appendages, and the vascular and nerve supply to the skin. For example, although the epidermis is only about 0.06 mm thick over much of the body, it may be several millimeters thick on the palms and soles. As a result of these variations, percutaneous absorption differs. The pattern of most toxic skin responses is influenced by both differences in percutaneous absorption and the distribution of target structures. Once these factors are understood, the pattern of occurrence of many skin diseases becomes much more explicable.

PERCUTANEOUS ABSORPTION

Because the major barrier function resides in the stratum corneum, percutaneous absorption is a critical determinant of the ability of a penetrant both to injure the underlying viable layers of the skin, causing skin disease, and to be absorbed into the bloodstream, causing systemic toxicity. There is a great range of rates of percutaneous absorption of different substances, from very rapid to negligible. Percutaneous absorption also is substantially influenced by the state of the skin and the vehicle in which any penetrant is applied to the skin.

Penetration across the stratum corneum occurs by passive absorption.[19] The appendages (hair follicles, sebaceous glands, and sweat glands) are relatively unimportant in this process and indeed constitute much less than 1% of the cross-sectional area of skin presented to any potential penetrant, although in the case of lipophilic substances, there may be a transient, rapid phase of diffusion through hair follicles and sebaceous glands before a steady state is established.

Much of the barrier property of the stratum corneum is attributable to its complex composition and structure. Polar and nonpolar substances appear to have different molecular pathways through this layer. Polar substances may diffuse through the outer surfaces of the protein filaments of the hydrated stratum corneum cells. The water content of the stratum corneum varies greatly, depending on humidity and surface water conditions; increased hydration may result in increased absorption of polar substances. Nonpolar molecules preferentially diffuse through the nonaqueous lipid matrix. Absorption seems to take place around rather than through the cornified cells.

Once through the epidermal barrier, substances diffuse through the living layers of the epidermis and dermis to the skin vessels. Relatively little barrier is presented at these levels, especially for polar substances. The circulation is the limiting factor for only a few exceptional substances that penetrate the stratum corneum very rapidly, such as helium, or that severely damage the stratum corneum.

In vitro studies with homologous series of molecules such as aliphatic alcohols have shown that percutaneous absorption across the stratum corneum follows Fick's law of diffusion. According to Fick's law

$$J_s = K_p \times C$$

where

J_s = the steady-state flux of the substance
K_p = the permeability constant for the substance
C = the concentration difference of the solute across the membrane

When the substance is applied to skin in a solvent

$$K_p = \frac{K_m \times D}{\delta}$$

where

K_m = the solvent-membrane partition coefficient for the substance
D = the average diffusion coefficient for the substance
δ = the thickness of the membrane

Thus the determinants of absorption through the stratum corneum are the solvent–stratum corneum partition coefficient, the diffusion constant, the thickness of the stratum corneum, and the concentration difference between the two sides of the stratum corneum.

There are some situations in which the simple application of Fick's law does not appear to hold well. These situations include the application of high concentrations or amounts of substances such as highly lipid-soluble materials to the skin. In this case, the presence of significant amounts of these substances in skin may increase the further penetration of lipid-soluble materials. Another exception occurs when the penetrant actually damages the stratum corneum, destroying part of the barrier function.

In practice a number of factors substantially affect percutaneous absorption. These factors are conveniently grouped as the nature of the substance, properties and state of the skin, and the vehicle. The state of the skin and vehicle effects may be of overriding importance in determining the rate and amount of absorption in specific circumstances.

Nature of the substance

As a general rule, water and polar nonelectrolytes penetrate poorly. Ionization of weak electrolytes reduces their permeability. Nonpolar substances and gases penetrate relatively well.

Organic liquids fall into two main categories, depending on whether they damage the barrier tissues. Lipid solubility is an important determinant for nondamaging solvents. Damaging solvents remove lipids from the skin, producing functional interstices that serve as low-energy diffusion pathways, resulting in a fairly porous, nonselective membrane.

There may be an interrelationship between metabolism within the skin and the rate of penetration of certain compounds that undergo metabolism within the epidermis. Both the rate of penetration and the cutaneous enzyme activity can determine the amount of a topically applied compound metabolized during its percutaneous penetration.[20]

Properties and state of the skin

There is a profound regional variation in absorption. For example, for hydrocortisone in humans there is a 300-fold difference between the permeability of the scrotum (the most permeable area) and the plantar foot arch (the least permeable area). In large measure this variation is determined by the thickness of the stratum corneum, but other anatomic features may also play a role.

The amount of substance absorbed depends on the applied dose, the time before contact is terminated (as by washing or removal), the concentration applied, and the surface area of application. Studies show that the efficacy of absorption can rise or fall as the concentration applied increases, although the total amount absorbed into the body always seems to increase.

Physical damage to the stratum corneum from abrasion or skin disease can greatly increase absorption. Poor skin contact in hair areas can reduce absorption (Fig. 15-2).

The penetration of polar substances is increased by hydration of the stratum corneum. Increased surface temperature also increases absorption; this relationship may be nonlinear with lipids, perhaps reflecting changes in viscosity. Occlusion of the site of application increases both hydration and skin temperature and greatly increases absorption; this property has been used to advantage in dermatologic therapy, for example, to increase the penetration of topically applied corticosteroids.[8]

Sweat may dissolve or leach substances from solid or porous objects, leading to absorption.

Vehicle

The composition and properties of the vehicle or solvent may affect percutaneous absorption of a solute in several ways. The nature of the vehicle governs the vehicle–stratum corneum partition coefficient, which determines absorption according to Fick's law. The vehicle may contain a solvent damaging to the barrier. The pH may influence the degree of ionization of electrolytes. Anionic and cationic surfactants such as soaps and detergents, even in dilute concentrations, increase the permeability of water and other polar substances.

Accordingly, differences in vehicles can lead to marked differences in effects.[21]

Experimental measurement of percutaneous absorption

Percutaneous absorption may be studied experimentally by the use of in vitro or in vivo techniques. There appears to be fairly good agreement between results obtained from equivalent in vitro and in vivo techniques when special care is taken to duplicate experimental conditions, but divergent results may be obtained if this duplication is not performed.[6] In vitro techniques generally involve diffusion through cells in which separated epidermis is used as the membrane. The compound for which absorption is to be studied is placed in a suitable vehicle on one side of the membrane. The fluid on the other side is usually physiologic saline, which is assayed at regular intervals for the presence of the compound under study.[5]

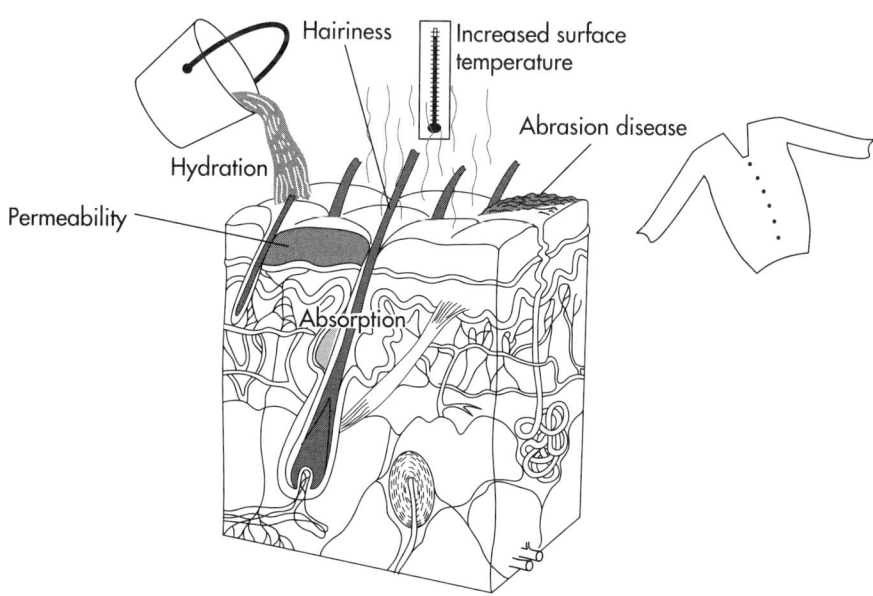

Fig. 15-2. Factors affecting percutaneous skin absorption of a dermal toxicant.

In vitro studies generally involve topical application of radiolabeled substances for a defined period. The radiolabel may subsequently be measured in excreta or tissues. Comparison with the results obtained after intraperitoneal or intravenous administration may be made. Detection of radiolabel indicates absorption but, unless speciation of radiolabeled material is performed, does not indicate the chemical nature of the absorbed material, which may have been biotransformed. Other methods include the use of a biologic response to indicate absorption and remainder analysis.

There is substantial species variation in percutaneous absorption. Results in rhesus monkeys are reasonably similar to those in humans. Guinea pigs, rats, and rabbits, in that order, show increasingly higher permeability than that in humans.

BIOTRANSFORMATION IN THE SKIN

The skin, particularly the viable epidermis, contains metabolically active cells that have a wide range of capacities to biotransform xenobiotics.[3,12] As a result, many compounds penetrating the stratum corneum may be biotransformed before entering the bloodstream.

One of the most studied activities is that of arylhydrocarbon hydroxylase. This activity, which is reversible, metabolizes a number of polycyclic aromatic hydrocarbons, including benzo[a]pyrene, to metabolites, including epoxides.[4] Other systems metabolize some topically applied drugs, such as glyceryl trinitrate.[22]

PHOTOCHEMICAL TRANSFORMATION AND PHOTOSENSITIVITY

Foreign substances not only may be biotransformed within the skin but may be subject to photochemical reactions on or in the skin. These reactions may lead to photosensitivity, an abnormal adverse reaction to ultraviolet or visible radiation, or may enhance other adverse reactions such as the development of skin cancers and of selective defects in immunologic functioning (Table 15-1).

Photosensitivity reactions may be produced by artificial sources of nonionizing radiation, including those used for cosmetic purposes such as tanning, but are more commonly caused by sunlight. The portion of the solar spectrum of major toxicologic interest is from 290 to 700 nm. Shorter wavelengths are absorbed by the atmosphere, mostly by the ozone layer of the stratosphere, whereas longer wavelengths may cause tissue heating but generally lack the energy to cause photochemical changes. In practice, most reactions are due to the solar ultraviolet component (290 to 400 nm).

The first law of photochemistry states that to produce an effect, radiation must be absorbed. Absorption of specific radiation by a chromophore (a molecule that can absorb that wavelength of radiation) results in electronically excited molecules, with subsequent emission of light (fluorescence or phosphorescence), emission of heat, or photochemical reactions. It is this that produces toxicologically significant effects.

Photosensitivity reactions resulting from exogenous chemicals may be conveniently classified as phototoxic, in which the increased reactivity to skin occurs primarily on a nonimmunologic basis, or photoallergic, in which a delayed-hypersensitivity reaction similar to that responsible for allergic contact dermatitis occurs.[10,15]

Most phototoxic reactions are oxygen dependent; either an excited triplet state is reduced, leading to the generation of highly reactive free radicals that subsequently attach to biologic substrates, or the excited molecule transfers its energy to O_2, generating singlet oxygen, an active oxidizing agent. In a limited number of cases, the excited-state molecule may react directly with a target molecule. An example

Table 15-1. Some examples of dermal toxicants

Irritation or burns	Allergic reactions	Photosensitization	Photoallergic reactions	Chloracne
Acids	Nickel salts	8-Methoxypsoralen	Halogenated salicylanilides	PCDFs
Alkali	Chromium salts	Tribromosalicylicanilide	Sulfonamides	PCBs
Phenolics	Organomercurials	p-*tert*-Butylphenol	Phenothiazides	PCNs
Nitrogen mustards	Plant sensitizers	Hexachlorobenzene	Coumarin	TCAOB
Organotins	Rubber additives	Procainamide	Musk ambrette	cmTCAB
Hydrogen fluoride	Epoxy oligomers	Isoniazid	Sunscreen components	
	Methyl methacrylate	Quinidine	Ragweed	
	Acrylic monomers		Australian bush	
	Diisocyanates			
	DNCB			
	Formalin			
	Aliphatic amines			
	Benzocaine			

PCDFs, polychlorinated dibenzofurans; *PCBs*, polychlorinated biphenyls; *DNCB*, dinitrochlorobenzene; *PCNs*, ; *TCAOB*, tetrachloroazoxybenzene; *TCAB*, 3,3'4,4'-tetrachloroazoxybenzene.

of the last is the reaction of furocoumarins such as 8-methoxypsoralen with specific sites on DNA to form a covalent bond between the pyrimidine base and the furocoumarin. On absorption of another photon, a second cycloaddition reaction can take place, resulting in cross-linked DNA and thus photosensitivity in the short term and mutagenesis or carcinogenesis in the longer term. A number of assay systems, including in vitro assays, are available to detect phototoxicity.

In photoallergic-type reactions, the main role of radiation appears to be in converting the hapten to a complete allergen. (See section on the mechanism of allergic contact dermatitis.)

The skin and external eye thus have a unique place in toxicology because of the important potential for both photochemical transformation and biotransformation to alter the toxicity of xenobiotics within the tissue.

EXCRETION FROM THE SKIN

Foreign substances or their metabolites may be lost from the skin in sweat, hair, nails, or desquamated cells. Certain metals, including arsenic, cadmium, and lead, are incorporated into the matrix of growing hair and remain in the hair tissue until they are eventually lost. Both metals and a number of water-soluble drugs are lost in sweat.[7] In the case of drugs, the excretion in eccrine sweat is consistent with partitioning between plasma at pH 7.4 and a fluid of pH near 5.[11]

CONTACT SENSITIVITY: ALLERGIC CONTACT DERMATITIS

Allergic contact dermatitis, a relatively common toxicologic reaction, occurs as a result of cell-mediated or type IV immune reactions.[2] Important features include the specificity of the reaction to a particular chemical, the possibility of cross-reactions with related substances, and the small amounts of allergen that may elicit a reaction (Table 15-1).

The mechanism of contact sensitivity

Allergic contact dermatitis is a biphasic phenomenon. During the induction, or afferent phase, sensitization is initiated, and in the elicitation, or efferent phase, after subsequent exposure to the same chemical, a cutaneous hypersensitivity reaction occurs.[13] The induction phase generally takes from 10 to 21 days. The elicited reaction is seen after a characteristic delay of roughly 12 to 48 hours (hence the name *delayed hypersensitivity*). Once induced, the sensitivity persists for a varying period, possibly for a lifetime.

Contact allergy may be produced infrequently by a large number of antigens; however, there is a great range in the potency to induce sensitization among different substances. A relatively small number of strong sensitizers have been identified experimentally or in humans. Strong allergens are often highly aromatic substances with a molecular weight of less than 500; they also tend to be highly lipid soluble and quite reactive with proteins. Certain metals, including nickel, chromium, and cobalt ions, also are strong sensitizers. It is not always clear why some exposures, and not others, initiate sensitization, but it is known that there is immunoregulation of contact sensitivity and that ultraviolet radiation and other factors modulate the functioning of the immune system in the skin.

Induction phase. As mentioned, cutaneous antigens (haptens) are generally of low molecular weight. The first step in the allergic process, after absorption of the hapten into the epidermis, appears to be covalent binding of the hapten to a carrier protein to form a complete antigen. This complete antigen appears to be bound to cell surfaces, especially those of the epidermal Langerhans' cells or macrophages. These cells process the antigen by altering the configurational arrangement and present it by holding it at the cell surface for subsequent interaction with histocompatible T lymphocytes. Either Langerhans' cells or T lymphocytes migrate from the skin to the regional lymph node. The antigen-bearing lymphocytes settle in the paracortical area of the node, where clonal proliferation occurs. Two populations of sensitized lymphocytes are formed: effector T lymphocytes, which travel through the bloodstream to the skin surface, and long-lived memory cells, which proliferate to form new populations of sensitized lymphocytes on recontact with the antigen.

Elicitation. Once the induction phase is complete, elicitation can begin as a result of either persistence or reintroduction of the antigen. The hapten again complexes with protein to form a complete antigen and associates with skin components, including Langerhans' cells. On recognition of the hapten-protein complex, effector T lymphocytes enlarge and undergo blast transformation. The activated lymphocytes and other cells synthesize and release a variety of substances (cytokines) that mediate the allergic response. These substances include interleukin-6 and various chemotactic, macrophage-, macrophage-activating, leukocyte-inhibiting, and lymph-node-permeability factors; lymphotoxins; transfer factors; and others. Other lymphocytes, monocytes, macrophages, and possibly mast cells and B lymphocytes play a role in the response.

Cross-sensitization may occur when two or more potential antigens share common groups so that sensitization to one also induces sensitization to the other. For example, substances with a primary para amine ($R-NH_2$) attached directly to an aromatic ring frequently cross-react. Cross-sensitization might be explained by the formation of similar reaction products in vivo or by the induction of similar changes in carrier proteins.

Predictive testing

A number of predictive tests have been developed to identify potential sensitizers. All require the use of intact mammals with functioning immunologic systems. Humans, certain strains of guinea pigs, and, more recently, mice have been used in these tests. The induction period in animals usually consists of a number of epicutaneous applications or intradermal injections, or both. After a rest period, a challenge test is performed with closed or open epicutaneous testing. Increased reactivity in comparison with presensitization or with results in control animals is considered to indicate sensitization.[14] Test procedures in human volunteers generally follow a similar pattern, with exposures to multiple epicutaneous occlusive patches followed by a rest period and subsequent challenge testing with nonirritating concentrations of the putative allergen.[16]

REFERENCES

1. Bassett F, Soler P, Hance AJ: The Langerhans cell in human pathology, *Ann N Y Acad Sci* 465:324-339, 1986.
2. Bergstresser PR: Contact allergic dermatitis—old problems and new techniques, *Arch Dermatol* 125:276-279, 1989.
3. Bickers DR: Drug, carcinogen and steroid hormone metabolism in the skin. In Goldsmith LA, editor: *Biochemistry and physiology of the skin,* New York, 1983, Oxford University Press.
4. Bickers DR: Metabolic activation of carcinogens by keratinocytes, *Ann NY Acad Sci* 548:102-107, 1988.
5. Bronough RL, Maibach HI: In vitro percutaneous absorption. In Marzulli FN, Maibach HI, editors: *Dermatoxicity,* ed 2, Washington, DC, 1983, Hemisphere.
6. Bronough RL et al: Methods for in vitro percutaneous absorption studies. I. comparison with in vivo results, *Toxicol Appl Pharmacol* 62:474-480, 1982.
7. Cohn JR, Emmett EA: The excretion of trace elements in human sweat, *Ann Clin Lab Sci* 8:270-275, 1978.
8. Feldmann RJ, Maibach HI: Absorption of some organic compounds through the skin in man, *J Invest Dermatol* 54:339-404, 1969.
9. Hammer S: Langerhans cells, *Pathol Annu* 23:293-328, 1988.
10. Harber L, Bickers DR: *Photosensitivity diseases,* Philadelphia, 1981, WB Saunders.
11. Johnson HC, Maibach HI: Drug excretion in human eccrine sweat, *J Invest Dermatol* 56:182-188, 1971.
12. Kao J, Carver MP: Skin metabolism. In Marzulli FN, Maibach HI, editors: *Dermatotoxicology,* ed 4, New York, 1991, Hemisphere.
13. Kimber I: Contact sensitivity. In Miller K, Turk J, Nicklin S, editors: *Principles and practice of immunotoxicology,* London, 1992, Blackwell.
14. Klecak G: Identification of contact allergens. In Marzulli FN, Maibach HI, editors: *Dermatotoxicology,* ed 4, New York, 1991, Hemisphere.
15. Kornhauser A, Wamer WG, Lambert LA: Light-induced dermal toxicity: effects on the cellular and molecular level. In Marzulli FN, Maibach HI, editors: *Dermatotoxicology,* ed 4, New York, 1991, Hemisphere.
16. Marzulli FN, Maibach HI: Contact allergy: predictive testing in humans. In Marzulli FN, Maibach HI, editors: *Dermatotoxicology,* ed 4, New York, 1991, Hemisphere.
17. Matolsky AG: Concluding remarks and future directions in the molecular and developmental biology of keratins, *Curr Top Dev Biol* 22:255-264, 1987.
18. Nordlund JJ et al: Pigment cell biology: an historical review, *J Invest Dermatol* 92(suppl 4):53-60, 1989.
19. Schaefer H, Zesch A, Stuttgen G: *Skin permeability,* Berlin, 1982, Springer-Verlag.
20. Storm JE et al: Metabolism of xenobiotics during percutaneous penetration: role of absorption rate and cutaneous enzyme activity, *Fundam Appl Toxicol* 15:132-141, 1990.
21. Stoughton RB: Percutaneous absorption of drugs, *Annu Rev Pharmacol Toxicol* 29:55-69, 1989.
22. Wester RC et al: Estimate of nitroglycerin percutaneous first pass metabolism, *Pharmacologist* 23:203, 1981.

Chapter 16

NEUROBEHAVIORAL TOXICITY AND TESTING

Nancy Fiedler
Joanna Burger
Michael Gochfeld

Brief history of neurobehavioral testing
Target components of the nervous system
 Autonomic nervous system
 Peripheral nervous system
 Central nervous system
Neurobehavioral toxicants
Neurobehavioral studies in animals
 Overview
 Primates
 Avian and rodents
 Learning
 Conditioning
 Naturalistic studies
Clinical consideration for the practitioner
 Overview
 Clinical interview
 Physical examination
 Vision
 Color vision impairment
 Hearing
 Olfaction
 Taste
 Touch
 Vibration
 Temperature
 Position sense
 Motor function
 Vestibular function
 Basal ganglia
 Cerebellar function
 Electrophysiologic studies
Pathophysiology
Psychometric testing
 Overview
 Rationale for testing
 Confounders of testing

 Testing protocols
 Testing for intellectual ability
 Testing for attention and concentration
 Testing for psychomotor functions
 Testing for memory and learning
 Testing personality, mood, affect
Developmental neurobehavior
Conclusion

Many organic and inorganic chemicals cause neurotoxic effects on the central and/or peripheral nervous system. Nervous system alterations by chemicals may manifest in a general way, such as the central nervous system (CNS) depression produced by a general anesthetic gas; or the response may also be very specific, such as the reported effect of MPTP (1-methyl-4-phenyl-1,2,3,6-tetrahydropyridine) on the substantia nigra causing irreversible parkinsonism. Agents with anticholinesterase activity such as organophosphate pesticides interfere with synaptic transmission; lead can cause a peripheral neuropathy, and organic mercury poisoning causes a cerebral-palsy-like birth defect.[77] Of the 220 environmental chemicals that have documented systemic toxicity in humans, 149 are known to affect the nervous system. Common neurotoxic symptoms include irritability, memory loss, difficulty concentrating, and incoordination. Many of these signs and symptoms of neurotoxicity are nonspecific,[34,39] and therefore, the practitioner may find that establishing the causation of a neurotoxic disorder poses a major challenge. Impairment of concentration and loss of memory are frequent CNS manifestations that are poorly identified by routine neurologic examination. Just as subclinical damage to the peripheral nervous system can be detected by nerve conduction studies, specialized techniques designed to provide quantitative measurements of behavioral and cognitive deficits are imperative for documenting subtle neurobehavioral changes.

This chapter will (1) provide a brief historical understanding of neurobehavioral testing, (2) emphasize the target locations of the nervous system that may be affected by neurotoxins, (3) discuss the animal and human scientific information concerning neurobehavioral effects from neurotoxicants, and (4) address the clinical approach for evaluating patients with suspected neurobehavioral disorders.

BRIEF HISTORY OF NEUROBEHAVIORAL TESTING

The potential of neurobehavioral testing as an effective clinical modality was brought to the medical community's attention in late 1973 when NIOSH held a Behavioral Toxicology Workshop.[86] Subsequently, substantial progress was made in developing experimental and clinical applications for neurobehavioral testing.[3,6,76] Major clinical syntheses were published,[3,38,82] and an entire journal, first published in 1979, was devoted to the field.[58]

Neurobehavioral manifestations result from the subtle CNS injury caused by a neurotoxicant that produces its effects at a concentration that is lower than the concentrations that usually cause neurologic symptoms.[78,83,86,88] A central theme of neurobehavioral toxicology is that neurotoxins may affect higher CNS centers of function and cognitive integration in humans and animals without obvious anatomic and physiologic modifications.[33,35]

In the past, clinical psychologists evaluated populations exposed to a neurotoxicant by applying standard instruments such as the Wechsler Adult Intelligence Scale and the Halstead-Reitan test battery. These tests have traditionally been used to evaluate brain-injured patients. Important early neurobehavioral investigations of solvent-exposed industrial populations took place in Scandinavia.[37] More recently the field has become more sophisticated, incorporating information and techniques from various disciplines, including the field of cognition and memory. Neurobehavioralists emphasize the importance of using a standardized battery of neurobehavioral tests for examining exposed populations. In 1985 the World Health Organization convened a special panel to develop a standard battery of tests to be used cross-culturally in epidemiological studies.[84] The Agency for Toxic Substances and Disease Registry (ATSDR) ran a similar workshop for environmental health field studies.[4]

While the effort to standardize the neurobehavioral testing for epidemiological studies is to be applauded, relatively less progress has been made on techniques for evaluating individual patients. Extensive data has been generated using the Neurobehavioral Evaluation System,[47] a computerized test battery but this battery was not intended to be used for the evaluation of individual patients. Therefore, normative data to be used for individual patient evaluation is not available. For the practitioner who wishes to refer a patient for neurobehavioral testing, it is imperative that appropriate methodology be employed by the neuropsychologist to provide the best normative data.

TARGET COMPONENTS OF THE NERVOUS SYSTEM

The major anatomic divisions in the nervous system that could potentially be affected by neurotoxins include (1) the *autonomic nervous system* (composed of parasympathetic and sympathetic), (2) the *peripheral nervous system* (composed of sensory receptors and integrators, sensory nerves, and motor nerves), and (3) the *central nervous system* (composed of the brain, including cerebral cortex, cerebellum, basal ganglia, brainstem, and spinal cord). The following discussion will relate to each of these components.

Autonomic nervous system

A number of chemicals cause manifestations that mimic neurotransmitter effects and therefore enhance or inhibit the normal function of either the parasympathetic or sympathetic nervous systems. The parasympathetic system controls certain normal physiologic activities (for example, peristalsis), while the sympathetic system mediates the body's "emergency response" system.

Peripheral nervous system

Neurotoxicant effects on the peripheral nervous system may lead to a sensory, motor, or mixed neuropathy. The specific anatomical aspect of the peripheral nerves affected may be the axon itself or the myelin sheath. For example, N-hexane induces a "dying-back" axonopathy that can lead to drastic slowing of nerve conduction. Sensory nerve fibers seem to have lower thresholds for damage than motor fibers.[71] Loss of vibration, temperature, and light touch sensation usually occur before motor weakness can be appreciated. The *Vibration II* and other instruments have been developed to assess peripheral vibratory sensation and are sensitive to the neurotoxic effects of solvents.[21] Normative values are developed for the Vibratron II to allow individual patient interpretation.[79]

Central nervous system

Neurobehavioral impairment can be related to interference of nerve transmission or synaptic communication between different areas of the brain. For example, organic and inorganic lead produce effects on microtubule assembly in the CNS. Substantial progress has been made in understanding what parts of the brain accomplish so-called higher functions (learning, memory, creativity, cognition, etc.), and evidence points to the role of numerous neuronal interconnections as the essential anatomic substrate.

NEUROBEHAVIORAL TOXICANTS

The textbook of neurotoxicology by Spencer and Schaumberg[72] catalogues neurotoxins. Anger and Johnson[2] reviewed many of the important issues in neurobehavioral toxicology. Tables 16-1 and 16-2 summarize causative agents and effects caused by some of the more common neurotoxins. A widespread CNS depression or general anaesthesia response is attributable to many compounds, including most industrial solvents, whether aliphatic or aromatic, chlorinated or not. Motivation, memory and learning, mood, and impulse control are endpoints found to be impaired in some studies.[59]

The concept that chronic CNS effects due to a long-term solvent exposure has been championed by a number of investigators, particularly in Scandinavia. Central nervous system syndromes due to solvent exposure have been classified as follows: type 1 = organic affective syndrome; type 2 = mild chronic toxic encephalopathy; type 3 = severe chronic toxic encephalopathy.[59] Type 1, or the organic affective syndrome, presents with symptoms of fatigue, memory impairment, irritability, and mood disturbance; type 2 responses may be subtle and are best defined through the use of neurobehavioral testing. Type 3 falls into the category of dementia or chronic deterioration of the overall intellectual and memory function which may be irreversible.[59] A critical question is whether the CNS effects are truly permanent in nature. The actual occurence of type 3 chronic solvent syndrome has been questioned because of confounding influences (for example, chronic alcohol use) and inadequacies in the experimental design of investigations.[26,30] However, it is clear that chronic solvent exposure does produce abnormal neurobehavioral testing, and its effects need careful examination. It is an important public health issue since NIOSH estimates that more than 9.8 million persons are exposed to organic solvents each year.

Carbon disulfide influences numerous components of the central and peripheral nervous systems, with peripheral neuropathy (paresthesia, numbness), cranial neuropathy, dementia (confusion), parkinsonism, acute psychoses, irritability, and memory loss being attributed to this compound.[17,73,80] Furthermore, abnormalities in regional cerebral blood flow have been discerned in a worker exposed to carbon disulfide.[1] Carbon monoxide exposure at relatively low levels (equivalent to COHb <10%) impairs vigilance, tracking, and ability to drive.[45,61] Among metals, inorganic and organic mercurials, manganese, arsenic, and particularly lead are known neurotoxins, but produce different effects (Table 16-2). Lead and mercury produce a wide spectrum of effects on the CNS.[5,75] Organic mercurials are much more neurotoxic than inorganic mercury, but the latter is associated with a peculiar CNS syndrome called *erethism*, characterized by emotional lability, pathologic shyness, depression, uncontrollable blushing, and outbreaks of temper tantrums. Organic tin compounds, which to a large extent have replaced methyl mercury as a component in paints used for boats, are potent neurotoxic compounds while inorganic tin is much less toxic.

A tragic event befell hundreds of persons who abused a byproduct of an illicit home synthesis of meperidine (demerol) which was contaminated by MPTP during its manufacture. MPTP exerts specific toxicity on the substantia nigra and leads to an irreversible parkinsonian-like syndrome. Another investigation documented an increased prevalence of nervous system symptoms among asphalt workers;[60] a good correlation was noted between CNS symptoms and the presence of 1,2,4 trimethylbenzene, a volatile emission from asphalt. As asphalt temperature increases, the level of asphalt fumes also increases. Keeping the temperature below 150° C and fumes below a level of 400 μg/m$_3$ was recommended as a preventive measure. It is clear that prolonged

Table 16-1. Common causes of neurobehavioral disorders

Metals	Solvents	Pesticides	Gases	Substances Related to Abuse
Lead	Xylene	Organophosphate	Carbon monoxide	Ethyl alcohol
Arsenic	Styrene	Organochlorine	Nitrous oxide	Hallucinogens
Mercury	Toluene	Pyrethroids	Hydrogen sulfide	Cocaine
Manganese	Carbon disulfide			Mood alterers
Thallium	Trichloroethylene			MPTP
Tin	Perchloroethylene			
	Methylene chloride			
	Acrylamide			
	n-Hexane			
	Methyl alcohol			
	Ethylene oxide			
	Ethylene glycol			

Table 16-2. Example to behavioral impairments associated with various toxic substances*

	Lead	Arsenic	Manganese	Mercury	Carbon disulfide	Organic solvents	Organo phosphates
Acute psychosis			+		+	+	
Emotional lability			+	+	+		
Memory impairment	+	+	+		+	+	
Psychomotor	+			+	+	+	+
Neurasthenia	+	+	+	+		+	+
Extrapyramidal			+		+		
Neuropathy	+	+					
Tremor			+	+	+		
Behavioral teratology	+						

*From Gochfeld M, Fiedler N, Burger J: Neurobehavioral toxicology. In Last JM, Wallace RB eds: *Maxcy-Rosenau-Last's public health and preventive medicine,* ed 13, Norwalk, Conn, 1992, Appleton Lange, p. 325.

exposure to neurotoxicants, such as organic solvents, mercury, lead, and petroleum products, lead to a "toxic encephalopathy" characterized by excessive fatigue, memory difficulties, irritability, depression, inability to maintain attention, headache, general slowness, and loss of interest.

While occasionally a neuropathy may worsen over time following cessation of exposure to a neurotoxin (carbon disulfide, carbon monoxide), encephalopathies generally improve within several weeks or months. Because the data on the neuropsychological prognosis following solvent exposure are limited, Morrow et al.[55,56] addressed whether a poor prognosis is expected with a solvent encephalopathy; whether there are exposure-related variables influencing the results; and finally, whether the affected state (for example, depression) or subjective feeling of improvement influence prognosis. The results of the study suggest that about 50% of workers with solvent induced encephalopathy improves neuropsychologically over time, and persons who do not recover are those who suffer a higher peak exposure and are more likely to require medical treatment at the time of the exposure. Hydrogen sulfide also causes hypoxic brain damage with a variety of subsequent symptoms, including anosmia, memory loss, motor dysfunction, and even dementia.[74] Ronnback and Hansson[67] focused on the cellular and molecular mechanisms to explain chronic encephalopathies, using mercury and lead exposure as a model.

NEUROBEHAVIORAL STUDIES IN ANIMALS
Overview

In 1973 three pioneers in studies of animal behavior,[50] Karl von Frisch, Konrad Lorenz, and Niko Tinbergen, were awarded the Nobel Prize in Biology and Medicine in recognition of their pioneering research in animal behavior, which contributed to our understanding of human behavior. Subsequently many studies of neurotoxicity have been conducted in animals, although no animal model adequately mimics the human mind, especially in the intellectual domain.

Primates

There has been a strong interest in studying the great apes and monkeys, our closest relatives in the animal kingdom and many interesting studies have been performed.[65,66] However, despite genetic similarities, it is precisely in the domain of neurobehavior that there is substantial divergence between the apes and humans. Although valuable information has been gained from ethologic and sociobiologic studies of primates in the wild, their most important function in the neurobehavioral laboratory has been to confirm that results obtained with rodents and birds are also true for primates. The cost and availability of primates has been a major limitation to their use in the laboratory, and concern for dwindling populations in the wild and for animal welfare has seriously curtailed primate research, even those involving only conditioning paradigms.[46] Among the questions concerning neurobehavioral studies in primates is that the stress of captivity may have much greater effects on cognitive performance than the toxicant being investigated.

Avian and rodents

The use of avian and rodent models to understand neurobehavioral toxicity is progressing rapidly. Large sample sizes and adaptation to laboratory conditions favor the use of such animals for studies. Like humans, birds rely primarily on vision and hearing for communication, and results obtained with birds are often analogous to those for humans, despite striking differences in brain structure.

Neurobehavioral toxicology has made important contributions to our understanding of changes in humans, even though there are vast differences between the functional capabilities of humans and our closest relatives. Certain chemicals, for example those that affect learning in a wide range of animals, must be studied for their effect on human learning as well. Despite differences, the basic structure of the CNS is similar among mammals, albeit with very different space devoted to the cerebral cortex. Testing animals is challenging, and the approaches used differ from testing humans, who can be asked to read instructions and respond verbally or manually to tasks. However, eye-limb coordination and learning are common to all vertebrates, and even cognition may be identified in many so-called lower organisms.[36] There is substantial and relevant literature on neurobehavioral studies in animals where learning, discrimination, locomotion, vigilance, and memory are studied.[14,46,64]

Learning

Learning is a basic task of the CNS and has been extensively studied. It occurs both in the short term and in the long term and offers an opportunity to test several modalities. Animals have traditionally been tested in mazes or on discrimination tasks, and the speed of learning or of relearning after a challenge is a common measure.[12,62,87] Animal studies have also helped develop paradigms applicable to humans.

Conditioning

Many studies of psychomotor performance in animals involve training by operant conditioning, using either positive or negative reinforcements. One paradigm involves comparing the ability to condition exposed and control animals, while another involves the degradation of performance after exposure to a neurotoxin.[18,46] Alterations in response to visual or acoustic stimuli are used to detect subtle chemical effects, even in animals that appear quite normal. Performance can be useful endpoints in conditioned animals.[46,66]

Naturalistic studies

Laboratory conditions are readily controllable and reproducible, but one must translate testing data obtained with real-life situations. What does it mean when mice reduce their wheel-turning behavior? Animals manifest behavior that is adaptive in nature for finding food, seeking shelter, avoiding predators, finding mates, and caring for young. These behaviors can be quantified through neurobehavioral testing and studied under both field and laboratory conditions, with and without chemical treatments. Young birds, for example, must maintain their balance while running to avoid predation, and balance should be a conservative function, for testing.[14,29] Substances such as lead may impair learning, learning retention, and performance. Some behaviors examined include accuracy and pecking rate of pigeons,[27] activity rates in mice[70] or rats,[69] nest site defense in falcons,[29] monkey behavior,[16] begging behavior and food manipulation in terns,[14] and web-weaving in spiders.[85]

The advantage of examining naturalistic behaviors is that the behaviors are important for fitness and have been shaped and perhaps optimized by evolution as has human behavior. Natural behaviors such as locomotion,[64] exploration, righting ability, depth perception, thermoregulation, aggression, avoidance,[7] learning, and parental recognition are all amenable to laboratory and field experimentation where variables can be controlled.[14,15] Although operant conditioning paradigms afford tighter control of experiments, Laties and Cory-Slecta[44] recommend cautions regarding confounding factors that may influence behavioral outcome in laboratory studies.

While some animal neurotoxicology studies examine the direct effect of exposure, multigenerational studies also yielded important results,[8,11] and show that children and even grandchildren of treated animals manifest behavioral deficits. Exposure of one or both parents can affect behavior in offspring. If both parents are exposed, the impact is greater than if either one is exposed alone.[11] Animal models used for behavioral research will continue to play an important role in developing an understanding of human behavioral function and its clinical applications.

CLINICAL CONSIDERATION FOR THE PRACTITIONER
Overview

An adequate neurobehavioral examination requires an interdisciplinary endeavor of the physician, neurologist, psychologist, and electrophysiologist. A complete examination includes an interview, a physical examination, and one or more neurobehavioral tests, supplemented when necessary by electrophysiology studies.

Clinical interview

The interview provides the examiner with an important opportunity for observing the mood, affect, and behavior of the patient being assessed. This interview can expand to include a more structured psychiatric interview and/or mental status examination. However, when there are time constraints, a mental status examination represents the best alternative, since structured psychiatric interviews require as long as 2 hours to complete. The clinical interview allows the examiner to explore the contribution of ''organic'' and ''psychologic'' pathology, and to detect anxiety, depression, changes in intellectual function, and other performance. Screening protocols are available to the practitioner to use for assessing for depression[8] and other psychological manifestations;[22] normative data is available for comparison. Such instruments help the clinician make a decision regarding referral for more specialized testing and evaluation.

Physical examination

The practitioner performs the neurologic examination by focusing on posture and gait; tests of cerebellar and cranial tests of nerve functions and gross peripheral sensation determine muscle strength and mass; and detect evidence of alterations in reflex responses. Some complex tasks such as resisting sway, heel-to-toe walking, or heel-to-shin maneuvers are really quite sensitive in detecting subtle neurologic deficits. More detailed discussions on interpreting the neurologic examination and diagnosis are provided in Chapter 26. A few areas of emphasis is necessary. The sensory system—vision, hearing, touch, taste, and smell—provides information about position, food, mates, and danger. All points along the pathways from the peripheral receptor to the brain and the central integration and responses can be affected by certain chemicals.

Vision. Neuroophthalmologists, neurologists, and ophthalmologists can evaluate the visual system for evidence of damage. A variety of electrophysiologic tests, such as electrooculography and visual evoked potentials are available. Neurobehaviorists test visual perception, eye-hand coordination, the ability to control eye movement, receptiveness of the eye, and processing of visual information. Behavioral toxicants affect visual acuity, visual fields, color hue sensitivity, and flicker fusion. The ability to detect pattern from noise can be evaluated by an embedded figures test.[76] Visuoperceptual tasks involve visual function along with higher-order cognitive function and integration.

Color vision impairment. Although color blindness is inherited, the ability to detect subtle differences in color saturation (dyschromatopsia) is sensitive to certain chemicals,[54] such as carbon disulfide[63] and styrene.[32] A common testing approach is the Lanthony 15 Hue Desaturated Panel in which subjects rank 15 colored pegs by chromatic sequence. Although most exposed subjects perform in the normal range, a significant proportion (9 of 41 styrene-exposed workers, Gobba et al.[32]) were reported to perform worse than control. This seldom-used panel may be a valuable way of documenting changes in the visual system.

Hearing. Acoustic thresholds at frequencies from 500 to 8000 Hz can be measured with audiometry. However, even with normal thresholds, performance of tasks involving auditory reaction time or auditory memory may be impaired. Antibiotics such as streptomycin and kanamycin damage the auditory nervous pathway, but more subtle changes in our ability to detect loudness, pitch, and timbre are the domain of the psychoacoustician, and in special cases can be evaluated as part of a neurobehavioral assessment. Since many patients exposed to neurotoxins work in industrial settings where hearing may be affected by noise, it is important to identify a pre-existing dysfunction. Hearing is required for administration of many neurobehavioral tasks. Recent evidence suggests that body sway, a neurologic function, may be compromised by hearing loss.[59]

Olfaction. Olfaction plays an important role in human appetite and sexual development and behavior.[13] Loss of smell (hyposmia or anosmia) can be disabling because of its profound impact on taste and nutrition. Chemicals may impair olfaction or lead to unusual and unpleasant smells, *cacosmia,* in two different ways. Cadmium, for example, lowers olfactory function.[68] The University of Pennsylvania Test (scratch test) provides a multiple choice battery of 40 odors that must be identified correctly.[23] While this olfactory battery of tests can be adapted for individual patient evaluation, it may not be sensitive for subtle impairment. Presently, odor threshold testing with dilutions of chemicals is generally confined to research.

Cacosmia is a rare condition that may or may not be associated with changes in olfactory threshold. Patients may complain of unusual sensitivity to odors and identify these as unpleasant. In actuality, when these patients are examined, they may not reveal decrements in their odor recognition ability or an actual enhanced odor threshold.[25] A possibly related condition is the entity of "multiple chemical sensitivity syndrome," a condition in which patients report developing various symptoms in response to very low-level exposures to chemicals at concentrations that most "normal" persons find tolerable (e.g., car fumes, perfumes).[19,28] In many instances, these patients report a heightened awareness of odors, although this alteration may not be reproducible with laboratory testing.

Taste. This sensory modality has seldom been incorporated into neurobehavioral testing. Some chemicals cause abnormal tastes such as the metallic taste that characterizes lead poisoning (but is not a lead taste), and the garlic-like taste that occurs with selenium (but is not a selenium taste). Olfaction and taste are closely linked, albeit different peripheral receptors, and diminished olfactory sensitivity or discrimination interferes with taste appreciation. Taste actually lends itself to more objective studies than does olfaction because one can control and determine the concentration of a substance in solution more easily than in air.

Touch. The sensory component of the physical examination can be elaborate and time consuming, but when administered properly will detect subtle nervous system malfunctions. The sensation of touch is a complex process because in addition to skin receptors, there are receptors in underlying tissues and muscle. The traditional ways of testing for touch sensation involve detecting light touch using a soft brush or hairs; there is also a test of two-point discrimination. A variation of the above procedures includes the ability to identify numbers that are traced on the skin of the palm or the ability to detect the shape of objects placed in the hand (for example, Sensory Perception on the Halstead-Reitan).

Vibration. The threshold for vibration sensation is a sensitive indicator of peripheral nerve damage by a neurotoxin. Quantification of vibratory sensation has been utilized for investigations of industrial populations.[10] Devices developed for assessing vibratory sensation include the *Optacon* and the *Vibratron.* The testing procedure involves having the subject press a fingertip or other body part against a detector and indicating when vibration is appreciated. The amplitude and frequency of the vibration can be adjusted. While the pressure applied to the detector by the patient may potentially influence a measurement, using a forced-choice paradigm[10] compensates for this factor.

Temperature. The ability to discriminate changes in temperature can be used as a testing maneuver for neurotoxicants. Devices that provide objective control of temperature combined with a forced-choice paradigm allow the clinician or researcher to evaluate this modality.[10] Currently, this type testing is used mainly in a research setting.

Position sense. The dorsal columns of the spinal cord relay information on position sense to the brain; the sensorimotor system compensates by adjusting tone. Tests for postural sway,[42] straight-line walking, and the Romberg tests are traditional ways of measuring the performance of these tasks. In addition to testing position sense, these tests are dependent on intact motor and vestibular functions.

Motor function. Neuromuscular function provides the organism with its main mode of manipulating its environment or manipulating within its environment. Motor deficits may be due to (1) muscle disease, (2) disorders of the motor cortex or pathways, (3) changes in the reflex pathways controlling tone, or (4) central disorders that interfere with volition, fine tuning, and coordination of motor function. Obvious changes in muscle mass (particularly asymmetry) and physical weakness can usually be detected by physical examination. In contrast, neurobehavioral testing for motor system dysfunction focuses on eliciting a CNS response, for example in terms of reaction time (see below), rapid alternating movements, and fine muscle control. Many compounds cause acute intoxication (such as alcohol) and affect sensory-motor interrelationships; consequently they produce alterations of gait and posture. Some neurotoxins cause a motor neuropathy and affect the motor branches of peripheral nerves leading to reduced strength, coordination, and fine muscle control. A loss of ability to perform previously learned motor sequences (apraxias) may be an indicator of neurotoxicity.

Vestibular function. The labyrinth, vestibular apparatus, and semicircular canals maintain equilibrium and awareness of position. Toxicity or inflammation of the vestibular system may result in disabling vertigo. Visual and proprioceptive impulses feed this system, and certain toxicants such as ethanol direct a specific impact. A postural sway test has been utilized as procedure to evaluate vestibular and proprioceptive functions.[42]

Basal ganglia. The extrapyramidal motor system (cerebellum, basal ganglia) may be targets of neurotoxicants. Interference with the cortico-striatal-pallidal-thalamic-cortical loop causes ataxias, tremors, and dystonia. MPTP is an example of a specific toxicant that affects the substantia nigra[43] and produces an irreversible Parkinson syndrome.

Cerebellar function. The cerebellum, in conjunction with the cortex and basal ganglia, refines motor function, and its role can be viewed as a quality control influence. It contributes to balance, posture, tone, repetitive movement, coordination, and spatial location. Gross cerebellar dysfunction manifests as ataxia with staggering gait, swaying, and/or stumbling; ataxias manifest as alterations of movements of specific limbs in which the timing of contraction of antagonistic muscle groups is disrupted and there is loss of controlled rapid alternating movements, (dysdiadochokinesia).

Electrophysiologic studies. In addition to electroencephalograms, electromyography, and nerve conduction studies, a variety of specific electrophysiologic techniques have been employed clinically, including electronystagraphy, electrooculography, and evoked potentials.

PATHOPHYSIOLOGY

Neurobehavioral testing measures CNS-dependent tasks such as vigilance, time and accuracy of perception and task performance, simple and complex reaction times, visual-motor coordination, and intellectual functions such as vocabulary, arithmetic skills, memory, learning, and associative functions. One of the more subtle measures of a neurobehavioral alteration involves the slowing of CNS function. Thus, complex perceptual-motor tasks take longer to complete; neurobehavioral testing evaluate, this slowing of central functions. Whether this can be thought of as an "increased resistance" in the central nervous system, or the need for adaptation wherein alternative pathways are sought for particular functions, is not known. It is not clear whether neuronal cells actually die, interconnections shrink or wither, or biochemical communication is inhibited; possibly all of these mechanisms apply.

A recently proposed mechanism to explain neuropsychologic changes involves impairment of astrocyte function.[67] The astrocytes in the brain are intimately associated and intermingle with other neuroglia and with neurons and appear to regulate the extracellular microenvironment of the brain and can thus influence neuronal excitability and metabolism. These cells support and protect neurons and can regulate their volume. The astroglia are targets for nonadrenergic and serotoninergic activation and, because they perform such function, regulate the extracellular milieu of neurons in the brain (i.e., amino acids like glutamate and ions such as $Ca2+$, $K+$, $Cl-$, $Na+$). Impairment of astroglia function, especially impeding the high-affinity glutamate uptake by certain neuronal cells by a neurotoxin, might lead to a lesser glutamate uptake and consequential glutamate "overflow," which then leads to clinical symptoms. When there is a higher neurotoxin concentration and more of an effect, glutamate uptake may be impaired even more, thus causing more of a buildup of extracellular glutamate; glutamate may reach concentrations that are cytotoxic to neurons at this stage. It is conceptualized that some regions of the brain, such as areas of the hippocampus, are especially vulnerable, as demonstrated by their high density of N-methyl-D-aspartate receptors. In any event, this cascade of biochemical events is translated clinically as neurobehavioral changes.

PSYCHOMETRIC TESTING
Overview

While a patient interview and mental status examination may divulge gross abnormalities, psychometric testing provides quantitation and a greater level of sensitivity for identifying subtle and possibly subclinical manifestations. Psychometric tests that have been validated with broad database of normative scores are especially useful. Many newly introduced tests may lack such normative data and therefore are more difficult to interpret on an individual patient basis;

these tests may be more appropriate for large-scale screenings or epidemiologic studies.

Rationale for testing

The use of neurobehavioral testing is based on the premise that subtle behavioral changes are sensitive indicators of neurotoxicant CNS effects.[78] Levels of exposure formerly thought safe are now known to have far-reaching consequences on important behavioral functions; for example, low-level lead exposure leads to hyperactivity and impaired intellectual development in children.[49,57] Patients with significant neurotoxic chemical exposure often show loss of cognitive functioning, and may manifest as memory impairment and a difficulty in concentration. However, these findings also are frequent among patients with depression and other psychologic illnesses. Neurobehavioral testing provides a way for the clinician to objectively standardize and quantitate complaints and may help differentiate memory and concentration difficulties due to emotional or psychological factors from similar abnormalities caused by a neurotoxin.

Confounders of testing

A number of variables influence the administration and interpretation of neurobehavioral testing results. A subject's innate capability prior to exposure, the so-called pre-morbid ability, is a major factor. Subject cooperation and motivation are essential to accomplish a valid assessment. Patients being assessed for legal purposes present special motivational circumstances that need to be taken into account. Neuropsychologists have addressed this problem, and methods are available for detecting response biases. In addition, there are other factors that may influence neurobehavioral performance, such as medication and alcohol use, fatigue, preexisting familiarity with the tests, underlying neurologic conditions such as head trauma, and medical conditions such as diabetes mellitus. While many factors will be recognized during the course of an examination, assistance may be gained by having the patient fill out a self-administered questionnaire prior to neurobehavioral testing to ascertain factors (such as fatigue) that might affect the test results. Additionally, neurobehavioral performance is also affected by education and intellectual level, age, ethnicity, and gender. It is imperative that the test results obtained on an individual patient be compared to appropriate normative group values from a population of similar educational status, age, ethnicity, and gender. Most neurobehavioral tests are strongly influenced by educational achievement and intellectual ability. Patients with minimal education (less than eighth grade) may not be able to perform neurobehavioral tests. Grandjean[34] points out that neurobehavioral tests, suitable for persons who have completed a high school education, may not be applicable to a majority of the working population of United States. On the other hand, tests such as the pegboard and reaction time are relatively independent of educational level.

An increasingly common concern, especially for today's working population, is English language ability; however, many tests also have Spanish and French versions. Thus, if a population study is proposed, it may actually be impractical to test large populations of mixed-origin persons that include workers from eastern and southern Europe, Asia, and Latin American countries.

Testing protocols

The following is a discussion of the core functions that must be assessed for neurobehavioral testing. The tests cited illustrate various neurobehavioral functions and importantly have validated normative data to allow proper interpretation of performance. In contrast to making group comparisons, an individual assessment of neurobehavioral dysfunction depends upon using reliable normative values for comparison. The comparison values can represent results of previous testing on the same person, but more often normative population values are used. A test result can be considered abnormal if an individual's performance on a test is more than two standard deviations below the mean value of normative data for peers (similar age, sex, race, and socioeconomic status). Confronted by a poor test performance, the clinician must ascertain that the standard against which the individual was being compared is reasonably similar to the individual patient's demographic profile. It is particularly necessary to be alert to cultural biases inherent in many of the tests. The interpretation of neurobehavioral testing requires observing a *pattern* of poor performance. For example, testing may represent administering several different tests to examine for one specific neurobehavioral function (for example, concentration). The neuropsychologist then examines the various test results and tries to document that there is a consistent pattern of poor performance present for several tests. An isolated poor performance on only one test may not be a strong enough indicator of a cognitive problem.

Testing for intellectual ability. Familiar tests of cognitive verbal ability include the Vocabulary and Information components of the revised Wechsler Adult Intelligence Scale (WAIS-R).[81] These tests are regarded as more insensitive to the effects of neurotoxins since they reflect abilities that are well-rehearsed and longstanding.[48] When an individual's verbal abilities are shown to be significantly abnormal, this finding generally indicates serious or chronic CNS damage. Such deficits are noted in persons who sustained head trauma or suffered a stroke; they are not usual aftermaths of a neurotoxic exposure unless the exposure was chronic over a number of years and present at high levels,[38] thus causing a well-defined dementia. The patient's performance on a vocabulary test can usually be used to estimate premorbid ability. Relatively poor performance on tests of other functions such as memory or concentration more likely indicate deficits due to neurotoxins.

More complex tests of cognitive nonverbal functions, indicative of overall ability, integrate spatial perceptual skills with some form of motor response. Probably the best known of these tests is the Block Design subtest of the WAIS-R.[81] This timed test requires the patient to assemble blocks to replicate a two-dimensional picture of a design. Thus, it requires perceptual and motor skills of a more complex nature than the simpler psychomotor tests previously described. Ravens Progressive Matrices is another nonverbal test of overall ability that does not rely on verbal skills. Such tests may be more appropriate as measures of premorbid ability among patients where, due to educational background, verbal skills provide an underestimate of premorbid ability. Clearly the best estimates of premorbid ability are the achievement and aptitude tests taken in high school. Thus, if possible, patients should be encouraged to get their high school records to estimate ability prior to exposure.

Testing for attention and concentration. Attention and perception are processes that influence performance on most neurobehavioral tests.[40] The individual must be oriented to the verbal and/or visual stimuli, concentrate while inhibiting irrelevant stimuli, and then use conceptual tracking to sustain attention over a period of time.[48] Ideally, a neurobehavioral evaluation will include tests of both visual and verbal attention and perception. At the most simplistic level, auditory and visual reaction time reflect the ability to sustain attention. As for all neurobehavioral tests, no single function can be assessed in isolation. That is, even for a simple reaction-time task, motor movement as well as sustained attention is required. More complex tests of attention involve not only orientation to stimuli and sustained concentration but active inhibition of irrelevant stimuli. For example, the Stroop Color Word test requires that the patient read the color of the ink in which different colored names are printed; (i.e., the word ''Red'' written in blue ink must be read as blue); the word is highly distracting. Another visual perceptual task in which irrelevant stimuli must be disregarded is the Embedded Figures task.[76] For this task the patient must pick out recognizable figures from a complex design with overlapping figures. Tasks of simple attention processes, such as simple reaction time have probably been the most sensitive to the effects of neurotoxins.[31] In addition to these tests, Digit Span from the WAIS-R also is frequently used as a measure of attention. It requires that the patient repeat an increasing string of digits both forward and backward. Again sustained auditory attention is required, but immediate memory is also involved in performance.

Testing for psychomotor functions. Tests of psychomotor function include tasks that require continuous processing and integration of sensory inputs with motor responses. The tests include visual and auditory reaction time, in which the patient responds as quickly as possible to either a visual or an auditory stimulus. The Grooved Pegboard and the Santa Ana pegboard tests measure how quickly a person can insert pegs into grooved holes; the test has been shown to be sensitive to the effects of various neurotoxicants that affect perception and dexterity.[31,52]

Testing for memory and learning. Short-term memory loss is a frequent clinical complaint of patients exposed to neurotoxins.[38] Tests of memory and learning assess a patient's short-term memory by presenting stimuli (for example, words, digits, pictures) visually or aurally and asking the individual to either recall or recognize the stimuli immediately or within a short period of time. Tests of verbal and visual memory usually involve immediate recall followed by delayed recall (usually a 30-minute delay). The Wechsler Memory Scale-Revised provides both verbal and visual memory subtests; there is also the Delayed Recall index to allow comparison of various aspects of memory. Memory may be impaired at different levels. For example, one patient may have difficulty encoding or learning information; another patient may note difficulty maintaining information after it is learned (that is, forgetting). The California Verbal Learning Test presents a string of words that the patient is asked to recall over five trials.[20] This test assesses short- and delayed-recall learning efficiency and recognition memory. Other memory tests present pictures of abstract drawings or actual objects and require the subject to recognize the picture from a set (such as the Benton Visual Retention Test[9]). If a patient's performance on a short-term memory task is abnormal as assessed by a vocabulary test, then complaints of memory difficulty are probably reliable.

Testing personality, mood, affect. A number of epidemiologic studies report that personality changes are important manifestations of some neurotoxicants. Erethism attributable to inorganic mercury is a classic example of this phenomenon. Mood changes are reported to result from exposures to solvents[56] and formaldehyde;[41] classroom behavior problems have been attributed to lead.[57] It is important to point out that mood and personality alterations may occur in the absence of neurologic abnormalities noted on physical examination. While a number of psychometric instruments are available to document personality and mood alterations (for example, Minnesota Multiphasic Personality Inventory-2), in the final analysis, these abnormalities are difficult to prove. The manifested symptoms may represent a premorbid or pre-existent state, or could be due to exposure to a neurotoxicant. For example, it is not uncommon for patients exposed to neurotoxins to exhibit a profile on the MMPI-2 that is consistent with psychiatric disorders known as somatoform disorders.[56] The Profile of Mood States[53] and the Symptom Checklist-90[22] both document levels of mood disturbance. The factors to which these symptoms can be attributed require a clinical assessment of other potential agents and/or stressors in an individual's life that could be causing mood disturbance (for example, divorce).

DEVELOPMENTAL NEUROBEHAVIOR

One major development of the 1980s was the focus on the developing nervous system. Both before birth and after, there are dramatic changes in CNS structure and function, particularly during the first 2 years of life. These include increasing size of the brain, changes in neuronal myelinization, and modifications of the neural connections; this leads to the child being able to expand his/her abilities for complex motor behavior, improve his/her coordination, and enhance his/her intellectual functioning, including such features as concept formation, pattern recognition, speech, and communication.

There are critical developmental periods when certain anatomic changes occur and when certain physiologic and cognitive processes become fixed. There may be critical periods for language development, as well as for other functions.[14,51] An infection developing during the first trimester of gestation will have a different impact on the child than a similar infection incurring later. After birth, there appears to be critical periods for development of certain skills such as acquisition of language. The boundaries of these periods are not sharply defined but there are times when learning proceeds more efficiently. For example, animals and humans that are isolated from normal sounds of their species during a critical period may fail to develop normal vocalizations or speech. Birds that suffer acoustic isolation develop songs that do not carry the normal species-specific sounds;[51] isolated infants, in addition to other psychologic dysfunction, will babble unintelligibly (idioglossia) and learn language only with great difficulty. As organisms mature, their locomotory ability, learning, and knowledge increases appropriately for their age. There is evidence that even low-level neurotoxicant exposures may produce a profound impact on the orderly acquisition of nervous system function. The magnitude of such changes is not fully appreciated, and the field of behavioral teratology is in a rapid growth phase.

The best example of behavioral teratology comes from lead exposure in infants and children. Depressed learning, reduced cognitive functions, and behavioral disturbances are documented to occur even in children whose blood lead levels are below 25 μg/dL, a value formerly believed "normal."[5,57,77] Teachers rated elementary school children having higher body burdens of lead as being less independent and organized, less attentive, more hyperactive, and more easily frustrated.[57] Needleman's publication shows remarkable dose-response relationships between dentine-lead levels and poor ratings. Children with higher lead levels had poorer performance on verbal and digit span components of IQ tests.[57]

CONCLUSION

Both anatomic and biochemical changes lead to impairment in the nervous system. New approaches involve early detection of functional decrements and perhaps biomarker assays specific to the CNS. Ethologists, clinical toxicologists, neuropathologists, and toxicologists will continue to expand our understanding of this most complicated organ system.

Neurobehavioral testing covers a broad range of CNS and peripheral functions, and subtle deficits can be measured. However, as with most clinical testing, lack of a baseline or premorbid test result makes it difficult to interpret subtle deviations from normal. Some scientists are of the opinion that neurobehavioral testing is best used as an epidemiologic tool to evaluate population groups and is not yet ready to be used for evaluating individual patients. However, clinical psychologists have a long history of evaluating individuals using this technique and have accumulated normative data that allows reliable characterizations when applied to an individual patient, particularly when deficits are severe.

As more tests are validated on groups of normal people, the opportunity to detect subtle abnormalities in individuals will improve. Neurobehavioral testing can be part of any evaluation where exposure to neurotoxins and CNS symptoms are reported or suspected.

REFERENCES

1. Aaserud O et al: Regional cerebral blood flow after long-term exposure to carbon disulfide, *Acta Neurol Scand* 85:266, 1992.
2. Anger WK, Johnson BL: Human behavioral neurotoxicology: workplace and community assessments. In Rom WN, ed: *Environmental and occupational medicine,* Boston, 1992, Little, Brown.
3. Annau Z, ed: *Neurobehavioral toxicology,* Baltimore, 1986, Johns Hopkins University Press.
4. Agency-Toxic Substances & Disease Registry: Neurobehavioral test batteries for use in environmental health field studies, U.S. Department of Health and Human Services, December 1992.
5. Agency of Toxic Substances & Disease Registry: The nature and extent of lead poisoning in children in the United States: a report to Congress, U.S. Department of Health and Human Services, 1988.
6. Baker EL, Letz R, Fidler A: A computer-administered neurobehavioral evaluation system for occupational and environmental epidemiology, *J Occup Med* 27:206, 1985.
7. Barthalamus GT et al: Chronic effects of lead on schedule-controlled pigeon behavior, *Toxicol Appl Pharmacol* 42:271, 1977.
8. Beck A, *Depression inventory,* 1978, The Psychological Corporation.
9. Benton A: *Visual retention test manual,* New York, 1974, The Psychological Corporation.
10. Bove F et al: Quantitative sensory testing in occupational medicine, *Seminars in Occup Med* 1:185, 1986.
11. Brady K, Herrera Y, Zenick H: Influence of parental lead exposure on subsequent learning ability of offspring, *Pharmacol Biochem Behav* 3:561, 1975.
12. Brown DR: Neonatal lead exposure in the rat: decreased learning as a function of age and blood lead concentration, *Toxicol Applied Pharmacol* 32:628, 1975.
13. Burger J, Gochfeld M: A hypothesis on the role of pheromones on age of menarche, *Med Hypoth* 17:39, 1985.
14. Burger J, Gochfeld M: Early postnatal lead exposure: behavioral effects in common tern chicks (Sterna hirundo), *J Toxicol Environ Health* 16:869, 1985.
15. Burger J, Gochfeld M: Lead and behavioral development: effects of varying dosage and schedule on survival and performance of young common terns (Sterna hirundo), *J Toxicol Environ Health* 24:173, 1988.
16. Bushnell PJ et al: Scotopic vision deficits in young monkeys exposed to lead, *Science* 333:167, 1977.
17. Cavanaugh JV: Peripheral neuropathy caused by chemical agents, *CRC Crit Rev Toxicol* 2:365, 1980.
18. Cory-Slechta DA, Weiss B, Cox, C: Delayed behavioral toxicity of lead with increasing exposure concentration, *Toxicol Appl Pharm* 71:342, 1983.

19. Cullen MR, ed: Workers with multiple chemical sensitivities, Philadelphia, 1987, Hanley & Belfus.
20. Delis D et al: *California verbal learning test manual,* New York, 1987, The Psychological Corporation.
21. Demers R, Markell B, Wabeke R: Peripheral vibratory sense deficits in solvent-exposed painters, *JOM* 33:1051, 1991.
22. DeRogatis LR: *SCL-90-R Manual II,* Towson, Md, 1983, Clinical psychomatric research.
23. Doty RL, Gregor T, Monroe C: Quantitative assessment of olfactory function in an industrial setting, *J Occup Med* 28:457, 1986.
24. Doty RL et al: Smell identification ability: changes with age, *Science* 226:1441-1443, 1984.
25. Doty RL et al: Olfactory sensitivity, nasal resistance and autonome function in patients with multiple chemical senactivities, *Arch Otolaryngol Head Neck Surg* 114:1422, 1988.
26. Errebo-Knudsen EO, Olsen F: Organic solvents and the presenile dementia (the Painters Syndrome): a critical review of the Danish literature, *Science Total Environment* 48:45, 1986.
27. Evans KI, Garman RH, Laties VG: Neurotoxicity of methylmercury in the pigeon, *Neuro Tox* 3:21, 1982.
28. Fiedler N, Maccia C, Kipen H: Evaluation of chemically sensitive patients, *J Occup Med* 34:529, 1992.
29. Fox GA, Donald T: Organochlorine pollutants, nest-defense behavior and reproductive success in merlins, *Condor* 82:81, 1980.
30. Gade A, Mortensen EL, Bruhn P: Chronic painters syndrome: a reanalysis of psychological test data in a group of diagnosed cases based on comparisons with matched controls, *Acta Neurol Scand* 77:293, 1988.
31. Gamberale F: Use of behavioral performance tests in the assessment of solvent toxicity, *Scand J Work Environ Health* 11(suppl 1):65, 1985.
32. Gobba F et al: Acquired dyschromatopsia among styrene-exposed workers, *J Occup Med* 33:761, 1991.
33. Gochfeld M, Fiedler N, Burger J: Neurobehavioral toxicology. In Last JM, Wallace RB, eds: *Maxcy-Rosenau-Last's public health and preventive medicine,* ed 13, Norwalk, Conn, Appleton & Lange, 1992.
34. Grandjean P: Application of neurobehavioral methods in environmental and occupational health, *Environ Res* 60:57, 1991.
35. Grandjean P: Applications of neurobehavioral methods in environmental and occupational health, *Environ Res* 60:57, 1993.
36. Griffin DR: *The question of animal awareness: evolutionary continuity of mental experience,* New York, 1976, Rockefeller University Press.
37. Hanninen H et al: Behavioral effects of long-term exposure to a mixture of organic solvents, *Scand J Work Environ Health* 2:240, 1976.
38. Hartman DE: *Neuropsychological toxicology,* New York, 1988, Pergamon Press.
39. Johnson BL ed: *Prevention of neurotoxic illness in working populations,* New York, 1987, Wiley.
40. Kagan J: The determinants of attention in the infant, *Amer Scient* 58:298, 1970.
41. Kilburn KH, Seidman BC, Warshaw R: Neurobehavioral and respiratory symptoms of formaldehyde and xylene exposure in histology technicians, *Arch Environ Health* 40:229, 1985.
42. Kilburn KH, Warshaw RH, Hanscom B: Are hearing loss and balance dysfunction link in construction iron workers? *Br J Indust Med* 49:138, 1992.
43. Langston JW et al: Chronic parkinsonism in humans due to a product of meperidine-analog synthesis, *Science* 219:979, 1983.
44. Laties V, Cory-Slechta DA: Some problems in interpreting the behavioral effects of lead and methylmercury, *Neurobehav Toxicol* 1(suppl 1):129, 1979.
45. Laties VG, Merigan WH: Behavioral effects of carbon monoxide on animals and man, *Ann Rev Pharmacol Toxicol* 19:357, 1979.
46. Laties VG: How operant conditioning can contribute to behavioral toxicology, *Environ Health Perspect* 26:29, 1978.
47. Letz R, Baker L: *NES2,* Neurobehavioral Evaluation Systems, June 1988.
48. Lezak M: *Neuropsychological assessment,* New York, 1983, Oxford University Press.
49. Lin-Fu JS: The evolution of childhood lead poisoning as a public health program. In Chisholm JJ, O'Hara DM, eds: *Lead absorption in children: management, clinical and environmental aspects,* Baltimore, 1982, Urban & Schwartzenberg.
50. Lorenz K: *On aggression,* New York, 1966, Harcourt, Brace & World.
51. Marler P: Bird song and speech development: could there be parallels, *Amer Scient* 58:669, 1970.
52. Matthews CG, Klove H: *Instruction manual for the Adult Neuropsychology Test Battery,* Madison, Wis, 1964, University of Wisconsin Medical School.
53. McNair D, Lorr M, Droppleman L: *Profile of mood states,* San Francisco; 1981.
54. Mergler D et al: Chromal focus of acquired chromatic discrimination loss and solvent exposure among printshop workers, *Toxicology* 49:341, 1988.
55. Morrow LA et al: Risk factors with persistence of neuropsychological deficits with organic solvent exposure, *J Nerv Ment Dis* 179:540, 1991.
56. Morrow LA et al: A distinct pattern of personality disturbance following exposure to mixtures of organic solvents, *J Occ Med* 31:743, 1989.
57. Needleman H et al: Deficits in psychologic and classroom performance of children with elevated dentine lead levels, *N Engl J Med* 300:689, 1979.
58. *Neurobehavioral toxicology,* 1:1979.
59. NIOSH: Organic solvent neurotoxicity, *Current Intelligence Bull* 48:1, 1987.
60. Norseth T, Waage J, Dale I: Acute effects and exposure to organic compounds in road maintenance workers exposed to asphalt, *Am J Indust Med* 20:737, 1991.
61. O'Hanlon JF: Preliminary studies of the effects of carbon monoxide on vigilance in man. In Weiss B, Laties VG, eds: *Behavioral toxicology,* New York, 1975, Plenum.
62. Ogilvie DM: Sublethal effects of lead acetate on the Y-maze performance of albino mice (Mus musculus L), *Canad J Zool* 55:771, 1977.
63. Raitta C et al: Impaired color discrimination among viscose rayon workers exposed to carbon disulfide, *J Occ Med* 23:189, 1981.
64. Reiter L: Use of activity measures in behavioral toxicology, *Environ Health Perspect* 26:9, 1978.
65. Rice DC, Gilbert SG, Willes RF: Neonatal low-level lead exposure in monkeys: locomotor activity, schedule-controlled behavior, and the effects of amphetamine, *Toxicol Appl Pharmacol* 51:503, 1979.
66. Rice DC: Behavioral deficit (delayed matching to sample) in monkeys exposed from birth to low levels of lead, *Toxicol Appl Pharmacol* 75:337, 1984.
67. Rennback L, Hansson E: Chronic encephalitis induced by mercury or lead: aspects of underlying cellular and molecular mechanisms, *Br J Indust Med* 49:233, 1992.
68. Rose CS, Heywood PG, Costanzo RM: Olfactory impairment after chronic occupational cadmium exposure, *JOM* 34:600, 1992.
69. Sauerhoff M, Michaelson GK: Hyperactivity and brain catecholamines in lead-exposed developing rats, *Science* 182:1022, 1973.
70. Silbergeld E, Goldberg A: A lead-induced behavioral disorder, *Life Sciences* 13:1275, 1973.
71. Singer R, Valciukas JA, Lilis R: Lead exposure and nerve conduction velocity: the differential time course of sensory and motor nerve effects, *Neutoxicol* 4:193, 1983.
72. Spencer P, Schaumberg HH: *Experimental and clinical neurotoxicology,* Baltimore, 1980, Williams & Wilkins.
73. Teisinger J: New advances in the toxicology of carbon disulfide, *Am Industr Hyg Assoc J* 35:55, 1974.
74. Tvedt B et al: Brain damage caused by hydrogen sulfide: a follow-up study of six patients. *Am J Ind Med* 20:91, 1991.
75. Valciukas JA et al: Central nervous system dysfunction due to lead exposure, *Science* 201:465, 1978.

76. Valciukas JA, Singer RM: An embedded figures test in environmental and occupational neurotoxicology, *Environ Res* 28:183, 1982.
77. Valciukas J: *Foundations of environmental and occupational neurotoxicology,* New York, 1991, Van Nostrand Reinhold.
78. Valciukas JA, Lilis R: Psychometric techniques in environmental research, *Environ Res* 21:275, 1980.
79. Physitemp Instruments: Vibratron II operating manual, Clifton, NJ, 1991.
80. Vigilani EC: Carbon disulfide poisoning in viscose rayon factories, *Brit J Industr Med* 11:235, 1954.
81. Wechsler D: *WAIS-R manual,* New York, 1981, The Psychological Corporation.
82. Weiss B, Laties VG: *Behavioral pharmacology: the current status,* New York, 1985, Alan R Liss.
83. Weiss B: Tools for the assessment of behavioral toxicity. In Xinteras C, Johnson BL, de Groot I, eds: *Behavioral toxicology: early detection of occupational hazards,* Washington, DC, 1974, U.S. Department of Health, Education and Welfare, NIOSH.
84. WHO: Chronic effects of organic solvents on the central nervous system—core protocol for an international collaborative study, Environmental Health Series No. 36, 1989.
85. Witt PN: Drugs alter web-building of spiders: a review and evaluation, *Behav Sci* 16:98, 1971.
86. Xinteras C, Johnson BL, de Groot I: *Behavioral toxicology: early detection of occupational hazards,* Washington, DC, 1974, U.S. Department of Health, Education and Welfare, NIOSH.
87. Zenick H et al: Influence of prenatal and postnatal lead exposure on discrimination learning in rats, *Pharmacol Biochem Behav* 8:347, 1978.
88. Zenick H, Reiter LW: *Behavioral toxicology: an emerging discipline,* U.S. Research Triangle Park, 1977, Environmental Protection Agency.

Chapter 17

BONE MARROW TOXICOLOGY

Robert Snyder

Bone marrow structure and function
    Components of bone marrow
    Colony-forming units
Chemically induced aplastic anemia
    Benzene
    Chloramphenicol
    Aplastic anemia caused by other agents
    Nonsteroidal antiinflammatory agents
    Phenothiazines
    Antithyroid drugs
    Salts of gold and other heavy metals
    Anticancer alkylating agents
    Other reports of bone marrow depression
    Lead-induced anemia
Chemically induced leukemia
    Benzene and leukemia
    Leukemia associated with cancer chemotherapy

The adverse effects produced by drugs and other chemicals on bone marrow, the blood-forming organ, are a major concern of clinicians and toxicologists. Swanson and Cook[67] published a compendium listing approximately 800 compounds that were claimed, mainly in case reports, to produce some form of blood dyscrasias. Few epidemiologic studies are available for most of these chemicals, but some have been intensively studied, and the database supports a cause-and-effect relationship between a number of chemicals and bone marrow damage. This chapter will emphasize chemicals that are thought to cause aplastic anemia and its related conditions and will also discuss the induction of leukemia by chemicals. Although it has been recognized for many years that chemicals can produce blood dyscrasias, studies of the mechanisms by which these effects are produced have been hampered because of our lack of understanding of the bone marrow. However, modern techniques for investigating bone marrow function and the application of molecular biologic approaches to study growth factors have accelerated the rate at which our knowledge of the mechanisms of hematopoiesis has expanded. This chapter discusses bone marrow function, chemical induction of aplastic anemia and leukemia, and causal relationships and risk estimations in hematotoxicity.

BONE MARROW STRUCTURE AND FUNCTION
Components of the bone marrow

Marrow is found in the central hollow segment of bones throughout the body and has a total volume about twice the size of the liver. Roughly half of the marrow volume is engaged in hematopoiesis. Early in prenatal life the liver and spleen act as hematopoietic organs. By the fifth fetal month the marrow reaches sufficient maturity to begin to assume the primary role in hematopoeisis, and by birth it is totally responsible for maintaining the supply of circulating blood cells. During the early years of life, the growth of the body and the expansion of blood volume demand a high level of hematopoiesis in marrow cavities throughout the body. With maturity a lower level of activity is required, and hematopoiesis in adults involves primarily vertebrae, ribs, sternum, and the proximal epiphyses of the long bones.

Early in the study of bone marrow, it became clear that the marrow must supply the body's need for red cells, white cells, and platelets. However, it was also clear that the total body requirement for blood cells for a lifetime could not be stored from birth in the bone marrow. The most reasonable hypothesis to explain how the marrow can provide blood cells for a lifetime is based on the concept of the stem cell. It is thought that all circulating cells derive from a primordial cell type in the bone marrow that, depending upon its microenvironment and a variety of stimulating factors, can become committed to the production of a single cell type, such as an erythrocyte, a thrombocyte, or one type of leucocyte. The process involves maturation through several morphologically distinct stages that can be characterized functionally in culture using colony-forming techniques, immunologic responses to specific antibody markers, responses to growth factors and cytokines, and tests specific to various cell types. Very few stem cells are needed since they yield one replacement stem cell and one committed cell at the time of mitosis. Thus the stem cell is described as "self-renewing." The committed daughter cell that derives from this initial mitotic event begins the process of development and proliferation to yield the requisite number of mature circulating cells.

The cells of the bone marrow that lead to the emergence of circulating cells in the blood are shown in hierarchic order in Fig. 17-1 and are termed (1) the pluripotential, or multipotential, stem cell, the most primitive stem cell that can lead to the production of any blood cell type, (2) the committed stem cell, the other cell resulting from the mitotic event in which the pluripotential stem cell renews itself but which is now sensitive to factors leading it to the production of a specific blood cell, (3) progenitor cells, those cells in the process of maturation and proliferation that eventually produce the circulating cells in the requisite numbers, and (4) mature blood cells, which are released into the circulation.

For these events to occur in the bone marrow, a separate and distinct group of cells is needed to play a supporting role in bone marrow functions. Endosteal cells, fibroblasts, reticuloendothelial cells, fat cells, the sinusoids and bone itself, and monocytes and macrophages all act to support and promote the development of blood cells in the bone marrow. Each of these cells are morphologically distinct and have specific assignments in the process of supporting hematopoiesis. As a group they are termed the bone marrow stroma or the hematopoietic microenvironment. Thus, from the toxicological viewpoint, the bone marrow offers two types of targets for adverse responses to chemicals: the stem and progenitor cell population, and the cells of the hematopoietic microenvironment.

Colony-forming units

Attempts to describe the series of events from the stem cell to the mature circulating cell were difficult when based solely on the morphologic evaluation of bone marrow smears because of the many cell types observed in a smear and the morphologic changes that occur during maturation, some of which are readily identified and others that are relatively subtle and more difficult to characterize. Nevertheless, through the use of specific staining techniques, pioneers in bone marrow biology such as Ehrlich[15] and Pappenheim[53] described cells of related morphology and suggested that gradual maturation from early primitive cells occurred in marrow.

Eventually the concept of the multipotential stem cell from which any blood cell could develop began to be appreciated.[43] Critical studies by Till and McCullough[69] showed that transplantation of bone marrow from normal mice to mice whose marrow was inactivated by x-irradiation, yielded spleen colonies of immature blood cells. Some were purely erythroid colonies, whereas others contained cells of more than one lineage. The conclusions were that (1) spleen colonies could be derived from a single bone marrow cell from the donor mouse, (2) some of these cells were multipotential because they yielded more than one cell type in a single colony, and (3) these colonies also contained stem cells because upon further transplantation in a similar system they could give rise to spleen colonies in the recipient mice. The spleen colony-forming unit technique, termed CFU-S, is now often used to study the effects of chemicals on early stem cells.

The precise series of events leading to the production of specific blood cells is somewhat different for each cell line. In recent years functional evaluation of bone marrow has been based on the study of colony-forming units, which originated from the concept of the CFU-S described. However, most colony-forming units are not now studied in vivo using x-irradiated animals, but are grown in tissue culture dishes using bone marrow cells treated with appropriate growth stimulants. The results have led to functional characterization of stem cells and intermediate progenitors and to the discovery of a series of growth factors controlling the development of each cell type.

Analysis of the bone marrow cells reveals that a small number of cells are stem cells and progenitors that initiate the development of cells that eventually, upon maturation, become the functional cells of the blood. The vast majority of cells in the marrow are constantly undergoing maturation and proliferation to reach the stage at which they will be released into the circulation. Fig. 17-2 shows the stem and early progenitor cells, bearing acronyms indicative of their status and their relationship to one another, but is not intended to reflect the relative numbers of cells in each com-

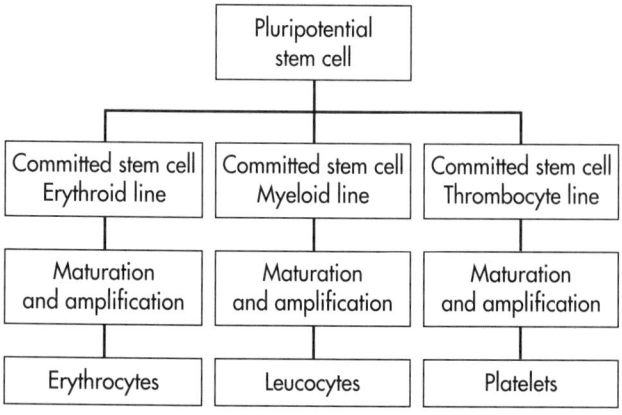

Fig. 17-1. General scheme for bone marrow cell maturation.

partment. The most primitive stem cell, the CFU-S, is normally in a resting state termed Go. It undergoes mitosis to yield another quiescent cell, plus a cell (CFU-SG$_1$/M) from which each of the lineages may develop. Either of two cells may emerge from this stage: CFU-L, which gives rise to the B and T lymphocyte lines, or CFU-GEMM, which gives rise to the granulocytes, erythrocytes, macrophages, and megacaryocytes. CFU-GEMM can give rise to BFU-E, the progenitors of the erythroid line, BFU-MK, the progenitors of the platelet line, CFU-Eo, the progenitors of the eosinophil line, and CFU-Ba, the progenitors of the basophil line. CFU-GEMM can also lead to CFU-GM, the granulocyte/macrophage lines, to yield either CFU-G or CFU-M, each of which in turn lead to circulating neutrophils or monocytes, respectively.

The controls of these developmental pathways are highly complex and are largely a function of the hematopoietic microenvironment. Various cells contribute growth factors that modulate the development of each cell lineage. This continues to be a rapidly developing field, and, therefore, the descriptions of the events in hematopoietic control must be considered tentative. Bagby and Segal[6] have characterized these as direct-acting lineage-specific factors; for example, erythropoietin (EPO), granulocyte colony stimulating factor (G-CSF), monocyte/macrophage stimulating factor (M-CSF), and interleukin-7 (IL-7), which induced the growth of B and T lymphocyte progenitors.

There are also direct-acting factors that act on multipotential progenitors and stem cells. These include interleukin-3 (IL-3) and granulocyte macrophage colony-stimulating factor (GM-CSF). Some factors such as interleukin-1 (IL-1) and tumor necrosis factor (TNF) act indirectly to cause other cells to release direct-acting factors. Finally, there is a series of interleukins (IL-2, IL-4, IL-5, IL-6) that can act to stimulate developing cells in several lineages.

The practitioner must have an understanding of the sequence of events leading to the production of circulating blood cells because many diseases of the blood may be related to specific steps in these processes. The concern of the toxicologist is that chemicals that produce blood dyscrasia may inhibit blood cell development by attacking stem or progenitor cells, may disturb the production of growth factors, or may damage other functions of the hematopoietic microenvironment.

CHEMICALLY INDUCED APLASTIC ANEMIA
(see box on p. 204)

People who have normal hematopoietic function can develop aplastic anemia as a result of exposure to certain chemicals. A bone marrow aspirate is required to confirm the diagnosis of aplastic anemia. Aspirates from patients with marrow aplasia contain excessive fat and are hypocellular. Few erythroid cells are usually seen, and megakaryocytes may be absent. Remaining granulocyte precursors may appear to be normal, although reduced in number. Residual macrophages may appear to have ingested iron and other cellular debris in the course of phagocytosis. It is not unusual to find islands of relatively normal hematopoietic activity. To fully evaluate the marrow, more than one aspirate may be necessary, and a trephine bone marrow biopsy is also recommended. Aplastic marrow biopsies show fatty replacement of hematopoietic cells and the presence of many non-hematopoietic cells, such as lymphocytes, plasma cells, and macrophages.

The designation ''severe aplastic anemia'' is indicated when the peripheral blood count displays two of the following three values: granulocytes <500/µl, platelets <20,000/µl, or reticulocytes (last stage in erythroid cell development prior to the mature erythrocyte) <1% (corrected for hematocrit), and a bone marrow biopsy demonstrating <25% cellularity.

Epidemiologic evaluation of the incidence of aplastic anemia in the United States and Europe suggests that it occurs at the rate of about 3 to 6 cases per million population.

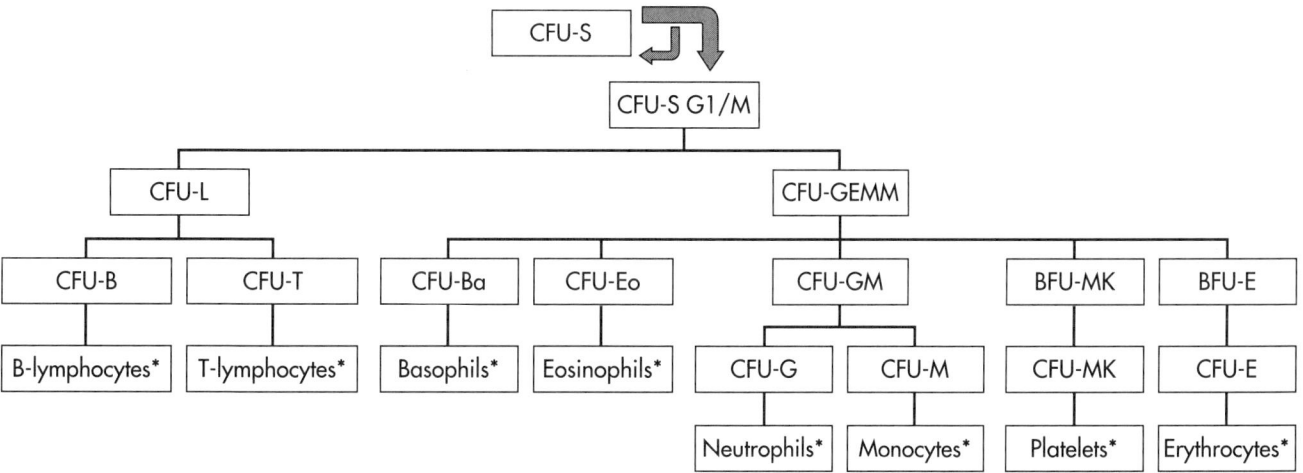

Fig. 17-2. Colony-forming unit based on description of bone marrow cell maturation.

Some causes of bone marrow toxicity

Aplastic anemia

COMMON CHEMICALS

Benzene	Chloamphenicol

NONSTEROIDAL ANTIINFLAMMATORY AGENTS

Amidopyrine	Aminopyrine
Dypirone	Phenylbutazone

PHENOTHIAZINES

Chlorpromazine	Mepazine
Perphenazine	Prochlorperazine
Promazine	Thioridazine
Triflupromazine	

ANTITHYROID DRUGS

Thiourea	Thiouracil
Propylthiouracil	Methimazole

GOLD AND HEAVY METAL SALTS

Aurothioglucose	Gold sodium thiomalate
Auranofin	

ANTICANCER ALKYLATING AGENTS

Cyclophosphamide	Chlorambucil
Mechlorethamine	Bisulfan
Carmustine	Lomustine
Semustine	Streptozotocin
Decarbazine	

OTHERS

Tolbutamide	Quinacrine
Indomethacin	Phenytoin
Quinidine	

Leukemias

Benzene	Nitrosureas
Procarbazine	Cyclophosamide
Mechlorethamine	Chlorambucil
Armustine	Lomustine
Semustine	Ionizing radiation

Higher incidences have been observed in the Far East, perhaps because of the higher prevalence of viral infections, or exposure to drugs and other chemicals. Attempting to sort out the etiology of aplastic anemia in various populations has been exceedingly difficult. More difficult still have been attempts to relate exposure to a specific chemical with aplastic anemia or other bone marrow diseases. Although many chemicals are claimed to cause aplastic anemia, evidence will be presented here only for some examples of well-documented cases in which there is good evidence that exposure to the chemical resulted in bone marrow depression.

Benzene

Benzene is one of the most heavily used industrial chemicals in the world. Approximately 12 billion pounds of benzene are produced each year, mostly during petroleum refining, and smaller quantities from coal during the process of coke formation in the steel industry. Benzene is used for many purposes in chemical synthesis, with a large percentage going into the eventual preparation of polystyrene plastics. Many other industries use benzene as a starting substance for chemical production. Although there are many less toxic replacements available, benzene continues to play an important role as a solvent on a worldwide basis. Exposure of the general public to benzene occurs most frequently when adding gasoline to automobile fuel tanks and during the smoking of cigarettes.

The association between benzene exposure and aplastic anemia was established early in this century. The studies of Santesson[59] and Selling[62] demonstrated that people exposed to benzene in industry, largely by inhalation, demonstrated weakness, hemorrhages, decreased blood levels of circulating cells and, eventually, marrow aplasia. These results were reproduced in inhalation studies in rabbits.[72,73]

A number of studies in industrial situations, for example, Santesson,[59] Selling,[62] Hunter,[37] Goldwater,[27] and Helmer[33] have shown that worker populations exposed to benzene exhibit different stages in the development of aplastic anemia; some demonstrate more severe depressions in blood cell counts than others. Early bone marrow damage may manifest as decreases in erythrocytes, platelets, or leucocytes. With continued exposure, greater bone marrow damage results and decrements in more than one cell type may be observed. Eventually if benzene exposure is not controlled pancytopenia occurs. The extent to which benzene toxicity of varying severity is observed in a given workplace is controlled by several factors. Ultimately the air concentration of benzene is the most important single factor in estimating the severity of the disease in a worker population. Closely related additional factors include the duration of exposure and nature of the job. The longer a worker works at a job that entails benzene exposure, and the greater the number of hours per day that exposure occurs, the greater will be the likelihood of developing benzene toxicity. Location in the plant may be a critical factor. Benzene levels may be higher in some areas than others. Nevertheless, all areas of a plant should be monitored since benzene may accumulate in unlikely locations such as offices removed from plant operations.

The most difficult factor to deal with is the possibility of individual susceptibility. Most workers will demonstrate adverse hematologic effects of benzene when exposed chronically to high concentrations. Although community or household exposure to benzene has been the subject of risk assessments and although clusters of leukemia have been investigated, the link between low-level exposure to benzene and leukemia has not been rigorously demonstrated. At present it is not possible to determine which individuals might be most sensitive to benzene. Earlier suggestions that women and children may be more susceptible than mature

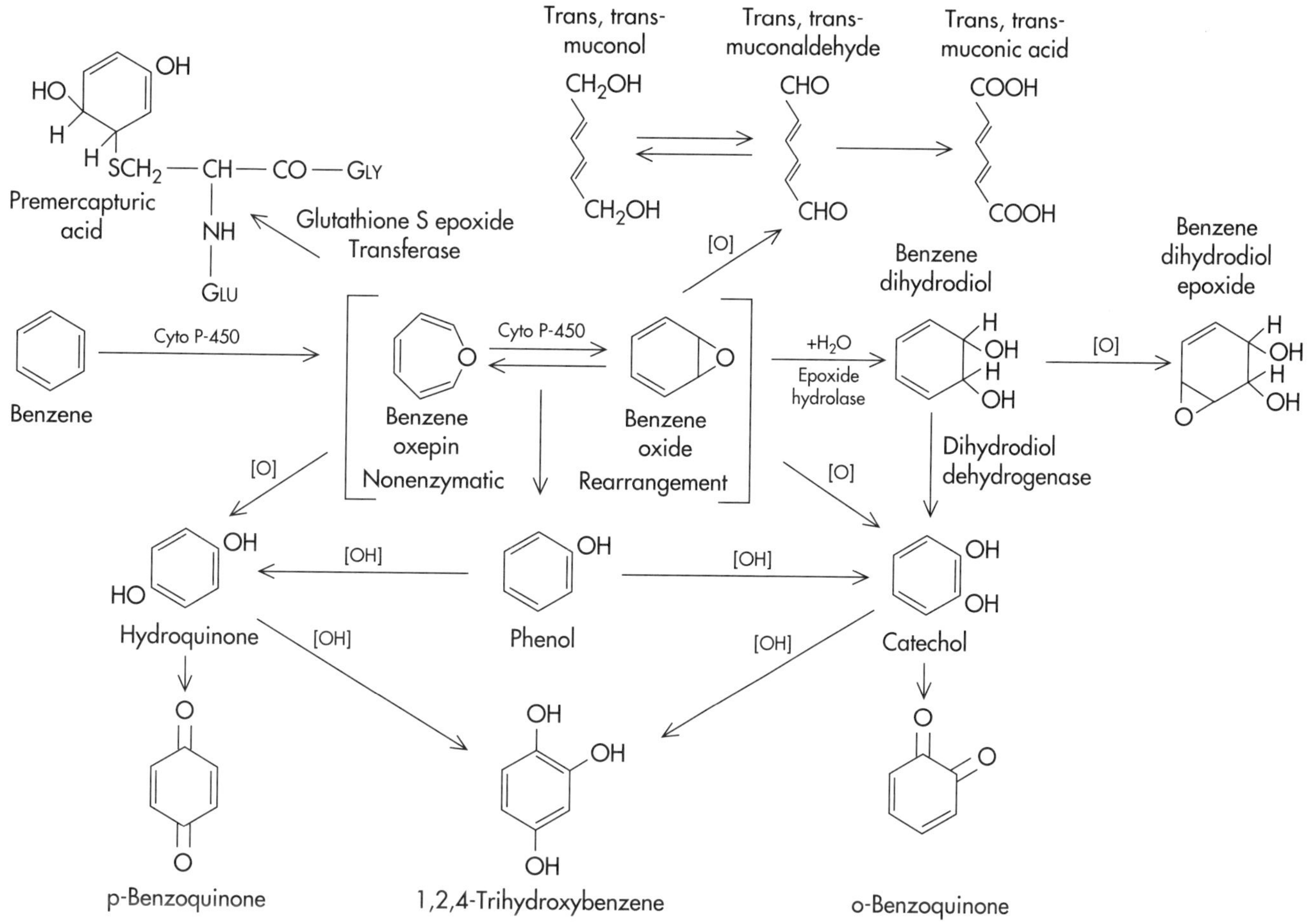

Fig. 17-3. Hepatic metabolism of benzene.

males have not been supported. The possibilities that polymorphisms, with respect to generation of toxic metabolites or excessive sensitivity of the bone marrow, may account for differences in susceptibility have yet to be established. Regardless of differential sensitivity, vigorous efforts are underway in many laboratories to develop biomarkers of exposure to benzene because it is thought that they reflect more accurately the exposure of individuals to benzene than the monitoring of air levels of the chemical.

The mechanism by which benzene produces marrow aplasia is exceedingly complex because it appears to involve several metabolites of benzene, their transport from liver to bone marrow, further metabolism in bone marrow, and the interaction of the metabolites with more than one target in bone marrow. Fig. 17-3 shows the pathway of benzene metabolism in the liver. Benzene is converted to benzene oxide, which is in equilibrium with its oxepin. Cytochrome P 450 2E1 appears to be most active in catalyzing this reaction. The most rapid subsequent reaction is the nonenzymatic rearrangement of the epoxide-oxepin tautomers to yield phenol, which can be further hydroxylated to hydroquinone and catechol. Further hydroxylation may yield 1,2,4-trihydroxybenzene.

Fig. 17-3 shows arrows that postulate the direct conversion of the benzene oxide-benzene oxepin tautomers to hydroquinone and catechol. This proposal is based on the report of Gilmour et al.,[25] which suggested that it was possible to convert some of the oxidized benzene metabolites to hydroquinone without the formation of free phenol. For example, a second hydroxylation may occur with either the oxepin or the oxide, which might then rearrange to give either hydroquinone or catechol.

The phenolic compounds may be conjugated with ethereal sulfate or glucuroic acid. In theory, the conjugates are considered detoxication products because they hasten the excretion of the benzene metabolites. However, in some cases conjugates may serve as mechanisms for the transport of metabolites to target organs.

Other metabolites that may be formed from benzene via the epoxide-oxepin pathway are premercapturic acid, which results from the conjugation of glutathione with the epoxide, and benzene dihydrodiol, which is mediated by the enzyme epoxide hydrolase. The fate of the dihydrodiol lies either in its oxidation via dihydroliol dehydrogenase to yield catechol or its further epoxidation to yield a diol epoxide, which is a postulated but unproven metabolite.[9] Ring opening to yield muconaldehyde, the precursor to the urinary metabolite muconic acid, occurs via an as-yet-unproven mechanism. Further metabolism of muconaldehyde may yield any of several oxidation or reduction products. The figure shows the reduction of the dialdehyde to the dialcohol.

Benzene has been shown to inhibit the formation of CFU-S,[23,28,32,71] CFU-C,[28,70] CFU-E, and BFU-E.[5,61] Studies of the effects of benzene on erythropoiesis suggest that it is also detrimental to maturation at the level of pronormoblast and normoblast, two early erythroid cells, but has little effect on the reticulocyte.[44]

The role of benzene metabolites in mediating these effects has been extensively examined. Studies of erythropoiesis have shown that hydroquinone or catechol given alone to animals reduces red cell production.[29,30] Muconaldehyde and p-benzoquinone, an oxidation product of hydroquinone, are more potent bone marrow toxins than the hydroxylated compounds. Mixtures of phenol with dihydroxylated compounds or muconaldehyde with hydroquinone result in severe bone marrow depression. These results suggest that benzene toxicity is mediated by the action of an array of metabolites rather than by a single metabolite.

Studies of the hematopoietic microenvironment have revealed several effects of benzene metabolites. Gaido and Weirda[20,21] reported that hydroquinone, p-benzoquinone, catechol, and 1,2,4-trihydroxybenzene depressed the ability of bone marrow stromal cells to support the growth of GM-CFU-C cells. In stromal macrophages, hydroquinone and p-benzoquinone inhibit both RNA synthesis[55] and the conversion of IL-1 to mature cytokine.[56] One aspect of the mechanism of benzene toxicity that has yet to be fully explored is the impact of benzene metabolites on the synthesis of key regulatory proteins in bone marrow, such as interleukins and cytokines. Benzene and its metabolites inhibit both nuclear and mitochondrial replication and transcription.[41] Benzene metabolites covalently bind to DNA[45,58] and decrease RNA synthesis. How these effects may play a role in the synthesis of regulatory proteins has yet to be explained.

Thus it appears that the mechanism by which benzene produces aplastic anemia involves inhibition of stem cell and early blast cell maturation. The effects may be due to the activity of several metabolites, such as polyhydroxylated or ring-opened metabolites, working additively or synergistically. Covalent binding of metabolites to DNA may result in inhibition of the synthesis of RNA and of key proteins. DNA replication is inhibited as well.[60] Thus benzene inhibits both maturation and proliferation of cells in the bone marrow.

Chloramphenicol

Chloramphenicol, first developed in the late 1940s, is a broad-spectrum antibiotic.[80] It inhibits protein synthesis in bacterial cells by binding to ribosomal RNA, thereby preventing the reaction with t-RNA to add amino acids, which extend the peptide chain in the course of protein synthesis.

An early sign of toxicity observed in most patients treated with chloramphenicol is an inhibition of erythropoiesis. The effect is concurrent with therapy, is dose-related, and is reversed upon cessation of treatment. The therapeutic blood level of chloramphenicol for treatment of infections is in the range of 20 to 60 µg/ml of blood ($0.5\text{-}2 \times 10^{-4}$M). Significant inhibition of mitochondrial protein synthesis occurs at 10 µg/ml. Because mitochondrial ribosomes bear a resemblance to bacterial ribosomes, chloramphenicol inhibits mitochondrial protein synthesis and, thereby, reduces the availability of ferrochelatase, the enzyme essential for inserting iron into the porphyrin ring system to form heme. The result is a decrease in hemoglobin synthesis and ineffective erythropoiesis. Other heme-containing enzymes such as cytochrome oxidase and cytochrome b are also reduced. The result is inhibition of cellular respiration and decreased ability of erythroid progenitors to proliferate. The selection of the erythroid cell for depression appears to be based on the sensitivity of early stem cells to chloramphenicol. It was shown that chloramphenicol inhibited the growth of CFU-GM cells in culture, but the inhibition was overcome by the addition of colony-stimulating factor (CSF). In contrast, CFU-E cells were inhibited at much lower doses than CFU-GM and erythropoietin did not overcome the effect of chloramphenicol. It appears that the erythroid cells are more sensitive than the myeloid elements to the effects of chloramphenicol.

Early reversible effects on red cells, which can be termed diserythropoiesis, are less severe than chloramphenicol-induced aplastic anemia.[79] Chloramphenicol is the drug that most frequently produces aplastic anemia. Several hundred cases were reported within a few years of its introduction into therapy. As a result, the use of chloramphenicol was restricted and a decrease in reported cases of aplastic anemia was observed. Although diserythropoiesis can be observed in most patients given chloramphenicol, relatively few develop aplastic anemia. However, whereas it appears that the two conditions are not related, it has not been ruled out that sensitivity to early reversible bone effects may predispose to more severe, irreversible effects.

The usual approach to antibiotic therapy is to administer the drug repetitively over a finite time period to ensure against relapse infection by surviving bacteria. The total dose may be great and, in the case of chloramphenicol, may predispose the patient to toxicity. Early stages in bone marrow suppression have been observed, including anemia and leukopenia, but the most common effect is pancytopenia and bone marrow aplasia. The time between treatment and appearance of pancytopenia is in the range of 2 months. Delayed responses are not usually observed.

Chloramphenicol has also been shown to inhibit bone marrow colony-forming activity. Hara et al.[31] studied effects of chloramphenicol using bone marrow preparations from C57B16 male mice where the animals were either treated in vivo and the bone marrow removed for study, or the extracted marrow was treated with the drug. They also used spleen cells and human bone marrow samples. In mice chloramphenicol reduced circulating reticulocytes and inhibited the growth of CFU-E and BFU-E but had no effect on CFU-C. When added in vitro, all three cell types failed to grow. Significant reductions in these colonies was also observed in the human samples of bone marrow in vitro.

Bostrom et al.[8] reported that the growth of human bone marrow stem cells committed to the granulocyte-macrophage cell line (CFU-GM) was stimulated by chloramphenicol at doses in the range of 10 μg/ml in the culture, which is 10 to 100 fold lower than the doses used by Hara et al.[31] When higher doses were used, cell growth was inhibited. Chloramphenicol stimulates at levels below 10 μg/ml in culture. In studies cited above, the levels were about 10 to 100 times greater and showed depression, as did higher levels in the Bostrom[8] study.

It is significant that chloramphenicol, like benzene, also causes adverse effects on bone marrow stromal function. Nara et al.[50] demonstrated that chloramphenicol inhibited fibroblast cultures, CFU-F, which were representative of stromal cells, as well as CFU-C. Thus production of aplastic anemia may well be potentiated when the chemical damages both progenitor cells and microenvironmental cells.

It has been suggested that there is a genetic susceptibility to chloramphenicol-induced bone marrow aplasia. Whereas all treated patients develop some impairment in red cell production, a smaller percentage develop rapidly fatal aplastic anemia. The genetic hypothesis is also supported by the finding of aplastic anemia in twins treated with chloramphenicol. Further studies are needed to verify this hypothesis.

The mechanism by which chloramphenicol acts has not been fully explained. It has been know for many years that in humans most of an administered dose is recovered in the urine as the side chain glucuronide formed at the hydroxymethyl group.[80] In humans products of the reduction of the ring nitro group can be found in the feces, probably due to reduction by intestinal bacteria, but these account for less than 1% of the metabolism. In contrast, the rat excretes much of the dose via the biliary system, thereby presenting the intestinal bacteria with high levels of substrate for reduction of the nitro group. As a result, as much as 25% of the dose may be recovered as aryl nitro and amine derivatives in the feces. Thus, attempts to describe the mechanism of action in humans based on studies in the rat must take differences in metabolism into account.

In a search for other possible toxic metabolites, Yunis and coworkers[80] examined bacterial degradation products of chloramphenicol and suggest that chloramphenicol may be converted into dehydrochloramphenicol (Fig. 17-4), perhaps by intestinal bacteria, re-enter the intestinal tract, and be transported to the bone marrow where the nitro group is reduced to yield a reactive metabolite. Thus Fig. 17-4 shows (1) chloramphenicol, (2) nitrosochloramphenicol, and (3) dehydrochloramphenicol. The postulated reactive intermediate, which has not yet been identified in these systems, would be nitrosodehydrochloramphenicol. Since the nitroso derivative of chloramphenicol can inhibit DNA synthesis, induce strand breaks, and possibly cause DNA degradation, this might be the basis for chloramphenicol-induced aplastic anemia. It must be explained, however, why some people are likely to show this effect whereas most people do not demonstrate aplastic anemia after chloramphenicol treatment.

Aplastic anemia caused by other agents

Textbooks of hematology or reviews of aplastic anemia invariably present long lists of chemicals claimed to have caused marrow aplasia. However, sufficient rigor to establish the cause-and-effect relationship has often been lacking. Epidemiologic studies need to firmly establish the control levels of the diseases within the population in question and to

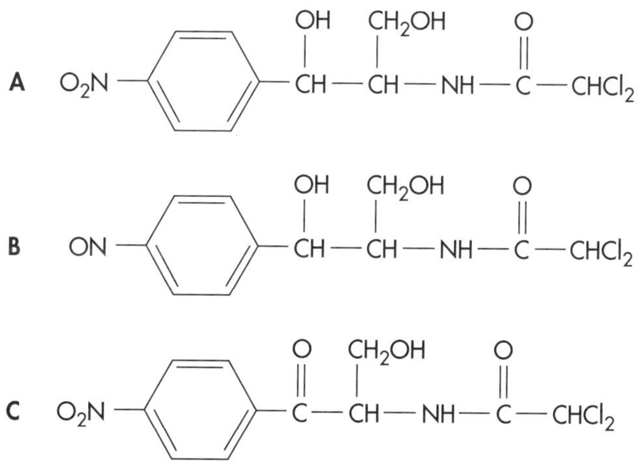

Fig. 17-4. **A,** Chloramphenicol. **B,** Nitrosochloramphenicol. **C,** Dehydrochloramphenicol.

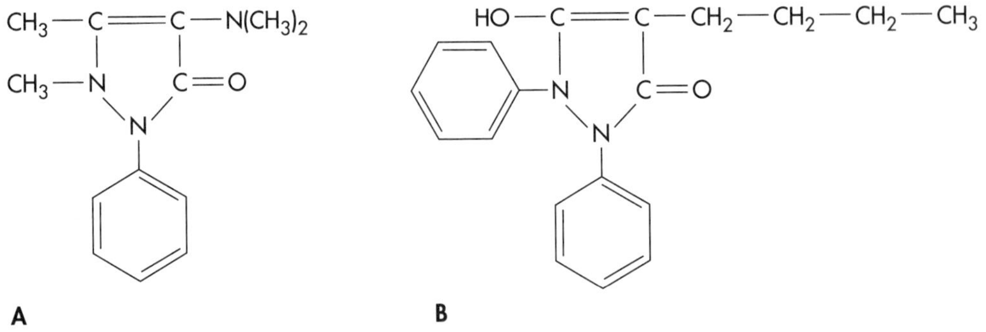

Fig. 17-5. **A,** Aminopyrine **B,** Phenylbutazone. Oxyphenbutazone is structured identically to phenylbutazone except that there is a hydroxyl group where the asterisk is located in the figure.

have a sufficient number of both controls and cases to demonstrate that the study has reasonable statistical power. In a complex society where people often take drugs and are exposed to many chemicals, these studies become very difficult. Nevertheless, some examples of drugs that appear to have the capacity to induce aplastic anemia will be cited.

Nonsteroidal anti-inflammatory agents. Pyrazoline derivatives such as amidopyrine, aminopyrine, antipyrine, and dypirone have been shown to have excellent properties, including analgesic, antipyretic, and antiinflammatory activity. Their use has been either discontinued or severely limited because of their well-documented bone marrow depressant activity. Phenylbutazone, another member of this family of compounds, remains in use because of its excellent antiinflammatory properties, but its use is usually only temporary and must be accompanied by frequent evaluation of circulating blood cell values. The structures of aminopyrine and phenylbutazone are shown in Fig. 17-5.

Early evidence[54] suggested that prior exposure to these compounds may induce an adverse immunologic response to subsequent treatment with the drug. Neutropenia may be observed within 7 to 10 days after beginning therapy with these drugs, but if there has been prior exposure the effects may be seen immediately: precipitous drops in white cell counts may occur, accompanied by chills, fever, tachycardia, anxiety, headache and, occasionally, mild shock. The basis of the neutropenia is the immunologically mediated destruction of circulating neutrophils.

Inman[39] reported that phenylbutazone and its metabolite, oxyphenbutazone, were responsible for a large number of cases of aplastic anemia. A comparison of the effects of phenylbutazone, oxyphenylbutazone, and γ-hydroxyphenylbutazone on human CFU-GM cells[64] revealed that their growth was inhibited by each compound and that prior exposure to phenylbutazone by the individuals whose bone marrows were sampled rendered them more sensitive to the effects on the CFU-GM.

It would appear that the mechanisms by which the pyrazoline congeners cause leukopenia involve both peripheral destruction of white cells and depression of bone marrow functions responsible for leucocyte generation.

Phenothiazines. Phenothiazines are known to produce a mild, transient leukopenia, as well as mild leucocytosis and eosinophilia. In some patients treatment results in agranulocytosis. Because of the rarity of the effect, it would ordinarily be difficult to associate phenothiazine treatment with the occurrence of agranulocytosis. However, for many years people with severe mental diseases, such as schizophrenia, were kept in mental hospitals and given large doses of phenothiazines. An example shown in Fig. 17-6 is chlorpromazine. Given that their health was regularly evaluated, their blood counts done frequently, and the dose and frequency of drug administration were well recorded, and they could be followed for years, it was possible to accurately estimate the development of bone marrow depression in these people and to associate it with phenothiazine treatment. Thus in the United States in 1965, prolonged treatment at high doses resulted in 163 cases of agranulocytosis in people taking chlorpromazine, mepazine, perphenazine, prochlorperazine, promazine, thioridazine, and triflupromazine.[54] A more benign form of mild leukopenia is observed in about 1 in 11 patients given lower doses. It usually disappears even when therapy continues. Those who develop agranulocytosis do so after a latency of about 20 to 40 days and a total dose in the range of 10 to 20 gm of phenothiazine. It was suggested that if a patient does not develop agranulocytosis after 3 months on rigorous therapy, he is unlikely ever to develop the disease. These observations suggest genetic variability in susceptibility to phenothiazines.

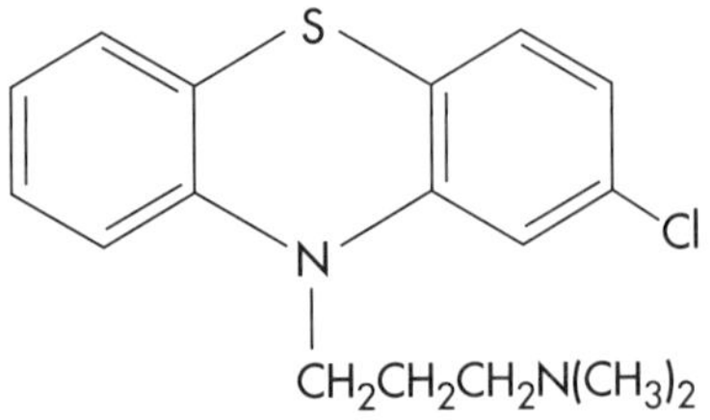

Fig. 17-6. Chlorpromazine, an example of a phenothiazine structure.

Mechanistic studies[54] suggested that chlorpromazine, but not its sulfoxide metabolite, inhibit colony-forming units in human bone marrow. Cessation of treatment results in regrowth of bone marrow cells, suggesting that whereas progenitors may be inhibited, microenvironmental cells may continue to function and allow for recovery of marrow function. It was also suggested that some individuals may display an inherent susceptibility to phenothiazines. In a comparison of the effects of chlorpromazine on granulocyte precursor cells in vitro, using marrow samples taken from controls versus chlorpromazine-sensitive individuals, chlorpromazine inhibited cell replication in both groups but was effective at lower doses in the sensitive group.[54]

Serious effects of phenothiazines apparently occur only after prolonged treatment with high doses. The reduction in the intensive use of these compounds in large numbers of patients in mental hospitals has considerably reduced the incidence of phenothiazine-induced agranulocytosis.

Antithyroid drugs. The very earliest reports on the use of thiourea and thiouracil to treat hyperthyroidism commented on the likelihood that agranulocytosis might accompany therapy. The development of propylthiouracil and methimazole resulted in more effective antithyroid agents that were also less damaging to the bone marrow. Many patients taking these compounds may experience a mild, transient decrease in white cells. However, authorities[24] warn against the potential for bone marrow depression in 3% of patients taking propylthiouracil and 7% of patients taking methimazole. Frank agranulocytosis, a more severe effect, is estimated to occur at an incidence of about 1 in 500 for either agent. Reactions are most likely to occur within the first few weeks or months of therapy. Thus far all antithyroid drugs of this class have displayed some potential for these effects, but for the less severe forms discontinuance of the drug leads to rapid recovery.

Salts of gold and other heavy metals. Gold containing compounds such as aurothioglucose, gold sodium thiomalate, and auranofin act as nonsteroidal anti-inflammatory agents and may be used in patients suffering from rheumatoid arthritis who are refractory to salicylate-type compounds. Their mechanism of action, while not completely elucidated, may be through their inhibitory effects on mononuclear phagocytes, which tend to otherwise accumulate in arthritic joints as part of the inflammatory response.

The most serious adverse response to gold salts has been the high rate of fatal aplastic anemia. The rate of bone marrow depression has been estimated at 1.6 per 10,000, with dozens of cases of aplastic anemia reported. Thrombocytopenia has been reported in 1% of cases, and many cases of leukopenia and agranulocytosis have been reported. Although the mechanism of inhibition is not known, it is significant that several reports have appeared suggesting that immunosuppressive therapy may be effective in preventing the effects of gold on the bone marrow.

Anticancer alkylating agents. Perhaps the most predictive bone marrow suppression occurs in patients receiving alkylating agents to treat various neoplastic diseases. One of the principles of cancer chemotherapy is that cells actively undergoing mitosis are most susceptible to treatment. By the same token however normal body cells, which undergo frequent mitotic events, are equally sensitive to these agents. Among the most rapidly proliferating cells in the body are the bone marrow cells. Therefore cancer chemotherapy patients are usually at risk for bone marrow depression.

The alkylating agents used for cancer chemotherapy are divided into several classes. Among the nitrogen mustards are cyclophosphamide, chlorambucil, and mechlorethamine. Busulfan is a frequently used example of the alkyl sulfonates, and thiotepa is an example of the ethylenimines. The nitrosoureas include carmustine (BCNU), lomustine (CCNU), semustine (methyl-CCNU), and streptozotocin. Other examples of alkylating agents include cisplatin and mitomycin. Finally, dacarbazine is an example of the triazenes. Most are direct-acting agents but some, such as cyclophosphamide, require metabolic activation in the liver.

The fundamental action of the alkylating agents is to react with bases of DNA to produce any of several types of changes. The first reaction is to covalently bind at nucleophilic sites on guanine, cytosine, thymine, or adenine. Some compounds, such as mechlorethamine (Fig. 17-7), may bind to a single site on DNA; others such as a busulfan are bifunctional alkylating agents and may bind two separate bases. If the adduct remains bound, there is a likelihood that DNA replication cannot occur and mitosis will be impaired. Thus growth of the tumor by replication of the cancer cells is retarded. Failure of cancer cells to continue to undergo mitosis is an indication that the cancer is in remission. Survival of cancer cells can lead to recurrence of the disease through the outgrowth of the surviving clone.

The same mechanism of action can occur in bone marrow cells, thereby inhibiting the normal process of maturation and amplification. Alkylating agents, in general, inhibit colony-forming unit activity. Drugs such as busulfan can attack CFU-S and other stem and progenitor cells and result in severe bone marrow depression. Others may produce less severe results during usual therapy, but if the dose is increased or the time of treatment extended, more severe depression can result. It is significant that in addition to the effects on maturation and amplification of bone marrow cells, many of these agents, such as cyclophosphamide, also act as immunosuppressants.

Other reports of bone marrow depression. Many other drugs have been associated with adverse effects on bone marrow, such as tolbutamide, quinacrine, indomethacin, phenytoin, quinidine, and carbimazole. The list is very long and the cause-and-effect relationship between treatment and bone marrow suppression may or may not be well established. If bone marrow depression is observed during the course of drug development, it is frequently well docu-

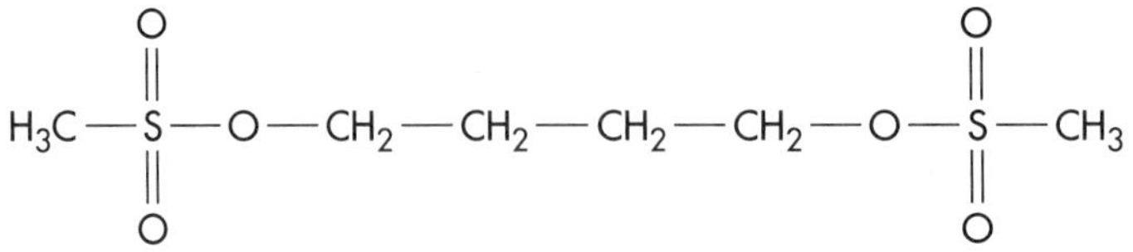

Fig. 17-7. **A,** Mechlorethamine **B,** Busulfan.

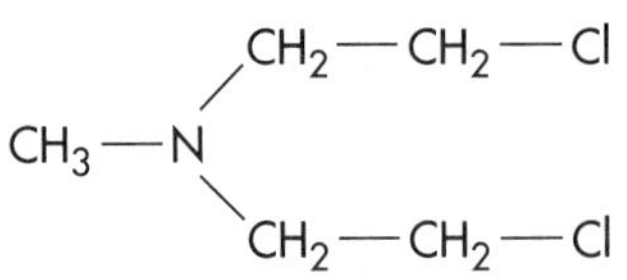

mented. The alternative course of events is for physicians to treat patients with a drug and then report some demonstrated examples of bone marrow depression ranging from simple neutropenia to aplastic anemia. In these cases it is important for the physician to distinguish between the effects of the drug and the possibility that one component of the underlying disease may have been bone marrow depression. Many of these relationships are based on case reports, not necessarily substantiated by epidemiologic or animal studies.

In the case of chemicals claimed to be bone marrow suppressants in the workplace or in the environment at large, establishment of the cause-and-effect relationship is much more difficult because of confounding factors. In the case of drugs, the patient is under the care of a physician who knows the dose that was given, the number of doses, and whether other drugs were also taken. In the case of environmental chemicals, the dose is rarely known, confounding exposures are usually not known, and the physician sees the patient only after the disease has developed. The physician may make the diagnosis and suggests the etiology of the disease on the basis of an interview with the patient and laboratory testing. Epidemiologic studies are needed to validate the association. Usually only chemicals used very extensively, to which many people are exposed, can be shown to have caused bone marrow depression. Whereas there is no question regarding the effect of benzene, the claims of bone marrow suppression by other solvents have been disputed, and it has been claimed that they may have been contaminated with benzene.

Thus, there have been many claims for the production of aplastic anemia by chemicals and drugs. Good data establishing drugs and chemicals as causative agents is frequently lacking. Since many of the claims cannot be ruled out, prudence demands that caution be used when using the chemical or the drug. Periodic monitoring of individuals at risk for bone marrow suppression is warranted. These concerns can only be addressed by thorough evaluation of the effects of these chemicals on bone marrow in the laboratory.

Lead-induced anemia. Lead poisoning, or plumbism, was recognized as a human disease in antiquity.[17,73] Ancient physicians were aware that ingested lead could cause colic and inhaled lead fumes might lead to paralysis. Lead-containing cooking vessels, the enhancement of wine fermentation by lead, the use of lead paint on a variety of forms of pottery, and other uses of lead resulted in reports of palsy, insanity, blindness, weight loss and wasting, and sterility among those who were exposed occupationally and those who were exposed as users of the finished products. In time the appreciation of the dangers of lead and technologic changes have resulted in decreased exposure to lead at high doses in both industry and in the environment.[26,76] The most important recent advances in the control of lead were the introduction of no-lead gasoline and no-lead paint.

Historically, one of the manifestations of lead toxicity has been lead-induced anemia. Attempts to explain the hemotoxic effects of lead have largely focussed on the inhibition of heme synthesis by lead. There is a large body of literature devoted to the mechanism of heme synthesis[68,49] as well as to the study of the mechanism by which lead inhibits heme synthesis.[48,14] Heme is essential to the synthesis of hemoglobin, and decreases in hemoglobin synthesis can be an underlying factor in anemia. The rate-controlling enzyme in the synthesis of heme is the mitochondrial enzyme δ-aminolevulinic acid (ALA) synthetase, which mediates the condensation of glycine and succinyl coenzyme A to yield ALA. Several subsequent steps occur extramitochondrially. Thus, the enzyme ALA dehydratase catalyzes the condensation of two molecules of ALA to form porphobilinogen, the basic building block of all tetrapyrroles. Four molecules of porphobilinogen are assembled by the enzyme uroporphyrinogen I synthetase to form hydroxymethylbilane, which is then cyclized to form the basic tetrapyrrole ring by the enzyme uroporphyrinogen III cosynthase. A series of modifications of the tetrapyrrole ring system then ensues. Uroporphyrinogen III is converted to coproporphyriogen III by uroporphyrinogen decarboxylase; coproporphyrinogen oxidase converts coproporphyringen III to protoporphyrinogen III, which is oxidized in turn to protoporphyrin III by protoporphyrinogen oxidase. Thus the biosynthetic steps leading to protoporphyrin involve uroporphyrinogen, coproporphyrinogen, and protoporphyrinogen. At any stage these can be converted to uroporphyrin, coproporphyrin, or protoporphyrin, respectively, through an oxidative step in which the methylene ($-CH_2-$) groups that link the pyrroles are oxidized to methine (—CH=) groups. (The latter are the forms most likely to be observed in excreta.) The insertion of iron into protoporphyrin III by ferrochelatase in the mitochondrion yields heme. When produced in sufficient quantities heme, acting through a negative feedback loop, decreases the activity of ALA synthetase, thereby reducing the activity of the entire heme synthetic pathway.

Lead intoxication may be associated with elevated levels of ALA in blood, coproporphyrin in urine, and protoporphyrin in erythrocytes. ALA dehydratase is inhibited by low concentrations of lead,[22,3] thereby decreasing the rate of production of substrates for each of the subsequent steps in heme synthesis. Ultimately, less heme is formed, releasing the negative feedback control on ALA synthetase, with the result that ALA synthetase activity increases and more ALA is formed and, in the absence of ALA dehydratase, accumulates.

Although it has been speculated that lead inhibits coproporphyrinogen oxidase and ferrochelatase, there are alternative mechanisms that might explain the increases in urinary coproporphyrin and erythrocyte protoporphyrin. For example, the data suggest that lead may not be a very effective inhibitor of ferrochelatase.[22] The efficiency of ferrochelatase, however, depends upon having available sufficient iron as substrate. A confounding factor is the appreciation that among children of lower socioeconomic status, where lead intoxication is most likely to be observed, there may be a prevalence of iron deficiency.[10,11,63,78] Thus the coupling of lead poisoning and iron deficiency may lead to an increase in unutilized protoporphyrin. The entire metabolic pathway may then back up as manifested by the increase in urinary coproporphyrin derived from coproporphyrinogen, which like protoporphyrin cannot participate in eventual heme synthesis in the absence of iron.

In lead-induced anemia the cells exhibit basophilic stippling and the life span of the erythrocyte is shortened. It has been suggested that enzymes critical to the maintenance of the red cell membrane, such as pyrimidine 5′-nucleotidase,[51] glucose-6-phosphate dehydrogenase, and pentose shunt activity, are reduced.[42] Other authors have suggested that lead may impair globin synthesis.[52] It would appear then that lead-induced anemia may result from a complex series of involvements of lead in both hemoglobin synthesis and the maintenance of erythrocyte membrane integrity.

Strenuous efforts to reduce exposure to lead have reduced the incidence of the anemia of lead poisoning. Current concerns regarding lead have been directed to low blood levels in the range of 15 to 25 µg/dl,[4,57] which appear to have implications relating to central nervous system functions but are below the levels likely to cause impairment of erythropoiesis.

CHEMICALLY INDUCED LEUKEMIA

Chemical carcinogenesis is a field devoted on the one hand to studies aimed at determining whether or not a chemical is a carcinogen and on the other hand to determining the mechanism by which chemicals cause cancer. Carcinogenic mechanisms are thought to include those that originate genetically, usually as a result of a specific mutagenic change in a somatic cell caused by a chemical or one of its metabolites, and those considered epigenetic, that is, they relate to other properties of a chemical, such as alterations in hormonal control of cell replication and changes in receptor function. Most kinds of cancers involve the transformation of a specific cell type to a related cancer cell. In the case of cancers of the blood, which are mostly termed leukemias, the varied nature of bone marrow cells yields a complex picture of cell types. The most frequently described form of leukemia associated with exposure to environmental chemicals or drugs is a group of related diseases that fall under the general heading of acute nonlymphatic leukemia (ANLL), which is also referred to as acute myeloid leukemia (AML). In these diseases large numbers of immature hematopoietic cells proliferate in the bone marrow, where they tend to replace normal progenitor cells of each of the lineages. Furthermore, the circulating blood usually displays large numbers of these cells. In the absence of the usual maturational processes blood contains inadequate numbers of mature erythrocytes, leucocytes, and thrombocytes, and the signs of the disease are in large measure the result of the deficiency of these cells. Untreated ANLL may be fatal within weeks or months.

The diagnosis of the disease requires evaluation of peripheral blood smears to count and characterize the circulating cells. Special attention should be paid to the appearance of immature cell forms. Peripheral white counts are usually elevated but may appear to be in the normal range. Thus examination of bone marrow aspirates and bone marrow biopsy material is needed to fully quantitate and identify the neoplastic cells.

The nomenclature of the ANLL subtypes was established by a French-American-British (FAB) Cooperative group[7] and has helped to allow comparisons between diagnoses made in diverse locations. It is based on morphologic examination and specificity of staining. The first two groups (M1 and M2) refer to the extent to which cells have matured to the myeloblast stage and are called AML with or without maturation to the myeloblast. Other types of leukemia are referred to as acute promyelocytic (M3), acute myelomonocytic (M4), and at least two types of acute monocytic (M5a,M5b). Acute erythroleukemia (M6) and acute megakaryocytic leukemia (M7) are characterized by the presence of immature cells of these lineages. This classification is revised periodically and other forms of leukemia have been described.

ANLL is thought to be a clonal disorder in which one cell, either a stem cell or an early progenitor cell, is transformed and gives rise to a line of neoplastic cells. Although some cells may predominate and give rise to the specific name of the disease, in fact the neoplastic cells may be heterogeneous. AML stem cells have the capacity to self-renew. Attempts to establish colony-forming units (AML-CFU) from neoplastic bone marrow demonstrate that some cells have a high proliferative potential and form large colonies, some have a lower proliferative potential and form small colonies, and others do not proliferate. The cells that arise from these colonies may be more mature than the starting cells but do not reach full maturity, suggesting that maturational block is an important component in the neoplastic process.

It is important to bear in mind that these cells do not grow in vitro in the absence of intercellular mediators. Various growth factors and cytokines active in normal cell maturation are needed to demonstrate leukemic colony-forming units. Furthermore, characterization of these cells on the basis of cell surface immunologic markers has helped to demonstrate their heterogeneity. Clearly a complex series of events ensue from the initial attack of the etiologic factor leading to excessive proliferation of immature cells.

Benzene and leukemia

Although there have been suggestions since the 1930s that benzene induces leukemia,[66] the studies of leukemia in benzene-exposed workers by Vigliani and coworkers[72] in Italy and France, by Aksoy and his colleagues[1] in Turkey, and by Infante et al.[38] in the United States have served to establish the association and have led to stricter controls of benzene exposure in the workplace. Indeed control of exposures to benzene in the workplace was initially established to prevent aplastic anemia. When prevention of leukemia became the major aim, the workplace standards were lowered significantly. The current value is 1 part per million for an 8-hour time-weighted average.

The mechanism by which benzene may cause leukemia has not been well studied because unlike aplastic anemia, there is no convenient animal model for benzene-induced leukemia. Success in demonstrating benzene-induced neoplastic diseases in rodents occurred only after many years of unsuccessful attempts and only through the use of very high doses of benzene for a lifetime. Early studies by Snyder et al.[65] suggested a leukemogenic effect of benzene. More definitive studies by the National Toxicology Program[36] in the United States and Maltoni[47] in Italy suggested that benzene was carcinogenic to the Zymbal gland, a wax-producing gland in the ear of the rat, produced several other solid tumors, and provided some evidence of leukemogenesis.

The demonstration of leukemia in animals is complicated by several factors. In the first instance the major effect of benzene on bone marrow cells is to inhibit cell replication. Leukemia is a disease involving rapid cell replication. At one time benzene was used to treat leukemia because it inhibited leukemic cell replication. Therefore the use of continuous benzene treatment in animals to produce leukemia presents a problem. Cronkite et al.[12] suggested that leukemia might be induced by treating animals for a given period of time and then withdrawing exposure with the intent of allowing the leukemia to express itself. The net effect was the demonstration of a leukemia/lymphoma in mice, which was analogous to leukemia. However this promising model has not been fully pursued to establish a mechanism for benzene-induced leukemia.

Two lines of mechanistic evidence have been developed. The first assumes that either aplastic anemia is a necessary precursor of acute benzene-induced leukemia or that the initial stages in both benzene-induced leukemia and aplastic anemia are the same with a branch point leading either to either aplasia or neoplasia. Thus one effect of benzene may be to inhibit cell replication, leading to aplastic anemia. Alternatively, the effect of benzene may be to cause transformation of and uncontrolled growth of an immature cell type. In either case the study of benzene metabolism, as discussed above, and its effects on bone marrow impairment lends itself to the study of either disease process.

The other approach is based on the finding by Forni et al.[18,19] that benzene-exposed workers display chromosomal aberrations in circulating white cells, which may persist for many years. For those in whom they disappear, there is not likely to be subsequent leukemia. In those who progress to leukemia, the aberrations have usually persisted. Other forms of chromosome damage, such as sister chromatid exchange[16] and micronuclei, have also been reported in benzene-treated animals.[34]

Thus the study of the interaction of benzene with DNA may lead to understanding of the mechanism of benzene-induced chromosome damage as well as the mechanism of benzene-induced leukemia. Indeed there is evidence that benzene metabolites can covalently bind to DNA.[45] However, whether the covalent binding to DNA underlies the mechanism of leukemogenesis has not been established.

The mechanism by which benzene induces leukemia has been difficult to study. If one assumes that carcinogenesis results from the mutation of a gene in a somatic cell, it should be possible to demonstrate the mutagenic activity of the chemical. Benzene has not been shown to be a mutagen in the in vitro test systems commonly used.[13] On the other hand, there has not been adequate examination of the mutagenic properties of its metabolites.

Other chemicals that are well known for their ability to produce aplastic anemia have been related to the production of AML. These include chloramphenicol and phenylbutazone. There are likely to be other chemicals capable of inducing a leukemogenic response, often associated with a period of bone marrow aplasia, but these are difficult to prove in the absence of a well-controlled study of sufficient statistical power to demonstrate the association. The problem is exemplified by attempts by the International Agency for Research on Cancer to determine whether or not some of these compounds are carcinogenic. Thorough literature searches are performed, panels of experts from around the world gather to evaluate the literature, and a consensus is reached based on the strength of the evidence. For example, chloramphenicol has been termed a suspected human carcinogen. Nevertheless whenever leukemia is reported in a patient who has been treated with a bone marrow depressant, it is common for the assumption to be made that the drug was also the cause of the leukemia. This has led many investigators to suspect that leukemia may be a response to bone marrow depression as opposed to a direct initiating effect of the drug. This remains a controversial issue.

Leukemia associated with cancer chemotherapy

It is possible that most chemical-induced AML is the result of treating patients with anticancer alkylating agents. Many patients treated with alkylating agents for lung cancer, ovarian cancer, germ cell tumors, breast cancer, non-Hodgkin's lymphoma, chronic lymphocytic leukemia, multiple myeloma, and other cancers later develop AML. The nitrosoureas, procarbazine, cyclophosphamide, mechlorethamine, chlorambucil, busulfan, armustine, lomustine, and semustine treatment have been related to subsequent leukemia in patients who exhibited remission of the original neoplastic disease and survived long enough to develop leukemia. It is not surprising that radiation therapy potentiates the neoplastic effect, given that radiation exposure of people at Hiroshima and Nagasaki resulted in excessive leukemia. In studies of patients given combined chemotherapy, a comparison of those given MOPP, which includes mechlorethamine, Oncovin (vincristine sulfate), procarbazine, and prednisone and is clearly rich in alkylating agents, with a group given adriamycin, bleomycin, vinblastine, and dacarbazine (ABVD), a mixture that is not rich in alkylating agents, demonstrated that the MOPP group developed a much greater percentage of subsequent leukemia than the ABVD group.

It is important to appreciate that it is not the preexisting neoplastic disease that drives these subsequent neoplastic events. Patients who have been treated for noncancerous diseases such as nephritis, rheumatoid arthritis, psoriasis, multiple sclerosis, systemic lupus erythematosus, and Wegner's granulomatosis with alkylating agents have demonstrated an increased rate of AML. Thus it appears that the alkylating agents are at the root of increased AML in patients treated either for neoplastic or nonneoplastic diseases.

It has been estimated that 10% to 15% of all cases of AML are related to previous treatment with alkylating agents, and the disease may occur as early as 3 years after treatment or after 7 years or more. Treatment of these secondary leukemias is often characterized by resistance to chemotherapy, and the prognosis is generally poor.

REFERENCES

1. Aksoy M, Erdem S, Dincol S: Leukemia in shoe workers exposed chronically to benzene, *Blood* 44:837, 1974.
2. Amdur MO, Doull J, Klaassen CD: *Casarett and Doull's toxicology, the basic science of poisons,* ed 4, New York, 1991, Pergamon.
3. Astrin KH et al: δ-Aminolevulinic acid dehydratase isozymes and lead toxicity, *Ann NY Acad Sci* 514:23, 1987.
4. Agency for Toxic Substances and Disease Registry: The nature and extent of lead poisoning in children in the United States: a report for congress. Atlanta, 1988, U.S. Department of Health and Human Services.
5. Baarson K, Snyder CA, Albert RE: Repeated exposures of C57B16 mice to 10 ppm inhaled benzene markedly depressed erythropoietic colony formation, *Toxicol Lett* 20:337, 1984.
6. Bagby GC Jr, Segal GM: Growth factors and the control of hematopoiesis. In Hoffman R et al: *Hematology, basic principles and practice,* New York, 1991, Churchill Livingstone.
7. Bennett JM et al: Proposed revised criteria for the classification of acute myeloid leukemia, *Ann Intern Med* 103:626, 1985.
8. Bostrom B, Smith K, Ramsay NKC: Stimulation of human committed bone marrow stem cells, (CFU-GM) by chloramphenicol, *Exp Hematol* 14:146, 1986.
9. Busby WF et al: Lung tumorigenicity of benzene oxide, benzene dihydrodiols and benzene diolepoxides in the BLU:Ha newborn mouse assay, *Carcinogenesis* 11:1473, 1990.
10. Clark M, Royal J, Seeler R: Interaction of iron deficiency and lead and the hematologic findings in children with severe lead poisoning, *Pediatrics* 81:247, 1988.
11. Cohen AR, Trotzky MS, Pincus D: Reassessment of the microcytic anemia of lead poisoning, *Pediatrics* 67:904, 1981.
12. Cronkite E, et al: Benzene inhalation produces leukemia in mice, *Toxicol Appl Pharmacol* 75:358, 1984.
13. Dean BJ: Recent findings on the genetic toxicology of benzene, toluene, xylenes and phenols, *Mutation Res* 154:153, 1985.
14. de Bruin A, Hoolboom H: Early signs of lead-exposure, *Br J Industr Med* 24:203, 1967.
15. Ehrlich P: Uber die specifischen granulationed des blutes, *Arch Anat Physiol Abt* 2:571, 1879.
16. Erexson GL, Wilmer JL, Klingerman AD: Induction of sister chromatid exchanges and micronuclei in male DBA/2 mice after inhalation of benzene, *Environ Mut* 6:408, 1984.
17. Finkel AJ: Lead. In *Hamilton and Hardy's industrial toxicology,* ed 4, Littleton, Mass, 1983, PSG Publishing.
18. Forni A, Pacifico E, Limonta A: Chromosome studies in workers exposed to benzene or toluene or both, *Arch Environ Hlth* 22:373, 1971.
19. Forni A et al: Chromosome changes and their evolution with past exposure to benzene, *Arch Environ Hlth* 23:385, 1971.
20. Gaido KW, Weirda D: In vitro effects of benzene metabolites on mouse bone marrow stromal cells, *Toxicol Appl Pharmacol* 76:45, 1984.
21. Gaido KW, Weirda D: Modulation of stromal cell function in DBA/2J and B6C3F1 mice exposed to benzene or phenol, *Toxicol Appl Pharmacol* 81:469, 1985.
22. Gibson SLM, Goldberg A: Defects in haem synthesis in mammalian tissues in experimental lead poisoning and experimental porphyria, *Clinical Science* 38:63, 1970.
23. Gill D et al: The importance of pluripotent stem cells in benzene toxicity, *Toxicology* 16:163, 1980.
24. Gillman AG et al: *The pharmacological basis of therapeutics,* ed 7, New York, 1985, Macmillan.
25. Gilmour SK, Kalf GF, Snyder R: Comparison of the metabolism of benzene and its metabolite in rat liver microsomes. In Kocsis JJ et al, eds: *Biological reactive intermediates III: mechanisms of action in animal models and human disease,* New York, 1986, Plenum.
26. Goldberg A: Annotation: lead poisoning and haem biosynthesis, *Br J Haematol* 23:521, 1972.
27. Goldwater LJ: Disturbances in the blood following exposure to benzene, *J Lab Clin Med* 26:957, 1941.
28. Green JD et al: Acute and chronic dose/response effects of inhaled benzene on multipotential hemopoietic stem (CFU-S) and granulocyte/macrophage progenitor (GM CFU-C) cells in CD-1 mice, *Toxicol Appl Pharmacol* 58:492, 1981.

29. Guy RL et al: Interactive inhibition of erythroid [^{59}Fe] utilization by benzene metabolites in female mice, *Chem-Biol Interact* 74:55, 1990.
30. Guy RL et al: Depression of iron uptake into erythrocytes in mice by treatment with the combined benzene metabolites p-benzoquinone, muconaldehyde and hydroquinone, *J Appl Tox* 11:443, 1991.
31. Hara H et al: Effect of chloramphenicol on colony formation from erythrocytic precursors, *Am J Hematol* 5:123, 1978.
32. Harigaya K et al: The detection of in vivo liquid bone marrow cultures, *Toxicol Appl Pharmacol* 60:346, 1981.
33. Helmer KJ: Accumulated cases of chronic benzene poisoning in the rubber industry, *Acta Med Scand* 118:254, 1944.
34. Hite M et al: The effect of benzene in micronucleus test, *Mut Res* 77:149, 1980.
35. Hoffman R et al, eds: *Hematology, basic principles and practice,* New York, 1991, Churchill Livingstone.
36. Huff JE et al: Multiple-site carcinogenicity of benzene in Fischer 344 rats and B6C3F1 mice, *Env Hlth Persp* 82:125, 1989.
37. Hunter FT: Chronic exposure to benzene (benzol). II. The clinical effects, *J Ind Hyg* 21:331, 1939.
38. Infante PF et al: Leukemia in benzene workers, *Lancet* 2:76, 1977.
39. Inman WH: Study of fatal bone marrow depression with special reference to phenylbutazone and oxyphenbutazone, *Br Med J* 1500, 1977.
40. Jimenez JJ et al: Chloramphenicol-induced bone marrow injury: possible role of bacterial metabolites of chloramphenicol, *Blood* 70:1180, 1987.
41. Kalf GF: Recent advances in the metabolism and toxicity of benzene, *Crit Rev Toxicol* 18:141, 1987.
42. Lachant NA, Tomoda A, Tanaka KR: Inhibition of the pentose phosphate shunt by lead: a potential mechanism for hemolysis in lead poisoning, *Blood* 63:518, 1984.
43. Laitha LC: The common ancestral stem cell. In Wintrobe MW, ed: *Blood, pure and elegant,* New York, 1980, McGraw-Hill.
44. Lee EW, Kocsis JJ, Snyder R: The use of ferrokinetics in the study of experimental anemia, *Env Hlth Perspect* 39:29, 1981.
45. Lutz WK, Schlatter CH: Mechanism of the carcinogenic action of benzene: irreversible binding to rat liver DNA, *Chem-Biol Interact* 18:241, 1977.
46. Mahaffey Six K, Goyer RA: The influence of iron deficiency on tissue content and toxicity of ingested lead in the rat, *J Lab Clin Med* 79:128, 1972.
47. Maltoni C, Conti B, Cotti G: Benzene: a multipotential carcinogen; results of long-term bioassays performed at the Bologna Institute of Oncology, *Am J Ind Med* 4:589, 1983.
48. Moore MR, Goldberg A: Health implications of the hematopoietic effects of lead. In Mahaffey KR, ed: *Dietary and environmental lead: human health effect,* Amsterdam, 1985, Elsevier.
49. Murray RK et al: Porphyrins & bile pigments, In *Harper's biochemistry,* ed 22, Norwalk, Conn, 1990, Appleton & Lange.
50. Nara N et al: Effects of chloramphenicol on hematopoietic inductive microenvironment, *Exp Hematol* 10:20, 1982.
51. Paglia DE, Valentine WN, Dahlgren JC: Effects of low-level lead exposure on pyrimidine 5'-nucleotidase and other erythrocyte enzymes, *J Clin Invest* 65:1164, 1975.
52. Pagliuca A et al: Lead poisoning: clinical, biochemical and haematological aspects of a recent outbreak, *J Clin Pathol* 43:277, 1990.
53. Pappenheim A: Abstammung und einstehung der roten blutzelle, *Archiv für Anatomie und Physiologie Anatomische Abt,* 22:89, 1898.
54. Pisciotta AV: Immune and toxic mechanisms in drug-induced agranulocytosis, *Sem in Hemat* 10:279, 1973.
55. Post GB, Snyder R, Kalf GF: Metabolism of benzene and phenol in macrophages in vitro and the inhibition of RNA synthesis by benzene metabolites, *Cell Biol Toxicol* 2:231, 1986.
56. Renz JF, Kalf GF: A role for interleukin-1 in benzene-induced hematotoxicity: inhibition of the conversion of pre-IL-1X to mature cytokine in murine macrophages by hydroquinone and the prevention of benzene-induced hematotoxicity in mice by interleukin-1, *Blood* 78:938, 1991.
57. Ritchey AK, Zaboy KA: Hematologic manifestations of childhood illness. In Hoffman R, eds: *Hematology, basic principles and practice,* New York, 1991, Churchill Livingstone.
58. Rushmore T, Kalf G, Snyder R: Covalent binding of benzene and its metabolites to DNA in rabbit bone marrow mitochondria in vitro, *Chem-Biol Interact* 49:133, 1984.
59. Santesson CG: Chronic poisoning with coal tar benzene: four deaths, *Arch Hyg (München)* 31:336, 1897.
60. Schwartz C, Snyder R, Kalf G: The inhibition of mitochondrial DNA replication in vitro by metabolites of benzene, hydroquinone and p-benzoquinone, *Chem-Biol Interact* 53:327, 1986.
61. Seidel HJ, Barthel E, Zinser D: The hematopoietic stem cell compartments in mice during and after long-term inhalation of three doses of benzene, *Exp Hematol* 17:300, 1989.
62. Selling L: Benzol as a leukotoxin; studies on degeneration regeneration of blood and hematopoietic organs, *Johns Hopkins Hospital Rep* 17:83, 1917.
63. Six KM, Goyer RA: The influence of iron deficiency on tissue content and toxicity of ingested lead in the rat, *J Lab Clin Med* 79:128, 1972.
64. Smith CS, Chinn S, Watts RWE: The sensitivity of human bone marrow granulocyte/macrophage precursor cells to phenylbutazone, oxyphenbutazone and γ-hydroxyphenylbutazone in vitro, with observations on the bone marrow colony formation in phenylbutazone-induced granulocytopenia, *Biochem Pharmacol* 26:847, 1977.
65. Snyder CA et al: The inhalation toxicology of benzene: incidence of hematopoietic neoplasms and hematotoxicity in AKR/J and C57BI/6J mice, *Toxicol Appl Pharmacol* 54:323, 1980.
66. Snyder R, Kocsis JJ: Current concepts of chronic benzene toxicity, *CRC Crit Revs Toxicol* 3:265, 1975.
67. Swanson M, Cook R: Drugs, *chemicals and blood dyscrasias,* Hamilton, Ill, 1977, Drug Intelligence Publications.
68. Tait GH: General aspects of haem synthesis. In Goodwin TW, ed: *Porphyrins and related compounds,* London, 1968, Academic Press.
69. Till JE, McCulloch EA: Direct measurement of the radiation sensitivity of normal mouse bone marrow, *Radiat Res* 14:213, 1961.
70. Toft K et al: Toxic effects on mouse bone marrow caused by inhalation of benzene, *Arch Toxicol* 51:295, 1982.
71. Uyeki EM et al: Acute toxicity of benzene inhalation to hemopoietic precursor cells, *Toxicol Appl Pharmacol* 40:49, 1977.
72. Vigliani EC, Saita G: Benzene and leukemia, *N Engl J Med,* 217:872, 1964.
73. Waldron HA: The anaemia of lead poisoning: a review, *Brit J Industr Med* 23:83, 1966.
74. Weiskotten HG, Shwartz SC, Steinsland HS: The action of benzol on blood and blood forming tissues, *J Med Res* 35:63, 1916.
75. Weiskotten HG et al: The action of benzol. VI. Benzol vapor leucopenia (rabbit), *J Med Res* 41:425, 1920.
76. White LM, Selhi HS: Annotation: Lead and the red cell, *Br J Haematol* 30:133, 1975.
77. Williams WJ, *Hematology,* ed 2, New York, 1977, McGraw-Hill.
78. Yip R, Norris TN, Anderson AS: Iron status of children with elevated blood lead, *J Pediatr* 98:922, 1981.
79. Yunis AA: Chloramphenicol: relation of structure to activity and toxicity, *Ann Rev Pharmacol Toxicol* 28:83, 1988.
80. Yunis AA: Chloramphenicol toxicity: 25 years of research, *Am J Med* 87:3-44N-3-48N, 1989.

Part III

CLINICAL ENVIRONMENTAL MEDICINE

Chapter 18

CLINICAL APPROACH AND ESTABLISHING A DIAGNOSIS OF AN ENVIRONMENTAL MEDICAL DISORDER

Mark R. Cullen
Linda Rosenstock
Stuart M. Brooks

Concerns of the patient and the practitioner
    The patient's perspective and concerns
    The physician's perspective and concerns
    Reasons for which a patient is referred to a physician
The clinical approach in environmental medicine
Step 1: Establishing the clinical characteristics of the medical condition
Step 2: Characterizing exposure
Step 3: Demonstrating a correlation between exposure and clinical manifestations
Step 4: Establishing the diagnosis of an environmental medical condition
Summary

Diagnosis of an environmental medical condition demands an approach similar to that used by physicians for diagnosis of other medical conditions. The physician practicing environmental medicine interviews the patient, inquiring about clinical symptoms, potential risk factors, and details of exposures indices; additional information includes past medical information, family history, hobbies, habits, and a review of systems. The clinical approach to an environmental medical problem requires the kinds of expertise that physicians have learned through medical and residency training and years of practice experience; however, because many practitioners are not familiar with the science of environmental medicine (which is rarely taught in medical school, residency training, or postgraduate education programs), this chapter addresses the matter more comprehensively.

The practitioner is compelled to play several roles as the care provider. First, the environmental medicine professional must acquire the skills necessary to define and diagnose environmentally-related medical conditions, which require education and experience, and it is anticipated that this text will assist in the process. The novice environmental medicine practitioner may gain experience by consulting with experts or using other resources (see Appendix 3) and by spending concentrated time practicing the medical specialty. Second, the physician must become adept at treating the patient and providing preventive strategies. (See Section 6.) Finally, the physician must be a skillful communicator. Because environmental medicine deals with disease risks in populations, it may not be possible to establish with certainty that disease seen in an individual patient has been caused by an environmental exposure. The physician or other health-care professional must communicate information about the probability that a disease was caused by an environmental exposure. There is often a dichotomy between what the patient believes to be an environmental health issue and what is supported by facts. The practitioner must be able to communicate the scientific information about risks in a way that is understandable to the patient. (See Chapters 4 and 67.)

CONCERNS OF THE PATIENT AND THE PRACTITIONER

The patient's perspective and concerns

The patient may be concerned about an environmental exposure or an environmentally induced illness. For example, the patient or some other party may suspect that some medical symptoms, signs, or laboratory abnormalities are due to an environmental factor. Alternatively, the patient may suspect that his or her actual disease is related to an environmental factor. Finally, a patient who has been exposed to a known environmental hazard may be concerned about the possibility of developing a disease.

The physician's perspective and concerns

When a clinical problem exists, the physician must weigh the possibility that it may be due to an environmental exposure. To address the concern thoroughly, the practitioner must search the scientific literature and other informational resources to determine whether the exposure or exposures can lead to the observed health effect and whether the temporal course of events from exposure to clinical manifestations is consistent with the information presented. If the exposure is capable of causing the observed effect, the next question is, how likely is the possibility of disease based on the exposure assessment and the presenting clinical pattern? This question can be posed in another manner. Given a hypothetical person who is similar to the patient and who suffers an exposure of similar duration and dose, how likely is it that a disease will occur? In other words, what is the risk for disease given the exposure indices (dose and duration)? Finally, the physician must decide what further studies or tests offer the best chance of determining whether the disease is environmentally induced. It is important to apply laboratory tests that best pertain to the patient's exposure or exposures and then explain the results of these laboratory tests in an epidemiologic sense, that is, the likelihood of a positive test result among persons having exposures similar to the patient's. In this context, of particular interest are specialized tests with high levels of predictive value.

Reasons for which a patient is referred to a physician

Individuals may seek the services of an environmental specialist for reasons that are dissimilar from those in other clinical practices. The evaluation of a patient suspected of having an environmental medical problem is not usually a straightforward differential diagnosis resulting in clearly recognized pathophysiologic processes. Other concerns, including social factors, must be considered. The sources of referral may include employers, lawyers, community groups, insurance companies, and governmental agencies as well as physicians. The mixture likely depends on the type of practice setting and perhaps factors unique to the practitioner or the institution. In some cases, the relationship between the patient and the practitioner is affected by the demands of third parties. What does the referring party expect from the examination? What do they want? How will they use the information? These issues are often clear to the patient and must be understood by the physician. Even when a patient is referred by another physician, there may be a hidden agenda, that is, interests of someone who has encouraged the referral, such as a lawyer or an insurance company.

In some cases the patient is a self-referral, and such patients may embody a different set of questions and conceptions. What has induced the patient to seek the consultation? Why now? What does the patient want? These expectations have important implications. Whatever the source of the patient and whatever the agendas of the patient and other parties, the ultimate diagnosis may well have clinical, economic, legal, and social consequences for both the patient and other parties. Importantly, these consequences may not be initially grasped by all the parties. Therefore, these nonmedical factors must be elicited and evaluated along with the diagnostic information that forms the technical basis for decisions. These nonmedical factors may be as important as the technical issues in the final explanation of the case and any eventual therapeutic decisions.

Health perceptions. Patients usually search for health care because they are experiencing symptoms or because they are concerned about future health problems. A patient's perception of a possible health risk might be a reason for the visit. There is currently both an increased consciousness and yet more confusion about environmental risks. The new awareness of environmental hazards comes from changes in our societal view about chemicals and other hazards, notification requirements of new laws, and wide public attention to certain environmental hazards. Most people have insufficient knowledge to discriminate between possibilities and probabilities and are unsophisticated about the concept of dose and risk. For example, many patients believe that a minor exposure may confer imminent risk of serious disease. At the other end of the spectrum, some people seriously underestimate major risks and neglect to act properly.

Misunderstanding of risk per se is not formidable to deal with and should not influence the diagnostic assessment. The environmental medical evaluation, however, demands that the physician have a sophisticated appreciation of the sources of patient misunderstanding, which may be deep-seated and linked to broader issues that bring the patient to the practitioner's office. The perception of risk and harm may be connected to social or family problems, such as a community's fight against a toxic waste site or distress over a child's physical development or behavior. The patient's information may have been obtained from a highly respected source within the patient's circle, including poorly informed physicians; the latter situation may be difficult to unravel.

Finally, a patient's personality traits can be important; this includes such factors as personality style (for example, anxious, paranoid, or obsessive) or general viewpoint about health (for example, those who externalize all misfortune, in contrast to those who internalize it).

For these reasons, it is important to establish not only what the patient believes might be going on but also the basis for that belief, which may have a substantial impact on diagnostic decision making. Sometimes, more testing may need to be performed than might have been necessary in another situation. Sometimes, it may be necessary for the clinician to talk with others to better understand the patient's perceptions. In environmental medicine, the basis for a diagnostic determination can be as important as the determination itself.

Exploring the home and family situation. In environmental medicine the family takes on a special dimension. The home itself may sometimes be the focus of the environmental exposure because of a hazard thought to be present in the air, walls and furnishings, or water supply (for example, see Chapter 38). This jeopardy to family health may have symbolic importance that surpasses health risk or impact. Grasping the significant role of the home and how a poison within the home threatens the family's sense of well-being is basic to the practice of environmental medicine. Not only is the home important symbolically, it is often the basis for a family's social and economic security. People do not easily leave their homes, even under the most formidable of environmental threats. This lesson was painfully learned at Love Canal and Times Beach, where forced relocations led to social disruption of many families. The likelihood that a hazard may lower property values based on environmental risk heightens the sense of threat.

The knowledge that an environmental risk may be smaller than other exposure situations must never cause the physician to dismiss concerns about that risk. This concept is reflected in environmental laws, in which far lower orders of risk are accepted in residential air and water than in occupational settings. On the other hand, the fundamental principles of dose-response hold true, irrespective of setting. Although a hazard in the home may affect persons at special risk, such as pregnant women, children, the elderly, and patients with chronic diseases, and may provide unusual opportunities for exposure during daily activities such as bathing and cleaning, there is nothing biologically special about the home to correspond to its social and psychologic significance. Actual risks and disease likelihoods are assessed as for any other environment. What differs is the need to develop a special appreciation for the information and concerns presented by the patient.

Agendas of third parties. In environmental medicine many patients are referred by lawyers, insurance companies, or governmental agencies. The interests of these outside parties must not significantly influence how the physician approaches the patient's diagnostic work-up or attributes environmental risks; however, these parties may limit access to information or even misrepresent facts and could interfere with the clinician's ability to make the correct diagnosis or risk estimation. Although some of the methods used are subtle, such as the provision of highly selected information, others are very direct, such as withholding necessary information about exposure or others with disease. Outside parties may expect diagnostic studies that are otherwise unnecessary or possibly confusing, further entangling diagnosis. For all these reasons, the potential interest of each of any third parties should be appraised as part of the diagnostic evaluation.

Lawyers. Many practitioners find the adversarial nature of the law distasteful. It is important to remember that attorneys present the facts of a situation in a way that maximizes the economic or legal benefit of their client. It is not the lawyer's role to establish the ultimate truth. This responsibility falls to the judge, administrator, or jury who has had the opportunity to hear the case, adversarial by design, of opposing parties. Obviously, legal truth may differ from medical truth.

For these reasons, the clinician should establish whether lawyers are involved in an environmental health issue under evaluation and then understand that attorneys will attempt to serve the best interests of their clients. The lawyer's view is not intended to be balanced or is it necessarily designed to protect the patient's health. It must be recognized that the information obtained from attorneys may represent biased information. The physician must question its completeness and balance; however, the physician's attitude about information supplied by the attorney must not seriously jeopardize the physician's relationship with the patient and lead to suspicion or derision of the patient because of the behavior of a lawyer. The physician must deal with many concerns and issues of the patient, of which the legal case is just one.

Employers. Generalizations about employers are difficult because they differ enormously in their knowledge and concern about environmental health issues. Nonetheless, it is important to appreciate several aspects common to all. In the vast majority of cases, risks, however great, are usually inadvertent aftermaths of industrial processes. However concerned an employer may be, environmental health affairs rarely advance business considerations. Managers rarely lose sight of their priorities and the ''bottom line'' as they process information and react to recommendations for change. On the other hand, employee or community health problems may become business considerations because of liability or serious community or worker concern about their activities.

For these reasons, physicians function most effectively with a uniform, factual, yet professionally dispassionate relationship with employers. Patient information that is relevant legally and ethically can be shared promptly to facilitate legitimate business needs. The physician must not allow business concerns to impede obtainment of the information necessary for patient evaluation and management, but must appreciate the fact that economic considerations affect employer responses.

A somewhat less clear issue is the relationship with employer-paid professional consultants. Many companies, especially smaller ones, employ no environmental professionals and may not be aware that they are creating an environmental hazard. If an employer employs medical or environmental health personnel, it is reasonable to assume a far higher level of knowledge and competence. Medical personnel, including nurses and physicians, are generally knowledgeable about the ethical and legal guidelines that require them to act in the best health interest of a patient. The same is not uniformly true of environmental professionals who are not health oriented. Although such personnel are often the most knowledgeable about environmental information needed for evaluation or treatment decisions, they may not feel bound by the same code of ethical responsibility that distinguishes physicians and nurses from their employer. For this reason, special care to protect confidentiality is requisite when information is exchanged with these otherwise invaluable sources.

The physician's agenda. Rarely in clinical medicine is the physician's own role in the patient's care a consequential source of bias in the evaluation; however, in environmental medicine this possibility merits express consideration along with the agendas of the patient and the third parties. There are at least three grounds on which conscious or subconscious physician influence may occur. The first is philosophic. Physicians often have well-developed viewpoints about the environment, one of the most widely discussed social issues of our time. The physician's philosophy on this subject could influence his or her perception of a difficult case, be it a strong conviction that polluters are destroying the planet (and human health) or the contrary belief that environmental concerns are interfering with necessary progress and development. As already mentioned, many physicians have negative feelings about lawyers and lawsuits, which may be a source of subconscious bias against litigants, whatever the merit of their case.

Social relationships are also a basis for subtle or not so subtle influences. Physicians may be friends, neighbors, or fellow club members with important players in environmental medical cases. This party may be the patient, family member, corporate manager, or attorney. These relationships can engender a sense of trust that could obscure professional judgment when the facts on which a diagnosis is made are weighed.

Last, and perhaps most deplorably, is the potential for direct financial interference in the diagnostic process. Often lawyers or corporations are prepared to pay substantial sums of money for opinions that protect their interests. Physicians who have been sympathetic in the past stand to be consulted again, which in some circumstances could constitute a serious conflict of interest. Conversely, physicians who sympathetically but uncritically support their patients' beliefs that their illness results from environmental exposures may find that this support is a source of lucrative referrals. There are, of course, no easy solutions to these sources of bias or influence. It is best to recognize that they occur and that they may influence various parties, including the physician.

THE CLINICAL APPROACH IN ENVIRONMENTAL MEDICINE

There are four steps in the diagnosis of environmental medical condition. The first step is to establish the characteristics of the medical condition. Second, the physician carefully defines the environmental exposure. The third step is to demonstrate a correlation between the exposure and the clinical manifestations. Finally, the diagnosis should be based on aggregation and interpretation of all available data (Fig. 18-1).

The more information available, the clearer the diagnostic puzzle becomes. When several pieces of the puzzle have been assembled, it becomes more apparent when a piece does not fit. This is most obvious when symptoms seem out of proportion to other findings. Thus, there is a need for more than one piece of information to interpret the full significance of individual pieces of the puzzle. Unless the physician uses all available information, an accurate or definitive diagnosis cannot be made. It cannot be emphasized strongly enough that relying only on symptoms and taking an incomplete environmental history are inadequate for making a decision on an environmental disease. Once the physician has obtained the necessary medical, environmental, and toxico-

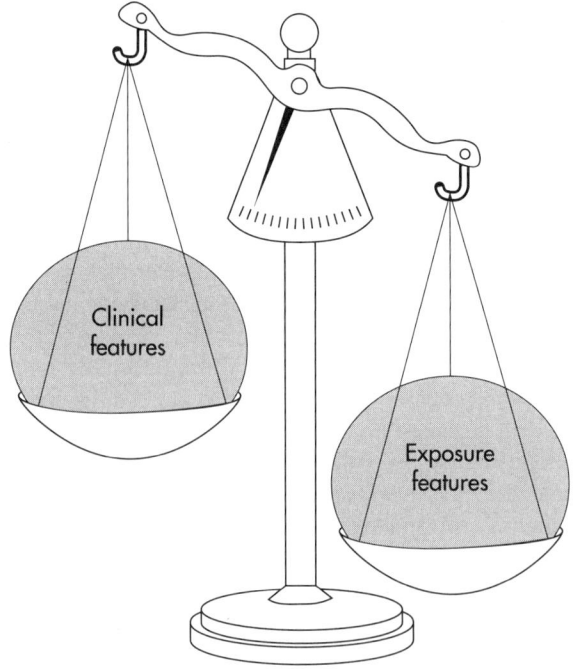

Fig. 18-1. The physician must clearly weigh illness and the exposure parameters. Too much emphasis on the exposure side of the balance and not enough focus on understanding the clinical presentation may lead to an inaccurate diagnosis. The alternative situation is also true.

logic information, a decision can generally be made about whether a specific environmental exposure plays a role in a medical disorder. It may be added that the environmental exposure may be only a contributing factor to disease and need not be the sole cause. Indeed, most disease is multifactorial, and the exposure may represent only one factor contributing to disease pathogenesis.

Step 1: Establishing the clinical characteristics of the medical condition

Chapters 2, 4, and 19 have emphasized the importance of exposure information in the evaluation of an environmental medical problem. Of much greater clinical significance is the need to characterize the clinical manifestations and determine the extent and nature of the patient's complaints, which require spending sufficient time for a proper work-up of the patient. Sometimes the patient presents with a list of subjective complaints for which no objective pathologic entity or biochemical alterations are identified. Because such an illness may seem perplexing, it may be labeled an environmental illness because the physician is unable to develop a more specific diagnosis. We wish to emphasize that the physician has an obligation to define the characteristics of the illness clearly, not only the symptoms, but also the functional and biochemical alterations that characterize the illness. The exposure history alone cannot establish a diagnosis. An exposure does not equate to disease, just as disease presence does not necessarily indicate there was an environmental exposure.

For all practical purposes, a correct diagnosis in environmental medicine is made by relating a health effect to an exposure. Although exploring the exposure details is often challenging, it is most important to establish on a pathophysiologic basis for what is wrong with the patient. The formulation of the pathophysiologic basis for complaints logically precedes consideration of causes. Although knowledge of potential causes, such as a history of exposure to a particular hazard or membership in a group with a high rate of a certain disease, may alter the strategy, the logical flow is to proceed from evaluation of health to evaluation of the environmental and other causal factors.

Environmental diseases are not unique. The clinical and pathologic expressions of most environmentally caused diseases cannot be distinguished from those of nonenvironmental origin. The belief that diseases of environmental origin are distinctive is widespread among health care providers and the public. As a consequence, consideration of environmental causes during the work-up of a complaint is often deferred until after more common disease possibilities are excluded. The idea that the environmental diseases caused are distinctive leads to the clinical practice of anticipating that specialists will recognize these special features and call them to the primary clinician's attention. In reality, diseases caused by hazards in the environment are neither rare nor distinctive, given their clinical presentations and usual laboratory findings. Typically such disorders are commonplace in appearance. Most, such as the cancers, not only resemble counterparts caused by other factors but are completely indistinguishable except by documentation of the relevant exposure. Other environmental diseases, such as asthma or dermatitis, may be distinguished clinically only with the use of specialized testing based on suspicion of the diagnosis; however, these specialized procedures are often not needed when a good history of exposure is combined with sound clinical reasoning, described later in this chapter. Only a few environmental diseases, such as heavy metal poisoning, are sufficiently distinctive that they can be diagnosed by exclusion or unusual features recognized on radiographs or a routine laboratory testing. Only by early consideration of environmental factors and the collection of exposure information are environmental diagnoses appropriately made. It is not the subspecialist but the primary care physician who has the highest likelihood of doing so, a fact well substantiated by the experience of environmental and occupational medicine consultants.

How an environmental illness may be manifest. It is critical that the physician successfully reach a diagnosis in cases being considered. It may be a formidable challenge. Although each environmental exposure and subsequent disease usually has its own clinical patterns and the basic diagnostic strategy is similar to other medical diagnostic strategies: obtaining a thorough medical history and performing a physical examination, gaining precise and unambiguous environmental exposure information, identifying all specific hazardous materials, and conducting some simple laboratory tests; the latter might include complete blood count, urinalysis, and standard blood chemistry analysis.

An environmental illness may be manifest in a variety of manners, and documentation of the objective manifestations is paramount to characterizing the disease. The illness may present as a newly developed clinical syndrome or an aggravation or change in a preexisting condition. Consequently, environmental illnesses can be classified according to various clinical features, such as the presence or absence of a preexisting condition, reported symptomatology, and observed objective findings. One way of classifying these variables is as follows: (1) a new condition defined both by symptoms and by objectively documented single-organ involvement; (2) a new condition defined by symptoms and objectively documented multiple-organ involvement; (3) a new condition without symptoms but with objectively documented single- or multiple-organ involvement; (4) new complaints but a stable preexisting medical condition and no change in laboratory test results; (5) new complaints but an altered preexisting medical condition and a change in laboratory test results. Of course, a clinical dilemma is the patient who presents with multiple symptoms and shows no evidence of organ involvement.

What organ system is affected? It is necessary to ensure that the medical disorder is completely and accurately characterized. Importantly, what organ systems are affected, as reflected by the patient's complaints? What damage does laboratory testing reflect? Are the two clinically consistent with each other? Unfortunately, some patients present with multiple complaints, but a work-up reveals no obvious pathologic abnormality or biochemical alteration. This patient often requires more time and effort than does a patient with documented disease. In such cases, the physician must determine whether there is objective evidence of disease. Ideally, there should be documentation of organ system involvement by objective laboratory biochemical alterations or pathologic findings. When a condition is characterized only by symptoms without documented organ involvement, reaching a definitive conclusion is more difficult.

The medical history. An accurate medical history is indispensable for identifying nonenvironmental illnesses and alternative medical conditions. The medical work-up should focus on the organ system that is affected and the extent of the organ damage. It is imperative that any injury or organ damage be documented accurately. When did the symptoms begin? Previous medical illnesses, including infections; hospitalizations; use of drugs; pets at home; allergic background; and hobbies should be described. The quantity and duration of cigarette smoking must be established because of its significance in causing disease. Knowledge of specific symptoms, particularly their onset and type of expression, is necessary. For example, a history of cough, sputum production, exertional shortness of breath, morning wheezing, and chest discomfort may suggest asthma, and ankle swelling, exertional shortness of breath, nocturnal attacks of wheezing; weight gain with fluid retention may indicate congestive heart failure. Subtleties in the temporal relationships and the aggregation of symptoms help characterize the medical condition.

Ordering laboratory tests. Although the major source of clinical information is obtained by direct communication with the patient, laboratory tests may be needed. The use of sophisticated laboratory investigations are ordered for specific reasons and are not necessary for all evaluations. For example, if a respiratory condition is suspected, tests may include exercise, arterial blood gas studies, and carbon monoxide diffusion capacity determination; sophisticated radiographic techniques such as computerized tomography, magnetic resonance imaging, and various scanning techniques have been advocated as diagnostic procedures. Elucidation of an airway disorder may require noting a response to an inhaled bronchodilator, the employment of methacholine or histamine challenges, or bronchial challenge testing to specific antigens. Bronchoalveolar lavage (BAL) has been shown to be of advantage in such disorders as pulmonary berylliosis; BAL-obtained lung lymphocytes respond to beryllium antigen and confirm sensitization to beryllium salt. Immunologic studies help conform the diagnosis of allergic alveolitis (precipitin antibodies) or asthma (specific immunoglobulin E). Sputum examination may demonstrate ferruginous bodies in an asbestos worker or cancer cells in a patient suspected of having cancer. Recognition of specific material in biologic fluids or tissue may be indispensable. Unusual cases of pulmonary fibrosis may require lung biopsy (transbronchial or open) and tissue analyses. Microprobe analysis with scanning electronmicroscopy and X-ray diffraction analyses have been used to identify specific causative agents, especially for mineral dusts and metals.

Whatever the circumstances of a diagnostic work-up, two warnings must be noted. First, it is important during the investigation stage of diagnostic work-up to cause no harm to the patient. To protect the patient's confidentiality, the physician must always discuss strategies for obtaining outside information with the patient. The second warning is that the diagnostic work-up of the patient should never be indefinitely delayed by the need for more environmental information. Suspect medical conditions that would merit urgent treatment should never be deferred while less life-threatening possibilities are explored. Frequently the information that the clinician would like to have is either unavailable or unobtainable in time to meet the needs for reaching clinical diagnostic and treatment choices.

Rationale for laboratory testing. Some clinicians are under the impression that the laboratory can substitute for proper exposure information and thorough medical evaluation. There has been remarkable progress of clinical toxicology, especially for the evaluation of drug and poison ingestions, and many laboratories are able to measure contaminants to the parts-per-trillion level in body tissues. It is important to point out that in environmental medicine, laboratory tests are often of limited diagnostic value.

Because of the potential for confusion about the value of laboratory tests in the diagnosis of environmental medicine disorders, a discussion on certain issues relevant to organ systems and environmental exposure is appropriate. Most laboratory tests serve one of three general purposes in the diagnostic process. First, the tests may define pathophysiologic mechanisms. These tests better clarify disease status and have value in determining causality or effect but, in and of themselves, rarely evaluate exposures. This category includes common tests such as imaging studies, standard chemistry profiles, and blood counts. There may be a role for specialized radiographic techniques, such as high-resolution computerized tomographic scanning.

A second use of laboratory testing is for estimation of exposures. The tests may establish the presence of a suspect causal agent in the body; such tests may indirectly measure exposure such as the serum cholinesterase levels or levels of other enzymes inhibited by toxicants. These tests are often called biologic monitoring tests because, to put it simply, they use the body as a sampling device to assess exposure (see Chapter 63). Examples are testing blood and urine to determine heavy metal levels or using polarizing light microscopy on a lung biopsy to identify crystalline silicates. These studies may lead to inferences about actual health;

however they measure exposure, not health effects. Although there may be a value, for public health reasons, to use measurements of exposure as a basis for identifying cases of disease (for example, considering a child with a lead level above 25 µg/dl lead poisoned for surveillance purposes), the actual measurement of a toxin in body fluids or tissue is not tantamount to demonstration of an effect attributable to its presence.

A third reason for laboratory testing may be to better substantiate the relationship between an exposure and an effect. Very few tests available specifically measure causal events. A common example is demonstration of an antibody to a sensitizing agent. The presence of antibody confirms both that exposure has occurred and that an immunologic effect has occurred, although not necessarily whether a disease such as asthma or rhinitis can be attributed to the exposure. Similarly, patch testing and specific bronchial inhalation challenges can document both an exposure and a sensitization and may even verify the relationship between the exposure and a specific health effect. Often, these distinctions may be oversimplified. For example, in a tissue biopsy, both fibrosis and a toxic material itself may be found. In this situation, both effect and exposure information may be inferred. Additionally, a high level of a toxicant in a body fluid may be so clearly associated with an effect that effect from an exposure level, such as high blood lead in a child, can be directly inferred; however, these situations are rare. There are also situations in which a test of one type is used to infer information of another. For example, zinc protoporphyrin in red cells, a measure of the blockade of the enzyme heme synthetase, is used as a surrogate measure of lead exposure; the results of the test are not used to prove poisoning at the clinical level but as a measure for lead itself. Correct interpretation demands that this logical inversion be appreciated. Similarly, measurement of the urine cadmium level, a good index of recent exposure, also is a measure of the renal effect of cadmium in individuals who have not had recent exposure, because the diseased kidney leaks stored cadmium but the intact kidney does not. In this case, a usual measure of an exposure is used to document an effect. These examples notwithstanding, the logical use of laboratory tests is straightforward. No test should be ordered without understanding to which part of the diagnostic equation the result will be applied.

Technical limitations of laboratory testing. Even when the logic is clear, there remain problems in interpreting laboratory tests. Some of these problems are caused by technical aspects, others by the circumstances of obtaining the test in the particular patient, and others by uncritical interpretation for diagnosis. The factors that may render data misleading include the sensitivity of the laboratory test to detect a substance or an effect, that is, how low a concentration can be detected by the technique; the reliability of the laboratory test to measure a result, that is, if the same test were redone at another time on the same sample, how closely would the results agree? the validity of results, that is, how does the laboratory test compare to a reference laboratory? the precision of results, that is, can the laboratory test differentiate results to the level of detail that may be desired? and the standardization of results, that is, does the laboratory test provide evidence of the results of the test in the same laboratory performed on a reference population?

Timing of laboratory tests. Although many tests in medicine do not depend intimately on timing or circumstances, such as chest radiographs, others can be interpreted only with the benefit of careful planning, such as measurement of blood glucose or plasma triglyceride levels. There are numerous situations in which the strategy for sampling is essential to interpretation of results for an environmental medical problem. For tests of effects, the timing of tests must be considered to avoid either missing the effect or confounding the effect with another. An example is the use of spirometry to detect environmentally induced asthma. Because the effect is ephemeral, the patient may have normal spirometry results if the test is not timed to coincide with expected effect or patient symptoms. Conversely, an audiogram performed shortly after high noise exposure documents the temporary effects of noise but cannot be used to determine hearing function.

For tests of exposure, the timing of samples may be even more problematic. Many toxicants are short-lived in the body and can be detected only shortly after an exposure. Knowledge of the kinetics of the agent of interest is essential before tests are ordered. Further, because exposures may be intermittent, samples must be timed to coincide with parts of the cycle of interest, such as peaks or troughs, much as is done with therapeutic drug monitoring. Failure to document the relationship between exposure or health events and the laboratory test results will lead to misinterpretation. Failure to consider testing strategy carefully may also vitiate interpretation of tests that measure the relationship between an exposure and effect. For example, in the course of environmental asthma, sensitization to agents such as isocyanates may reverse after a period away from exposure. Therefore, specific challenge with the agent may fail to induce bronchoconstriction in the laboratory if the patient had not been exposed for a long time before testing.

Interpretation of normal and abnormal laboratory results. It is common practice by even reputable laboratories to provide results with a statement about whether that result is normal. By convention, these statements are taken to mean that a test result falls within or outside the range of 95% of the healthy population, although for a few tests other guidelines are used. Although these interpretations may be of great value for range finding or other clinical purposes, it is very important that they not be used to dismiss a case prematurely or to overreact. For example, an accidental exposure to a chlorine leak may lead to mild reductions in flow rates that are considered normal but are not normal for this victim. Conversely, because incidental excursions outside the normal range of liver transaminase levels frequently occur, a small elevation in a person exposed to a hepatotoxin must not by itself be construed as proof of an effect, let alone a clinically important effect.

Particular attention should be paid to whether any specialized tests may refine the initial diagnostic impression. Biologic tests of exposure may be available to confirm that an exposure of interest has occurred and, in certain cases, quantify it. On the effect side, the literature may provide reason to believe that a certain test has good positive or negative predictive value when performed on exposed individuals. An example is the lymphoblast transformation test for beryllium hypersensitivity, which predicts the occurrence of chronic beryllium disease. Dynamic tests that directly relate exposures to effects, such as patch testing, frequently assist in diagnosis when they are available, but few are available.

Step 2: Characterizing exposure

General concepts. Once the physician has obtained the necessary and appropriate medical information, a decision about whether a specific environmental exposure plays a role in a medical disorder can be considered. It may be added that the environmental exposure may be only a contributing factor to disease and need not be the sole cause. Indeed, most disease is multifactorial, and the exposure may represent only one factor contributing to disease pathogenesis.

The environmental history. Many physicians view obtaining information about an unknown environmental exposure as comparable to finding a needle in a haystack. The clinician may envisage spending valuable time quizzing the patient on former environmental, work, and home exposures while the patient narrates in detail the specific information that can be recollected. The practitioner may not be adequately motivated, interested, or educationally prepared for this exercise. The most important information about environmental exposures is obtained from a detailed environmental history. (See Chapter 19 for a detailed discussion of the subject.) A complete environmental history may take 30 to 60 minutes to complete, but pertinent information can usually be procured in 10 to 15 minutes if the history taker is able to focus on exposures that are most likely related to the patient's disorder. The practitioner should not discount important exposure information or limit the scope of the environmental history but must be prepared to focus as much as possible on the most relevant parts. Information furnished by a self-administered questionnaire, including home audits and jobs held in the past (see Chapter 20), can be a starting point. A survey of past and present jobs in a chronologic order is necessary to authenticate all potential risks. Because of the latency period between exposure to a carcinogenic agent and disease development, identification of earlier exposures and jobs has merit. After reviewing the self-completed survey with the patient, the physician may be able to focus better on one or more past environmental exposures of importance.

It is important to understand why the environmental history alone may be insufficient for accurate assessment of an exposure. Such is the case because patients are often unaware of the hazards to which they have been exposed; patients do not usually have information on dose; patient recollection of historic events, especially those that may long precede the clinical evaluation, are often incomplete; and patient reports of exposures tend to be influenced by their own understanding of the connections between health and the environment. For example, agents that are acutely irritating or bothersome or have been labeled as hazardous are better remembered than are others that may be more important. Social and other factors may obscure or bias patient accounts of environmental exposures and prior health status, such as anger over economic consequences posed by a hazard or fear of disease. For all of these reasons, it is often necessary to obtain additional exposure information, to verify the chemical or physical hazards to which the patient has been exposed, to establish the dose of exposure, and to corroborate or modify the information that has been obtained directly from the patient.

Cardinal exposure indices. There are four cardinal pieces of exposure information: (1) The material or agent in the environment should be identified. (2) The duration of the exposure should be determined, that is, whether the exposure was short-term and lasted a few days, weeks, or months or was long-term and lasted for years. A longer duration of exposure is more likely to generate an injury than a brief exposure. A transient exposure, unless to a very toxic material and in high concentrations or possibly to an agent causing an immunologic response, rarely causes significant chronic disease. Agents present in low concentrations generally take months or years of exposure to cause disease to develop. Duration of exposure can be carefully scrutinized in the context of the type of disease presented. (3) The magnitude or extent of an exposure should be estimated. A basic toxicologic premise is one of dose and response. The intensity of an exposure represents the dose part of the relationship. It is important to determine whether an exposure is consequential. An example is asbestos in an office building; its presence does not generally pose high risk for cancer unless there is a substantial exposure. (4) If possible, the relationship between the environment and clinical manifestations should be explored.

A number of strategies have been proposed as means for estimating or inferring an exposure dose and type. This information is presented in detail in Chapters 2 and 4 and summarized here.

Use of company records. By law in the United States, companies that use or transport hazardous materials are obligated to maintain material safety data sheets (MSDSs) for each material that may result in worker or community exposure. Further, under federal and a variety of state laws, the employer is obligated to make this information available to anyone who might have been exposed or to his or her physician. Although these laws have increased the accessibility of information, there are difficulties in implementation. First, the MSDSs themselves are often of very limited usefulness. Much potentially useful information, such as minor ingredients that may be responsible for health effects such as allergic responses, is omitted. The health information included is often presented in uncritical lists without adequate discussion. For many of these MSDSs, the most useful information listed is the telephone number to call for emergency toxicologic information.

It may also be very difficult for patients or their physicians to know exactly what to ask for. Except in the case of a direct leak or spill, materials leaving the facilities as waste may be complex and may differ considerably from those purchased as raw materials or handled as finished products. For these reasons, exposure information is often best obtained directly from plant professionals such as company physicians, industrial hygiene personnel, or environmental managers. This procedure may be especially useful in an active exposure situation, about which these professionals may be well aware. The variable backgrounds of these professionals often produce perspectives that differ from the patient's and this suggests that information obtained from such sources must be interpreted cautiously.

Use of information from health and regulatory agencies. Often a factory, toxic waste site, or environmental hazard has been inspected by some governmental authority. The results of these inspections are generally available to physicians and may be excellent sources of information. As with other sources, the limitations must be appreciated. Most inspections are conducted for the purpose of determining compliance with various regulations, not for the purpose of assessing the exposure pattern to a particular person. Regulatory limits may not always prevent harm that can occur at levels lower than the acceptable limits. Conversely, many exposed to illegally high levels under some regulation may be at minimal or almost no health risk from the hazard regulated. Therefore, although regulatory information may be valuable for establishing exposure and estimating the dose, the conclusion that a person's exposure was above or below a standard should not be used for clinical diagnosis without further interpretation.

Direct site visit. When information on current exposures is obtained, direct on-site inspection may be valuable because it offers the advantages of contact with managers and health professionals involved and the chance to relate the history with observable facts and direct assessment of the potential for exposure and dose. Direct assessment of exposures is a specialized set of skills requiring the assistance of an industrial hygienist, an environmental engineer, or a comparably trained professional. Even with such consultants, the visit must be scheduled to ensure that typical activities are observed. Obviously, the biggest limitation is obtaining the assistance and cooperation of supervisors or others with responsibility for the site. Without them, a meaningful visit is either impossible or unlikely to be revealing.

Role of community groups. Although they may not have access to as much information as company officials or governmental regulators do, some community organizations take environmental health issues seriously and obtain substantial amounts of exposure information. Although their information may be limited, the quality may be very good and the motivation to cooperate a distinct advantage.

Step 3: Demonstrating a correlation between exposure and clinical manifestations

Clinical approach. Once the exact environmental agent is identified, the exposure estimated, and the duration of the exposure acknowledged, the clinician can determine whether the material is known to cause the injury noted. Are the clinical manifestations widely known and universally accepted as an adverse reaction to the suspected chemical or environmental exposure? Are the clinical manifestations known to occur at the exposure dose received in the suspected case? Library sources, reference texts, governmental agencies, data bases, and university expertise are resources for obtaining specific toxicologic information on the exposure. The information needed is "what is it?" and "what does it do?" Information on the specific hazardous material and its toxicologic consequences are key to making a diagnosis of an environmental disease. Without this basic information, causal relationships between exposure and disease cannot be determined accurately. In some cases there has not been sufficient clinical experience with the exposure to judge the significance of the noted clinical manifestations; this fact must be acknowledged and weighed for the final decision.

Use of exposure-assessment data bases. Often it is difficult to confirm an exposure or estimate its dose, especially for exposures that occurred long before the clinical evaluation. Fortunately there are some resources for obtaining at least semiquantitative estimates about exposure and dose. Texts such as this book may summarize the hazards and exposures typically associated with particular settings. Environmental surveys reported in public documents are another source. Scientific reports can provide valuable summaries of the ranges of exposures and doses in particular situations, which may be relevant to the patient at hand and allow prediction about dose.

Use of epidemiologic data bases. Although they differ in quality and in relevance to any particular patient, epidemiologic studies form the strongest basis for belief that an exposure causes an effect in humans (see Chapter 5). These studies may establish limits for an association between exposure and disease by demonstrating how long after exposure that increases in disease risk become evident. Existing epidemiologic investigations that show a strong association between exposure and health outcome provide useful information for clinical assessment. It must be understood that in any individual case epidemiologic data may or may not be relevant (that is, there may be other causes), but, in itself, the epidemiologic review process is a valuable educational process and fortifies the health professional's understanding of the subject matter. Furthermore, these kinds of data are well suited for a quantitative inference of individual risk. When comparably exposed individuals have been studied, quantitative determination of risk is straightforward. It is often possible to extrapolate from the range of reported exposures to estimate the patient's risk, even when they are occupational, not environmental, exposures. Access to such epidemiologic studies is easy through computerized literature searches; however, the relevance of these epidemiologic studies to the patient at hand is not always obvious. First, the exposure dose in the patient must be reasonably similar to the exposure dose of at least a portion of the study population. Although the practitioner can extrapolate results to lower doses (which is often done for risk-assessment purposes), it is not always valid. The population under study ideally should resemble the patient demographically; it is hazardous to apply results in occupational populations to environmental settings without some consideration of other health differences between them. Because most studies have focused on worker populations because they are much easier to perform, there is often no choice but to use the data and modify the interpretation. The same sort of modification may be needed when there are other differences between the patient and the study population, such as intercurrent disease or unusual susceptibility factors.

Use of toxicologic data bases. Epidemiologic data often are not available or are poor. In this situation the effects of the toxicant in animal tests (see Chapter 6) may be helpful. Such studies may provide evidence of dose-related effects of hazards and suggest that an association is biologically plausible. They may also provide clues to certain laboratory abnormalities, such as biochemical changes or histopathology. Toxicologic studies can be identified easily by computer searches. Summaries may also be available in texts or monographs such as the toxicologic profiles complied by the U.S. Agency for Toxic Substances and Disease Registry located in Atlanta.

Toxicologic studies may not always be relevant. In addition to potential differences among species, toxicologic studies often use routes of exposure that are convenient, such as intravenous exposure or gavage (tube feeding), but differ from the ways in which a patient may have been exposed. Further, most animal studies are performed at high doses of single toxins, which may not be applicable to a clinical case, especially in assessing the likelihood of an effect after exposure. These problems notwithstanding, animal tests can anticipate effects in humans. Such observations have prompted recognition of many serious environmental hazards, such as vinyl chloride. For this reason, similarities between animal effects and effects in patients exposed to hazards must be given significant weight. Toxicologic investigations that show an association between an exposure and health outcome provides useful information for clinical assessment. It must be understood that in any individual case toxicologic data may or may not be relevant and there may be other causes to explain the alterations.

Use of clinical studies and case reports. Clinical reports describing effects of exposures are scientifically limited because they lack controls, subjects with similar exposures who may not have any effects. For this reason, they must be reviewed with the understanding that the frequencies of features described are impossible to establish. Case studies, however, may be very useful for clinicians. Compared with epidemiologic studies, very detailed information about the patients, their exposure, and the dose is often available. Specific clinical information, such as the results of a wide array of tests, severity of illness, clinical course, and response to various treatments, is often provided. Of particular value is that the use of particular diagnostic tests is often described.

At their best, clinical reports and case studies are so relevant that they may provide a basis for all subsequent steps. At their worst, these reports may create the illusion of causal relations between events that cannot be proven and may be highly misleading. Therefore, although all case reports relevant to an exposure should be reviewed carefully, the weight given them should be proportional to the degree to which other evidence, such as some toxicologic or epidemiologic studies, can corroborate or refute them.

Use of clinical experience. Often a physician has examined similar patients or knows colleagues who have. Plant-based physicians often develop extensive experience with certain industrial hazards. Local health authorities, environmental medicine referral centers, and specialists may become experienced with a local environmental problem. These specialists may suffer from biases of perception, because they are more likely to have seen exposed individuals with problems than those without problems; however, their experience offers a great relevance, allowing comparison of a patient with others of comparable background and specific exposures. The specialist may also have some population information on the group from which the patient comes, such as results of surveys, which reduce the likelihood of clinical bias. This kind of clinical experience should be weighed heavily among the available resources for drawing inferences about likelihood of effects. Although not drawn from the scientific literature, the relevance in terms of exposure profile and personal characteristics makes this source extremely valuable. For this reason, the practitioner should always attempt to identify local physicians who may have previous experiences with patients like their own.

Objective evidence of overexposure. Evidence of very high exposure is beneficial for establishing the presence of an environmental disease. A number of questions can be posed. For example, is the clinical manifestation a dose-related phenomenon? This relationship would suggest a correlation. Can an exposure be documented by biomarkers? Is there evidence that excessive exposure occurred? Taking timing into consideration, do the results of diagnostic tests and pathologic findings or measurements of the breath, tissue, serum, urine, or other body fluid levels of the chemical exposure or metabolite of the chemical support the diagnosis of a toxic exposure for the patient? Alternatively, is the level reported strongly against the diagnosis of excessive exposure, or does the clinical manifestation in this patient represent an idiosyncratic overreaction to the chemical or chemicals?

Removal from exposure. An important consideration is whether the clinical manifestations improved substantially after removing the patient from exposure. Of course it is possible that the clinical manifestations do not improve substantially when the patient is removed from exposure, but generally the patient's clinical course should not worsen substantially after cessation of an exposure. It is also possible that the clinical manifestations improved but the degree or rate was unexpected or there was auxiliary treatment or maneuvers that make interpretation impossible. In fact, it may not be possible to remove the patient from the exposure or the time sequence is such that it is not possible to assess the effect of removal accurately. It is important to consider and weigh these various alternative clinical scenarios.

Reexposure relationship. Although it is often not possible or ethical to reexpose a patient, such important information may exist historically. An important query is whether the clinical manifestations recurred or exacerbated on reexposure. If they did not, an alternative diagnosis might be considered. Often, there was no rechallenge, or the response of the clinical manifestations was obscured or not interpretable because of auxiliary treatments or maneuvers. Each alternative holds different significance in a final diagnosis.

Preexisting illness. In some instances the patient may be suffering from a condition present before the environmental exposure occurred, and the question of whether the clinical manifestations represent a change (exacerbation, recurrence, or complication) or a new manifestation in the preexisting clinical condition arises. Several questions must be addressed. For instance, is the preexisting condition commonly followed by the type of change noted? Are there any new alternative diseases that could explain the change? Is the clinical manifestation consistent in quality and severity with any new alternative disease other than a preexisting condition? Were the clinical manifestations consistent in timing with any of the alternative diseases, and is the clinical manifestation noted with the alternative condition? Does the clinical manifestation commonly occur in this type of patient in the absence of recognizable etiologic candidates?

Multiple causes. The recognition of another cause of a disease does not necessarily reduce the possibility of an environmental cause. Most chronic diseases and many acute ones have multiple causes that are not mutually exclusive. For example, lipid disorders, diabetes, and hypertension do not mitigate the importance of smoking as a cause of arteriosclerotic cardiovascular disease. In fact, underlying disease or risk may accentuate the importance of controllable environmental exposure in patients with multiple risks. For example, asbestos-exposed workers who smoke have a far greater likelihood of developing lung cancer than do nonsmokers. Alcohol consumption potentiates the effects of some hepatotoxins in causing hepatic necrosis or steatosis. The extent and basis for some of these interactions are explored in Chapters 27 and 28, which covers general principles on susceptibility. The important consequence to practice is that the effect of an environmental agent is not necessarily reduced because another pathogenic factor is present. This is especially important for the most common environmentally related clinical complaints, such as irritation and sensitization of the skin and respiratory tract. Too often, environmental possibilities are ignored because symptoms and signs can be related to smoking, viral infection, or common allergy. The possibility of interaction is another reason why environmental diseases are not diagnoses of exclusion.

Temporal relationships. Examination of temporal relationships is often meaningful. Was the timing consistent with an environmental exposure? Was the timing not only consistent with but expected for an adverse reaction to the environmental exposure? Was the timing of the appearance of the clinical manifestation relative to the exposure difficult or impossible to assess, because the clinical course represented an equivocal change in a preexisting clinical condition? Is the association between the exposure and the clinical manifestation so unusual as to prevent knowledge of the timing to expect for the reaction observed?

Clinical effects of environmental exposures occur after a predictable latent interval between the onset of exposure and the occurrence of disease. With toxins that cause direct and acute injury to an organ, such injury typically occurs immediately after an exposure or after a period of build-up. Clinically, onset in such cases occurs early in the course of exposure, which allows simpler exploration of possible environmental connections. With factors that act via the immune system, such as many of those that cause dermatitis or asthma, effects are manifested after months or a few years, after the immune process has been stimulated; however, given the nature of the immune system, the disease invariably begins while exposure is still ongoing, despite the delay.

Chronic effects, such as organ scarring or destruction, become clinically apparent after a long latent interval, often of many years from the causal exposure. Such is the case for carcinogens, which typically cause cancer years after first exposure. The exposure itself in these cases may have long since ceased, or the patient may have left the environment of concern. There is no uniform relationship between these late outcomes and any earlier effects. For example, leukemia may occur in a worker exposed to benzene at daily levels of exposure far below those that would cause acute bone marrow injury or any other noticeable health effect. For this reason, individuals who seem resistant to the early effects may be at the highest risk for the later effects because they are likely to tolerate higher doses.

Although the search for a cause for a disease with long latency, such as cancer or pulmonary fibrosis, may be a challenge to the clinician, knowledge of latency can be used to advantage. In these cases, current or very recent exposures are not as important, so consideration can be focused on former activities, where the yield will be greatest.

Clinical evaluation of dose-response. The dose of exposure to a hazard predicts the likelihood of an effect. Toxins resemble drugs in that there is a clear relationship between dose of exposure and subsequent effects. Although individuals may differ in their susceptibility to disease (see later), knowledge of these relationships and estimated exposures is central to diagnosis in environmental medicine. Although detailed knowledge of the toxicology of specific hazards is invaluable in applying this concept, three generic patterns cover most situations. (1) For direct-acting toxins, such as some metals, organic solvents, or pesticides, there is typically a threshold dose of exposure below which there is no adverse effect. As the dose increases above this level, the severity increases. For these direct-acting toxins, the dose-response relationship is fairly straightforward. (2) Other harmful agents such as those that cause asthma or dermatitis, act by eliciting an immunologic response. Many individuals experience no effect from these hazards at any dose; they are not susceptible, for genetic or other reasons. In individuals who are susceptible, increasing the dose increases the likelihood of sensitization. Once sensitization occurs, however, the severity of reactions may not have any relationship to dose. Such reactions often occur at very low levels of

---

Categories for making a diagnosis of an environmental medical condition

Factors	Diagnostic impact	Factors	Diagnostic impact
Clinical toxicology of chemical or exposure		2. Alternative medical conditions are possible, but no definitive ones have been diagnosed	Neutral
1. Clinical manifestation is widely known and universally accepted as an adverse reaction to the suspected environmental exposure or chemical	Support environmental diagnosis	3. Clinical manifestations are consistent in type, quality, severity and timing with a new and alternative disease and do not represent a preexisting condition	Suggest alternate diagnosis
2. Clinical manifestations is not widely known and universally accepted as an adverse reaction to the suspected environmental exposure or chemical	Suggest alternate diagnosis	*Temporal relationship*	
3. There is not enough information accumulated about the chemical or exposure so that most adverse clinical manifestations to the environmental exposure or chemical are likely to have been reported	Neutral	1. The temporal relationship (timing) of the clinical manifestation is not only consistent with but is expected for the type and extent of exposure	Support environmental diagnosis
Alternative etiologic considerations		2. The temporal relationship (timing) of the clinical manifestation is not consistent with nor is expected for the type and extent of exposure	Suggest alternate diagnosis
1. A preexisting condition (that is, a condition present before exposure to the suspected environmental agent) exists, and the clinical manifestations observed are well explained as representing a change, recurrence, complication, or new manifestation of the established underlying clinical condition	Suggest alternate diagnosis	3. The temporal relationship (timing) of the clinic manifestation is equivocal or nonassessable for the type and extent of exposure or because the clinical manifestations represent an equivocal change in a preexisting clinical condition	Neutral

Categories for making a diagnosis of an environmental medical condition–cont'd

Factors	Diagnostic impact	Factors	Diagnostic impact
Objective evidence of overexposure		**Removal from exposure**	
1. The results of diagnostic tests and pathologic findings or measurements of the breath, tissue, serum, urine, or other body fluid levels of the chemical exposure or metabolite of the chemical support the diagnosis of a toxic exposure for the patient	Support environmental diagnosis	1. The clinical manifestations improved substantially after removal of the patient from exposure	Support environmental diagnosis
2. The results of diagnostic tests and pathologic findings or measurements of the breath, tissue, serum, urine, or other body fluid levels of the chemical exposure or metabolite of the chemical do not support the diagnosis of a toxic exposure for the patient	Suggest alternate diagnosis	2. The clinical manifestations did not improve substantially after removal of the patient from exposure	Suggest alternate diagnosis
		3. The clinical manifestations improved, but the degree or rate is unexpected or auxiliary treatment or maneuvers make interpretation impossible	Neutral
3. The results of diagnostic tests and pathologic findings or measurements of the breath, tissue, serum, urine, or other body fluid levels of the chemical exposure or metabolite of the chemical were not obtained, are unknown, or are equivocal for supporting the diagnosis of a toxic exposure for the patient	Neutral	4. It is not possible to remove patient from the exposure or the time sequence is such that it is not possible to assess accurately	Neutral
		Exposure relationship	
		1. Clinical manifestations recur or exacerbate on reexposure	Support environmental diagnosis
		2. Clinical manifestations do not recur or exacerbate on reexposure	Suggest alternate diagnosis
		3. There was no rechallenge attempted or ethically indicated, or the response of the clinical manifestations was obscured or not interpretable because of auxiliary treatments or maneuvers	Neutral

exposure. Usually the history reveals an occasion in which a significant dose of exposure did occur, probably the basis of sensitization. (3) For chemicals that interact with DNA to cause mutations or initiate cancers, even the smallest dose creates a finite chance of the harmful effect, a chance that will increase as the dose of exposure increases. If the disease occurs, the dose that caused it becomes irrelevant in terms of disease severity, but increasing dose increases the likelihood of the disease.

Variation in susceptibility. Individual susceptibility to noxious exposures is highly variable, perhaps because of genetic differences, age, gender, size, simultaneous exposures to environmental substances that interact, preexisting diseases, or behavioral factors. Unfortunately, knowledge of the factors that determine this variability is highly limited, which complicates evaluation of the relationship between environmental exposure and health effects. For example, in an accidental community exposure the occurrence of a health problem in only one exposed person would generally suggest an alternative explanation, but it is possible that only that individual was at risk at the dose of exposure. Although the pattern of occurrence of illness in a population may be a vital clue and should always be carefully assessed, variability of susceptibilities within the population must be considered before an environmental cause is ruled out.

Step 4: Establishing the diagnosis of an environmental medical condition

Assessing the exposure details and correlating them with the medical condition require various testing procedures and lead to a logical conclusion based on the information available. The necessary criteria for diagnosis of an environmental medical condition include obtaining a detailed medical and environmental history with the specific identification of an offending agent. There must be scientific documentation that the agent can plausibly cause the observed medical condition. Furthermore, the medical condition identified should be one that is acknowledged as being environmentally induced (see Step 3). Preferably there should be documentation of organ system involvement by objective laboratory biochemical alterations or pathologic findings. Finally, because of the different significance of the various clinical and exposure possibilities, weighing of the information is helpful in determining the probability that the exposure caused the environmental condition. Usually, the first three steps generate some information but may not be enough to provide a quantitative estimate of disease likelihood. In such cases, one might be able to estimate likelihood on a semiquantitative basis such as "occurs commonly in similarly exposed people" or "possibly" or "rarely occurs in similarly exposed people." This estimate becomes the foundation for quantitative diagnostic decision making.

Various pieces of the overall work-up are helpful in determining the probability that the exposure caused the en-

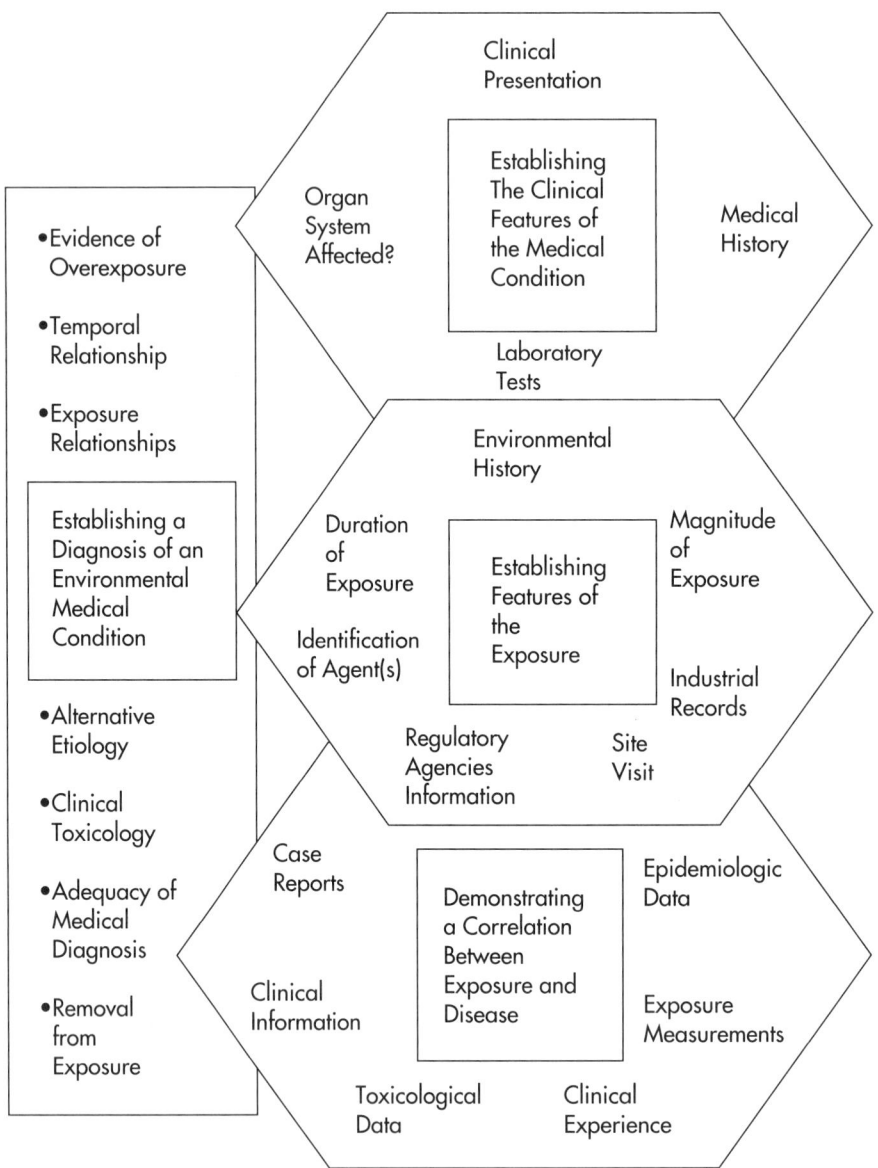

Fig. 18-2. The four steps required to establish the diagnosis of the environmental medical condition dictates that the physician carefully define the features of the medical condition and environmental exposure. There needs to be a way of demonstrating a correlation between the exposure and the clinical manifestations. Reaching a final diagnosis is analogous to fitting together a puzzle—the more pieces fitted into the puzzle, the clearer the picture becomes and thus the more conclusive the diagnosis. Important considerations relate to exposure indices, clinical toxicology, strength of medical diagnosis, and alternative possibilities. An estimate based on a semiquantitative basis may become the foundation for a more quantitative diagnostic decision making.

vironmental condition. The box on pp. 228 and 229 lists factors that may assist the physician in reaching a more objective clinical diagnosis of an environmental medical condition. For each category, factors that support an environmental cause are listed along with others that favor other alternatives; some possibilities are not informative (neutral). If all these factors are taken under consideration and the data do not suggest that an environmental effect is very likely, the most likely interpretation is that the patient's problem is nonenvironmental. Only if the presentation is very compelling—for example, the patient is symptomatic only in a particular environment, or symptoms' onset coincides with an unusual exposure—is the possibility of a previously unrecognized association between a hazard and disease worth considering.

The penultimate step is consideration of alternative possibilities that could explain the signs, symptoms, and laboratory results. When environmental causes have been considered only after other possibilities had been excluded, this step is generally moot; however, when the concern of the patient or a referring party has prompted early consideration of an environmental cause, this is a vital step before reaching the correct diagnosis, especially because disease features for environmental diseases are rarely unique. Fig. 18-2 summarizes the approach.

Once a list of alternatives has been generated, the final task is to use all available evidence to arrive at the most likely diagnosis. The process is orderly. Very rare conditions can generally be ruled out with probability reasoning, except for infectious or malignant possibilities, which may require specific tests for exclusion because of their clinical ramifications. When less rare considerations remain, quantitative clinical reasoning can be used to decide whether more invasive tests are indicated. In the end, the process is little different from general bedside (Bayesian) reasoning in medicine. Two principles must be remembered. First, the evaluation process may not result in a certain diagnosis; likelihood, not certainty, is the reasonable goal. Second, once significant exposure to a hazard has been established, the occurrence of adverse consequences from it is not unlikely; in fact, it is much more likely than is the occurrence of almost any other new disease.

SUMMARY

The process of diagnostic problem solving in environmental medicine remains part science, part art form. Although the basic approach is highly structured and scientific, the remarkable incompleteness of the existing data and their heterogeneity in quality and type provide a huge realm for individual judgment by the clinician. To exercise it well, the physician must also be aware of the complexity of the clinical context and the biases that the physician brings. Nonetheless, the fact remains that a firm, if imperfect, diagnosis must be rendered in every case.

Chapter 19

THE ENVIRONMENTAL HISTORY

Arthur Frank

The case for the environmental history
Classification of environmental disease
Understanding the origin of the problem: exposure information
Physical examination
Laboratory information
Sources of exposure at home: the home audit
Case studies
Personnel and information resources
References

THE CASE FOR THE ENVIRONMENTAL HISTORY

Physicians are trained, beginning in medical school, to recognize the important elements of diagnosis so that therapy can be started and prognosis accurately assessed. Of the three main elements of patient assessment—history, physical examination, and laboratory tests—the first is of critical and major importance. It has been suggested that the medical history makes up the bulk of the information to be collected by the physician, and if it has been properly conducted, the physical examination and laboratory tests usually only confirm what has been learned from the history. There are only a few diagnoses that absolutely require physical or laboratory findings or both for their determination.

There is nothing different in the approach to making diagnoses related to environmental exposures. The basic approach to the patient was laid down by Hippocrates several centuries ago and has varied little over time. The only significant addition to this approach was a question added by Bernadino Ramazzini, a physician who in 1700 wrote that it was important for physicians to ask their patients what they did for a living; in our society, we need to extend question that to environmental exposures. In 1713 the last edition of *De Morbis Artificium*[3] (On the Diseases of Workers) was published posthumously, and in it Ramazzini both laid out the approach to making environmental and occupational assessments and cataloged for the first time numerous specific occupational and environmental diseases. In some areas, this classic document has been little improved on over the centuries.

In addition to the paramount importance of the history, the physical examination and laboratory studies have a role to play in environmental medicine. There are at least two reasons to obtain an accurate and complete environmental and occupational exposure history from a patient. Given the nature of the interaction of a medical encounter, there are few things that the patient thinks that he or she knows better than the physician does; however, asking about the home, environment, and workplace gives the patient some small area of the encounter in which he or she is master. A proper approach to asking these questions can accomplish much in putting patients at ease and can truly facilitate the medical interaction.

In addition, the historical nature of the information may be critical to the proper and complete assessment of the patient and his or her condition and may suggest an ongoing screening program for that patient. It is only by such a historical review, virtually covering the patient's complete lifetime, that causal relationships can be truly understood.

CLASSIFICATION OF ENVIRONMENTAL DISEASE

Environmentally related diseases, when they are appreciated as such, may affect virtually every organ system. Although traditionally much has been learned from workplace exposures leading to the development of disease, it is increasingly necessary to consider environmental exposures away from the workplace as sources of disease among individuals. Traditionally there are two ways to classify disease, and this method also applies to environmental diseases.

First, one could look at the array of organ systems and consider how environmental exposures might produce disease in each of those systems. This system allows some manageable classification. The second approach is to take individual toxic agents or exposures and look to what problems might arise after such exposures. A case study in environmental medicine entitled *Taking an Exposure History*,[1] developed by the Agency for Toxic Substances and Disease Registry (ATSDR), uses both these approaches. The major organ systems that need to be considered include the respiratory, dermatologic, liver, kidney, cardiovascular, reproductive, hematologic, and neuropsychologic systems.

With respect to respiratory disorders, a variety of environmental pollutants, including both ambient and indoor air pollution, radon, cigarette smoke, asbestos, and chemicals released from adhesives and household products, can affect the lungs. The skin can be damaged by a large number of exposures, especially to certain chemicals and metals, which may commonly be found in the home, in jewelry, or at sites other than workplaces. Liver and kidney toxicity are often related to solvents or heavy metals or both. Cardiovascular disease is traditionally related to tobacco smoke as well as to a wide variety of other substances, including gases such as carbon monoxide and nitrates in drinking water. At one time there was a problem with heart disease related to the addition of cobalt as a foaming agent to Canadian beers.

Reproductive hazards are an especially difficult area to evaluate, but exposure to carbon monoxide, lead, and other heavy metals and chemicals may alter reproductive outcomes. The hematologic effects of benzene, a common constituent in gasoline, radiation, or other substances, may be found in nonworkplace environments and ultimately can cause disease. Similarly, neuropsychological difficulties after a variety of exposures, including metals, organics, and noise can be related to the environment.

The ATSDR document goes on to consider a variety of other sources of exposure, the classification of which resides with the nature of the material. One should always consider the basics, which are taken to be food, water, air, and soil, and the potential each might have to expose individuals in a manner that may adversely affect their health. In addition, a variety of other exposures commonly found in the home, including household products, pesticides and lawn applications, lead, and other hazards, could be the source of environmental disease.

With regard to air pollution, there are both ambient air and work-related difficulties in certain communities with local industry or acute exacerbations after temperature inversions. We are increasingly becoming aware of indoor air pollutant issues, including secondhand tobacco smoke, wood stove and kerosene heater vapors, and the contribution of building materials, new furniture, and new carpet, which contribute to what is sometimes called *tight* or *sick building syndrome*. In addition, microbiologic organisms can accumulate in heating and cooling systems to a point at which they can sensitize individuals and cause disease. The Environmental Protection Agency (EPA) has estimated that more than 730,000 public buildings contain potentially friable asbestos, as do approximately one third of all public schools. Given the increasing number of reports of asbestos-related disease among individuals whose only exposure was employment in such buildings, this finding gives rise to appropriate concern for the future. For example, the reports of teachers' developing mesothelioma, documented by Lilienfeld,[2] points to valid reasons for concern about this ongoing public health problem.

In 1987 the EPA found that the concentrations of 12 common organic pollutants are two to five times higher inside of homes than they are outside, because of the use of household products. Paint thinners, dry-cleaning solvents, air fresheners, toilet-bowl deodorizers, and moth crystals all contribute to the mixture of chemicals that can concentrate in the home. Increasingly, Americans are turning to pesticides and other lawn-care products. With more than 1400 active ingredients found in more than 34,000 preparations, this clearly may be a difficult area to assess. Lead enters the home through drinking water, having been brought into the home through lead plumbing or lead-soldered pipes. In addition, the use of ceramics with lead-containing glazes to store acidic substances such as juice may leach lead and add to the risk of individuals' becoming ill from exposures inside their home.

Last, one should consider what some have termed recreational hazards, which may be as simple as fishing or swimming in contaminated water, filling sand boxes with sand containing asbestos, or arts and craft hobbies that can expose the individual to talc, solvent, heavy metals, or other potential elements. Even musicians may not be spared the difficulties of environmentally related disease through either lung problems after years of playing wind or brass instruments or noise-induced hearing loss from exposure to loud music.

When information about environmental exposure gleaned from a patient is sifted through, the proximate nature of the problem makes the understanding of the problem easier. The onset of diabetic symptoms or shortness of breath associated with congestive heart failure can be relatively easily diagnosed with careful attention to what the patient says. There is a similar ease of diagnosis after environmental exposures; however, it should be noted the patient's illness may much more often have a relationship to an exposure that does not have the immediacy that is generally encountered in clinical medicine.

In some settings an immediate cause-and-effect relationship can be noted. Ammonia is inadvertently added to certain household cleansers to form a toxic gas; in such cases the cause-and-effect relationship of the exposure and the patient's symptoms is quickly recognizable. These circumstances, however, occur only infrequently. Much more common is a situation in which there is a gap between the exposure and the development of disease, and this gap can span decades. In environmental medicine, the categories with regard to time frame and cause and effect can be put into five headings: (1) immediate, (2) soon, (3) delayed, (4) latent, and (5) generational.

As noted previously, immediate cause-and-effect relationships are rarely difficult to understand. A valve breaks, a bee stings, a chemical is used, and the consequences occur almost immediately. The patient can readily share this information with the physician, and the ease of diagnosis is assured; however, any delay brings increasing levels of complexity.

The category *soon* means a short delay in the effect of exposure, from several hours to perhaps days. An excellent example is the matter of metal fume fever, which is a distinct possibility in individuals who weld with galvanized steel. Steel coated with zinc is termed galvanized, and the use of a torch on this material aerosolizes the zinc coating on the steel, rendering it into a form that can be easily inhaled. No illness may be noted at the time of exposure to the fumes, but hours later, perhaps in the evening at the end of a day, the individual with exposure may feel the onset of a flulike illness. Such individuals may experience fever and muscle fatigue and often go to bed with such symptoms; after a night's rest, they awaken without symptoms, which may cause them to repeat the process, unless and until they make the association of the hazard or complete the task.

Delayed effects may occur weeks or months later. A classic example is that of lead poisoning; previously workers who used leaded paints or had worked with nonorganic lead, became ill after a period of many months. The neurologic damage, such as wristdrop, would be such a delayed effect.

Similarly, hematologic problems would take place in this kind of time frame. Increasingly, the presence of lead in the home and school environment in drinking fountains and water pipe is being recognized as a source of potential medical problems.

Some disease is best considered latent. The best example is the carcinogenic potential of many environmental or occupational exposures. In general, it is convenient to think of the "20-year rule." For recognized human carcinogens, cancer does not occur within days, weeks, months, or even several years after first exposure but generally occurs decades after the onset of exposure. Generally, excess human cancers seen with various carcinogens begin to appear about 20 years after such exposure. Classically, disease due to cigarette smoking exhibits this pattern, as does exposure to a variety of other well-documented human carcinogens, including asbestos, arsenic, vinyl chloride, and others. When a patient has developed a malignancy, the history of exposures occurring 20, 30, or more years previously becomes critical in establishing such a cause-and-effect relationship.

Last, and with greatest difficulty, one must be able to recognize that disease may affect only those of a subsequent generation from those who actually had the exposure. An excellent example of this is use of diethylstilbesterol (DES), a drug formerly used to stop premature births. This drug had been used extensively in the 1950s for the treatment of women with histories of spontaneous miscarriage. Ultimately, this drug demonstrated no clinical efficacy, but a legacy was passed on to the next generation in terms of disease, the most critical problem being that of the development of clear cell carcinomas of the vagina in daughters of women who had taken DES. The drug had obviously demonstrated transplacental carcinogenesis, with the development of these cancers late in the second decade of life. The determination of this problem highlights the necessity for careful and complete historical data, even with consideration of parental exposures.

Other examples of parental exposures leading to illness in the next generation are the increase in ear infections among children whose parents smoke and exposure to lead during pregnancy's leading to subsequent effects due to placental transfer.

UNDERSTANDING THE ORIGIN OF THE PROBLEM: EXPOSURE INFORMATION

Most physicians learn to develop medical information from a standardized format. The items of this history, which may vary slightly in content or order from physician to physician, include (1) chief complaint, (2) history of present illness, (3) past medical history, (4) family history, (5) social history, (6) environmental and occupational history, (7) home environmental history, (8) review of systems, (9) physical examination results, and (10) laboratory test results.

In obtaining an environmental history, it should be recognized that although a few minutes may be all that is needed for a cursory examination, a detailed evaluation of environmental or workplace exposures or both may take considerably longer. Therefore, it is important to focus on the symptoms and try to relate them to the number of specific organ systems. Development of exposure information has certain essential pieces that need to be considered.

There should be as precise a determination as possible of the material or agent thought to be the cause of health problems. The practitioner must be quite specific with patients about exposures they may have had and should be knowledgeable about trade names and identifying them with specific chemicals. Sources of information in this area are discussed later in this article.

Next, in addition to identifying a potential chemical, the physician should obtain information about exposure duration and time since exposure onset. Given the previous discussion regarding the time intervals from exposure to disease, the duration since onset is important, depending on the nature of the problem. Clearly, the total duration of exposure to specific agents is also an important piece of information to obtain to properly weigh the likelihood that such exposure has caused disease. Brief exposure to many agents does not cause long-lasting disease, but occasionally with especially toxic substances, even exposures of short duration can lead to problems years later. Such an example might be that of a farmer who enters a silo and is quickly affected by oxides of nitrogen given off as silage gas but does not seek medical attention at the time and demonstrates radiographic changes and possible pulmonary function impairment many years later. Therefore, the duration, intensity, and specific nature of the exposure all come together in allowing a physician to make an appropriate diagnosis.

When this constellation of information is available, better judgments are made. Often, however, the physician may need to obtain specific knowledge about the toxicity of specific chemicals. There are too many chemicals and too many potential exposures for any physician to be completely knowledgeable about such information.

It is also useful to ask the patient whether anyone else in a similar environment is experiencing the same symptoms. Family members, others living in the same neighborhood, or co-workers may be having similar health problems. This classic public health approach may lead to consultation with local health authorities, which may be a potentially important aspect of such determinations.

Under certain circumstances, it may also be necessary to make a special assessment at the site of exposure. Just as industrial hygienists assess workplaces, it may be necessary to involve individuals with such expertise to assess homes or other environmental settings. Industrial hygienists, laboratory testing services, and others are available to perform on-site inspections and testing. There may be a need to test water, soil, air, food, or household utensils in the search for sources of toxic exposure. Assessment of heating and cooling systems also may be necessary, as may special microbiological testing.

In addition to assessment of such environmental exposures for toxins, it is necessary to consider other personal factors that may have a relationship to the exposure. Examples include the synergistic effect between smoking and other environmental exposures, such as asbestos and radiation, or the effect of alcohol with certain chemicals. It is necessary to obtain such information and to consider it in relation to environmental exposures.

PHYSICAL EXAMINATION

The signs and symptoms associated with environmental or occupational exposure can be specific but often are extremely general and of a nonspecific nature. Such diffuse symptoms as nausea, vomiting, headache, parasthesias, development of a chronic cough, and similar common complaints may be the first sign of an environmentally or occupationally induced illness. The physician must always be sensitive to the possibility of a specific problem related to these nonspecific symptoms.

In conducting the physical examination, the physician must also be sensitive and vigilant for certain changes. Listed herein are several possibly environmentally or occupationally connected physical findings that may be seen in a patient:

Skin: Areas of depigmentation, multiple small burns, Mees' lines on fingernails, and toenails, discoloration of the gingiva, areas of cellulitis.

Head, eyes, ears, nose, and throat: Areas of alopecia, perforated eardrums, decreased hearing, cataracts, perforated nasal septum, inflamed or diseased-appearing vocal cords.

Chest and heart: Gynecomastia, crepitant rales, increased anteroposterior diameter, abnormal cardiac rhythms, hypertension.

Abdomen: Diffuse discomfort, dysphasia, rectal mass, enlarged or painful liver.

Musculoskeletal system: Swollen joints, decreased range of motion, back spasms, muscle atrophy.

Nervous system: Central or peripheral manifestations of neurologic disease.

These are but a few examples of conditions that may be related to environmental or occupational exposures of a specific nature.

LABORATORY INFORMATION

A number of laboratory tests are useful in the full assessment of potential environmental exposure problems. Perhaps the most commonly used are pulmonary function tests, especially simple spirometry. The assessment of obstructive and restrictive changes can be made with this modality.

Screening chest radiographs are rarely specifically indicated among groups of individuals exposed, except when there is a particularly high risk of the development of cancer such as that in asbestos workers and uranium miners. Otherwise, there is little value in routine chest radiographs among exposed populations.

Routine blood tests for liver function, electrolytes, and hematologic status are indicated only for a few specific exposures such as leukemogens—for example, benzene—or liver toxins such as carbon tetrachloride. As a routine screening test for liver or kidney disease, these tests are of little value and generally detect disease only at a relatively advanced stage.

Specific tests for specific indications, such as heavy metal screenings or specific urinary metabolite levels, may be justified on the basis of the exposure history given by the patient.

Federal or other requirements may dictate testing for specific exposures according to some specified-interval testing. In general, the philosophic approach is to test only for in exposures for which such screening has been thought to be useful.

In general, justified screening includes that for organ-specific cancers, such as lung cancer in the case of exposure asbestos, coke oven emissions, and radiation; blood analysis for leukemogens when there has been exposure to benzene or radiation; and a variety of other screens that correspond with specific exposures. Another example is urinary cytology after workplace exposure to benzidene and β-naphthylamine, both bladder carcinogens.

Other types of screening, such as for chronic exposure to lead, becomes justified when there are certain levels of exposure. Also, given the potential for hearing loss connected with high noise exposures, a hearing conservation program including screening tests for hearing is justified or may be required by law if certain threshholds of noise are exceeded.

SOURCES OF EXPOSURE AT HOME: THE HOME AUDIT

A document called the home audit has been developed to assist in the assessment of exposures at home, especially as they relate to children. This document has been designed specifically for the pediatrician but has relevance to other physicians. There are three objectives related to its use: (1) The physician should review topics to be covered in a home audit. (2) The physician should be able to obtain information about a child's home environment by use of a home audit questionnaire completed by the parents. (3) It is expected that physicians would be able to provide anticipatory guidance about a child's home environment.

Among the topics covered in a home audit are indoor air pollution, pesticides and lawn-care products, lead, playground hazards, arts-and-crafts hazards, and electromagnetic fields. It is clear that children of different ages are affected differently by each of these categories.

Among the areas to be reviewed regarding the subject of indoor air pollution are environmental tobacco smoke, the use of wood and gas stoves, formaldehyde, radon, asbestos, and other toxins. Again, a complete smoking history, including details of the amount and sites of smoking, should be obtained. Smoking cessation should be encouraged, but if parents will not stop smoking, other suggestions can be made, such as smoking in isolated areas, not smoking in the car, and not leaving full ashtrays around as counterproductive influences for children.

The use of wood stoves, fireplaces, and gas stoves is of concern with such matters as carbon monoxide, oxides of nitrogen, and polycyclic aromatic hydrocarbons as well as respirable particulates. Studies have shown that children living in homes heated by wood stoves have a significant increase in respiratory symptoms. In some inner-city homes, gas stoves are frequently used for heat and pots of water simmer for humidification, providing an additional risk for children.

Formaldehyde is a common problem in certain settings, especially mobile homes, and this substance can off-gas from particle board, insulation materials, carbon adhesives, and other products used in the manufacture of mobile homes. Radon, a naturally occurring, colorless, odorless gas, is a by-product of uranium decay. Radon exposure has been environmentally linked to lung cancer.

Also part of the home audit is the problem of asbestos. The issue at hand, given the usually lower levels of exposure in households, is not so much the problems of lung fibrosis, known as asbestosis, but the risk of malignancy with regard to lung cancer (especially with concomitant cigarette smoking), mesothelioma, and a variety of other cancers, such as those of the gastrointestinal tract. Exposure to asbestos in schools is another pressing national issue in the United States.

Other toxins include a variety of organic hydrocarbons with which individuals may come into contact. Methylene chloride may be found in paint thinners and adhesive removers, perchlorethylene may come home on improperly dry-cleaned clothing, and paradichlorobenzene may be found in room air fresheners and toilet bowl deodorizers. These are among the many potential hydrocarbons to which children can be exposed in the home environment.

Another area of concern is that of pesticides and lawn-care products. Exposure may occur through the skin, respiratory tract, or gastrointestinal tract. A great deal of pesticide exposure may be taking place in unknown ways, because the Food and Drug Administration tests relatively little of the food supply of the United States and certain pesticides banned for use in this country are still widely used overseas, with subsequent importation of food that may contain these otherwise banned products. Teaching a child the proper use of insect repellants and household pesticides and proper preparation of food, especially fruits and vegetables, can help preserve health.

Lead poisoning continues to be a problem in the household. Continued lowering of lead acceptable levels has been the trend in recent years, and additional lowering of the standard is expected. Lead can occur in the household through the use of lead paint, from lead dust arising from sanding or scraping, or in drinking water, especially in older cities that used lead pipes. In addition, lead may be present in food, and of special concern is imported pottery; lead sometimes leaches from the glaze if acidic liquids such as juice are stored in it. In addition, lead occurs in the air, which has been reduced in large part because of the replacement of leaded gasolines, and it must be remembered that parents can bring lead into the household if they work in certain manufacturing situations, perform demolition work, or have other similar exposures.

Special attention has been paid in recent years to potential health hazards at playgrounds. Wooden playground structures may contain preservatives with potential health hazards, such as arsenic, pentachlorphenol, or creosote. Some play sands have been reported as containing asbestos fibers, and certain clay materials for children's use have also been shown to contain asbestos. There is increasing concern about playground safety with regard to placement of rubber mats to help minimize injury. Potential arts-and-crafts hazards also are important. In addition to asbestos, as noted earlier, other potentially toxic materials are used, among them certain dusts, such as silica or talc; solvents, including organic solvents; and heavy metals, including lead.

A last area of significant concern, in addition to potential radon exposure, is the increasing evidence of potential health effects of a variety of electromagnetic hazards, including microwave, radiofrequency, and extremely-low-frequency) (ELF) exposures. ELF refers to the normal 60-Hz exposures received from household current. Some data associate a higher risk of childhood leukemia with increasing ELF exposure, and there continues to be concern about high-tension power lines.

CASE STUDIES

To help illustrate the range and complexity of environmental exposures, a series of case studies is offered.

Case study 1

A 42-year-old man is referred for evaluation of arsenic poisoning. He has been ill for approximately 5 months, and several weeks ago one of his treating physicians, after performing a heavy-metal screen because of the development of Mees' lines (white lines in fingernails), makes the diagnosis of arsenic poisoning.

An occupational history reveals that the man works as a manager of a convenience store that also sells gasoline. He has recently moved into a new mobile home with his family. He has built an outdoor deck with specially treated wood, has applied pesticides to his new lawn, and has begun using a new ceramic coffee cup. At work there has been no spraying for pests.

The diagnosis of arsenic poisoning is confirmed, and detailed evaluation shows that the ceramic glaze on the coffee cup does not contain arsenic. The deck wood had been treated with arsenic, and excess pieces were burned outside; however, the patient did not do the burning, nor did he handle the ashes. It was done by other family members, none of whom exhibit signs of arsenic poisoning. The patient apparently has good relations with his wife. (Spousal poisoning should always be included in suspected or documented cases of arsenic poisoning.)

It is determined at the time of a home visit that he mixed large quantities of pesticides containing arsenic in a glass taken from the kitchen, and on several occasions returned the unwashed glass to the kitchen. The glass in question was used by no other family member except the patient. His arsenic poisoning was from the residue of pesticide being measured into the glass.

Case study 2

A middle-aged art-gallery owner in New York City usually lived in a small apartment near the gallery but also had a large house in Connecticut. After playing tennis in early spring she developed lower back pain and to save walking steps in the Connecticut house moved into a daughter's bedroom on the first floor. Approximately 10 days later, while continuing to have back pain, she also experienced a severe case of dizziness. She returned to New York, was examined by her doctor, and was told to continue to rest her back and to take a nonsteroidal antiinflammatory drug.

That weekend she went to the Connecticut house for bedrest and continued to take the medication. She then developed diarrhea that was blamed on the nonsteroidal inflammatory drug, so its use was discontinued. She stayed at the country house, and approximately 1 week later she experienced a severe case of diarrhea and stomach cramps, with generalized weakness. This syndrome continued over the weekend, and the intestinal symptoms worsened. Her weakness progressed, and she developed transient pain in her hands and legs. She began to lose weight and became very thirsty. It became difficult to walk or stand.

She again consulted her internist approximately 1 month after the onset of symptoms. A chest radiograph at that time revealed no abnormality, although she had developed a dry cough with wheezing. She continued to lose weight, and a gastroenterologist found only rapid motility in her gastrointestinal tract.

She continued to experience a pulling sensation in her legs, associated with twitching and severe pain along the nerve distribution in her abdomen. She began to experience memory loss, diplopia, and other visual disturbances. She also experienced speech difficulties. On two occasions 1 month apart she was again seen by her physician, who found nothing abnormal in her laboratory test results.

She was referred to a psychiatrist, who determined that this syndrome was not totally due to depressive symptoms but believed that the cause was physical in nature. She then underwent a series of medical evaluations by a gynecologist, an endocrinologist, and an infectious disease specialist. These evaluations ruled out diabetes and multiple sclerosis. Parasitic infection was considered but could not be proven.

At this point the patient spent a month-long summer vacation consisting mainly of rest on the west coast, and her symptoms disappeared. On return to the east coast the patient lived in her New York City apartment and continued to feel well. At this time a colleague showed her a magazine article about pesticide poisoning.

On calling her exterminator, she found that an organophosphate had been sprayed twice at the Connecticut home prior to the onset of symptoms, once in great quantity in the bedroom in which she stayed, to combat fleas. Spraying had occurred on the carpet, drapes, bed, and other furniture. Later, when symptoms once again worsened, they were associated with monthly spraying, not only in the house but with additional organophosphates on the lawn.

At this point, armed with this information, her physician diagnosed her illness as a hypersensitivity to organophosphates, and slowly her symptoms resolved.

Case study 3

A scientist at a government laboratory, knowledgeable about potential health effects of toxic materials, enjoyed competitive pistol shooting as a hobby. He was noted to use hearing protection at the range, but further discussion revealed that he made his own bullets in an unventilated basement, using a heated cauldron to melt the lead. Although he had no clinical symptoms, measurement of the blood lead level revealed a markedly elevated value of 50 µg/dL. His levels returned to normal after he stopped manufacturing his own bullets.

Case study 4

A 38-year-old high school physical education teacher and football coach was diagnosed with a mesothelioma. A detailed exposure history revealed that for 2 to 3 months one summer while he was in college, about 20 years earlier, he was actively involved with handling materials containing asbestos while working with a construction crew.

Case study 5

A 28-year-old accountant went to his doctor with dull chest pain that on evaluation over the next several months, including thoracotomy, was found to be a malignant mesothelioma. Lung tissue taken during thoracotomy revealed the presence of two forms of asbestos. A detailed occupational and environmental history at first failed to reveal any potential source of asbestos exposure. The young man had been a college student, had never worked in any environment with known asbestos exposure, and had always worked as an accountant. Being under 30, the development of mesothelioma seemed unusual, given the usual latency period for development of this disease.

A further review of a map of his two places of residence during his lifetime revealed that both sites were within three blocks of a naval shipyard, and one of the types of asbestos found in his lung was of a type most commonly used aboard U.S. naval vessels. His exposure had been environmental during his childhood, and his 28-year latency period now seemed appropriate.

PERSONNEL AND INFORMATION RESOURCES

A large number of resources are available to the interested health care provider to obtain assistance in assessment of environmental diseases. Resources with well-trained personnel include professional organizations such as the American College of Occupational and Environmental Medicine, the American Board of Medical Toxicology, and the Association of Occupational and Environmental Clinics. In addition, there are a number of federally funded educational resource centers in the areas of occupational and environmental health, along with a variety of individually funded programs geographically distributed in the United States. The National

---

Sources of technical information

Material safety data sheets (available from agencies and companies)
Poison-control centers
State and local health departments
Academic institutions (National Institute for Occupational Safety and Health–sponsored Environmental Resource Centers and Program Projects)
Medical libraries

Technical data bases

MEDLARS: Medical Literature Analysis and Retrieval System (operated by the National Library of Medicine, 1-800-538-8480)
TOXLINE: Toxicology Information Line
TOXLIT: Toxicology Literature
CHEMLINE: Chemical Dictionary On-LINE
TOXNET: Toxicology Data Network (operated by the National Library of Medicine, 1-301-496-6531)
HSDB: Hazardous Substances Data Bank
CCRIS: Chemical Carcinogenesis Research Information System
RTECS: Registry of Toxic Effects of Chemical Substances
DBIR: Directory of Biotechnology Information Resources
ETIC: Environmental Teratology Information Center
TRI: Toxic Chemical Releases Inventory (operated by the National Library of Medicine, 1-800-496-6531)

Organizations concerned with environmental and occupational health

American College of Occupational and Environmental Medicine
American College of Preventive Medicine
American Lung Association
Association of Occupational and Environmental Clinics
American Public Health Association
Agency for Toxic Substances and Disease Registry
Collegium Ramazzini
Consumer Product Safety Commission
Department of Energy
Department of Transportation
Environmental Protection Agency
International Labour Office
National Cancer Institute
National Institute for Environmental Health Sciences
National Institute for Occupational Safety and Health
Nuclear Regulatory Commission
Occupational Safety and Health Administration
Society for Occupational and Environmental Health

Institute for Occupational Safety and Health can identify the nearest such resource. Other organizations such as state and local health departments, poison-control centers, and others the like can provide assistance. The box on p. 238 gives a fuller list of sources for technical information.

In addition to such resources, a number of computerized data bases can be relatively easily abstracted. The second box on p. 238 lists data bases that serve as an excellent source of information. The box above gives a relatively comprehensive list of organizations concerned with occupational or environmental health and can serve as a resource for those seeking additional information.

Of special note is the current availability of documents called material safety data sheets (MSDS). Relatively new in terms of federal regulation, the MSDS reviews toxicologic aspects of all chemicals currently manufactured and distributed. These documents are available through some of the agencies noted previously or the supplier of such chemicals. They provide an initial insight to the toxicologic aspects and potential hazards associated with a wide variety of chemicals.

A bibliography appended to this chapter lists additional reading materials regarding the environmental and occupational history as well as texts and journals for consultation in environmental disease.

REFERENCES

1. Agency for Toxic Substances and Disease Registry: *Case studies in environmental medicine: taking an exposure history,* Washington, DC, 1992.
2. Lilienfeld DE: Asbestos-associated pleural mesothelioma in school teachers: a discussion of four cases, *Ann NY Acad Sci* 643:454, 1991.
3. Ramazzini B: *De morbis artificum (Diseases of workers),* New York, 1964, Hafner (Translated from 1713 edition by WC Wright).

BIBLIOGRAPHY

American College of Physicians: Position paper: Occupational and environmental medicine: the internist's role, *Ann Intern Med* 113:974, 1990.
Becker CE: Key elements of the occupational history for the general physician, *West J Med* 137:581, 1982.
Clayton GD, Clayton FE, eds: *Patty's Industrial Hygiene and Toxicology,* 3, New York, 1978-1985, Wiley.
Ellenhorn MJ, Barceloux DG: *Medical toxicology: diagnosis and treatment of human poisoning,* New York, 1987, Elsevier.
Finkel AJ: *Hamilton and Hardy's industrial toxicology,* ed 4, 1983, PSG.
Goldman RM, Peters JM: The occupational and environmental health history, *Ann Intern Med* 246:2831, 1981.
Himmelstein JS, Frumkin H: The right to know about toxic exposures: implications for physicians, *N Engl J Med* 312:687, 1985.
LaDou J: Approach to the diagnosis of occupational illness. In LaDou J, ed: *Occupational medicine,* 1990, Lange.
Levy BS, Wegman DH: *Occupational health: recognizing and preventing work-related disease,* ed 2, Boston, 1988, Little, Brown.
Occupational and Environmental Health Committee of the American Lung Association: Taking the occupational history, *Ann Intern Med* 99:641, 1983.
Proctor NH, Hughes JP, Fischman ML: *Chemical hazards in the workplace,* 2, Philadelphia, 1988, JB Lippincott.
Raffle PA et al: *Hunter's diseases of occupations,* ed 7, Boston, 1988, Little, Brown.
Rom WN, ed: *Environmental and occupational medicine,* ed 2, Boston, 1992, Little, Brown.
Schwartz DA et al: The occupational history in the primary care setting, *Am J Med* 90:315, 1991.
Zenz C, ed: *Occupational medicine: principles and practical applications,* ed 3, Chicago, 1993, Mosby–Year Book.

SUGGESTED JOURNALS

American Industrial Hygiene Association Journal
American Journal of Epidemiology
American Journal of Industrial Medicine
American Journal of Public Health
American Review of Respiratory Diseases
Archives of Environmental Health
Occupational and Environmental Medicine
Chest
Environmental Health Perspectives
Journal of Occupational and Environmental Medicine
Scandinavian Journal of Work, Environment, and Health
Yearbook of Occupational and Environmental Medicine

TOPICS IN CLINICAL SYSTEMS

Chapter 20

THE EYES AND VISION

Pete Casten
K. Loftfield

Anatomy and physiology
Exposure sources and clinical presentations
    Eye irritants
    Chemical burns
    Systemic toxicity
    Electromagnetic radiation
Patient management and prevention

This chapter focuses on various responses of the eye to chemical agents and electromagnetic radiation. Widespread use of chemicals both at home and at work make chemical eye injuries a common problem confronting physicians. Depending on characteristics of the chemical agent, concentration, and duration of exposure, effects can range from mild irritation to severe chemical burns with loss of vision. Additionally, a variety of systemically absorbed neurotoxic substances have the potential for ophthalmic toxicity. This toxicity is due to damage of the neuro-optic pathways. The eye is also constantly exposed to the full spectrum of electromagnetic radiation. Various ocular structures respond to this exposure in different ways, resulting in a variety of distinct clinical entities. Knowledge of potential eye damage from these environmental exposures can help physicians appropriately educate patients in preventive measures.

ANATOMY AND PHYSIOLOGY

The eye, although relatively small, is a complex sensory organ. It has three main layers: the outer structural layer (cornea and sclera), the middle vascular layer (uvea), and the inner neurosensory layer (retina and retinal pigment epithelium). Internally, it is divided into three chambers: anterior chamber, posterior chamber, and vitreous chamber. It is derived from the interaction of multiple embryologic tissues. The corneal epithelium, conjunctiva, and lens are surface ectodermal in origin. The iris, choroid, ciliary body, nonepithelial cornea, and sclera are primarily mesodermal, while the retina, retinal pigment, epithelium, and optic nerve are true neural tissue. It contains two avascular structures (lens and cornea) bounded by unique active transport systems, which maintain a steady state of relative dehydration and thus transparency. The aqueous system (analogous to the cerebrospinal fluid system in the CNS) is produced by the ciliary body and drains through the trabecular meshwork (see Fig. 20-1).

The globe is housed in the bony orbit. The eyelids are modified folds of skin that cover the eye, distributing tears, regulating the amount of light admitted, and protecting the eye from foreign objects. The associated lacrimal system is composed of the lacrimal glands (main and accessory) and the drainage passages (puncti, canaliculi, lacrimal sac, and nasolacrimal duct). The extraocular muscles rotate the globes and when functioning normally maintain the alignment of the eyes with respect to one another.

The eye is unusual in that, like the skin, it is directly exposed to the environment. The conjunctiva, the corneal epithelium, and their associated tear film are the portions of the eye directly exposed to external insult. In addition, because the eye is an optical system, many internal structures (cornea, lens, retina, and retinal pigment epithelium) are exposed to light and other forms of electromagnetic radiation.

The conjunctiva is a mucous membrane consisting of nonkeratinizing squamous epithelium and globlet cells on its surface, and a thin, richly vascularized substantia propia. It is continuous with the dermis at the lid margin and with the corneal epithelium at the limbus. The three portions, the tarsal, fornical, and bulbar conjunctiva, together create a

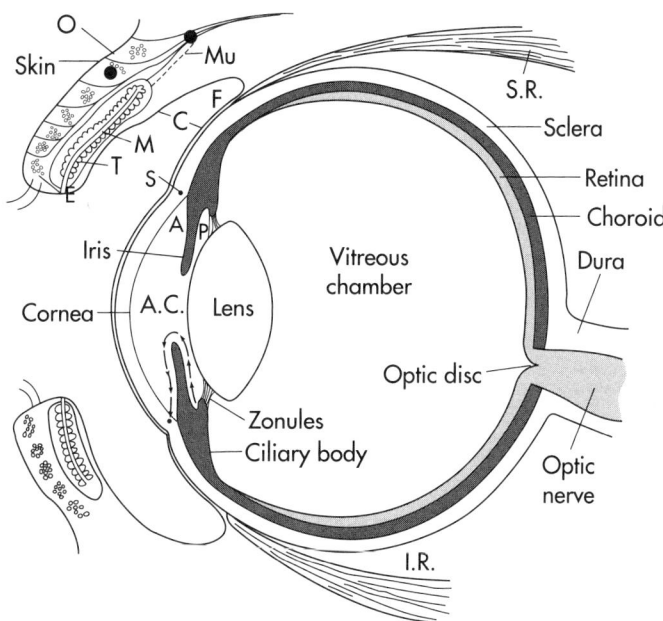

Fig. 20-1. Anatomic cross-section of the eye showing the cornea, conjunctiva and lens as well as other structures. (A.C. = anterior chamber; A = aqueous humor; C = conjunctiva; F = fornix; S = sclera; M = meibomian glands; Mu = muscle; P = posterior chamber; S.R. = superior rectus muscle; I.F. = inferior rectus muscle; T = tarsal) (From Goldberg S: *Ophthalmology made ridiculously simple,* Miami, 1982, MedMaster, Inc.)

smooth surface for nonirritative opening and closing of the lids. The mucous of the conjunctival globlet cells make up one of the three layers of the tear film, the others being lipid from the meibomian glands of the eyelid and the aqueous from the lacrimal glands. Abnormal degenerative changes of the conjunctiva can occur (pengueula), while mild inflammatory reactions result in conjunctivitis. More extensive injury can lead to destruction of tissue with scar formation (symblepharon).

The sclera and the cornea make up the outer structural layer of the eye. The sclera is made up of collagen fibrils and is opaque white in color. The cornea, the window of the eye, is composed of tissue much like the sclera. However, the arrangement of collagen fibers is much more regular. The cornea is steeply curved, which enables it along with its tear film to perform most of the refraction (bending and focusing) of the light entering the eye. (The lens also focuses light but to a much lesser degree.) Although only about 1 mm thick, the cornea is a relatively tough tissue. Following ocular trauma, the outer corneal epithelial layer regenerates quickly with little or no scarring. If the tough Bowman's membrane just below the epithelium is breached and the corneal stroma is involved, scarring does occur. This impairs vision, particularly if the central cornea over the pupillary aperture is involved. Corneal transparency is based primarily on the geometric array of collagen fibers in its stroma. Damage to the corneal endothelium affects the water balance in the stromal collagen meshwork and will result in corneal clouding (see Fig. 20-2).

The middle layer of the globe, the pigmented vascular uveal layer, consists of the iris, ciliary body, and choroid. The ciliary body processes are the site of aqueous production and maintain the blood-aqueous barrier. The aqueous exits the eye through the trabecular meshwork system. This fluid fills the posterior and anterior chambers, bathing the anterior lens capsule and corneal endothelium, and is the primary source of nutrition for these avascular structures. It is optically empty because of a relative absence of cells and protein. Inflammation (iritis) results in a breakdown of the blood-aqueous barrier with an increased amount of protein and cells in the aqueous. This gives the clinical sign of cells and flare in the anterior chamber (the hallmark of iritis). This is clinically associated with pain, photophobia, and blurred vision. The ciliary body also supports the lens behind the iris via the zonules. Contraction of the ciliary body muscle allows rounding up of the lens, the process of accommodation.

The lens embryologically is a piece of skin that is folded into the eye and upon itself. The basement membrane of the lens epithelial cells completely surround it, forming the lens capsule. New lens cell fibers (formed by the lens epithelial cells) are constantly being formed from an early embryonic stage, and this continues throughout life. Thus with aging, the lens increases in size and decreases in elasticity, resulting in loss of accommodation (presbyopia). With time, fibers undergo degenerative changes that result in opacification. All opacities in the lens, regardless of etiology, are called cataracts and may obstruct vision. Those located posteriorly

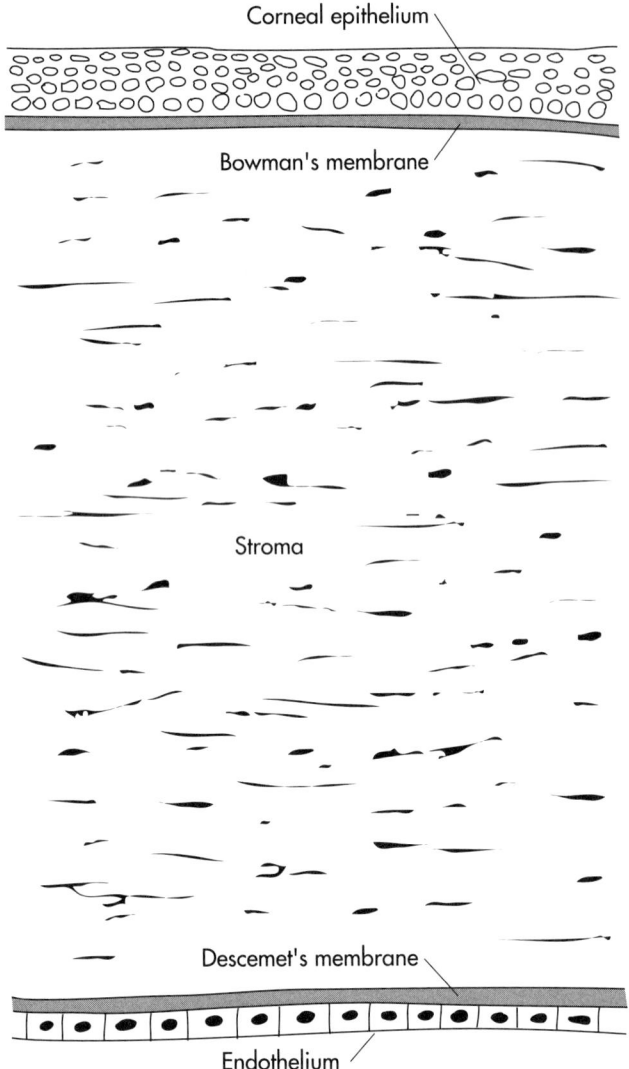

Fig. 20-2. Diagramatic representation of microscopic cross-section through cornea. (From Goldberg S: *Ophthalmology made ridiculously simple,* Miami, 1982, MedMaster, Inc.)

and centrally impair vision to a greater degree than anterior and more peripheral opacities.

The third and innermost layer of the eye is the retina and its associated retinal pigment epithelium. After light passes through the cornea, anterior chamber, pupil, posterior chamber, lens and vitreous chambers, it strikes the retina. Light is received by the sensory retina and is transformed photochemically into an electric impulse ready for transmission through the optic nerve and to the brain. All other components of the eye actually exist to support this photoreceptive function, serving primarily as refractive media (cornea and lens), for nourishment (uvea and retinal pigment epithelium), or for protection (cornea and sclera). The retina is transparent, and light passes through the entire thickness of the retina before striking the rods and cones. These photoreceptors then initiate a chain of neuronal impulses from photoreceptor to bipolar to ganglion cells. The ganglion cells become the optic nerve, which extends to the brain (see Fig. 20-3).

The associated retinal pigment epithelium is sandwiched between the choriocapillaris and the photoreceptors. While much of the retina receives its nourishment from the branches of the central retinal artery, the photoreceptors are dependent on diffusion from the choroid. This places considerable metabolic demands on this important cell layer, and an intact, healthy retinal pigment epithelium is vital to the continued health and function of the photoreceptors. When a retinal detachment occurs and the retina is separated from the retinal pigment epithelium, irreversible damage to the photoreceptors can occur after several days, presumably from hypoxia. There can be little doubt that the etiologies of many retinal disorders may have their primary origin in a malfunctioning retinal pigment epithelium. Age-related macular degeneration is one significant disease felt to have retinal pigment epithelium dysfunction as a major component.

EXPOSURE SOURCES AND CLINICAL PRESENTATIONS
Eye irritants

The eyes are susceptible to injury from a wide variety of chemical substances. However not all chemical injuries result in severe ocular damage or scarring. For example, exposure to low-dose vapor concentrations of respiratory tract irritants often results in conjunctival membrane irritation in addition to upper respiratory tract irritation. Respiratory tract irritants represent a diverse spectrum of compounds, usually in the gaseous or vapor state, that cause irritation to mucous membranes manifested as nonspecific inflammation.[2] Ammonia, hydrogen chloride, phosgene, sulfur dioxide, and chlorine gas are examples. In low-dose exposures, self-limited "chemical conjunctivitis" without residual sequelae can be expected. However, exposures to these same substances in high concentrations can result in severe damage and opacification of the cornea. In most cases the higher the level of exposure, the more severe is the conjunctival membrane irritation. Therefore knowledge of the extent of acute eye irritation occurring at the time of a respiratory irritant exposure may provide additional insight when trying to retrospectively assess the level of respiratory irritant exposure that may have occurred.

Environmental tobacco smoke, volatile organic compounds, ventilation system problems, and various building materials have been implicated in the sick building syndrome. This syndrome consists of mucous membrane complaints (eye, nose, and throat irritation), odor complaints, and diffuse symptoms such as headaches, dizziness, difficulty concentrating, and fatigue.[25] The eye complaints include eye

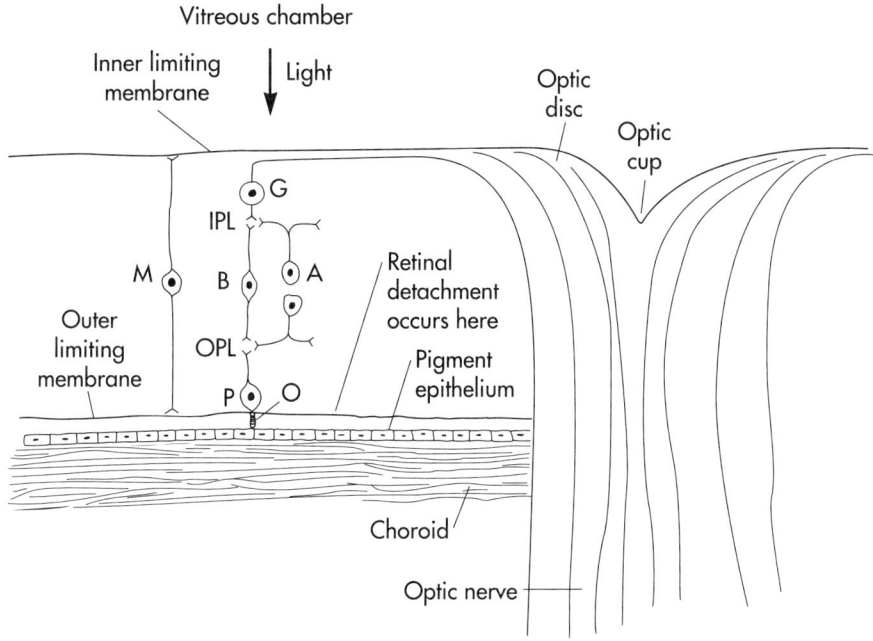

Fig. 20-3. Diagramatic representation of microscopic cross-section through retina and optic nerve (G = ganglion neuron; B = bipolar neuron; P = photoreceptor neuron; A = axon). (From Goldberg S: *Ophthalmology made ridiculously simple,* Miami, 1982, MedMaster, Inc.)

dryness, irritation, and inability to wear contact lenses.[28] Although most clinical investigations have not demonstrated physical or laboratory abnormalities, one study has shown these eye complaints to be associated with decreased stability of the precorneal tear film.[12] In cases where patients complain of persistent eye irritation, the physician should inquire about exposure to environmental tobacco smoke, and whether or not symptoms can be localized to a particular indoor or outdoor environment. If symptoms predominate indoors, inquiry should be made about air ventilation quality. Use of nonprescription lubricating drops (artificial tears) is recommended and usually sufficient in alleviating symptoms.

Godish[17] has described eye irritation as one of the most prevalent effects of outdoor air pollution. The ocular effects often precede problems of asthma, sinus problems, and bronchitis. Unfortunately there is little information on specific physiologic changes from air pollution beyond immediate tearing.[28] Many patients will present with symptoms of hyperemia, mucous discharge, and foreign body sensation. During the eruption of Mount St. Helens in 1980 the primary ocular complaints due to volcanic ash exposure in the surrounding areas were irritative conjunctivitis and foreign-body sensations with or without retained conjunctival or corneal foreign bodies composed of ash particles. Patients with contact lenses or sicca syndrome had the most frequent ocular complaints, but no long-term ocular effects have been noted secondary to volcanic ash exposures.[13] The condition is usually mild and self-limited once the exposure has ceased. Again, supportive therapy with frequent artificial tear use often minimizes symptoms.

Red, itchy, watery eyes are typical features of allergic conjunctivitis.[15] This common form of conjunctivitis results from the interaction of IgE on conjunctival mast cells with the pollen of airborne allergens. Since either allergic or irritant phenomena may lead to eye irritation with similar presenting complaints by patients, determining the etiology of eye irritation requires, as a first step, a careful environmental history to assess where and when symptoms occur. Additionally, the most prominent symptom of allergic conjunctivitis is itching, and eosinophils can usually be recovered on conjunctival scrapings.[16] Other immunologic eye conditions, such as contact sensitivity, atopic keratoconjunctivitis, and vernal keratoconjunctivitis should also be considered when attempting to differentiate irritant from allergic eye conditions. The true allergic conjunctivitis typically runs a chronic recurrent clinical course, in contrast to the irritant conjunctivitis, which typically resolves once the irritant exposure has ceased.

Chemical burns

Injuries to the cornea may result from direct contact with acids, alkalis, organic solvents, metallic salts, and inorganic agents. Accidental splashing of highly concentrated acids or alkalis generally produce the most severe corneal burns, often also involving the sclera and even lens and iris. Immediate recognition and emergency medical management of these injuries are vital to limiting the severity of injury. The most severe chemical burns often produce little pain, due to destruction of the sensory nerves in the cornea, whereas relatively superficial injuries involving the corneal epithelium may cause great discomfort due to nerve ending irritation rather than destruction.[20]

The corneal epithelium and endothelium provide a barrier to water-soluble substances, while the corneal stroma is a barrier to lipid-soluble substances. Therefore, substances with both water and lipid solubility penetrate the cornea with greater ease than substances that are only water- or lipid-soluble.[41] Solubility, duration of contact, and pH of the substance are the most important factors in determining the extent of any chemical eye burn. The rapid destruction of tissues can be minimized only by immediate copious irrigation. Identification of the substance will aid the physician in anticipating the ocular complications that will follow.

The corneal epithelium offers moderate protection against penetration of dilute acids; therefore, little damage occurs unless the acid pH is below 2.[20] If the epithelium has been disrupted, however, tissue destruction can occur, even when the pH is more than 2.5.[41] In mild acid burns, superficial erosion of the corneal epithelium and hyperemia of the conjunctivae completely resolve without serious sequelae. The transient defects seen on fluorescein staining rapidly return to normal within a few days. In more severe burns, thrombosis of conjunctival and episcleral blood vessels produces ischemia of surrounding tissues and pallor of the cornea.[20] Severe iritis, opacification of the cornea, and even opacification of the lens may result.

Acidic substances are commonly found both at home and at work. For example, sulfuric acid is used in fertilizing and is also found in automobile batteries. Many eye injuries have resulted from explosions of automobile batteries containing 20% to 25% sulfuric acid.[38] Hydrochloric acid and nitric acid are commonly found in chemical manufacturing. Hydrofluoric acid (commonly used in the chemical refining and semiconductor industries) is a potent and extremely damaging acid due to the high reactivity and penetrating ability of the fluoride ion in tissues.[35] When injury due to hydrofluoric acid occurs, healing is generally prolonged, and late complications such as ulceration or perforation are likely to arise.

While tissue proteins tend to buffer and localize the effects of many acid substances, hydroxyl ions of alkaline compounds combine with fatty acids in cell membranes and cause saponification leading to extensive tissue destruction, thus allowing alkali to penetrate rapidly and cause damage to intraocular structures.[48] Common household alkali chemicals include household bleaches (sodium, potassium, or calcium hypochlorite), household ammonia (7% ammonium hydroxide), drain cleaners containing lye (sodium hydroxide), and lime (calcium hydroxide).[41] Contact with an alkali solution of pH greater than 11.5 generally results in immediate destruction of corneal epithelial cell membranes with denaturation of intracellular enzymes.[14] Significant alkali burns may produce opacification of the cornea. Two to 3 minutes after the burn, the anterior chamber pH dramatically rises, giving rise to damage of all adjacent tissue, including trabecular meshwork, iris, lens, and ciliary body.[43,44] The inflammatory reaction (iritis) involving the aqueous humor may lead to secondary glaucoma, or damage to the ciliary body by alkali may cause permanent ocular hypotony with irreversible visual loss.[44] Other complications of severe alkali burns include the possibility of cataract formation and retinal damage.[47] Based on the appearance of the cornea and conjunctiva 24 hours after alkali injury, prognosis for recovery or later ulceration can be estimated.[30]

Systemic toxicity

A variety of systemically absorbed toxins have significant ocular manifestations. Extraocular muscle palsies with diplopia, pupillary abnormalities, or visual dysfunction secondary to optic neuropathy, retrobulbar neuropathy, and papilledema have been described from exposure to various metals (including lead, mercury, and arsenic), organic solvents (including methanol, benzene, toluene, and trichloroethylene), gases (including carbon disulfide and carbon monoxide), and pesticides (including organophosphates, DDT, and other insecticides).[18]

Since this is an ocular manifestation of a systemic toxin, bilateral symmetrical involvement of both eyes is particularly characteristic for the long list of substances capable of causing optic neuropathy, optic neuritis, or optic atrophy. The finding of optic atrophy does not establish whether the primary site of toxic action was at the ganglion cell in the preretinal nerve fiber layer, the optic disc, or some site behind the eye. Neither does it indicate if it is a direct toxic effect or secondary to a disruption of blood supply. For example, the initial insult from carbon disulfide is a retrobulbar optic neuritis, which in some cases progresses to a nonspecific, nonlocalizing optic atrophy.[20] Additionally, there is still little known about why some substances cause peripheral visual field constriction and other substances produce central scotomas. Most victims of methylmercury toxicity at Minimata showed bilateral concentric constriction of visual fields with relative preservation of central vision.[54] Postmortem exams revealed widespread lesions throughout the cerebral and cerebellar cortices, including the occipital visual cortex. Histologically, the neurons in the anterior portion of the visual cortex seemed to be selectively affected, and this pattern was felt to correspond to the observed concentric peripheral visual field defect.[50]

Carbon disulfide, used in the past as a solvent in the viscose process for rayon and cellophane, causes central vision defect and retinal involvement. In addition to pallor of the optic disc seen on ophthalmoscopic examination, fluorescein angiography reveals microaneurysms, dot hemorrhages, and small exudates.[49] Other neurotoxic solvents with potential for ophthalmic toxicity include trichloroethylene, xylene, toluene, and methylene chloride.[36] Chronic exposure to trichloroethylene has been reported to produce double vision, changes in color perception, optic neuropathy, and blindness.[7,20] Xylene, toluene, and methylene chloride have been associated with visual disturbances and, in cases of severe exposures, optic neuropathy or visual hallucinations.*

In cases of organic solvent toxicity, it has been suggested that altered integrity of neuro-optic pathways is not necessarily reflected by diminished visual acuity.[36] Rather, loss of color vision and contrast sensitivity may be early clinical indicators of retinal disease, optic neuropathy, or both, even when visual acuity remains intact.† Mergler et al.[36] demonstrated significantly lower contrast sensitivity in former microelectronics assembly workers, and it was suggested that exposure to ophthalmotoxic chemicals was the most probable risk factor for the visual dysfunction found.

*References 6, 10, 36, 42, 59.
†References 1, 4, 21, 22, 26.

Electromagnetic radiation

Electromagnetic radiation consists of waves of radiant energy classified according to specific wavelengths that vary in size from very short cosmic rays to long radio waves. Visible light is a narrow band in the spectrum. Longer wavelengths have less energy (infrared, radiowaves, and microwaves), while shorter wavelengths have higher energy (ultraviolet, gamma, and cosmic radiation). The majority of radiation reaching the Earth from the sun lies in the ultraviolet, visible, and infrared regions. These regions, in addition to ionizing and microwave radiation, have special significance in relation to the eye. Different structures in the eye may be adversely affected by exposure to different regions of the spectrum, resulting in a variety of clinical lesions (see Table 20-1).

Ultraviolet light is divided into three bands, each with its own relevance to biologic adverse effects. UV-A (400-320 nm) is the closest to visible blue. UV-B (320-290 nm) is shorter. UV-C (290-100 nm) is the shortest and most powerful. Ultraviolet A induces the browning or tanning effect on skin, whereas ultraviolet B causes sunburn, blistering, and skin cancer.

Almost all of the UV-C is filtered out by the ozone. The remainder of what little UV-C gets through the atmosphere

Table 20-1. The electromagnetic spectrum*

Wavelength (mm)		Major common sources		Photon energies (ev)	Effects when absorbed
10^{12}	Long-wave	Radio			
10^{13}	Medium-wave				
10^{10}	Short-wave	Diathermy			Rotational and vibrational
10^{9}					
10^{8}		Television			
10^{7}	Microwave	Radar		0.001	
10^{4}					
10^{3}				0.01	
10^{4}	Infrared	Sun	Blast furnaces	0.12	
10^{3}			Carbon		
750--------			Xenon arc lamps		
	Visible	Sun	Incandescent lamps	1.14	Electronic excitation and molecular dissociation
100--------		Sun	Fluorescent lamps	2.06	
280--------	Ultraviolet		Germicidal lamps	3.10	
10^{2}				4.90	
10^{1}				6.20	
10^{0}	Soft x-radiation		Isotopes	12.50	Ionization (bond breakage)
10^{-1}	(grenz)				
10^{-2}	Hard x-radiation	Radioactive minerals	x-ray apparatus		
10^{-3}	Gamma radiation				
10^{-4}					
10^{-5}	Cosmic radiation		Isotopes		

*From Lermans: *Radiant energy and the eye*, New York, 1980, Macmillan, p 2.

is filtered out by the cornea. The cornea increasingly transmits longer wavelengths of electromagnetic radiation, with over 60% UV-A being transmitted. The lens absorbs almost all UV-B, and more than 99% of radiation below 320 nm. The lens increasingly transmits longer wavelengths of UV-A, with 50% wavelength 400 nm (visible blue light region) being transmitted. The retina will absorb any radiation that reaches it.[31,51-53]

Numerous epidemiologic studies have shown that people with high sun exposure (for example, sailors and farmers) get more nonmelanoma skin cancers, particularly on the sun-exposed skin, such as face, neck, and hands.[51] Basal cell carcinomas of the eyelids are quite common. When these lesions involve the lid margins, skilled excision with proper reconstruction of the lid is necessary. Basal cell carcinomas that occur in the medial canthal area are particularly treacherous, as they tend to go deep and often recur after previous excision.

There is a high correlation between UV light exposure and pterygium formation. Cameron[5] found pterygia to be more prevalent between 40 degrees north and 40 degrees south latitude. Island populations seemed particularly at risk, and he concluded that ultraviolet radiation was responsible. Other studies supporting the UV light correlation included a large rural Australian study that showed less pterygium in southern Australia, and a Japanese welder study demonstrating that pterygium was much more common in welders.[27,39] There is considerable circumstantial evidence for the role of sunlight, but irritation from dust or ice particles seems to be an additional factor and in some populations may be the major factor. The highest prevalence of pterygium is found in areas that are both sunny and dusty.[29] Evidence for the importance of ocular irritation is also provided by the high prevalence of pterygium in sawmill workers in British Columbia, northern India, Taiwan, and Thailand compared with control groups in the same areas.[8] In all four studies, pterygium was much more common in sawmill workers even when compared with outdoor workers. Most mild-to-moderate pterygia are well tolerated, although cosmetically unattractive, and may even play an adaptive role in these warm climates by decreasing ocular irritation secondary to profuse sweating.[37] Large pterygia can impinge on the visual axis, interfering with vision, and must be surgically removed. Unfortunately, there is a significant recurrence rate.

The cornea filters wavelengths below 295 nm while transmitting wavelengths of 295 to 400 nm.[31] The epithelial layer has two absorption peaks, one at 289 nm and the other at 254 nm. Fortunately the ultraviolet intensity required to induce photochemical damage is higher than ordinarily encountered, except in polar regions. This is the classic "snow-blindness" of polar explorers and snow skiers. Ordinary glass filters almost all wavelengths less than 300 nm, and therefore ordinary glasses offer protection. Arc welders' keratitis is essentially the same process. The condition is self-limited and disappears within 48 hours after complete repair of the corneal epithelium.

Because the cornea effectively filters all UV radiation shorter than 295 nm, we need only consider the effects of longer wavelengths on the interior of the eye. The lens absorbs 99% of UV-B, but increasingly transmits longer wavelengths.

Cataract refers to any opacity of the biologic lens. There are many etiologies: genetic, congenital, nutritional, diabetic, and advancing age. Although only small amounts of UV light enter the eye under normal conditions, the cumulative effect of many years of exposure could be significant, particularly when considering man's ever increasing life span. Epidemiologic studies provide strong support for the thesis that sunlight plays a role in some types of cataracts.[3,51-53,62]

Experimentally, the lens is most susceptible to damage to radiation in the UV-B band.[52] Initial epidemiologic studies reveal a clear association between cortical and posterior subscapsular cataracts.[3,51-53,57] No association with UV-A or visible light was found. The association with UV-B revealed a linear dose-response relationship.[52] There was no evidence of an absolutely safe dose. Thus, a little bit of UV-B is bad for the lens and a lot is worse.[51]

The final answer is not in. Further studies are needed to confirm these epidemiologic findings. Also, further studies are needed to determine the role of antioxidants (such as vitamins A, C, and E) in modifying the UV-light-induced cataract. However, there is also biochemical and experimental evidence to suggest that UV-B is associated with cataracts, and epidemiologic studies to date also point in that direction.

Infrared radiation has also been associated with cataract formation. Man-made sources of infrared radiation are the major culprits with respect to potential ocular damage. The extreme heat in certain industrial processes, particularly steel making and glass blowing, was a major source of infrared radiation. This resulted in lenticular damage, the classic glass blowers' cataract, considered to be a thermally induced injury. This has been mostly eliminated by shorter workdays, furnace shields, and protective eyewear. There is still a slight increase in cataract development at a slightly younger age in these workers.[46]

Microwave has also been associated with cataracts. At present 100 to 150 mW/cm^2 is considered to be the cataractogenic dose.[31] Appleton feels that microwave-induced acute lens damage in humans is extremely unlikely, as the amount of energy needed would also result in associated facial burns.[31] This is consistent with animal studies in which cooling blankets were needed to keep the animals from expiring from heat before cataracts could be produced.[46] However, Cleary disagrees and notes that over 40 cases of cataracts in humans have been attributed to microwave exposure.[31] There is now some indication that repeated lower doses may eventually cumulate in tissue damage. If this bears out, a mechanism other than the well-known thermal effects of microwaves must exist. Cleary has proposed a molecular mechanism termed dielectric dispersion as a possible explanation.[31]

Ionizing radiation is associated with cataract formation and has been recognized since the initial reports in 1928.[31] The delay in fully appreciating this association can be attributed to the relatively long latency of 1 to 20 years.[31] The lens is extremely sensitive to ionizing radiation, and this can be appreciated by the fact that in some survivors of the Hiroshima and Nagasaki atomic explosions, cataract development was the only sign of radiation damage.[31] Presently, ionizing radiation therapy to the eye is advocated for intraocular tumors such as retinoblastoma and malignant melanoma, when the risk to life far outweighs the cataractogenic hazard. Some types of ocular lymphomas and skin tumors can be successfully treated with radiation without cataract formation if the eye is properly shielded.[31]

The normal adult lens blocks almost all wavelengths less than 400 nm. However, in a young person, the lens transmits a band between 310 and 320 nm.[33,34] This transmission decreases with age as the lens acquires more light-absorbing pigment. Obviously, this crystalline lens filter is absent in aphakes and in pseudophakes with non-UV absorbing intraocular lenses. Most intraocular lenses implanted now have built-in UV filtering properties.

The retina has a number of built-in defenses against light exposure. But these defenses can be overcome by brief intense exposure. One extreme is the thermal damage of laser retinal photocoagulation. A less extreme example is solar retinopathy induced by solar eclipse viewing. Because acute light exposure can damage the retina, it has long been questioned whether the cumulative effect of chronic light exposure might also be damaging.

Retinal photocoagulation occurs when retinal irradiance is high enough to cause a temperature increase great enough to produce thermal trauma and subsequent coagulation and scarring. Phototoxicity or photoretinopathy takes place with a more prolonged exposure to lower light levels.[34] Photoretinopathy has been studied extensively. Blue light is more hazardous than longer wavelengths. Ultraviolet light is potentially even more hazardous because of its even shorter wavelength and therefore higher energy. Phototoxicity can be divided into two categories.[34] Type 1 is mediated by the photoreceptor pigment and may be involved in the blue color contrast deficiency reported in long-term users of argon blue-green photocoagulators.[34] Type 2 phototoxicity involves light levels that are higher but still well below photocoagulation thresholds. This type primarily affects the retinal pigment epithelium and is felt to be important in solar retinopathy and injury from ophthalmic operating microscopes.

Eclipse blindness has been known since ancient times. In 1916, Verhoeff and Bell demonstrated that the concentration of the sun's rays on the retina resulted in thermal damage to the tissue.[31] This solar retinopathy was felt to result from the magnification of the sun's rays, visible and particularly infrared, on the retina, resulting in acute thermal injury. More recently, Ham et al. have proposed that solar retinopathy is not a thermal injury, but a thermally enhanced photochemical effect of the short-wave visible components of the sun's spectrum.[31] Mainster maintains that looking directly at the sun with a normally constricted pupil produces only a 3° to 4°C temperature increase, well below the 10° to 20°C increase needed for retinal photocoagulation.[34] He also feels it is a phototoxic and not a thermal retinal injury. He notes that while solar retinopathy is usually associated with direct sun gazing, young patients who are sunbathing but not sun gazing while at the beach can also develop solar retinopathy. He feels this is associated with the relative enhanced transmission through the younger person's clear crystalline lens, associated with the high reflectivity of the sand. An acute solar injury is a yellowish lesion that fades over several weeks. But a severe injury can produce long-term foveal distortion or even a macular hole.[34] Similar nonsolar retinal burns can be produced from exposure to high-intensity light, such as xenon arc lamps, prolonged indirect ophthalmoscopy, and exposure to lasers emitting in the infrared region.[31]

There has also been some concern that light exposure may be a factor in age-related macular degeneration.[60] As early as the 1920s, it was noted that macular degeneration was more common in aphakic patients and less common in patients with cataracts.[34] This suggests that light may play a role in macular degeneration. Evidence linking the two is still circumstantial. Laboratory investigations in which intense light exposure has been applied in animal models has resulted in extensive damage to photoreceptor cells and the retinal pigment epithelium.[34,55,60] The possibility that long-term exposure to light may be a factor in age-related macular degeneration has been raised, but as yet little conclusive evidence is available.[34,55] In one recent study with phakic subjects, even with high levels of sunlight exposure there was no evidence of increased risk of age-related macular degeneration associated with UV-B or UV-A exposure.[58] This finding was also supported in a subsequent study by Taylor et al.[53] However, Taylor et al.[53] did find that patients with advanced age-related macular degeneration (geographic atrophy or disciform scarring) had significantly higher exposure to blue (400 to 500 nm) or visible (400 to 700 nm) light over the preceding 20 years, compared with age-matched controls. It was concluded that exposure to blue or visible light may be related to the development of age-related macular degeneration.[53] However, there are clearly many other factors involved that affect macular aging.

The retina is susceptible to a variety of of laser-induced injuries. Because of its unique composition, morphology, and optical properties, the eye is the most susceptible of all body tissues to damage from exposure to laser radiation. The mode of operation of the instrument determines the type of exposure. There are three types: the continuous-wave mode in which exposure can vary from milliseconds to minutes, the normal multiple-spike mode with exposure times from 100 microseconds to 2 milliseconds, and the Q-switched mode, with an exposure time less than 100 nanoseconds. The type and degree of laser-induced retinal damage depends on the power density of the laser, the time exposure, the wavelength, and the size of the image on the retina. The continuous-wave- and multiple-spike-mode lasers cause primarily thermal and photochemical damage, which is wavelength to a considerable extent. However, the high-intensity Q-switch laser can create shock waves and even vaporization of tissue. These shock waves formed by thermal expansion could be of sufficient intensity to disrupt cellular organelles at a significant distance from the site of absorbed energy. This is why the industrial and military Nd-YAG laser is so treacherous. It is a significant source of severe eye injury, with associated visual loss. In recent years, between 20 to 100 severe ocular injuries involving these lasers have been documented.[46] Most injuries could be prevented by use of appropriate protective eyewear that are laser-type-specific.

Video display terminals present no significant radiation hazard to the eyes. A misunderstanding of the emission of these devices has led to much overconcern in the press. By comparison to any other type of electromagnetic source, the video display terminal is contributing an extraordinarily small dose rate of any form of nonionizing radiation. Video display terminals can be associated with eye strain. This can be minimized by proper lighting to minimize glare and reflections, by keeping the display monitor clean of dust, and by taking periodic rest breaks. Proper optical correction is also important, and as many video display terminal users prefer a viewing distance a little further away than that at which they normally read, a separate pair of glasses can often be helpful.

PATIENT MANAGEMENT AND PREVENTION

Proper eye protection with goggles when working with toxic chemicals is obviously the key to preventing serious chemical eye injuries. Safe work practices should be emphasized both at home and at work. However, when injuries do occur, immediate treatment can limit the severity of injury. The emergency response to a chemical eye injury should be irrigation at the accident site with the first available nontoxic fluid and continued irrigation en route to the nearest medical facility.[41] In the emergency department, intravenous solution with tubing can be set up to provide continuous irrigation. Topical anesthetics may be applied, followed by complete inspection of upper and lower conjunctival fornicies to remove any foreign bodies. The pH of the conjunctiva should be monitored with litmus paper, and irrigation should continue until the pH is neutral (pH 7). The pH portion of a combination urine chemistry reagent strip (for example, Combistix, Labstix) can also be used to monitor the pH.[41]

Irrigation should be continued until a stable pH in the range of 7 is achieved. In the case of acid burns, the pH generally remains stable once it has neutralized. However, in the case of alkali burns, irrigation may be required for several hours prior to the pH returning to the neutral range. For prolonged continuous irrigation, use of a Morgan Therapeutic Lens connected by intravenous tubing to normal saline, lactated Ringer's, or 5% dextrose has been one very effective technique described.[40]

Any significant chemical eye injuries require prompt evaluation by an ophthalmologist who is knowledgeable about chemical burns to the eyes. In the case of severe alkali burns, many ophthalmologists will recommend an anterior chamber tap (paracentesis) and irrigation with a balanced salt solution if the patient is seen within 2 hours of sustaining the injury. [Nelson] Mydriasis, cycloplegia, and antibiotic therapy will usually be continued as long as an epithelial defect is present. Subsequent complications include chronic ocular surface abnormalities associated with a poor tear film, persistent corneal epithelial defects, corneal opacification and vascularization, elevated intraocular pressure with secondary glaucoma, cataract, and incomplete lid closure (lagophthalmos) with chronic exposure.

Since the sun's radiant energy is capable of various effects on the eyes, including UV keratitis and solar retinopathy, and most likely plays a major role in other conditions, such as pterygium formation and cataract formation, protection from the sun by wearing hats and sunglasses may reduce ocular exposure and possibly reduce the risk of disease.[3] Sunglasses can be used to minimize the potential for photochemical damage to the eye from various electromagnetic radiation sources, and particularly from ultraviolet rays. The sale of sunglasses is a several-billion-dollar industry in the United States. Over 2 million pairs per year are sold worldwide, and over one half of these are sold in the United States.[11] Unfortunately, there are no guidelines for lenses considered as cosmetic or fashion wear. Many lenses are not labeled at all or are poorly labeled with respect to their transmission characteristics. It seems reasonable to note the effectiveness in filtering UV and visible (especially short blue wavelengths). A large number of lenses transmit near UV, visible, and infrared portions of the spectrum. Lens composition, color, and cost were not good indicators of effectiveness.[11] The rule of ''buyer beware'' applies here. The American Academy of Ophthalmology has taken the stand that the public has the right to know the transmission characteristics of the sunglasses they buy.

The ideal lens might filter out almost all infrared and UV bands. Blue light up to 470 nm or possibly up to 530 nm should also be highly absorbed.[11] Reasonable color discrimination, especially of red and green for traffic safety, should be permitted by the lens. Ideally, the frames should have side shields to cut down on oblique incident light. The glasses should meet flamability, durability, and impact-resistant standards. When possible, they should also allow for refractive correction.

REFERENCES

1. Arden GB: Testing contrast sensitivity in clinical practice, *Clin Vis Sci* 2:213, 1988.
2. Barkman HW: Respiratory tract irritants. In Rom WN, ed: *Environmental and occupational medicine,* Boston, 1992, Little, Brown.
3. Bochow TW et al: Ultraviolet light exposure and risk of posterior subscapsular cataracts, *Arch Ophthalmol* 108:369, 1989.
4. Bodis-Wollner I: Methodological aspects of contrast sensitivity measurements in the diagnosis of optic neuropathy and maculopathy, *Doc Ophthal Proc Ser* 35:225, 1983.
5. Cameron ME: *Pterygium throughout the world,* Springfield, Ill, 1965, Charles C Thomas.
6. Channer KS, Stanley S: Persistent visual hallucinations secondary to chronic solvent encephalopathy, *J Neurol Neurosurg Psychiat* 46:83, 1983.
7. Department of Labor: Occupational exposure to trichloroethylene, *Fed Reg* 40:49032, 1975.
8. Detels R, Dhir SP: Pterygium: a geographic study, *AMA Arch Ophthal* 78:485, 1967.
9. Duke-Elder S, MacFaul PA: Radiation injuries: action on the lens. In Duke-Elder S et al: *System of ophthalmology,* vol XIV, part 2, St Louis, 1972, Mosby.
10. Ehya A, Freeman FR: Progressive optic neuropathy and sensorineural hearing loss due to chronic glue sniffing, *J Neurol Neurosurg Psychiat* 46:349, 1983.
11. Fishman GA: Sunglasses and other protective devices, *Ophthalmology* 89(suppl 9A):109, 1992.
12. Franck C: Eye symptoms and signs in buildings with indoor climate problems (''office eye syndrome''), *Acta Ophthalmol* 64:306, 1986.
13. Fraunfelder FT: Ocular effects following the volcanic eruptions of Mount St. Helens, *Arch Ophthalmol* 101:376, 1983.
14. Friedenwald JS, Hughes WF, Herriman H: Acid base tolerance of the cornea, *Arch Ophthalmol* 31:279, 1944.
15. Friedlaender MH: Immunologic aspects of diseases of the eye, *JAMA* 268:2869, 1992.
16. Friedlaender MH, Okumoto M, Kelley J: Diagnosis of allergic conjunctivitis, *Arch Ophthalmol* 102:1198, 1984.
17. Godish T: *Air quality,* Chelsea, Mich, 1985, Lewis Publishers.
18. Goetz CG: *Neurotoxins in clinical practice,* New York, 1985, Spectrum Publications.
19. Goldberg S: *Ophthalmology made ridiculously simple,* Miami, 1982, MedMaster.
20. Grant WM: *Toxicology of the eye,* ed 3, Springfield, Ill, 1986, Charles C. Thomas.
21. Harmor MF: Contrast sensitivity and retinal disease, *Ann Ophthalmol* 13:1069, 1981.
22. Hart WM: Acquired dyschromatopsias, *Surv Ophthalmol* 32:10, 1987.
23. Hiller R, Giacometti L, Yuen K: Sunlight and cataract: an epidemiologic investigation, *Am J Epidemiol* 105:450, 1977.
24. Hiller R, Sperduto RD, Ederer F: Epidemiologic associations with cataract in the 1971-72 National Health and Nutrition Examination Survey, *Am J Epidemiol* 118:239, 1983.
25. Hodgson MJ: Clinical diagnosis and management of building-related illness and the sick-building syndrome, *Occupational Medicine: State of the Art Reviews* 4:593, 1989.
26. Hyvarien L, Laurinen P, Rovamo J: Contrast sensitivity function in evaluation of visual impairment due to macular degeneration and optic nerve lesions, *Acta Ophthalmol* 61:161, 1983.
27. Karai I, Horiguchi S: Pterygium in welders, *Br J Ophthal* 68:347, 1984.
28. Klopfer J: Effects of environmental air pollution on the eye, *J Am Optom Assoc* 60:773, 1989.
29. Editorial, Pterygium and its causes, *Lancet* 1:1392, 1984.
30. Lempe MA: Cornea and sclera, *Arch Ophthalmol* 92:158, 1974.
31. Lerman S: *Radiant energy and the eye,* New York, 1980, Macmillan.
32. Mackezie FD et al: Risk analysis in the development of pterygia, *Ophthalmology* 99:1056, 1992.
33. Mainster MA, Ham WT, Delori FC: Potential retinal hazards: instrument and environmental light sources, *Ophthalmology* 90:927, 1983.
34. Mainster MA: Sunlight as a factor in macular degeneration, *Ophthalmology* 89(suppl 9A):109, 1992.
35. McCulley JP et al: Hydrofluoric acid burns of the eye, *J Occup Med* 25:447, 1983.
36. Mergler D et al: Visual dysfunction among former microelectronics assembly workers, *Arch Env Health* 46:326, 1991.
37. Miller D: Solar risks to the skin and ocular surface, *Ophthalmology* 89(suppl 9A):109, 1992.
38. Minatoya HK: Eye injuries from exploding car batteries, *Arch Ophthalmol* 96:447, 1978.
39. Moran DJ, Hollows FC: Pterygium and ultraviolet radiation: a positive correlation, *Br J Ophthalmol* 68:343, 1984.
40. Morgan LB: A new drug delivery system for the eye, *Ind Med Surg* 40:11, 1971.
41. Nelson JD, Kopletz LA: Chemical injury to the eyes, *Postgrad Med* 81:62, 1987.
42. O'Donaghue JL, ed: *Neurotoxicity of industrial and commercial chemicals,* vol 1, Boca Raton, Fla, 1985, CRC Press.
43. Paterson CA, Pfister RR, Levinson RA: Aqueous humor pH changes after experimental alkali burns, *Am J Ophthalmol* 79:414, 1979.
44. Pfister RR, Koski J: Alkali Burns of the eye: pathophysiology and treatment, *South Med J* 75:417, 1982.
45. Sasaki K, Hockwin O, eds: Distribution of cataracts in the population and influencing factors, *Dev Ophthalmol* 21:120, 1991.
46. Sliney DH: Risks from non-solar radiation, *Ophthalmology* 89(suppl 9A):109, 1992.
47. Smith RE, Conway B: Alkali retinopathy, *Arch Ophthalmol* 94:81, 1976.
48. Stern AL, Pamel GJ, Benedetto LG: Physical and chemical injuries of the eyes and the eyelids, *Dermatol Clin* 10:785, 1992.
49. Sugimoto K et al: Ocular fundus photography of workers exposed to carbon disulfide: a comparative epidemiologic study between Japan and Finland, *Int Arch Occup Environ Health* 37:97, 1979.
50. Takeuchi T et al: Grade and distributions of pathological lesions in the nervous system in Minimata disease, from observations of 72 autopsy and 6 biopsy cases, *J Kumamoto Med Soc* 51:216, 1977.
51. Taylor HR: Sunlight as a factor in cataracts, *Ophthalmology* 89(suppl 9A):109, 1992.
52. Taylor HR et al: Effect of ultraviolet radiation on cataract formation, *N Engl J Med* 319:1429, 1988.
53. Taylor HR et al: The long-term effects of visible light on the eye, *Arch Ophthalmol* 110:99, 1992.
54. Tokuomi H, Okajima T: Clinical Minimata disease, *Adv Neurol Sci* 13:69, 1969.
55. Tso MO, Woodford BJ: Effects of photic injury on the retinal tissues, *Ophthalmology* 90:952, 1983.
56. Van Heyninger R: The human lens. I. A comparison of cataracts extracted in Oxford (England) and Shikarpur (W. Pakistan), *Exp Eye Res* 13:136, 1972.
57. West SK et al: Senile eye changes: ultraviolet light and risks of cataract, *Invest Ophthalmol Vis Sci* 28(suppl):397, 1987.
58. West SK et al: Exposure to sunlight and other risk factors for age-related macular degeneration, *Arch Ophthalmol* 107:875, 1989.
59. Wyse DG: Deliberate inhalation of volatile hydrocarbons: a review, *Can Med Assoc J* 108:71, 1973.
60. Young RW: Pathophysiology of age-related macular degeneration, *Surv Ophthalmol* 31:291, 1987.
61. Zhang JD: An investigation of aetiology and hereditary of pterygium, *Acta Ophthalmologica* 65:413, 1987.
62. Zigman S, Datiles M, Torczynski E: Sunlight and human cataracts, *Invest Ophthalmol Vis Sci* 18:462, 1979.

Chapter 21

DISORDERS OF THE EAR AND HEARING

Doug Swift
Tim Molon

Cochlear disorders
    Introduction
Anatomy of the ear
    External and middle ears
    Inner ear
Physiology of the ear
    Introduction
    Nature of noise-induced hearing loss
Causes of nonoccupational hearing loss
    Environmental
    Chronic exposure to noise
    Ototoxic drugs and chemicals
Nonenvironmental causes of hearing loss
    Congenital
    Presbycusis
    Other causes
Clinical evaluation of hearing
    Audiogram
    Air conduction
    Bone conduction
    Masking
    Speech reception threshold
    Speech discrimination
    Brainstem evoked-response
    Other screening tools
    Clinical examination
Vestibular Disorders
Anatomy
Physiology
Pathology
Vestibular evaluation and testing
    Medical diagnosis
Specific environmental causes of vestibular disorders
    Solvents
    Heavy metals
    Salicylates
    Alcohol
    Trauma

Diagnosis and management
Future directions

COCHLEAR DISORDERS
Introduction

We live in a noisy world! Noise is America's most widespread nuisance. Excessive noise exposure annoys individuals, produces stress, impairs the ability to communicate, interfers with work and play activities, and in high enough doses produces permanent damage to the auditory system, which leads to a significant hearing loss. In 1980, the most recent year for which U.S. census figures are available, there were 14,953,000 hearing-impaired persons in the United States, of whom 1,977,000 were functionally deaf. Only 10% of Americans older than 65 have "normal" hearing, and 60% of those with impaired hearing are deaf.[42,59]

ANATOMY OF THE EAR

There are three parts to the human ear: the external, middle, and inner ears, plus the internal auditory canal.

External and middle ears

The external ear is the only part of the ear that grows after birth. There are two parts to the external ear: the pinna (auricle) and the external auditory canal. The pinna consists of an irregular plate of fibrocartilage tightly covered by skin and a thin layer of subcutaneous tissue. The external auditory canal is a tortuous composite tube with an average length of

3.7 cm in the adult male. The tympanic membrane forms a common wall between the external canal and the middle ear. The middle ear is a flat, air-filled chamber enclosed by five bony walls. The sixth and lateral wall is the tympanic membrane. The lumen, which is lined by a delicate, ciliated mucous membrane, is traversed laterally to medially by a chain of three small interarticulated bones—the malleus (hammer), the incus (anvil), and the stapes (stirrup)—and posteriorly to anteriorly by the slender chorda tympani nerve.[29]

Inner ear

The inner ear is composed of a system of channels and chambers (bony labyrinth) hollowed into the densest bone in the body (oticcapsule) (Fig. 21-1). These channels are filled with fluid (perilymph), the composition of which is similar to that of cerebrospinal fluid. In the perilymph a corresponding closed system of delicate membranous tubes and sacs (membranous labyrinth) is suspended; these sacs are filled with fluid (endolymph) that contains a high level of potassium. The inner ear is anatomically and functionally divided into two parts: the more primitive superior and posterior vestibular labyrinth (balance) and the anteroinferior cochlea (hearing).[29]

In the human the cochlea is a channel coiled into half turns around a central bony axis, the modiolus, which contains the spiral ganglion, whose component cells are the cell bodies of the cochlear nerve. The cochlear channel is subdivided into three compartments, called scalae (Fig. 21-1). A central membranous cochlear duct or scala media contains endolymph. The two surrounding compartments, the scala vestibuli and the scala tympani, contain perilymph and communicate with each other at the apex of the cochlea. The scala vestibuli opens into the vestibule. At the basal end of the scala tympani there is a defect in the bony wall called the round window, which is sealed by the round window membrane. The cochlear duct is the essential hearing apparatus. It is roughly triangular when seen in cross-section. The base of the triangle is the basilar membrane, which is comprised of fibers that extend from a tiny, hollow, bony partition to the spiral ligament (Fig. 21-2). The oblique side of the triangle is the delicate Reissner's membrane, which is two cells thick. The third side of the triangle contains a bed of capillaries, the stria vasculares. The sensory cells of the hearing apparatus are massed together in the organ of Corti, which sits on the scala media surface of the basilar membrane. The organ of Corti is divided by a tunnel that is lined

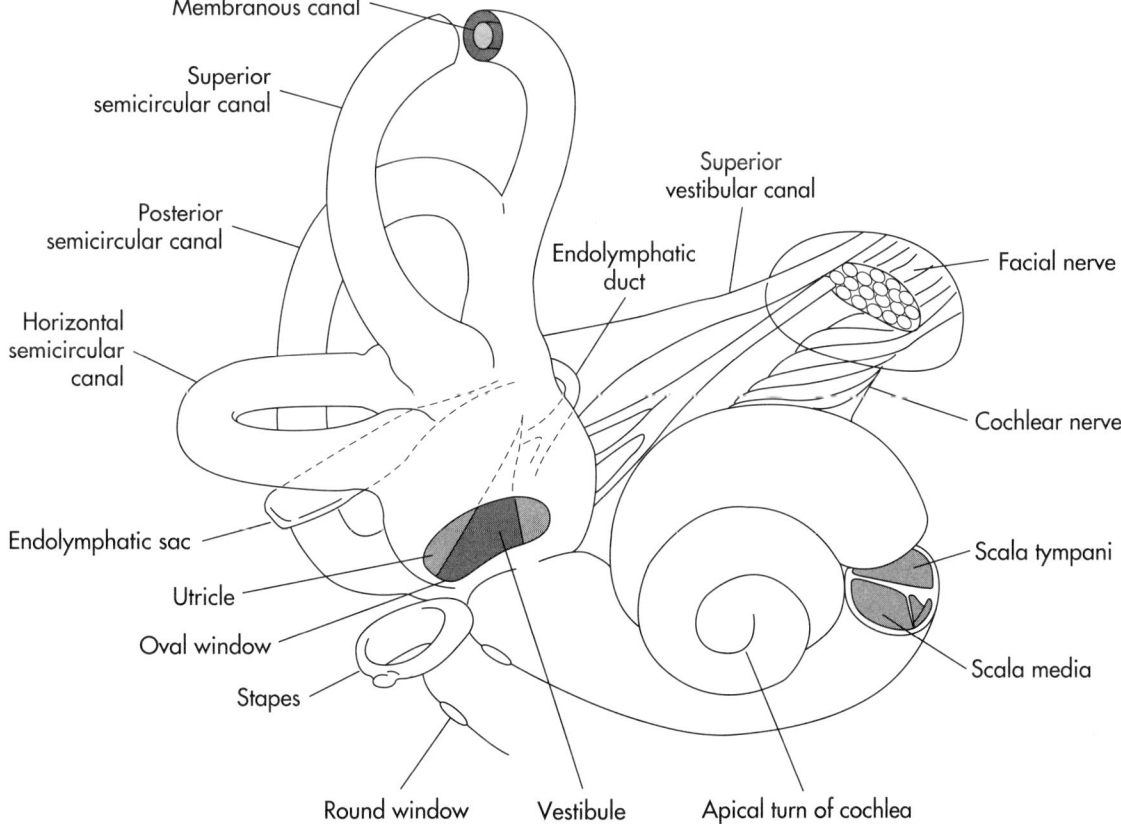

Fig. 21-1. Stylized diagram of inner ear. There are two areas of deficit in the bony capsule of the inner ear that faces the middle ear: the oval window, into which fits the footplate of the stapes, and the round window, which is sealed by the round winsow membrane. (From Karmody CS: Anatomy and physiology of the ear. In Bradford LJ, Hardy WG, eds: *Hearing and hearing impairment,* New York, 1979, Grune & Stratton).

by two pillars of acellular material. On the inner side of the tunnel is a single row of hair cells, which is the inner hair cell; on the strial side of the tunnel are three rows of outer hair cells. In the human ear there are about 12,000 hair cells and 25,000 to 30,000 cell bodies in the spiral ganglion. The base of the hair cells is flanked by the endings of the afferent and efferent nerves. The cilia are in contact with the undersurface of the tectorial membrane, a gelatinous structure that is firmly anchored to the limbus and draped over the organ of Corti, forming a barrier between the organ and the endolymph. An efferent system exists in the cochlea, in which cell bodies are in the superior olivary nucleus. Their axons form the olivocochlear bundle of Rasmussin, which follows the vestibular and cochlear nerves, passes through the spiral ganglion, and then crosses the tunnel of Corti to arborize around the bases of the outer hair cells. Blood supply to the inner ear is provided by a single small vessel, the internal auditory artery. This is an end artery and has no anastomosis with neighboring blood vessels. The vestibular labyrinth is an essential part of the balancing system of the body. There are three semicircular canals disposed in the three dimensions of space, two vertical and one horizontal, and all are at right angles to each other.[29]

PHYSIOLOGY OF THE EAR
Introduction

Sound creates vibrations in the air somewhat similar to the ''wave'' created when a stone is thrown into a pond. The outer ear collects these sound waves and funnels them down the external ear canal to the tympanic membrane. As sound waves strike the membrane, they are transmitted by mechanical action through the middle ear over the bony bridge formed by the malleus, incus, and stapes. These vibrations cause the membranes over the openings to the inner ear to vibrate, setting in motion the endolymph in the inner ear. Sound waves stimulate the organ of Corti by exciting movements of the endolymph, which in turn causes motion in the basilar membrane and concomitant distortion of the hair cell to produce a chemical mediator. [This initiates nerve impulses in axons of the spiral ganglion cells which then are transmitted along the cochlear nerve to the cochlear nuclei.] The cochlea acts as a transducer, converting sound energy into neural activity for transmission to the brain, where it excites the sensation of hearing.[51] The cochlea is frequency-specific, with pitch differentiation occuring at the site of maximal stimulus. Higher frequencies stimulate the basal cochlea, near the oval window, and lower frequencies stimulate the apical cochlea. A 4000-Hz source of noise will stimulate hair cells at the first turn of cochlea from the oval window.

Nature of noise-induced hearing loss

There are many known causes, but only two basic types, of hearing loss: conductive and sensorineural. Conductive hearing loss is caused by any condition that interferes with the transmission of sound through the external and middle to the inner ear. If it is in the middle ear, the damage may involve the footplate of the stapes, as in otosclerosis, or the mobility of the eardrum and ossicles caused by fluid. Conductive hearing losses are generally correctable.

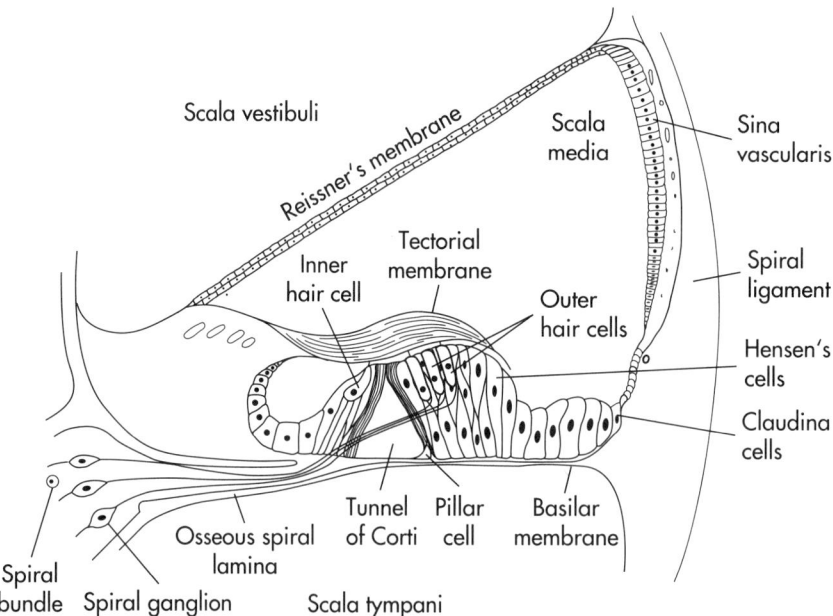

Fig. 21-2. The cochlear duct. The stria vascularis consists of fine capillaries and is probably responsible for homeostasis of the endolymph. There are three rows of outer hair cells and one row of inner hair cells in the organ of Corti. (From Karmody CS: Anatomy and physiology of the ear. In Bradford LJ, Hardy WG, eds: *Hearing and hearing impairment,* New York, 1979, Grune & Stratton.)

Sensorineural hearing loss is due to the damage that lies medial to the stapedial footplate in the inner ear, the auditory nerve, or both. The cochlea has approximately 30,000 hearing nerve endings (hair cells). These hair cells and the nerve that connects them to the brain are susceptible to damage from a variety of causes. Noise-induced hearing loss is sensorineural. The prognosis for restoring a sensorineural hearing loss with presently available therapy is poor.

CAUSES OF NONOCCUPATIONAL HEARING LOSS
Environmental

There are numerous sources of noise in the environment that have the potential to produce noise-induced hearing loss. Some of the significant sources and maximum levels of nonoccupational noise are given in Table 21-1.

The acoustic impulses produced by handguns and rifles can cause mild-to-severe sensorineural hearing loss. Reported peak sound levels from rifles and shotguns have ranged from 132 dBA for .22 caliber rifles to more than 172 dBA for high-powered rifles and shotguns.[43] If the instantaneous peak sound pressure level (PSPL) exceeds 140 dB, the acoustic energy in the signal can stretch the delicate inner ear tissues beyond their elastic limits and tear them apart. This type of damage is called acute acoustic trauma, and results in an immediate and usually permanent hearing loss. The hearing loss is often accompanied by tinnitus, which may subside within a few hours or days after the exposure. Because the impulsive noises mechanically damage the ear, the duration of the signal is of little significance; the most important variable is the peak sound pressure level. Animal studies have suggested that certain pathologic features are consistent within species, especially the acute mechanical failure associated with acute acoustic trauma. Consistent findings include separation of the organ of Corti from the basilar membrane and disturbances in function of the typanic membrane and ossicles.[9] The audiometric evaluation in acute acoustic trauma usually reflects damage in the high frequencies at about 4000 to 6000 Hz.

Chronic exposure to noise

The situation is not so equivocal with respect to the damage associated with years of exposure to more moderate noise. Exposure to noise primarily damages the inner ear, especially the organ of Corti.[7] The hair cells, cochlear blood vessels, stria vascularis, and nerve endings can be damaged also. Initially, the basal turn of the cochlea is affected and eventually disruption of the media and apical areas occurs. Long-term, noise-induced hearing loss may represent a gradual accumulation of noise microtrauma. Noise is characterized by irregularity, so some high-dB level of noise will occasionally occur, and these infrequent peaks may irreversibly injure a hair cell; after several years of noise exposure, the cumulative hair cell loss from these microtrauma becomes significant.

An alternative point of view, and one historically much older, is that long-term NIHL is the outcome of a slowly accumulating exhaustion of metabolites at the cytochemical or enzymatic level not involving direct gross tissue destruction. It is believed that biochemical changes eventually produce widespread hair cell destruction only indirectly.

Studies have indicated that the vascular supply of the basilar membrane tends to be disrupted secondary to high noise levels. Some early studies had shown that noise stimulation produced a decrease in the oxygen tension in the cochlea duct. A variety of animal investigations have been performed that confirm the above finding. However, in studies of direct observation of blood flow in the cochlea, neither vasoconstriction nor vasodilation can be found until the sound level reached 120 dB B SPL.

In a transmission electron microscopic study, edema and swelling of the afferent nerve endings below the inner hair cells were found.[18] In general, most investigators agree that a combination of mechanical, metabolic, and vascular factors are involved in causing the destructive changes that lead to noise-induced hearing loss (NIHL). In contrast to acute acoustic trauma, NIHL is cumulative and insidious, growing slowly over years of exposure. Eventually, the organ of Corti

Table 21-1. Sources and maximum levels of nonoccupational noise

Category	Range maximum sound pressure levels (DBA)
Recreational	
Shooting	>120
Cap pistol	>108
Model airplane	>105
Motorcycle/snowmobile	>80
Auto "boom box"	>110
Hobbies/workshop	
Chain saw	>105
Power saw	>95
Lawn mower	>80
Household	
Garbage disposal	>65
Vacuum cleaner	>60
Air conditioner	>50
Music	
Personal stereo	>95
Rock concert	>90
Symphony concert	80
Home stereo	>90
Transportation	
Automobile (50 feet)	>60
Passing truck at 50 feet	>70
Train at 50 feet	>80

breaks down, leading to elimination of sensory structures and replacement by a single flat cell layer.[9]

Ototoxic drugs and chemicals

Tinnitus, hearing loss, and vertigo are the cardinal symptoms resulting from the detrimental effect of drugs and chemicals on the inner ear. The box below illustrates the variety of substances that cause damage and highlights the ototoxic drugs encountered most frequently in clinical practice.

Hearing impairment resulting from ototoxic agents is almost always sensorineural. Ototoxicity from aminoglycoside antibiotics may be cochleotoxic or vestibulotoxic. Hearing loss produced by aminoglycoside antibiotics ranges from minimal to severe. It usually starts at high frequencies and progresses to low frequencies. Tobramycin and amikacin are considered more cochleotoxic, whereas streptomycin and gentamycin are considered more more vestibulotoxic. Cochlear toxicity from aminoglycoside antibiotics affects the inner row of outer hair cells first, followed by the outer rows or hair cells, then by the inner hair cells.[16] The pathology has also been localized to the stria vascularis, spiral ligament, and spiral prominence. Several theories of the mechanism of damage have been proposed, including direct damage to the hair cells and disruption of the metabolism in the stria vascularis and spiral ligament, which lead to changes in cationic differences of the perilymph.[16] The mechanism of vestibular damage remains poorly defined.

Ototoxic agents

Chemicals

Carbon monoxide	Lead
Mercury	Arsenic
Oil of chenopodium	Aniline dyes
Nicotine	Alcohol
Gold	Potassium

Drugs

Antibiotics	*Diuretics*
Aminoglycosides	Furosemide
streptomycin	Ethacrynic acid
Neomycin	Bumetanide
Gentamicin	Acetazolamide
Kanamycin	Mannitol
Tobramycin	
Amikacin	

Other antibiotics	*Miscellaneous*
Vancomycin	Analgesics and Antipyretics
Erythromycin	Salicylates
Polymyxin B	Quinine
Ampicillin	Chloroquine
Viomycin	Antineoplastics
Pharmacetin	Pentobarbital
Colistin	Practolol

A close relationship exists between renal and cochlear physiology; similarly most nephrotoxic agents are also ototoxic. Two diuretics in particular depress auditory function: furosemide causes a temporary sensorineural hearing loss, and ethacrynic acid causes a permanent hearing loss. However, ototoxicity only occurs when high doses are given intravenously and is heightened by concomitant renal dysfunction. Small doses of quinine (antimalarial) can cause tinnitus in susceptible individuals. Permanent deafness is rare. Chloroquine (another antimalarial) has caused permanent deafness.

Girardi et al. (1967) studied the effects of carbon disulfide, carbon monoxide, lead, benzene, carbon tetrachloride, and other compounds and found that both vestibular and cochlear disturbances occurred, with vestibular effects predominating. It is concluded that the lesions caused by these poisons were located in the nucleoreticular substance of the brainstem. Carbon monoxide poisoning occurs only too frequently, and one of the most disturbing sequences of survivors is sensorineural hearing loss. Attention has been drawn to the hearing loss occurring in children following exposure to environmental arsenic, usually the result of burning coal with a high arsenic content.[6] The arsenical atoxyl produces damage to the stria vascularis, followed inevitably by hair cell degeneration in experimental animals.[1] Potassium bromate is a constituent of the neutralizer of permanent hair waving sets. Accidental ingestion of this compound is toxic to the ear and the kidney, producing severe hearing loss and renal failure.

A large number of viral infections have been associated with sensorineural hearing losses. Rubella and mumps are the classic examples. Hearing loss with mumps is usually unilateral, whereas the loss with rubella is bilateral. In both cases the temporal bone pathology includes extensive degeneration of the sensory cell, stria vasculares, and tectorial membrane as well as the nerve supply.[35,36,52] Other viruses that have been implicated in both the gradual and sudden onset of sensorineural hearing loss include influenza, adenovirus, and herpes hominis.[26] Most viral infections of the inner ear are described as "endolymphatic labyrinthitis," with a pathology consisting of degeneration of the stria vascularis, organ of Corti, and tectorial membrane. Bacterial infections of the external and middle ears can also affect hearing; however, they are usually conductive hearing loss.

NONENVIRONMENTAL CAUSES OF HEARING LOSS
Congenital

Congenital aplasia (absence of external auditory canal) is a defect in fetal development. It can cause conductive hearing loss. Congenital cochlear defects cause sensory hearing loss. Hereditary hearing loss can be either conductive or sensorineural. Congenital ossicular defects are a variety of defects that may arise in the ossicular chain during fetal development and produce a conductive hearing loss of 60 to

70 dB, even though the eardrum and middle ear appear to be normal. Congenital syphilis can cause sudden bilateral hearing loss. More often, it causes unilateral sudden hearing loss.[51]

Presbycusis

This form of deafness is caused by aging and is the most prevalent cause of sensorineural hearing loss. Around the age of 40 years all humans begin to lose their hearing, initially in the higher frequencies because of selective degeneration of the organ of Corti. As a matter of fact, the process of presbycusis starts quite early in life. Children can hear up to about 20,000 Hz; however, many adults can hear only up to 14,000, 12,000, or 10,000 Hz. With advancing years the ability to hear the higher frequencies becomes less acute, and by the age of 70 most people do not hear frequencies above 6000 Hz. The rate at which presbycusis advances and the degree to which the individual becomes affected vary widely. To some extent heredity plays a role, for early or premature presbycusis is often found in several members of the same family. Presbycusis can be classified as sensory, neural, or metabolic, caused by degeneration of the organ of Corti, Cochlear nerve, and stria vascularis, respectively. Degeneration of the stria vascularis is reflected by a flat audiometric curve with comparatively good speech discrimination.[51]

Other causes

Although a great deal of attention has been paid to hereditary diseases associated with hearing loss, relatively little emphasis has been placed on recognizing the many nonhereditary diseases that are linked with deafness.

Oxygen deprivation in the neonatal period may produce sensorineual hearing loss. This connection may explain the increased incidence of deafness associated with traumatic, cyanotic, or premature birth, although the causal relationship has not been proven.

The AIDS clinical syndrome is characterized by immunodeficiency, frequently complicated by opportunistic infection and neoplasia. AIDS-related diseases may affect every body system, including the head and neck. Patients with AIDS are particularly susceptible to infectious agents, including viruses, bacteria, and fungi. Pneumocystic carinii infection has been found in the external and middle ears. These infections are associated with mixed conductive and sensorineural hearing loss. Hearing loss of patients with AIDS can also result from drug-induced ototoxicity.[51]

A significant percentage of patients with inner ear disease have been found to have hyperlipoproteinemia.[55] Studies found that hypertension plus an atherogenic diet alone does not produce significant hearing loss at any frequency. The role of an atherogenic diet in genetically predisposed hypertensive animals has been linked to an increased susceptibility to hearing loss with exposure to intermediate levels of chronic noise. This also supports findings that diet alone did not produce hearing loss in humans. However, hypertension, a chronic atherogenic diet, and chronic noise is devastation, even when the noise is of a moderate intensity.[41,46]

It has been suggested that cigarette smoking increases the risk of noise-induced hearing loss. Dangerous noise levels produce high levels of metabolism and capillary vasoconstriction in the cochlea resulting in a decrease in oxygen tension and lactate accumulation. Smoking is associated with rheologic changes in hematocrit, fibrinogen, and blood viscosity. Perhaps smoking imposes rheologic changes in the blood that have adverse effects on the microcirculation. This situation could significantly worsen the already compromised metabolic demand of the noise-exposed ear.[27]

At least 6 million diabetics live in the United States and up to 40% of diabetics develop hearing loss, although estimates vary from study to study. The hearing loss generally is sensorineural, progressive, bilateral, most severe in the high frequencies, and tends to be worse in the elderly diabetic. Laboratory research also supports the association of diabetes and hearing loss.*

CLINICAL EVALUATION OF HEARING

People are exposed to many kinds of environmental noise that can be distinguished according to the source of the noise or to its physical characteristics such as intensity, frequency spectrum, and variation in time. In evaluating a hearing-impaired person, the physician is advised to review the results of pure tone audiometric testing or other special hearing testing.

Audiogram

An audiogram is a written record of a person's hearing level measured with certain pure tones. The pure tones generally used are the frequencies 250, 500, 1000, 2000, 3000, 4000, 6000, and 8000 Hz; these tones are generated electronically by the audiometer.

With 0 dB representing average normal hearing, a 50-dB hearing threshold level also can be called a 50-dB "hearing loss." It was found that the threshold of a person with normal hearing ability fluctuated over approximately a 15-dB range. An average was reached at 0 dB of hearing. Average normal hearing, or 0 dB, is the reference level on the audiometer. A hearing loss at some specific frequency is expressed and recorded as the number of decibels by which a tone must be amplified for a patient to hear it.

Air conduction

Air conduction denotes the ear's ability to receive and conduct sound waves entering the external ear canal. When air conduction is impaired as a result of damage to the outer or middle ear and the sensorineural mechanism of the inner

---

*References 5, 6, 20, 32, 39, 40.

ear is intact, the maximum difference between air and bone conduction thresholds is about 60 dB.[51]

Bone conduction

Bone conduction is a measure of the patient's ability to hear sound vibrations that are transmitted directly to the cochlea through the bones of the skull, bypassing the outer and middle ear. Bone conduction is unimpaired in simple conductive hearing loss. When the bone conduction and the air conduction curves or levels are of the same magnitude, there is no air-bone gap. However, if the bone conduction level is better, air-bone gap is said to exist.[51]

The typical pattern of noise-induced permanent threshold shift (NIPTS) usually involves a maximum loss at 4000 Hz. Because the loss is sensorineural, it is seen in both air and bone conduction audiograms. Persons entering a very noisy area may experience a measurable loss in hearing sensitivity but recover sometime after returning to a quite environment. This phenomenon, called noise-induced temporary threshold shift (NITTS), can be measured as a shift in audiometric thresholds.

Masking

It is difficult to test hearing in only one ear because sound waves travel in all directions and are not stopped easily by merely plugging the opposite ear. The only way to keep the other ear from participating in the test is to keep it busy with a masking noise. Generally, masking should be used whenever there is a difference of 40 dB or more between the air conduction reading in the poorer ear and the bone conduction threshold in the better ear. It should be used if there is a difference of 40 dB or more between the left and right ear when bone conduction testing has not been performed. Unlike the 40-dB criteria in air conducting testing, in most cases, masking should be used routinely when doing bone conduction testing.[51]

Speech reception threshold

This is a measure of a person's ability to hear speech, using a speech audiometer that controls the intensity of the speech output. A person who hears normally can hear and repeat words at a level of about 15 dB or less. The higher the number of decibels, the greater the hearing loss. SRT should approximate PTA (500 Hz+1000 Hz+2000 Hz/3).

Speech discrimination

Speech discrimination testing is a measure of a person's ability to understand speech when it is amplified to a comfortable level. The testing usually is done at 30 or 40 dB above the Speech Reception Threshold (SRT). Only those words understood perfectly are counted as correct. Each word has a value of two points. Perfect score is 100 points. If 10 of the 50 words are repeated incorrectly, the patient has an 80% discrimination score. A discrimination score provides only a rough idea of the patient's ability to distinguish certain sounds in a quiet environment. Discrimination scores are moderately lower in patients with hearing loss due to presbycusis or congenital causes. Severe reductions in discrimination are associated with disorders medial to cochlea (eighth nerve and brainstem), that is, acoustic neuroma.

Brainstem evoked-response

Brainstem evoked-response audiometry (BERA) can be measured under general anesthesia or during deep coma. Absence or distortion of peaks, or delay between peaks, can help localize lesions in the audiotory pathway. BERA has become very popular because it is objective, consistent, and provides a great deal of valuable information. The test measures electrical peaks generated in the brainstem along the auditory pathways. The tests can be used on infants and children and have even been advocated for routine screening in newborn nurseries.[51]

Other screening tools

Audioscope is one of many other screening tools commonly used. It can be inserted into the ear and delivers a 40-dB tone at frequencies of 500, 1000, 2000, and 4000 Hz to assess the degree of hearing impairment. Hearing Handicap Inventory for the Elderly (HHIE) is a self-administered 10-item questionnaire designed to assess emotional and social problems associated with impaired hearing.[34]

W-22MAX assesses speech discrimination of words that are presented with a competing sound. This procedure determines a person's ability to communicate in everyday life by assessing both psychosocial impairment and biologic damage to the hearing mechanism. In W-22MAX, words are presented on an audiotape in the presence of background noise. W-22MAX appears to be a unique measure of both noise-related damage to the cochlea as well as a determinant of communication handicap.[49]

Clinical examination

Human hearing has a remarkable capability for differentiating sounds ranging from 20 to 20,000 Hz. In the early stages of noise-induced hearing loss, a person may complain only of tinnitus, muffling of sound, discomfort in the ears, or temporary hearing impairment, but improves after several hours away from the noise. The early symptoms of NIHL tend to be subtle and may not be readily recognized by the patient. People with NIHL initially have difficulty with various consonants. As NIHL progresses, the person's ability to distinguish becomes less intense.

The primary effect of NIHL is on the inner ear. A physician must be aware of other symptoms of inner ear disease, especially vertigo. Vertigo or dizziness also is a frequent companion of deafness. Because the hearing and the balance mechanisms are related so intimately and bathed in the same labyrinthine fluid, vertigo often accompanies hearing difficulties. Vertigo is often the first symptom of inner ear disorders. However, vertigo is seldom associated with NIHL or presbycusis.

NIHL rarely produces profound deafness, but the condition tends to be progressive. Hearing handicaps are usually noticed when the hearing level of important speech frequencies such as 500, 1000, 2000, and 3000 Hz averages more than 25 dB. The diagnosis of NIHL is straightforward when the physician incorporates occupational and nonoccupational history with the results of an audiometric evaluation.[59]

Early impairment due to NIHL tends to occur at 4000 Hz; preservation of hearing at higher frequencies (8000 Hz) is typical. The audiometric pattern has a similar deficit in the 4000-Hz range in persons with presbycusis; however, the loss tends to be greater in the 8000-Hz range (no notch is noted). The audiometric findings of hearing loss due to ototoxicity are similar to those of presbycusis. However, it is generally reversible. Repeated audiometric evaluations often show improvement following withdrawal of the medication.[49]

A hearing difficulty is quite different from the usual complaints presented to a physician. The patient with a hearing loss is likely to be in good health. Physical examination of the patient with otologic complaints should begin with a general assessment. Complete examination should include the nose, the neck, the throat, the presumably normal ear, and the impaired ear. Testing of hearing and balance function are fundamental in patients with otologic complaints. Metabolic tests must be selected on the basis of clinical need in each individual case. Neurotologic diagnosis has been revolutionized by modern radiologic technology. Magnetic resonance imaging (MRI) is the mainstay of radiologic evaluation of the neurotologic patient. MRI of the brain and internal audiotory canals is required for complete assessment.[51]

VESTIBULAR DISORDERS

Disorders of the vestibular system commonly give rise to the complaint of dizziness. It is important to mention, however, that not all dizziness is caused by vestibular disorders. The term *dizziness* can describe various sensations from giddiness, lightheadedness, wooziness, the sensation of moving or spinning, to syncope, fainting, and actual loss of consciousness. The terminology in this area can be confusing, and it is important to define specific sensations because they have important diagnostic implications. Dizziness is a nonspecific term referring to any feeling of disorientation. Vertigo is a specific sensation defined as the hallucination of motion. This motion is often a spinning sensation, but it can also be other nonrotatory sensations such as moving in various planes. Unsteadiness refers to a sensation of abnormal balance and lightheadedness that often accompanies this as well as other nonvestibular-related disorders. Syncope with loss of consciousness is generally not due to vestibular disorders and has a different differential diagnosis.

Evaluation of a patient with a complaint of dizziness begins with a complete history with a description of the sensations, temporal patterns with origins and occurrences, and provoking situations. This is followed with a complete otologic as well as a neurologic examination, and, if necessary, clinical testing.

ANATOMY

The vestibular system can be divided into two basic systems; the labyrinth and the vestibular nerve are commonly referred to as the peripheral vestibular system. The brainstem, with its connections to the ocular motor, cerebellar, vestibular spinal, and cortical systems, forms the central vestibular system. The peripheral vestibular system can be subdivided further into the labyrinth and vestibular nerve. The labyrinthine vestibular system consists of the three semicircular canals: horizontal, vertical, and posterior, as well as the utricle and the saccule. The semicircular canals are rotational sense organs. The utricle and the saccule sense gravity and linear acceleration. The most peripheral sensory component of the vestibular system is the hair cell, which has multiple short stereocilia and a single, long kinocilia, which are the actual motion-sensitive receptors. Electrical discharges are created at the level of the hair cells, which then pass through their respective vestibular nerves to synapse in the Scarpa's ganglion and are carried via the vestibular nerve through the internal auditory canal and through the cerebellopontine angle to the vestibular nuclei in the brain stem. These vestibular nuclei are bilateral divisions of the brain stem with four divisions (superior, lateral, medial, and descending). From these nuclei, neural projections go to several centers as well as to synapse in the reticular formation. Connections go to the cortex as well as to the ocular motor system, the sympathetic nervous system, cerebellum, and the anterior horn cells of the spinal column. The peripheral vestibular system consists of paired organs lying in the temporal bone. The labyrinth consists of a bony component lined by endosteum containing perilymph, which is a physiologic correlate to cerebrospinal fluid (high sodium, low potassium). Suspended in the bony labyrinth is the membranous labyrinth containing endolymphatic fluid, a physiologic correlate to intracellular fluid (high potassium, low sodium). The three semicircular canals lie at 90-degree angles to each other and have saccular dilatations on their ends that house the cristae (sensory epithelium). These cristae are located anterior on the horizontal and superior canals and posteriorly on the posterior semicircular canal. The hair cells in the utricle and the saccule are located in the maculae. The macula sacculi lies in a vertical plane. The macula utriculi lies in the horizontal plane. These organs are made up of a membrane composed of a mucopolysaccharide gel containing the otoconia, which are calcium deposits. The weight of the otoconia make the utricle and the saccule sensitive to acceleration as well as to gravity.

PHYSIOLOGY

Each of the paired vestibular end organs has a resting electric discharge. In the normal vestibular system this electric discharge at rest is equal and continuous from the right and left vestibular systems. In the condition of motion, whether it is rotation, acceleration, or deceleration in any plane, the resting electric discharge is altered due to deflection of hair cells in the semicircular canals, utricle, or saccule. Under normal conditions, motion will cause accentuation of discharge from one side and deattenuation of discharge from its paired opposing side. In condition of disease, these electric discharges are altered, giving rise to the pathologic sense of motion or rotation commonly described as vertigo. The sensation of vertigo can arise from abnormal discharge from either the peripheral or the central vestibular system. Common causes of vestibular pathology include viral infections, trauma, and toxic exposures.

The vestibular system has a plasticity that enables it to recover from damage to the peripheral vestibular sense organ. When one side is damaged from any source, the initial sensation is one of vertigo. A phenomenon known as a "cerebellar clamp" occurs immediately when it is recognized at a cortical level that the information emanating from the vestibular system is in error. This spontaneously suppresses discharge from the normal side via processes that go on in the central vestibular system, enhancing the remaining discharge from the diseased side. This is a phenomenon known as "vestibular compensation," responsible for recovery after significant vestibular end organ injuries. The initial injuries associated with the sensation of vertigo with the accompanying nystagmus as well as autonomic symptoms consist of nausea and vomiting, pallor, and clamminess. Over the ensuing 72 hours, strong compensatory factors arise, rapidly decreasing the sense of vertigo. Symptoms remain, however, for many weeks as the central vestibular system completes its compensation. Compensation is much more rapid in younger individuals than in older individuals. With time, this compensation in most patients is complete to the point where they feel as if they have normal balance. However, testing may show the vestibular system to be permanently inactivated. Various degrees of injury can cause various degrees of symptomatology, and vestibular disorders often take on an intermittent course. Patients with central vestibular disorders tend to have the most difficulty with recovery as compensation is primarily a function of the central vestibular system.

In summary, the anatomy of the vestibular system consists of paired vestibular sense organs tied into central connections, going from the level of the brainstem to the cerebellum, ocular motor nuclei, and anterior horn cells of the spinal column. At rest the system has a steady state discharge that is altered when movement takes place. Under normal conditions, this motion agrees with visual as well as proprioceptive signals, and one feels as if he has normal balance. Conditions of disease of the vestibular sense organ or the central vestibular centers lead to the sensation of vertigo. Disorders of the other components of the balance system, the eyes, cervical proprioceptors, and peripheral proprioceptors, can also lead to the sensation of vertigo, but more often lead to the sensations of lightheadedness and unsteadiness. The vestibular system is plastic and has the ability to compensate for injuries to the peripheral vestibular system. Injuries and disorders of the central vestibular system do compensate, albeit much more slowly.

PATHOLOGY

Altered sense of balance can be caused by disorders anywhere in the vestibular system. Disorders of the peripheral vestibular system cause abnormal discharges to occur, which are sensed at the brain stem and cortical level as being pathologic. This gives rise to the sensation of vertigo or the hallucination of motion. The differential diagnosis of vestibular system pathology can be divided into three separate sections. These sections are the labyrinth, vestibular nerve, and central vestibular system with its ocular, cerebellar, and proprioceptive connections. Table 21-2 provides a differential diagnosis for disorders that can affect the labyrinth, vestibular nerve, or central vestibular system.

Table 21-2. Differential diagnosis of vestibular system pathology

Category	Examples
Infections	Viral, bacterial, mycotic, fungal, syphilitic
Vascular	Vertebral, basilar, internal auditory, vestibular artery, microcirculation-spasm or occlusion, subclavian steal syndrome, migraine, hypotension AVM aneurysm
Neoplastic	Carcinoma primary or metastatic, sarcoma glomus tumor, acoustic neuroma, meningioma, astrocytoma, ependymoma, epidermoid cyst
Traumatic	Concussion, CHI, fracture barotrauma
Metabolic	Diabetes, otosclerosis, Paget's disease, uremia, familial ataxia, thiamin deficiency
Developmental	Genetic defects, Arnold Chiari malformation, syringobulbia
Toxic	Aminoglycosides, salicylates, ETOH, chemotherapeutic agents, heavy metal, solvents
Unknown	Meniere's disease, cupulolithiasis, seizure disorders
Autoimmune	Cogan's syndrome, autoimmune inner ear disease, allergic-mediated vestibulopathies

VESTIBULAR EVALUATION AND TESTING
Medical diagnosis

An appropriate history will produce an accurate diagnosis in 90% of cases. In evaluating the "dizzy" patients, the clinician must first determine whether the problem is of a vestibular or nonvestibular origin. As mentioned previously, vestibular disorders—disorders of the peripheral vestibular system as well as the central vestibular system—typically cause the hallucination of motion, vertigo. Other sensations, such as loss of consciousness, presyncope, and weakness, are not generally vestibular in origin. The sensation that the patient is describing must be characterized with regard to its origination, rapidity of onset, frequency, and enciting factors as well as length of symptomatology and exacerbating activities. In general, episodic vertigo is peripheral, whereas chronic vertigo is most often central in nature. Motion tends to exacerbate vestibular disorders but may actually improve affective disorders (anxiety). Disorders that occur in conjunction with meals suggest hyper- or hypoglycemia. Specific antecedent incidents such as recent viral illnesses, head trauma, or specific exposure to toxins or allergens should be elicited. Past medical history with the emphasis on metabolic disorders is important. Hypertension, circulatory disorders, psychiatric disorders, and metabolic problems can aid in the diagnosis. Medication history should be taken as dizziness is one of the most common side effects of drugs affecting the neurologic as well as vascular system. Family history points to disorders such as otosclerosis and Meniere's disease. Social history with regard to smoking and alcohol ingestion are important.

A complete otologic as well a neurologic examination must be done. This includes inspection of the ears, nasal passages, and throat. Cranial nerve examination, as well as cerebellar function testing, should be done. The Romberg test with eyes opened and closed, as well as observation of the gait, should be performed. Tests for positional nystagmus and vertigo may be helpful in the patient complaining of episodic positional vertigo. The Dix-Hallpike test or Barany maneuvers are simple and rapid to perform. They consist of sitting the patient on the end of an examination table. The patient's head is turned to one side and he is asked to lie down on his back rapidly with the eyes open and the head extended. A positive test is noted by the onset of rapid rotary nystagmus with the fast phase down, which fatigues after multiple attempts. This is classic benign paroxysmal positional vertigo and is caused by vestibular pathology in the undermost ear. Etiology may be due to multiple causes, including trauma, toxic exposure, or viral and vascular disorders of the inner ear.

Audiometric testing consists of air and bone pure tone averages with speech reception threshold testing. Discrimination as well as tympanometry and reflex testing should also be done. If necessary, BAER testing is available. Vestibular lesions are often associated with audiometric abnormalities, any of which have subtle manifestations and may not be aware to the patient. Vestibular testing at the present time consists of three modalities. Electronystagmography is a test of the peripheral vestibular system with its connection to the ocular motor system. This consists of tests of eye tracking, gaze testing, and positioning testing. The patient's eye motions are monitored in the dark to limit visual suppression. The eye is a dipole with a positive and negative charge. Deflection in the eye movements can be sensed electrically by electrodes placed to the sides as well as above and below the eyes. Typical vestibular-generated nystagmus has a fast and slow phase. The direction of the fast phase identifies the conventional direction of the nystagmus. The slow phase is generated at the level of the peripheral vestibular system, while the fast phase is generated in the central ocular motor nuclei to provide visual fixation in a rapidly turning environment. Warm and cool irrigation is directed into the external auditory canal to stimulate the lateral semicircular canal. Irrigations cooler than body temperature cause nystagmus that has its fast phase beating toward the opposite ear. Irrigations warmer than body temperature beat with their fast phase toward the irrigated ear.

The response of each ear is compared, and a determination can be made on ENG testing whether there is an abnormality of the peripheral vestibular system, the central vestibular system, or an abnormality that cannot be localized to either. Limitations of a conventional ENG are significant. They only test the peripheral vestibular system at a small range, and in general only large abnormalities can be detected. Rotary chair testing consists of similar monitoring apparatus to ENG testing that is linked into a computer. The vestibular stimulus is supplied by a rotating chair in the vertical axis. The results of this testing are helpful in differentiating between peripheral and central disorders. In general, laterality of disease is more difficult to determine. Computerized platform posturography tests the patient's equilibrium in a static and dynamic state. The patient stands on force plates that are linked to weight-sensitive sensors. The patient is examined in various conditions where proprioceptive, visual, and vestibular inputs are manipulated. This can assist in a diagnosis of central versus peripheral disorders as well as monitor progress or lack of progress in vestibular compensation. A separate part of the test examines long loop reflex responses in the lower extremities and can help determine whether the patient will benefit from balance and gait training with physical therapy.

Hematologic testing may be indicated in specific circumstances. Sedimentation rate, tests for syphilis, fasting blood sugar, 5-hour glucose tolerate test, and heavy metal screening with solvent biologic standards can be performed.

SPECIFIC ENVIRONMENTAL CAUSES OF VESTIBULAR DISORDERS

Environmental causes of disorders of the vestibular system generally fall into two categories: toxicities and trauma. Toxicities are most often caused by solvents around the home,[44] heavy metal exposure due to contamination of the water supply, and exposure to toxic levels of pesticides.[50] Environmental exposures to trauma are most often in the form of barotrauma, head injuries, and blast or noise trauma. Barotrauma occurs with flying or diving. Head injuries can occur through accidents around the home or falls. Blast and noise trauma is associated with power tools, recreational exposure to excessively loud music, fireworks, or guns.

Solvents

Solvents, particularly xylene, are found in the home in various solvent mixtures. These can be found in paints, varnishes, and thinners. Acutely, solvent exposure causes a sensation of intoxication with headache, vertigo, dysequilibrium, nausea, and possibly euphoria. If exposure continues, subacute and later chronic symptoms may develop.[33] Long-standing symptoms in particular can cause dysequilibrium. This problem, when associated with other signs and symptoms of chronic solvent exposure, is known as chronic toxic encephalopathy (CTE). Toluene is commonly found in numerous consumer products. They are also commonly abused by "glue sniffers." Both xylene and toluene are found to be ototoxic and cause hearing loss in experimental settings.[13] Similar injuries that correlate with long-term difficulty with dysequilibrium and other balance disorders may develop in the vestibular system.[17] Objective testing includes audiometry, electronystagmography, posturography, rotary chair testing if available, and MRI. Abnormalities on the smooth pursuit test on ENG and the visual suppression test on rotary testing have been shown to be helpful in the diagnosis.[47] Computerized platform posturography reveals impaired equilibrium testing on the sensory organizational test. Auditory testing revealed abnormalities of the auditory brainstem responses and tests of cortical function. Computerized tomography (CT) has not been helpful in the diagnosis of chronic toxic encephalopathy. MRI in CTE has demonstrated brain atrophy in the posterior fossa structures, the parietal lobes, and the pericisternal white matter.

Initial exposure causes problems such as dysequilibrium, nausea, headaches, and irritability, whereas long-term exposures develop similar symptoms in addition to intellectual impairment and significant personality changes. The development of chronic toxic encephalopathy is initially slow and potentially reversible. Long-term exposure is associated with permanently impaired function.

Heavy metals

Heavy metal exposure occurs primarily in the water supply. Exposures to toxic levels of tin, lead, triethyl tin (TET), mercury, arsenic, and manganese have all been reported as causing specific cochlear and vestibular lesions.* Mercury poisoning en masse has presented clinically as the Hunter-Russell syndrome. This has been diagnosed as Minamata disease. This is a severe neurologic disorder first recognized in people living in the vicinity of Minamata, Japan, in 1953. The onset of Minamata disease is associated with ataxic gait, clumsiness, dysarthria, dysphagia, blurring of vision, and deafness. Up to 80% of patients with Minamata disease suffer hearing loss. The transmission of mercury was via toxic dumping into an adjoining bay with ingestion of fish and shellfish. Animal studies in the Guinea pig have revealed that damage to the labyrinthine blood vessels occurs with endothelial cell swelling, mitochondrial disintegration, and protrusion of the endothelial cell cytoplasm herniating into the blood vessel lumen.[1,14,31]

Environmental lead exposure is common. Elevated blood lead levels in children are associated with delays in development, including the ability to sit up, walk, and speak. Lead-intoxicated guinea pigs showed segmental demyelination of the eighth nerve which resembled peripheral nerve lesions of lead-poisoned animals. In this study, the sensory cells of the inner ear were not affected by exposure to lead.†

Salicylates

Patients receiving high-dose salicylate therapy often complain of tinnitus, ear fullness, hearing loss, and vertigo. Caloric testing reveals bilateral caloric hypoactivity.[8,23,37] Cessation of salicylate ingestion usually leads to rapid improvement (within 24 hours). Salicylates are concentrated in the perilymph, and it has been suggested that they interfere with enzymatic activity of the hair cells and the cochlear neurons.[54]

Alcohol

The signs and symptoms of acute alcohol ingestion are well known to most physicians. Alcohol ingestion will cause specific characteristic abnormalities on ENG testing.[2] Chronic alcohol toxicity is associated with cerebellar disorders with abnormality of gait and motor control.

Trauma

Trauma is another major source of environmental vestibular pathology. This can occur with barotrauma due to sudden pressure changes in diving or flying. Closed head injuries from falls or accidents around the home can lead to inner ear concussions or temporal bone fractures.[11,23] Blast injuries have similar effects. All three areas of the vestibular system, peripheral, eighth nerve, and central, can be affected by trauma.[19]

Typically, barotrauma causes injury to the peripheral end organ and can be associated with loss of perilymph due to oval window or round window fistulas.[15] Closed head injuries as well as direct injury to the end organ can affect the central vestibular system at the level of the cortex and brain stem.[24] Vestibular dysfunction frequently follows blows to the head that do not result in temporal bone fracture. The

---

*References 3, 25, 28, 48, 51, 58.

†References 10, 21, 22, 45, 53.

most common symptom of labyrinthine concussion is positional vertigo.[4] The patient develops sudden brief attacks of vertigo precipitated by changes in head position. Specific injuries to the eighth nerve and brainstem have been poorly documented. Severe head blows produce petechial hemorrhages and focal infarction in the brainstem, but these pathologic changes are always associated with alteration in level of consciousness or other neurologic signs. Mitchell and Adams studied sections in the brainstem in 100 cases of fatal blunt head injury.[38] Seven had abnormalities in the brainstem attributable to the primary impact. This suggests that "primary brainstem injury" does not exist, but rather is one aspect of diffuse brain damage.

Fistula of the oval and round windows results from blunt head injury, blast noise, diving, and possibly barotrauma while flying.[7] Sudden negative or position pressure change in the middle ear cavity or CSF is transmitted to the inner ear via the cochlear aqueduct. High-pressure differentials lead to the sudden onset of vertigo, hearing loss, or both. Management of these patients is controversial, as a high percentage of patients with labyrinthine fistula will spontaneously heal.[52]

DIAGNOSIS AND MANAGEMENT

Significant exposures to solvents, heavy metal, and toxins will often cause specific abnormalities on the mentioned tests. The history will suggest the antecendent exposure. The physical exam may show alterations of cerebellar function as well as abnormalities on Romberg testing. Positional testing is often abnormal in posttraumatic cases. Vestibular testing may show abnormalities. Solvent exposures typically cause ENG tracking abnormalities when chronic and will often show nonlocalized abnormalities when acute. Computerized platform posturography may show disorders of the central and peripheral vestibular system. Trauma may cause mixed central as well as peripheral disorders, as well as combined central and peripheral disorders on computerized platform posturography and rotary chair testing. MRI examination may show alterations in posterior fossa structures with chronic solvent exposure. Blood testing can document exposure indices indicating acute and chronic exposures. Management is directed to limiting further toxic exposure as well as to rehabilitation. Vestibular rehabilitation is now directed by the physical therapist. Guided by results of the posturography testing, they can generate patient-specific programs to assist in balance retraining and gait training. Rehabilitation in posttraumatic patients is similar. The exception to this is the patient with an acute blast injury or barotrauma who after an adequate waiting period still has significant signs and symptoms of perilymphatic fistula. Surgical exploration and a closure of the fistula can be of assistance in these situations.

FUTURE DIRECTIONS

Many areas of vestibular physiology and pathology are poorly understood. The effects of solvents and heavy metals on the inner ear have not been adequately documented. In the future, diagnosis may be assisted by sophisticated techniques such as brain mapping, PET scanning, off-axis rotary chair testing, vestibular evoked response, and physiologic MRI evaluation. Evaluation of other semicircular canal function and otolith function is presently being researched with off-axis rotary chair testing and infrared ENG technology.

REFERENCES

1. Anniko M, Sarkady L: Morphological changes of labyrinthine blood vessels in following metal poisoning, *Acta Otolaryngol (Stockh)* 83:441, 1977.
2. Aschan G, Bergstedt M: Positional alcoholic nystagmus (PAN) in man following repeated alcohol doses, *Acta Otolaryngol* (suppl 330):15, 1975.
3. Axelsson A, Fagergerg SE: Auditory function in diabetes, *Acta Otolaryngol* 66:49, 1988.
4. Barber H: Positional nystagmus especially after head injury, *Laryngoscope* 74:891, 1964.
5. Bencko V, Symon K: Test of environmental exposure to arsenic and hearing changes in exposed children, *Environ Health Perspect* 19:95, 1977.
6. Bencko V et al: Health aspects of burning coal with a high arsenic content. II. Hearing changes in exposed children, *Environ Res* 13:386, 1977.
7. Berger EH et al eds: *Noise and hearing conservation manual,* Akron, Oh, 1986, A 1 HA.
8. Bernstein JM, Weiss AD: Further observations on salicylate ototoxicty, *J Laryngol Otol* 81:915, 1967.
9. Bohne AB: Mechanisms of noise damage in the inner ear. In Henderson D, et al, eds: *Effects of noise on hearing,* New York, 1976, Raven Press.
10. Ciurlo E, Ottoboni A: Variations of the internal ear in chronic lead poisoning, *Minerva Otorinolaringol* 5:130, 1955.
11. Clark WW: Hearing: the effects of noise, *Otol Head and Neck Surgery,* 106:669,
12. Davey LM: Labyrinthine trauma in head injury, *Conn Med* 29:250, 1965.
13. Ehyai A, Freeman FR: Progressive optic neuropathy and sensorineural hearing loss due to chronic glue sniffing, *J Neurol Neurosurg Psychiatry* 46:349, 1983.
14. Falk SA et al: Acute methyl mercury intoxication and ototoxicity in guinea pigs, *Arch Pathol* 97:297, 1974.
15. Fee G: Traumatic perilymphatic fistulas, *Arch Otolaryngol* 88:477, 1968.
16. Fee WE: Aminoglycoside toxicity in the human, 1980, Lindsay, J.R. 1959.
17. Fornazzari L et al: Cerebellar, cortical, and functional impairment in toluene abusers, *Acta Neurol Scand* 67:319, 1983.
18. Fredelius L: Time sequence of degeneration pattern of the organ of Corti, *Actaotolaryngology* 106:373, 1988.
19. Friedman AP, Brenner C, Denny-Brown D: Post-traumatic vertigo and dizziness, *J Neurosurg* 2:36, 1945.
20. Gerstner HB, Huff JE: Clinical toxicology of mercury, *J Toxicol Environ Health* 2:491, 1977.
21. Goyer RA: Lead toxicity: from overt to subclinical to subtle health effects, *Environ Health Perspect* 86:177, 1990.
22. Gozdzik-Zoinierkiewicz T, Moszynski B: Eighth nerve in experimental lead poisoning, *Acta Otolaryngol (Stockh)* 68:85, 1969.
23. Graham J, Parker W: The toxic manifestations of sodium salicylate therapy, *Quart J Med* 18:153, 1948.
24. Hart CW: Traumatic vestibular impairment in the nervous system. In *Human communication and its disorders,* New York, 1975, Raven Press.
25. Ishii EK et al: Is NIDDM a risk factor for noise-induced hearing loss in an occupationally noise exposed cohort? *Science of the Total Environment* 127:155, 1992.

26. Jaffe BF, Maasab HF: Sudden deafness associated with adenovirus infection, *N Engl J Med* 276:1406, 1967.
27. Jogn A, Barone DO, Peters JM, Garabrant DH, MD, Bernstein L, Krebsbach R: Smoking as a risk factor in noise-induced hearing loss, *J Occ Med* 29:741, 1987.
28. Jorgensen M, Buch N: Studies on inner ear function and cranial nerves in diabetes, *Acta Otolaryngol* 53:350, 1964.
29. Karmody CS: *Textbook of otolaryngology,* Philadelphia, 1983, Lea & Febiger.
30. Kelemen G: Fractures of the temporal bone, *Arch Otolaryngol* 40:333, 1944.
31. Konishi T, Hamrick PE: The uptake of methyl mercury in guinea pig cochlea in relation to its ototoxic effect, *Acta Otolaryngol (Stockh)* 88:203, 1979.
32. Kurland LT, Faro SN, Siedler H: Minamata disease: the outbreak of a neurologic disorder in Minamata, Japan, and its relationship to the ingestion of seafood contaminated by mercuric compounds, *World Neurol* 1:370, 1960.
33. Ledin T et al: Chronic toxic encephalopathy investigated using dynamic posturography, *Am J Otolaryngol* 12:96, 1991.
34. Lichtenstein MJ: Validation of screening tools for identifying hearing-impaired elderly in primary care, *JAMA* 259:2875, 1988.
35. Lindsay JR, Hemenway WG: Inner ear pathology due to measles, *Ann Otol Rhinol Laryngol* 63:711, 1954.
36. Maasab HF: The role of viruses in sudden deafness, *Adv Otol Rhinol Laryngol* 20:229, 1973.
37. Mc Cabe P, Dey F: The effect of aspirin upon auditory sensitivity, *Ann Otol Rhinol Laryngol* 74:312, 1965.
38. Mitchell DE, Adams JH: Primary focal impact damage to the brainstem in blunt head injuries: does it exist? *Lancet* 2:215, 1973.
39. Mizukoshi K et al: Neurotological studies upon intoxication by inorganic mercury compounds, *ORL J Otorhinolaryngol Relat Spec* 37:74, 1975.
40. Mizukoshi K et al: Neurotological follow-up studies upon Minamata disease, *Acta Otolaryngol (Stockh)* suppl 468:353, 1989.
41. Morizono T, Paparella MM: Hypercholesterolemia and auditory dysfunction: experimental studies, *Ann Otol* 87:804, 1978.
42. National Association of the Deaf, National Information Center on Deafness, Gallaudet College: *Estimate of hearing loss,* Washington, D.C., 1980, Office of Demographic Studies.
43. Ocless JS: A caustic trauma of sportsman hunter due to gunfiring, *Laryngoscope* 82: 1971, 1972.
44. Odkvist LM, Moller C, Thuomas KA: Otoneurologic disturbances caused by solvent pollution, *Otolaryngology—Head and Neck Surgery* 106:687, 1992.
45. Otto D et al: Five-year followup of children with low-to-moderate lead absorption: electrophysiological evaluation, *Environ Res* 38:168, 1985.
46. Pillsbury HC: Hypertension, hyperlipoproteinemia, chronic noise exposure: is there synergism in cochlear pathology? *Laryngoscope* 96:1112, 1986.
47. Poulsen P, Jensen JH: Brain-stem response: audiometry and electronystagmographic findings in chronic toxic encephalopathy (chronic painter's syndrome), *J Laryngol Otol* 100:155, 1986.
48. Proctor C: *Hereditary sensorineural hearing loss,* Rochester, Minn, 1978, American Academy of Ophthalmology and Otolaryngology.
49. Rom WN: *Environmental and occupational medicine,* ed 2, Little, Brown.
50. Rybak LP: Hearing: the effects of chemicals, *Otolaryngology—Head and Neck Surgery* 106:677, 1992.
51. Sataloff RT, Sataloff J: *Occupational hearing loss,* ed 2,
52. Schuknect HF: *Pathology of the ear,* Cambridge, Mass, 1974, Harvard University.
53. Schwartz J, Otto D: Blood lead, hearing thresholds, and neurobehavioral development in children and youth, *Arch Environ Health* 42:153, 1987.
54. Silverstein H, Bernstein J, Davies D: Salicylate ototoxicity: a biochemical and electrophysiological study, *Ann Otol Rhinol Laryngol* 76:118, 1967.
55. Spencer JT, Jr: Hyperlipoproteinemia in the etiology of inner ear disease, *Larygoscope,* 83:639, 1973.
56. Sudden deafness due to virus infection, *Arch Otolaryngol,* 69:13,
57. Taylor PH, Bicknell PG: Rupture of the round window membrane, *Ann Otol Rhinol Laryngol,* 85:105, 1976.
58. Triana RJ et al: Inner ear damage secondary to diabetes mellitus, *Arch Otolaryngol Head Neck Surg,* 117:635, 1991.
59. U.S. Department of Health and Human Services: Hearing ability of persons by sociodemographic and health characteristics, Washington, D.C., DHHS Publication no. (PHS) 82-1568.

Chapter 22

COMMON ENVIRONMENTAL DERMATOSES

David T. Harvey
Daniel J. Hogan

Factors that influence percutaneous absorption
    Concentration and area of exposure
    Skin thickness, anatomic site, and cutaneous integrity
    Occlusion and skin permeability
    Vehicle composition
The mechanisms of environmentally induced skin disease
Overview of some common environmental dermatoses
    Dermatitis
    Acne lesions
    Photosensitivity reactions
    Pigmentary changes
    Urticaria
    Scleroderma
    Infectious disorders
    Cutaneous malignancy
An overview of specific environmental factors that can affect the skin
    Mechanical factors
    Physical factors
    Chemical agents
    Biologic agents
The approach used to diagnose environmental dermatoses
    Historical aspects of environmental dermatoses
    Clinical aspects of environmental dermatoses
Prevention and treatment
    Personal protection and avoidance
    Hygiene
    Education
    Regulation
    Motivation
Conclusion

Environmental skin diseases may occur as a manifestation of exposure to various environmental chemicals and to physical stimuli such as sunlight. The skin protects against the toxic effects of such exposures by providing an important barrier function. Despite its defense function, the skin also serves as a selected portal of entry for agents found in our environment, both naturally occurring and manufactured. Consequently, a number of adverse cutaneous responses can result from such exposures. The exact type of reaction and the morphologic features of each response depend on a multitude of factors such as exposure time, immunocompetence, and age of the patient. We review herein the mechanisms of environmentally induced skin disease, the presenting symptoms of these disorders, and effective investigation and diagnosis of these conditions.

FACTORS THAT INFLUENCE PERCUTANEOUS ABSORPTION

A number of readily recognizable factors influence the ability of a compound to be absorbed through the skin. The dermal toxicity elicited depends on the degree to which an environmental chemical can penetrate the skin. We focus on factors that are believed to play an important role in percutaneous penetration.

Concentration and area of exposure

Absorption of a particular compound into the dermis depends on both the concentration of the applied dose and the surface area of application, which can be mathematically demonstrated with Fick's law of diffusion, which states that for a single vehicle, the absorption rate is directly proportional to the applied agent's concentration such that

$$J \propto C_v$$

where J is the absorption rate per area (flux) and C_v is the concentration of the penetrant in the vehicle.[54] The equation does not hold here, however, if there is a concentration-dependent adverse effect of the penetrant on the stratum corneum (SC) or solvent properties of the vehicle.[54] If the area of skin on which the agent is applied is increased, there is a corresponding increase in direct absorption; thus an environmental chemical that has made contact with the skin over a large surface area in a concentrated fashion is absorbed more than is one that has contacted the skin locally and in a dilute form.

Skin thickness, anatomic site, and cutaneous integrity

Skin thickness is another significant factor in percutaneous absorption. The primary permeability barrier resides within the SC, which is the outermost layer of the epidermis (Fig. 22-1). The loss of cutaneous barrier function through either skin disease or direct environmental insult enhances percutaneous absorption.[68] It has been shown that removal of the SC with cellophane tape allows enhanced penetration of some agents by as much as fourfold.[54]

Certain anatomic regions also demonstrate variability in percutaneous absorption. This variability is thought to be due to differences of SC thickness in selected areas. For example, skin on the palms and soles has a thicker SC layer, with consequently lower percutaneous penetration than in areas with a thin layer of SC, such as the genitalia, where the greatest percutaneous absorption is found. (Table 22-1)[25] Any disruption of the SC allows enhanced percutaneous permeability. Structures such as the epidermal basement membrane and epidermal cells possess some protective function because complete removal of the SC does not allow 100% penetration of external agents.[54]

Occlusion and skin permeability

Topical occlusive or dressings are known to enhance percutaneous absorption. In part this enhancement is thought to occur secondarily to the dressing's effect of increasing both the hydration and the temperature of the intact skin.[91] Occlusive dressings also serve as a mechanical barrier to prevent the accidental removal or evaporation of a compound. In clinical practice, occlusive dressings are useful to ensure that a topical medication is maximally absorbed. Occlusion also increases cutaneous injury due to noxious chemicals and percutaneous absorption of both therapeutic and toxic compounds; for example, a pesticide spray leaking into a glove is more damaging than is pesticide contact on nonoccluded skin.

Vehicle composition

It is known that lipids and lipid-soluble materials penetrate more readily into the SC but water and ionized compounds permeate with more difficulty.[91] When an agent is mixed within a vehicle or other material, the absorption of the compound depends on its partition coefficient. For example, a material with a low solubility in a carrier vehicle tends to penetrate readily into the skin, whereas material that is soluble in the carrying vehicle tends to remain in the vehicle. The vehicle also may have properties that can be damaging to the SC,[62] and expectedly, a disrupted epidermal barrier allows enhanced absorption of the material. Finally, some compounds affect percutaneous absorption by having special properties or containing certain agents, e.g., dimethylsulfoxide or azone (see Box). This may be important in assessing certain environmental materials, because a naturally occurring substance may be contained in more than one vehicle.

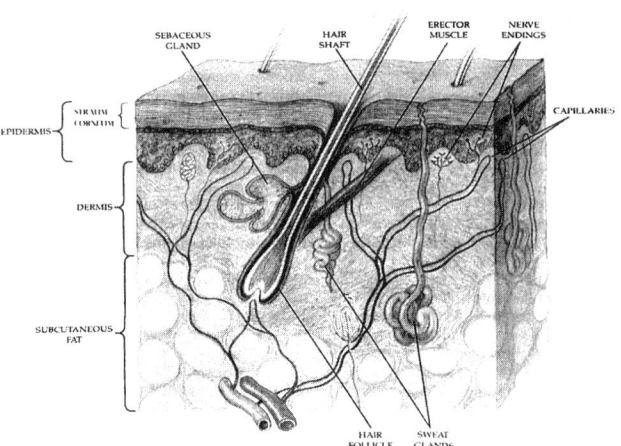

Fig. 22-1. Stratum corneum—the most superficial layer of the epidermis.

Table 22-1. Penetration of hydrocortisone in humans in various anatomic sites

Anatomic site	Penetration ratio
Palm	0.83
Back	1.7
Axilla	3.6
Forehead	6.0
Genitalia	42.0

Modified from Wester RC, Maibach HI: In vivo percutaneous absorption. In Marzulli FN, Maibach HI, editors: *Dermatotoxicology,* ed 3, New York, 1987, Hemisphere.

Factors affecting percutaneous absorption

Concentration and area of exposure
Skin thickness
Cutaneous integrity
Vehicle properties
Occlusion
Anatomic site

Environmentally induced skin disorders

Dermatitis
   Irritant
   Allergic

Acne lesions
   Chloracne
   Oil acne

Pigmentary changes
   Hyperpigmentation
   Hypopigmentation
   Absence of pigment

Photosensitivity reactions
   Phototoxic reactions
      Porphyria cutaneous tarda
      Actinic damage

Photoallergic reactions

Urticaria

Scleroderma

Infectious disorders

Cutaneous malignancy
   Nonmelanoma skin cancer
   Malignant melanoma

Environmental factors that induce skin disease

Mechanical factors
   Friction
   Pressure
   Vibration

Physical factors
   Heat
   Cold
   Humidity
   Water
   Sunlight
   Ultraviolet light
   Ionizing radiation

Chemical agents
   Primary irritants
   Sensitizers
   Photoirritants
   Photosensitizers

Biologic agents
   Parasites
   Bacteria
   Rickettsiae
   Fungi
   Viruses
   Irritant and sensitizing plants and woods

Modified from Webster RC, Maibach HI: *Principles and practice of environmental medicine,* New York, 1992, Plenum.

THE MECHANISMS OF ENVIRONMENTALLY INDUCED SKIN DISEASE

Environmental stimuli can manifest toxic effects on the skin in a multitude of ways.

These effects have been described and classified primarily on the basis of readily demonstrable cutaneous disorders[91] (see box). Mechanical, physical, chemical, and biologic environmental factors (see box)[40] are responsible for the induction of such changes. Most responses are not well understood, but we are gradually gaining strides in understanding areas such as sunlight (ultraviolet B)–induced non-melanoma skin cancer (NMSC) formation[23,29] and immune-mediated allergic responses.

OVERVIEW OF SOME COMMON ENVIRONMENTAL DERMATOSES

Manifestations of common environmental dermatoses include contact dermatitis, urticaria, scleroderma, and pigmentary disorders (see box). Although the list is broad, we attempt to define the more readily seen environmentally induced skin conditions and discuss those clinical characteristics that are important for the practicing physician to recognize.

Dermatitis

Dermatitis is the most commonly[53] seen cutaneous response to environmental chemical exposure. This form of cutaneous reaction is due to a reaction produced by contact of a chemical with various cellular and noncellular elements of the skin. The condition generated is referred to as contact dermatitis (CD). CD is defined as inflammation of the skin with spongiosis (intercellular edema) which occurs after the direct contact of the skin with a chemical agent.[56] Clinically, acute dermatitis is characterized by vesiculation and weeping. Chronic dermatitis tends to have more scaling, lichenification, and pigmentary changes (Fig. 22-2). CD can be either due to irritation from direct exposure with a substance (irritant contact dermatitis [ICD]) or as a result of a delayed cell-mediated immune reaction (allergic contact dermatitis [ACD]).

Irritant contact dermatitis. ICD is the predominant type of contact dermatitis seen, accounting for 80% of all eczematous reactions.[53] Typical ICD is limited to the area of exposure and can range in presentation from mild erythema to frank necrosis and ulceration. Chemicals that adversely cause this reaction can induce first pain and burning and later pruritus.[53] Unlike ACD, the effects from the chemical exposure do not depend on specific immunologic mech-

Chemical agents associated with irritant and allergic contact dermatitis	
Irritant dermatitis	*Allergic dermatitis*
Solvents	Benzocaine
Acids	Nickel
Alkalis	Chromium
Metal salts	Neomycin
Oxidants	Formaldehyde

Modified from Webster RC, Maibach HI: Disorders of the skin. In *Principles and practice of environmental medicine*, New York, 1992, Plenum.

Table 22-2. Irritant versus allergic contact dermatitis

Feature	Allergic	Irritant
Burning	++	+++(early)
Erythema	++++	++++
Vesicles	++++	+
Itch	++++(early)	+++
Fissuring	++	++++
Reaction time	Days	Minutes to hours

Modified from Marks J, Deleo V: *Contact and occupational dermatology*, St Louis, 1992, Mosby–Yearbook.

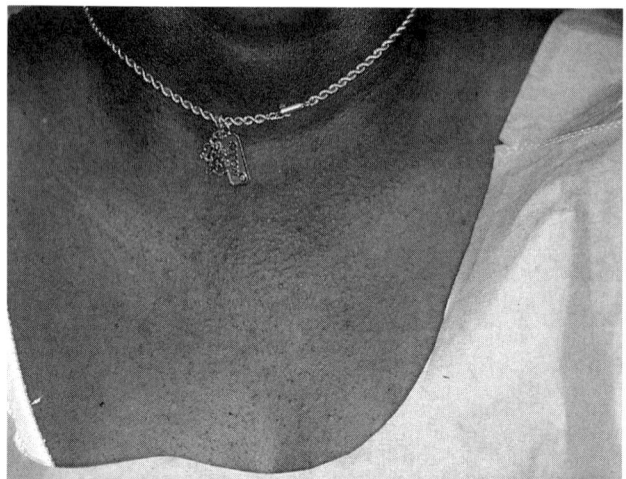

Fig. 22-2. Contact dermatitis—illustration of nickel contact allergy as manifested by a vesiculopapular eruption and postinflammatory hyperpigmentation.

anisms (Table 22-2). Often, ICD is due to exposure to acidic or alkaline substances.

Allergic contact dermatitis. Allergically mediated reactions are specific, requiring a history of prior sensitization to a particular agent. ACD can occur with exposures to low concentrations of environmental antigen. In the environment, certain plants such as *Toxicodendron* (poison ivy) can produce ACD. Only previously sensitized individuals develop ACD after exposure to a nontoxic concentration of an allergen. ACD arises from a cell-mediated delayed hypersentivity reaction. Sensitization is initiated after the environmental agent or the hapten combines with skin proteins to form a complete antigen. This antigen is then processed by epidermal Langerhans' cells,[79] where it is made ready for presentation to host T lymphocytes. The T lymphocytes, which interact with Langerhans' cell–processed antigen, provide a specialized function in that only certain T-cell lines possess the capability to recognize the modified antigen via their receptors. Some of these T cells (effector cells) circulate peripherally in the blood, where they release biochemical signals in the form of lymphokines such as interleukin.[24,57] Lymphokines (cytokines) serve in many instances as mediators of inflammation. They are small protein molecules[64] that are released when T lymphocytes are reexposed to an antigen. T cells that do not circulate peripherally are important because of their memory functions. Such cells generate new populations of sensitized lymphocytes when they are reexposed to the same or closely related antigen.[91]

Initial contact with an allergen without sensitization is termed the refractory period and lasts a few days on average. Later, in the latent stage, dermal sensitization is completed. This stage lasts from approximately 4 days to several weeks. After sensitization has been completed, reexposure to a sensitizing antigen provokes acute dermatitis within 48 to 72 hours. This period is known as the reaction time and is the rationale behind patch testing for cases of suspected ACD. Some examples of common environmental agents that cause ACD are nickel, neomycin, and formaldehyde (see box on this page).

Acne lesions

Acneiform lesions are another manifestation of environmental exposures. Contact with oil or exposure to warm, humid environments can induce formation of comedonal plugs, papules, and pustules.

Tropical acne. Tropical acne due to heat and moisture was a cause of early military discharges from the Vietnam theater during that war.[63] It characteristically involves the back, buttocks, and neck to a greater degree than it does the face. This severe form of acne resolves when the individual affected returns to a temperate climate.

Chloracne. Chloracne is one of the most sensitive indicators of exposure to dioxin and related chemicals such as chlorinated or brominated aromatic compounds.[20] It is characterized by recalcitrant comedones and cysts, predominantly in the malar and postauricular areas.[32,97] It is discussed in greater detail in the section on environmental agent dioxin later in this chapter.

Photosensitivity reactions

Photodermatitis requires activation of a chemical substance on the skin surface by sunlight or ultraviolet radiation. Inflammation develops on cutaneous areas exposed to both light and the photosensitizing substance. Dioxin is a well known mediator of this type of acne as we shall discuss later. Involved areas usually include the face, pinnae of the ears, the back and sides of the neck, the V of the neck, and the dorsal aspects of the forearms, and the hands. Characteristically the eyelids, submental area of the chin and neck, retroauricular folds, and surfaces covered by clothing are spared.

Phototoxic reactions. Phototoxic reactions are analogous to ICD except for the additional requirement of ultraviolet radiation. The phototoxic chemical absorbs ultraviolet radiation, and the subsequent energy to the skin in such a way that cellular damage occurs. There is a direct dose-response relationship between a phototoxic reaction and both the concentration of the inciting chemical agent and the amount of specific radiation exposure.

Phototoxic reactions typically are associated with symptoms of stinging, burning, or smarting shortly after exposure to sunlight, and clinical inflammation resembles an acute sunburn more than eczematous dermatitis. So-called tar smarts caused by creosote or similar coal tar derivatives may be associated with urticarial swelling. Once this reaction has been initiated, subsequent exposures to small amounts of ultraviolet light can reproduce the symptoms for several hours.[19] This smarting sensation usually resolves rapidly once the affected skin is protected from sunlight.

Phototoxic reactions induced by psoralens are typically followed by hyperpigmentation; in mild cases, bizarrely patterned patches of hyperpigmentation may develop without apparent preceding inflammation. A variety of phototoxic reactions resulting from environmental exposures have been reported. Localized bullae and hyperpigmentation have been reported to occur on the hands and arms of workers who harvest celery and in grocery workers and chefs who trim and cut celery.[56,73] Subsequent exposure to natural ultraviolet light and high-intensity ultraviolet A lights (sunbeds) were the sources of radiation that produced the reaction.

Pigmentary changes

Hyperpigmentation. Repeated trauma and rubbing of the skin may produce hyperpigmentation in susceptible individuals. Chemical or thermal insults may initiate what is termed *postinflammatory pigmentary alteration* secondary to direct injury. Hyperpigmentaion (Fig. 22-3) can also result from ingestion, injection, or direct contact with photosensitizers. Phytophotodermatitis is one such example and is characterized by persistent hyperpigmentation. It may be caused by naturally occurring psoralens found in various vegetables and foods, such as celery and lime.[33,56,73] (See the section on phytophotodermatitis.)

Hypopigmentation. Loss of pigment can develop when the degree of cutaneous injury is sufficient to destroy melanocytes. These changes are seen with exposure to rubber additives, phenol compounds, and naturally occurring oils.

Exogenous discoloration of the skin. A wide array of chemicals may discolor the skin and nails. Environmental agents can modify normal skin color or affect melanization. Staining of the skin may also occur when naturally occurring dyes bind to the SC. Argyria (silver deposition in the skin from past medical and industrial use of silver) is a relatively rare occurrence today. It is important to recognize that systemic absorption of heavy metals such as mercury, silver, gold, and arsenic can induce diffuse discoloration of the skin.

Porphyria cutanea tarda. Porphyria cutanea tarda (PCT) is a disease process characterized by photosensitivity, hyperpigmentation, hypertrichosis, and bullous lesions (Fig. 22-4).[60] PCT can occur after exposure to various compounds such as dioxin[20] and particularly hexachlorobenzene (HCB)[16,17] The disorder is due to excessive amounts of porphyrin are aberrantly deposited in the skin. We shall discuss

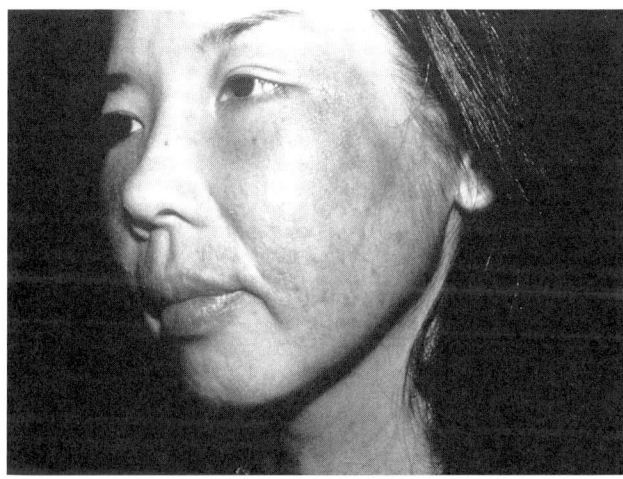

Fig. 22-3. Hyperpigmentation on face resulting from direct contact with a photosensitizer.

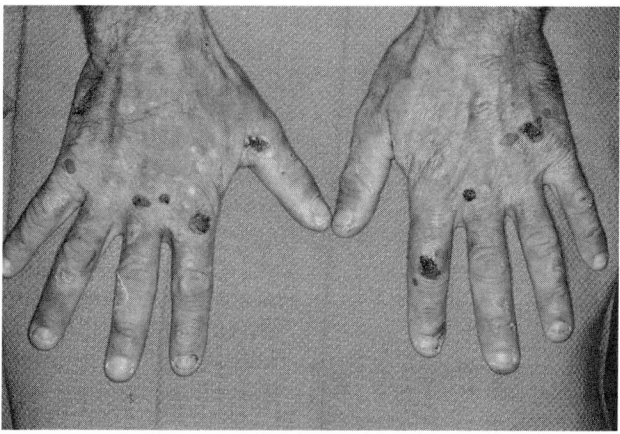

Fig. 22-4. Porphyria cutanea tarda—dorsal hand involvement, characterized by eroded bullae and multiple milia.

PCT and an epidemic that occurred in Turkey secondary to HCB exposure later in this chapter.

Actinic damage. Chronic ultraviolet B exposure induces a series of intriguing changes in the skin. Actinically damaged skin is skin that has received excessive cumulative sun exposure. Typically, this skin is coarse and leathery.[26] With continued exposure, the skin may take on a yellowish hue and lose its elasticity. Long-term ultraviolet B exposure can also lead to the development of precancerous lesions (actinic keratoses), which are erythematous flat-topped papules with sharp adherent scale (Fig. 22-5). Actinic keratoses are the precursors to squamous cell carcinoma, as discussed later in this chapter. Ultraviolet B exposure may also induce telangiectasias, elastotic nodules, comedones, pigmentary abnormalities, and sebaceous gland hyperplasia.[26] (See box on page 272.)

Photoallergic reactions. Photoallergic reactions are analogous to ACD in that a specific cell-mediated process is required.[53] This reaction usually occurs in relatively few individuals who have been previously sensitized by exposure to both the photosensitizing chemical and the appropriate ultraviolet radiation, usually in the 320-nm to 400-nm (ultraviolet A [UVA]) region.[60]

Photoallergic dermatitis typically presents as an acute eczematous reaction that may be followed by lichenified papules and plaques. Unlike phototoxic reactions, these lesions may extend beyond the areas exposed to the sun or other source of radiation. Exacerbations characteristically occur 1 to 2 days after sun exposure. Photoallergic contact dermatitis can be confirmed by the technique of photo patch testing.[53] Some individuals with environmentally induced photoallergic contact dermatitis develop persistent disabling cutaneous reactivity to UVA irradiation that persists for months or years after removal of the causative agent. Affected patients may also develop abnormal sensitivity to ultraviolet B and even visible light, such as persistent light reaction and actinic reticuloid.[35]

Urticaria

Urticaria occurs as a wheal-and-flare response to environmental stimuli. It may be induced by immunologic or nonimmunologic mechanisms. There are numerous portals of entry for such reactions. The generalized form of urticaria usually occurs secondary to the ingestion of an allergen. This type of urticaria may be associated with bronchial asthma, diarrhea, and pruritus. Conversely, localized urticaria usually manifests after a specific environmental agent is absorbed into the dermis. Many materials have been reported to produce contact urticaria in the environment (see box).

Allergic contact urticaria. Allergic contact urticaria may produce symptoms ranging from pruritus and edema to anaphylaxis and even death. The most severe reactions have occurred with exposure to rubber (*Hevea brasiliensis*); eggs; silk; and animal fur.

Nonallergic contact urticaria. Nonallergic contact urticaria does not require prior sensitization and may develop in a large percentage of exposed individuals. It is the most common type of contact urticaria and is caused by a wide variety of compounds, symptoms including nettles and certain caterpillar species. Immunologically, the urticaria does not depend on specific cell-mediated mechanisms.

Scleroderma

Scleroderma can also result from certain of environmental exposures. Typically, scleroderma patients have thickened, bound-down skin (Fig. 22-6) and sclerodactyly (Fig.

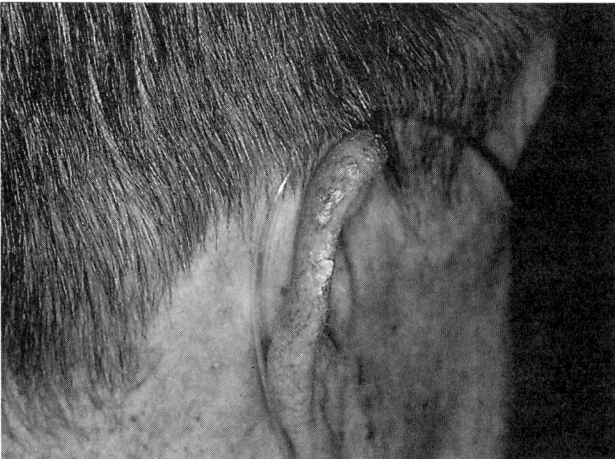

Fig. 22-5. Actinic keratosis—multiple flat-topped erythematous papules with adherent yellow scale (precancerous lesions) on the ear.

Examples of environmental agents that can induce contact urticaria

Medications
- Horse serum
- Streptomycin
- Cod liver oil

Physical agents
- Heat
- Cold
- Water (aquagenic)
- Light (ultraviolet and visible)

Textiles
- Wool
- Silk

Animals
- Dog and cat saliva
- Dander
- Anthropods
- Marine life

Plants
- Nettles
- Cactus
- Rubber

Foods
- Eggs
- Wheat
- Flour
- Spices
- Carrots
- Potato
- Raw beef
- Fish
- Pears
- Peanut butter
- Apples
- Kiwi

22-7), and polyarthralgia. If systemic disease is present, the heart, kidneys, and gastrointestinal tract may become involved. Cardiac conduction abnormalities or renal hypertensive crisis may ensue. Contacts with polyvinyl chloride, silica, dioxin, epoxy resins, rapeseed oil, solvents, and L-tryptophan have been documented to be associated with sclerodermatous conditions (see box). The latter (L-tryptophan) has also been associated with an eosinphilia-myalgia syndrome, as discussed later in this chapter. It is important to assess the duration of exposure and the degree of systemic compromise when patients who have had contact with these environmental agents are examined.

Infectious disorders

Environmental dermatoses may be produced by a wide array of infectious organisms. These may include fungi, viruses, or bacteria. Lesions may present as furuncles or pustules, as in the case of bacterial infections, or vesicles and crusted papules, in the case of virus-induced lesions. Herpesviruses, the orf poxvirus, *Sporothrix,* and dermatophytes are some of the more common infectious agents causing these types of dermatoses. The incidence of most common pyodermas and fungal infections increases with heat, humidity, and lower standards of living. We examine in detail some of these infectious conditions and the way in which they manifest later in this chapter.

Cutaneous malignancy

It is well known that skin cancers have been directly associated with a multitude of environmental stimuli (Table 22-3). Nonmelanoma skin cancer (NMSC), the most common type of cutaneous malignancy, have been associated with long-term ultraviolet B irradiation, as well as with aromatic hydrocarbon exposure. Basal cell carcinoma, the most common of the NMSC, typically presents with a pearly white rolled border and prominent telangiectasias (Fig. 22-8). Squamous cell carcinoma, which constitutes approximately 25% of NMSC, tends to have more metastatic potential and may take on the appearance of an nonhealing ulcerated plaque (Fig. 22-9) or a raised erythematous

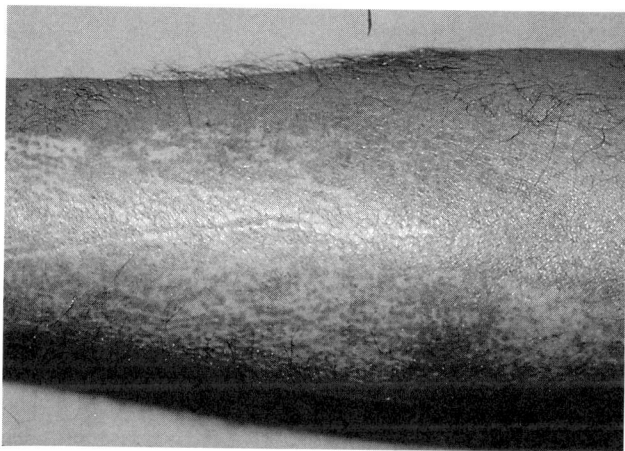

Fig. 22-6. Scleroderma—illustration of mottled hyperpigmentation and hypopigmentation with skin that appears "bound down" on the forearm. (Courtesy of T. Fotopoulos and N. Fenske)

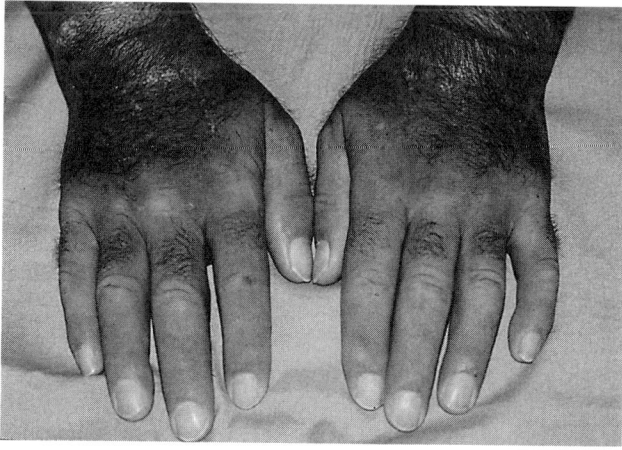

Fig. 22-7. Scleroderma—illustration of sclerodactly taut skin over the digits making mobilization difficult. (Courtesy of T. Fotopoulos and N. Fenske)

Environmental agents which have been associated with sclerodermatous conditions

Polyvinyl chloride
Dioxin
Silicosis
Epoxy resins
Rapeseed oil
L-Tryptophan
Solvents

Table 22-3. Environmental factors associated with cutaneous malignancy

Skin cancer type	Etiology
Nonmelanoma skin cancer	
Basal cell carcinoma (75%)	UVB exposure (cumulative)
Squamous cell carcinoma (25%)	UVB exposure (cumulative)
	Hydrocarbons (soot, coal tar, shale petroleum, paraffin, pipe smoking)
Melanoma	
Lentigo maligna melanoma	Long-term UVB exposure
Superficial spreading melanoma, nodular melanoma	Intermittent UVB exposure

UVB, ultraviolet B.

nodule. Lentigo maligna melanoma is the one subtype of malignant melanoma that is associated with cumulative long-term ultraviolet B exposure. It is characterized as an irregularly pigmented macule or plaque on a sun-exposed area, with variegation of color and ill-defined borders. This lesion, as other melanomas, follows the ABCD mnemonic in terms of its description (see box). Most other forms of melanoma, such as superficial spreading and nodular melanoma, are usually located on the trunk and are related to intermittent solar radiation.

The ABCDs of malignant melanoma

A = Asymmetry
B = Border irregularity
C = Multiple colors (red, white, blue)
D = Diameter > 0.5 cm

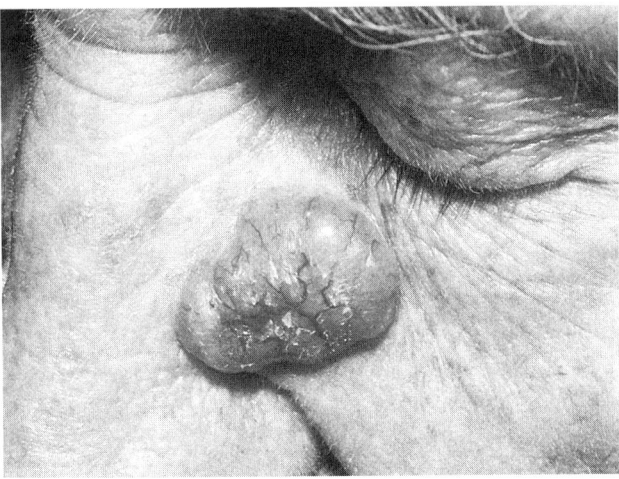

Fig. 22-8. Basal cell carcinoma—nodular type.

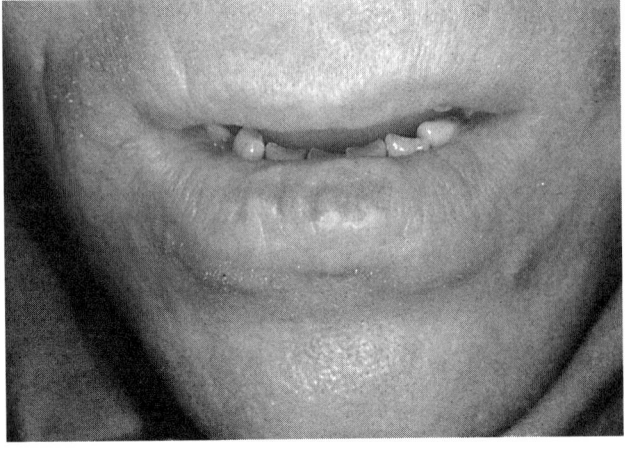

Fig. 22-9. Squamous cell carcinoma presenting as an ulcerative erythematous plaque on the lower lip.

AN OVERVIEW OF SPECIFIC ENVIRONMENTAL FACTORS THAT CAN AFFECT THE SKIN

As previously discussed, a myriad of environmental stimuli can induce cutaneous disease. In the previous section we attempted to define some of the more commonly seen dermatoses by their clinical presentation. We now turn our attention to the factors responsible for initiation of these disorders. We discuss the potentially adverse affects of the most common environmental agents that induce cutaneous reaction. It is important for the practitioner to be familiar with these agents and the way in which they cause disease. Although the list of environmental stimuli that can initiate disease is exhaustive, we have divided them into the following categories: mechanical, physical, chemical, and biologic.

Mechanical factors

A number of mechanical factors are known to provoke disease. Some place the patient at risk for secondary infection or trauma through the disruption of the intact SC. Friction, pressure, and vibration can cause callosities, contusions, and abrasions. Although some of these changes can induce further complications, others, such as a friction callus, may provide protection, particularly to the palms. Exposures to such abrasives as spicules of fiberglass or particulate dusts (including those from mineral or chemical sources) may rub against skin and produce severe itching, especially when particles are trapped beneath clothing. With fiberglass, the intensity of itching is inversely related to fiber diameter, and short fibers (less than 3.5 micron diameter) are least likely to cause symptoms.[38] Pinpoint excoriations are the principal clinical findings. Foreign-body reactions also can result from the penetration of splinters from thorns, accidentally introduced carbon products, or sand. Secondary infection can also set in.

Physical factors

Heat. High temperatures cause excessive sweating, miliaria, and maceration, which in turn predispose to secondary infection of the skin. Excessive exposure to heat also causes severe systemic symptoms and signs relative to heat cramps, heat exhaustion, and heat stroke.[48] Contact with radiation sources, hot metal or other solids, or molten substances can also produce burns of the skin.

Other specific dermatoses can be produced by excessive exposures to naturally occurring heat such as wood-burning fires. Erythema ab igne is one such condition and is characterized by mottled, reticulate hyperemia with melanoderma and telangiectasia. This disorder occurs after long-term and intense exposures to heat that are insufficient to produce a burn. After months or years of exposure, hyperkeratotic nodules and skin changes resembling those seen in chronic actinic exposure appear.[45] Occasionally, erythema ab igne leads to the development of NMSC.

Miliaria is another common skin disorder that occurs in

a warm and humid environment, particularly in the tropics. The lining of the distal sweat ducts swells because of high humidity, leading to obstruction of the sweat ducts and sweat retention. When sweating occurs proximally to an intraepidermal sweat duct obstructed in the superficial skin layer (SC), small, superficial, noninflammatory vesicles develop. These vesicles subside when sweating ceases or when the SC overlying the vesicles exfoliates. This condition is termed miliaria crystallina.

Miliaria rubra occurs when the sweat duct in the deeper layers of the epidermis is obstructed. It typically occurs in parts of the skin covered by clothing. These lesions are small pruritic papulovesicles surrounded by erythema. Widespread miliaria rubra can impair the ability of the individual to sweat normally and to withstand continued exposure to hot or humid conditions. Pustular lesions may contain gram-positive bacteria in addition to neutrophils. The primary treatment is to curtail further sweating to avoid continued damaging epidermal maceration. Natural desquamation of the skin clears the occlusion of the sweat ducts after several days. There is no dramatically effective topical or systemic treatment for miliaria.[41]

Cold. The skin's physiologic behavior can also be altered by low temperatures. Excessive exposure to cold water or cold and wet footwear, even in the presence of warm air temperatures, can lead to immersion or trench foot. Not only can blistering and ulceration occur but severe tissue damage can ensue, depending on certain factors such as the rate of chilling and rewarming of the involved areas.

Frostbite occurs when tissues have been overexposed to air temperatures lower than 10° F. It occurs with the actual formation of ice crystals in the viable epidermis, and dermis. Factors such as high altitude, strong winds, and contact with cold metal aggravate the effects of cold exposure on living cells. Outdoor workers and those exposed to arctic waters are more prone to suffer from cold injuries to their acral regions. Treatment consists of rest, systemic antibiotics, analgesics, and rapid rewarming of tissues.[90]

Chilblain, or pernio, is a recurrent localized effect of cold exposure noted particularly in those with vascular abnormalities. The hands, feet, nose, ears, and cheeks are the sites most commonly involved.

Water. In certain instances water can act as an irritant to the skin, especially if the cutaneous barrier has been disrupted. Hard water, which contains traces of lime, magnesium, and iron, can potentiate this irritation because of mechanical stimulation. Water can also be associated with other dermatoses (see box). Aquagenic pruritus is a condition that induces an intense pruritus in the area of water contact, without any visible cutaneous change. Histamine and acetylcholine mediators are thought to play a role in this disorder. Patients with polycythemia vera commonly are afflicted with aquagenic pruritus. These patients can often have elevations of histamine found in both their skin and serum.

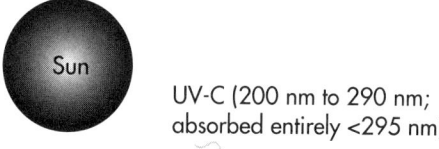

Water-related skin conditions

Cold urticaria
Aquagenic pruritus
Irritant dermatitis
Xerosis
Infectious diseases

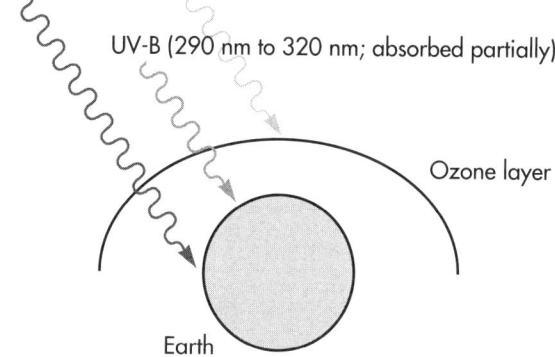

Fig. 22-10. Protective effects of ozone on ultraviolet absorption with respect to specific wavelengths of light.

The sun and ultraviolet irradiation. The sun is the main source of ultraviolet radiation exposure in our environment. Approximately 35% of the nonionizing radiation that reaches the earth is perceived as visible light; 60%, as heat; and 5%, as ultraviolet radiation. The actual solar spectrum that finally reaches the earth's surface represents a small fraction of the total energy emitted by the sun, in part because of the protective effects of many elements such as carbon dioxide, water, and the ozone layer (Fig. 22-10). Although solar radiation is beneficial to humans by providing warmth, light, vitamin D production, and photosynthesis, it also has several untoward effects.

Short-term ultraviolet exposure. Ultraviolet radiation absorption leads to acute and chronic cutaneous cell damage. In the short term, the release of various mediators such as interleukin-1 and tumor necrosis factors are important in the sunburn reaction, which occurs after intense ultraviolet B exposure. The acute signs of this reaction include erythema (rubor), warmth (calor), pain (dolor), swelling, and vesiculation.

Long-term ultraviolet exposure. Chronic ultraviolet exposure can manifest in several ways in the skin. There are several cutaneous signs of photoaging[26] (see box). These signs are well documented and include the noted changes of

> **Manifestations of long-term ultraviolet exposure**
>
> Rough, dry skin
> Skin with yellowish hue
> Comedones
> Thickened, coarse skin
> Pigmentary anomalies
>   Guttate hypomelanosis
> Vascular lesions
>   Telangiectasias
>   Ecchymoses
> Loss of cutaneous elasticity
> Premalignant lesions
>   Actinic keratoses
> Malignant lesions
>   Basal cell carcinoma
>   Squamous cell carcinoma

coarse, leathery skin, loss of cutaneous elasticity, deep wrinkling, and telangiectasia.[26] The primary causative agent of DNA mutagenesis within the electromagnetic spectrum is UVB irradiation.[28] Regular avoidance of exposure to ultraviolet radiation and the use of protective sunscreens with a sun-protection factor of 15 or higher help minimize chronic photodamage.[85]

Cutaneous malignancies. NMSC is the most common cancer in the United States.[10,65] Of the types of NMSC, basal cell carcinoma of the skin is most common[72] and is directly related to lifetime exposure to ultraviolet light, particularly in the ultraviolet B or sunburn spectrum (290 to 320 nm).[28] Recent increases in incidences may reflect both a progressively aging population[36] and the popularity of outdoor leisure time.[66] Those whose vocations require frequent exposure to ultraviolet B radiation, such as farmers and police officers, are at an elevated risk of developing NMSC.[41,43] The epidemiology of cutaneous malignant melanoma is more complex than is that of NMSC. It does not follow the same simple dose-response curve as does NMSC. Instead, most melanomas result from the combination of genetic susceptibility and intermittent intense exposure to UVR.

Trauma is less clearly defined as a risk factor for skin cancer, although it has been accepted in the past by regulatory and compensation agencies as a causative factor of skin cancer. In summary, some of the major causes of environmentally induced skin cancer are ultraviolet irradiation, aromatic hydrocarbons, arsenic, ionizing radiation, and trauma.*

Chemical agents

A variety of chemical agents has been implicated in the development of environmentally induced cutaneous diseases. These agents include such materials as solvents, preservatives, pesticides, and various resins. The number of man-made chemical products has increased during the past few decades. As previously mentioned, the effects of these agents on the skin can be dramatic, and cutaneous presentations may range from photosensitivity reactions and pigmentary disorders to chloracne and cutaneous malignancies. The following section focuses on some of the major environmental chemicals responsible for these changes and the impact that they have had on society.

Dioxin. Dioxin exposure has been associated with a myriad of cutaneous dermatoses. The structural name for dioxin is 2, 3, 7, 8-tetrachlorodibenzo-*para*-dioxin (TCDD).[13,20] TCDD has no real industrial uses[20] but is the by-product of several reactions involving chlorinated phenols.[32] Its use in the Vietnam War as the defoliant in Agent Orange has been well publicized.[15] TCDD can accumulate in humans by different mechanisms, which include direct contact with the agent and secondary dermal absorption, inhalation, and direct ingestion. TCDD has had significant untoward side effects in humans, usually resulting from large industrial accidents in which significant amounts of dioxin were released in small areas. One of the most publicized events occurred in Seveso, Italy, on July 10, 1976.[13,64] In this case, a technical accident involving sodium trichlorophenate processing occurred. TCDD was released in the form of a cloud that covered approximately 200 acres of land, including both urban and rural areas. As the large radius suggests, a significant number of children, adolescents, and adults were exposed to the agent.

Follow-up studies of these populations revealed a multitude of cutaneous lesions.[13] In the first few weeks after exposure, the sampled group demonstrated erythema, edema, and papulonecrotic lesions. Months after exposure, the populations studied developed acne lesions consisting of open comedones intermingled with pale yellow cysts that spared the central regions of the face. The term *chloracne* was used to describe this condition. Clinically chloracne is characterized by recalcitrant comedones and cysts located predominantly in the malar and postauricular areas.[32,97] With increasing severity, other regions of the head, neck, upper arms, chest, back, abdomen, outer thighs, and genitalia may become involved.

Chloracne is one of the most sensitive indicators of exposure to dioxin and related chemicals.[81,97] Lesions may continue to appear after all exposure to the inciting chemical has ceased. They usually last about 2 years after exposure ceases, but in some cases widespread scarring can result.[13,20] Other findings associated with TCDD exposure include hyperpigmentation, conjunctivitis, follicular hyperkeratosis, and actinic elastosis. If exposures to TCDD are extensive, the associated chloracne is typically more severe.[20] Highly exposed patients can develop milia and demonstrate changes consistent with PCT.[20] Other agents in the environment that

---
*References 23, 28, 42, 43, 65, 94.

may produce similar lesions include chlornaphthalenes, polychlorinated biphenyls, polybrominated biphenyls, polychlorinated dibenzo-*p*-dioxins, polychlorinated dibenzofurans, 3,4,3,4-tetrachlorazobenzene, and 3,4,3,4-tetrachlorazoxybenzene.

L-Tryptophan. L-Tryptophan is an amino acid found in most foods.[39] Its use has been popularized as an over-the-counter remedy for insomnia,[49] depression, weight loss,[77] and the discomfort associated with menstrual cramping.[39] Recently, an influx of reports has associated L-tryptophan ingestion with scleroderma-like skin abnormalities, eosinophilia, and fasciitis.[77] In one series,[77] nine patients who had ingested 1 to 3 g/day of L-tryptophan for 1 to 18 months developed rash and edema of the lower extremities, followed by scleroderma-like skin changes, myalgia, muscle weakness, eosinophilia, and peripheral neuropathy. Chemical evaluation of these patients revealed the increased presence of L-kynurenine and quinolinic acid, which are metabolites of L-tryptophan. Biopsies of involved areas revealed inflamed fascia with an infiltrate of lymphocytes, plasma cells, and macrophages. The exact mechanism of L-tryptophan–induced disease has not been elicited, but more than 1000 cases have been reported to the Centers for Disease Control.[86] Some have speculated that L-tryptophan could serve as a trigger that under the right set of environmental and host circumstances could initiate the features of the syndrome, including fibrosis, swelling, and polyinflammation.[39]

Vinyl chloride. Vinyl chloride (VC) is a synthetic resin used in industrial processes. Its use became prevalent in Germany and the United States in the 1930s. VC was first reported to be associated with pruritus and scleroderma-like lesions in 1963 in Romania.[80] Several workers were noted to be afflicted. Their clinical symptoms resolved upon their removal from the exposure site. *Occupational acroosteolysis* is the term used to describe the triad of Raynaud's phenomenon, sclerodermatous skin lesions, and osteolytic defects of the terminal phalanges that occurs in those exposed to the VC monomer.[62] Typically, workers who directly handle cleaning agents containing the VC monomer develop the triad of symptoms.

One possible method of entry of the VC monomer into the body is the aerosolized route. Once VC is absorbed, pruritus and erythema with swelling soon ensue. The scleroderma-like syndrome that is seen with VC exposure should be classified as being distinct from classic systemic sclerosis (Table 22-4).[62] Lesions induced by VC are usually located on the dorsal aspects of the extremities and consist of papules and plaques.[88] The usual atrophy and tapering of the fingertips seen with systemic sclerosis is not seen. Instead, fingertip shortening and osteolytic lesions of the distal phalanx are present. VC-induced changes additionally differ from those of systemic scleroderma in that telangiectasias, subcutaneous calcification, and visceral organ involvement are lacking.[50] Histologically these changes include the presence of a thinned epidermis, swollen collagen bundles, and preserved eccrine structures.

Table 22-4. Differences between VC-associated disease and scleroderma

Clinical sign	VC-associated disease	Scleroderma
Visceral involvement	No	Common
Telangiectasias	No	Common
Cutaneous changes	Hands and forearms	Diffuse
Hands	Hyperhydrosis, no ulceration, finger tip shortening, acroosteolysis (lytic bone lesions)	Anhydrosis, ulceration, fingertip tapering

Modified from Ostlere LS et al: Atypical systemic sclerosis following exposure to vinyl chloride monomer: a case report and review of the cutaneous aspects of vinyl chloride disease, *Clin Exp Dermatol* 17:208, 1992.

Although the etiopathogenesis of the scleroderma-like lesions has not yet been identified, a genetic component is thought to play a role, because human leukocyte antigen haplotypes HLA-DR5, -B8, and -DR3 are increased in those with VC-induced acroosteolysis.[62] Antinuclear antibody and other serologic markers of connective disease are usually not present. In addition to VC, silica dust,[37] rapeseed oil,[47] trichloroethylene,[18] cocaine,[46] L-tryptophan,[77] and silicone implants[87] have been reported to be associated with the development of scleroderma-like changes.[14] Further studies are under way to elucidate the exact mechanisms of some of these associations.

Hexachlorobenzene. One of the uses of HCB is as a fungicide for wheat seed storage prior to planting. In the early 1950s it was a common practice in southern Turkey to mix HCB with wheat to avoid vegetative infection with the wheat fungus *Tilletia tritrici*.[16] Between 1955 and 1961, more than 3000 cases of porphyria were noted to occur in a diverse population in Turkey during a famine in which people, mostly children, ingested protected seedlings.[69] Soon after ingestion, pigmentation, hirsutism, porphyrinuria, and bullae developed. The term *porphyria turcica* was coined to describe the syndrome in this population group.[16]

The average interval between ingestion of wheat treated with HCB and the development of symptoms was 6 months. Weakness, photosensitivity, and anorexia were the first symptoms to appear.[19] Facial hyperpigmentation, hypertrichosis, and bullae with mutilating scarring were a later finding. Frequently, children were described as having a monkeylike appearance. Twenty to 30 years after the exposure, the most common findings in one study of survivors[16] were hyperpigmentation (71%), dorsal hand scarring (86%), pinched facies (42%), hypertrichosis (47%), and painless arthritis (67%). Many of these patients still had elevated levels of porphyrins, especially uroporphyrin, in their urine or stool, or both.

The exact mechanism of HCB-induced porphyria has yet to be elicited. Some speculate that HCB or its metabolites inhibit uroporphyrinogen decarboxylase, thereby leading to a gradual accumulation of hepatic porphyrins.[26] In addition to HCB, dioxins,[8,20,70] polychlorinated biphenyls,[8] 2,4-dichlorophenoxyacetic acids,[8] ethanol,[8,20] iron,[8,21,51] and estrogens[21,67] may mediate induction of PCT.

Polycyclic hydrocarbons, alkylators, and aromatics. Polycyclic hydrocarbons are prevalent in the environment as by-products of the combustion of fossil fuels and organic materials.[23,91,94] These compounds are found in tar, soot, and pitch.[94] Alkylating agents such as nitrogen mustard and beta-propiolactone are sometimes used in medical treatments[14] but also are agents of war and scientific experimentation. Aromatic compounds such as phenol and anthralin are used in medicine and industry and may play a role in the formation of NMSC.[94,95] NMSC formation is thought to occur in three steps: initiation, tumor promotion, and malignant conversion.[94,95] Polycyclic hydrocarbons have been the most extensively studied initiators and often exert their effects through covalent interactions with epidermal deoxyribonucleic acid (DNA).[11] Such interaction allows the formation of a carcinogen-DNA adduct. Tumor promotion results from repeated exposures of initiated skin to agents that permit latent tumor phenotype expression.[94,95] Actinic keratoses are an example of such latent tumor phenotypes. Thousands of agents such as anthralin, benzoyl peroxide, and phorbol esters are thought to function as promoting agents.[94,95] The third stage, known as malignant conversion, results from the transition of a premalignant state to one that is cancerous. Although this transition often happens spontaneously, some speculate that the frequency is enhanced by repeated exposures to mutagenic agents such as those responsible for the initiation step.[104] The exact sensitivity of the malignant transformation step to particular exogenous agents has yet to be determined. Thus a variety of agents, through altering DNA sequencing, binding, and functional properties, can work in synergy with ultraviolet irradiation to induce cutaneous malignancies.

Halogenated hydrocarbons. Halogenated hydrocarbons are found in everyday devices such as refrigerators and air conditioners. Chlorofluoromethane (CF_2Cl_2) is one example of a halogenated hydrocarbon and is found in freon, hairspray, and deodorants.[14,78] These compounds have been thought to be responsible for the gradual catalytic losses of the ozone layer.[48] Ozone is the protective agent of the earth's stratosphere responsible for blocking ultraviolet rays with a wavelength of less than 290 nm (all of the ultraviolet C and part of the ultraviolet B region).[48] Interaction of the hydrocarbon with oxygen generates a chlorine monoxide monomer (ClO) that subsequently reacts with ozone and catalyzes it to oxygen (Fig. 22-11).

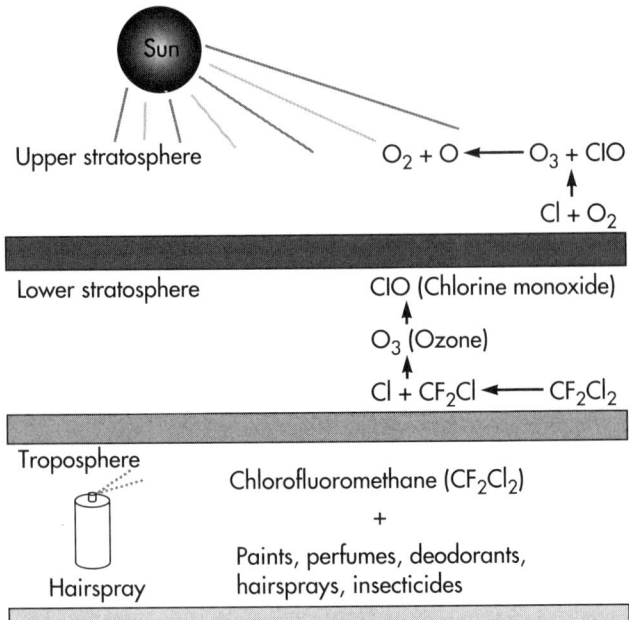

Fig. 22-11. Detrimental effects of chlorofluoromethane (CF_2Cl_2) on the ozone layer (O_3).

The depletion of the earth's ozone layer has directly correlated with increased uses of halogenated hydrocarbons over the past several years, especially over the North and South Poles. It has been estimated that for every 1% decrease in ozone concentration, there is a 2% increase of ultraviolet B radiation reaching the earth and a 3% increase in NMSC formation. Current efforts are being made to minimize ozone depletion through changes in industrial standards and elimination of halogenated hydrocarbons from toiletries and appliances.

Nickel. Nickel is a common environmental allergen. Nickel allergy can manifest in a variety of ways, including vesicular hand dermatitis and contact eczematous reactions in areas such as the belt-buckle region of the waist. Dermatitis most commonly affects females who become sensitized through ear piercing and use of nickel-containing earrings.[1] Nickel may be found in many devices such as cookware handles, doorknobs, paper clips, coins, and clothing studs.[17] Nickel exposure is often seen in the cosmetology trade, because of the use of nickel-plated hair clips and cutting shears. Dietary sources of nickel include vegetables, whole wheat, and shellfish (see box).[17] From 1% to 10% of ingested nickel is absorbed by the gastrointestinal tract, and it is excreted in high concentrations in sweat.[59]

Testing for nickel in metal objects can be performed in the physician's office with the dimethylglyoxime spot test.[1,27] After the reagents have been added, rubbing the article tested with a cotton-tipped applicator or gauze sponge often makes the red-pink color of a positive reaction more apparent. (This test may be purchased from Allerderm Lab-

Foods that commonly contain nickel
Herring
Oysters
Asparagus
Beans
Mushrooms
Onions
Corn
Wheat
Spinach
Tomatoes
Tea
Cocoa
Baking powder
Cooked pears

Potential sources for chromium exposure
Ceramics
Cements
Drilling muds
Fire retardants
Meat
Milk products and preservatives
Paper products
Photography materials
Tanned leather

Modified from Andersen K, Burrows D, White I: Allergens from the standard series. In Menné R, Frosch R, editors: *Textbook of contact dermatology,* Berlin, 1992, Springer-Verlag.

oratories, P.O. Box 931, Mill Valley, CA 94941.) Medical practitioners should advise nickel-allergic patients to consider purchasing a test kit for their own use when possible.

Chromium. Chromium occurs naturally as chrome iron ore or chromite. It is an alloy that consists of a combination of chromium oxides and iron.[17] The salts of this alloy are responsible for contact hypersensitivity reactions to chromate.[1,17] Chromium is commonly used in the manufacturing of cutting tools, cement, and printing products (see box).[1,12,17,55] Although chromium is better absorbed in its hexavalent state,[52] chromium allergy occurs from the element's trivalent form in which it can combine with epidermal proteins to function as a hapten.[1]

The dermatitis that results from exposure to chromium salts can be either localized or diffuse. Chrome ulcers[1,7,58] nasal perforations, generalized contact dermatitis, and pompholyx have been reported to occur after exposures to this agent.[1,17] Once diagnosed, chromate dermatitis has a bad prognosis, because many individuals endure severe, chronic dermatitis despite treatment.[1,30]

Biologic agents

A myriad of biologic agents have been implicated in the causation of environmental dermatoses. Organisms such as bacteria, viruses, parasites, rickettsiae, and various plants have be known to penetrate the percutaneous barrier either directly or through release of endogenous toxins. The clinical manifestations from biologic contacts are multiple, ranging in clinical presentation from the phytophotodermatitis associated with lime (*Citrus aurantiifolia*)[5,17] exposure to the painless digital ulceration or nodule seen in *Sporothrix schenckii* infections.[75] The following section reviews some of the more common biologic agents and attempts to illustrate how varied the clinical presentations can be.

Herpesvirus. Herpes lesions present as grouped vesicles on an erythematous base, usually on the lip or genital region. The lesions often have a pruritic or burning quality. It is important to remember that asymptomatic individuals may shed herpesvirus in the mouth or genitalia, particularly when they are febrile or severely ill.[40] Health care workers may develop herpetic whitlow when unprotected hands directly contact viral shedding lesions.

Other viruses. Orf and milker's nodules are poxvirus infections transmitted to humans by sheep, goats, and cows.[75] Their clinical manifestations, usually a single asymptomatic or slightly painful 1-cm nodule located most commonly on the finger, are very characteristic. In the case of milker's nodules, usually less than a half dozen lesions are confined to the hand and forearm.[75] These cases may be complicated by secondary erythema multiforme.[96] Differentiation of these lesions from herpetic whitlow, cutaneous tuberculosis, and syphilitic chancre can at times be clinically difficult.

Dermatophytes. Tinea pedis is a example of a cutaneous dermatophyte infection. Occluded moist skin is an ideal medium for their growth. Dermatophytes may also induce maceration, erythema, and scale (Fig. 22-12).[2] Secondary bacterial infections can ensue once the percutaneous barrier has been damaged and should be watched for.[2] *Trichophyton verrucosum* produces dermatophyte infection in cattle and may be transmitted to humans, provoking severe inflammatory skin lesions that frequently involve the face and often heal with scarring despite treatment with griseofulvin and prednisone.[40] The spores of *T. verrucosum* can produce lesions in those exposed even years after an infectious cattle source has left the area.[40]

Sporothrix. Sporotrichosis is produced by the dimorphic fungus *Sporothrix schenckii*.[2] The initial lesion is a painless papule or ulceration at the site of inoculation; secondary nodules develop along the draining lymphatics.[75] This disease is acquired by those exposed to a variety of soils and plants. Sporotrichosis may directly be inoculated by trauma from contaminated splinters, sticks, rosebush thorns, and sphagnum peat moss.[75] Protective measures to

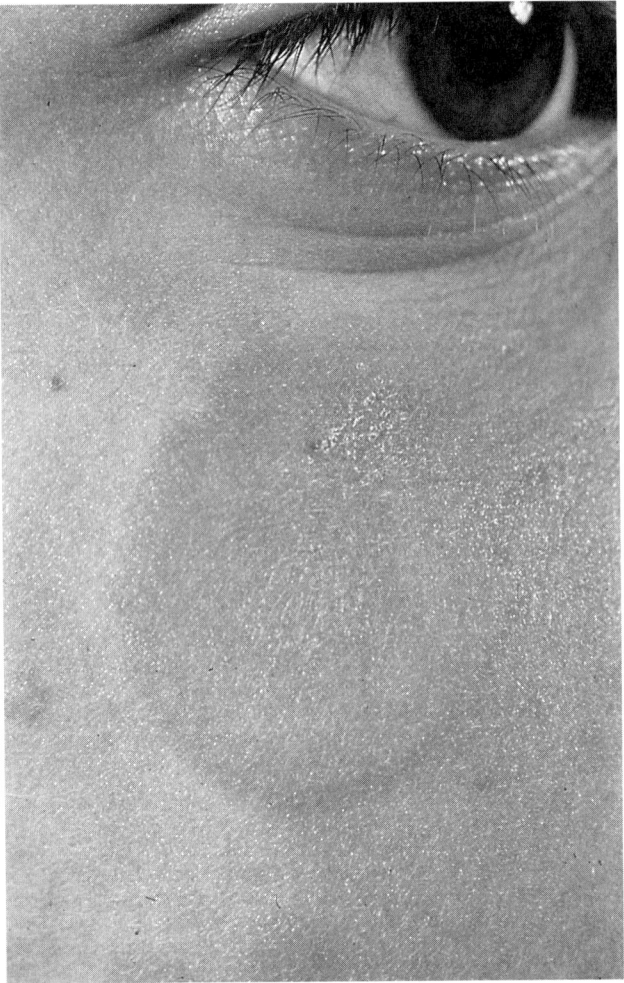

Fig. 22-12. Dermatophyte infection—*T. mentagrophytes* presenting as a well-circumscribed circinate plaque on the left cheek in this child.

avoid abrasions and skin punctures are recommended to prevent colonization by these organisms.

Bacteria. Individuals with dermatoses such as exudative dermatitis[74] and psoriasis[44] frequently are coinfected with group A *Streptococcus* or *Staphylococcus aureus*. The number of organisms usually decreases as the dermatitis or psoriasis clinically improves. The physician must be aware that a true pyoderma may require systemic antibiotics.[74] Pyoderma may develop in those who deal with fresh meat products, especially if the hands are inflamed or lacerated. Erysipeloid is an example of an infection which infests the skin of fresh water and salt water fish, shellfish, poultry, and decaying meat products.[74,93,98] This infection is produced by the gram positive bacillus bacteria *Erysipelothrix insidiosa* (formerly *rhusiopathiae*).[98] Organisms usually enter the skin through abrasions or puncture wounds of the hands.[74] Clinical infection develops 3 to 7 days after inoculation. The disorder is characterized by painful erythematous papules that enlarge to form red nodules and associated lymphangitis. Septicemia may occur if treatment with penicillin is not undertaken or the patient is immunocompromised.[31,34,74]

Parasites. The parasitic diseases of environmental origin occur with sufficient frequency to bear mention. In Florida, cutaneous larva migrans, or creeping eruption, is a common disease seen in those who come into contact with soil contaminated with *Ancylostoma braziliense*.[4] Lesions usually appear on the lower extremities as pruritic, thin wandering tunnel-like lesions which sometimes contain serous fluid.

Mites. Mites are another environmental parasite that can produce cutaneous lesions. Prior to the application of pesticides, farm handlers who harvested or processed grain products developed grain itch from the mite *Pyemotes ventricosus*.[7] Another example can be seen in grocers and longshoremen, who may contract eczematous lesions from the mites of the genus *Tyroglyphus*. These parasites have been known to infect cheese, cereals, and sugar cargoes. Finally, poultry processors occasionally have experienced epidemic outbreaks of dermatitis caused by the parasite *Dermanyssus gallinae*.[9] Lesions produced by these mites vary from bright red macules to papular urticaria and vesicular dermatitis.[76]

Plants and woods

Plants. Dermatoses due to plants and woods are commonplace in today's environment. Plants known to cause dermatitis are numerous, but in the United States, the genus *Toxicodendron* accounts for most cases. In California, *T. diversilobum* (poison oak) dermatitis accounts for almost 25% of all occupational skin disease claims per year.[3] The essential oleoresins of this plant family, Anacardiaceae, are phenolic in nature; thus they can serve as both irritants and sensitizers. A highly potent although less publicized substance within the Anacardiaceae family is the oleoresin produced in cashew shells. The extract from these shells can induce dermatitis in those exposed to the uncured resin.[71]

Additional plants reported[6] to be among the most troublesome for the induction of dermatitis (characterized acutely by vesiculation and chronically by lichenification) include castor bean pomace (*Ricinus communis*); chrysanthemum (*Chrysanthemum leucanthemum, Chrysanthemum indicum, Chrysanthemum coccineum, Chrysanthemum cineraraefolium*); hops (*Humulus lupulus*); hyacinth (*Hyacinthus orientalis*); jute (*Corchorus olitorius, Corchorus capsularis*); oleander (*Nerium oleander, Nerium odorum*); poison sumac (*Rhus vernix*); primrose (*Primula obconica*); ragweed oleoresin (*Ambrosia artemisiifolia, Ambrosia elatior*); tomato (*Lycopersicon esculentum*); and tulip bulb (*Tulipa gesneriana*). *Alstroemeria* species have also accounted for outbreaks of allergic contact dermatitis among florists.[84]

Phytophotodermatitis. Photoreactivity is an inherent quality of many plants, notably those of the Moraceae, Umbelliferae, and Rutaceae families (Table 22-5). The reactive material in many plant species that induces dermatitis is a naturally occurring psoralen. Some of the better-known

Table 22-5. Phytophotodermatitis

Family	Plant species
Compositae	Stinking mayweed, yarrow, great burdock
Umbelliferae	Celery, dill, parsnip, carrot
Rutaceae	Orange, lime, lemon
Moraceae	Fig, rubber plant, mulberry
Papilionaceae	

plants and fruits that cause phytophotodermatitis are *Ammi majus* (Umbelliferae), bergamot (Rutaceae), pink-rot celery (Umbelliferae), fig (Moraceae), lime (Rutaceae), parsley (Umbelliferae), parsnip (Umbelliferae), and rue (Rutaceae).[5,6] The reaction spectrum for many of these species is in the ultraviolet A range.[92] Reactions to these substances are characterized early by erythema and pruritis and later by hyperpigmentation, which can take months to fade.[2,61,92]

Woods. Contact dermatitis from naturally occurring wood is less frequent than that from plant species. Nonetheless, certain wood products have been classified as dermatologic hazards. Types of wood species known to cause contact dermatitis include acacia, alder, ash, beech, birch, chestnut, cedar, creosote bush, elm, maple, mesquite, oak, pine, poplar, prune, and spruce.[82] The presentation is similar to that of the lesions is of plant dermatitis. It is important for the medical practitioner to investigate the possibility of exposure to these species through either occupational or domestic contacts. We emphasize the importance of complete history-taking in the evaluation of these dermatoses in the next section.

THE APPROACH USED TO DIAGNOSE ENVIRONMENTAL DERMATOSES

To establish the diagnosis of environmental dermatoses, a detailed history to elicit potential exposure risks should be undertaken by the clinician. In addition, the practitioner must use clinical clues in concert with the history to substantiate his or her suspicions of what initiated the presenting lesions. We focus herein on those aspects of history and examination that we believe best serve the physician to elicit the source of the dermatoses.

Historical aspects of environmental dermatoses
Pertinent medical history

Exposure to a plausible agent. The amount of exposure to a environmental agent should be of a magnitude generally agreed as sufficient to cause the dermatosis in question. To a large extent, this criterion may be answerable only through personal and historical experience. For example, ICD from water is not likely to develop from a brief hand-washing once a day; however, washing 20 to 30 times a day would be a reasonable explanation for the noted irritation, especially in traumatized skin.[40]

Temporal relation to the presenting symptom. Environmental exposure must precede the onset of any dermatosis. Once exposure has occurred, the delay before onset of disease is extremely variable. With contact dermatitis, lesions often become noticeable within the first 3 to 6 months of regular exposure. Environmental skin infections may occur within a few days of exposure, depending on the organism. The onset of chloracne varies, depending on whether it results from a single large exposure or a series of repeated low-dose exposures. Once contact with the inciting agent has ceased, the risk of development of a environmental dermatosis (provided that it has not already occurred) diminishes quickly. For example, ICD usually does not appear suddenly 3 to 4 days after exposure but rather often occurs after minutes or hours.[53] Chloracne lesions are not likely to appear for the first time if more than 6 to 8 weeks have passed since the last exposure, although new lesions may continue to appear for months after the disease process has been initiated.[13,20,40,97] NMSCs have a variable latent period and may not develop for many years after ultraviolet B exposure.[39,72,98]

Work exacerbations. Many environmental dermatoses that occur with occupations, for example, grain tick infestation, typically improve or clear when the patient is away from work only to recur or worsen on his or her return to the previous occupational environment. When skin infections are attributed to work, the presence of a source of exposure by the offending organism in the workplace should be verified. In some instances, exposure to the causal agent may occur both within and away from the job site. In such cases, it should be demonstrated that most of the exposure actually occurred in the workplace. For example, it should be documented that at least 50% of an individual's lifetime cumulative exposure to sunlight was attained as a result of a specific outdoor employment setting before NMSC development can be attributed to occupation.[40]

With respect to contact dermatitis, most cases show significant improvement if exposure has been stopped for at least 1 week. Concomitant treatment during this timeframe may make this criterion difficult to evaluate. Palmar or plantar dermatitis typically improves more slowly and is prone to exacerbations, possibly because of underlying endogenous factors. Some chronic dermatoses (such as NMSC and infections) do not require persistent exposure to continue once the disease process has been initiated and do not improve away from work without appropriate treatment.[40]

Nonoccupational exclusions. Nonoccupational dermatoses (such as seborrheic dermatitis and nummular eczema) must be excluded from serious consideration by skillful history and clinical examination. Once the clinical type of dermatosis (for example, contact dermatitis) has been established, potential environmental exposures must be eliminated by careful history and investigation.

Family history and medications. Certain host factors such as the patient's ethnic background, family history, and medications also must be considered. A family history of history of atopy; food intolerance or reactions to cosmetics must be determined in the evaluation of these conditions.[91]

Immunocompetence. If the patient is immunocompromised because of acquired immunodeficiency syndrome, diabetes, or malignancy, routine infections may be more difficult to eradicate, as in the case of resistant pyodermas with infection with *Pseudomonas* or Methicillin-resistant *Staphylococcus aureus.*

Aggravating factors. The issue of aggravation of a preexisting dermatosis is complex. The physician should take the following questions into consideration before concluding that there has been substantial aggravation: (1) Is the dermatosis more subjectively severe (worse pain, itch, or impairment) because of an environmental exposure? (2) Is the dermatosis more clinically extensive (covers substantially more surface area) because of the same environmental exposure?[40]

Clinical aspects of environmental dermatoses

Pertinent physical examination results

Morphology. The observed morphology of the presenting dermatoses must be consistent with the clinical changes known to be caused by the putative agent. For example, the morphology of acute contact dermatitis appears vesicular rather than lichenified (the appearance of chronic dermatitis), and the lesions of chloracne are characterized by closed comedones and small cysts in a malar distribution, as opposed to common acne, which consists of inflammatory papules and pustules occurring on the trunk, back, and face.[83,97]

Anatomic site. The dermatosis should normally occur on a skin surface that has been exposed to an environmental agent. For example, ACD from poison ivy invariably occurs on the hands and arms, but NMSC should occur in sun exposed regions. If the route of exposure is thought to be ingestion, inhalation, or percutaneous absorption, then the areas involved may be different. Another example can be seen in the disorder cutaneous larva migrans, which could manifest on either the back or the lower extremities, depending on where there has been direct contact with the organism *Ancylostoma braziliense.*

Patch testing. The patch test is one of the most useful tools for identifying environmental dermatoses.[91] Patch testing makes use of the delayed hypersensitivity reaction to establish the diagnosis.[53] Typically, standard agents are dissolved in nonirritating vehicles such as petrolatum and then applied to easily accessible areas, such as the back. Regions are numbered to correlate the test site with the antigen. The areas are viewed at 48 and 96 hours to determine reactivity. Classically, reactions vary from trace erythema to frank vesiculation and edema. The relevance of a positive patch-test result depends on the clinician's awareness and the significance of the contact allergen in the patient's environment. It is important to correlate historical and clinical factors with the patch-test procedure. It must be recognized that

---

Important historical and clinical aspects in the workup of environmental dermatoses

History

Exposure to a plausible agent
Temporal relation to the presenting symptom
Work exacerbations
Nonoccupational exclusions
Family history and medications
Immunocompetence
Aggravating factors

Physical examination

Morphology of the lesion
Anatomic site

---

although it often is helpful, patch testing has its limitations. It is important to understand that false-negative and false-positive responses can occur during routine testing, the latter usually because of the use of irritating substances as test agents or vehicles.[53]

PREVENTION AND TREATMENT
Personal protection and avoidance

Once the causative agent has been identified, it is important to recognize and avoid potential allergen sources. If the source cannot be avoided, barrier protection, such as clothing or creams, may be used. The physical and chemical resistance properties of protective clothing are essential considerations to guide proper selection. Guidelines are available through various supply manufacturers and distributors. Some potential allergens are capable of penetrating protective clothing (such as rubber gloves) in small amounts without causing obvious physical deterioration of the material. The benefits of barrier creams as substitutes for protective clothing are a debated issue; some barrier creams do facilitate the removal of oil and grease from the skin and may be most useful when combined with good personal hygiene. Both protective clothing and barrier creams may aggravate dermatitis if worn or used over inflamed skin. Occasionally, patients may become sensitized to the ingredients in these products, which must be taken into account when such items are used.[44]

Hygiene

Personal hygiene has an added importance when skin contact with an adverse agent cannot be avoided.[40] Mild soap and water or lipid-free cleansers, for example, Cetaphil and Aquanil, are sufficient to remove most minor irritants. When they are unsatisfactory, waterless hand cleaners (which contain an organic solvent dispersed in a cream formulation) may be used to remove tenacious dirt, oil, or grease stains; any residual film of waterless cleaner left on the skin should then be removed by gentle cleansing with soap and water.

Abrasive soaps may be required to remove the most resistant stains from the palms; they work by stripping away the outermost stained layer of the SC but may contribute to irritation if used on the thinner skin of the dorsal hands and forearms. Neither waterless cleaners nor abrasives should be used to clean inflamed skin, because they are likely to aggravate dermatitis. Regardless of which personal hygiene product is used, it is a good practice to apply a moisturizer after washing. Hygiene efforts directed toward washing contaminated clothing are important if significant exposures are thought to occur from such sources.

Education

Educational efforts aimed at promoting an awareness of agents that can initiate environmental dermatoses are a key element of a comprehensive prevention program.[44] Such efforts should cover all relevant topics, that is, avoidance, potential sources, and treatment. Reference manuals and pocket-sized booklets are currently being developed for the purpose of educating the public about the many causative agents of environmental dermatoses.

Regulation

With few exceptions, no present state or federal regulatory requirements govern skin exposure to potential skin hazards.[40] For example, pesticide residues on crops have occasionally been used to establish safe reentry intervals to prevent dermatitis among agricultural field workers. Given the dynamic nature and wide range of variables that may be necessary to induce environmental dermatoses, however, it is unlikely that regulations based on exposure levels will be developed. Such regulations would have to be based on well-characterized dose-response relationships, which are extremely difficult to define at present.

Motivation

Motivation is an important but frequently neglected aspect of prevention programs.[40] Without adequate motivation, it is difficult for even a well-conceived idea to be successful. All motivational approaches must be based on both a true interest and a devotion to the patient's well-being. Communication and compassion are essential ingredients in the patient-physician relationship for these programs to be successful.

CONCLUSION

Cutaneous disorders are an important manifestation of the interaction between body and environment. The skin serves to protect against the toxic effects of exposures to chemicals, physical agents, and organisms through its barrier function properties. It is well documented that certain environmental stimuli are capable of inducing adverse cutaneous sequelae. The exact type of reaction and the morphologic features of each response depend on a multitude of factors such as exposure time, immunocompetence, and age of the patient.

It is important that the medical practitioner be familiar with these disorders and the various ways in which they can present. Knowledge, compassion, patience, and motivation are useful tools for the practitioner to employ in the successful diagnosis and treatment of these conditions.

REFERENCES

1. Andersen K, Burrows D, White I: Allergens from the standard series. In Roycroft R, Menné T, editors: *Textbook of contact dermatitis,* Berlin, 1991, Springer-Verlag.
2. Arnold et al: Diseases due to fungi and yeasts. In *Andrews' diseases of the skin: clinical dermatology,* ed 8, Philadelphia, 1990, WB Saunders.
3. Baginsky E: *Occupational skin disease in California,* San Francisco, 1982, California Department of Industrial Relations.
4. Barber TE, Husting EL: Biological hazards. In Key MM et al, editors: *Occupational diseases: A guide to their recognition.* DHEW (NIOSH) Publ No 77-181 ed, Washington, DC, US Government Printing Office.
5. Benezra C et al: *Plant contact dermatitis,* London, 1985, CV Mosby.
6. Benezra C et al: *Plant dermatitis,* Toronto, 1985, BC Decker.
7. Betz TG et al: Occupational dermatitis associated with straw itch mite, *JAMA* 247:2821, 1982.
8. Bickers D et al: The porphyrias. In Fitzpatrick T et al, editors: *Dermatology in general medicine,* ed 4, New York, 1993, McGraw-Hill.
9. Booth BH, Jones RW: Mites in industry, *Arch Derm Syph* 69:531, 1954.
10. Boring C, Squires T: Cancer statistics of 1992 CA 1:42, 1992.
11. Brookes P, Lawley P: Evidence for the binding of polynuclear aromatic hydrocarbons to the nucleic acids of mouse skin: relation between carcinogenic hydrocarbons and their binding to deoxyribonucleic acid, *Nature* 202:781, 1964.
12. Burrows D, Adams RM: Metals. In Adams RM, editor: *Occupational skin disease,* ed 2, Philadelphia, 1990, WB Saunders.
13. Caputo R et al: Cutaneous manifestations of tetrachlorodibenzo-*p*-dioxin in childrena and adolescents: follow-up 10 years after the Seveso, Italy incident, *J Am Acad Dermatol* 19:812, 1988.
14. *Causes and effects of stratospheric ozone reduction: an update,* Washington, DC, 1982, National Academy of Science.
15. Council on Scientific Affairs: Health effects of Agent Orange and dioxin contaminants, *JAMA* 248:1895, 1982.
16. Cripps DJ, Peters HA, Gocmen A: Porphyria turcica due to hexachlorobenzene: a 20 to 30 year follow-up study on 204 patients, *Br J Dermatol* 111:413, 1984.
17. Cronin E: Metals. In *Contact dermatitis,* Edinburgh, 1980, Churchill Livingstone.
18. Czirjak L et al: Systemic sclerosis and exposure to trichloroethylene, *Dermatology* 186:236, 1993.
19. Diette IM, Gange RW, Stem RS: Coal tar phototoxicity: characteristics of smarting reaction, *J Invest Dermatol* 84:268, 1985.
20. Dunagin WG: Cutaneous signs of systemic toxicity due to dioxins and related chemicals, *J Am Acad Dermatol* 10:688, 1984.
21. Elder GH: Porphyria cutanea tarda: a multifactorial disease. In Champion RH, Pye RJ, editors: *Recent advances in dermatology,* vol 8, Edinburgh, 1990, Churchill Livingstone.
22. Elder GH et al: The effect of the porphyrogenic compound, hexachlorobenzene, on the activity of hepatic uroporphyrinogen decarboxylase in the rat, *Clin Sci Mol Med* 51:71, 1976.
23. Epstein JC: Photocarcinogenesis, skin cancer and aging, *J Am Acad Dermatol* 9:487, 1983.
24. Feldmann M, Londei M, Haworth C: T cells and lymphokines, *Br Med Bull* 45:361, 1989.
25. Feldmann R, Mailbach H: Regional variation in C^{14} cortisone in man, *J Invest Dermatol* 48:181, 1967.
26. Fenske N, Lober C: Photoaging and the skin: differentiation and clinical response, *Geriatrics* 45:36, 1990.

27. Fisher AA: *Contact dermatitis,* ed 3, Philadelphia, 1986, Lea & Febiger.
28. Fitzpatrick T, Sober A: Sunlight and skin cancer, *N Engl J Med* 313:818, 1985.
29. Fraser MC, Hartge P, Tucker MA: Melanoma and nonmelanoma skin cancer: epidemiology and risk factors, *Semin Oncol Nurs* 7:2, 1991.
30. Fregert S: Occupational dermatitis in a 10 year material, *Contact Dermatitis* 1:96, 1975.
31. Garcia-Restoy E et al: Bacteremia due to *Erysipelothrix rhusiopathiae* in immunocompromised hosts without endocarditis, *Rev Infect Dis* 13:1252, 1991.
32. Gawkrodger DJ: Chloracne: causation, diagnosis and treatment, *J Dermatol Treat* 2:73, 1991.
33. Gellin GA: Pigment responses: occupational disorders of pigmentation. In Mailbach HI, editor: *Occupational and industrial dermatology,* Chicago, 1987, Year Book.
34. Grieco M, Sheldon C: *Erysipelothrix rhusiopathiae, Ann NY Acad Sci* 174:523, 1970.
35. Harber L, Bickers D: *Photosensitivity diseases: principles of diagnosis and treatment,* ed 2, Philadelphia, 1989, BC Decker.
36. Harvey DT, Fenske NA: Intrinsic aging and its relation to nonmelanoma skin cancer formation, *J Geriatr Dermatol* 1:121, 1993.
37. Haustein U: Silica-induced scleroderma, *J Am Acad Dermatol* 22:444, 1990.
38. Heisel ED, Hunt FE: Further studies in cutaneous reactions to glass fibers, *Arch Environ Health* 17:705, 1968.
39. Hertzman P et al: Association of the eosinophil-myalgia syndrome with the ingestion of tryptophan, *N Engl J Med* 322:869, 1990.
40. Hogan D, Mathias: Occupational dermatoses. In *Dermis,* Chapter X, 1994.
41. Hogan DJ, Tanglertsampan C: The less common occupational dermatoses, *State of the Art Reviews: Occup Med* 385, 1992.
42. Hogan DJ et el: Risk factors for basal cell carcinoma, *Int J Dermatol* 28:591, 1989.
43. Hogan D et al: Risk factors for squamous cell carcinoma in Saskatchewan, Canada, *J Dermatol Sci* 1:97, 1990.
44. Honig PJ: Guttate psoriasis associated with streptococcal disease, *J Pediatr* 113:1037, 1988.
45. Kanerva L: Physical causes of occupational skin disease. In Adams RM, editor: *Occupational skin disease,* ed 2, Philadelphia, 1990, WB Saunders.
46. Kerr HD: Cocaine and scleroderma, *South Med J* 82:1275, 1989.
47. Kilbourne EM et al: Clinical epidemiology of toxic oil syndrome: manifestations of a new illness, *N Engl J Med* 398:1408, 1983.
48. Kochevar I, Pathak M, Parrish J: Photophysics, photochemistry, and photobiology. In Fitzpatrick T et al, editors: *Dermatology in general medicine,* ed 4, New York, 1993, McGraw-Hill.
49. Lahmeyer HW: Tryptophan for insomnia, *JAMA* 262:2748, 1989.
50. Lelbach W, Marsteller H: Vinyl chloride–associated disease, *Adv Intern Med Ped,* 47:1, 1981.
51. Lundvall O: The effect of replenishment of iron stores after phlebotomy therapy in porphyria cutanea tarda, *Acta Med Scand* 189:51, 1971.
52. Mali J et al: Quantitative aspects of chromium sensitization, *Acta Derm Venereol* (Stockh) 44:44, 1964.
53. Marks J, DeLeo V: *Contact and occupational dermatology,* St Louis, 1992, Mosby–Year Book.
54. Marzulli F, Mailbach H: *Dermatotoxicology,* ed 3, New York, 1987, Hemisphere.
55. Marzulli F, Mailbach H: Contact allergy: predictive testing in humans. In *Dermatotoxicology,* ed 4, New York, 1991, Hemisphere.
56. Maso MJ et al: Celery phytophotodermatitis in a chef, *Arch Dermatol* 127:912, 1991.
57. McKenzie RC, Sauder DN: Keratinocyte cytokines and growth factors: functions in skin immunity and homeostasis, *Dermatol Clin* 8:649, 1990.
58. Meneghini CL: Cutaneous ulcers in workers exposed to chromium, *Rassegna di Medicina Industriale* 19:161, 1950.
59. Menné T, Maibach H: Systemic contact-type dermatitis. In Marzulli F, Maibach H, editor: *Dermatotoxicology,* ed 4, New York, 1991, Hemisphere.
60. Meola T, Lim H: The porphyrias, *Dermatol Clin* 11:583, 1993.
61. Mitchell JG: Plants. In Cronin E, editor: *Contact dermatitis,* Edinburgh, 1980, Churchill Livingstone.
62. Ostlere LS et al: Atypical systemic sclerosis following exposure to vinyl chloride monomer: a case report and review of the cutaneous aspects of vinyl chloride disease, *Clin Exp Dermatol* 17:208, 1992.
63. Plewig G, Kligman AM: *Acne: morphogenesis and treatment,* New York, 1975, Springer-Verlag.
64. Preliminary report: 2,3,7,8-tetrachlorodibenzo-*p*-dioxin exposure to humans, Sevaso, Italy, 1988, *MMWR* 37:733, 1988.
65. Preston D, Stern R: Nonmelanoma cancers of the skin, *N Engl J Med* 327:1649, 1992.
65a. Razsi L, et al: Painful annular plaques on the hand, *Arch Derm* 130(10):1311, 1994.
66. Richey H, Fenske NA: Nonmelanomatous skin cancer: new concepts in pathogenesis, *South Med J* 8:362, 1987.
67. Roenigk HH, Gottlob ME: Estrogen-induced porphyria cutanea tarda, *Arch Dermatol* 102:260, 1970.
68. Scheuplein RJ: Permeability of the skin, *Physiol Rev* 51:702, 1971.
69. Schmid R: Cutaneous porphyria in Turkey, *N Engl J Med* 263:397, 1960.
70. Schwartz BA et al: Toxicology of chlorinated dibenzo(*p*) dioxins, *Environ Health Perspect* 5:87, 1973.
71. Schwartz L, Tulipan L, Birmingham DJ: *Occupational diseases of the skin,* Philadelphia, 1957, Lea & Febiger.
72. Scotto J, Fears TR, Fraumenia JF: *Incidence of nonmelanoma skin cancer in the United States,* NIH Publ No 83-2443, Washington, DC, 1983, Government Printing Office.
73. Seligman PJ, Mathias CGT, Malley MJ: Phytophotodermatitis from celery among grocery workers, *Arch Dermatol* 123:1478, 1987.
74. Shadomy H, Utz J: Infections due to gram-positive bacteria. In Fitzpatrick T et al, editors: *Dermatology in general medicine,* ed 4, New York, 1993, McGraw-Hill.
75. Shadomy H, Utz J: Deep fungal infections. In Fitzpatrick T et al, editors: *Dermatology in general medicine,* ed 4, New York, 1993, McGraw-Hill.
76. Shadomy H, Utz J: Arthropods and stings. In Fitzpatrick T et al, editors: *Dermatology in general medicine,* ed 4, New York, 1993, McGraw-Hill.
77. Silver R: Scleroderma, fascitis, and eosinophilia associated with the ingestion of tryptophan, *N Engl J Med* 322:874, 1990.
78. Stern R: The epidemiology of cutaneous disease. In Fitzpatrick T et al, editors: *Dermatology in general medicine,* ed 4, New York, 1993, McGraw-Hill.
79. Stingl G et al: Immunologic functions of Ia bearing epidermal Langherhans cells, *J Immunol* 121:2005, 1978.
80. Suciu I, Derjman I, Valaskai M: Contributii la studiul imbolnaviril or produse declorina de vinil, *Medicine International* 15:967, 1963.
81. Suskind RR: The hallmark of dioxin intoxication, *Scand J Work Environ Health* 11:165, 1985.
82. Tan KS, Mitchell JC: Patch and photopatch tests in contact dermatitis and photodermatitis: a preliminary report of investigation of 150 patients with special reference to "cedar poisoning," *Can Med Assoc J* 98:252, 1968.
83. Taylor JS: Environmental acne: update and review, *Ann NY Acad Sci* 320:295, 1979.
84. Thiboutot DM, Hamory BH, Marks JG: Dermatoses among floral shop workers, *J Am Acad Dermatol* 22:54, 1989.
85. Thompson SC et al: Reduction of solar keratoses by regular sunscreen use, *N Engl J Med* 329:1147, 1993.

86. Update: eosinophilia-myalgia syndrome associated with ingestion of L-tryptophan: United States as of Jan. 9, 1990, *MMWR* 39:14, 1990.
87. Varga J et al: Systemic sclerosis after augmentation mammoplasty, *Ann Intern Med* 111:377, 1989.
88. Veltman G et al: Clinical manifestations and course of vinyl chloride monomer disease, *Ann NY Acad Sci* 246:6, 1975.
89. Vitaliano P, Urbach F: The relative importance of risk factors in non-melanoma carcinoma, *Arch Dermatol* 116:454, 1980.
90. Ward M: Frostbite, *BMJ* 1:67, 1974.
91. Webster RC, Maibach HI: *Principles and practice of environmental medicine,* New York, 1992, Plenum.
92. White I: Phototoxic and photoallergic reactions. In Fitzpatrick T et al, editors: *Dermatology in general medicine,* ed 4, New York, 1993, McGraw-Hill.
93. Woodbine M: *Erysipelothrix rhusiopathiae* bacteriology and chemotherapy, *Bacteriol Rev* 14:161, 1950.
94. Yupsa S: Cutaneous chemcial carcinogenesis, *J Am Acad Dermatol* 15:1031, 1986.
95. Yupsa S, Hennings H, Saffiotti U: Cutaneous chemical carcinogenesis: past, present, and future, *J Invest Dermatol* 67:199, 1976.
96. Zbitnew A, Hogan DJ: Milker's nodule (parapoxvirus) with erythema multiforme, *Can J Dermatol* 1:97, 1990.
97. Zugerman C: Chloracne: clinical manifestations and etiology, *Dermatol Clin* 8:209, 1990.

Chapter 23

DISORDERS OF THE UPPER AND LOWER RESPIRATORY TRACT

Henry L. Abrons
Daniel E. Banks
Lee A. Reed

Airway inflammation and hyperreactivity
    Pathogenesis
    Clinical and epidemiologic assessment
    Treatment
Granuloma formation
    Hypersensitivity pneumonitis
    Assessment of HP
    Treatment
Diffuse alveolar damage
    Pathogenesis
    Natural history of acute toxic gas exposure: selected examples
    Epidemiology
    Treatment
Interstitial fibrosis
    Approach to diagnosis
    Silicosis
    Coal workers' pneumoconiosis
    Asbestos-related respiratory disorders

Environmental factors are of singular importance in respiratory disease because of the direct contact of inhaled substances with the upper and lower respiratory tracts. The respiratory system is a portal of entry for potentially deleterious physical, chemical, and microbiologic agents the toxic effects of which may occur in distant organs or within the airways and the lung. Among the hazardous inhalants are inorganic and organic gases, vapors, fumes, and particulates. Exposure can occur in diverse settings and involve pollutants in ambient air, the workplace environment, and the home. There is substantial overlap between occupational and nonoccupational respiratory disorders with regard to causative agents as well as the mechanisms and manifestations of disease.

Although the variety of potential environmental insults is extensive, the respiratory system has only a limited repertoire of physiologic and pathologic responses. This chapter describes the pathophysiology of cellular, tissue, and organ responses that play an important role in the noninfectious and nonneoplastic environmental respiratory disorders frequently encountered in clinical and epidemiologic practice (Table 23-1).

AIRWAY INFLAMMATION AND HYPERREACTIVITY

The internal surface of the respiratory system in adults has an area of about 40 to 80 m^2, comparable with that of a tennis court. This large interface between the internal milieu and the external environment is in perpetual contact with dusts, chemical agents, microbes, ionizing radiation, and extremes of temperature and humidity. The airways are the first line of defense in the respiratory system. Five interrelated phenomena are important in understanding the effects of environmental exposures on the airways: inflammation, cough, bronchoconstriction, airway hyperreactivity, and asthma.

Airway inflammation is manifested by alterations in the

Table 23-1. Respiratory system responses to environmental insults

Response	Pathophysiology
Bronchitis	Airway inflammation
Asthma	Airway hyperreactivity
Hypersensitivity pneumonitis	Granuloma formation
Acute irritant gas exposure	Diffuse alveolar damage
Pneumoconiosis	Interstitial fibrosis

integrity of mucosal and submucosal structures. These alterations include edema and the proliferation and infiltration of inflammatory and immune effector cells (neutrophils, macrophages, lymphocytes, eosinophils, and mast cells). Mucus hydration and molecular composition are altered by inflammation, and the function of cilia may be deranged, resulting in the impaired clearance of secretions and inhaled matter. At the ultrastructural level, intercellular tight junctions separate and expose subepithelial nerve terminals and cells to environmental stimulation or injury. Chronic inflammation further alterates airway structures, which can be seen with light microscopy; this alteration includes hyperplasia of the mucin-producing goblet cells, hypertrophy of the mucus glands, epithelial cell metaplasia and desquamation, thickening of the basement membrane, and hypertrophy of airway smooth muscle.

Cough and bronchoconstriction are induced by irritants through nerve reflexes initiated by the stimulation of mucosal receptors. The afferent pathways of the cough reflex are vagal nerve fibers from receptors in the airways, pleura, ear canal, and gastrointestinal tract; glossopharyngeal nerve fibers from receptors in the pharynx; trigeminal nerve fibers from receptors in the nose and paranasal sinuses; and phrenic nerve fibers from the diaphragm and pericardium. From the cough center in the medulla, the efferent limb of the reflex activates the laryngeal, diaphragmatic, intercostal, and abdominal wall muscles. Cough can be provoked by exposure to irritants below levels that cause inflammation; however, in the presence of inflammation the threshold for stimulation of cough is greatly reduced.

The bronchoconstrictor reflex operates through parasympathetic pathways in response to the stimulation of mucosal receptors. Although bronchoconstriction and cough are often induced by the same stimuli, evidence suggests that the receptors or afferent pathways may be different.[99]

Airway hyperreactivity is a related phenomenon that frequently, but not always, accompanies inflammation. Bronchospasm refers to an exaggerated increase in the resistance of the airways on the basis of either constriction of the bronchial smooth muscle or encroachment on the lumen by edema or excessive secretions; in actuality, these alterations often occur in combination. Nonspecific airway hyperreactivity connotes hyperresponsiveness to multiple nonantigenic stimuli. Examples include exercise and the inhalation of histamine, cholinergic agonists such as methacholine, hypertonic or hypotonic saline aerosol, cold air, and sulfur dioxide (SO_2). Specific airway hyperreactivity connotes that there is an allergic reaction to a specific allergen. Nonspecific and specific hyperreactivity are not necessarily present together but may coexist. The onset of the asthmatic response may begin almost immediately after the stimulus (early response) and wane after several hours, or it may be delayed for 4 to 8 hours (late response); frequently, there is a combination of early and late responses (dual response). The early response is due to bronchial smooth muscle contraction producing transient constriction in the caliber of the airway lumen, and the late response is associated with the development of an inflammatory reaction in the airways.

A universally accepted definition of asthma remains elusive; however, one formulation is "the presence of intermittent symptoms, including wheeze, chest tightness, and cough, together with demonstrable bronchial hyperresponsiveness."[116] In asthmatics, increasing low doses of inhaled histamine or methacholine elicit increasing bronchoconstriction. In contrast, airway hyperreactivity in other disorders such as chronic bronchitis is characterized by a plateau in the dose-response relationship.[116]

Pathogenesis

Respiratory tract irritants elicit reactions in most subjects when exposure exceeds a certain threshold; however, host factors may influence the threshold for an irritant response (for example, tolerance develops with repeated exposure to ozone)[45] or lower it (for example, asthmatics have increased sensitivity to SO_2 inhalation).[97] Stimulation of mucosal nerve receptors by irritants produces cough; more severe irritation may induce reflex bronchoconstriction, even in individuals with normal airways. Individuals with airway hyperreactivity manifest cough and bronchoconstriction at exposure levels that are below the normal irritant threshold.

Inflammation of the airway mucosa occurs as a result of direct cell injury, activation of complement, release of proinflammatory mediators from tissue mast cells, or activation of the immune system. These mechanisms amplify one another. Direct cell injury can result from proteolytic enzymes or toxic oxygen molecules (such as superoxide anions and hydroxyl radicals). Activation of complement by complexes of antigen and preformed antibody (the classic pathway) leads to the generation of factors that cause contraction of bronchial smooth muscle, attraction of neutrophils and mononuclear phagocytes, direct cytotoxicity, and mast-cell degranulation. Mast cells activated by the reaction of antigen with membrane-bound specific IgE release proinflammatory mediators capable of causing smooth muscle contraction, increased capillary permeability, and mucus secretion. Immune system activation involves macrophages, which continually screen foreign material by phagocytosis and present antigens to lymphocytes for further processing by the immune system. Macrophages also play a key role in regulation

Table 23-2. Examples of agents that may cause environmental asthma

Agent	Exposures
Animal	
Small animals: rats, mice, guinea pigs	Pet owning
Domestic animals	Domestic animal owning
Wool	Wool working
Birds (feathers, serum, droppings)	Bird breeding
Sea squirt fluid	Oyster and pearl gathering
Culture oysters (marine organisms)	Oyster shucking
Glue (fish origin)	Bookbinding
Hog trypsin, pancreatic extract, amylase	Cystic fibrosis (both children and parents)
Bacillus subtilis, esperase	Detergent enzymes
Human hair products	Hairdressing
Beetles (coleoptera)	Insect collecting
Locusts	Insect collecting
Moths, butterflies	Butterfly collecting
Stick insects	Insect collecting
Cockroaches	Homes, insect collecting
Crickets	Outdoor work
Housefly maggots	Angling
River flies: sewerworm flies, sewage flies	Outdoor work
Ivory dust	Ivory carving
Vegetable	
Wood dusts of various types	Woodworking, carpentry
Latex	Use of latex gloves, condoms; spina bifida
Papain	Food technologists
Diastase	Food handling
Karaya gum	Food processing
Gum arabic, acacia, tragacanth	Printing
Alternaria, Aspergillus, spores of *Cladosporium*	Indoor air pollution
Verticillium, paecilomyces, Merulius lacrymans	Domestic work
Pink rot fungus	Celery picking
Mushroom molds	Mushroom picking
Potatoes	Homemakers
Alkaline hydrolysis derivative of gluten	Biscuit making
Chemical	
Trimellitic anhydride	Epoxy resins
Ammonium thioglycate	Hairdressing cosmetics
Dioazonium salt	Photocopying
Colophony	Soldering
Persulfate salts, extract of henna	Hairdressing
Reactive dyes	Textile dyeing
Paraphenylene diamine	Fur dying
Psyllium	Mixing laxative powders
Amprolium hydrochloride	Poultry feed mixing
Pesticides, insecticides	Application, fumigation
Sulphone chloramides	Home brewing
Hexamethaline diisocyanate	Auto body spray-painting
Toluene diisocyanate	Polyurethane

of the immune response through the secretion of cytokines and growth factors.

Recognized immunologic sensitizers include various naturally occuring antigens and manufactured products (Table 23-2). Other inflammatory processes can induce hyperreactivity; viral respiratory infections are well documented,[31] and there is evidence that ozone at concentrations occasionally reached in urban air can produce hyperreactivity in normal subjects;[42] however, SO_2 or nitrogen dioxide (NO_2) do not produce similar effects.

Clinical and epidemiologic assessment

Among individuals with underlying chronic respiratory disease or chronic exposure, it is difficult to determine the relationship of symptoms and signs to specific environmental factors. Exposures to an irritant sufficient to cause inflammation of the lower respiratory tract, almost invariably causes conjunctival, nasal, and pharyngeal mucosa effects. Manifestations of cough, sputum production, chest tightness, dyspnea, and wheezing may be elicited. Chest radiographs and computed tomography (CT) scans are not ordinarily informative in airway disorders unless bronchiectasis or associated parenchymal lung disease is suspected. Airway inflammation may or may not be accompanied by air-flow obstruction detectable by spirometry or measurement of airways resistance. Ongoing inflammation is often apparent bronchoscopically by visual inspection as well as by mucosal biopsy and analysis of the epithelial lining fluid recovered by bronchoalveolar lavage (BAL);[105] the latter has utility mainly as a research tool.

A diagnosis of asthma is based routinely on the history, clinical examination, and conventional spirometry, and does not require bronchoprovocation testing. However, this approach is not foolproof. Not all asthmatics wheeze; some have persistent cough as their only symptom. Moreover, the auscultatory findings associated with bronchospasm may be absent when the patient's asthma is quiescent, and spirometry may also be normal. However, when there is uncertainty about the diagnosis of asthma, determination of airway responsivenesss by provocation testing may be definitive.

Airway hyperreactivity is assessed in the laboratory by bronchoprovocation (bronchial challenge) testing. Care must be taken in monitoring the patient's respiratory status, as the goal is to induce a "controlled" episode of asthma. Airways resistance or the forced expired volume in the first second (FEV_1) are the most frequently assessed variables of pulmonary function and are measured serially under baseline conditions after the administration of the test stimulus in increasing levels of intensity. A dose-response relationship is plotted, with the results usually expressed as the provocative dose causing a 20% decrement in FEV_1 (PD20) or a 40% to 50% increase in airways resistance. The test is considered complete when either of these endpoints is reached or all doses of the agent have been provided. Procedures for assessing hyperreactivity must be reproducible;[47,84] the delivery of the stimulus or provoking agent must be precisely controlled; the dose must be below the irritant threshold; and the responses of nonhyperreactive subjects must be used for comparison. For nonspecific hyperreactivity, protocols using histamine or methacholine as the test stimulus are well standardized. For specific hyperreactivity, testing procedures using chemicals or particulate antigens to identify a cause for the development of airway hyperresponsiveness have also been devised but are methodologically challenging.

Attribution of mucosal inflammation or airway hyperreactivity to an environmental (or occupational) agent requires identification of exposure to a respiratory irritant or sensitizer. When the pathogenic potential of an agent is in doubt, the medical literature should be reviewed. Carefully performed experimental studies in humans provide the most convincing proof of pathogenicity; epidemiologic associations and case reports are helpful but cannot prove cause and effect. A temporal relationship between the exposure and the clinical manifestations should be sought, and the breathing zone or ambient air concentration of the suspected agent determined, if possible. Environmental causation is difficult to determine in the presence of other conditions capable of causing similar manifestations, such as acute respiratory infections, preexisting asthma, and chronic bronchitis due to cigarette smoking. Rarely, controlled blinded challenge in an exposure chamber performed in a properly equipped laboratory is necessary for reaching a diagnosis.

The recognition of an index case of environmental respiratory disorder should stimulate inquiry into whether other individuals are at risk or have been affected. A case definition of the disorder under study is necessary. For epidemiologic purposes reporting the numbers of individuals exposed and affected must keep in mind that the removal of susceptible individuals from the population may have occurred by a process of self-selection. Children, the elderly, asthmatics, and perhaps others with underlying lung disease may show increased susceptibility to irritants. Furthermore, adverse effects may be accentuated by exercise, as shown for healthy young adults exposed to ozone[53] and for asthmatics exposed to SO_2.[12] Finally, under specific conditions, combinations of inhaled irritants may have potentiating effects.[63]

Once exposure to the offending agent has ceased, mucosal inflammation is often self-limited. With continued exposure, tolerance to the effects of low-dose exposure to some irritants, for example, ozone[45] and SO_2,[98] may develop; however, after certain toxic exposures, airway hyperreactivity may persist. In the model of environmental asthma, allergic sensitization develops after a latency interval and, in some instances, may endure indefinitely. For example, isocyanate-induced asthma may persist for years after the cessation of exposure[82] or may recur on reexposure after many years of quiescence.[6] When sensitivity develops after what appears to be a short-term high-level irritant exposure, a nonallergic inflammatory response is presumed to be responsible. This has been termed the *reactive airways dysfunction syndrome* (RADS),[15] and a variety of irritating agents have been incriminated in its cause.[2]

Treatment

Removal from or abatement of exposure is important. Bronchodilator therapy usually offers symptomatic relief and inhaled β_2-adrenergic drugs are the agents of choice. Inhaled cromolyn is also effective in blocking the immediate allergic airway respone. The late response is inhibited by corticosteroids; for chronic treatment, inhaled steroids are preferred. In cases in which cholinergic reflex mechanisms are operating to produce cough or bronchoconstriction, inhaled ipratropium, an anticholinergic agent, is effective.

GRANULOMA FORMATION

The formation of granulomas is a manifestation of cell-mediated immunity at sites where antigen persists because of low solubility or resistance to degradation. Histologically granulomas are focal collections of histiocytes, lymphocytes, plasma cells, and epithelioid giant cells, sometimes associated with liquefaction necrosis. Pulmonary granulomas are the histologic hallmark of various respiratory infections (particularly those due to mycobacterial or fungal organisms), reactions to certain metals and organic particles, and several idiopathic disorders (such as sarcoidosis).

Environmental outbreaks of coccidioidomycosis[36] and histoplasmosis[114] results from the dispersal of fungal spores by wind or the excavation of soil. These infections are particularly virulent in individuals with impaired cell-mediated immunity, who form granulomas poorly and tend to develop disseminated disease.

Among illnesses due to metals, beryllium (Be) disease is a disorder that has become less common as exposure has been curtailed. Although new occupational cases still occur, most can be traced to exposure that occurred prior to the 1960s in industries that extracted or used Be. Cases of non-occupational Be disease were reported in the 1940s and 1950s in community residents exposed to industrial discharges before the institution of control measures.[30,50] Brief, high-level Be inhalation causes an acute tracheobronchitis and pneumonitis. Chronic pulmonary berylliosis is due to persistent exposure, usually for months or years, and is associated with an alveolitis characterized by the accumulation of Be-specific helper T cells in alveolar lining fluid, which can be recovered by bronchoalveolar lavage.[92] Histologically, there is a granulomatous interstitial pneumonitis with variable degrees of interstitial fibrosis that is indistinguishable from pulmonary sarcoidosis. Both diseases may have disseminated granulomas in lymph nodes, liver, spleen, skeletal muscle, and other sites; however, the two disorders can be differentiated by the presence, in berylliosis, of Be in tissues[103] and specific immunologic responses to Be;[90] the metal appears to function as an antigen or hapten.[92] The question has arisen whether sarcoidosis is similarly caused

Table 23-3. Selected causes of hypersensitivity pneumonitis

Antigen	Source	Disease
Thermophilic actinomycetes (various species)	Moldy hay Contaminated ventilation	Farmer's lung Ventilation pneumonitis
Avian proteins	Pigeons, turkeys, budgerigars	Bird fancier's lung
Mammalian urine proteins	Laboratory rats	HP
Isocyanates (various compounds)	Polyurethane foam	HP
Gold, amiodarone	Therapeutic drugs	HP

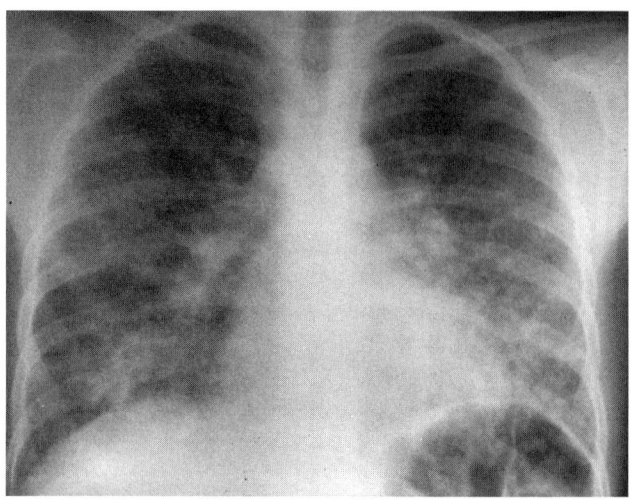

Fig. 23-1. Hypersensitivity pneumonitis in a 16-year-old boy exposed to moldy compost. The chest radiograph shows diffuse reticular and nodular infiltrates that cleared on a film taken 3 weeks later.

by an antigen, and various possibilities (mycobacteria, fungi, pollen, or an unidentified transmissable agent) have been proposed but none has been proven.

Hypersensitivity pneumonitis

Antigenic particles of respirable size are ubiquitous, but when inhaled by a sensitized host, hypersensitivity pneumonitis (HP) may ensue. This granulomatous immunologic disorder is of particular relevance to environmental medicine. Environmental or occupational sources initially associated with antigens causing HP have led to names such as farmer's lung, bird fancier's lung, ventilation pneumonitis, and other colorful appellations (Table 23-3). Although the immunopathogenesis of HP has not been elaborated in full detail, animal models and human studies have led to a better understanding than for many other pulmonary disorders. Typically, intense or prolonged inhalation of particles 1 to 3 μm in aerodynamic diameter results in alveolar deposition and induction of localized pulmonary immune responses of both the humoral and cell-mediated types. On repeated exposure, acute alveolitis develops in the sensitized host. Complexes of deposited antigen and preformed antibodies of the immunoglobulin M (IgM) and IgG classes activate complement, leading to increased vascular permeability, influx of neutrophils, and release of cytokines. Endotoxin, a microbial lipopolysaccharide with potent ability to activate complement by the alternate pathway, may accompany inhaled antigens and contribute to the release of cytokines. Sensitized macrophages and lymphocytes accumulate in the pulmonary interstitium and participate in granuloma formation.

Although about 50% of exposed individuals have demonstrable antibodies in surveys of populations exposed to various HP agents,[73] the attack rate of HP is only about 5% to 15%. The reasons why are not entirely clear, but exposure levels and host factors undoubtedly play a role. Some authors find an association between HP and human leukocyte antigen type,[89] but other studies fail to show a link.[34,78] Subtle features of immune regulation, for example, the balance between the suppressor and helper subsets of T lymphocytes in the immunized host, may influence host susceptibility.[10,62]

Assessment of HP

Clinically, HP presents in acute and chronic forms. Typically, the symptoms occur repeatedly without development of tolerance to the antigen; however, in perhaps 5% of patients tolerance evolves, or the symptoms are mild enough that repeated exposure leads insidiously to the development of chronic injury and pulmonary fibrosis. In acute HP, there is a close temporal association between exposure and the onset, 4 to 6 hours later, of fever, chills, malaise, myalgias, dyspnea, and dry cough. The patient appears acutely ill, with fever and tachypnea, and crackles are heard over the lung fields. Hypoxemia is often present, with hyperventilation (low partial pressure of carbon dioxide); the peripheral white blood cell (WBC) count is usually elevated, with moderate eosinophilia; and the chest radiograph typically shows diffuse alveolar and interstitial infiltrates (Fig. 23-1). Pulmonary function studies during the acute illness demonstrate restrictive ventilatory impairment and reduced diffusing capacity. The symptoms and signs resolve spontaneously over 4 to 6 days after removal of the offending antigen. In chronic HP, dyspnea, fatigue, and weight loss are prominent symptoms; fever, leukocytosis, and other signs of acute illness are usually absent, and the chest radiograph is remarkable for signs of fibrosis.

When a possible case of HP is confronted, both the patient and the environment need to be assessed. Every effort should be made to remove the patient from the suspected antigen while treatment is proceeding. A detailed description of the work and home environment should be obtained, seeking potential sources of exposure to materials (including those handled in hobbies), contaminated heating and ventilation systems, pets, and medications. A survey and sampling of the environment by a qualified industrial hygienist or environmental engineer can be of great value. Serologic panels are helpful in confirming the presence of immunologic sensitization, keeping in mind the limitations of sensitivity and specificity.

Confirmation that a patient has been immunologically sensitized to a suspected antigen can be obtained by demonstration of serum antibodies using several techniques: double immunodiffusion, complement fixation, radioimmunoassay, or enzyme-linked immunosorbent assay. The sensitivity of serology may be as high as 90%, depending on the antigen; however, the specificity is low because about 40% of exposed individuals without HP have elevated antibody titers. Cell-mediated immunity can be demonstrated by intradermal injection of antigen, but impure antigenic extracts produce nonspecific skin reactions; in vitro methods, such as the production by sensitized lymphocytes of macrophage migration-inhibition factor when stimulated by antigen, are preferred in laboratories with the capability to perform these studies. The cause of HP can best be proven by documentation of acute illness in a sensitized person on exposure to a recognized antigen, or by inhalation challenge with the antigen. The latter should be attempted with extreme caution, and intravenous steroids must be given to terminate the episode. Bronchoalveolar lavage demonstrates a marked increase in the population of T lymphocytes, primarily of the CD8 subset.[64] Lung biopsy in acute HP shows lymphocytic interstitial infiltration and granuloma formation (Fig. 23-2). In chronic HP the biopsy usually shows fibrosis without distinctive diagnostic features.

Acute HP must be differentiated from organic dust toxic syndrome,[28,29] viral infections, and sarcoidosis; in the latter two conditions, a temporal relationship and specific immunity to an environmental factor are lacking, and neither high fever nor WBC count elevation is prominent in sarcoidosis. Chronic HP is difficult to differentiate from other causes of pulmonary fibrosis except by historical clues such as exposure to a known causative agent or previous recurrent episodes suggestive of acute HP.

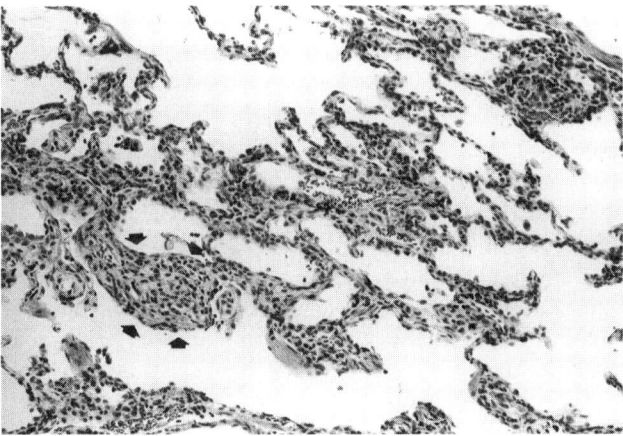

Fig. 23-2. Hypersensitivity pneumonitis. The lung interstitium is focally expanded by a granulomatous reaction (*arrows*) consisting of accumulations of macrophages and lymphocytes (16×).

When confronted with a potentially hazardous environment and an exposed population, serologic surveys should not be used for surveillance purposes, because the interpretation of serologic data is nonspecific. Symptom surveys can be helpful, keeping in mind the necessity of eliminating nonspecific and random occurrences by comparing the observed rates with a control survey of an unexposed but otherwise similar population. Periodic objective assays that may be useful include body temperature, WBC count, vital capacity, and diffusing capacity, with chest radiographs when suspicion of the illness is raised. Recently the use of a bronchial biopsy has been suggested as a useful diagnostic tool.

Treatment

Acute HP is a self-limited illness. Removal from exposure and supportive respiratory care with oxygen are usually all that is required in milder cases. In severe illness, mechanical ventilation may be necessary, and corticosteroids hasten recovery.

DIFFUSE ALVEOLAR DAMAGE

Diffuse alveolar damage (DAD) is a term that refers to the histologic changes induced by acute lung injury caused by toxic agents and also by factors associated with a variety of systemic illnesses, such as sepsis. Many of the toxic events occur in the chemical industry, where excessive exposures may occur. On the other hand, low-dose exposure to some of these agents may also be a part of daily life for the general population and do not result in DAD.

Pathogenesis

DAD is initiated by injury to capillary endothelial and alveolar epithelial cells. Of the many agents that can cause DAD, irritant gases are most relevant to this discussion (Table 23-4). The most important determinants of parenchymal lung injury are the dose of the exposure and the solubility of the gas in the aqueous layer of airway mucosa. Because of their high aqueous solubility, gases such as ammonia and SO_2 exert their effects primarily in the upper airways and only reach the lower airways when inhaled in very high amounts. In contrast, gases with low solubility, such as phosgene and NO_2, penetrate below the upper airways and adversely affect the lower airways and alveoli. If exposures fall within accepted permissible exposure limits, adverse respiratory effects are unusual or at least exceedingly subtle. If

Selected irritant gases causing diffuse alveolar damage
SO_2
NO_2
Ammonia
Chlorine
Phosgene
Hydrogen sulfide

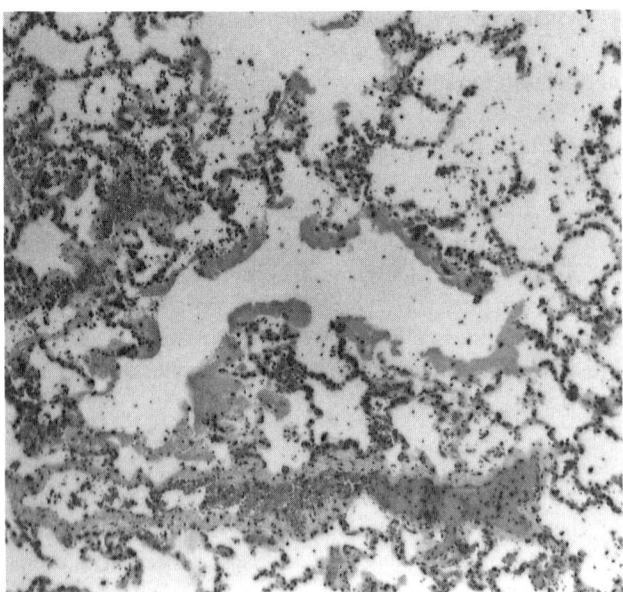

Fig. 23-3. Diffuse alveolar damage, early phase. Hyaline membranes line an alveolar duct (10×).

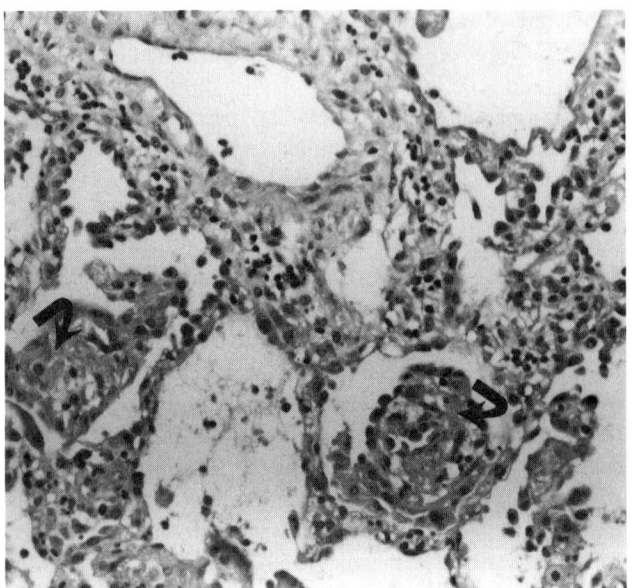

Fig. 23-4. Diffuse alveolar damage. The alveolar spaces are filled with fibrin deposits that are undergoing organization by fibroblasts (*arrows*). There is an interstitial infiltrate composed primarily of macrophages, and conspicuous hyperplasia of the type II pneumocytes lining the alveoli (20×).

exposures exceed these limits yet remain low, it becomes more difficult to determine the possible effects.

DAD begins with sloughing of type I pneumocytes into alveolar spaces and increased capillary permeability. The influx of serous fluid into the alveolar spaces results in edema and the formation of hyaline membranes, which line the alveolar spaces (Fig. 23-3). Surfactant changes, including altered composition, pool sizes, and metabolism and inactivation by serum proteins present in the interstitial space, may occur.[68] Within a few days, a reparative process is evidenced by hyperplasia and proliferation of type II pneumocytes and interstitial inflammatory infiltrate composed of macrophages and other effector cells (Fig. 23-4). The alveolar septa are thickened by proliferating fibroblasts (Fig. 23-5). For complete repair to occur, the epithelial basement membrane must remain intact to act as a framework for the restoration of alveolar structures. The organization of these changes influences whether death due to acute respiratory failure or recovery with or without fibrosis occurs. The eventual determinant of the outcome remains incompletely understood but most likely relates to the extent of the initial injury.

The clinical manifestations of DAD are referred to as the adult respiratory distress syndrome (ARDS).[4] When initiated by an excessive exposure to an irritant gas or vapor, ARDS is preceded by varying degrees of cough, sputum, dyspnea, and bronchoconstriction. Features found on clinical examination include inflamed mucous membranes, tachycardia, tachypnea, and wheezing. The onset of ARDS is heralded by diminished lung compliance, profound hypoxemia, and, often, the need for mechanical ventilation with high concentrations of supplemental oxygen. The volume of the lung diminishes, probably because of disturbance of surfactant;

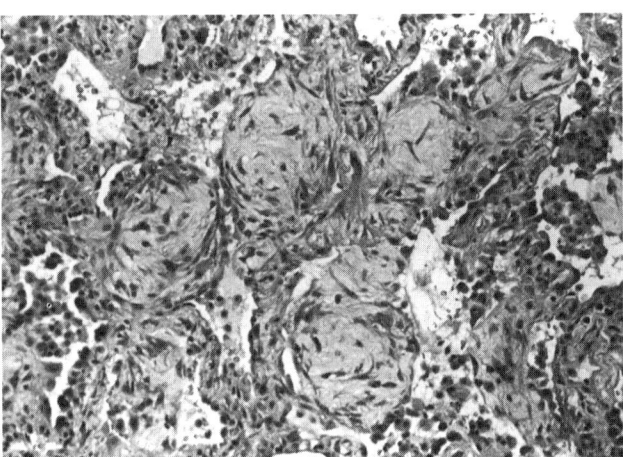

Fig. 23-5. Diffuse alveolar damage, reparative phase. There is delicate fibroblastic proliferation within the alveolar spaces, which eventually are incorporated into the interstitium (20×).

the collapse of lung units occurs as a consequence of the acute lung injury.

Bronchiolitis obliterans is another consequence of intense exposure to irritant gases. It results from an inflammatory process that develops 1 to 2 months after an acute toxic insult, leading to occlusion of the lumen of small airways.[5] It has been reported to occur after exposure to methyl isocyanate,[110] NO_2,[54] and a number of other toxic gases and fumes. Histologic examination reveals obstruction of the terminal and respiratory bronchioles by polypoid masses of connective tissue. The distal airspaces are overinflated or filled with cellular debris. The radiograph may appear normal or suggest an interstitial process. Diagnosis is confirmed by open lung biopsy. Bronchiolitis obliterans often responds to corticosteroid therapy if treatment is started early.

Natural history of acute toxic gas exposure: selected examples

Accidental exposures to high levels of irritant gases such as SO_2, chlorine, phosgene, NO_2, and methyl isocyanate provides experience in understanding the outcome of DAD. Inhaled SO_2 at concentrations exceeding 50 ppm causes fatal laryngotracheal and pulmonary edema. Several studies report the consequences of acute excessive SO_2 exposure.[16] Perhaps the most descriptive is a report of nine workers trapped in a mine after an explosion that resulted in exposure to toxic amounts of SO_2 for more than one half hour.[49] One worker died within hours of the accident. Autopsy showed a histologic appearance consistent with DAD. The survivors complained of chest pain and had rapid onset of cyanosis, dyspnea, cough, and conjunctival irritation. Chest auscultation revealed moist crackles. Three had chest radiographs consistent with ARDS. All received therapy with corticosteroids. The respiratory health of seven survivors was followed up for the next 4 years. All continued to complain of shortness of breath. Although their lung function improved, airways obstruction remained after 4 years in six workers, and in the seventh, borderline restriction was apparent. Although the diffusing capacity remained normal in all, four of the seven had increased airway responsiveness to histamine, implying continuing airway inflammation and possibly exaggerated responses of irritant receptors (or development of RADS).

Chlorine is intermediate in solubility among the gases; it has the potential to affect both the upper and the lower airways and to inflict DAD. Despite numerous reports of the respiratory health of workers exposed over the long term to low levels or short term to high levels of chlorine, disagreement about the outcome remains. Experience after World War I suggested that chlorine gas inhalation could cause chronic respiratory impairment, but most survivors were not disabled.[41] Recent reports of outcome after an acute chlorine exposure[58,112] showed no accelerated decline of lung function in the group (as a whole) at the time of long-term follow-up. Another report of follow-up lung function measurements 12 years after an acute excessive chlorine exposure showed results of spirometry remained stable but a decrease in the residual volume was observed.[93] The authors hypothesized that this finding was the result of small airway stiffening from peribronchial fibrosis.

Phosgene is a colorless gas heavier than air. Exposure produces a concentration dependent series of events. In some workers exposed to concentrations between 1 and 3 ppm, a transient vagal reflex produces rapid shallow breathing.[37] Exposures greater than 30 ppm have the potential to induce severe lung injury leading to ARDS after a period of several hours. At exposures exceeding 200 ppm, phosgene gas passes into the pulmonary capillaries and reacts with blood constituents, inducing hemolysis, thrombosis of the pulmonary vasculature, and death with acute cor pulmonale.[26] Sublethal exposure but subsequent ARDS has been reported to have a good prognosis; individuals with underlying lung function abnormalities at the time of the acute exposure may have a worse prognosis;[27] however, exertional dyspnea may persist, and normalization of lung function may take several years.

The experience with methyl isocyanate exposure after the disastrous industrial accident at Bhopal, India, in 1984 showed a gradation of toxic effects not dissimilar to the aforementioned description. There was apparent rapid suffocation in those most heavily exposed. ARDS developed in a high proportion of severely exposed individuals evaluated with chest radiographs.[96] A high prevalence of impaired ventilatory function, primarily of a restrictive pattern, was observed in survivors,[59] with persistence over months in some individuals and gradual improvement in others.[60]

Epidemiology

Perhaps the clearest and still the most reasonable criteria for linking the development of chronic respiratory disease to an acute toxic gas exposure were put forth soon after World War II.[83] First, there must be severe lung injury. This criterion can be judged best by the need for aggressive medical intervention. As a general rule, admission to the hospital with development of ARDS implies severe injury and the likelihood of long-term respiratory impairment. Alternatively, evaluation in the emergency department with discharge to home after the acute event suggests a lesser exposure that is not likely to induce long-term effects. Second, chronic impairment of lung function should persist. Third, there should be no other explanation for the development of pulmonary disease. When these criteria are met, it is very reasonable to attribute alterations in pulmonary physiology to a past excessive chemical exposure. When the relationship between lung injury and exposure is not clear, clinical judgement plays a larger role and the degree of confidence linking the exposure and the lung injury is less.

Treatment

When the manifestations are mild, recovery is usually rapid and requires relatively little medical intervention close observation for 24 to 48 hours is warranted because of occasional instances of deterioration due to delayed manifestations of the acute injury. More severe cases require monitoring and respiratory support in an intensive care unit. ARDS is managed with administration of supplemental oxygen and mechanical ventilation with added positive end-expiratory pressure. Despite more than 25 years' recognition of ARDS, the mortality rate continues to approximate 50%. When DAD is due to excessive environmental exposure to a chemical agent, the underlying plan for therapy should include measures to lessen the acute inflammatory response and provide symptomatic relief. Corticosteroids may diminish airway inflammation but have not been shown to affect alveolar permeability or improve the recovery from ARDS. Antibiotics may be necessary to treat superimposed infections. Aminophylline and inhaled β_2-adrenergic agonists may be helpful in treating acute airflow obstruction. The prognosis for ARDS is variable, encompassing full recovery, persistent residual impairment, life-threatening complications of associated multiple organ failure, and, in many severe instances, death from asphyxia. Investigational therapies such as intratracheal surfactant instillation may affect the outcome of ARDS in the future.[109,115]

INTERSTITIAL FIBROSIS

Although occurring mainly in occupational settings, the pneumoconioses represent an important group of environmental disorders in which the inhalation of certain inorganic dusts produces interstitial pulmonary fibrosis. The fibrogenic dusts that cause pneumoconiosis must be distinguished from nuisance dusts that cause nonobstructive bronchitis but are not fibrogenic (see box below). The three most prevalent pneumoconiosis in the United States, and probably throughout industrialized societies, are silicosis, coal workers' pneumoconiosis (CWP), and asbestosis. Silicosis and CWP are the least likely to be encountered apart from the occupational setting and are discussed herein only briefly; however, asbestos-related respiratory disorders occur as a consequence of nonoccupational environmental exposure. Clinical aspects of these disorders are covered in this chapter; and public health issues are discussed in Chapter 38.

Unlike interstitial lung diseases in which the cause of the pulmonary fibrosis is unknown (such as idiopathic pulmonary fibrosis and sarcoidosis), dust-induced interstitial lung diseases are a known initiator of fibrosis and there is a predictable relationship between the amount of exposure, fibrogenic potency of the dust, and the extent of fibrosis. As a rule, when the amount of inhaled dust exceeds the rate of clearance from the lung, an alveolitis begins and is the first step toward lung injury. If these events continue, the immune system responds nonspecifically by amplifying the inflammatory stimuli with an influx of effector cells into the alveolar and interstitial spaces. As the process proceeds, cellular and connective tissue alterations produce irreversible scarring that, in its severe form, leads to end-stage fibrosis.[38]

Approach to diagnosis

There are three requisites for the diagnosis of dust-induced interstitial lung disease. First, the patient must provide a history of dust exposure sufficient to cause the disease in question; second, the chest radiograph should show opacities consistent with the disease; and third, no underlying illness that radiographically or physiologically mimics pneumoconiosis should be present. Although respiratory symptoms and lung function impairment are commonly present, it is important to remember that neither is a necessary criterion for diagnosis; however, when symptoms and functional impairment exist, they occur in a relatively established pattern. In each type of dust-induced illness the rate of decline in lung function and progression of dyspnea depend on the amount of dust inhaled and the persistence of a burden of dust in the lungs;[56] latency, or the time from first exposure to the recognition of disease, also plays a role.

Whether inhalation of a fibrogenic dust results in lung fibrosis depends on the particle size, amount, and biologic properties of the dust. Respirable particles are capable of reaching the vulnerable region of the lung (the respiratory bronchioles, terminal bronchioles, alveolar ducts, and alveoli); typically they have a median aerodynamic diameter between 0.5 and 5 μm. Larger particles are efficiently trapped in the nose and upper airway, and those that are smaller ($<0.1\mu$) are exhaled without being deposited in the respiratory tract. Beach sand, for example, does not cause silicosis, because the particles are too large to be respirable; however, when silica particles are made smaller (as with sandblasting or drilling), they become respirable and potentially toxic. Coal mining also generates respirable dust. Friable asbestos, most often encountered in insulation, becomes respirable when the fibers are fractured.[39] There is no opportunity for asbestos fibers that remain undisturbed to be inhaled, and they are best left alone.

Determining whether the dose of fibrogenic dust is sufficient to cause interstitial lung disease may be difficult, requiring not only clinical judgement tempered by knowledge of the potential pitfalls in reaching this conclusion but also the help of a knowledgeable industrial hygienist.[51,102] Important determinants include the duration of exposure and the concentration of respirable dust. Actual measurements of respirable dust concentration, if available, are valuable but must be interpreted carefully. For example, acute silicosis occurred in surface coal mine drillers when reported dust levels were within recommended limits,[7] because the measurements were not representative of the overwhelming

---

Selected fibrogenic and nonfibrogenic inorganic dusts

Fibrogenic	*Nonfibrogenic*
Carbon (coal, graphite)	Limestone
Crystalline silica	Amorphous silica
Quartz	Glass
Cristobalite	Diatomite
Tridymite	
Silicates	
Asbestos	
Talc	
Kaolin	

dust exposures. On the other hand, the use of an effective respiratory protective device can reduce the inhaled dose if the device is designed and worn properly. Therefore, it is critical that the physician be aware of the conditions under which the dust samples were collected. Also important is the latency period between first exposure and the development of disease. Dust remaining in the lung represents a stimulus to fibrogenesis and can cause the progression or development of radiographic opacities even after exposure has ceased.[40,52] Finally, and perhaps most important, the clinician must be aware that the diagnosis of one individual with environmental lung disease means that other individuals may very likely have been exposed and that further investigation is needed.

When the three criteria for diagnosis are met, the diagnosis of pneumoconiosis can be accurately made on a clinical basis and additional investigations are unnecessary. On occasion the possibility of dust-induced lung disease is raised, but not all of the criteria are fulfilled and a clinical diagnosis is not possible. This case could occur when the exposure history is uncertain or the chest radiograph implicates other disorders in the differential diagnosis. In such instances, lung biopsy may be necessary. Bronchoscopic transbronchial biopsy is often inadequate in pneumoconioses, just as it is in idiopathic pulmonary fibrosis, because the small tissue sample may be insufficient for diagnosis. Furthermore, the risk of pneumothorax after transbronchial biopsy is increased in the presence of diminished lung compliance due to fibrosis. Therefore, when tissue for diagnostic analysis is required, an open lung biopsy with generous tissue sampling is preferred and allows specialized studies of dust in the lung.[7]

Silicosis

Silica (silicon dioxide) is the most abundant mineral in the Earth's crust. It is considered to be free when it is not bound to other minerals and combined when it is bound. Quartz (including granite), flint, chert, opal, chalcedony, and diatomite have high proportions of free silica. Combined forms of silica are termed *silicates* and may be fibrous in form. These forms include, among others, asbestos, talc, and kaolin. It is of biologic significance whether the physical structure of silica is crystalline or amorphous. Crystalline forms exist as quartz, cristobalite, and tridymite. Of these, quartz is diffusely distributed throughout the planet as sand. Cristobalite and tridymite occur in lava and are formed by heating quartz or amorphous silica. Cristobalite is more fibrogenic than quartz. Amorphous silica is noncrystalline by definition and is not fibrogenic. It occurs as vitreous silica (glass), formed by melting and then quickly cooling free crystalline silica, and diatomite (skeletons of prehistoric marine organisms). Heating diatomite, with or without alkali (a process known as *calcining*), converts it to crystalline cristobalite, imparting the potential for fibrogenesis.

The other major determinants of toxicity are the duration of the exposure, the silica content of the dust, and the concentration of respirable dust. Respirable particles between 0.5 and 5 μm in diameter are deposited most efficiently in the alveoli; those less than 1 μm in diameter are believed to be the most fibrogenic. Depending on particle size, as much as 80% of the silica dust is rapidly cleared, and the retained particles are responsible for fibrogenesis.

Workers and artisans engaged in crafts have many opportunities for exposure to respirable free crystalline silica. Some commonly encountered situations in which the risk of silicosis exists are reported in Table 23-4.

Silicosis typically develops slowly,[117] with a latency period averaging 10 to 30 years from initial exposure to the onset of clinical manifestations. Silicosis is categorized radiographically by the size of the opacities. Small, rounded opacities (less than 10 mm in diameter) denote simple silicosis and typically predominate in the upper lung zones, where, for reasons not well understood, the retention of silica particles is favored. Complicated silicosis or progressive massive fibrosis (PMF) results from the coalescence of small opacities and appears as unilateral or bilateral mass lesions greater than 10 mm in diameter, again typically distributed in the upper lung zones. The size and profusion of opacities, the areas of the lungs affected, and the presence and size of PMF lesions can be described with use of a classification system formulated by the International Labour Office (ILO).[57]

In unusual circumstances an acute form of silicosis (or silicoproteinosis) occurs within 5 years of initial exposure as the result of overwhelming dust inhalation. Radiographically, it appears as an alveolar filling pattern resembling pulmonary alveolar proteinosis.

There are two important respiratory risks to the individual with silica exposure. The first is the development of simple

Table 23-4. Occupations and crafts with silica exposure

Occupation	Exposure
Sandblasting	Ship building and repair, preparation of steel structures for painting (oil rigs, bridges, etc.)
Mining	Silica contamination of ore or overlying rock
Milling	Dry finely ground silica flour for abrasives and fillers
Boiler construction and repair	Exposure to refractory brick dust
Quarrying and stone work	Slate and granite dust
Foundry work	Fettling (chipping) to remove rough spots from castings made in silica molds
Pottery making	Crushing and chipping flint
Glassmaking	Sand used as an abrasive for polishing

silicosis, a disease typically causing little or no impairment of pulmonary function; however, the implication of the development of simple silicosis is that there is a subsequent risk of progression to PMF, which is associated with severe respiratory disability and a reduced life span.[33,113] Although a diagnosis of silicosis carries with it the recommendation that the individual cease exposure, there is no guarantee that this intervention will affect the outcome, because the disease may begin or progress after exposure has stopped. Unfortunately, there are no proven methods of halting the progression, although some unproven strategies have been suggested.[8]

The other risk is the predisposition of silica-exposed individuals to develop mycobacterial infection even in the absence of radiographically apparent silicosis.[22,100] This predisposition is thought to result from silica-induced impairment of local immunologic defenses.[13,23,24,69,71] Mycobacterial infection in a silicotic patient has the potential to increase respiratory impairment and reduce survival. The clinician must realize that changes over a relatively short time in the chest radiograph of a silicotic patient signify superimposed mycobacterial infection until proven otherwise. An acute chest illness, a new infiltrate, coalescence of nodules in the upper lung, or cavitation of a preexisting lesion are reasons for great concern and demand an aggressive search for mycobacterial organisms. It is reasonable to perform chest radiograph and tuberculin skin test surveillance in patients with silicosis, although this regimen has not been studied in a systematic fashion. If the tuberculin test converts to positive without clinical evidence of active tuberculosis, at least 1 year of isoniazid therapy is indicated.[9,21,101] Many advocate life-long preventive antituberculosis therapy in this setting.[75]

Coal workers' pneumoconiosis

Although clinically similar, CWP and silicosis are distinct disorders. It was previously believed that respiratory problems of coal miners were caused by the silica content of the dust; however, the observation that pneumoconiosis occurred in coal trimmers (workers exposed to washed coal essentially free of crystalline silica)[19] led to the understanding that disease attributable to coal dust could occur without silica exposure. Our understanding of the epidemiology of CWP comes mainly from radiographic surveys of British and American coal miners, using the ILO classification system.[33] The radiographic extent of simple CWP increases with the length of time spent underground, and deviations from this relationship are explained by the rank of coal mined (a higher prevalence of CWP occurs among miners who mine high-rank coal such as anthracite, and a lower prevalence occurred among miners who mine low-rank coal such as bituminous); differences in dust exposure; and, possibly, variation in radiographic technique and interpretation.

The term *black lung* should be considered in a different light from CWP, the former being a nonmedical colloquialism referring generically to an aggregation of respiratory complaints, including asthma, chronic bronchitis, and emphysema, in coal miners. The diagnosis of CWP requires a history of coal mining (usually 10 years or more), radiographic evidence of pneumoconiosis, and no other disorder that could mimic pneumoconiosis (such as sarcoidosis or pulmonary rheumatoid nodules). Individuals with simple CWP may have no symptoms or may complain of chronic cough and sputum production (chronic bronchitis), which reflect airway irritation by dust and should be distinguished from pneumoconiosis per se. As in silicosis, the chest is quiet on examination, although coarse airway sounds consistent with bronchitis are sometimes heard. End-inspiratory crackles and clubbing are not features of CWP and should impel the clinician to consider other interstitial lung diseases.

The signs of simple CWP on chest radiography begin as small, rounded opacities 10 mm or less in diameter, typically appearing in the upper lung zones. As the disease advances, the rest of the lung becomes involved and the opacities often enlarge. Complicated CWP or PMF is the result of coalescence of small, rounded opacities and is present when the chest radiograph shows opacities exceeding 10 mm in diameter. Pulmonary function studies generally show the forced vital capacity (FVC) and forced expiratory volume in 1 second (FEV_1) to be less than those of nonminers; in simple CWP the reductions are small and the values are usually within the normal range or only marginally decreased.[65,76,80] PMF can be associated with severe respiratory impairment. The relationship between airflow obstruction and mining suggests that coal dust inhalation can cause a decrease in lung function, but the decrement is small and related to associated industrial bronchitis.[104] A recent metaanalysis suggested that miners have a greater risk of developing emphysema when there is increased silica in the mine dust.[81]

The primary consequence of simple CWP is the potential to develop PMF, which often entails severe impairment of lung function. Unlike silicosis, no clear predisposition to develop mycobacterial disease has been shown; however, in miners with concurrent silica exposure the concern regarding mycobacterial infection remains relevant.

Asbestos-related respiratory disorders

Asbestos is virtually indestructible and remains in the environment indefinitely. It has been widely used because of its resistance to heat and chemicals, high tensile strength, and lower cost than that of man-made materials. Cause-and-effect relationships between environmental and occupational exposure to asbestos and the disorders listed in the box on p. 293 are well established. Of importance is the recognition that asbestos-related disease is the result of exposure beginning many years earlier. Prevention of future illness can be accomplished by limiting asbestos exposure through appropriate engineering controls and the use of safer materials.

Exposure occurs during the mining, milling, handling, and manufacturing of asbestos, and during the destruction of previously manufactured material. Once the fibers are in-

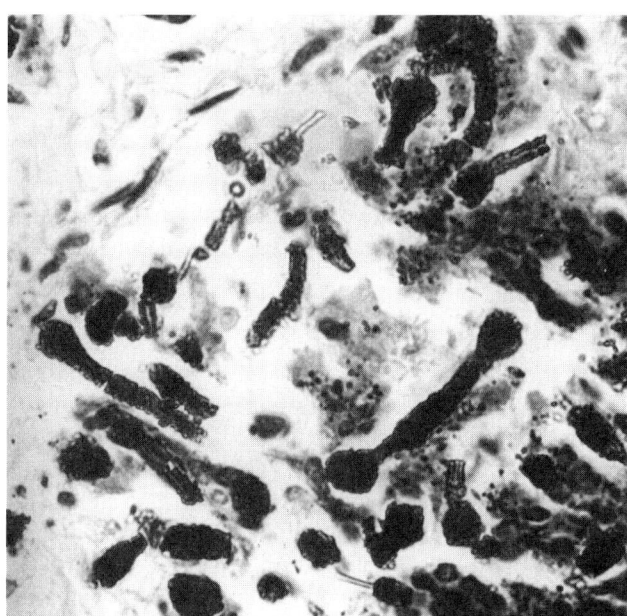

Fig. 23-6. Asbestos (ferruginous) bodies. The dumbbell-shaped structures are formed by asbestos fibers coated with iron-containing protein (40×).

Asbestos-related respiratory disorders

Asbestosis (asbestos pneumoconiosis)
Benign pleural effusion
Benign pleural thickening
Pleural mesothelioma
Bronchogenic carcinoma

---

corporated into manufactured items, there appears to be little health risk unless the item is disrupted.[39] The Occupational Safety and Health Administration has mandated strict workplace dust controls, worker protection, and annual examinations of exposed workers. Guidelines for minimization of worker and community exposure to asbestos installed in buildings have been issued by the Environmental Protection Agency.[32]

Asbestos fibers that escape clearance by airway cilia penetrate into the lung parenchyma. Parenchymal penetration is inversely proportional to fiber diameter. Fibers may remain imbedded in the lung for years despite the attempts of macrophages to engulf them; however, with time, the longest fibers (typically amphiboles) may become coated with acid mucopolysaccharides and iron.[74] Sometimes referred to as *asbestos bodies* (Fig. 23-6), the coated fibers are more appropriately termed *ferruginous bodies* because other inhaled fibers (such as talc, fibrous glass, cotton, and diatomaceous earth) are handled in like manner. Thus, although ferruginous bodies have most commonly been found to have an asbestos core,[17] coated fibers are not necessarily asbestos.

Although the coating of fibers within the lung is thought to decrease fibrogenicity, most fibers are not coated. The great majority of fibers in the lung exist as fragments visible only by electron microscopy. They are thought to represent chrysotile fibers that have been fragmented and perhaps dissolved by leaching.[44] As a marker of urban living, the lungs of nearly all urban dwellers over the age of 40 contained ferruginous bodies that were not routinely associated with pathologic abnormalities.[20]

Asbestosis Asbestosis is the parenchymal fibrosis associated with asbestos exposure. The signs and symptoms are identical to those of other forms of diffuse interstitial fibrosis. Like silicosis and CWP, the diagnosis is made by recognition of a history of asbestos exposure (most often 10 years or longer), typical radiographic appearance, and lack of another illness that confounds the diagnosis (see box below). Restriction of lung volumes is an early sign, and digital clubbing and late inspiratory crackles are findings but are not necessary for diagnosis.[79] Like silicosis and CWP, asbestosis may progress even after cessation of exposure;[43] however, there must be a large tissue fiber burden for asbestosis to occur. Recent analyses suggest that modern exposure limits have resulted in declining mortality from asbestosis in Great Britain[25] and the occurrence in the United States of few new cases among those first exposed since 1960.[40]

The chest radiograph classically shows small, irregular opacities (Fig. 23-7) that may progress to honeycombing. The appearance is identical to that of other diffuse fibrotic processes; specificity for asbestos-induced fibrosis is enhanced when pleural thickening and, in particular, pleural calcification are present.

The changes in lung function appear related to the amount of asbestos fibers inhaled. Asbestosis is associated with restriction of lung volumes; there is diminished gas transfer as evidenced by a decreased diffusing capacity. On occasion, small-airways changes may occur because of the peribronchial accumulation of asbestos dust.[11] Longitudinal follow-up of workers with asbestosis typically shows progressive and accelerated decline in lung function. Recent epidemiologic research has suggested that even exposed individuals without asbestosis appear to have a 2% decline in FVC and FEV_1 relative to the predicted values per decade from first exposure.[14]

Pleural effusion and thickening Asbestos may cause a benign exudative pleural effusion and diffuse pleural thick-

---

Clinical manifestations of asbestosis

History of sufficient asbestos exposure
Dyspnea
Restrictive impairment (FVC less than 80% of predicted level)
Digital clubbing
Late inspiratory crackles
Irregular basilar opacities on chest radiograph

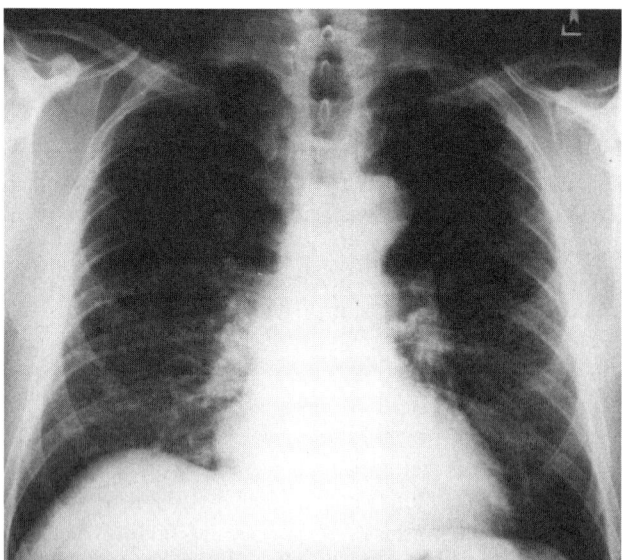

Fig. 23-7. Asbestosis in a 47-year-old construction worker. The chest radiograph shows irregular interstitial opacities with a predominantly basilar distribution.

ening, which can be identified on the chest radiograph by a blunted costophrenic angle and adjacent lateral chest wall thickening. Recent estimates suggest that pleural thickening is associated with a 4% reduction of FVC expressed as a percentage of the predicted value.[14]

Pleural plaques located on the parietal pleura are not associated with adhesions, and cause no disability. The early radiographic sign of a pleural plaque is a thin soft-tissue density, usually at the lateral margin of the seventh or eighth rib. This early change may be difficult to distinguish from normal companion shadows of the muscles that insert into the ribs. The routine chest radiograph defines only 8% to 15% of all pleural plaques.[55] Oblique views and CT scans may assist in their recognition.

The pathogenesis of pleural plaques is unclear. It has been suggested that inhaled fibers gradually migrate to the base and periphery of the lung by the continual motion of breathing,[106] which explains the usual distribution of plaques in dependent lung zones. Grossly the plaques are firm, raised deposits with a pale, glistening surface.[72] Microscopically, collagen fibers are oriented in a parallel fashion and covered by normal mesothelial cells. Thus, the plaque is actually extrapleural. This and the slow, nonexudative growth of the plaque may explain the lack of adhesions. Pleural calcification occurs in areas of collagen degeneration and implies that the plaque has been present for 20 or more years.[35] Plaques serve only as markers of asbestos exposure; there is no evidence to suggest that pleural plaques are premalignant lesions leading to the development of mesothelioma.

Malignant mesothelioma Of all the disorders caused by asbestos, mesothelioma may be the most intriguing and perhaps the most relevant to environmental asbestos exposure.

Unlike asbestosis, in which there is a clear dose-response relationship between inhaled fibers and the extent of disease, the relationship between amount inhaled and the development of mesothelioma is more complex.[77] First, the latency interval between first exposure and the development of disease is often 30 or more years. Second, it appears that crocidolite fibers, to a greater extent than chrysotile, induce mesothelioma, implying that the disease may depend on fiber type.[11]

Mesotheliomas may be benign or malignant. The terms *solitary* and *diffuse* are respective synonyms.[85] Benign, or solitary, mesotheliomas are unrelated to asbestos exposure. Diffuse mesothelioma has a gross appearance that is more diagnostic than is the variable histologic appearance.[61,91] In the early stages, it appears as multiple gray nodules on the pleural surface, spreading and encasing the lung and resulting in a loss of volume. Distant metastases beyond the regional lymph nodes occur with time and reflect advanced disease. The tumor has a predilection for growth along incision or biopsy sites. Microscopically, malignant mesothelioma may have one of three histologic patterns: epithelial, sarcomatous, or mixed. Usually one pattern predominates, but mixed elements may be present.[118]

Mesothelioma is exceedingly rare in the non–asbestos-exposed population. The relationship between malignant mesothelioma and asbestos exposure was first well documented in 1960.[108] More recently, a study of 17,800 asbestos insulators uncovered 66 mesotheliomas.[95] Persons having household contact with asbestos workers also are at increased risk for the development of mesothelioma.[3]

Symptoms develop insidiously and include progressive dyspnea, weight loss, and severe chest pain. The presenting sign is usually a unilateral pleural effusion. Lymphadenopathy and rib tenderness are signs of local tumor invasion. Superior and inferior vena cava obstruction can occur. Malignant mesothelioma should be considered in the differential diagnosis of unexplained exudative pleural effusion, particularly if there is a history of asbestos exposure with a latency of 25 or more years. Clinical clues suggesting past asbestos exposure include pleural plaques and calcification. Mesothelioma is commonly seen in the absence of radiographic evidence of asbestosis.[67]

In an attempt to diagnose the cause of a pleural effusion, thoracentesis is performed. With mesothelioma, it may be difficult to enter the pleural space because of thickened pleura. The effusion is viscous, exudative, and highly cellular, with a mixture of normal, inflammatory, and malignant cells. Cytologic examination is often of limited diagnostic value because of difficulty in the differentiation of benign from malignant mesothelial cells. The level of hyaluronic acid in the fluid may be elevated.[88] Needle biopsy may aid in the diagnosis, but thoracoscopic or open pleural biopsy is usually necessary to obtain adequate tissue for diagnosis.[86] Because of rapid fluid accumulation, repeated thoracenteses may be necessary to palliate dyspnea.

Treatment efforts have combined surgery, radiotherapy, and chemotherapy. Nevertheless, the average survival time from the onset of symptoms is only 12 to 15 months and has not changed since the mid-1970s.[66,85] There is no clear evidence that the outcome is significantly altered with more aggressive therapy.

Bronchogenic carcinoma An association between asbestos exposure and bronchogenic carcinoma was first suggested in 1935,[70] and many subsequent studies documented this relationship. Persistent retention of asbestos in the lung parenchyma results in continued exposure to its carcinogenic properties. In one series 60% of English workers disabled by asbestosis died of lung cancer.[70] In another series, a cohort of asbestos workers was evaluated 35 years after they began work.[94] Even workers with less than 1 month of work-related asbestos exposure had an increased probability of developing lung cancer; this probability increased with greater duration of exposure. Older workers and those employed longer developed lung cancer after a shorter latency period than other workers. Thus, the latency period from exposure to development of lung cancer depends on both the amount of exposure and the age at which exposure began.

In another study of the same workers, the risk of lung cancer in asbestos workers was compared with that of a group without asbestos exposure.[46] Asbestos workers who smoked cigarettes had 53 times the risk of developing lung cancer of that of nonsmoking, nonexposed controls. In nonsmoking asbestos workers, this risk was only fivefold. These data suggest a synergistic effect of asbestos and cigarette smoking in causing lung cancer.

REFERENCES

1. Abraham JL, Spragg RG: Documentation of environmental exposure using open lung biopsy, tranbronchial biopsy and bronchopulmonary lavage in giant cell pneumonia (GIP), *Am Rev Respir Dis* 119(suppl):A197, 1979.
2. Alberts WM, Brooks SM: Advances in occupational asthma, *Clin Chest Med* 13:281, 1992.
3. Anderson HA et al: Asbestosis among household contacts of asbestos factory workers, *Ann NY Acad Sci* 330:387, 1979.
4. Ashbaugh DG et al: Acute respiratory distress: adults, *Lancet* 2:319, 1967.
5. Baar HS, Galindo J: Bronchiolitis fibrosa obliterans, *Thorax* 21:209, 1966.
6. Banks DE, Rando RJ: Recurrent asthma due to toluene diisocyanate, *Thorax* 43:660, 1988.
7. Banks DE et al: Silicosis in surface coalmine drillers, *Thorax* 38:275, 1983.
8. Banks DE et al: Strategies for the treatment of silicosis, *Occup Med* 8:205, 1993.
9. Baras G: Silico-tuberculose en Suisse, *Schweiz Med Wochenschr* 100:1802, 1970.
10. Barquin N et al: Immunoregulatory abnormalities in patients with pigeon breeder's disease, *Lung* 168:103, 1990.
11. Begin R et al: Airway function in lifetime-nonsmoking older asbestos workers, *Am J Med* 75:631, 1983.
12. Bethel RA et al: Interaction of sulfur dioxide and dry cold air in causing bronchoconstriction in asthmatic subjects, *J Appl Physiol* 57:419, 1984.
13. Bowden DH, Adamson IYR: The role of cell injury in the continuing inflammatory response in the generation of silicotic pulmonary fibrosis, *J Pathol* 144:149, 1984.
14. Brodkin CA et al: Correlation between respiratory symptoms and pulmonary function in asbestos-exposed workers, *Am Rev Respir Dis* 148:32, 1993.
15. Brooks SM, Weiss MA, Bernstein IL: Reactive airways dysfunction syndrome (RADS): persistent asthma syndrome after high level irritant exposures, *Chest* 88:376, 1985.
16. Charan NB et al: Pulmonary injuries associated with acute sulfur dioxide inhalation, *Am Rev Respir Dis* 119:555, 1979.
17. Churg A, Warnock ML, Green N: Analysis of the cores of ferruginous (asbestos) bodies from the general population II: true asbestos bodies and pseudoasbestos bodies, *Lab Invest* 40:31, 1979.
18. Churg J, Rosen SH, Moolten S: Histological characteristics of mesothelioma associated with asbestos, *Ann NY Acad Sci* 132:614, 1965.
19. Collis E, Gilchrist J: Effects of dust upon coal trimmers, *J Ind Hyg Toxicol* 10:101, 1928.
20. Committee of the Scientific Assembly on Environmental and Occupational Health of the American Thoracic Society: Diagnosis of nonmalignant diseases related to asbestos, *Am Rev Respir Dis* 134:363, 1986.
21. Cowie RL, Langton ME, Becklake MR: Pulmonary tuberculosis in South African gold miners, *Am Rev Respir Dis* 139:1086, 1989.
22. Craighead JE, Vallyathan NV: Cryptic pulmonary lesions in workers occupationally exposed to dust containing silica, *JAMA* 244:1939, 1980.
23. Craighead JE et al: Diseases associated with exposure to silica and nonfibrous silicate minerals, *Arch Pathol Lab Med* 112:673, 1988.
24. Davis GS: Pathogenesis of silicosis: current concepts and hypotheses, *Lung* 164:139, 1986.
25. Davis JMG: The pathology of asbestos related disease, *Thorax* 39:801, 1984.
26. Diller WF: Pathogenesis of phosgene poisoning, *Toxicol Ind Health* 1:7, 1985.
27. Diller WF: Late sequelae after phosgene poisoning: a literature review, *Toxicol Ind Health* 1:129, 1985.
28. do Pico GA: International workshop on health effects of organic dusts in the farm environment, Skokloster, Sweden: 23-25 April 1985, *Am J Ind Med* 10:261, 1986.
29. do Pico GA: Hazardous exposure and lung disease among farm workers, *Clin Chest Med* 13:311, 1992.
30. Eisenbud M et al: Nonoccupational berylliosis, *J Ind Hyg Toxicol* 31:282, 1949.
31. Empey DW et al: Mechanism of bronchial hyperreactivity in normal subjects after upper respiratory infection, *Am Rev Respir Dis* 113:131, 1976.
32. Environmental Protection Agency: *Managing asbestos in place: A building owner's guide to operations and maintenance programs for asbestos-containing materials*, Washington DC, 1990.
33. Finkelstein M, Kusiak R, Suranyi G: Mortality among miners receiving compensation for silicosis in Ontario: 1940-1975, *J Occup Med* 24:663, 1982.
34. Flaherty DK et al: Serologically detectable HLA-A, B, and C loci antigens in farmer's lung disease, *Am Rev Respir Dis* 122:437, 1980.
35. Fletcher DE, Edge JR: The early radiological changes in pulmonary and pleural asbestosis, *Clin Radiol* 21:355, 1970.
36. Flynn NM et al: An unusual outbreak of windborne coccidioidomycosis, *N Engl J Med* 301:358, 1979.
37. Frosolono MF, Holzman BH, Scarpelli EM: Cardiopulmonary response to phosgene inhalation and the effect of vagotomy, *Am Rev Respir Dis* 117(suppl):A234, 1978.
38. Fulmer JD: An introduction to the interstitial lung diseases, *Clin Chest Med* 3:457, 1982.

39. Gaensler EA: Asbestos exposure in buildings, *Clin Chest Med* 13:231, 1992.
40. Gaensler EA, Jederlinic PJ, McLoud TC: Radiographic progression of asbestosis with and without continued exposure. In *VIIth international pneumoconiosis conference* (NIOSH-ILO), DHHS (NIOSH) pub no 90-108 part I, Rockville, MD, 1990, National Institute for Occupational Safety and Health.
41. Gilchrist HL, Matz PB: The residual effects of warfare gases: the use of chlorine gas, with report of cases, *Med Bull VA* 9:229, 1933.
42. Golden J, Nadel JA, Boushey HA: Bronchial hyperirritability in healthy subjects after exposure to ozone, *Am Rev Respir Dis* 118:287, 1978.
43. Gregor A et al: Radiographic progression of asbestosis: a preliminary report, *Ann NY Acad Sci* 330:147, 1979.
44. Gylseth B, Mowe G, Wannag A: Fibre type and concentration in the lungs of workers in an asbestos cement factory, *Br J Ind Med* 40:375, 1983.
45. Hackney JD et al: Adaptation to short-term respiratory effects of ozone in men exposed repeatedly, *J Appl Physiol* 43:82, 1977.
46. Hammond EC, Selikoff IJ, Seidman H: Asbestos exposure, cigarette smoking and death rates, *Ann NY Acad Sci* 330:473, 1979.
47. Hammad YY, Rando RJ, Abdel-Kader H: Considerations in the design and use of human inhalation challenge systems, *Folia Allergol Immunol Clin* 32:37, 1985.
48. Hargreave FE, Woolcock AJ, editors: *Airway responsiveness: measurement and interpretation,* Mississauga, Ontario, 1985, Astra Pharmaceuticals Canada.
49. Harkonen H et al: Long-term effects of exposure to sulfur dioxide: lung function four years after a pyrite dust explosion, *Am Rev Respir Dis* 128:890, 1983.
50. Hasan FM, Kazemi H: Chronic beryllium disease: a continuing epidemiologic hazard, *Chest* 65:289, 1974.
51. Hearl FJ, Hewett PJ: Problems of monitoring dust levels within mines, *Occup Med* 8:93, 1993.
52. Hodous TK, Attfield MD: Progressive massive fibrosis developing on a background of minimal simple coal workers' pneumoconiosis. In *VIIth international pneumoconiosis conference* (NIOSH-ILO), DHHS (NIOSH) pub no 90-108 part I, Rockville, MD, 1990, National Institute for Occupational Safety and Health.
53. Horstman DH et al: Ozone concentration and pulmonary response relationships for 6.6 hour exposures with five hours of moderate exercise to 0.08, 0.10, and 0.12 ppm, *Am Rev Respir Dis* 142:1158, 1990.
54. Horvath EP et al: Nitrogen dioxide-induced pulmonary disease, *J Occup Med* 20:103, 1978.
55. Hourihane DO'B, Lessof L, Richardson PC: Hyaline and calcified pleural plaques as an index of exposure to asbestos: a study of radiological and pathological features of 100 cases with a consideration of epidemiology, *Br Med J* 1:1069, 1966.
56. Hughes JM et al: Determinants of progression in sandblasters' silicosis, *Ann Occup Hyg* 26:701, 1982.
57. International Labour Office: *Guidelines for the use of ILO international classification of radiographs of pneumoconioses,* (Occupational Safety and Health Series no 22 [rev.]), Geneva, 1980.
58. Jones RN et al: Lung function after acute chlorine exposure, *Am Rev Respir Dis* 134:1190, 1986.
59. Kamat SR et al: Early observations on pulmonary changes and clinical morbidity due to the isocyanate gas leak at Bhopal, *J Postgrad Med* 31:63, 1985.
60. Kamat SR et al: Sequential respiratory changes in those exposed to the gas leak at Bhopal, *Indian J Med Res* 86(suppl):20, 1987.
61. Kannerstein M, Churg J, McCaughey WTE: Asbestos and mesothelioma: a review, *Pathol Annu* 13:81, 1978.
62. Keller RH et al: Immunoregulation in hypersensitivity pneumonitis: phenotypic and functional studies of bronchoalveolar lavage lymphocytes, *Am Rev Respir Dis* 130:766, 1984.
63. Koenig JQ et al: Prior exposure to ozone potentiates subsequent response to sulfur dioxide in adolescent asthmatic subjects, *Am Rev Respir Dis* 141:377, 1990.
64. Leatherman JW et al: Lung T cells in hypersensitivity pneumonitis, *Ann Intern Med* 100:390, 1984.
65. Legg S, Cotes J, Bevan C: Lung mechanics in relation to radiographic category of coalworkers' simple pneumoconiosis, *Br J Ind Med* 40:28, 1983.
66. Legha SS, Muggia FM: Therapeutic approaches in malignant mesothelioma, *Cancer Treat Rev* 4:13, 1977.
67. Legha SS, Muggia FM: Pleural mesothelioma: clinical features and therapeutic implications, *Ann Intern Med* 87:613, 1977.
68. Lewis JF, Jobe AH: Surfactant and the adult respiratory distress syndrome, *Am Rev Respir Dis* 147:218, 1993.
69. Lowrie DB: What goes wrong with the macrophage in silicosis? *Eur J Respir Dis* 63:180, 1982.
70. Lynch KM, Smith WA: Pulmonary asbestosis III: carcinoma of lung in asbesto-silicosis, *Am J Cancer* 24:56, 1935.
71. Martin TR et al: Leukotriene B$_4$ production by the human alveolar macrophage: a potential mechanism for amplifying inflammation in the lung, *Am Rev Respir Dis* 129:106, 1984.
72. Mattson S-B, Ringqvist T: Pleural plaques and exposure to asbestos, *Scand J Respir Dis* 51(suppl 75):3, 1970.
73. Moore VL, Fink JN: Immunologic studies in hypersensitivity pneumonitis: quantitative precipitins and complement-fixing antibodies in symptomatic and asymptomatic pigeon breeders, *J Lab Clin Med* 85:540, 1975.
74. Morgan A, Holmes A: Concentration and dimension of coated and uncoated fibers in the human lungs, *Br J Ind Med* 37:25, 1980.
75. Morgan EJ: Silicosis and tuberculosis, *Chest* 75:202, 1979.
76. Morgan WKC et al: Ventilatory capacity and lung volumes of US coal miners, *Arch Environ Health* 28:182, 1974.
77. Mossman BT et al: Asbestos: scientific developments and implications for public policy, *Science* 247:294, 1990.
78. Muers MF et al: HLA-A, B, C, and HLA-DR antigens in extrinsic allergic alveolitis (budgerigar fancier's lung disease), *Clin Allergy* 12:47, 1982.
79. Murphy RLH Jr et al: Diagnosis of "asbestosis": observations from a longitudinal survey of shipyard pipe coverers, *Am J Med* 65:488, 1978.
80. Nemery B et al: Impairment of ventilatory function and pulmonary gas exchange in non-smoking coal miners, *Lancet* 1:1427, 1987.
81. Oxman AD et al: Occupational dust exposure and chronic obstructive pulmonary disease: a systematic overview of the evidence, *Am Rev Respir Dis* 148:38, 1993.
82. Paggiaro P, Rossi O, Bacci E: Prognosis of occupational asthma, *Folia Allergol Immunol Clin* 32:61, 1985.
83. Penington AH: War gases and chronic lung disease, *Med J Aust* 1:1510, 1954.
84. Pepys J, Hutchcroft BJ: Bronchial provocation tests in etiologic diagnosis and analysis of asthma, *Am Rev Respir Dis* 112:829, 1975.
85. Pisani RJ, Colby TV, Williams DE: Malignant mesothelioma of the pleura, *Mayo Clin Proc* 63:1234, 1988.
86. Prakash UBS, Reiman HM: Comparison of needle biopsy with cytologic analysis for the evaluation of pleural effusion: analysis of 414 cases, *Mayo Clin Proc* 60:158, 1985.
87. Ramsdell JW, Hauer D, Nachtwey FJ: Bronchial provocation testing. In Clausen JL, ed: *Pulmonary function testing: guidelines and controversies.* New York, 1982, Academic Press, pp 205-214.
88. Rasmussen KN, Faber V: Hyaluronic acid in 247 pleural fluids, *Scand J Respir Dis* 48:366, 1967.
89. Rodey GE et al: A study of HLA-A, B, C, and DR specificities in pigeon breeder's disease, *Am Rev Respir Dis* 114:755, 1979.
90. Rossman MD et al: Proliferative response of bronchoalveolar lymphocytes to beryllium: a test for chronic beryllium disease, *Ann Intern Med* 108:687, 1988.

91. Saccone A, Coblenz A: Endothelioma of the pleura with a report of two cases, *Am J Clin Pathol* 13:186, 1943.
92. Saltini C et al: Maintenance of alveolitis in patients with chronic beryllium disease by beryllium-specific helper T cells, *N Engl J Med* 320:1103, 1989.
93. Schwartz DA, Smith DD, Lakshiminarayan S: The pulmonary sequelae associated with accidental inhalation of chlorine gas, *Chest* 97:820, 1990.
94. Seidman H, Selikoff IJ, Hammond EC: Short-term asbestos work exposure and long-term observation, *Ann NY Acad Sci* 330:61, 1979.
95. Selikoff IJ, Hammond EC: Asbestos-associated disease in United States shipyards, *CA* 28:87, 1978.
96. Sharma PN, Gaur KJ: Radiological spectrum of lung changes in gas-exposed victims, *Indian J Med Res* 86:39, 1987.
97. Sheppard D et al: Lower threshold and greater bronchomotor responsiveness of asthmatic subjects to sulfur dioxide, *Am Rev Respir Dis* 122:873, 1980.
98. Sheppard D et al: Tolerance to sulfur dioxide–induced bronchoconstriction in subjects with asthma, *Environ Res* 30:412, 1983.
99. Sheppard D et al: Mechanism of cough and bronchoconstriction induced by distilled water aerosol, *Am Rev Respir Dis* 127:691, 1983.
100. Sherson D, Lander F: Morbidity of pulmonary tuberculosis among silicotic and nonsilicotic foundry workers, *J Occup Med* 32:110, 1990.
101. Snider DE: The relationship between tuberculosis and silicosis, *Am Rev Respir Dis* 118:455, 1978.
102. Spooner CM: Air measurements of dusts, chemicals and fumes, *Clin Chest Med* 13:179, 1992.
103. Sprince NL, Kazemi H, Hardy HL: Current (1975) problem of differentiating between beryllium disease and sarcoidosis, *Ann NY Acad Sci* 278:654, 1976.
104. Stenton SC, Hendrick DJ: Airflow obstruction and mining, *Occup Med* 8:155, 1993.
105. Thompson AB, Rennard SI: Assessment of airways inflammation utilizing bronchoalveolar lavage, *Clin Chest Med* 9:635, 1988.
106. Thomson JG: The pathogenesis of pleural plaques. In Shapiro HA, ed: *Pneumoconiosis: proceedings of the international conference, Johannesburg, 1969.* Cape Town, 1970, Oxford University Press, pp 138-141.
107. Wagner JC: Asbestos carcinogenesis, *Br J Cancer* 32:258, 1975.
108. Wagner JC, Sleggs CA, Marchand P: Diffuse pleural mesthelioma and asbestos exposure in the North Western Cape Province, *Br J Ind Med* 17:260, 1960.
109. Weg J et al: Safety and efficacy of an aerosolized surfactant (Exosurf) in human sepsis-induced ARDS, *Chest* 100(suppl):S137, 1991.
110. Weill H: Disaster at Bhopal: the accident, early findings and respiratory health outlook in those injured, *Bull Eur Physiopathol Respir* 23:587, 1987.
111. Weill H, Hughes J: Asbestos as a public health risk: disease and policy, *Am Rev Public Health* 7:171, 1986.
112. Weill H et al: Late evaluation of pulmonary function after acute exposure to chlorine gas, *Am Rev Respir Dis* 99:374, 1969.
113. Westerholm P: Silicosis: observations on a case register, *Scand J Work Environ Health* 6(suppl 2):1, 1980.
114. Wheat LJ et al: A large urban outbreak of histoplasmosis: clinical features, *Ann Intern Med* 94:331, 1981.
115. Wiedemann H et al: A multicenter trial in human sepsis-induced ARDS of an aerosolized synthetic surfactant (Exosurf), *Am Rev Respir Dis* 145:A184, 1992.
116. Woolcock AJ: Asthma. In Murray JF, Nadel JA, editors: *Textbook of respiratory medicine,* Philadelphia, 1988, WB Saunders, pp 1030-1068.
117. Ziskind M, Jones RN, Weill H: Silicosis, *Am Rev Respir Dis* 113:643, 1976.

Chapter 24

GASTROINTESTINAL TRACT AND LIVER

Todd McCune
Stuart M. Brooks

Gastrointestingal defense mechanisms
    Overview
    Luminal defense
    Mucosal defense
    Xenobiotic metabolism
    Immunologic defense
Gastrointestinal absorption
Gastrointestinal nervous control
    Autonomic nervous system
    Sympathetic (adrenergic) system
    Parasympathetic (cholinergic) system
The liver
    Anatomy
    Enterohepatic circulation
Hepatotoxicity
    Predictable and unpredictable hepatotoxicity
    Direct and indirect hepatotoxins
    Drug-related hepatotoxicity
    Selective zonal hepatotoxicity
    Hepatocyte form and function
    Cytochrome P450
    Pathology of hepatotoxicity
    Pathophysiologic correlations
    Clinical correlations
Exposure types and sources
Clinical presentations of gastrointestinal-induced disorders
    Patterns of clinical response
    Acute poisoning
    Suspected subacute environmental toxicity
Biologic markers
    Overview
    Biomarkers of liver function
    Research needs
Cancer
Trial of therapy with an N of 1
    Overview
    Method for "N of 1" trial

Although it is not a leading organ system for occupational illness, the gastrointestinal system potentially serves as a major route of exposure for environmental toxins.[65] Consequently considerable scientific attention is focused on elucidating the pathophysiologic mechanisms, epidemiologic factors, and clinical experience of potential gastrointestinal chemical environmental hazards. It is anticipated that these efforts will enable more accurate public health risk assessments and improve the diagnostic, treatment, or prognostic judgments involving these substances.[68] As in many other aspects of environmental medicine however the practitioner and public health officials must have a clear conception of the empirical basis for decision-making in these matters. At one end of the spectrum our knowledge of pathophysiologic mechanisms may be sufficient to enable pinpoint diagnostic accuracy, efficacious treatment, sound prognostic accuracy, and clear public health policy recommendations.[60] Even without clear mechanistic models certain environmental stressors are sufficiently toxic and prevalent in the United States so that clinical experience enables practical guidance when one raises similar clinical or public health questions. When clinical experience is too infrequent the clinician may have enough epidemiologic evidence available to enable useful decisions in these areas.[25,85] All too often however even the epidemiologic experience with environmental toxins is inadequate to make the types of reliable, interpersonally consistent judgments that define scientific accuracy.[31] As our pathophysiologic or empirical knowledge decreases scientists and clinicians must rely more and more on philosophic arguments to answer these types of diagnostic, treatment, prognostic, and public health questions.[1,13,14,30,62] While the pathophysiologic and empirical understanding of environmental hazards to the gastrointestinal system is often quite limited,[32] the gastrointestinal system offers a unique opportunity to approach certain environmental exposures in a manner that is familiar to physicians and that complements their typical "reductionist" view of medical problems.[89]

Despite the enormous potential for exposure to environmental toxicants, the gastrointestinal tract is generally not regarded as a major target organ system for occupational chemicals.[24] The U.S. Department of Health and Human Services however reports that at least 20% of waterborne disease outbreaks are due to chemical poisoning. Furthermore they cannot identify an etiologic agent in approximately 50% of these outbreaks.[17] Although the overall number of national waterborne disease outbreaks is only about 13 per year, the number of chemical poisoning outbreaks have increased, particularly over the past 20 years.[101]

GASTROINTESTINAL DEFENSE MECHANISMS
Overview

Recent investigations have explored the complex interaction of host immune and nonimmune defense factors and their influence on xenobiotic substances, both natural and man-made.[36,37,61] Knowledge of these defense mechanisms and how they are influenced by diet, age, and sex should warn physicians about the importance of confounding factors when dealing with gastrointestinal illness.

Food and water enter the body and make contact with millions of projecting microvilli that present a massive mucosal surface area, some 200 times greater than the body's surface area.[36] The ingested material may contain biologic or infectious agents (for example, bacteria, viruses, protozoa, parasites); food or plant substances; or toxic agents or xenobiotics present in the food and water. The various components of the gastrointestinal defense system include intestinal secretions, enzymes, mucus, bacterial microflora, epithelium, and the immune system. There is also mucosal metabolism, excretion, and cell exfoliation.

The intestinal mucosa is an important entry site due to its vast numbers of islands of projecting intestinal microvilli that create a tremendous surface area for contact by an environmental chemical. In order for the foreign chemical (xenobiotic) to enter the body and pass into the circulation, the xenobiotic must prevail over a number of defense barriers. Fig. 24-1 depicts the various barriers an environmental chemical must pass through before it can be absorbed by the gastrointestinal mucosa and into the vascular space. The following discussion briefly explores each of the barriers.

Luminal defense

As the foreign chemical enters the gut lumen it mixes with large volumes of intestinal fluids and solids that may alter its properties and concentration or may cause chemical and enzymatic alterations to evolve (for example, changes in pH may alter a chemicals reactivity). The unstirred layer is the first layer that the xenobiotic or gastrointestinal toxi-

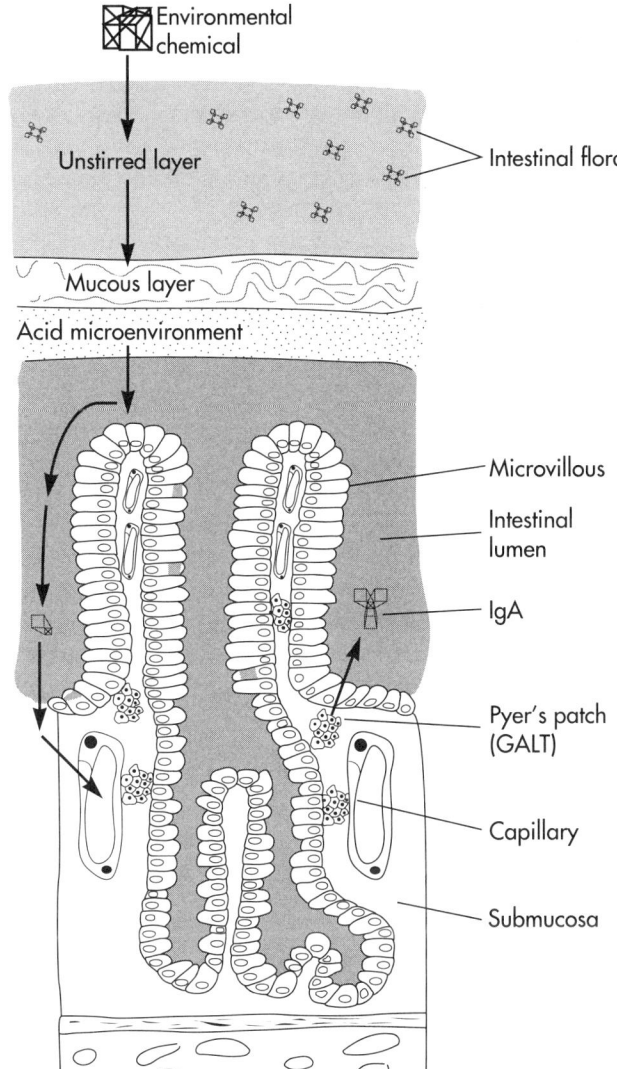

Fig. 24-1. The various barriers an environmental chemical must pass through before it can be absorbed by the gastrointestinal mucosa and into the vascular space.

cant must cross before reaching the mucosal surface, and its presence can retard intestinal absorption of some xenobiotics.[94,99] The "unstirred layer" is the name given to the layer of fluid abutting the mucosa and consists of a relatively immobile layer, a mucus component, and the glycocalyx or acidic mucopolysaccharides present directly on the surface of the microvilli. Gastrointestinal mucus consists mainly of water mixed with glycoproteins and small concentrations of salts, nucleic acids, and proteins; it forms a continuous gelatinous coat over the mucosal surface and is the second layer that xenobiotics must cross.[73] The mucus may act as a diffusion barrier for hydrogen ion. It is an important barrier to water electrolytes and small molecules, and may trap heavy metals.[36] It also provides a defense for biologic agents and furnishes a matrix for immunoglobulins. An acid microclimate composed of a proton-rich sheet, approximately 20 μm thick and acidic in nature (pH 5.9 vs. the higher pH of 7.3 noted elsewhere), makes up the third layer for passage and influences the permeability of weak acids and bases.[59] Microorganisms making up the intestinal flora within the intestinal lumen play an important role in the metabolism of foreign compounds.[87,92] The greatest change in intestinal flora numbers occurs between the proximal small intestine and the ileum, where concentrations increase several magnitudes; the most dramatic change is at the ileocecal valve, where bacterial counts of 10^9 to 10^{12} microorganisms per gram of feces are noted.

Mucosal defense

The mucosa of the microvilli presents the final hurdle for the xenobiotic before entry into the circulation. The intestinal epithelial cells perform a variety of functions, including the secretion of mucous, accomplishing metabolic functions, and achieving absorption. A chemical penetrates the epithelial surface cover (or glycocalyx). After the glycocalyx the xenobiotic passes through the cell's apical membrane, through the body of the cell, and finally through the cell's basolateral membrane. The apical membrane is composed of two molecular layers of lipids in opposition with fused outer layers (some 9.5 to 11.5 nm thick) that form a tight junction between adjacent cells and maintains an effective barrier between the intestinal content and the intercellular space.[12] The apical membrane contains a number of enzyme and transport systems that are capable of biotransforming various substances. The epithelial cell body itself also affords a barrier to the transfer of xenobiotics. Once the xenobiotic passes through the cell contents, it traverses the bilayer basal membrane of the epithelial cell and enters the narrow, water-filled extracellular space that separates the cell from its basement membrane. The chemical then passes through the basement membrane into the submucosa and penetrates the membrane of the villous capillary.[20] The capillary membrane contains pores or openings about 40 to 50 nm wide covered by a very thin mucoploysaccharide membrane that allows entrance into the circulation. The villus capillary endothelial cells incorporate fenestrae that comprise approximately 10% of the capillary surface area. The fenestrae membrane contains almost no lipid, thus enabling xenobiotic transport.

Xenobiotic metabolism

The intestinal mucosa has a metabolic enzyme capacity that is similar to the liver. It is able to metabolize xenobiotics and potentially has the capability to detoxify chemicals.[35,42] Phase I and phase II reactions occur, embodying the mucosal mixed-function oxidase system as well as other enzyme systems for metabolic conversion of xenobiotics, including uridine diphosphoglucuronyltransferase, sulfotransferases, and glutathione-S-transferases. An "intestinal first-pass effect" is a term used to differentiate intestinal cell metabolism from metabolism occurring as part of a "liver first-pass effect" or the metabolism by the intestinal microflora.[28] Like the liver, the gut metabolic enzyme system can lead to the bioactivation of a chemical and its increased toxicity or carcinogenicity.[5]

Age, diet, nutritional status, and exposure to other chemicals can change a xenobiotics intestinal biotransformation activity.[36] Mucosal secretions and shedding of mucosal cells are also valuable defense mechanisms.[56,58] The gut can function as an excretory organ and secrete such reactive agents as quaternary ammonium compounds and strong acids. Gastrointestinal epithelial cells have a rapid turnover rate approaching one cell per 100 cells per hour, and it has been estimated that the intestine sheds billions of cells per day.

Although the oxidative metabolism of xenobiotic compounds usually associated with the liver often begins within the intestinal mucosa, clinical assessment of its importance is not possible. Sensitive tests of liver metabolism exist that may enable early recognition of adverse effects before they progress to irreversible, chronic disease.[51] Because they swallow so many foreign agents, humans have evolved an elaborate gastrointestinal defense system.[103] The last "wall" in that defense is the immune system.

Immunologic defense

The gut-associated lymphoid tissue (GALT), which includes clusters of nodular lymphoid tissue (Peyer's patches), solitary mucosal lymphoid follicles, and solitary mucosal cells arranged throughout the entire gastrointestinal mucosa, protects individuals from biologic agents and xenobiotics.[91] Peyer's patches are aggregates of lymphoid tissue distributed just below the epithelium and are capable of absorbing macromolecules particulate. The lymphoid cells can migrate into the circulation via the mesenteric nodes and thoracic duct, and from the circulation they can migrate back to the mucosa or other tissue sites. Exchange of information between one mucosal site and another occurs through this migratory pathway of intestinal lymphoid cells, a common mucosa-associated lymphoid system (MALT) that is widely distributed in the gut, the lung, part of the urogenital tract, mammary glands, the conjunctiva, middle ear, and lacrimal and salivary glands has been identified.[8]

An important immunologic defense at the mucosal surface is the availability of IgA antibodies in the intestinal secretions.[61] The bimeric IgA with its secretory component detected in intestinal secretions is structurally different from monomeric IgA present in the serum. Intestinal antibodies function to bind antigens in the intestine and limit their absorption, prevent bacteria from adhering to the intestinal mucosal surface, control the proliferation and mucosal penetration of bacteria, neutralize viruses in the absence of complement, and protect the bowel mucosa from injury resulting from continuous antigen exposure. The intestine also contains IgG and IgM antibodies and is rich in IgE antibodies. The intestinal mucosa also demonstrates cell-mediated immunologic capabilities. Nutrition plays a critical role in the intestinal immunologic structure and function.

GASTROINTESTINAL ABSORPTION

The absorption area of the gastrointestinal tract is approximately 250 square meters. In addition, most particulate matter inhaled by the lungs eventually enters the gastrointestinal tract by way of the bronchial mucociliary system. Consequently substances that initially enter the lungs in particulate form may become absorbed once acted on by digestive processes. Clearly the potential for systemic absorption is of great interest when environmental toxins abound. The complexity of gastrointestinal physiology is augmented by its close interaction with the nervous system. These interactions enable gastrointestinal problems to occur through neurologic mechanisms ranging from conscious psychologic stress to peripheral nerve chemical blockade.

Xenobiotics enter the intestine in a manner similar to nutrients, by diffusion, facilitated diffusion, active transport, and pinocytosis.[36,42] Absorption is also influenced by a chemical's water solubility, degree of ionization, "solvent drag," and molecular size, as well as gastric emptying time, intestinal motility, surface area of the small intestine, intestinal blood flow, diet, genetic factors, and so on.[36,42,74] A significant volume of fluid is secreted each day that serves to dilute further whatever concentration of chemical exists in ingested food or drink.[86]

Gastrointestinal flora, although capable of diverse types of chemical transformations, often promote molecular transformations that facilitate systemic absorption rather than promote excretion. In other words, intestinal bacteria often convert poorly absorbed polar compounds into nonpolar lipophilic substances. The lipophilic substances can then cross cell membranes more easily and thereby enter the systemic circulation. Since diet affects intestinal bacterial enzyme activity, it is not surprising to find a correlation between colon cancer and certain types of diets, especially those rich in beef fat and low in fiber.[93] Diet can also affect the mucosa's ability to metabolize xenobiotics.

GASTROINTESTINAL NERVOUS CONTROL
Autonomic nervous system

The autonomic nervous system (ANS) supplies all structures of the body except skeletal muscles. Although it controls or influences many bodily functions such as respiration, circulation, metabolism, and temperature, we focus on its gastrointestinal effects. The ANS is divided into two subsystems called the sympathetic and parasympathetic nervous systems. In general, these two subsystems are physiologic antagonists, and the gastrointestinal system is innervated by both. The sympathetic fibers, acting through intermediate ganglia, utilize various catecholamines as neurotransmitters, whereas the parasympathetic system utilizes acetylcholine as a peripheral neurotransmitter, as do the peripheral somatic nerves that innervate skeletal muscle.

Sympathetic (adrenergic) system

The sympathetic nervous system uses a variety of adrenergic neurotransmitters such as epinephrine, dopamine, and norepinephrine. It is norepinephrine that innervates the gastrointestinal tract (along with the skin, eyes, heart, lungs, and exocrine glands). There are two basic types of adrenergic receptors, alpha and beta, which are differentiated on the basis of their response to catecholamines and various adrenoreceptor blocking agents.

Of the two basic types of adrenergic receptors the alpha receptors are the primary type found in the gastrointestinal tract. Alpha receptors are further divided into alpha 1 and alpha 2 receptors. Alpha 1 receptors are primarily located in the postjunctional location of nerves arising in the sympathetic ganglion. These alpha 1 receptors initiate postsynaptic smooth muscle contraction and exocrine gland activity. Alpha 2 receptors act primarily on the presynaptic release of norepinephrine, thereby inhibiting postganglionic nerve activity. In this way the alpha 1 and 2 receptors provide a feedback mechanism for controlling sympathetic system input into the gastrointestinal tract.

Parasympathetic (cholinergic) system

Any parasympathomimetic drug or toxin affects acetylcholine (cholinergic) receptors in the central nervous system, all autonomic ganglia, the somatic neuromuscular junction, all postganglionic parasympathetic fibers, and the adrenal medulla. Cholinergic receptors are further classified into muscarinic and nicotinic receptors. Muscarinic receptors are located in postganglionic parasympathetic fibers and autonomic ganglia as well as cortical and subcortical neurons. Consequently those compounds or drugs with muscarinic properties affect both the peripheral and central nervous systems. Signs of muscarinic stimulation include miosis, vasodilation, bradycardia, depressed myocardial contractility, bronchorrea, increased gut motility, micturation, and sweating. Atropine and the belladonna alkaloids inhibit muscarinic effects. In general, clinical effects resemble sympathomimetic actions (for example, elevated blood pressure and temperature, erythema, delirium, and mydriasis) except that parasympathetic agents produce silent bowel sounds and dry skin. Nicotinic actions primarily affect the neuromuscular junction and the muscarinic effects of the autonomic ganglion.

THE LIVER

The liver has many important functions that are essential to survival (Fig. 24-2). These include homeostasis of nutrients such as glucose, lipids, and amino acids. The liver is particularly important for preventing the body from having excessive levels of glucose after a meal and deficient levels

302 CLINICAL ENVIRONMENTAL MEDICINE

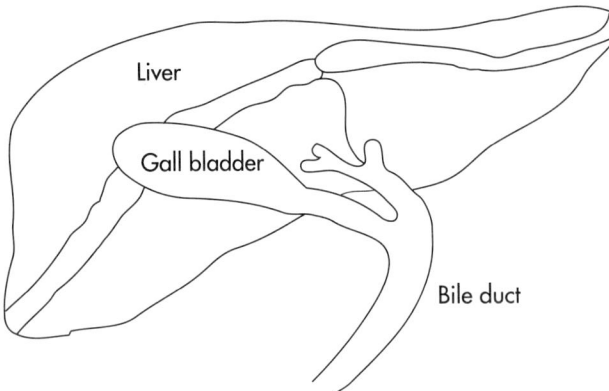

Fig. 24-2. The gross anatomy of the liver, gall bladder, and bile ducts. The liver's important functions include: maintenance of homeostasis of glucose, lipids, and amino acids; filtering intestinal bacterial products; manufacturing bile; synthesizing plasma proteins; and detoxifying xenobiotic compounds.

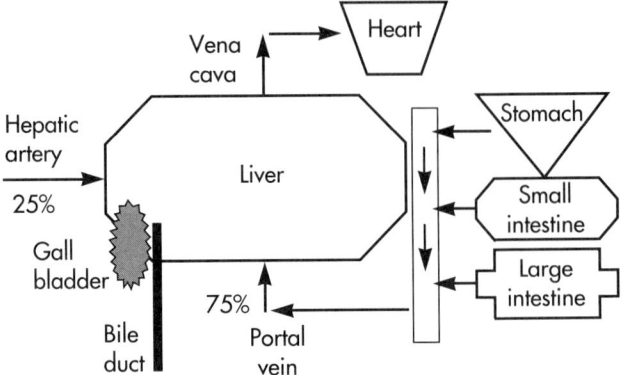

Fig. 24-3. The liver has a dual blood supply, with the hepatic artery supplying about 25% to 30% of the liver's blood and the portal vein supplying most of the liver's blood (70% to 75%). The portal vein derives its blood from the venous return from the gut and is rich in nutrients from the small intestine and waste products from the large intestine.

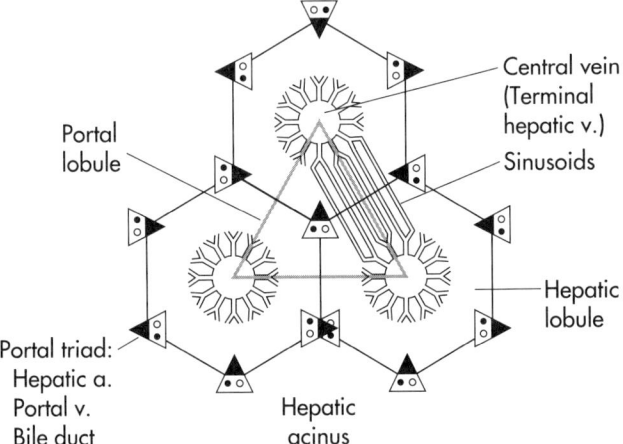

Fig. 24-4. The classic hepatic lobule is divided into the periportal area, which is around the portal triad; the mid-zonal region; and the centrilobular region, which is around the central vein. The portal vein and the hepatic artery enter the liver parenchyma together and both transport their blood into hepatic sinusoids. The blood eventually exits the sinusoids at the level of the terminal hepatic venules or the central vein.

between meals. The liver also filters intestinal bacterial products, manufactures bile, and synthesizes plasma proteins such as clotting factors and albumin. Of particular interest, however, is the liver's ability to detoxify a large number of endogenous and exogenous xenobiotic compounds.

Anatomy

An important anatomic feature of the liver is its dual blood supply (Fig. 24-3). The hepatic artery supplies about 25% to 30% of the liver's blood. This blood is well oxygenated, whereas the portal vein, which supplies most of the liver's blood (70% to 75%) is not as well oxygenated. The portal vein derives its blood from the venous output of the stomach, small and large intestine, and also, to some extent, the spleen. Consequently the portal blood is rich in nutrients taken up from the small intestinal and waste products taken up from the large intestine.

The portal vein and the hepatic artery enter the liver parenchyma together, and both transport their blood into hepatic sinusoids (Fig. 24-4). The blood eventually exits the sinusoids at the level of the terminal hepatic venules or the central vein. Until relatively recently the hepatocytes were believed to perform the vast majority of liver functions. There is increasing evidence, however, that the endothelial cells that line the sinusoid, and the Kupffer's cells, which are liver macrophages, also play a significant role reacting with certain types of endogenous and xenobiotic substances. The blood, once it enters the sinusoids, flows toward the central vein, where it eventually leaves the liver through the hepatic vein and enters the systemic circulation via the inferior vena cava.[83]

Two models are used to describe the liver's microanatomy (Fig. 24-4). The first is called the classic hepatic lobule, which is centered around the central vein and is divided into three units: the periportal area, which is around the portal triad; the mid-zonal region; and the centrilobular region, which is around the central vein. The hepatic "acinus" is a more contemporary anatomical conception of the liver's functional anatomy (Fig. 24-5), which better describes liver function in relation to its blood supply. The acinus is centered around the portal tract instead of the central vein. Zone I is the region closest to the portal triad. Zone III is the region furthest from the portal triad, which corresponds to the classic model's centrilobular region. The intermediate area, between these two zones, is Zone II. As Fig. 24-5 demonstrates, the classic and acinar models closely resemble each other in that Zone III of the acinar model is very similar to

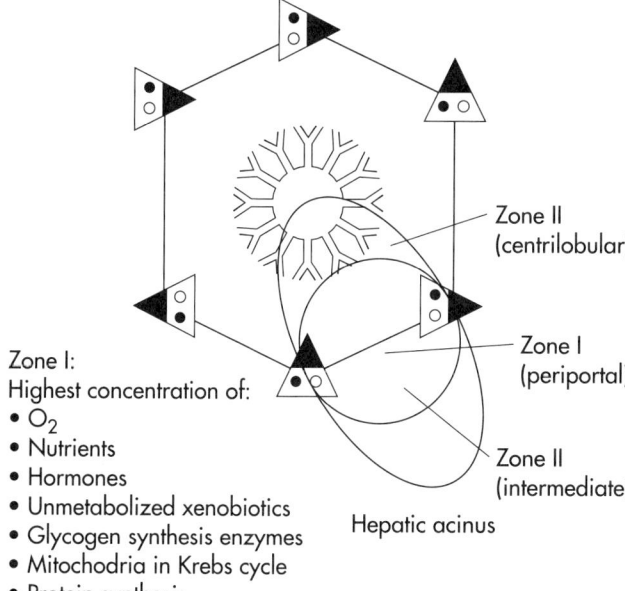

Fig. 24-5. The hepatic "acinus" is an anatomic conception of the liver's functional anatomy that is centered around the portal tract and describes liver function in relation to its blood supply. There are various functional zones identified, including Zone I, which is the region closest, and Zone III, the region farthest from the portal triad.

the centrilobular region of the liver, and Zone I is very similar to the periportal region. Certain toxins damage specific regions of the liver depending on their pathophysiology.[4,15,49] There are also relatively specific biomarkers of damage for Zones I and III.[33] These are discussed in more detail later.

Enterohepatic circulation

The liver first forms then secretes bile into the bile ductules, which lead to the bile ducts and eventually the gall bladder for storage. The bile is released into the duodenum in response to ingested fat. Bile salts are the major component of bile and enable the uptake of lipids present in the diet. After bile acids are released into the intestine, their uptake process begins and is eventually completed when the bile acids reach the end of the small intestine. At the ileum they are removed from the intestine and reenter the portal blood. On their return to the hepatocytes these bile acids are rapidly extracted then transported through the hepatocyte back into the bile ductules. The process just described is called the enterohepatic circulation.

The liver forms bile through a number of pathways, including (1) uptake of bile salts at the sinusoidal or plasma membrane, (2) the vesicular endocytosis and translocation of proteins, (3) the pericellular diffusion pathway, and (4) the uptake and secretion of organic ions such as bilirubin. Bilirubin is picked up by a transporter and conjugated inside the cell with glucuronide. Other important pathways of bile formation involve the excretion of metals such as copper, iron, and manganese. In some cases, for example, in copper and manganese, this mechanism is very important for the removal of these toxic metals from the body.

HEPATOTOXICITY
Predictable and unpredictable hepatotoxicity

A number of xenobiotic compounds have a predilection for damaging one particular zone (using the acinar model) (Table 24-1 and Fig. 24-5). Hepatotoxicity can also be classified according to intrinsic (predictable) and idiosyncratic (unpredictable) categories.[107] An intrinsic hepatotoxin usually affects the hepatic lobule in a pharmacologic manner. That is to say, the predictable hepatotoxin damages the liver in a way that is dose-dependent. It appears that reactive metabolites cause injury either directly.[77,81] Either way, larger doses cause more damage. Intrinsic toxins are consequently more predictable in their effect on animals or human beings. Histologically, liver injury is further classified by the presence of cholestasis, steatosis, necrosis, cirrhosis, and fibrosis (Table 24-1). More recent attention has focused on the role of inflammatory cells (i.e., macrophages) in hepatotoxicity.[55]

Direct and indirect hepatotoxins

As mentioned, intrinsic hepatotoxins are further subdivided into "direct" and "indirect" hepatotoxins. Apparently, reactive metabolites cause injury directly by covalently altering cellular macromolecules or indirectly by oxidizing cellular components through reactive intermediates such as hydrogen peroxide, hydroxyl radicals, or lipid peroxides.[77,81] Examples of direct hepatotoxins are carbon tetrachloride, chloroform, and acetaminophen. Both direct and indirect hepatotoxins cause necrosis- or steatosis-type injury patterns, but dose-dependent cholestatic (biliary stasis) injury patterns are more likely secondary to indirect hepatotoxins.

Drug-related hepatotoxicity

Many drugs and chemicals produce hepatic damage *unpredictably* in a small number of those exposed to these substances. In fact, the majority of drugs that cause hepatotoxicity appear to act in an idiosyncratic manner.[77] There are two hypothesized explanations for the unpredictable, idio-

Table 24-1. Pathological changes associated with various hepatotoxicants

Pathology	Agent
Necrosis (Centrilobular—Zone 3)	Aspirin, acetaminophen, carbon tetrachloride, mycotoxins, tetrachlorethane, phalloidin, isoniazid, methyldopa, halothane, papaverine, propylthiouracil, sulfonamides, polychlorinated biphenyls (PCBs)
Periportal (Zone 1)	Allyl alcohol, iron, manganese, N-hydroxy-2-acetylaminofluorene
Cholestasis (Biliary tract)	Chlopromazine, erythromycin estolate, arsenic, methylenediamine, dinitrophenol, chromium, anabolic steroids, estrogens, a-napthyliosthiocyanate (ANIT) 4,4'-methylene dianiline (MDA), 1-(2-chloroethyl)-3-cyclo-hexyl-1-nitrosurea (CCNU)
Fatty	Ethanol, corticosteroids, organochlorine pesticides, 2,3,7,8-tetrachlorodibenzodioxin, chlordecone
Fibrosis	Ethanol, methaotrexate, aflatoxins, arsenic
Vascular	Oral contraceptives, anabolic steroids, radiation
Granuloma	Beryllium
Carcinoma	Oral contraceptives, aflatoxin, ethanol, thorium dioxide, vinyl chloride, anabolic steroids, arsenic
Angiosarcoma	Vinyl chloride, arsenic thoratrast, copper sulfate
Adenoma	Oral contraceptives, androgens

syncratic nature of these reactions. The mechanism thought most prevalent is an allergic- or hypersensitivity-type immunologic reaction.[18] There are well-known examples of drug hypersensitivity (fever, rash, eosinophilia developing 1 to 5 weeks after initiation of therapy and recurring after one or two challenge doses) that support an immune mechanism. However, the absence of these signs does not exclude an immunologic etiology, since cell-mediated immunity may be involved. The alternative explanation for idiosyncratic hepatotoxicity involves the variable biochemical makeup of different individuals. An individual might have "abnormally" high or low levels of enzymes that activate or deactivate absorbed toxins. We will briefly discuss the evidence supporting the immunologic and biochemical explanations for idiosyncratic liver toxicity after elaborating on the zonal biochemical specificity of the liver.

Selective zonal hepatotoxicity

There are a number of physiologic reasons for zonal selectivity. (1) There is a difference in the nutrient concentration experienced by Zone I hepatocytes in comparison to those in Zone III. (2) Hepatocytes in Zone III have glutathione transferase, which is absent from hepatocytes in Zone I. (3) There is also an oxygen gradient as the blood flows from Zone I toward Zone III (Fig. 24-5). In fact, within a distance of 10 hepatocytes there is a drop in oxygen concentration of 280 torr using an isolated perfused liver model.[100] This oxygen gradient is of particular interest in understanding the liver's response to various toxicants. (4) The hepatocytes in Zone I remove bile salts as they enter the sinusoid, so well that under normal circumstances very little if any bile salts reach Zone III, and essentially none leaves the liver.[5,22] (5) Zone III have higher concentrations of cytochrome P450 enzymes.

Hepatocyte form and function

Hepatocytes possess contractile ability and can partially contract around the bile canaliculi. These contractions "milk" the bile salts down the canalicular lumen toward the biliary tract. This milking action is the result of a cytoskeletal network of actin and myosin arranged around the bile canaliculi. There are several hepatotoxins, particularly the mushroom toxin phalloidin, that alter or impair the function of this contracting ability of the canaliculus.

There are a variety of differences between Zone I and Zone III hepatocytes (Fig. 24-5). Several of these have already been mentioned, such as the higher oxygen tension, glutathione levels, and others. Examples of Zone I toxins also include iron overload. The toxicity of iron involves stimulation of lipid peroxidation. The Zone I cells are more affected by this process because they store more iron than Zone III hepatocytes. Allyl alcohol's toxicity involves the oxidation to acrolein. This process is oxygen-dependent and hence the conversion is more efficient in Zone I cells.

In contrast, Zone III hepatocytes have higher concentrations of many different P450 cytochrome isozymes and glutathione transferase enzymes. The classic Zone III toxicant is carbon tetrachloride. Its mechanism of injury begins with activation of cytochrome P450 to a carbon tetrachloride free radical. The explanation for why it is a Zone III toxin, besides the high level of cytochrome P450 enzymes, is the relatively low level of oxygen in these cells. Oxygen is a competitive inhibitor of the P450 activation process. The primary effect of ethyl alcohol is in Zone III. Once again this selective toxicity is believed to be secondary to the relatively low oxygen tension in this area. The explanation of why acetaminophen is a Zone III hepatotoxin involves an imbalance between its activation by cytochrome P450 and detoxification by glutathione-dependent processes. In the case of acetaminophen, toxicity results from the lack of cytochrome P450 enzymes in Zone III combined with the relative lack of glutathione.[70]

Cytochrome P450

Hepatic injury often involves bioactivation and oxidative processes.[34,70,71,76] Many of the oxidative bioactivations can be attributed to cytochrome P450, although there are a number of other oxidative mechanisms. An important concept involves the multiplicity of P450 forms.[79] An understanding of such P450 mechanisms helps explain the clinical situation where an apparent idiosyncratic reaction affected a handful of individuals who developed life-threatening side effects from combining terfenadine and ketoconazole.[75,106]

It may not be appropriate to classify cytochrome P450 enzymes according to reaction type. With the right substrate P450 can catalyze a multitude of different types of chemical reactions. Structural features of the enzyme also dictate whether an appropriately oriented substrate can actually be oxidized. For example, although the structure of cytochrome P450 enzymes may be quite similar between different species, the function of these enzymes may be quite different. Recent investigations have divulged that altering a single amino acid can drastically alter an enzyme's catalytic properties. Consequently two enzymes can maintain a considerable amount of structural similarity but have just enough dissimilarity so that they no longer resemble each other functionally. Conversely, one can take two enzymes with very low structural similarity and they may still catalyze the same chemical reaction.

Cytochrome P450s are considered part of the same family if they are greater than 40% identical in amino acid sequence. If they are identical in greater than 55% of the same amino acid sequences, they will be placed into the same subfamily.[69] As a result of the above structural variability in cytochrome P450 enzymes it is not possible to predict with certainty how a human cytochrome P450 will function based on activities of its counterpart in another species. Although one isozyme often predominates in the metabolism of a substrate, more than one isozyme may contribute to a chemical's biotransformation. The complexity is magnified when one considers toxin interactions (such as induction or inhibition), hormonal influences, and the effect of diet, age, etc. Toxicologists are still a long way from being able to rationalize and predict all toxic reactions for individual patients.

Pathology of hepatotoxicity

Hepatic histotoxicity is expressed in a limited number of ways morphologically. The morphologic patterns of liver damage include steatosis (fatty liver), necrosis, cholestasis, fibrosis/cirrhosis, vascular, and neoplasia[107] (see Table 24-1). Zone III, or pericentral, necrosis is the hallmark of a number of chemicals, including acetaminophen, aflatoxins, botulinus toxins, carbon tetrachloride, and phalloidin. Examples of Zone I, or periportal, toxins include allyl alcohol, ferrous sulfate, N-Hydroxy-2-acetylaminofluorene, and manganese. There are also a number of toxicants that particularly damage the biliary tract. These include a-Napthylisothiocyanant (ANIT), 4-4-methylene dianiline (MDA), and the chemotherapeutic agent CCNU.[4,15,49]

Pathophysiologic correlations

One can anticipate an intrinsic toxicant to some extent if (1) there is evidence of preferential accumulation of toxicants in the cells of one zone or the other, (2) there is a difference in the acinar distribution of enzyme processes or transport mechanisms responsible for converting a toxicant into intermediates that cause cell damage, and (3) glutathione, which helps repair the damage from lipid peroxidation, is in much lower concentration in Zone III cells than in Zone I cells. When the location of different types of biochemical reactions vary within a single organ, the result can be distinctive patterns of hepatocellular damage. These distinctive patterns may facilitate diagnosis of environmental disease if (1) one suspects exposure to a chemical known to produce dose-dependent selective zonal effects, (2) there are adequate biomarkers to selectively detect biochemical alterations in the different zones, (3) there are no significant confounding factors that might better account for biomarker alterations, and (4) your preliminary conclusions are confirmed by further investigation. Fig. 24-6 diagrammatically illustrates the metabolic routes of a xenobiotic and its metabolite(s).

Clinical correlations

Idiosyncratic reactions are more likely immunologically determined but may reflect an inborn or acquired metabolic deficiency or excess of enzyme activity. In such cases the

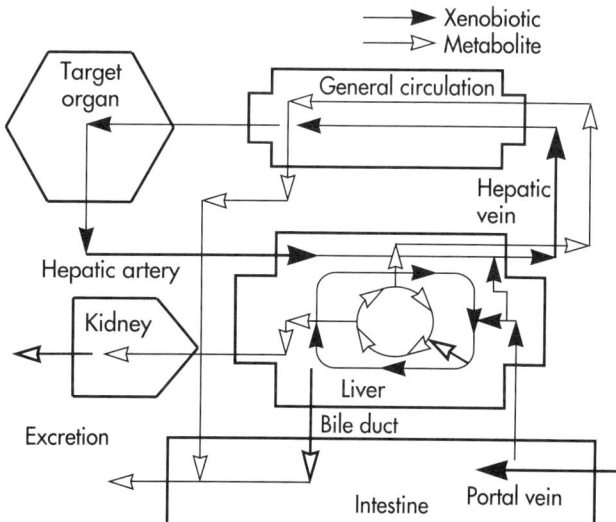

Fig. 24-6. Schematic illustration of the metabolic routes of a xenobiotic and its metabolites (see text).

diagnosis depends on satisfaction of the following criteria[18]: (1) the disappearance of symptoms after removal of the toxin(s), (2) the reappearance of symptoms on reexposure to said toxin(s), (3) the correspondence of symptoms with well-known allergic reactions, (4) identification of the reaction-producing substance through the results of specific allergy and immunologic tests (usually skin or blood tests) or measurement of toxin levels or its metabolites in body fluids. There is significant interindividual biochemical variability that may explain some of the idiosyncratic hepatotoxic reactions known to occur.

EXPOSURE TYPES AND SOURCES

From the perspective of gastrointestinal illness one might intuitively suspect contaminated water or food as the most likely point of exposure. Surprisingly, several studies have pointed out the possibility of indoor air pollution as a source for volatile organic compound exposure.[2] Ground water and surface water exposure other than through the water supply might be of concern if natural springs, sink holes, or ground water-supplied swimming pools are extensively used. Consider ingestion of soil-borne contaminants in those families that consume plants, animals, or other food products that come from one particular location such as a local garden or farm. As might be expected, the type of food ingested varies widely depending on the region of the country and individual preferences for eating wild game or vegetation such as rabbits, crayfish, and mushrooms. A review of the many parameters affecting internal dose[57] might convince practitioners that their time is better spent measuring the effects of environmental changes on the patient's illness or evaluating surrogate indicators of exposure, that is, biological markers of exposure (see Chapter 2 for more discussion on exposure types and sources).

CLINICAL PRESENTATIONS OF GASTROINTESTINAL-INDUCED DISORDERS
Patterns of clinical response

Practitioners can approach the diagnosis of an environmental illness by classifying the clinical gastrointestinal response using a modified classification convention first proposed by Hoigne et al.[43] An immediate reaction is any illness that occurs within 60 minutes of exposure. An acute illness begins between 1 and 24 hours of exposure. A subacute reaction is within 1 day to several months of first exposure. By default a chronic clinical response takes greater than a year to manifest. Evaluation of a chronic clinical response (such as cancer) is best done by clinicians with extensive experience in the fields of epidemiology and toxicology.

Acute poisoning

What about patients with suspected immediate, acute, or subacute environmental gastrointestinal toxicity? Immediate and acute poisonings pose few methodologic problems for physicians familiar with emergency problems. Based on the diagnostic assessment one can decide whether to provide (1) supportive care alone, (2) specific antidotal therapy, and (3) active poison removal therapy, or all three.[29]

Suspected subacute environmental toxicity

Suspected subacute adverse chemical effects involve situations where the primary care physician may make a reasonable diagnosis of environmental illness. The following generally accepted criteria exist to guide physicians in these types of determinations. (1) The symptoms, signs, and laboratory tests are consistent with the diagnosis. (2) The temporal pattern of exposure and disease onset is coherent, that is, exposure precedes disease onset or aggravation. (3) The exposure, if known, was sufficient to cause the disease. (Biologic monitoring for the assessment of exposure or specific end-organ effects, if available, is consistent with dose-response characteristics. Epidemiologic data, if available, support the effects at exposures comparable to those experienced by the individual.) (4) No other condition or exposure more readily explains the disease. These general criteria may be insufficient to enable physicians to make causal determinations with a high degree of interpersonal reproducibility. Further criteria for determining causal relationships between a given agent and a disease have been proposed. Bradford Hill revised the Koch-Henle criteria so that they would be useful for environmental illnesses.[39]

BIOLOGIC MARKERS
Overview

A biologic marker or biomarker is any cellular or molecular indicator of toxic exposure, adverse health effects, or susceptibility (see Chaper 54).[67] Clinicians have used biomarkers for many years, for instance, blood lead to measure exposure and alkaline phosphatase as a measure of toxic effect of chlorinated hydrocarbons. More recently protein products of oncogenes have been used as a potential measure of cancer susceptibility.[11,10] What makes the latest generation of biomarkers unique is their remarkable sensitivity, which enables measurement of events from initial exposure to clinically significant disease.[88] Sensitivity has drawbacks, however, from both scientific and philosophic perspectives. High sensitivity is usually accompanied by a large number of confounding factors, other than environmental toxins, that can affect biomarker results. Various hereditary and acquired host factors can magnify or blunt biomarker response in a given individual. There are few if any biologic makers that fulfill the criteria developed by the CDC and ATSDR that measures a marker's usefulness.[16] From the philosophic perspective increased test sensitivity brings with it an increased risk of drawing causal inferences from perceived associations that, in truth, do not really exist.[54]

Biomarkers of liver function

There are at least three biologic markers of liver function that may prove useful in the workup of individuals who claim ill effects from environmental hepatotoxins. These tests may also be useful if you know the individual is exposed to low concentrations of potential hepatotoxins but their symptoms come from other organ systems. In such a situation the biomarker serves as a measure of whether significant exposure exists. Unfortunately such markers usually do not exist if the patient is complaining of gastrointestinal ailments that are not mediated by the liver. A glaring exception to this statement is pesticide exposure where the pesticide causes an cholinesterase deficiency (anticholinesterase effect). In general, however, one will have to depend more on reported symptoms as a measure of illness severity rather than objective biological markers.

The usual liver function tests, aspartate aminotransferase (AST or SGOT), alanine aminotransferase (ALT or SPGT), gamma glutamyl transferase (GGT), and alkaline phosphatase (AP), generally provide an inexact picture of overall liver function and do not reflect specific chemical exposures.[41] Alkaline phosphatase is an exception to this if the chemical exposure involves a substance that targets the biliary tract, but in general the statement holds. The CDC/ATSDR report on hepatobiliary biomarkers recognized the limits of the usual liver function tests and included fasting bile acids in the recommended panel of basic screening tests for hepatotoxicity. Several studies indicate that widely used chlorinated hydrocarbon solvents such as trichlorethylene interfere with bile acid uptake.[7] The interference is a physiologic process as described earlier in the section on liver physiology. Significant pathologic effects on liver cells do not appear to occur at exposure levels detectable by bile acid assay so long as more common liver tests are normal. Similar sensitivity seems to exist with carbon tetrachloride and chloroform exposure.[6,19] One widely used methodology for measuring bile acids was developed by Wang.[104] A recent advance using evaporative light-scattering mass detection promises to considerably shorten assay time.[82]

The second tier of recommended testing consists of an indocyanin green (ICG) dye clearance measurement. This test should be considered if any of the first tier tests are confirmed abnormal; that is, repeat and confirm any abnormal test first before considering it "truly" abnormal. Although anionic dye clearance testing (like the ICG test) has been used clinically for over 30 years, many providers have little experience using them. Sulfobromophthalein (BSP), another dye clearance test, developed an unfavorable reputation after experience revealed problems with anaphylactic reactions, phlebitis, and local skin reactions.[97] The strength of ICG clearance tests are their safety and sensitivity to mild chemical liver injuries.[63,96] Conventional aminotransferase tests perform best when acute liver cytotoxicity occurs as commonly happens with infectious hepatitis or exposure to high doses of hepatotoxins. Chronic low-level liver injury such as one might find with certain chlorinated hydrocarbons leads to progressive fibrosis and vascular injury, not acute widespread hepatocellular damage. Consequently the ICG test in combination with a bile acid assay provides the best sensitivity and specificity in patients whom you suspect have low-level exposure to hepatotoxins.[98]

Research needs

Evidence has been accumulating that in many animal models and human subjects a chemical's ability to induce P450 I and II enzymes correlates with the toxic potential of several chemicals.[38,78] Human research in this area requires a safe, sensitive, and reproducible method to monitor specific forms of P450 I and II enzymes in large numbers of people. Out of this need came development of various carbon dioxide breath tests,[50] including the caffeine breath test (CBT), which specifically measures P450 IA2 activity. The CBT has been used in numerous epidemiologic field studies[53] and appears to be a measure of toxic susceptibility, at least for those chemicals whose toxicologic mechanism of injury depends on activation of P450 IA2 enzymes.[52]

What about one's susceptibility to cancer? Are relatively simple, inexpensive tests available that could be used to screen for chemically induced cancer susceptibility? The answer to that question is not clear yet, but exciting developments over the past 20 years hint that the answer might be yes. The accuracy of such tests will depend on the accuracy of the proposed carcinogenic mechanism that one monitors. One such mechanism involves a specific cytochrome P450 family, namely the P450 I family. Evidence implicating this specific family of enzymes in xenobiotically induced disease, including cancer, has been accumulating since the early 1970s.[23,48,51,80]

CANCER

Chronic illnesses include those especially feared by the general public, such as cancer. Publications on environmental illness often focus considerable attention on epidemiologic associations between various types of gastrointestinal cancer and suspected environmental agents.[84] Several human epidemiologic studies have raised the possibility of gastrointestinal cancer. Several studies in the 1970s of occupational exposure to vinyl chloride fumes confirmed the association of such exposure with angiosarcoma of the liver,[9,44] finding a clear association between liver angiosarcoma and residents living near vinyl chloride polymerization or fabrication plants.[9] The scientific community, however, has had trouble clearly elucidating and communicating the risks involved from low-dose exposure to potentially carcinogenic substances.[64] Cancer risk analysis is severely hampered by the uncertainty inherent in missing or ambiguous scientific data, gaps in scientific theory, and the need for inferences beyond existing data.[26] The traditional philosophic approach used by epidemiologists to derive inferences on causal relationships focuses on statistically significant human epidemiologic studies.[39,102] Contemporary philosophers of science argue that no one can disprove that any particular substance can cause a disease,[13] and conversely such a relationship can never be absolutely proved.[14] For practical purposes, however, a causal relationship truly exists if careful, systematic, and repeated observations demonstrate a recurring association between a suspected agent and disease. This is where an N-of-One clinical trial can prove useful to the clinician attempting to evaluate subacute environmental gastrointestinal illness.

TRIAL OF THERAPY WITH AN N OF 1
Overview

In everyday practice clinicians often conduct a "trial of therapy" to help guide their selection of a treatment most likely to help a specific patient. Using the same rationale, clinicians often rely on the effect of drug removal (dechallenge) and readministration (rechallenge) for determinations of adverse drug reactions. This same method can be extended in a modified form to help determine adverse reactions to occupational and environmental chemicals.[40] "For patients where there is a question of environmental toxicity one can usually determine which exposure route (dermal, gastrointestinal, or respiratory) is the most likely source of chemical absorption. The respiratory or gastrointestinal tracts are the usual routes of environmental exposure. If the exposure is gastrointestinal the most likely source is tap water, especially if this water comes from a well. By substituting bottled water for tap water one can measure the "treatment's" effect on the patient's objective and subjective clinical manifestations. An association between these clinical manifestations and such a trial of "therapy" would reinforce one's suspicions of environmental toxicity. A causal association would be inappropriate based on such meager data, but notification of public health officials would be warranted. The local or state public health department could then determine if further data are needed or if the local public's health is threatened.

Method for "N of 1" trial

A summary of one method for conducting such an "N of 1" clinical trial follows:*

1. A clinician and patient agree to modify the patient's usual (baseline) environment to determine the intervention's (intervention environment's) ability to improve or control the patient's symptoms, signs, or body measurements of chemical exposure.
2. The patient then undergoes pairs of intervention periods organized so that one period of each pair involves removal of the suspected environmental contamination exposure route (establishes the intervention environment) and the other period restores the suspected route (re-challenges the patient with the baseline environment). The order of these two periods within each pair should be randomized in a manner that ensures that each period has an equal chance of applying the environmental intervention.
3. Whenever possible, both the clinician and the patient are "blind" to the treatment being given during any period.
4. The clinical manifestations of disease are monitored (using a patient diary if necessary) to document the effect of the intervention environment or the baseline environment.
5. Pairs of treatment periods are replicated until the clinician and patient are convinced that the two environments clearly affect or clearly do not affect the clinical manifestations.

*Adapted from Sackett DL et al, eds: *Clinical epidemiology: a basic science for clinical medicine,* Boston, 1991, Litte Brown.

REFERENCES

1. Adler MJ: *The 4 dimensions of philosophy,* New York, 1993, Macmillan.
2. Andelman JB: Exposure to volatile chemicals from indoor uses of water. Proceedings of the EPA/AWMA specialty conference: total exposure assessment methodology, Pittsburgh, Air & Waste Management Association, 1990.
3. Andelman JB, Couch A, Thruston WW: Inhalation exposures in indoor air to trichlorethylene from shower water. In Kopler FC, Craun GF, eds: *Environmental epidemiology,* Chelsea, Mich, 1986, Lewis.
4. Ansari GAS et al: Methylene chioniline; toxicity, metabolism and effects on biliary function, *The Toxicologist* 11:608A, 1991.
5. Autrup H: Carcinogen metabolism in human tissues and cells, *Drug Metab Rev* 13:603, 1982.
6. Bai CL, Canfield PJ, Stacey NH: Individual serum bile acids as early indicators of carbon tetrachloride- and chloroform-induced liver injury, *Toxicology* 75:221, 1992.
7. Bai CL, Stacey NH: Mechanism of trichlorethylene-induced elevation in individual serum bile acids II. In vitro and in vivo interference of trichlorethylene with bile acid transport in isolated rat hepatocytes, *Toxicol Appl Pharmacol* 121:296, 1993.
8. Bienstock J et al: Mucosal immunology, *Monogr Allergy* 16:1, 1980.
9. Falk H et al: Epidemiology of hepatic angiosarcoma in the United States: 1964-1974, *Environ Health Perspect* 41:107, 1981.
10. Brandt-Rauf PW: New markers for monitoring occupational cancer: the example of oncogene proteins, *J Occup Med* 30:399, 1988.
11. Brandt-Rauf PW, Niman HL: Serum screening for oncogene proteins in workers exposed to PCBs, *Br J Ind Med* 45:689, 1988.
12. Bretcher M: Membrane structure: some general principles, *Science* 181:622, 1973.
13. Buck C: Popper's philosophy for epidemiologist, *Int J Epidemiol* 4:159, 1975.
14. Bunge MA: *Causality: the place of the causal principle in modern science,* Cleveland, 1963, World.
15. Cullen JM, Ruebner BH: A histopathologic classification of chemical-induced injury of the liver. In Meeks RG, Harrison SD, Butt RJ, eds: *Hepatotoxicotogy,* Boca Raton, Fla, 1991, CRC Press.
16. Center for Disease Control & Agency for Toxic Substances and Disease Registry (CDC/ATSDR) Subcommittee on biomarkers of organ damage and dysfunction: Summary report, Atlanta, 1990.
17. Cruan GF: Surface water supplies and health, *J Am Water Works Assoc* 80:40, 1988.
18. De Weck AL: Immunological mechanisms and clinical aspects of allergic reactions to drugs. In de Weck AL, Bundegaard H, eds: *Allergic reactions* to drugs. Berlin, 1983, Springer-Verlag.
19. Dirscoll T et al: Concentrations of individual serum or plasma bile acids in workers exposed to chlorinated aliphatic hydrocarbons, *Br J Indus Med* 49:700, 1992.
20. Eade M: Gut circulation and absorption, a review. part I, *N Z Med J* 84:10, 1976.
21. Reference deleted in proofs.

22. Erlinger S: Secretion of bile. In Schiff L, Schiff ER, eds: *Diseases of the liver,* Philadelphia, 1993, JB Lippincott.
23. Felton JS, Nebert DW: Mutations of certain activated carcinogens in vitro associated with genetically mediated increase in monooxygenase activity and cytochrome P 1 450, *J Biol Chem* 250:6769, 1975.
24. Fleming LE: Unusual occupational gastrointestinal and hepatic disorders, *Occupational Medicine: State of the Art Reviews* 7(3):433, 1992.
25. Fletcher RH: Three ways of knowing in clinical medicine, *Southern Med J* 83(3):308, 1990.
26. Foster KR, Bernstein, DE, Huber PW, eds: *Phantom risk: scientific inference and the law,* Cambridge, 1993, MIT Press.
27. Wallace LA: The TEAM study: Personal exposures to toxic substances in air, drinking water, and breath of four hundred residents of New Jersey, North Carolina, and North Dakota, *Environ Res* 43:290, 1987.
28. Gibaldi M, Perrier D: Route of administration and drug disposition, *Drug Metab Rev* 3:185, 1974.
29. Goldberg MJ et al: An approach to the management of the poisoned patient, *Arch Intern Med* 146:1381, 1986.
30. Greenland S: Probability versus Popper: an elaboration of the insufficiency of current Popperian approaches for epidemiologic analysis. In Rothman KJ, ed: *Causal inference,* Chestnut Hill, Penn, 1988, Epidemiology Resources.
31. Grinnell F: *The scientific attitude,* ed 2, New York, 1992, Guilford Press.
32. Grisham JW, ed: *Health aspects of the disposal of waste chemicals,* New York, 1986, Pergamon.
33. Groothuis GMM, Hardonk MJ, Meyer DK: Hepatobiliary transport of drugs: do periportal and perivenous hepatocytes perform the same job? *Trends in Pharmacol Sci* 6:322, 1985.
34. Guengerich FP: Enzymatic oxidation of xenobiotic chemicals, *Crit Rev Biochem Mol Bio* 25:97, 1990.
35. Hartiala K: Metabolism of hormones, drugs and other substances by the gut, *Physiol Rev* 53:496, 1973.
36. Hartmann F, Jenss H: The gastrointestinal tract. In Tarcher A, ed: *Principles and practice of environmental medicine,* New York, 1992, Plenum.
37. Heyworth MF, Jones AL, eds: *Immunology of the gastrointestinal tract and liver,* New York, 1988, Raven Press.
38. Hidetoshi Y et al: Possible correlation between induction modes of hepatic enzymes by PCBs and their toxicity in rats, *Ann NY Acad Sci* 320:179, 1979.
39. Hill AB: *Principles of medical statistics,* ed 8, London, 1987, The Lancet Limited, chapter xxiv.
40. Hodgson MJ: N-of-one clinical trials, *J Occup Med* 35:375, 1993.
41. Hodgson MJ, Goodman-Klein BM, van Thiel DH: Evaluating the liver in hazardous waste workers, *J Occup Med* 5:67, 1990.
42. Hoensch H, Swenk M: Intestinal absorption and metabolism of xenobiotics in humans. In Schiller C, ed: *Intestinal toxicology,* New York, 1984 Raven Press.
43. Hoigne R, Stocker F, Middleton P: Epidemiology of drug allergy: drug monitoring. In deWeck AL, Bundgaard H, eds: *Allergic reactions to drugs,* Berlin, 1984, Springer-Verlag.
44. Infante PF: Observations of the site-specific carcinogenicity of vinyl chloride to humans, *Environ Health Perspects* 41:88, 1981.
45. Jo WK, Weisel CP, Lioy PT: Chloroform exposure and the health risk associated with multiple uses of chlorinated tap water, *Risk Anal* 10:581, 1990.
46. Jo WK, Weisel CP, Lioy PJ: Routes of chloroform exposure and body burden from showering with chlorinated tap water, *Risk Anal* 10:575, 1990.
47. Kilburn KH: How should we think about chemically reactive patients? *Archiv Environ Health* 48:4, 1993 (editorial).
48. Kouri RE: Relationship between labels of aryl hydrocarbon hydroxylase activity and susceptibility to 3-methylcholanthrene and benzo(a)pyrene-induced cancers in inbred strains of mice. In Freundenthal RI, Jones PW, eds: *Polynuclear aromatic hydrocarbons: chemistry, metabolism, and carcinogenesis,* New York, 1976, Raven Press.
49. Kretschmer NW et al: Studies on the mechanism of 1-(2-chloroethy) 3 cycloherxyl-1-nitrosourea (CCNU)-induced hepatotoxicity III. Ultrastructural characterization of bile duct injury, *Cancer Chemother Pharmacol* 19:109, 1987.
50. Lambert GH, Kotake AN, Schoeller D: The CO2 breath test as monitors of the cytochrome P-450 dependent mixed function mono-oxygenase system, *Prog Biol* 119:119, 1983.
51. Lambert GH, Nebert DW: Genetically mediated induction of drug metabolizing enzymes associated with congenital defects, *Teratology* 16:117, 1977.
52. Lambert GH et al: Cytochrome P450IA2 in vivo induction: a potential biomarker of polyhalogenated biphenyls and their related chemical's effects on the human, *Chemosphere* 23:197, 1992.
53. Lambert GH et al: The caffeine breath test and caffeine urinary metabolite ratios in the Michigan cohort exposed to polybrominated biphenyls: a preliminary study, *Environ Health Perspect* 89:175, 1990.
54. Langmuir I: Pathological science, *Physics Today* 42:36, 1990.
55. Laskin DL: Nonparenchymal cells and hepatotoxicity, *Semin Liver Dis* 10:293, 1990.
56. Lauterbach F: Intestinal secretions of organic ions and drugs. In Kramer M, Lauterbach F, ed: *Intestinal Permeation,* Amsterdam, 1974, Excerpta Medica.
57. Lioy PJ: Assessing total human exposure to contaminants: a multidisciplinary approach, *Environ Sci Technol* 24:938, 1990.
58. Lipkin M: Proliferation and differentiation of normal and diseased gastrointestinal cells. In Johnson L, ed: *Physiology of the gastrointestinal tract,* New York, 1987, Raven Press.
59. Lucas M: The association between acidification and electronic events in the rat proximal jejunum, *J Physiol* (Lond) 257:645, 1976.
60. Marshall E: Toxicology goes molecular, *Science* 259:1394, 1993.
61. McNabb P, Tomasi T: Host defense mechanisms at the mucosal surface, *Ann Rev Microbiol* 35:477, 1981.
62. Miettinen OS: *Theoretical epidemiology: principles of occurrence research in medicine,* New York, 1985, Wiley.
63. Miller B, Liss G, Tamburro CH: The safety of indocyanin green clearance as a screening and diagnostic test for hepatic disease, *Clin Res* 31:765A, 1983.
64. Moore M, ed: *Health risks and the press: perspectives or media coverage of risk assessment and health,* Washington, DC, 1989, The Media Institute.
65. MMWR: prevention of leading work-related diseases and injuries, Washington, DC, 1991, #648-004/40813, U.S. Government Printing Office.
66. National Research Council: *Environmental epidemiology,* vol 1, *Public health and hazardous wastes,* Washington, DC, 1991, National Academy Press.
67. National Research Council: Biologic markers in environmental health research, *Environ Health Perspect* 74:39, 1987.
68. National Research Council: Human exposure to airborne pollutants, Washington D.C., 1991, National Academy Press.
69. Nebert DW et al: The P-450 superfamily: update on new sequences, gene mapping, and recommended nomenclature, *DNA* 10:1, 1991.
70. Nelson SD: Molecular mechanisms of the hepatotoxicity caused by acetaminophen, *Semin Liver Disease* 10:267, 1990.
71. Nelson SD, Pearson PG: Covalent and noncovalent interactions in acute lethal cell injury caused by chemicals, *Ann Rev Pharmacol Toxicol* 30:169, 1990.
72. Nethercott JR, Davidolf LL, Curlow B: Multiple chemical sensitivities syndrome: toward a working case definition, *Arch Environ Health* 48:19, 1993.
73. Neutra M, Forstner J: Gastrointestinal mucous: synthesis, secretion, and function. In Johnson L, ed: *Physiology of the gastrointestinal tract,* New York, 1987, Raven Press.

74. Ochsenfahrt H, Winne D: The contribution of solvent drag to the intestinal absorption of the basic drug amidopyrine and antipyrine from the jejunum of the rat, *Arch Pharmacol* 281:175, 1974.
75. Peck CC, Temple R, Collins JM: Understanding consequences of concurrent therapies, *JAMA* 269:1550, 1993 (editorial).
76. Pessayre D, Larrey G: Acute and chronic drug-induced hepatitis, *Baillieres Clin Gastroenterol* 2:385, 1988.
77. Pohl LR: Drug-induced allergic hepatitis, *Semin Liver Dis* 10:305, 1990.
78. Poland A, Knutson JC: 2,3,7,8-Tetrachlorodibenzo-p-dioxin and related halogenated aromatic hydrocarbons: examination of the mechanism of toxicity, *Ann Rev Pharmacol Toxicol* 22:517, 1982.
79. Porter TD, Coon MJ: Cytochrome P-450: multiplicity of isoforms, substrates, and catalytic and regulatory mechanisms, *J Biol Chem* 266:13469, 1991.
80. Potter WZ et al: Acetaminophen-induced hepatic necrosis. III Cytochrome P-450 mediated covalent binding in vitro, *J Pharmacol Exp Ther* 187:203, 1973.
81. Reed DJ: Glutathione: toxicological implications, *Ann Rev Pharmacol Toxicol* 30:603, 1990.
82. Roda A et al: Determination of free and amidated bile acids by high-performance liquid chromatography with evaporative light-scattering mass detection, *J Lipid Res* 33:1393, 1992.
83. Rubin E, Farber JL: The liver and biliary system. In Rubin E, Farber JL, eds: *Pathology,* Philadelphia, 1988, JB Lippincott.
84. Rubin E, Farber JL: Environmental diseases of the digestive system, *Med Clin N Am* 74:413, 1990.
85. Sackett, DL et al, eds: *Clinical epidemiology: a basic science for clinical medicine,* Boston, 1991, Little, Brown.
86. Schedl HP: Water and electrolyte transport: clinical aspects, *Med Clin North Am* 58:1429, 1974.
87. Scheline R: Metabolism of foreign compounds by gastrointestinal microorganisms, *Pharmacol Rev* 25:451, 1980.
88. Schulte PA: Contribution of biological markers to occupational health: keynote address, 23rd International Conference on Occupational Health, Montreal, Canada, Sept. 1990.
89. Seitz F: *The science matrix,* New York, 1992, Springer-Verlag.
90. Sharma R, ed: *Immunologic considerations in toxicology,* vols 1 and 2, Boca Raton; Fla, 1981, CRC Press.
91. Shorter R, Tomasi T: Gut immune mechanisms, *Ann Intern Med* 27:247, 1982.
92. Simon G: Intestinal flora in health and disease, *Gastroenterology* 86:174, 1984.
93. Simon GL, Gorbach SL: Intestinal flora in health and disease. In Johnson LR, ed: *Physiology of the gastrointentinal tract,* ed 2, New York, 1987, Raven Press.
94. Smithson V et al: Intestinal diffusion barrier: unstirred layer or membrane surface mucous coat, *Science* 214:1241, 1981.
95. Reference deleted in proofs.
96. Tamburro CH, Greenburg RA: Effectiveness of federally required medical laboratory screening in the detection of chemical liver injury, *Environ Health Perspect* 41:117, 1981.
97. Tamburro CH, Liss GM: Tests for hepatotoxicity: usefulness in screening workers, *J Occup Med* 28:1034, 1986.
98. Tamburro CH et al: Report on implementation and assessment of a demonstration cancer control detection and prevention program in a cohort of industrial workers, National Cancer Institute, contract NO-1-CN55212, 1978.
99. Thomas A: Unstirred water layer: a basic mechanisms of gastrointestinal mucosal cell cytoprotection. In Harmon J, ed: *Basic mechanisms of gastrointestinal mucosal cell injury and protection,* Baltimore, 1981, Williams & Wilkins.
100. Thurman RG et al: Is hypoxia involved in the mechanism of alcohol-induced liver injury? *Fund Appl Tox* 4:125, 1984.
101. United States Department of Health and Human Services: Healthy People 2000, Washington, DC, 1990.
102. United States Department of Health and Human Services: The health consequences of smoking: report of the Surgeon General, Washington, DC, 1976, pub. no. CDC 78-8357.
103. Walker W: Host defense mechanisms in the gastrointestinal tract, *Pediatrics* 57:901, 1976.
104. Wang G, Stacey NH, Earl J: Determination of individual bile acids in serum by high performance liquid chromatography, *Biomed Chromatog* 4:136, 1990.
105. Winne D: Rat jejunum perfused in situ: effects of perfusion rate and intraluminal radius on absorption rate and effective unstirred layer thickness, *Naunyn-Schmiedebergs Arch Pharmacol Exp Path* 307:265, 1979.
106. Woosley RL et al: Mechanism of the cardiotoxic actions of terfenodine, *JAMA* 269:1535-1559, 1993.
107. Zimmerman HJ: Classification of hepatotoxins and mechanisms of toxicity. In Zimmerman HJ *Hepatotoxicity: the adverse effects of drugs and other chemicals on the liver,* New York, 1978, Appleton-Century-Crafts.
108. Zimmerman HJ, Maddrey WC: Toxic and drug-induced hepatitis. In Schiff L, Schiff ER, eds: *Diseases of the liver,* Philadelphia, 1993, JB Lippincott.

Chapter 25

KIDNEY AND URINARY TRACT

David Parkinson
Stuart M. Brooks

Renal anatomy
Renal physiology
Nephrotoxicity
Clinical presentations
Lead
Cadmium nephrotoxicity
Mercury
Other metals
Silica
Hydrocarbons

It is somewhat surprising that the occupational medical literature is not replete with reports of renal damage caused by occupational and environmental toxins, as the kidney serves to eliminate and in many cases concentrate such toxins. Recently more sophisticated tests of renal function have become available, and evidence is beginning to accrue that subtle changes indicating renal damage may occur at levels of exposure that were previously considered to be without hazard.

The problems of identifying a relationship between renal disease and environmental exposure parallel those in occupational diseases. Of these perhaps the most important is identifying exposure. In the case of heavy metals, such as lead and cadmium, estimates of body burden may be made if these agents are suspect, but for volatile toxins (which do not accumulate), such as solvents, such measurements are not possible. This places great reliance on a history of exposure from which it may be very difficult to assign even qualitative measurements of exposure. Additionally, there is significant renal reserve and thus toxicity may not be identified using traditional measurements of renal function. This also means that prevention of nephrotoxic disease at a stage when it is still reversible is not possible using traditional tests of renal function such as blood urea and serum creatinine. Measurements of low-level exposure must be combined with the use of sensitive tests of cytotoxicity to prevent renal nephropathy.

High exposures may lead to acute renal disease sometimes leading to renal failure, and in these instances the relationship to exposure is usually clear. It is the low-level exposure that provides a challenge both in measurement of exposure and the development of subtle renal disease. Although case reports of many chemicals causing nephrotoxic effects can be found, there are few compounds in which sufficient evidence exists for definitive assignment of a relationship between exposure and renal disease. These compounds generally fall into two groups: heavy metals and organic chemicals, particularly halogenated solvents.[58]

RENAL ANATOMY

The kidney may be divided anatomically into two major parts, the medulla and the cortex (Fig. 25-1). The primary vascular elements are located in the cortical region. Much of the renal blood flow passes through the cortex, making this area more susceptible to chemical effects. Although the medullary area has a lesser blood flow, because of its anatomic arrangement with the loops of Henle, a chemical can become concentrated in the medullary region.

The functional unit of the kidney is the nephron, which consists of (1) the renal capsule composed of a glomerulus and Bowman's capsule, (2) at least 12 morphologically and functionally distinct tubular portions, and (3) the blood supply via the afferent and efferent arterioles. It has been estimated that the human has about 1 million functioning nephrons.[55] As shown in Fig. 25-1, the nephron contains a glomerulus, a proximal convoluted tubule, and vascular units, which are usually located within the cortex. The me-

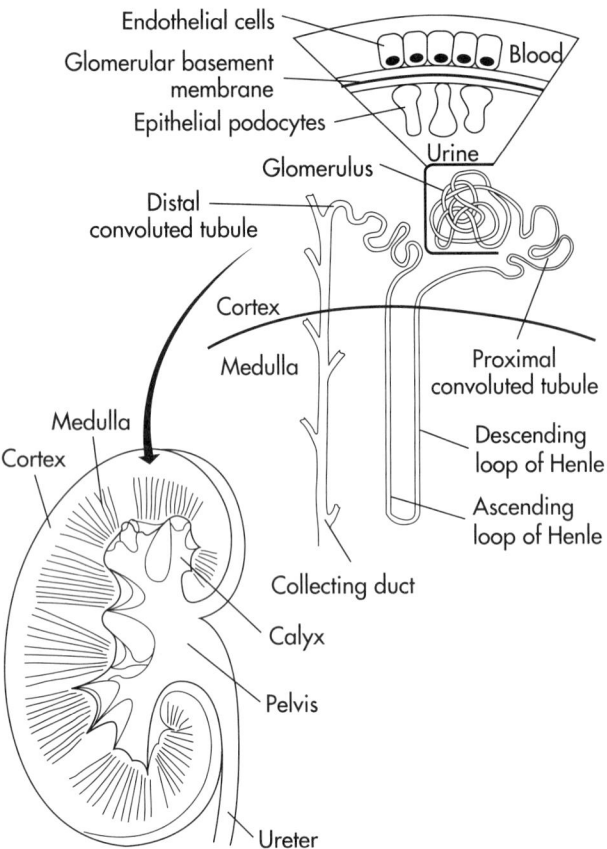

Fig. 25-1. The kidney may be divided anatomically into two major parts, the medulla and the cortex. The functional unit of the kidney is the nephron, which consists of a glomerulus, a proximal convoluted tubule, and vascular units that are usually located within the cortex, whereas the medulla contains the straight portion of the proximal tubule, loops of Henle, and collecting ducts. Glomerular filtration is carried out by three cell types—endothelial, mesangial, and the epithelial cells of the visceral layer or podocytes. There is also the glomerular basement membrane sandwiched between the endothelial and epithelial cells.

dulla receives the straight portion of the proximal tubule, loops of Henle, and collecting ducts. However, depending on the location of a glomerulus (that is, nearer or farther from the medulla), the corresponding loops of Henle will burrow deeper into the medulla (for example, if juxtapositioned near the medulla) or actually be contained in the cortex (for example, if positioned closer to the kidney's outer surface).

RENAL PHYSIOLOGY

A detailed discussion of renal physiology is beyond the scope of this text. The kidney regulates extracellular fluid volume and composition of the body by filtering and reabsorbing large quantities of water and electrolytes. However, the nephron can be viewed as a functional unit performing several essential physiologic functions. The glomerulus is a specialized capillary bed uniquely positioned between two vasoactive arterioles (afferent and efferent arteriole). It contains a capillary that allows selective filtering of plasma. Whether a material is filtered through the porous capillary will depend on its molecular size, net charge, and shape.[30]

The renal blood flow in humans is about 3 to 5 ml/min/g of kidney weight.[10] The normal human blood pressure is influenced by the kidney's vascular supply with prominent sympathetic innervation and its capacity to secrete renin. A normal human man weighing about 150 pounds has a kidney weight of approximately 290 grams and a renal blood flow of 1160 ml/min; this represents about 20% to 25% of the total cardiac output. This accomplishment is in contrast with the fact that the kidneys constitute only about 0.5% of the total body mass.[30] This inordinate relationship is necessary to maintain the very high blood flow through the kidneys and the high glomerular filtration rate. Approximately 20% to 40% of the plasma entering the glomeruli is filtered, about 180 liters per day. The glomerular filtrate represents an ultrafine, protein-sparse filtrate of plasma since the glomerular capillary restricts passage of macromolecules of greater than 20 Å or molecular weight higher than 40,000 (that is, plasma proteins). At the nephron level the afferent arterioles deliver blood to the glomerular capillary encased in its Bowman's capsule; the efferent arteriole removes the residual of the filtered plasma. Thus these vascular units serve several functions: the afferent arteriole presents waste and other materials that are filtered by the glomerulus and delivered to the tubules for excretion; the efferent arteriole returns reabsorbed and synthesized materials to the systemic circulation; and it delivers oxygen and metabolic substrates to the nephron.[30] The glomerular filtration is carried out by three cell types: endothelial, mesangial, and epithelial cells of the visceral layer or podocytes. There is also the glomerular basement membrane sandwiched between the endothelial and epithelial cells.

The tubular cells function by reabsorbing, secreting, and metabolizing the filtered plasma. About 60% to 80% of solute and water filtered by the glomerulus is reabsorbed within the proximal tubule, which reabsorbs sodium, potassium, bicarbonate, chloride, phosphate, calcium, and magnesium ions, as well as glucose, amino acids, and certain organic acids. The tubular unit as a whole selectively reabsorbs 98% to 99% of the salts and water presented to it. Likewise almost all of the sugars and amino acids are also reabsorbed. The proximal tubule especially helps maintain acid balance by actively secreting organic compounds, hydrogen, and potassium ions and generating ammonia formation. The tubules also promote activation of vitamin D. Because of its prominent transport system and high energy and substrate requirements, the proximal tubule is the portion of the nephron most often affected by nephrotoxic agents or ischemia.

NEPHROTOXICITY

An environmental chemical can lead to a nephron injury in several ways. First, vasoconstriction may reduce renal blood flow and glomerular filtration rate and subsequently decrease urine output. There may also be tissue ischemia with cellular death. Second, the toxicant may damage the glomerulus and lead to increased permeability with compromised filtration. Third, there may be direct tubular damage influencing tubular reabsorptive and secretory capacities. The nephrotoxic chemical may cause biochemical changes affecting active transport systems and accumulate within cellular compartments and binding of the chemical or metabolite to cellular macromolecules such as membranes and enzymes.[18] The nephrotoxic agents can lead to alterations that result in precipitation of material or toxicant within the tubular lumen, causing blockage of urine flow. There may be an immunologic mechanism operating as a result of deposition of circulating immune complexes in the glomerulus with subsequent activation of complement, recruitment of leukocytic cells and release of their proteases, activation of reactive oxygen species, and generation of prostaglandins and other mediators. Alternatively the immunologic reaction within the glomerulus may be between circulating glomerular component(s) antibodies and glomerular antigen(s). In this latter situation an immunofluorescence pattern of linear or granular nature may ensue. Other important influencing determinants are host factors, such as age and diet.

CLINICAL PRESENTATIONS

There are several clinical presentations that may result from an acute or prolonged exposure to a nephrotoxicant[8,35]; these are summarized in Table 25-1. The diagnosis is directly dependent on the practitioner's ability to obtain an appropriate exposure history and whether the individual has or could have absorbed sufficient amounts of a nephrotoxicant to develop renal disease. Sources of exposures may include history of receiving a nephrotoxic drug (analgesics, antibiotics), occupational and home exposures (solvents, metals), ingestion of contaminated food or drink (ethylene glycol), exposure to environmental chemicals (lead in children), and drug addiction (glue sniffing).[8] A clue to the diagnosis is noting the manifestations of associated organ systems, especially the nervous system and liver. Thus halogenated hydrocarbons such as carbon tetrachloride produces profound liver and kidney damage; mercury causes renal and neurobehavioral alterations. A diagnosis is strengthened if a suspected chemical is found to be elevated by urine, blood, tissue biopsy, or gastric fluid analyses. Of course it is important to rule out other medical conditions (for example, diabetes, hypertension) that can be accounted as the cause of the renal disease.

There are sensitive biomarkers reported for renal injury that may be used for screening purposes, which includes the finding of albuminuria for glomerular disease and retinol-binding and β2-microglobulin proteins for detecting tubular injury.[7] Enzymuria, such as β-N-acetylglucosaminidase, may help identify early proximal tubular damage. Destruction of renal tissue may cause release of renal antigens detected by quantitative immunochemical methodology such as, ligandin, carbonic anhydrase, and alanine aminopeptidase-binding proteins.

The box on p. 314 presents some examples of nephrotoxic chemicals. The text following discusses the important agents. Table 25-2 lists carcinogenic agents.

LEAD

There is little question of the relationship between high lead exposure and renal disease. Wedeen[59] reports that Lancereaux provided the first description of occupational lead nephropathy in an artist using lead-based paints. Legge[36] found an excess of renal failure due to chronic interstitial nephritis. Henderson[28] identified a group of young adults in

Table 25-1. Clinical presentations and causes of renal disease

Clinical types				
Acute renal failure	Chronic renal failure	Tubulointerstitial nephritis	Nephrotic syndrome	Rapidly progressive glomerulonephritis
Manifestations				
Azotemia	Azotemia	Aminoaciduria	Heavy proteinuria	Hematuria
Oliguria	Acidosis	Urine acidosis	Hypoproteinemia	Oliguria
	Anemia	Glucosuria	Edema	Renal failure
	Hypertension	Concentrating defect	Hyperlipidemia	
Uremia	Salt wasting	Hyperlipiduria		
Examples				
Solvents	Heavy metals	Heavy metals	Mercury	Petroleum
Heavy metals	Silicon	Radiation		Hydrocarbons
Pesticides	Solvents			
	Pesticides			
	Uranium			

Some examples of nephrotoxic chemicals

Halogenated hydrocarbons	Volatile hydrocarbons	Organic solvents	Metals	Others
Carbon tetrachloride	Petroleum	Ethylene glycol	Lead	Mycotoxins
Chloroform	Hydrocarbons	Toluene	Cadmium	Paraquat
Trichloroethylene		Styrene	Mercury	Pentachloro-
Tetrachloroethylene		Diethylene glycol	Gold	phenol
Bromobenzene			Nickel	Silicon
Bromodichloromethane			Uranium	Organophosphates
Dibromochloropropane			Chromium	
Dibromomethane			Arsenic	
Hexachlorobutadiene				

Table 25-2. Examples of some urinary-tract-cancer-causing agents

Kidney	Bladder/ureters
Nitroso compounds	β-Naphthyline
Alkylating agents	Benzidine
Cadmium	4-Aminodiphenyl
Lead	Auramine
Hydrazine	Magenta
	Cigarette smoke

Queensland, Australia, who had sustained acute lead intoxication in childhood and subsequently developed renal failure. In all these reports lead exposures were very high, and a report by Malcom[37] concluded that renal failure was likely to occur in groups with episodes of clinical poisoning. Acute lead exposure has its main effect on tubular transport mechanisms with the development of Fanconi syndrome (proximal tubular defect: proteinuria, glycosuria, aminoaciduria, phosphaturia altered calcium metabolism). This is usually associated with a characteristic histologic appearance in which degenerative changes in tubular epithelium and nuclear inclusion bodies containing lead/protein complexes are seen.[26] Goyer,[25] in animal studies, documented a sequence of histologic changes leading from inclusion bodies of diffuse interstitial fibrosis. Similar histologic changes on renal biopsy were reported by Cramer[14] in a small group of workers with heavy occupational lead exposure from a shipwrecking operation. In the earlier studies of lead-exposed workers later studied again by Malcom,[37] Dingwall-Fordyce and Lane[19] showed a significant excess of cerebrovascular accidents, and it has been suggested that hypertension subsequent to renal disease could explain the excess. Subsequent studies in other groups of lead workers[46] have not confirmed any excess of hypertension, but studies at much lower levels of lead in the general population have identified a relationship.[27] A pathologic mechanism for the biphasic effects of lead on blood pressure has recently been suggested by Khalil-Manesh et al.,[38] which proposes that low lead levels produce an increase in endotheli and a decrease in endothelium-derived relaxing factor (EDRF).

The use of the EDTA disodium calcium-lead mobilization test to measure lead body burden enabled Wedeen[60] to identify lead nephropathy in workers who lacked routine laboratory evidence of renal disease. Reduced glomerular filtration was found in 21 of 57 workers with excessive lead body burdens. Kidney biopsy in 12 of these workers showed tubular interstitial nephritis. Similarly, Batuman[4] identified lead as a cause of renal disease with gout. More recently Staessen[52] reported blood lead levels in association with renal insufficiency in a large European population. Blood lead ranged from 23 to 725 µg/l, and a tenfold increase in blood lead was associated with a decrease in glomerular filtration of 13 ml/min in men and 30 ml/min in women. The question of whether this decrease in clearance is reversible with reduction in blood lead level was not investigated. It is clear however that renal dysfunction occurs at lower levels of lead than previously reported. New methods for evaluating early renal damage described by Cardenas et al.[11] suggest that biochemical changes, such as decreased renal excretion of Prostaglandin E_2 and increased excretion of thromboxane and some tubular antigens, should alert the practitioner to the possibility of potential renal damage. Combining these new measurements of renal function with more sophisticated measurements of lead body burden, such as in vivo x-ray fluorescence,[3] may allow the relationship of lead body burden and renal nephropathy to be explored and strategies for prevention of toxic effects to be developed.

CADMIUM NEPHROTOXICITY

In 1948 Friberg[20] first described chronic cadmium nephropathy. In the years since this pioneering work, elucidation of the stages of renal damage has emerged. The first sign of renal damage by cadmium is a tubular proteinuria with the excretion of low-molecular-weight proteins such as B_2 micro-globulin and retinol binding protein. This may be followed by excretion of high-molecular-weight proteins, suggesting glomerular damage.[34] Along with proteinuria, glycosuria, and aminoaciduria, other signs of Fanconi syndrome, such as phosphate wasting and altered calcium metabolism, may appear.[33] Glomerular function may also be affected as noted by Friberg,[21] who performed insulin clearances on cadmium-exposed workers in 1950. The kidney, like the liver, synthesizes a low-molecular-weight protein, metallothionein, and this complex is also filtered through the glomerulus and reabsorbed by tubular cells. It is thus possible that cadmium does not exert a toxic effect until the capacity for metallothionein production is exceeded.[15] Friberg and co-workers also sought and found evidence of disturbances of calcium metabolism. Several workers in his 1950 report[21] had renal stones, and a 1961 study showed that 44% of workers exposed for more than 15 years had renal stones.[1]

Friberg, because of a report of a French alkaline battery plant,[44] looked for but found no evidence of osteomalacia. This suspicion of an impact on calcium metabolism-causing osteomalacia is supported by the Japanese reports of Itai-Itai disease in villages where rice was heavily contaminated with cadmium.[56] Nogawa[45] has suggested that a decreased level of dihydroxy vitamin D may be involved in this phenomenon, and Friberg[22] proposed that cadmium in the proximal tubule depresses conversion of 25(OH) vitamin D to $\alpha(OH)_2$ vitamin D. Further studies of this proposal are lacking, but the impact on phosphorus and calcium metabolism is well documented by Thun et al.[54] This study also has good estimates of the cumulative dose of cadmium that produces effects. These estimates are similar to those in previous studies such as Ellis,[16] and Thun[53] recommends a cumulative exposure below 225µg/M3/years. Thun[54] also demonstrated a correlation between rising serum creatinine concentration and cumulative exposure. The level of cadmium exposure below which no impact on glomerular filtration occurs must be sought, as it is clear that persistent microproteinuria is not reversible and may be the forerunner of a progressive deterioration in renal function.[47] A recent study of a large battery of markers in cadmium-exposed workers supports a urinary level of 5 µg Cd/1 g creatinine as an exposure limit to prevent tubular proteinuria.[48]

However, increased levels of other biochemical markers, such as urinary prostanoids, were still present. The significance of these changes for predicting tubular proteinuria or decrement in glomerular filtration is still unknown.

MERCURY

Metallic mercury vapor and salts of mercury, particularly mercuric salts, are excreted through the kidney, and the kidney develops the highest levels.[13,29] As a result the kidney is a primary target for acute renal toxicity with proximal tubular necrosis and renal failure occurring rapidly.[6] At lower concentrations both glomerular and tubular effects have been reported. Typically proximal tubular defects are seen with renal glycosemia and other elements of the Farconi syndrome. In addition, enhanced excretion of enzymes such as n-acetyl-glucosominidase and low-molecular-weight proteins such as a retinol binding protein occur.[49]

Immunologic glomercular disease may also develop, and nephrotic syndrome has been reported.[24] It is also possible that early immune glomerular disease progresses to interstitial immune complex nephritis.[57] A recent study by Cardenas et al.[12] investigated a variety of markers of renal change in low-level worker exposures. Three types of markers were studied: functional markers such as creatinine and low-molecular-weight proteins; markers of cytotoxicity such as tubular antigens and enzymes in urine; and biochemical markers such as the excretion of eicosanoids and thromboxane. At urine levels of mercury above 50 µg Hg/g creatinine changes indicative of cytotoxicity were seen. The relationship of these changes to alterations in renal function is not known; their use in medical surveillance requires further investigation.

OTHER METALS

Many other metals are reported to produce nephropathies similar to those already described for lead, cadmium, and mercury. Proximal tubular dysfunction is very common and several, such as gold and bismuth, may produce immune complex glomerulonephropathy. For all these metals high concentrations will produce renal failure.

SILICA

It is surprising that the multiplicity of studies of silica exposure and its impact on the lung have not previously identified kidney toxicity. There have been case reports that suggested a relationship.[23,42,51] A recent epidemiologic study[43] of silica-exposed workers compared with age-matched, nonexposed controls demonstrated significantly higher urinary excretion of albumin and α-1-microglobulin. Seven silicotics also had significantly higher excretion of albumin, α-1-microglobulin, and β-N-acetylglucosominidase even though they had ceased exposure 3 to 17 years before the study. This suggested that silica exposure may produce irreversible nephrotoxicity.

HYDROCARBONS

Many organic compounds have been identified as nephrotoxic agents. Hewitt et al.[31] list a wide variety of pharmaceuticals, pesticides, herbicides, mycotoxins, solvents, and other hydrocarbons. In view of their wide use, nephrotoxicity associated with solvents and other hydrocarbons are explored in greater depth.

Anderson[2] first reported a case of nephritis due to turpentine exposure, and since then there have been many reports of acute renal failure produced by a variety of hydrocarbons, chlorinated, aromatic, and aliphatic.[50] It is likely that the acute effects seen at high exposure levels are due to a direct toxic action on the tubule with resultant acute tubular necrosis. The relationship between lower-level hydrocarbon exposures and glomerular nephritis is gradually becoming clear. In 1972 Beirne et al.[5] reported on six cases of antiglomerular basement membrane (GBM) glomerulonephritis in individuals with recent hydrocarbon exposure. Similar reports such as that of Zimmerman[62] are summarized in Nelson et al.[41] It seems likely that many cases of glomerular nephritis in association with hydrocarbon exposure are caused by GBM-antibody-mediated glomerulonephritis. Case reports of a relationship between Goodpastures syndrome and hydrocarbon exposure,[32,40] which involves auto antibodies cross-reactive to alveolar and glomerular basement membrane support the idea of an autoimmune-related phenomenon with hydrocarbon exposures. The relationship between Goodpastures syndrome and hydrocarbon exposure has recently been reviewed by Bombassei and Kaplan.[9] Case-control studies, such as that of Finn,[17] who investigated 87 patients with end-stage renal failure and found that 59% of patients with glomerular nephritis had significant contact with hydrocarbons, support the relationship. Eight case-control and two cross-sectional studies are reviewed in Nelson et al.,[41] and these studies are relatively consistent in suggesting a relationship between hydrocarbon exposure and glomerulonephritis. Two recent cross-sectional studies of workers exposed to hydrocarbons[39,61] find early renal changes with excretion of enzymes and other markers of tubular cytotoxicity. The relationship of these changes to progressive nephropathy is unknown. The recent development of these sensitive measures of renal dysfunction do however provide an opportunity for further elucidation of the development of nephropathy and may lead to the identification of more renal disease associated with occupational and environmental exposure. This could lead to prevention of those renal diseases identified with occupational and environmental toxins.

REFERENCES

1. Ahlmark A et al: Further investigations into kidney function and proteinuria in chronic cadmium poisoning, *Int Congress Occ Health* 201, 1961.
2. Anderson K: Acute nephritis due to turpentine absorbed by the skin, *Br Med J* 3:881, 1912.
3. Armstrong R et al: Repeated measurements of tibia lead concentrations by in vivo x-ray fluorescence in occupational exposure, *Br J Ind Med* 49:14, 1992.
4. Batuman V et al: The role of lead in gouty nephropathy, *N Eng J Med* 304:520, 1981.
5. Beirne GJ, Brennam JT: Glomerulonephritis associated with hydrocarbon solvents, *Arch Env Health* 25:365, 1972.
6. Berlin M: Mercury. In Friberg L, Nordberg GF, Vouk VB, eds: *Handbook on toxicology of metals,* vol II, ed 2, Amsterdam, 1986, Elsevier.
7. Bernard A, Lauwery R: Epidemiologic application of early markers of nephrotoxicity, *Toxicol Lett* 46:293, 1989.
8. Bernard A, Lauwerys R: Renal toxicity from hazardous chemicals. In Sullivan J, Krieger G, eds: *Hazardous materials toxicology,* Baltimore, 1992, Williams & Wilkins.
9. Bombassei GJ, Kaplan AA: The association between hydrocarbon exposure and anti-glomerular basement membrane antibody mediated disease (Goodpastures syndrome), *Am J Ind Med* 21:141, 1992.
10. Brenner B, Zatz R, Ichikawa I: The renal circulation. In Brenner B, Rector F Jr., eds: *The kidney,* Philadelphia, 1986, WB Saunders.
11. Cardenas A et al: Markers of early renal changes induced by industrial 3 pollutants II. Application to workers exposed to lead, *Br J Ind Med* 50:28, 1993.
12. Cardenas A et al: Markers of early renal changes induced by industrial pollutants I. Application to workers exposed to mercury vapour, *Br J Ind Med* 50:17, 1993.
13. Clarkson TW, Klipper RW: The metabolism of inhaled vapor in animals and man. In Clarkson TW ed: *Heavy metals as environmental hazards to man,* Rochester, 1978, EHS Center Program Project.
14. Cramer K et al: Renal ultrastructure, renal function and parameters of lead toxicity, *Br J Ind Med* 31:113, 1974.
15. Elinder CG, Norderg C: Metallothioneine. In Friberg L et al: *Cadmium and health: a toxicological and epidemiological appraisal,* vol 1, Boca Raton, Fla, 1986, CRC Press.
16. Ellis KJ, Cohn SH, Smith TJ: Cadmium inhalation exposure estimates: their significance with respect to kidney and liver cadmium burden, *J Toxicol Environ Health* 15:173, 1985.
17. Finn R, Fennerty AG, Ahmad R: Hydrocarbon exposure and glomerulonephritis, *Clin Nephrol* 14(4):173, 1980.
18. Ford S, Hook J: Biochemical mechanisms of toxic nephropathies, *Semin Nephrol* 4:88, 1984.
19. Dingwall-Fordyce I, Lane RE: A followup study of lead workers, *Br J Ind Med* 20:313, 1963.
20. Friberg L: Proteinuria and kidney injury among workmen exposed to cadmium and nickel dust, *J Ind Hyg Toxicol* 30:32, 1948.
21. Friberg L: Health hazards in the manufacture of alkaline accumulators with special reference to chronic cadmium poisoning, *Acta Med Scand* 138(suppl 240):1, 1950.
22. Friberg L, eds: *Cadmium and health—a toxicological and epidemiological appraisal,* vols I and II, Boca Raton, Fla., 1986, CRC Press.
23. Giles RD et al: Massive proteinuria and acute renal failure in a patient with acute silica proteinosis, *Am J Med* 64:336, 1978.
24. Goyer R: Environmentally related disease of the urinary tract, *Med Clin North Am* 74(2):377, 1990.
25. Goyer RA: Lead and the kidney, *Cur Top Pathol* 55:147.
26. Goyer RA: Renal changes associated with lead exposure. In Mahaffey KR et al: *Dietary and environmental lead: human health effects,* Amsterdam, 1985, Elsevier.
27. Hanlon WR, Landis JR, Schmouder RI: The relationship of blood lead and blood pressure in adolescent and adult population, *JAMA* 253:530, 1955.
28. Henderson DA: The etiology of chronic nephritis in queensland, *Med J Aust* 1:377, 1958.
29. Hersh JB et al: The effect of ethanol on the fate of mercury vapor inhaled by man, *J Pharmacol Expr Ther* 3:520, 1980.
30. Hewitt W, Goldstein R, Hook J: Toxic responses of the kidney. In Amdur M, Doull J, Klaassen C, eds: *Toxicology: the basic science of poisons* New York, 1991, Pergamon.
31. Hewitt WR, Goldstein RS, Hook JB: Toxic responses of the kidney. In *Casarett and Doull's toxicology,* New York, 1991, Pergamon.
32. Keogh AM et al: Exacerbation of Goodpastures syndrome after inadvertent exposure to hydrocarbon fumes, *Br Med J* 288:188, 1984.
33. Kiellstrom T: Renal effects. In Friberg L et al, *Cadmium and health: a toxicological and epidemiological appraisal,* vol 2, Boca Raton, Fla, 1986, CRC Press.
34. Lauwerys RR et al: Characterization of cadmium proteinuria in man and rat, *Environ Health Perspect* 54:147, 1984.
35. Leaf A, Cortran R: *Renal pathophysiology,* Oxford, 1985, Oxford University Press.
36. Legge TM, Goadby KW: *Lead poisoning and lead absorption,* London, 1912, Arnold.
37. Malcolm O, Barnett HAR: A mortality study of lead workers, *Br J Ind Med* 39:404, 1982.

38. Khalil-Manesh F et al: Effects of chelation treatment with dimercaptosuccinic acids (DMSA) on lead related hypertension, *Environ Res* 1993 (in press).
39. Mutti A et al: Nephropathies and exposures to perchlorethylene in dry cleaners, *Lancet* 340:189, 1992.
40. Nathan AW, Toseland PA: Goodpastures Syndrome and trichloroethane intoxication, *Br J Clin Pharmacol* 8:284, 1979.
41. Nelson NA, Robins TG, Port FK: Solvent nephrotoxicity in humans and experimental animals, *Am J Nephrol* 10:10, 1990.
42. Newberne PM, Wilson RB: Renal damage associated with silicon compounds in dogs, *Proc Nat Acad Sci USA,* 65:872, 1970.
43. Ng TP et al: A study of silica nephrotoxicity in exposed silicotic and non-silicotic workers, *Br J Ind Med* 49:35, 1992.
44. Nicaud O, Lafitte A, Gros A: The problem of chronic cadmium intoxication, *Arch Mal Prof Med Trav Secur Soc* 4:192, 1942.
45. Nogawa K et al: Mechanism for bone disease found in inhabitants environmentally exposed to cadmium: decreased 1,25 dihydroxy vitamin D level, *Int Arch Occup Environ Health* 59:21, 1987.
46. Parkinson DK et al: Blood pressure and occupational lead exposure, *Br J Ind Med* 44:744, 1987.
47. Roels H et al: Health significance of cadmium induced renal dysfunction: a five year follow-up, *Br J Ind Med* 46:755, 1989.
48. Roels HY et al: Markers of early renal changes induced by industrial pollutants III. Applications to workers exposed to cadmium, *Br J Ind Med* 50:37, 1993.
49. Rosenman KD et al: Sensitive indicators of inorganic mercury toxicity, *Arch Env Health* 41:208, 1986.
50. Roy AT, Brautbar N, Lee DBN: Hydrocarbons and renal failure, *Nephron* 58:385, 1991.
51. Sherson D, Jorgensen F: Rapidly progressive crescenteric glomerulonephritis in a sandblaster with silicosis, *Br J Ind Med* 46:675, 1989.
52. Straessen JA et al: Impairment of renal function with increasing blood Pb concentrations in the general population, *N Engl J Med* 327:151, 1992.
53. Thun MJ, Elinder GG, Friberg L: Scientific bases for an occupational standard for cadmium, *Am J Ind Med* 20:629, 1991.
54. Thun MJ et al: Nephropathy in cadmium workers: assessment of risk from airborne occupational exposure to cadmium, *Br J Ind Med* 46:689, 1989.
55. Tischer C, Madsen K: Anatomy of the kidney. In Brenner B, Rector F, Jr., eds: *The kidney,* Philadelphia, 1986, WB Saunders.
56. Tsuchiya K, ed: *Cadmium studies in Japan: a review,* Amsterdam, 1978, Elsevier/North Holland Biomedical Press.
57. Tubbs RR et al: Membranous glomerulonephritis associated with industrial mercury exposure, *Am J Clin Pathol* 77:409, 1982.
58. Wedeen RP: Occupational renal disease, *Am J Kidney Dis* 3:291, 1984.
59. Wedeen RP: *Poison in the pot: the legacy of lead,* Carbondale, Ill, 1984, Southern Illinois University Press.
60. Wedeen RP, Mallik DK, Batuman V: Detection and treatment of occupational lead nephropathy, *Arch Intern Med* 139:53, 1979.
61. Yagoob M et al: *Quart J Med* 86(3):165, 1993.
62. Zimmerman SW, Groehler K, Beirne GL: Hydrocarbon exposure and chronic glomerulonephritis, *Lancet* 2:199, 1975.

Chapter 26

NERVOUS SYSTEM

Yuen T. So

Hallmarks of neurotoxic disorders
    Dose-response relationship
    Temporal relationship between exposure and symptoms
    Coasting
    Chemical structure
    Neurotoxicants
    Neurologic recovery
    Remote exposure
General approach to patients
    Importance of history
    Characterization of complaints
    Confounding influences
    Temporal sequence
Peripheral nervous system
    Complaints
    Physical examination
    Laboratory testing
Central nervous system
    Complaints
    Physical examination
    Laboratory testing
Selected neurologic disorders due to neurotoxins
    Lead
    Organophosphates
    Organic solvents

Neurologic symptoms are common presenting complaints in patients seen by occupational and environmental health professionals. Evaluation of these patients is a formidable task despite recent advances in neurodiagnostic techniques. Cognitive difficulties, headaches, fatigue, dizziness, and limb paresthesias are frequently encountered complaints but are nonspecific and seldom point to a single disease. The problems are compounded by the presence of a large and growing number of chemicals in our environment. Few of these agents are fully tested for their neurotoxic effects. Even for chemicals proven to be neurotoxic, there is considerable controversy about the safe limits of exposure duration and level. Reliable data on the neurologic hazards of long-term low-level exposure are especially difficult to obtain. The problem is further compounded by the difficult establishment of the intensity of exposure in individual patients. With notable exceptions, such as lead and some heavy metals, a reliable marker of exposure is not available for many substances. Finally, litigation and other potential sources for secondary gains frequently complicate environmental or occupational exposures that come to medical attention. This is particularly problematic for neurologic disorders, because psychologic factors may have profound effects on the patient's perception of neurologic symptoms, even in those with genuine organic disease. Failure to recognize the emotional issues may lead to errors in diagnosis and treatment.

HALLMARKS OF NEUROTOXIC DISORDERS

A number of common clinical features are shared by the better-characterized neurologic disorders due to environmental toxins. Some of these observations are useful as a conceptual framework in approaching these diseases, and some are useful in the daily evaluation of patients. Our knowledge of these diseases is rudimentary at best. The following discussion considers the limitations and uses of these generalizations.

Dose-response relationship

Although susceptibility to neurotoxins depends to some extent on the biologic state of the individual, there is a strong dose-response relationship in nearly all the neurotoxic disorders. Neurologic symptoms appear only after the acute or cumulative exposure reaches a certain level. Known exceptions are limited to idiosyncratic reactions to several medications, for example, prolonged muscle paralysis to succinylcholine in individuals with abnormal pseudocholinesterase. Unfortunately, a reliable adverse-effect threshold has not been established for many toxins. Further problems arise when the extent of exposure is unknown or multiple toxins are involved. Even if known, the adverse-effect threshold serves only as an approximate guideline in the clinical evaluation of patients.

Temporal relationship between exposure and symptoms

The mode of onset of neurologic symptoms after exposure depends on the underlying pathophysiologic mechanisms. Symptoms that appear immediately after acute exposure are usually due to the physiologic effects of the agent (for example, the cholinergic effects of organophosphates and the narcotizing effects of some organic solvents). These symptoms subside with cessation of exposure and elimination of the compound from the body. By contrast, delayed neurologic disorders are generally a result of pathologic alterations of the nervous system. Symptoms appear in a subacute manner over days or weeks after short-term exposure. In the case of long-term exposure, symptoms may appear insidiously and progress over many weeks or months. Recovery can be expected after cessation of exposure, but the recovery is slow and depends on the extent of neuronal damage.

Coasting

Coasting is the phenomenon of continuing clinical progression of neurologic deficits after the removal of the offending toxin. It is best characterized in the toxic neuropathies, especially those due to *n*-hexane[1,16] or pyridoxine intoxication.[6] Weakness or sensory deficits of these neuropathies often worsen for as long as 4 or 5 months after cessation of exposure, reflecting the delayed neuronal death or degeneration induced by the toxin.

Chemical structure

The chemical structure of an agent does not predict neurotoxicity. This observation underscores our rudimentary understanding of the pathogenetic mechanisms that lead to neuronal death and probably will be proven incorrect with improvement in the understanding of these diseases. There has already been some progress in a few areas, most notably in our understanding of the delayed neurotoxicity of organophosphates.[23]

Neurotoxicants

Neurotoxicants do not cause focal (asymmetrical) neurologic syndrome. This is probably one of the most useful rule of thumb in the clinical evaluation of patients. Neurotoxins reach the nervous system by the systemic route and cause neurologic symptoms and deficits in a diffuse and symmetric manner. Any significant asymmetry in the presentation, such as weakness or numbness affecting one limb or one side of the body, should suggest an alternative cause.

Multiple neurologic syndromes are possible from a single toxin. Although the effects of neurotoxins are symmetric, neurons from different parts of the nervous system react differently to the agent. The differential effect depends on the level and duration of exposure as well as other physiologic factors.

Neurologic recovery

One of the hallmarks of the nervous system is its plasticity or ability to adapt to injury. Peripheral sensory and motor nerve fibers have a remarkable capacity to regenerate after removal of the neurotoxin. Even though neurons in the central nervous system lack the ability to multiply, surviving neurons may eventually take over the function of degenerated neurons and partially restore neurologic functions. When given sufficient time, partial clinical improvement is therefore demonstrable in the majority of cases.

Remote exposure

A caveat in our concept of neurologic recovery is the possibility that a toxic exposure in the remote past may induce neurologic symptoms many years later. Such a mechanism has been hypothesized in the pathogenesis of Parkinson's disease and amyotrophic lateral sclerosis.[8] Proponents have suggested that the degree of neuronal death during exposure to a neurotoxin may not be sufficient to cause immediate neurologic symptoms. The exposure, however, may deplete the functional reserve of that part of the nervous system such that, with further depletion of neurons from normal aging, symptoms eventually appear years or decades later.

GENERAL APPROACH TO PATIENTS

It is important to recognize that very few neurotoxic disorders present with pathognomonic symptoms, signs, or laboratory findings. The clinical syndrome may mimic a wide range of psychiatric, metabolic, nutritional, inflammatory, or degenerative diseases. The diagnosis of a neurotoxic disorder depends therefore on documentation of an appropriate neurologic syndrome after a sufficient exposure and exclusion of other neurologic disorders that can account for a patient's symptoms and clinical signs. A full discussion of the neurologic history and examination is beyond the scope of this chapter. Excellent discussions of the subjects are widely available.[9,15] Only aspects directly relevant to environmental medicine are discussed here.

Importance of history

As is the case in other environmental disorders, the key to diagnosis is a focused history of environmental or occupational exposure. This exposure may be either chemical (for example, metals or pesticides) or physical (for example, noise or radiation), although the majority of neurologic disorders are due to the former type. Unsuspected toxic exposure may arise from household products, hobbies, or a contaminated home environment. When a potential toxin is identified, it is important to ascertain the duration and frequency of contact. The potential routes of entry into the body and the intensity of exposure should be considered. Inquiries about similar symptoms in co-workers or family members who may have similar exposures should be made. When the nature of the toxin or the intensity of exposure is unknown, clustering of cases may be the only initial clue in establishing a common environmental cause. Unfortunately, clustering of reports can also be a result of mass hysteria, especially in settings in which the potential toxicity is widely publicized.

Characterization of complaints

The nature of the neurologic complaints needs to be characterized as fully as possible. Commonly used descriptions, such as weakness, dizziness, forgetfulness, pain, and numbness, have different meanings to different individuals and should never be accepted without further inquiry. For example, weakness should be distinguished from fatigue or asthenia; the latter implies a disinclination for physical activity rather than a disorder of the motor system. One should always inquire about the functional consequences of the patient's neurologic symptoms. Drawing from concrete examples of everyday life is particularly useful, both to understand the patient's complaints better and to provide a more objective assessment of the severity of the problem.

Confounding influences

A number of physiologic and psychologic factors greatly influence a patient's perception and report of symptoms. An obvious example is depression, either directly or indirectly related to the neurologic injury. Another example is the neuropathic pain commonly encountered in patients with peripheral neuropathies. The severity of this pain sometimes bears little relationship to the severity of neuropathy. Pain may intensify during a period of recovery, or it may remit paradoxically as the neuropathy progresses (with further loss of sensation of the extremities). Pain is therefore not a reliable indicator of neurologic progression or recovery.

Temporal sequence

As in most neurologic disorders, the temporal course of neurologic symptoms in environmental disorders is important to scrutinize. The mode of symptom onset has important implications in pathogenesis. Symptoms may appear within seconds (abrupt), within minutes to days (acute), over several weeks (subacute), or over many months or years (chronic). Fluctuating symptoms may suggest recurrent exposures or other superimposed factors. Recovery after discontinuation of exposure helps to implicate the exposure. By contrast, continuation of neurologic deterioration more than a few months after cessation of exposure argues against a causative role for the exposure.

PERIPHERAL NERVOUS SYSTEM

Environmental diseases of the peripheral nervous system primarily manifest as a disorder of the peripheral nerve, or neuropathy. Myopathy is uncommon. Because systemic toxins simultaneously affect many nerves, the resultant clinical syndrome is commonly referred to as a polyneuropathy, in contrast to mononeuropathy or focal neuropathy, which is seldom the result of neurotoxin. Focal neuropathies (for example, carpal tunnel syndrome) are frequently the consequence of localized mechanical or inflammatory injuries.

Complaints

In patients with toxic polyneuropathy, the distal limbs are affected first, reflecting the greater vulnerability of the longest nerve axons. Sensory disturbances are usually reported as a tingling or burning sensation distributed in a stocking-and-glove pattern (Fig. 26-1). The toes and the feet are affected first, and hand symptoms are seldom present during the early stage. Bilateral hand tingling or numbness without lower-extremity symptoms is more commonly due to bilateral carpal tunnel syndrome than to a systemic polyneuropathy. Involvement of the motor nerve fibers, if present, manifests first as atrophy and weakness of the intrinsic foot and hand muscles. More severe cases may present with foot drop or wrist drop, reflecting degeneration of motor axons to the lower leg and forearm muscles.

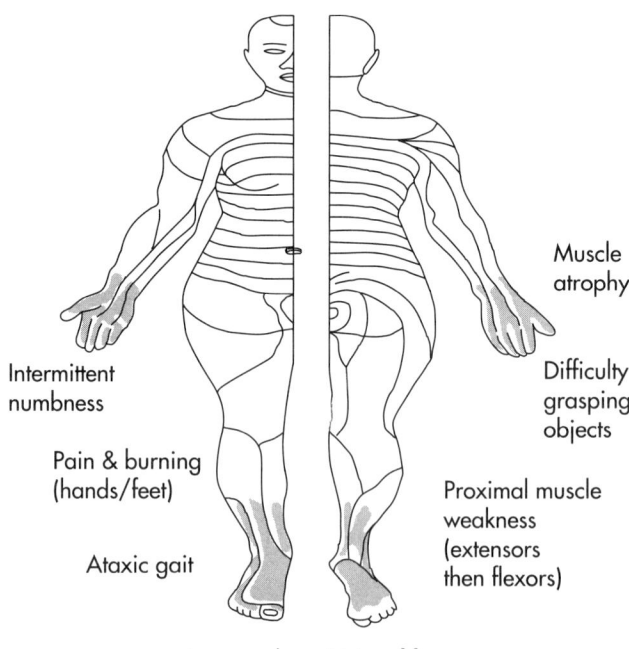

Fig. 26-1. In most polyneuropathies the limbs are affected in a length-dependent manner. Sensory symptoms typically begin in the toes and soles. Lower extremity symptoms spread proximally as the disease progresses. Tingling and numbness generally spread beyond the feet and ankles before symptoms appear in the hands.

Physical examination

Physical examination should include testing of muscle strength, sensation, and tendon reflexes. Because the common neuropathies often manifest first in the longest axons, symptoms and signs typically begin in the feet before spreading to the lower legs and hands. Testing of the tendon reflex at the ankles and the sensation at the toes is useful means of documenting early neurologic deficits. Sensation to vibration depends on the function of large-diameter sensory fibers and can be readily assessed at the bedside by determining the sensory threshold to vibration of a 128-Hz tuning fork. Sensation to pain is mediated by small-diameter nerve fibers and can be assessed partly by the patient's report of pain to a pinprick stimulus.

Laboratory testing

There has been a recent surge in interest in the application of quantitative sensory testing in the occupational health setting.[3,21] Quantitative sensory testing uses specialized equipment to deliver reproducible, precisely calibrated sensory stimuli. Vibrating instruments such as the Bioesthesiometer and Optacon are among the most widely used in clinical practice. Other sensory modalities, such as temperature and light-touch discrimination, can be tested with available equipment. Like all sensory testing, success of quantitative testing depends on proper patient cooperation. It is sometimes difficult to assure the reliability of the patient's reported sensory threshold. The proven value of these tools is in the reduction of variability among observers. They are thus valuable in the longitudinal follow-up of patients and in the therapeutic trials in treatment of neuropathies.

Nerve conduction studies and electromyography (EMG) are the primary tools for the laboratory evaluation of neuromuscular disorders. These two tests are often performed together and can provide diagnostic and prognostic information when properly performed and interpreted.[2]

Nerve conduction studies record the electrical response of a nerve or muscle to electrical stimulation at different sites along the course of a nerve. Nerve conduction velocity and the amplitude of response can be measured and serve as a quantitative assessment of peripheral nerve function. A toxic polyneuropathy is characterized by a diffuse and relatively symmetric pattern of abnormalities. The abnormalities can be further subdivided into those of either axonal or demyelinating neuropathy. The subdivision narrows the diagnostic possibilities, even though nerve conduction studies alone never identify the specific cause of a polyneuropathy.

In EMG, a needle electrode is inserted to record the electrical activities of skeletal muscle fibers. Characteristic abnormalities are seen in acutely denervated muscles, muscles undergoing chronic reinnervation, and those affected by primary muscle diseases. The most frequent use of EMG is in the diagnostic evaluation of clinical weakness. For example, it is helpful when strength testing is difficult because of the presence of either pain or malingering.

There are several drawbacks to conventional electrodiagnostic studies. Specialized training and expensive electronic equipment are generally needed for the proper performance and interpretation of these tests. Furthermore, these tests are uncomfortable at best, and patient compliance is occasionally a problem. Although simplified devices have been used with varying success (e.g., in screening for carpal tunnel syndrome), they invariably result in some compromise in diagnostic sensitivity and specificity.

The relative degree of sensory and motor involvement in patients with toxic neuropathy depends largely on the agent and the nature of the exposure. This clinical pattern is important in identifying the cause of a neuropathy (see box). Many toxins manifest as a nonspecific syndrome of distal sensorimotor impairment that is indistinguishable from the neuropathies due to common systemic diseases (for example, diabetes mellitus, vitamin B_{12} deficiency, alcoholism, and uremia). In such cases, the common causes of neuropathy should be excluded before a diagnosis of toxic neuropathy is considered. Toxins such as lead have a striking predilection for motor fibers and usually produce minimal sensory symptoms. The differential diagnosis of a predominantly motor neuropathy is relatively narrow and encompasses many of the hereditary and immunologic neuropathies. These neuropathies are uncommon and generally require the expertise of a specialist.

Agents associated with a toxic polyneuropathy

Sensorimotor polyneuropathies (weakness if any is mild)

Metal: arsenic (long-term exposure), mercury
Ethylene oxide
Methyl bromide
Polychlorinated biphenyls
Acrylamide

Neuropathies with significant and sometimes severe weakness

Metal: lead, arsenic (acute), mercury
Hexacarbons: n-hexane, methyl n-butyl ketone
Organophophates: triorthocresyl phosphate, leptophos, mipafox, chlorpyrifos, parathion, and others

Cranial neuropathy

Trichloroethylene (trigeminal)

Prominent autonomic dysfunction

n-Hexane (glue-sniffing)
N-(3-pyridinylmethyl)-N'-(4-nitrophenyl) urea (Vacor)

Possible association with neuropathies (mostly anecdotal)

Methyl methacrylate
Dioxin
Carbon monoxide
Benzene
Pyrethrins

CENTRAL NERVOUS SYSTEM
Complaints

The differential susceptibility of different types of neurons in the central nervous system (CNS) accounts for the diverse manifestations of toxic exposure by the brain and spinal cord. Symptoms and deficits depend on which group of neurons is most affected, which in turn depends on the nature of toxin and the intensity and duration of exposure. Diffuse cortical or subcortical injury may lead to an encephalopathy characterized by personality change and cognitive dysfunction. Cerebellar or vestibular deficits manifest predominantly as a disorder of equilibrium, with vertigo and gait stability as the chief symptoms. A syndrome of parkinsonism, with bradykinesia, tremor, and limb rigidity, may result from injury to the basal ganglia or other parts of the extrapyramidal motor system. As mentioned earlier, focal deficits do not result from systemic exposure to toxins. Thus ataxia or weakness limited to one side of the body and isolated cortical deficits such as aphasia should suggest another cause of the disorder.

Physical examination

The physical examination should be tailored to the clinical syndrome in question. In patients with cognitive symptoms the minimal bedside examination includes a mini–mental state evaluation.[12] More extensive evaluation is necessary in patients with predominantly cognitive complaints. Formal neuropsychologic testing, if necessary, provides further insights into the pattern and severity of the cognitive deficits. Quantitative assessment of deficits is meaningful only if there is patient cooperation, and interpretation of neuropsychologic test results depends largely on the expertise of the neuropsychologist. Thus, each test report should always be considered in light of the overall clinical picture.

Examination of patients with complaints of gait unsteadiness, dizziness, or vertigo should include careful observation of cranial nerve and cerebellar functions. The examiner should observe the patient's gait, including the ability to walk heel-to-toe. The presence of nystagmus or other abnormalities in extraocular movements, hearing deficits, limb ataxia, sensory deficits or Romberg's sign should be noted.

Laboratory testing

Despite advances in neurodiagnostic techniques, laboratory investigation in suspected toxic injury of the CNS is revealing only infrequently. Diffuse abnormalities on magnetic resonance imaging (MRI) have been reported in a few cases of massive exposure to organic solvents, typically in the setting of recreational abuse.[27] Computed tomography (CT) or MRI is more typically normal in the majority of patients with environmental or occupational exposures. Electroencephalography (EEG) and other electrophysiologic studies are likewise of little value in most patients. Two factors contribute to the low incidence of abnormal results from traditional neurodiagnostic tests. First, MRI and EEG assess gross neuroanatomy and physiologic function, respectively. Most affected patients encountered in developed countries have a relatively mild injury that cannot be detected with these methods. Second, a significant number of patients are brought to medical attention because of ongoing litigation or emotional problems and do not actually have neurologic disease. The current neurodiagnostic methods provide little help to clinicians in the differentiation between organic and functional disorders. Rather, the main value of neuroimaging and neurophysiologic studies is in the diagnosis of unrelated neurologic diseases that may mimic a neurotoxic disorder.

Under the appropriate setting, the use of toxicologic or biologic markers of exposure, such as serum lead level and red blood cell acetylcholinesterase level, is more helpful. These studies are discussed in detail in the chapters dealing with the specific toxins.

SELECTED NEUROLOGIC DISORDERS DUE TO NEUROTOXINS

It is impossible to provide a comprehensive review of the major neurotoxic disorders in this chapter. The better-known syndromes are summarized in Table 26-1. Only three neurotoxins are selected for further discussion. They illustrate some of the issues discussed in this chapter as well as the unique diagnostic difficulties of occupational and environmental diseases.

Lead

Despite the ban on leaded fuel and lead-based paints in the United States, lead is widely found in contaminated soils and old paint and still represents a significant environmental hazard. High-level exposures, typically from accidental ingestion or industrial exposure, result in a subacute syndrome of abdominal colic and intermittent vomiting. Microcytic hypochromic anemia, basophilic stippling of erythrocytes, and lead lines at the metaphyses of long bones may be seen but are too inconstant to be reliable. Neurologic symptoms such as headache, apathy, and lethargy occur with blood lead levels of 50 μg/dl or higher. More massive intoxication, especially in children, may lead to brain edema, stupor, and, eventually, transtentorial herniation. Overt encephalopathy is far less common in adults; the usual presenting symptoms are abdominal pain, anemia, and peripheral neuropathy.

Lead poisoning in adults manifests commonly as a motor neuropathy with minimal or no sensory complaints. The classic patterns of focal weakness of wrist extensors (wristdrop), shoulder girdles, or peroneal muscles (footdrop) are now extremely rare. More recent reports outlined a syndrome of generalized weakness and reflex loss.[7] In studies of exposed workers, significant slowing in peripheral nerve conduction velocity was demonstratable in those with blood lead levels around 35 to 60 μg/dl.[34] Conduction slowing was especially common in those with levels of 50 to 70 μg/dl or above.[7,33] Significant peripheral neuropathy has also been

Table 26-1. Neurologic syndromes associated with various neurotoxins

Neurotoxins	Neurologic syndromes	Common sources
Metals		
Arsenic	Polyneuropathy, encephalopathy, headache	Contaminated shellfish, paints, pigments, pesticides, electroplating industry
Lead	Encephalopathy, headache, polyneuropathy	Old paints, ceramics, contaminated soil, batteries, foundries, smelters, soldering
Manganese	Parkinsonism, encephalopathy	Welding, iron industry, mining of manganese, paints, fireworks, fertilizers
Mercury	Encephalopathy, headache, cerebellar ataxia, choreoathetosis, polyneuropathy	Amalgams, electroplating industry, photography
Pesticides and fungicides		
Organophosphates	Acute: cholinergic symptoms Chronic: polyneuropathy, encephalopathy	Gardening and farming use, pesticide manufacturing
Organotin	Encephalopathy, cerebellar ataxia	Fungicides, paints, plastic stabilizers
Solvents		
Carbon disulfide	Polyneuropathy, encephalopathy, parkinsonism	Insecticides, solvents for industrial use
n-Hexane, methyl butyl ketone	Acute: dizziness, encephalopathy Chronic: polyneuropathy, encephalopathy	Glue-sniffing, other abuse, shoe and rubber industries, paints, lacquers, varnish, cleaning solvents
Trichloroethylene	Acute: CNS depression Chronic: polyneuropathy, trigeminal neuropathy, encephalopathy	Industrial solvents, glues, adhesives, paints, varnish
Toluene	Acute: euphoria Chronic: encephalopathy, cerebellar ataxia	Industrial solvents, glues, paints, lacquers

shown in children with chronic exposure and blood lead levels as low as 20 to 40 μg/dl.[29]

Acute lead encephalopathy and motor neuropathy from lead poisoning undoubtedly represent only the tip of the iceberg. Long-term, low-level lead exposure has been linked to a chronic and more subtle encephalopathy. The typical symptoms are behavioral disturbances and neuropsychologic impairment. This neurotoxicity is dose related. Overt symptoms, such as memory loss, hallucinations, lethargy, and disorientation, appear in individuals with exposure for more than 6 months and blood levels over 40 μ/dl.[5] There is increasing evidence that neurobehavioral problems may be encountered at levels as low as 20 μ/dl. Especially disturbing are studies that suggest that long-term, low-level exposure in children may lead to a decreased global intelligence quotient as well as a wide range of behavioral disturbances. An increased incidence of poor self-confidence, impulsive behavior, and shortened attention span has been reported as occurring in exposed children.[10,20,26]

Organophosphates

Organophosphorous agents are widely used as pesticides. The immediate neurologic effects are due to the antagonistic effect of these compounds on acetylcholinesterase. Abdominal cramps, blurred vision, miosis, and increased salivation and sweating are manifestations of cholinergic excess and are readily reversed by atropine. Coma, loss of pupillary reflexes, muscle fasciculations, paralysis, and even respiratory arrest may occur with more severe intoxication. Unless complicated by anoxia or other secondary insults to the brain, rapid recovery generally follows metabolism and excretion of the agent; however, there may be subtle residual neurologic deficits, as suggested by a study showing persistent neuropsychologic impairment 2 years after an episode of acute poisoning.[28] Moreover, long-term low-level exposure to organophosphates has been linked to a chronic encephalopathy with symptoms of forgetfulness and other cognitive dysfunction.[19]

A striking delayed polyneuropathy has been reported to occur with exposure to several organophosphates (see box on p. 321). The onset of symptoms is variable, with most patients presenting 3 to 4 weeks after exposure. Symptoms are those of a distal symmetric motor polyneuropathy. Sensory loss is relatively mild. Recovery is slow and incomplete and depends on the degree of axonal loss as well as the involvement of the spinal cord in some cases. Of the organophosphates that can cause a neuropathy, triorthocresyl phosphate is the most extensively studied and probably has caused the largest number of toxic neuropathies. Several famous outbreaks have been well documented. The so-called jake paralysis in the Prohibition era was traced to drinking the extract of contaminated Jamaican ginger.[4] Other outbreaks include contamination of cooking oil in Morocco and gingli oil in Sri Lanka.[30,35]

The pathogenesis of this delayed neuropathy probably involves binding and inhibition of neuropathy target esterase (NTE), an esterase that is distinct from acetylcholinesterase.[18,24] A second step, aging of the inhibited phosphoryl–NTE complex, is necessary to produce neuropathy. Organophosphate compounds that age the NTE complex lead to delayed neuropathy, whereas those that do not age are safe. NTE screening has suggested that many compounds previously regarded as safe may be toxic to the peripheral nerves.[23] It remains to be seen whether monitoring of lymphocyte NTE in exposed individuals may be useful in detection of subclinical neurotoxicity and eventual prevention of neuropathy.

Organic solvents

Organic solvents, which are volatile liquid compounds, are commonly used in our environment. Clinically important exposures occur primarily as a result of industrial contact and volitional abuse. Brief exposure at extremely high concentrations causes an acute and reversible encephalopathy, underscoring the acute narcotizing properties possessed by most organic solvents. Long-term exposure to moderate or high levels of solvent can cause either CNS disease or a peripheral polyneuropathy. The better delineated agents and clinical syndromes are outlined in the box on p. 321 and Table 26-1. The levels necessary to cause neurologic deficits are generally higher than that likely to be encountered in environmental exposures.

Considerable controversies surround a syndrome attributed to long-term, low-level solvent exposure, variously termed painters' syndrome, chronic toxic encephalopathy, or psychoorganic syndrome. These patients were typically exposed to a mixture of several solvents at concentrations below currently accepted occupational standards. It has been argued cogently that the usual concept of threshold limit value (TLV) applies only to exposure involving a single solvent and that adverse effects to a mixture of solvents may occur at a level much lower than the individual TLVs. The neurologic symptoms described in the psychoorganic syndrome are diverse and include headache, dizziness, asthenia, mood and personality change, inattentiveness, forgetfulness, and depression.

Most of the literature regarding the psychoorganic syndrome originated from Scandinavian investigations using extensive neuropsychologic testing in exposed workers. Despite a lack of uniformity in the methods of testing, the studies consistently suggest a diffuse pattern of performance impairment.[14,22] Additionally, in both symptomatic and asymptomatic subjects, a high incidence of electrophysiologic abnormalities[25,31,32] and cerebral atrophy on CT[17] has been reported. It is common practice for many occupational and environmental health physicians to make the diagnosis of toxic encephalopathy if some of the typical symptoms of psychoorganic syndrome are present and another organic disease is not identified by laboratory evaluations.

Other investigators, on the other hand, are less willing to embrace the idea of a psychoorganic syndrome due to low-level solvent exposure. Many have pointed out that the neurologic complaints in this syndrome are nonspecific and are typical of other neurologic or psychiatric illnesses. Moreover, in the vast majority of these patients, the results of physical examination and laboratory evaluation are uniformly negative. Many of the studies supporting the painters' syndrome have also been criticized because of methodologic problems and failure to account for confounding factors such as psychiatric diseases or alcohol abuse.[11] Furthermore, several studies using control groups matched for age, education, and socioeconomic status have failed to identify a significant difference between exposed subjects and controls with regard to neuropsychologic performance and CT and electrophysiologic findings.[13,36]

REFERENCES

1. Altenkirch H et al: Toxic polyneuropathies after sniffing a glue thinner, *J Neurol* 214:137-152, 1977.
2. Aminoff MJ: Electrophysiologic recognition of certain occupation-related neurotoxic disorders, *Neurol Clin* 3:687-697, 1985.
3. Arezzo JC, Schaumberg HH: The use of the Optacon as a screening device, *J Occup Med* 22:461-464, 1980.
4. Aring CD: The systemic nervous affinity of triorthocresyl phosphate (Jamaican Ginger Palsy), *Brain* 65:34, 1942.
5. Baker EL et al: Occupational lead neurotoxicity: a behavioral and electrophysiological evaluation: study design and year one results, *Br J Ind Med* 41:352-361, 1984.
6. Berger AR et al: Dose response, coasting, and differential fiber vulnerability in human toxic neuropathy: a prospective study of pyridoxine neurotoxicity, *Neurology* 42:1367-1370, 1992.
7. Buchthal F, Behse F: Electrophysiology and nerve biopsy in men exposed to lead, *Br J Ind Med* 39:135-147, 1979.
8. Calne DB et al: Alzheimer's disease, Parkinson's disease and motor-neuron disease: abiotropic interaction between aging and environment, *Lancet* 2:1067-1070, 1986.
9. DeJong RN: *The neurologic examination,* New York, 1979, Harper and Row.
10. de la Burde B, Choate MS: Early asymptomatic lead exposure and development at school age, *J Pediatr* 87:638, 1975.
11. Errebo-Knudsen EO, Olsen F: Organic solvents and presenile dementia (the painters' syndrome): a critical review of the Danish literature, *Sci Total Environ* 48:45-67, 1986.
12. Folstein MF, Folstein SE, McHugh PR: "Mini-mental state": a practical method for grading the cognitive state of patients for the clinician, *J Psychiatr Res* 12:189-198, 1978.
13. Gade A, Mortensen EL, Bruhn P: "Chronic painter's syndrome": a reanalysis of psychological test data in a group of diagnosed cases, based on comparisons with matched controls, *Acta Neurol Scand* 77:293-306, 1988.
14. Grasso P et al: Neurophysiological and psychological disorders and occupational exposure to organic solvents, *Food Chem Toxicol* 10:819-852, 1984.
15. Greenberg DA, Aminoff MJ, Simon RP: *Clinical Neurology,* ed 2. Norwalk, Conn, 1993, Appleton and Lange.
16. Huang CC et al: Biphasic recovery in n-hexane polyneuropathy: a clinical and electrophysiological study, *Acta Neurol Scand* 80:610-615, 1989.
17. Jensen PB et al: Chronic toxic encephalopathy following occupational exposure to organic solvents: the course after cessation of exposure illustrated by a neurophysiological follow-up investigation, *Ugeskr Laeger* 146:1387-1390, 1984.

18. Johnson MK: Organophosphates and delayed neuropathy: is NTE alive and well? *Toxicol Appl Pharmacol* 102:385-399, 1990.
19. Korsak RJ, Sato BA: Effects of chronic organophosphate pesticide exposure on the central nervous system, *Clin Toxicol* 11:83-95, 1977.
20. Lee WR, Moore MR: Low level exposures to lead: the evidence for harm accumulates, *Br Med J* 301:504-506, 1990.
21. Le Quesne PM, Fowler CJ: Quantitative evaluation of toxic neuropathies in man, *Electroencephalogr Clin Neurophysiol* (EEG suppl 39):347-354, 1987.
22. Lindstrom K: Behavioral effects of long-term exposure to organic solvents, *Acta Neurol Scand* 66(suppl 92):131-141, 1982.
23. Lotti M: The pathogenesis of organophosphate polyneuropathy, *Crit Rev Toxicol* 21:465-487, 1992.
24. Lotti M et al: Inhibition of lymphocytic neuropathy target esterase predicts development of organophosphate-induced delayed neuropathy, *Arch Toxicol* 59:176-179, 1986.
25. Mutti A et al: Neurophysiological effects of long-term exposure to hydrocarbon mixtures, *Arch Toxicol* 5:120-124, 1982.
26. Needleman HL: The neurobehavioral consequences of low lead exposure in childhood, *Neurobehav Toxicol Teratol* 4:729-732, 1982.
27. Rosenberg NL et al: Toluene abuse causes diffuse central nervous system white matter changes, *Ann Neurol* 23:611-614, 1988.
28. Rosenstock L et al: Chronic central nervous system effects of acute organophosphate pesticide intoxication, *Lancet* 338:223-227, 1991.
29. Schwartz J et al: Threshold effect in lead-induced neuropathy, *J Pediatr* 112:12-17, 1988.
30. Senanayake N, Jeyaratnam J: Toxic polyneuropathy due to gingli oil contaminated with tricresyl phosphate affecting adolescent girls in Sri Lanke, *Lancet* 1:88, 1981.
31. Seppalainen AM: Neurophysiological findings among workers exposed to organic solvents, *Acta Neurol Scand* 66(suppl 92):109-116, 1982.
32. Seppalainen AM: Neurophysiological aspects of the toxicity of organic solvents, *Scand J Work Environ Health* 11:61-64, 1985.
33. Seppalainen AM, Hernberg S, Kock B: Relationship between blood lead levels and nerve conduction velocities, *Neurotoxicology* 1:313-332, 1979.
34. Seppalainen AM et al: Subclinical neuropathy at "safe" levels of lead exposure, *Arch Environ Health* 30:180-183, 1975.
35. Smith HV, Spalding JMK: Outbreaks of paralysis in Morocco due to orthocresylphosphate poisoning, *Lancet* 2:1019, 1959.
36. Triebig G et al: Cross-sectional epidemiological study on neurotoxicity of solvents in paints and lacquers, *Int Arch Occup Environ Health* 60:233-241, 1988.

Chapter 27

DISORDERS OF THE IMMUNOLOGIC SYSTEM

Clement A. Maccia
Andor Szentivanyi
Khalid Ali
Christine Abarca
Stuart M. Brooks

Introduction and classification
Description of various immunologically mediated disorders
    Type I reactions (immediate hypersensitivities)
    Examples of type I hypersensitivity disorders
    Type II reactions (cytotoxic tissue injury)
    Type III reactions (immune complex tissue injury)
    Type IV reactions (cell-mediated immune tissue injuries)
    Clinical features
    Mixed immunologic reactions
    Disorders of autoimmunity
    Immunodeficiency disorders
    Tests for antibody formation following active immunization

INTRODUCTION AND CLASSIFICATION*

In the past decade there has been a tremendous explosion of knowledge in the field of immunology. This chapter will focus on the immunologically mediated diseases, with special emphasis on immunologic problems that arise from environmental exposures or from acquired syndromes of deficit or altered immunity. The immune system has the dual ability to react to foreign molecules (antigens) and to be tolerant to self-molecules of the body's own tissues. There are humoral and cellular compartments that possess a complex interdependence, and there are nonspecific components, including the complement and kinin cascade, the acute-phase response, and the phagocytic cell system.

Immunologically mediated disease may be viewed as three general types, depending upon whether the offending antigen is exogenous, allogeneic, or autologous. Failure of the immune system is based on the following factors: (1) an enhanced immune response, which produces more damage than it prevents; (2) failure of self-recognition leading to autoimmunity; and (3) failure of adequate production of an immune response translated clinically as immunodeficiency. The various types of immunopathologic processes have also been subdivided by the classification by Coombs and Gell[19a] into the following four basic types: (1) type I—immediate hypersensitivities; (2) type II—cytotoxic tissue injury; (3) type III—immune complex tissue injury; and (4) type IV—cell-mediated immune tissue injuries. This classification is oversimplified because of the complex interrelationships that exist between the several events that constitute an inflammatory response. Nevertheless this view represents the closest approximation of the various basic patterns of immune tissue injury, and the classification does not depend on the host species or on the method of antigen exposure. Another valuable feature of the classification is its integrated emphasis on the important central point that in these various patterns of immune injury the tissue damage results from the

---
*References 4, 7, 8, 10, 24, 26, 43, 57, 60, 71.

immune activation of cellular and biochemical mediator systems of the host. The combination of the immune reactants produces only minimal direct effects, but as a trigger mechanism it sets the destructive factors into play. A fifth category of conditions not included in the Gell and Coomb classification are the immunodeficiency disorders, either congenital or acquired. The following discussion deals with the various categories of immunologic disorders.

DESCRIPTION OF VARIOUS IMMUNOLOGICALLY MEDIATED DISORDERS*

Type I reactions (immediate hypersensitivities)

Overview. The term *immediate hypersensitivity* denotes an immunologic sensitivity to antigens that manifests itself by tissue reactions occurring within minutes after the antigen combines with its appropriate antibody. Such a reaction may occur in any member of a species (nonatopic immediate hypersensitivity) or only in certain predisposed or hyperreactive members (atopic immediate hypersensitivity). The prototype of the nonatopic immediate hypersensitivity is local or generalized anaphylaxis, whereas manifestations of atopic immediate hypersensitivity include bronchial asthma, hay fever, allergic rhinitis, chronic urticaria, and atopic dermatitis.

Terminology. *Anaphylaxis* is defined as a manifestation of immediate hypersensitivity resulting from the in vivo interaction of cellular sites with antigen and specific antibody. *Generalized anaphylaxis* refers to a shocklike state occurring within minutes following an appropriate antigen-antibody reaction. Upon the first exposure of an animal to an antigen, a cytotropic antibody may form that sensitizes mast cells, basophils, and other cells, storing and/or synthesizing pharmacologically active effector molecules in tissues and in blood. After a second exposure to the antigen, the animal so sensitized reacts with the explosive release of the foregoing effector molecules, resulting in the hemodynamic, bronchial, and cutaneous manifestations of shock. In this particular example, we are referring to *active anaphylaxis,* since the final clinical manifestation is dependent on the active production of cytotropic antibodies by the test animal. If, however, the test animal is the recipient of cytotropic antibodies produced by a donor animal, the condition of the test animal resulting from exposure to the antigen is called *passive anaphylaxis.* Another term, *local anaphylaxis,* is used for describing the anaphylactic response of a specific target organ (for example, the bronchial tree, gastrointestinal tract, nasal mucosa, or skin). Under experimental conditions such a reactivity may be induced by passive sensitization of the tissue in question with antibody-containing serum obtained from a sensitized donor; subsequent intravenous or local administration of the corresponding antigen will then result in a local anaphylactic reaction. An illustrative example of this kind of reactivity is the so-called *passive cutaneous anaphylaxis (PCA)* in which an animal is injected intracutaneously with serum from a sensitive animal of the same or another species. After a certain latent period required for the cutaneous fixation of the antibody, the antigen is administered intravenously along with Evans blue dye, which will react with the skin-fixed antibody, causing the release of histamine from cutaneous mast cells. The histamine release results in local vasodilation and leakage of albumin to which the blue dye is attached, producing a blue spot. The latter indicates that an anaphylactic reaction has taken place in the skin. For experimental purposes, several in vitro tissue models of anaphylaxis have also been developed.

Anaphylaxis. Theoretically any immunogen should be able to elicit anaphylaxis in a properly sensitized host. These may be proteins, chemical haptens such as drugs attached to proteins, carbohydrates, or, occasionally, nucleic acids. Cellular antigens such as red cells or bacteria usually cause weak and inconsistent sensitization. Cytotropic antibodies—primarily the IgG and IgE classes, but in special circumstances IgA and IgM—may also be involved in anaphylactic sensitization. Nevertheless homocytotropic antibodies (antibodies that will sensitize an animal of the same species) are cardinal in such reactions, and these are of the IgE class in all species so far examined. In general, 10 to 14 days are required after immunization before IgG antibodies result in active anaphylactic sensitization, whereas IgE sensitization may occur earlier. Passive sensitization has a latent period (the time needed for the antibody to attach to the cells storing or synthesizing the pharmacologically active effector molecules) of 3 to 6 hours for IgG antibodies, and it is short-lived because the IgG molecules become detached from these cells within 12 to 14 hours. However, passive sensitization with IgE antibody, although it may occur within 6 hours, becomes strong by 24 to 72 hours. Consequently, anaphylactic reactions occurring after 48 to 72 hours are practically exclusively due to IgE antibodies, since IgG antibodies are already detached from the target cells and, therefore, do not participate in such a reaction. IgE antibodies remain fixed to the target basophils and mast cells for about 6 weeks in humans.

Following the initiation of antibody production, the cytotropic antibodies (primarily IgE) that are formed disseminate throughout the circulation to become almost selectively and uniquely attached to the cell membranes of basophils in the circulation and mast cells in the tissues. The attachment occurs through a structural area in the Fc part of the antibody molecule to a specific receptor on the basophil or mast call membrane. Although some evidence indicates that subpopulations of monocytes, macrophages, and lymphocytes also express Fc receptors for IgE antibody, of all mammalian cells only basophils and mast cells exhibit an extraordinary binding affinity for this antibody. There is a relative abundance of these IgE molecules bound along the membrane, and they are located close to each other physically. When the IgE becomes attached, the cells are said to be sensitized

---
*References 3, 13, 55, 64, 66.

and the individual is now in a sensitive state for reactivity on subsequent exposure to the antigen.

A second or subsequent exposure can occur via many routes such as inhalation, ingestion, or injection. The immunogen (antigen, allergen) must move across membrane and tissue barriers in order to come to the surface of the sensitized cells. When this close encounter occurs with an immunogen of sufficient size to react with the immunogen-binding sites of two closely adjacent IgE molecules, it produces a "bridging" effect. In this molecular interaction one immunogen molecule combines with two antibody molecules to form a bridge. This bridging brings together two IgE receptor molecules, which results in distortion of the cell membrane, triggering an enzymatic cascade that causes the release of pharmacologically active effector molecules responsible for the clinical symptomatology of anaphylaxis (Fig. 27-1). These agents include amines, peptides, lipid substances, Hageman factor pathway and other enzymes, and proteoglycans. Collectively they produce an increase in blood flow, capillary permeability, constriction of smooth muscles, and secretion of mucous glands. These varied effects account for the sudden tissue changes characteristic of local and systemic anaphylactic reaction.

The particular tissue site of the reaction depends on the portal of entry (route of exposure) of the antigen. Antigens that are inhaled make contact with mast cells by crossing the mucous membranes of the nose, the sinuses, and the lower respiratory tract. The local effects in these tissues are characterized by a marked increase in mucus secretion with congestion and edema of the mucous membranes. The effect on bronchi and bronchiolar smooth muscle causes constriction with impairment of air flow, severely restricting pulmonary exchange and usually associated with the sudden onset of wheezing respirations.

Ingestion of antigens in food substances or oral medications can cause local and diffuse reactions in the gastrointestinal tract. Such exposure may produce symptoms of acute onset, commonly in the form of intestinal hypermotility, dyspepsia, colicky pain, and a sensation of fullness and bloating. These symptoms occur because of local release of pharmacologically active effector molecules by the immune reaction along the submucosa of the gastrointestinal tract. Antigens may also be absorbed into the circulation from the gastrointestinal tract and disseminate throughout the body, resulting in generalized systemic reactions or localized reactions in the skin and viscera or both. In the skin the acute reactions can present as edematous papules or larger urticarial lesions. Acute systemic reactions can occur following the injection of an antigen such as a drug or vaccine in individuals with marked sensitivity. The condition of acute anaphylaxis can lead to shock, respiratory insufficiency, and death unless there is immediate treatment. Such profound systemic reaction is due to the massive intravascular release of effector molecules from the circulating basophils.

Allergic and atopic disorders. Manifestations of atopic immediate hypersensitivity include bronchial asthma, hay fever, allergic rhinitis, certain forms of chronic urticaria, and atopic dermatitis. Only a minority of the population shows some form of atopic disease in spite of the fact that by and large identical conditions of antigen exposure must be presumed to exist for all members of the population. Many theories of the constitutional basis of atopy have been proposed. Two general ideas, are prominent: (1) the perception of atopy as a primary disorder of the immune system with sequelae in the various effector tissues; and (2) a concept of atopy as a primary autonomic imbalance, essentially beta-adrenergic in character, with sequelae in effector cells, including those engaged in the production of antibodies. The autonomic imbalance is perceived as being caused not by some disorder of the autonomic nervous system itself but by a defective functioning of its effector cells. There are critically important nonimmune differences between the imme-

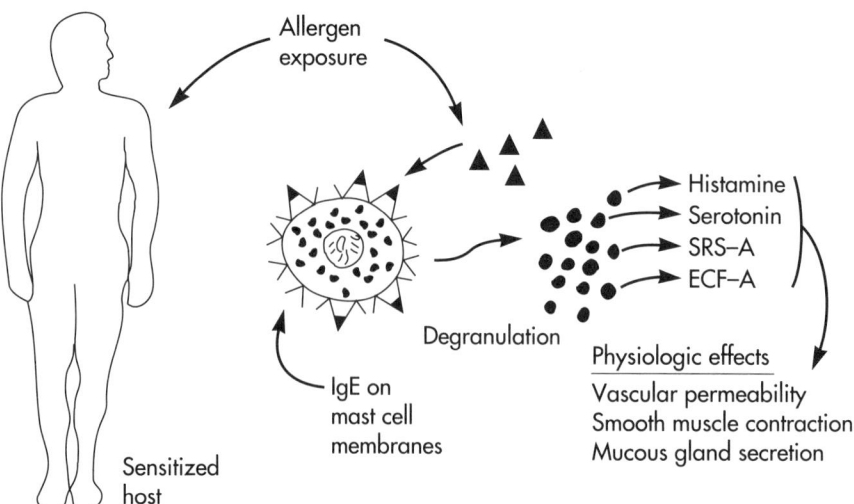

Fig. 27-1. Pathogenic events in anaphylaxis.

diate hypersensitivities of the atopic and nonatopic type. Thus it appears that in anaphylaxis we are dealing with a normal (physiologic) antibody response to an unnatural exposure to antigen, whereas in atopic allergy an "abnormal" antibody response to natural antigenic exposure seems to be involved. Anaphylactic reactivity of the sensitized individual depends on the release of an amount of pharmacologically active effector molecules sufficient to be toxic for most members of the same species. In contrast, individuals with atopic disease possess a quantitatively and qualitatively abnormal reactivity to otherwise nontoxic concentrations of endogenously released or exogenously administered pharmacologic mediators. Another essential difference between atopic and nonatopic varieties of immediate hypersensitivities is the major contributory role played by infection in atopy, whereas infection has not been shown to be causally related to anaphylactic allergy—anaphylaxis, the Arthus reaction, or serum sickness. Moreover, atopic conditions can be precipitated by a number of totally unrelated stimuli, whereas anaphylaxis can be brought about only by the specific antigen. Finally, the latter conditions may be produced artificially, but atopic disease, with its spontaneous pattern of familial occurrence, cannot be induced at will. Acute human pulmonary anaphylaxis, which can include asthmatic features, for example, has never been reported to lead to the development of bronchial asthma or other atopic disease.

Clinical features of allergic disease.[17,35,46,65] Allergic diseases or type I reactions provide clinical manifestations primarily by influencing three target organs: the respiratory tract, the gastrointestinal tract, and the skin. Clinical disease requires both genetic predisposition and environmental exposure. Allergic rhinitis and asthma are the most common manifestations of clinical disease following exposure to environmental allergens. Genetic studies of identical twins document that environmental factors are crucial in the expression of the atopic predisposition, and the expression and manifestations are dependent upon specific and nonspecific factors enhancing antigen entry and IgE responsiveness. Some specific and nonspecific factors of importance are listed in Table 27-1.

Takafuji et al.[65] reported that particulates from diesel exhaust act as a powerful adjuvant for IgE production. Environmental air pollutants (for example, SO_2, NO_2) and tobacco smoke reportedly enhance antigen entry and IgE production. Furthermore, epidemiologic data documents that allergic parents appear to be more likely to have children who develop allergic disease, and the presence of elevated serum IgE levels is considered to represent an important risk factor for the future development of an allergic disorder.

Examples of type I hypersensitivity disorders

Allergic rhinitis.[50] Allergic rhinitis is the most common allergic disease, believed to affect some 15% of the population of the United States. The disease influences both sexes equally and causes considerable morbidity when one takes into account the loss of time from school and work. Allergic rhinitis may be seasonal or perennial. The patient complains of a watery rhinorrhea, sneezing, nasal and palate itching, and nasal stuffiness. The observation that nasal symptoms disappear on weekends suggests an occupational etiology. On physical examination of the nasal passages there is swelling of the mucosa. The affected person may exhibit "allergic shiners" and evidence of blepheroconjunctivitis. Severe attacks may be accompanied by malaise, fatigue, and weakness. The diagnosis of allergic rhinitis is established by the history and physical examination. Eosinophils may be found in the nasal secretion, but this is not exclusive to allergic rhinitis. The documentation of a specific allergy can be strengthened by the detection of specific IgE employing skin or in vitro testing. The specific allergens to be tested are determined by the patient's history and local environmental exposures. The practitioner uses the allergy history obtained from the patient to confirm relationships between serum rast (radio-allergosorbent test) or skin test identified allergy for specific allergic diagnosis. Perennial symptoms, seasonal variations, and perennial with seasonal variations in symptoms, provide extremely important information to help identify the allergens. Table 27-2 is an example of the type of allergens found in the New Jersey area according to the month. A detailed survey of the home, work, or school environment can be extremely helpful. Fluctuation in allergic

Table 27-1. Enhancement of antigen entry and IgE production

Nonspecific factors:
- Environmental pollutants (SO_2, NO_2)
- Diesel fumes
- Smoking (low consumption)

Specific factors:
- Pollens
- House dust mites
- Foods
- Drugs
- Molds
- Animals
- Insects
- Serum
- Occupational exposures

Table 27-2. New Jersey allergy seasons

Month	Allergen peaks
March–May	Tree pollen
May–June	Grasses
July–August	Outdoor molds
August–October	Ragweed and other weeds
November–February (and perennial)	Dust mites, animals, household molds, cockroaches

Table 27-3. Differential diagnosis of allergic rhinitis

	Eosinophils/ nasal smear	Skin test
Allergic rhinitis/seasonal	+	+
Allergic rhinitis/perennial	+	+
Vasomotor rhinitis	−	−
NARES*	+	−
Rhinitis medicamentosa	−	−
Infectious rhinitis	−	−

*Nonallergic rhinitis with eosinophils.

symptoms during the week or on weekends may be helpful in elucidating the etiologic agent. Primary irritants should be identified, such as paints, perfumes, hair sprays, colognes, and other strong odors. The number of days of restricted activity at work and school loss should be documented to help judge the severity of the condition. Individuals with allergic rhinitis may also show concurrent vasomotor rhinitis symptoms. Because the specific diagnosis of rhinitis may not be clear, Table 27-3 provides a differential diagnosis of vasomotor rhinitis, nonallergic rhinitis with eosinophilia syndrome (NARES), rhinitis medicamentosa, and infectious rhinitis. The basic therapeutic techniques for treating seasonal or perennial allergic rhinitis include (1) avoidance of the offending allergens, (2) use of appropriate pharmaceutical agents, and (3) allergy immunotherapy.

Bronchial asthma.* Bronchial asthma is characterized by reversible airway obstruction and airway hyperresponsiveness. The pathophysiologic abnormalities in asthma include smooth muscle contraction, mucous hypersecretion, mucosal and submucosal edema, and bronchial hyperresponsiveness. There appears to be an increase in mortality and morbidity worldwide despite advances in recognition and symptomatic therapy of asthma. In fact, asthma is the leading cause of absenteeism from school and work. The America College of Chest Physicians and American Thoracic Society[1] have defined bronchial asthma as "a disease characterized by an increased responsiveness of the airways to various stimuli and manifested by slowing of forced expiration which changes in severity, either spontaneously, or as a result of therapy." Among patients with bronchial asthma, symptoms may vary from patient to patient and even in the same patient at different times.

Asthmatics may be conventionally divided into extrinsic (allergic) and intrinsic (nonallergic). Pollat et al.[56] demonstrated that in adults younger than 50 years of age, the prevalence of IgE antibodies was fourfold greater among subjects with asthma than among control subjects, suggesting that the presence of serum IgE antibodies to common inhalant allergies is a major risk factor for acute attacks of asthma. Approximately 90% of the asthmatics younger than 30 years are found to be allergic when tested, while about 50% of asthmatics older than 30 years are allergic. It is clear, however, that specific antigens and nonspecific factors are instrumental in precipitating asthma attacks. Clinically, patients may describe the presence of wheezing that can be intermittent or constant. On auscultation, wheezing may be absent, especially in children who present with persistent coughing and for whom a diagnosis of "bronchitis" is made. Adults may also present in this fashion and are diagnosed as having "cough-variant asthma." An important clinical manifestation is what can be termed "bronchial irritability." The subject describes an increased sensitivity to many and varied nonspecific airborne irritants and odorants. The airway's responsiveness to a specific allergen after a bronchial challenge presents in a number of ways. There may be an immediate reaction with documented reductions in forced expiratory volume at one second (FEV1), in 5 to 20 minutes, and return to original levels within 1.5 to 3 hours. A late-phase reaction begins within 3 to 4 hours and peaks between 8 and 12 hours, and may last 24 to 36 hours. The early and late phases may be present as a dual response. There is good correlation between the results of allergy skin tests, in vitro allergy tests, and the presence of bronchial provocation status. The stronger the skin test reaction, the greater the chances of a positive bronchial provocation test. Bronchial challenges are not necessary for the diagnosis of asthma in the vast majority of patients but may be appropriate for patients who present with isolated cough, atypical dyspnea, or negative physical findings and normal spirometry. It is important to document the presence of nonspecific airway hyperresponsiveness, a characteristic feature of asthma. This finding can be documented by performing inhalation challenge testing with methacholine, histamine, ultrasonic nebulizer with distilled water, or cold air hyperventilation challenge. A negative challenge encourages the practitioner to consider other causes of bronchial disease.

Gastrointestinal allergy.[31,36,47] The clinical manifestations of food allergy usually occur as an immediate type I reaction within minutes to an hour after ingestion of an allergen. Symptoms include perioral erythema, lip swelling, oral irritation, tongue and pharynx swelling, nausea, and vomiting. Severe reactions may be followed by anaphylaxis. The most common food allergies are to eggs, cow's milk, wheat, fish, and nuts. In adults, shellfish is also common. The food may not only affect the gastrointestinal tract, but also may target other organs such as the skin and lungs. Avoidance is the specific treatment of food allergy.

Atopic dermatitis.[52,58,62,73] The primary defect in atopic dermatitis is unknown. The incidence is higher in children and may approach 3% to 5%. Atopic dermatitis can be divided into infantile, childhood, and adult forms, but there is predilection for different areas of the skin for different age groups. Approximately one half of individuals with atopic dermatitis develop asthma or rhinitis. The cause of atopic

---
*References 1, 12, 15, 22, 44, 56, 67, 68.

dermatitis is not predictable, but about 50% of the patients do not have symptoms after reaching 15 years of age. Numerous studies have defined the immunologic features of atopic dermatitis, which include elevated serum IgE levels, decreased blood lymphocyte numbers bearing CD3, CD4, and CD8, increased CD4+/CD8+ lymphocyte ratio, decreased cutaneous delayed hypersensitivity manifestation, decreased numbers of NK (natural killer) cells, increased blood, but not tissue eosinophils counts, and increased histamine releasing factors. There is no single or multiple diagnostic test useful in the diagnosis of atopic dermatitis. Over 50% of the patients with atopic dermatitis are known to have elevated IgE. Of atopic dermatitis patients in a study reported by Rajka,[58] 75% had a positive immediate cutaneous reaction to common aeroallergens or food. Sampson et al.[62] have reported that more than half of children with atopic dermatitis had positive food challenges. Six foods accounted for 90% of the positive reactions and included soy, milk, wheat, egg, peanut, and fish.

Urticaria. The exact incidence of urticaria is not known, but it has been stated that about 20% of the U.S. population will have urticaria at some time in their life. Acute urticaria has been defined as persisting for less than 6 weeks, while chronic urticaria lasts more than 6 to 8 weeks; the latter is more frequent in middle-aged adults. IgE-mediated mechanisms are important in the activation of skin mast cells and production of hives. IgE-mediated causes of urticaria include food, drugs, insects, and transfusion reactions. IgG4 subclass is another class of antibody that has been shown to bind weakly to mast cells and circulating immune complexes and may activate inflammatory cells such as platelets and lymphocytes. There are other operative immunologic mechanisms occurring in hives, including release of histamine from mast cells and basophils, possibly as the result of activating the classical pathway of complement and the formation of anaphylatoxins (C3a, C4a, C5a); these events may lead to cutaneous vasculitis. Activation of the alternative pathway of complement also produces anaphylatoxins and produces histamine release and mediator formation. The plasma kinin system seems to play a critical role in urticaria development, although not through histamine release. Nonimmunologic mechanism causes of urticaria due to histamine release occur after administration of certain drugs and chemical agents such as morphine, codeine, d-tubocurarine, polymyxin antibiotics, and thiamine.

Type II reactions (cytotoxic tissue injury)

Overview. Type II reactions are cytotoxic and involve the combination of IgG or IgM antibodies with antigenic determinants on a cell membrane. A free antigen or hapten also may be absorbed by a tissue component or cell membrane, and antibody subsequently combines with this adsorbed antigen. Complement fixation frequently occurs in this situation and leads to cell damage. The usual sequelae of attachment of circulating antibody to either a tissue antigen or membrane-adsorbed antigen are, therefore, as follows: (1) cell lysis or cell inactivation with activation of complement; (2) phagocytosis of the target cells with or without activation of complement; and (3) lysis or inactivation in the presence of effector killer cells.

Complement-dependent antibody lysis.[25,39,49] The target for the cytotoxic reaction may be either a formed blood element or a specific cell type within a particular tissue. This form of injury follows immune reactions of antigen and antibody in which the antibody is of the IgG or IgM class; these two classes are the only immunoglobulins that activate the complement system. Immune complexes formed by IgG, IgA, and IgD do not exhibit complement-activating effects, and indeed among the four subclasses of IgG only subclasses IgG1 and IgG3 exhibit substantial complement activation.

The conditions of sensitivity in complement-dependent disorders are that the individual has been exposed to the antigen previously and has produced an antibody response of IgM or IgG or both. Subsequent exposure to the reactive antigen then results in immune complex formation, which initiates activation of the complement system. The antigens in this form of hypersensitivity are often derived from infections with microorganisms (for example, bacteria, fungi, and viruses), injections or inoculations in the course of immunization or blood transfusion, or drug therapy.

Red cell lysis is an illustrative example of type II cytotoxic reaction involving the lysis of red blood cells by a complement-dependent antibody-lysing process or phenomenon that classically occurs during transfusions with grossly incompatible blood. Platelets, polymorphonuclear leukocytes, and lymphocytes can also be lysed by similar mechanisms under certain conditions. Type II reactions can occur in any tissue by inducing heterologous antibodies to different tissue components. Deposition of antibodies may occur in a linear pattern along the human glomerular basement membranes in three groups of diseases, as follows. (1) Abnormalities related to renal transplantation—In earlier years of renal transplantation people were treated with antilymphocyte antisera. Today, these antisera are known to have contained antibodies against glomerular basement membranes that deposited along the glomerular basement membrane of the transplanted kidney. This situation is analogous to classic nephrotoxic serum nephritis. (2) Goodpasture's syndrome, in which there is deposition of antibodies directed against glomerular and pulmonary basement membranes, accounting for the symptoms of hematuria, renal failure, and recurrent hemoptysis. (3) Several other diseases, such as scleroderma, diabetic glomerulonephritis, systemic lupus erythematosus, malignant hypertension, polyarteritis nodosa, and toxemia of pregnancy—In these situations the primary disease leads to renal damage, which in turn sensitizes the patient to glomerular basement membrane. In the skin, type II reactions caused by linear deposition of antibody against the basement membrane at the dermal-epidermal junction occur in pemphigoid disorders.

Another type of complement-dependent cell destruction occurs as a result of immune adherence. In this situation there is immune activation of complement along a cell surface that generates abundant C3b, and C3b molecules attach to the cell surface. They act as specific receptors that facilitate rapid phagocytic clearance of the coated cells from the circulation by immune adherence. This causes the C3b-covered cells to attach to receptors on reticuloendothelial cells (Fig. 27-2). Phagocytosis occurs and is followed by intracellular destruction of the engulfed cell or particle. When the cells affected are erythrocytes, chronic severe reactions of this type can lead to profound anemia and are incorrectly termed *hemolytic*. *Phagocytic anemia* would be a more appropriate diagnostic term. If leukocytes or platelets are the target cells, they are cleared from the circulation in a similar manner. Commonly, these reactions are due to an immune reaction with antigens intrinsic to or linked to the cell surface.

Antibody-mediated killer cell toxicity. Another mechanism of antibody-dependent cell injury is called *antibody-dependent cytotoxicity* or *natural killer (K)-cell destruction* (Fig. 27-3). A target cell that possesses antigens along the cell surface, either as part of the cell membrane or linked to the cell membrane, binds antibody through the Fab region along the surface. Following this the small mononuclear (natural killer) cells of the circulation that have a receptor site for the Fc portion of IgG come close to the antibody-coated target cell and contact the cell by receptor-binding with the Fc portion of the antibody molecules. This cell contact is then followed by release of a biochemical factor that kills the target cell, which then undergoes fragmentation and

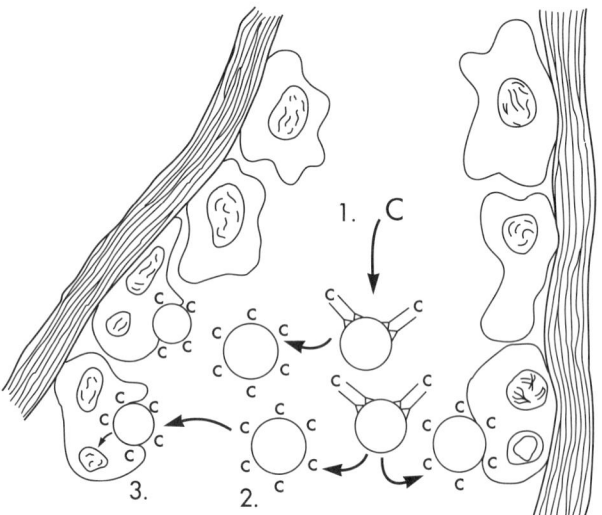

Fig. 27-2. Pathogenic sequence in complement-depended cytotoxicity. **1,** Complement activation by antigen-antibody reactions of erythrocyte surface. **2,** Complement (C3b) on cell surface. **3,** Phagocytosis and intracellular destruction of erythrocyte facilitated by complement (C3b) on cell surfaces.

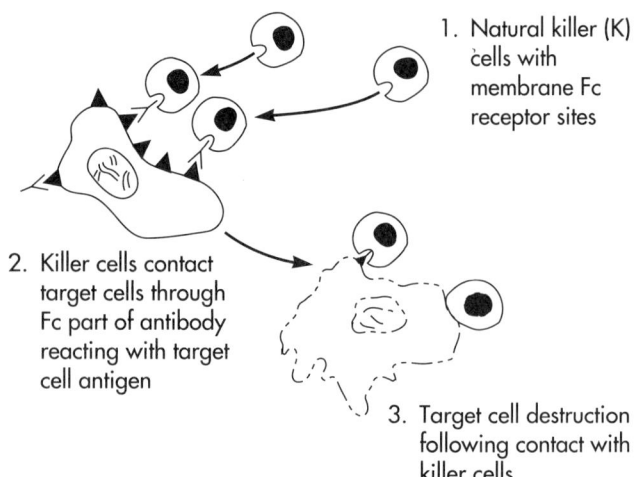

Fig. 27-3. Mechanism of antibody-dependent killer (K) cell destruction of target cell.

dissolution. In this reaction, the specificity derives from the antigen-antibody reaction, whereas the killer cell (K cell) effect is essentially nonspecific. It is attracted to the target antigens by reaction of its Fc receptor with the antibody molecule bound to cell antigens. This mechanism of destruction appears to be due to release of a biochemical factor via an energy- and calcium-dependent reactions contingent upon microtubule function in the K cell. These K-cell reactions appear to be of importance in conditions in which cells develop virus-associated, drug-induced, or tumor-associated antigens closely linked to HLA antigens on the cell membranes. It also promises to provide the basis for an important therapeutic approach to the specific immunologic treatment of neoplasms.

Clinical Presentations. Alloantigens are antigens genetically present on cells of a given species. These antigens differentiate one member of a given species from another. The process of alloimmunization occurs when these antigens become involved in immunologically mediated disease. There are three broad categories of disorders associated with these antigens: (1) blood incompatibility encountered in transfusion or pregnancy, (2) organ transplantation, and (3) tumor antigens.

Blood incompatibility.[76] Mismatched blood transfusion of the ABO and other blood groups systems may have preformed antibodies present in a blood transfusion. Such an event will cause an immediate and severe reaction in the recipient. There may also be a delayed type of reaction associated with a late-onset hemolytic anemia. The immediate-type mismatch reaction is due to the presence of circulating specific IgM or IgG antibodies that bind to the infused erythrocytes and consequently causes activation of the complement system, subsequent lysis of the red cells, and intravascular hemolysis. Delayed reactions may occur in patients immunized by previous pregnancy or transfusion. Pretransfusion testing does not detect the presence of the previous antigen, but with reexposure to the incompatible antigen, an anamnestic reaction occurs and there is production of IgG antibodies, destroying the transfused cells.

Another example of a severe cytotoxic reaction is hemolytic disease of the newborn, which is caused by Rh incompatibility. In the United States, individuals are classified as being Rh positive (85%) or Rh negative (15%) depending on the presence of the D antigen. Rh antibodies are a result of alloimmunization from previous transfusions or pregnancy. These Rh antibodies are usually IgG in type and do not fix complement. Anti-D antibodies are the most important clinically and there has been a great deal of success using anti-D prophylaxis. Other Rh antibodies, such as Rh(C,E), Kell, Duffy, and Kidd, are less common, but may also cause transfusion reactions and hemolytic disease of the newborn. The Coomb's test is used to demonstrate the presence of the IgG antibody on red cells. The direct Coomb's test is used to demonstrate in vitro attachment of antibodies to red cells, as in autoimmune hemolytic anemia and alloimmune hemolytic disease of the newborn. In the indirect Coomb's test, red cells are first incubated with serum in vitro and then tested with antihemoglobulin. Antigen systems on platelets and neutrophils have also been defined, and the clinical significance of these platelet and neutrophil antibodies need to be better delineated. The development of antibodies to IgA globulins has been reported to account for approximately 80% of nonhemolytic transfusion reactions.

Organ transplantation.[33,38,75] Self-reactivity is critical to normal immune response and immune regulation. Transplantation is a technologically advanced form of therapy from what was once an experimental and lifesaving emergency procedure. The widespread use of renal transplantation beginning in the 1960s provided the basis of genetics and immunology for transplantation to become relevant to today's patient care. Before proceeding to organ transplantation, a consideration of ABO compatibility, HLA antibody shared by the prospective donor and recipient, and previous graft or blood transfusions must be investigated. A major barrier to successful organ transplantation is the status of the recipient's immune response toward the antigens of the MHC (major histocompatibility locus) expressed by the allograft. It has been adequately documented that matching for the HLA-B and DR antigens leads to a better chance for graft survival. Control of the host's responses against HLA incompatibility can be managed by employing induced immunosuppression using chemical suppressors, antibody-mediated suppressors, and total lymphoid irradiation.

The stages of rejection in renal transplantation are hyperacute, acute, and chronic. Hyperacute rejection occurs within minutes to hours of transplantation in the presensitized host. It is noted with both heart and kidney transplants. In hyperacute rejection the specific antibody binds to vascular endothelium and then activates complement formation. Consequently, the graft's vasculature is severely injured by this mechanism.[49] In the acute form of rejection HLA antigens present on the surface of cells of the transplanted organ, and the recipient's bloodborne antigenic cells provide the primary stimulus. The antigen-presenting cell (APC) represents an antigen in the format lymphocytes can recognize. Interleukins aid in activating the lymphocytes. Both CD4+ and CD8+ subclasses of effector lymphocytes are directly involved in destroying graft cells by way of classic T-cell mechanisms. Other lymphokines, especially gamma interferon (IFN-γ generated by T-cell activation), generate two important effects. Interferon gamma induces greater expression of HLA-A, -B, and -DR antigens on graft tissue, making the graft more vulnerable to injury. Additionally, monocytes are activated, promoting a detrimental delayed hypersensitivity response against the graft. Interleukins IL-4 and IL-5 direct B-cell production of antibody with resultant antibody-mediated damage on the target organ. Chronic rejection is more serious because generally this situation is refractory to immunosuppressor therapy and there may be vascular obliteration and extensive scarring. Transplant outcomes have become more successful as understanding in molecular immunology improves.

Type III reactions (immune complex tissue injury)

Overview. Type III reactions are characterized by localization of antigen-antibody complexes in tissues and an associated inflammatory response. Typical manifestations of this group are the Arthus phenomenon, serum sickness, and immune complex diseases (Fig. 27-4).

The Arthus phenomenon. In the classic form of the Arthus phenomenon, following the intradermal injection of antigen into a sensitized rabbit, the area shows local swelling

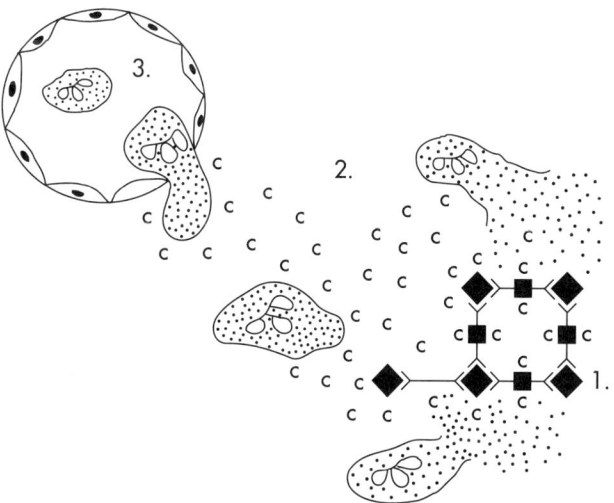

Fig. 27-4. Immune complex tissue injury—pathogenic sequence. **1,** Complement activation by antigen-antibody complex lodged in tissue. **2,** Complement chemotaxis of neutrophils into tissue site of immune reaction with release of destructive lysosomal enzymes. **3,** Migration of neutrophil from blood vessel due to chemoattraction.

and erythema in 1 to 2 hours, which increases to a maximum within 3 to 6 hours and disappears within 10 to 12 hours. The Arthus phenomenon was originally believed to be a local variant of systemic anaphylaxis but is now regarded as a prototype of an inflammatory lesion due to immune complex disease as described below. One human clinical example of an Arthus reaction is hypersensitivity pneumonitis or extrinsic allergic alveolitis, which is caused by inhalation of organic dusts.

Serum sickness. In the early decades of the twentieth century patients frequently developed serum sickness after treatment with horse serum as an antiserum to diphtheria, tetanus, or other organisms. It is seen today only in underdeveloped countries in which alternative methods of active immunization may not be available. In developed countries today it occurs only as a reaction to drugs such as penicillin or consequent to renal allotransplantation in patients who receive heterologous antilymphocyte serum. Like the Arthus phenomenon, serum sickness was for a long time regarded as a manifestation of immediate hypersensitivity, but now we know that its key pathogenetic feature is the formation of antigen-antibody complexes in the bloodstream and their subsequent deposition throughout the body.

Immune complex diseases.* Disorders associated with significant clinical features secondary to formation and deposition of immune complexes are now collectively termed *immune complex diseases*. The critical pathologic feature of these diseases is that formation of the immune complex is followed by entrapment of the complex in the tissue. This provides the focus for development of the lesion. Complement activation occurs on the immune complex in the tissue, yielding chemotactic factors that specifically attract the neutrophils. Once in the tissue, the neutrophils release destructive hydrolytic enzymes from their lysosomal granules. The degradative action of these enzymes produces the necrotic destructive lesion at the site of immune complex localization. Some examples of disseminated immune complex disease in humans include systemic lupus erythematosus, various forms of acute and chronic glomerulonephritis, polyarteritis nodosa, Hashimoto's thyroiditis, rheumatoid arthritis, dermatitis herpetiformis, Crohn's disease, and disorders associated with a variety of infectious and neoplastic diseases.

Type IV reactions (cell-mediated immune tissue injuries)

Overview. Cell-mediated immune reactions occur as the result of the interactions between actively sensitized lymphocytes and specific antigens. They are mediated by the release of lymphokines or by direct cytotoxicity or both. Historically, the classic lesion of a cell-mediated immune reaction is the delayed skin-hypersensitivity reaction (the tuberculin reaction). The cell-mediated reactions can be most effectively arranged around (1) the T-cell–dependent reaction, leading to granulomatous injury, and (2) the T-lymphocytecytotoxic reactions.

T-cell reactions with granulomatous injury.[49] In the type of T-cell–dependent reaction resulting in the formation of a granuloma, the T cell reacts with the stimulating antigen through specific receptors on the cell surface (Fig. 27-5). Consequent to this contact, the T lymphocyte is stimulated to increased metabolic activity and exhibits nuclear enlargement with cytoplasmic basophilia, a change described as *blast formation*. Along with the increased metabolic activity, there is production of many soluble biochemical factors or *lymphokines* that cause certain physiologic and biologic effects and are the primary mediators of this reaction sequence: (1) stimulation and activation of blood monocytes and transformation to macrophages, (2) a chemotactic effect on monocytes to attract them specifically into tissue, and (3) a migration inhibition effect that limits motility of monocytes and macrophages once they have arrived at the tissue site.

---
*References 2, 19, 32, 41, 45.

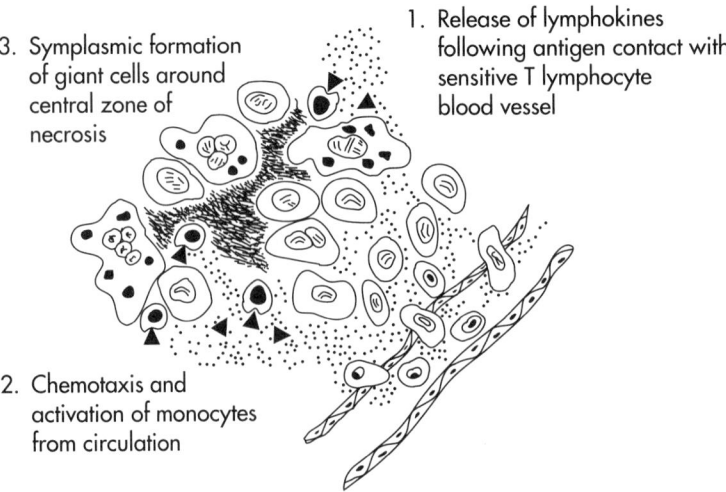

Fig. 27-5. Events in the development of T-lymphocyte–dependent hypersensitivity granulomatous lesion.

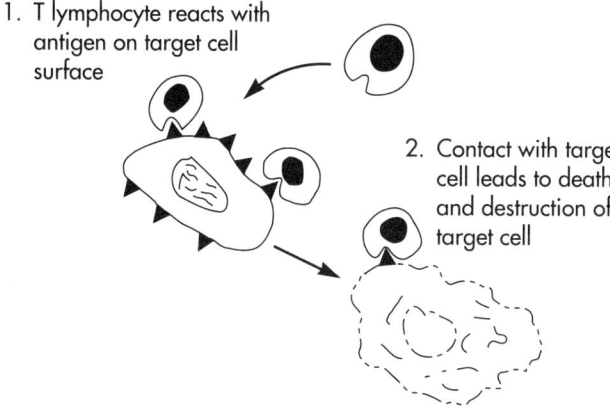

Fig. 27-6. Events in cytotoxic T-lymphocyte reaction.

These lymphokines mediate the cellular events that produce a characteristic histopathologic lesion known as a *granuloma*. Individual macrophages cluster and fuse around a central site of antigen concentration that may show focal necrotic change due to leakage of proteolytic enzymes and give rise to the typical appearance of a granuloma with multinucleate giant cells surrounding a central area of necrotic change bounded by a mantle of mononuclear cells. Such a necrotic or cellular granuloma is a characteristic lesion of delayed hypersensitivity reactions. It is often observed in certain infectious diseases in which there is antigen persistence with marked T-cell reactivity, as in tuberculosis and in fungal and viral infections.

T-lymphocyte cytotoxic reaction. A variant of immune injury produced by T lymphocytes in a role as effector cells is called *cytotoxic*, or killer (K)-cell infiltrative reaction (Fig. 27-6). This type occurs as a result of contact by the effector lymphocyte with histocompatibility-linked antigens on the surface of target cells. The T cell contacts the antigen directly, rather than through antibody linkage as in the antibody-dependent form of injury, and the killing effect appears to be due to release of a biochemical factor from the T lymphocyte. Some examples of such tissue reactions in human disease are the acute phase of homograft rejection, autoimmune tissue lesions, viral infections, and some forms of dermatitis. The granulomatous and cytotoxic forms of T-cell reactivity can occur together, although one usually predominates as the primary form.

Clinical features

Allergic contact hypersensitivity.[34] Allergic contact dermatitis is a manifestation of delayed-type hypersensitivity. Contact dermatitis refers to both allergic contact dermatitis and primary irritant dermatitis. Primary irritant contact dermatitis is more common than allergic contact dermatitis. There are no familial tendencies in humans toward the development of allergic contact dermatitis. The interval between exposure to the responsible agent and the occurrence of clinical manifestations in a sensitized subject is usually 12 to 24 hours. On initial exposure the development of skin sensitivity may be as short as 2 to 3 days. The appearance of allergic contact dermatitis depends on the stage at which the patient presents. The acute stage presents with erythema, papules, and vesicles with edema and occasionally bullae. In the subacute phase vesicles are less pronounced, and crusting, scaling, and lichenification may be present. In the chronic phase papulovesicular lesions are fewer, with thickening, lichenification, and scaling predominating. Diagnosis is based on a good history. Information should include occupation, hobbies, clothing, cosmetics, jewelry, outdoor exposures, and treatments used on the skin. The pattern of involvement may provide a clue to the etiology. Contact dermatitis to the face, for example, may be due to cosmetics; other possibilities include hair dye, shampoo, and hair styling preparations. Eyelid dermatitis may be caused by eye shadow, mascara, eye liner, and nail polish. It is extremely important that the physician be familiar with the distribution patterns of contact dermatitis that occur with particular allergens. Certain contact allergens may be airborne. Examples include ragweed and the oleoresin of poison ivy plants. Another means of exposure to poison ivy without direct contact is by contact with clothing or animal fur containing the oleoresin. The five most common causes of allergic contact dermatitis in the United States are toxicodendron (poison ivy, poison oak, poison sumac), paraphenylenediamine, nickel, rubber compounds, and ethylenediamine hydrochloride. Sometimes patch testing is necessary to confirm the association or to identify one of the several possible agents. A patch test of the substance is used for this purpose and inspected at 48 and 72 hours. A positive reaction consists of pruritus, erythema, swelling, and vesiculation. The patch test is safe and reliable if properly performed by qualified individuals using appropriate materials. Most recently with the increased usage of latex gloves by medical personnel, allergic contact dermatitis has been increasingly recognized. This is related to the accelerators, antioxidants, stabilizers, or vulcanizers rather than to the natural latex protein. There are also type I hypersensitivity reactions to latex, and evidence indicates that the chemical additives are not responsible for these reactions. The latex allergen appears to be a mixture of proteins in a molecular weight range from 10 to 67 Kd. A coexistence of type I allergy to latex and a type IV allergy to chemicals has also been described.

The differential diagnosis includes seborrheic dermatitis, atopic dermatitis, and primary irritant dermatitis. Another contact skin condition is photocontact dermatitis. This is caused by the interaction between a chemical and ultraviolet light. The diagnosis is based on the location of the reaction where the body is exposed to UV light. Sensitizers include drugs (tetracycline, griseofulvin, or sulfa compounds). Certain drugs and chemicals produce dermatitis in sun-exposed areas of skin in all individuals, causing cell damage on the first exposure to sunlight. This is a phototoxic reaction and is not mediated immunologically. Avoidance of sensitizing agents and sunlight are recommended as the usage of topical corticosteroids.

Mixed immunologic reactions

Allergic bronchopulmonary aspergillosis (ABPA).[37,42,60] Mixed immunologic reactions in the lung are classically represented by bronchopulmonary aspergillosis (types I and III) and extrinsic allergic alveolitis (types I and IV). ABPA is a subacute inflammatory reaction elicited by both IgE- and IgG-mediated immune responses directed at aspergillus species growing in the respiratory tree. The incidence in the United States is unknown. Diagnostic criteria include allergic asthma, eosinophilia, positive skin test to Aspergillus antigen, IgG antibodies to Aspergillus antigen, marked increase in IgE level, pulmonary infiltrates, and central saccular bronchiectasis. Minor criteria include Aspergillus in sputum, expectoration of brown plugs, and late-phase (or Arthus reaction) skin test results to Aspergillus antigen. Corticosteroids are the treatment of choice, and the patient is monitored with chest x-rays and serial IgE levels.

Extrinsic allergic alveolitis (hypersensitivity pneumonitis).[28,29,69] The inhalation of organic dusts, thermophilic actinomycetes, molds, and proteinaceous materials have been implicated in the immunologic inflammatory reaction involving the bronchioles, alveoli, and lung interstitium. These agents are usually encountered in the home, at work, or by hobby exposures. The prevalence of hypersensitivity pneumonitis is estimated to be between 7% and 15% of exposed individuals. The presentation may be acute, subacute, or chronic depending on the duration, frequency, and intensity of the exposure and the host's response. The pathology is dependent upon the stage of the disease at the time of biopsy. The early stage reveals granulomatous interstitial pneumonitis with lymphocytic infiltration and vasculitis. The alveolar spaces contain foamy macrophages, giant cells, and neutrophils. Scattered eosinophils and collagen may be deposited in the alveolar walls. With repeated exposure and development of subacute and chronic phases of disease, diffuse interstitial fibrosis may develop.

Serum precipitins are considered to be markers of exposure to antigen. Lymphocyte transformation to specific antigens has been demonstrated in patients during acute illness. Bronchoalveolar lavage fluid reveals a lymphocytosis, increased NK cells and CD8+ T-cell predominance, and impaired suppressor cell function. Inflammatory cytokines such as IL-1, IL-6, tumor necrosis factor, and granulocyte macrophage colony stimulating factor are involved. Arachidonic metabolites and immune complexes are also present. Extrinsic allergic alveolitis therefore represents an exaggerated immune response with cellular and humoral hypersensitivity processes that produce pulmonary inflammatory disease.

Disorders of autoimmunity[69,70,72]

Overview. Some autoimmune diseases exhibit both T-cell–dependent and antibody-dependent injury, but others are not associated with a clearly defined pathogenesis. We are now much closer to understanding the autoimmune phenomenon than before, but we still lack the needed information to define with assurance all the factors in the developmental mechanism of autoimmunity. The puzzle is not how we develop an immune response to our own tissues as antigens but rather how we develop and normally maintain a state of unresponsiveness. Key answers will no doubt be forthcoming from current and future research.

Definitions of autoimmunity. Autoimmunity can be defined as an organism's failure to recognize its own tissue, and includes any immune response to the host's own tissue, whether it is humoral (for example, circulating autoantibodies) or cellular (for example, delayed hypersensitivity). Autoimmunity is a concept that may explain the pathogenesis of a number of diseases and is a major immunologic phenomenon in clinical medicine.

The body is endowed with mechanisms to distinguish self from nonself. However, as will be discussed, there are many pathways for the breakdown of the control mechanisms underlying self-recognition. Such breakdowns result in an autoimmune response. Autoantibodies that react with the tissue antigens of the host may or may not cause tissue injury and produce disease. The term *autoimmune disease* has been generally assigned to those conditions in which an immune mechanism of injury has contributed to the pathogenesis of the disease. In certain diseases, such as organ-specific autoimmune thyroiditis, the autoimmune response is the major factor in initiating the tissue injury. However, there are many other diseases in which the immunologic response is notably secondary to the initial tissue injury. Detection of autoantibodies may be of equal value in the diagnosis of the latter group of diseases. Autoimmunity may play a role in a wide range of clinical situations, including aging, response to viral and other microbial infections, organic-specific immunologic diseases, and generalized systemic immunologic diseases such as systemic lupus erythematosus.

The term *autoallergic* is often used interchangeably with the word *autoimmune*. The term *allergy* was originated by von Pirquet in 1906 to describe an altered reaction to repeated injections of heterologous gamma globulin to diphtheria toxin. Thus allergy is often used to mean harmful altered reactions secondary to immune mechanisms. Today, the term *allergy* is most commonly applied to diseases characterized by hypersensitivity reactions, such as hay fever and asthma, which are mediated by cytophilic IgE antibodies. Hypersensitivity has been used to describe immune reactions similar to allergy and also to describe nonimmunologic reactions such as nonimmune hypersensitivity to drugs.

Autoimmunity that is observed in clinical and experimental circumstances can be defined as an apparent termination of the natural unresponsive state to self. Immunologic tolerance is the result of an active physiologic process and is not simply the lack of immune response. There are two types of immunologic tolerance: one results in a central unresponsive state characterized by an irreversible loss of competent lymphocytes; the other is a peripheral inhibition in which competent cells are present but suppressed. A definition of *unresponsiveness* is the inability to make a detectable immune response to an antigenic challenge, as distinguished from so-called *tolerance,* which is a term commonly used in transplantation immunology in addition to nonimmunologic events to describe endurance without ill effects of substances such as endotoxins and drugs. However, for the purposes of the section, the terms unresponsiveness and tolerance will be used interchangeably since the discussion will be confined to immune mechanisms.

Concept of unresponsive state or tolerance and relation to autoimmunity.[14,63] Currently it is believed that a person becomes unresponsive to his own tissue antigens during fetal development and that the natural unresponsive state develops as a result of direct contact between the self-constituents and receptor sites on the surface of lymphocytes reactive to these antigens (Fig. 27-7). This is a phenomenon that was first predicted by contact of antibody-forming cells with their respective antigens during fetal or early postnatal life, leading to destruction or inactivation with elimination of the corresponding clones. The mode of induction of the natural unresponsive state is probably by two mechanisms: (1) the clones are immunocompetent cells capable of reacting to self-antigens and are eliminated by a mechanism of the clonal theory of Burnet[14] (contact of antibody-forming cells with their respective antigens during fetal or early postnatal life leads to destruction or inactivation with elimination of the corresponding clones), and (2) antigen-producing cells are made unresponsive by early exposure to self-antigen. It is now clear that the T cells and B cells interact in the production of autoantibodies and that the mechanisms of induction of the unresponsive state at the cellular level of the T cells and B cells are different.

In the cellular aspects of unresponsiveness the cells involved are macrophages, B cells, T cells, and antibody-producing B cells from the bone marrow. When specific antigen-sensitive cells interact for production of antibodies, specifically reactive T cells and B cells must both interact. Although macrophages play a major role in the establishment of the unresponsiveness, they appear to be nonspecific and under genetic control.

Both T and B lymphocytes can become unresponsive or tolerant. However, the kinetics of tolerance in these two lymphocyte populations differ greatly. When there are limited concentrations of these self-components, the unresponsive state is maintained only in the T cells, not in the B cells. The natural unresponsive state to antigens is maintained because of the lack of T-helper cell signal, and autoantibody production is *not* initiated (Fig. 27-8). High doses of antigen can induce unresponsiveness in both T and B lymphocytes. Even with high doses of antigen, the unresponsive state of B lymphocytes is often incomplete and some antibody of low affinity can still be formed. Several studies have demonstrated the existence of antireceptor or antiidiotypic antibodies that may arise as a result of various T-cell bypass mechanisms. These antibodies may block the expression of an immune response and produce a tolerance-like situation to self-antigen. When an animal makes an immune response to a given antigen, autoantibodies directed to the antibody made as the result of the antigenic stimulus also may be produced. The autoantibody to the idiotype may block or suppress the immune response to a given antigen, and the loss of the control mechanism could lead to expression of an autoimmune response to self-antigen.

Genetic factors in autoimmunity.[5,21,23,27] The genetic basis of immunologic regulation is an important area of research today. A group of genes located within the major histocompatibility locus (MHC) plays an important role in immunologic regulation. The differences and susceptibility to various viruses and the intensity of the cellular immune response of graft-versus-host reaction is also controlled within the cluster of genes located within the major histocompatibility region.

Genetically determined cell surface antigens termed *Ia* are important immunologic factors involved in antigen recognition, cellular interaction, and cellular cooperation. Much evidence suggests that genes associated with the major his-

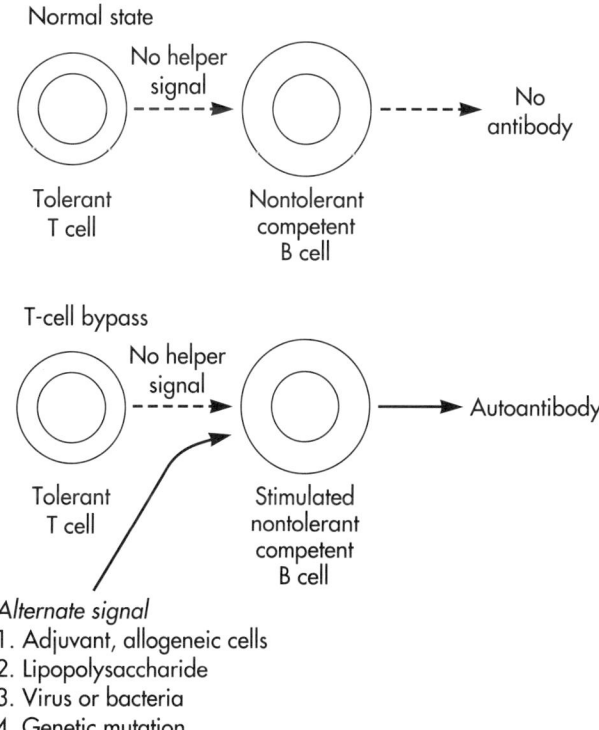

Fig. 27-8. T-cell bypass mechanism of autoimmunity.

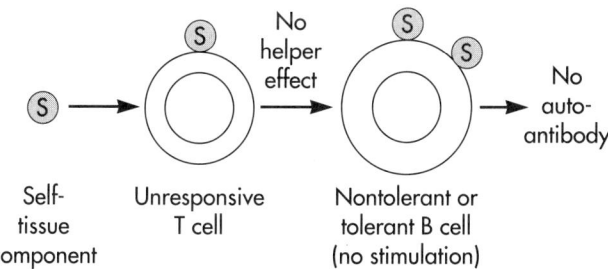

Fig. 27-7. Natural unresponsive state.

tocompatibility locus in humans (HLA) may be important in the immune regulation and in the pathogenesis of autoimmunity. The association of HLA antigens has been found to be marked in cases of ankylosing spondylitis, in which as many as 90% of patients are found to possess HLA-B27 antigens. It should be noted that the association does not imply that the disease is caused by possession of the HLA-B27 antigen. Certain autoimmune diseases, particularly the organ-specific disorders such as idiopathic hepatitis and Sjögren's syndrome, occur more frequently in individuals who have HLA-B8. Other diseases, such as multiple sclerosis and rheumatoid arthritis, appear to be associated with lymphocyte-defined genetic loci whose products on the cell membranes are responsible for mixed lymphocyte reactivity. Although the exact mechanisms by which genetic factors and autoimmunity are related are unclear, it is likely that the immune response (Ir) genes, lymphocytic surface antigen, and possible receptors for specific viruses are involved. Viruses and other infectious agents are often associated with autoimmunity. Many virus buds from cell surfaces can incorporate normal membrane constituents as part of their viral envelope. Such combinations of viral and host tissue antigens may become immunogenic and give rise to autoimmune responses.

General theories and mechanisms of autoimmunity. Numerous mechanisms may initiate an autoimmune response. The autoimmune reaction is the result of disruption of the normal pathways of interaction of T cells and B cells with autoantigens. Autoimmunity may arise whenever there is a state of immunologic imbalance in which B-cell activity is excessive and suppressor T-cell activity is diminished (Fig. 27-9). This imbalance may occur as a consequence of genetic, viral, and environmental mechanisms acting singly or in combination (Fig. 27-10). Manipulation of autoantigens in a way to stimulate helper T-cell functions, such as the use of adjuvants, immunogenic carriers, or cross-reactive antigens, also induces the autoimmune phenomenon (Fig. 27-11). Furthermore, the decrease in normal suppressor cell activity caused by aging, cancer, or other disease mechanisms may permit self-reactive cells to proliferate, resulting in the production of autoantibody and autoreactive lymphocytes.

Classification of human autoimmune disease.[72] The autoimmune disorders can be broadly separated into three main groups: (1) organ-specific diseases, (2) nonorgan-specific diseases, and (3) diseases with nonorgan-specific autoantibodies but with lesions restricted to one or only a few organs (Table 27-4).

Organ-specific autoimmune disease. These disorders are characterized by chronic inflammatory changes in a specific organ. The autoantibodies in this group of diseases exhibit specificity for antigens of the diseased organ. Such autoantibodies may demonstrate species specificity, and familial clustering of diseases within this group occurs with remarkable frequency. Examples of this group are (1) Hashimoto's autoimmune thyroiditis, (2) primary hypothyroidism, (3) thyrotoxicosis (Graves' disease), (4) chronic atrophic gastritis, (5) primary adrenal atrophy, (6) post–rabies vaccination encephalomyelitis, and (7) autoimmune hemolytic anemia.

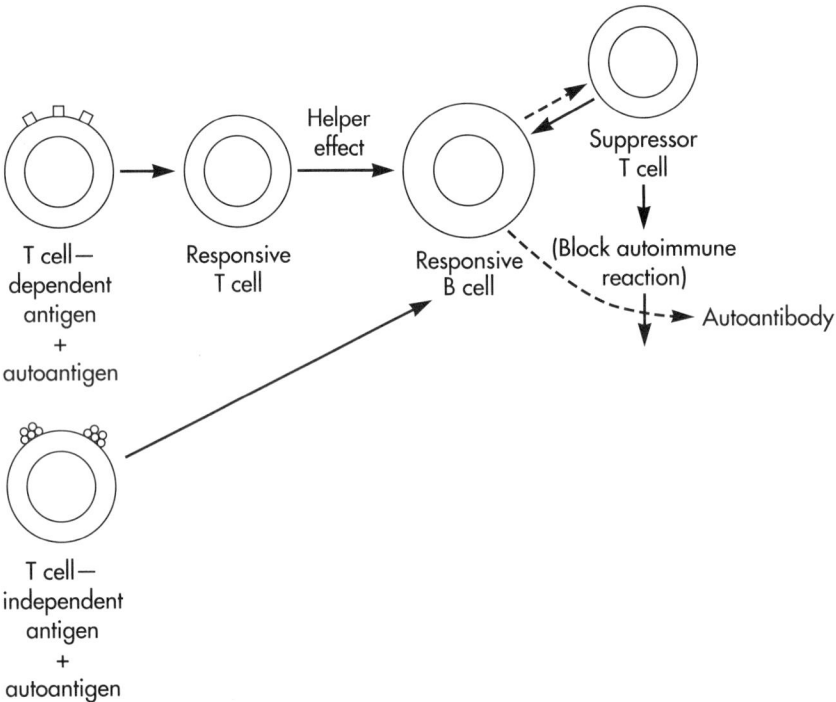

Fig. 27-9. Suppressor T cells in the prevention of autoimmune reactions.

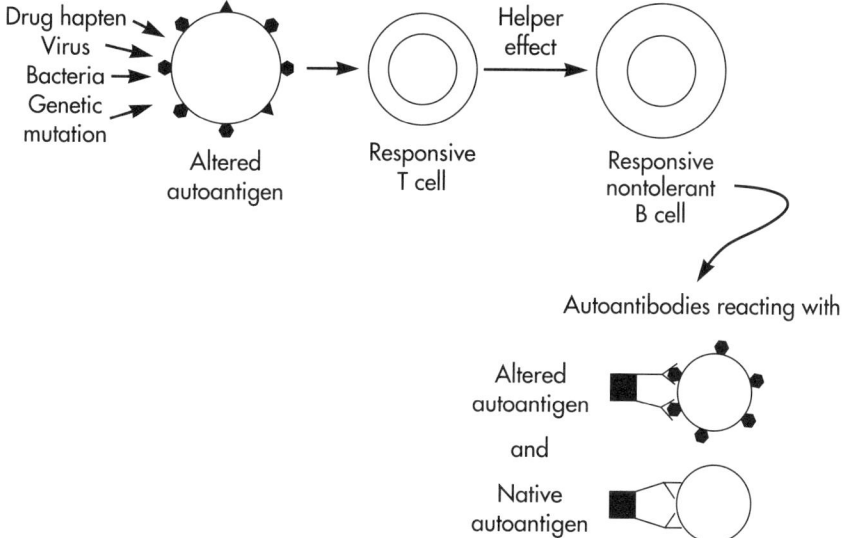

Fig. 27-10. Autoantibody formation in certain organ-specific autoimmune diseases.

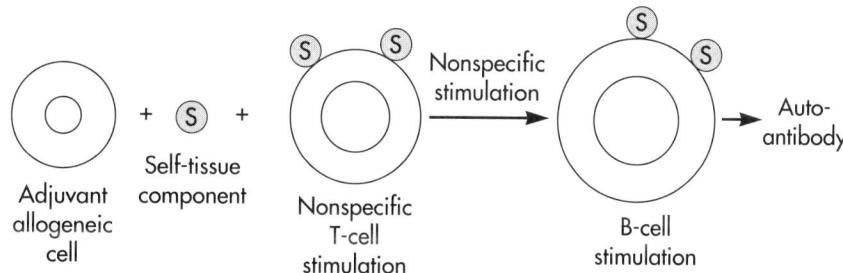

Fig. 27-11. Autoimmunity following adjuvant and allogeneic cell stimulation.

Non–organ-specific autoimmune diseases. These diseases are characterized by widespread pathologic change in many different organs and tissues throughout the body. Furthermore, the associated serum autoantibodies often lack organ and species specificity and experimental lesions are not readily produced; however, similar diseases arise spontaneously in certain inbred animal strains. Examples of this group are (1) systemic lupus erythematosus, (2) rheumatoid arthritis, and (3) various other connective tissue disorders such as progressive systemic sclerosis (scleroderma). In the group of non–organ-specific autoimmune diseases the primary mechanism of injury is by immune complexes. In systemic lupus erythematosus the pathogenic complex is the DNA–anti-DNA complex. The factors involved in production of anti-DNA antibody are probably complex, with an abnormal imbalance and interaction of viral, genetic, and immunologic factors.

Disorders with non–organ-specific autoantibodies and with lesions restricted to one or few organs. By definition these diseases combine the features of both organ-specific and non–organ-specific categories. Examples of this group are (1) primary biliary cirrhosis and (2) chronic aggressive hepatitis. The autoimmune liver disorders are characterized by the production of non-organ-specific and non-species-specific antibodies, such as antimitochondrial and anti–smooth-muscle-cell antibodies. The relationships of these antibodies to immune injury and the lesion are unknown, and the levels of the antibodies do not correlate with the severity or duration of the disease.

Clinical observations that indicate autoimmune pathogenesis. Autoimmune disorders are frequently associated with malignancies, immune deficiency syndromes, and aging. Possible autoimmune pathogenesis in a given disease is indicated when one observes (1) the existence of autoantibodies, (2) amyloid deposits of denatured gamma globulin, (3) hypergammaglobulinemia with elevation of various immunoglobulins, (4) vasculitis, serositis, and glomerulonephritis, which suggest an immune complex disease, and (5) existence of other diseases, such as endocrinopathies, known to be associated with autoimmune disorders.

Systemic lupus erythematosus (SLE).[19,32] SLE is the prototype for autoimmune disease. The presence of auto-

Table 27-4. Organ and clinical criteria for classification of SLE

Organ system	Criteria
Skin	Malar rash
	Discord rash
	Photosensitivity
Mucous membranes	Oral or nasopharyngeal ulceration
Joints	Arthritis (two or more joints)
Pleura pericardium	Serositis
Renal	Renal proteinuria
	Cellular casts
CNS	Neurologic seizures, psychosis
Blood	Hematologic-hemolytic anemia
	Leukopenia
	Lymphopenia
	Thrombocytopenia
Immune	Immune disorder
	(+) LE cell preparation
	DNA antibody to native DNA in abnormal titer
ANA antibody	Anti-Sm; false positive serologic test for syphilis
	ANA titer abnormal by immunofluorescence, abscence of drug-induced lupus

Table 27-5. Specific antibodies for diagnosis of SLE

Staining pattern	Antigen
Peripheral	• Double-stranded DNA (ds-DNA)
Homogeneous	• DNA histone complex
Speckled	• Smith (Sm) antigen—renal, CNS involvement
Speckled	• RNP (ribonucleoproteins)—SLE, Sjögren's syndrome
Speckled	• Robert (Ro) (SS-A)—Skin disease, neonatal SLE, Sjögren's syndrome
Speckled	• Lane (La) (SS-B)—Sjögren's syndrome
Drug-induced lupus	
Homogenous	• DNA histone complex

antibodies is important for its diagnosis and clinical manifestation. The prevalence rate is one in 2000, but one in 700 for women between the ages of 20 and 64 years and one in 245 for black women in the same age group. The etiology of SLE is unknown. Genetic studies have revealed that those SLE patients with HLA-DR2 are more likely to develop anti–ds-DNA (double-stranded DNA) antibodies and those with HLA-DR3 produce anti–SS-A and anti–SS-B antibodies. HLA-DR4 and HLA-DR5 produce anti-Sm (Smith) and anti-RNP (ribonucleoprotein) antibodies. The immunological features of SLE include the lupus erythematosus cell, antinuclear antibodies, complement level depression, tissue deposition of immunoglobulins and complement, circulating anticoagulants, and other autoantibodies.

Antinuclear antibodies, detected by the immunofluorescent technique, are highly sensitive, but not specific for the diagnosis of SLE. High titers are often associated with SLE, and a negative test is strong evidence against the diagnosis of SLE. Table 27-5 demonstrates the antinuclear antibodies related to SLE. Complement-mediated tissue injury in SLE is initiated by immune complex deposition in various sites. Decreased levels of complement are associated with greater risk of renal and central nervous system involvement. Genetic deficiency of the early components of complement (C1, C4, C2) are associated with SLE and other rheumatic diseases. Immune complex deposition along the glomerular basement membrane and at the dermal-epidermal junction can be detected by direct immunofluorescence and electron microscopy. The presence of antibodies to ds-DNA has predictive value in immune-complex–mediated renal disease. Almost 90% of patients with SLE have immunoglobulin and complement deposition in the dermal-epidermal junction of noninvolved skin. The IgG or IgM appears as brightly stained homogeneous or granular bands. In discoid lupus, the immune complex deposition is found only in involved skin. Anticoagulants and autoantibodies circulating to red blood cells and causing a hemolytic anemia are present in patients with SLE. Autoantibodies to neutrophils and platelets may also be present. The clinical features of SLE consist of multisystem involvement. SLE does not present a single clinical pattern, and the onset can be acute or insidious. The diagnosis can be established in a patient with multisystem involvement with the aid of the criteria for diagnosis of SLE and a high-titer positive ANA test. A patient with four or more of the 11 criteria can be said to have SLE. Treatment has significantly affected the mortality and morbidity with a 90% survival of at least 15 years. Antiinflammatory drugs, steroids, antimalarials, cyclophosphamide, and plasmapheresis have been employed to control the disease.

Drug-induced lupus. [69] The most common drugs that cause drug-induced lupus include procainamide hydrochloride, hydralazine hydrochloride, anticonvulsants, and chlorpromazine hydrochloride. Drug-induced lupus does not affect the kidneys or central nervous system. The antinuclear antibodies (ANAs) in the drug-induced syndrome are histone dependent, while in idiopathic SLE, histone dependence is found in only 30% of patients. There is resolution of signs and symptoms after these drugs have been discontinued.

Rheumatoid arthritis. [40,42] In rheumatoid arthritis (RA) the synovial lining of the joints is the frequent site of inflammatory injury. RA may involve multiple organ systems. Inheritance appears to be polygenic with an increased incidence of HLA-DR4. The etiology of RA remains unknown.

Immunologic features include rheumatoid factors, ANAs, immune complexes, and complement levels. Rheumatoid factors are antibodies with specificity for the Fc fragment of IgG. Latex agglutination detects 19S IgM rheumatoid factors, but 7S IgM, IgG, and IgA may have rheumatoid factor activity. Latex agglutination is positive in 80% of patients who fit the ARA criteria for RA. The criteria for RA include morning stiffness, pain on motion or tenderness in a least one joint, swelling of at least one joint, swelling of at least one other joint, symmetrical joint swelling of the same joint right and left, subcutaneous nodules, x-ray changes typical of RA, positive serum test for rheumatoid factors, poor mucin clotting to synovial fluid, and characteristic histologic changes in RA. ANAs are found in 14% to 28% of patients with RA. Positive tests for mixed cryoglobulin indicate a large amount of immune complexes (IgG and 7S IgM rheumatoid factors) and are associated with an increased incidence of extraarticular manifestations, especially vasculitis. In general, RA patients have normal complement. However, in RA patients with vasculitis the complement levels are depressed.

The therapy in RA requires a multimodality approach involving the primary care physician, consulting physician, physical therapist, psychologists, and surgeon. Rest, physical therapy, salicylates, and nonsteroidal antiinflammatory agents are given for the patient with mild to moderate RA. Progressive RA may require gold, antimalarials, d-penicillamine, steroids, and/or cytotoxic drugs.

Sjögren's syndrome (SS).[30] Sjögren's syndrome is a chronic inflammatory disease of unknown etiology that affects lacrimal, salivary, and other excretory glands, leading to keratoconjunctivitis sicca and xerostomia. There is a strong association with histocompatibility antigens HLA-B8 and HLA-DR3. The immunologic features include hypergammaglobulinemia in 50% of patients. This may lead to hyperviscosity syndrome. Antinuclear antibodies may be in a speckled or homogeneous pattern and are present in 65% of patients. A primary form of Sjögren's is not associated with other diseases, and a secondary form is associated with RA and other connective-tissue diseases. Antibodies to SS-A antigen have been associated with vasculitis in primary SS. Antibodies to SS-B antigen are nearly always found in association with SS-A and only occur in SLE and SS. Rheumatoid factors are present in 90% of both primary and secondary Sjögren's. Antibodies to salivary duct antigens are frequently detected in patients with secondary SS. A strong association of SS with RA and SLE suggests that in SS the etiologic factors that should be considered are infection, abnormalities of the immune regulation, and genetic factors. Clinical manifestations include dry eyes, dry mouth, and recurrent salivary gland pain and swelling. Chronic cough and hoarseness may develop. Dysphagia and atrophic gastritis result from involvement of the gastrointestinal tract. Renal tubular acidosis may be present and vasculitis involving peripheral nerves of the CNS. There is a forty-four-fold increase in the development of lymphoma in patients with SS with the possibility of a pseudolymphoma preceding the lymphoma. The laboratory aids for diagnosis of SS include characteristic patterns on scialography and radionuclide scanning of the salivary gland demonstrating decreased function. Schirmer's test for ocular secretions are abnormal and there is a decrease in oral secretions. Treatment includes usage of artificial tears. Oral hygiene is essential, and water must be drunk to help the teeth. Systemic steroids are used in severe cases with involvement of lungs, kidneys, CNS, or vasculitis.

Progressive systemic sclerosis (scleroderma).[11,59] Scleroderma is a collagen vascular disease of unknown origin. The disease is associated with smooth muscle atrophy and fibrosis of internal organs. Renal involvement with accelerated hypertension is most likely to be fatal. It is three times more common in females than males and occurs in the third and fourth decade of life. The subtypes of the disease may be classified as follows: (1) diffuse scleroderma and systemic sclerosis; (2) sclerodactyly, CREST syndrome, and related variants; (3) overlap syndrome featuring scleroderma; (4) limited forms such as morphea (localized and diffuse) and linear scleroderma; (5) scleroderma-like diseases, for example chronic GVHD and eosinophilic fasciitis; (6) chemically induced scleroderma variants due to vinyl chloride, bleomycin, trichloroethylene, pentazocine; (7) scleroderma mimics such as porphyria cutanea tarda, carcinoid syndrome, amyloidosis, progeria, Werner's syndrome, and lipoatrophy. In scleroderma antinuclear antibodies are formed to extractable nuclear antigens, the nucleolus, the centromere, and Scl-70. Antinuclear antibodies are detected in 40% to 90% of patients with scleroderma. A speckled ANA pattern with antibodies to n-RNP (ribonuclear protein) antigen suggests mixed connective tissue disease (overlap of the clinical features seen in SLE, scleroderma, and polymyositis). Since 80% of these patients usually develop scleroderma or remain undifferentiated, the preferable nomenclature should be "undifferentiated connective tissue syndrome."

Antinucleolar pattern is considered most specific for scleroderma. Antibodies to the PM-Scl antigens produce a homogeneous nucleolar pattern. The patients have clinical features of scleroderma and a high frequency of myositis. Anticentromere antibody is specific for patients with CREST syndrome (calcinosis, Raynaud's phenomenon, esophageal dysfunction, sclerodactyly, and telangiectasia). Patients with CREST syndrome can develop pulmonary fibrosis, hypertension, and biliary cirrhosis. Patients with antibodies to Scl-70 have been associated with diffuse truncal skin involvement, increased frequency of pulmonary interstitial fibrosis, and digital pitting scars, but not renal involvement. The clinical features include Raynaud's phenomenon in 50% of the cases. Skin manifestations go through three stages: (1) nonpainful pitting edema; (2) a sclerotic "hidebound" stage during which skin becomes tight, smooth, and waxy, skin folds disappear, and patient develops typical facies; and (3) atrophy or softening and a return toward normal. Articular complaints with contracture are common, and the patient may develop inflammatory myopathy. There is almost always lung fibrosis, which may be asymptomatic and accompanied by pulmonary hypertension. The kidney and heart may be involved. Kidney involvement may be life-threatening. There may be wide mouth diverticula in the colon. The diagnosis may be obvious by the clinical appearance. The diagnosis is difficult in the early stages when there is no skin involvement above the wrist and there is only sclerodactyly or pitting edema of the hands. The ANA can be helpful. Antibodies to the centromere are evident early in the course of CREST. Esophageal hypomotility can be demonstrated early in the course of the disease. The treatment modalities include corticosteroids, colchicine, d-penicillamine, and immunosuppression.

General laboratory tests to detect autoimmune disorders. The most commonly used tests for the diagnosis of autoimmune disorders involve the detection of circulating antibodies. Tests for cellular sensitivity are done in the larger centers primarily on an investigative basis. See Table 27-6 for methods of antibody detection.

Immunofluorescence, enzyme-labeled antibody, and radioimmunoassay methods utilize primary antigen-antibody binding reactions and, because of their high sensitivity, are preferred for the detection of circulating and tissue-bound antibodies and antigens. Tests that involve secondary antigen-antibody preparations such as complement fixation, agglutination, and precipitation in agar gel, may not be as sensitive as immunofluorescence or radioimmunoassay in some circumstances, but may be technically more suitable for the identification of certain autoantibodies. The indirect immunofluorescence test (IFT) and the more recently developed peroxidase-labeled antibody method are the most widely used immunohistochemical procedures for the detection of serum autoantibodies in the clinical laboratory. Both methods can be used to demonstrate (1) autoimmune antibodies in serum, (2) tissue localization and fixation of autoantibody, and (3) deposition of antigen-antibody complexes in kidney, vessels, and other tissues.

In addition to tissue autoantibody detection, numerous other methods have proved useful in the evaluation of patients with suspected autoimmune disorders. These include various assays for cell-mediated immunity that have potential usefulness in studying patients with autoimmune thyroiditis, certain liver diseases, and rheumatoid arthritis. Still other, less cumbersome methods are frequently employed, such as (1) rheumatoid factors, (2) immune complexes in serum or joint fluid, (3) quantitation of serum immunoglobulins, (4) immunoelectrophoresis of serum and other body fluids, (5) cryoglobulins, (6) complement assays, and (7) biopsy of kidney, vessel, or joint for immunofluorescence location of antibody and immune complexes.

Interpretation of serum autoantibody levels. In general, the level of antibody is high in patients with autoimmune disorders and low in apparently healthy persons. A very high titer of autoantibody is significant, but a low or absent titer of autoantibody does not rule out the possibility of an autoimmune disorder. Therefore the level, or titer, of a given antibody must be interpreted in relation to the stage or treatment of a particular disease. When adults are tested for rheumatoid factor and the antibodies to nuclear cell, parietal cell, thyroglobulin, thyroid epithelial cell, reticulin, mitochondria, and smooth muscle, the incidence of autoantibodies in the general adult population to one or more antigens at a level of 1:10 titer or greater varies from approximately 21% to 27%, with a higher incidence in females. The incidence of certain autoantibodies increases with advancing age. In one study, 50% of subjects over 60 years of age demonstrated low titers of one or more autoantibodies.

The antinuclear, antiparietal cell, and antithyroid antibodies are age- and sex-dependent, with an increasing incidence in females and older persons. However, the incidences of smooth muscle antibody and rheumatoid factor do not correlate with age and sex. The incidences of smooth muscle antibody and rheumatoid factor are similar in males and females.

Autoimmunity and neoplasia.[40,51,69] Autoimmune reactions to damaged or altered tissue may facilitate malignant degeneration with adoptive loss of cellular components. Human cancer and autoimmunity may be related, since (1) certain autoimmune diseases may be considered precancerous and are associated with a higher incidence of cancer than occurs in the control population, and (2) the host immune response to the invading cancer may initiate immunologic injury with formation of nonmetastatic distant lesions. There may be a step-by-step developmental sequence from normal immunologic regulation through autoimmunity and benign lymphoproliferation, leading ultimately to lymphoid neoplasia. Considerable evidence from studies in humans and animals suggests that autoimmunity, monoclonal immunoglobulin production, and malignant lymphocytic and plasma cell proliferation may be related events. There is a clear association between autoimmunity and the lymphoma that occurs in Sjögren's syndrome. Sjögren's syndrome represents a lymphocytic attack on the salivary and lacrimal glands, and the disease is associated with rheumatoid arthritis in almost 50% of cases. Sjögren's syndrome is often benign, leading to progressive oral and ocular dryness. However, some patients exhibit an aggressive course, demonstrating lymphocytic infiltrates with lymphadenopathy. The term pseudolymphoma has been applied to this condition, and some patients with this abnormality develop malignant lymphomas without necessarily passing through the pseudolymphoma state. The lymphomas are often highly undifferentiated and may be associated with hypogammaglobulinemia and loss of antibodies.

A pathologic entity termed *immunoblastic lymphadenopathy* has been described, a lesion that has been confused with

Table 27-6. Antibodies in various autoimmune diseases

Diseases	Antigen involved	Methods for detection of antibody
Organ-specific endocrine diseases		
Autoimmune thyroiditis, primary myxedema, thyrotoxicosis	Thyroglobulin	Immunofluorescent test (IFT) (indirect)—methanol-fixed human thyroid
		Passive hemagglutination
		Latex agglutination
	Cytoplasmic microsome	IFT (indirect)—unfixed human hyperplastic thyroid tissue
		Passive hemagglutination
		Complement fixation
Thyrotoxicosis	Thyroid cell surface antigen	Bioassay—mouse thyroid stimulation in vivo
		Radioimmunoassay with inhibition of TSH on human thyroid tissue receptor
Addison's disease	Adrenal cell cytoplasm	IFT (indirect) on unfixed human adrenal cortex
Parathyroid	Parathyroid cytoplasmic antigen	IFT (indirect) human parathyroid gland
Early-onset diabetes	Islet cell	IFT on human or guinea pig pancreas
Non–organ-specific diseases		
Lupus erythematosus	Nuclear antigens	
Dermatomyositis		
Periarteritis nodosa		
Scleroderma		
Rheumatoid arthritis	Altered gamma globulin	Latex agglutination (rheumatoid factor)
		Rose test, sheep cell agglutination
	Rheumatoid arthritis precipitin	Immunodiffusion
Sjögren's syndrome		
Polymyositis		
Other collagen diseases		
"Autoimmune" liver diseases		
Alimentary tract diseases		
Atrophic gastritis	Parietal cell microsomes	IFT (indirect)—human or mouse gastric mucosa substrate
Pernicious anemia	Intrinsic factor	Radioactive vitamin B_{12}–binding assay
Sjögren's syndrome	Salivary duct cells	IFT (indirect)—unfixed human salivary gland
Ulcerative colitis	Colon, lipopolysaccharide	IFT (indirect)—human or rat colon
Celiac disease	Reticulin	IFT (indirect)—rat kidney, liver
Crohn's disease	Reticulin	IFT (indirect)—rad kidney, liver
Liver diseases		
Chronic aggressive hepatitis	Smooth muscle (actin)	IFT (indirect)—rat gastric mucosa, human cervical tissue
	Liver/kidney microsomal	IFT (indirect)—rat kidney and liver
Primary biliary cirrhosis	Mitochondrial	IFT (indirect)—rat kidney, unfixed
Other		
Myasthenia gravis	Skeletal or heart muscle	IFT (indirect)—rat skeletal muscle and calf thymus
	Acetylcholine receptor	Radioimmunoassay
Goodpasture's syndrome	Glomerular and lung basement membrane	IFT (direct)—biopsy of patient's kidney
		IFT (indirect)—patient's serum on kidney substrate
		Radioimmunoassay on serum
Pemphigus vulgaris	Prickle cell desmosomes	IFT (direct and indirect)—human skin
		Peroxidase-labeled antibody
Bullous pemphigoid	Epithelial basement membrane	IFT (direct and indirect)—human skin
		Peroxidase-labeled antibody
Cicatricial pemphigoid	Epithelial basement membrane	IFT (direct) on biopsy of mucous membrane—indirect on human skin
Dermatitis herpetiformis	Reticulin	IFT (indirect)—rat kidney, liver
Autoimmune hemolytic anemia	Red cell	Coombs' antiglobulin test (direct and indirect)
Central nervous system demyelinating diseases (i.e., multiple sclerosis)	Myelin	IFT (indirect)—mammalian spinal cord

From Nakamura RM, Tucker ES: In Henry JB, editor: *Clinical diagnosis by laboratory methods,* ed 16, Philadelphia, 1978, WB Saunders.

Hodgkin's disease. The lymph node shows immunoblastic proliferation in the B-lymphocyte plasma cell series, with proliferation of small vessels and deposits of amorphous interstitial material. The cellular proliferation is considered benign; however, the clinical course is associated with a poor prognosis. Many of the patients show hypersensitivity reaction to drugs; this entity supports the concept that there is uncontrolled immunoblastic proliferation following an antigenic stimulus, and a true neoplasm may develop.

Immunodeficiency disorders*

Overview. Four major aspects of the immune system involved in the defense against various viral, bacterial, and other injurious stimuli consist of (1) B-cell or antibody-mediated immunity, (2) T-cell or cell-mediated immunity, (3) phagocytic mechanisms, and (4) the complement system. Each of these systems can act independently or in conjunction with one or more of the others. The immunodeficiency disorders can be classified under five major categories: (1) antibody- or B-cell deficiency diseases, (2) cellular or T-cell immunodeficiency diseases, (3) combined B- and T-cell immunodeficiency diseases, (4) diseases with a phagocytic dysfunction, and (5) complement abnormalities and immunodeficiency diseases. Primary immunodeficiency diseases are genetic disorders and result from a failure of proper development of the humoral or cellular immune system or both. Secondary, or acquired, immunodeficiency diseases occur in patients in association with a variety of diseases and include immunodeficiency states associated with intestinal lymphangiectasia, protein-losing enteropathy, X-irradiation, immunosuppressive and cytotoxic agents or drugs, lymphoreticular malignancies, and so forth. More details of some specific immunodeficiency disorders are discussed in greater detail in the Chapter Immunotoxicology.

Diagnosis and laboratory evaluation of immunodeficiency disorders. Because immunodeficiency has been proposed as a mechanism for some types of environmental illnesses, the discussion will focus on the clinical manifestations of acquired immunodeficient states. Classically, recurrent infection is the hallmark of the immunodeficient patient. The following types of infection may suggest an immunologic defect: (1) recurrent infection caused by bacteria of high-grade virulence, (2) those caused by low-grade virulence or unusual organisms, and (3) those caused by fungi and unusual reactions to vaccines. The nature of the immunodeficiency determines the spectrum of infections that may be encountered. The primary T-cell deficiencies demonstrate an unusual susceptibility to intracellular infections, which may be caused by viruses, fungi, and certain bacteria such as *Mycobacterium tuberculosis.* B-cell deficiencies allow infections by organisms that are largely disposed by opsonization (for example, pneumococci, staphylococci, and streptococci).

In the evaluation of patients suspected of immunodeficiency diseases one should obtain a detailed history. Some of the important points to be investigated are as follows: (1) history of allergy and tests completed in past; (2) prior surgery, particularly tonsillectomy and adenoidectomy as well as appendectomy; results of pathologic examination on excised tissue may help in the assessment of the immune system; (3) radiation therapy to the thymus or nasopharynx; (4) sites of infection and organisms recovered; age at onset of infections; (5) previous immunizations and reactions; (6) prior gamma globulin treatment; and (7) family history of collagen diseases, endocrine disorders, tumor, or early death. The box on page 345 shows the various diagnostic tests commonly used to evaluate immunodeficiency states.

Evaluation of the T-cell deficiency.[74] Generally, a T-cell deficiency is indicated by increased susceptibility to infection by fungi, viruses, atypical acid-fast organisms, and some of the so-called lower-grade pathogens. Various organisms that are involved include *Candida albicans,* vaccinia and mumps virus, *Mycoplasma,* and *Pneumocystis carinii. Pneumocystis carinii* is frequently involved and produces pulmonary lesions in patients with a combined B- and T-cell deficiency. In these patients, the pneumonia shows characteristic accumulations of foamy, pink-staining exudate containing many *Pneumocystis* organisms. The following tests are used for the evaluation of the T-cell system: (1) absolute lymphocyte count, (2) delayed-type skin reaction, (3) lymphocyte stimulation test, (4) migration inhibitory factor test, (5) examination of circulating lymphocytes for T-cell markers, and (6) radiologic evidence of normal lymphoid tissues. Skin tests for delayed hypersensitivity to common antigens may be of little help in young children who have not had the opportunity to develop a cell-mediated immune reaction to the antigens. However, a negative skin test to *Candida* antigens in children suffering from infection with this fungus has diagnostic usefulness. Morphologic analysis of the small lymphocytes in the peripheral blood and the deep cortical areas of biopsy lymph nodes provides some information about the adequacy of the T-cell system.

Evaluation of the B-cell system.[48,74] The deficiency of the B-cell system is generally indicated by frequent bouts of infections with pathogenic organisms causing otitis media, pneumonia, meningitis, and other infections. Such organisms include pneumococcus, *Streptococcus, Hemophilus, Meningococcus,* and hepatitis virus. A variety of immunologic tests are available for quantitation of the immunoglobulin levels. The antibody tests for humoral immunity can be divided into two groups: (1) tests for the presence of immunoglobulin and existing antibodies to common antigens, and (2) tests for antibody formation following active immunization. The immunoglobulin levels can be quantitated by various techniques, including radial immunodiffusion, immunofluorescence, and other immunoprecipitin techniques. There should be some caution in the evaluation of

---
*References 6, 16, 20, 53, 54.

Diagnosis of immunodeficiency disorders

T-cell deficiency	B-cell deficiency
Evaluation of T-cell Functions	*Evaluation of B-cell Functions*

1. Absolute lymphocyte count
2. Delayed-type skin reaction
3. Lymphocyte stimulation test
4. Migration inhibitory factor test
5. Assessment of T-cell markers
6. Radiologic evaluation of lymphoid tissue
	Immunoglobulin assays to common antigensImmunoglobulin assays following active immunization with
	   Diphtheria (Schnick test)
	   Pertussis
	   Tetanus
	   Typhoid vaccine
	A & B isohemaglutinnins assays
	The absent isohemaglutinnins titer in the first two years of life indicate IgM deficiency
	Rectal mucosal biopsy for immunoglobulin localization
	
	The methods of immunoglobulin assay
	   1. Immunoelectrophoresis
	   2. Immunodiffusion
	   3. Immunofluorescence
	   4. Immune-precipitin techniques
	   5. Rectal mucosal biopsy

---

immunoglobulin levels in adult sera as they may vary greatly among individuals. The measurements may not be reliable in the case of quantitation of various monoclonal gamma globulins owing to the nature of the specificity of the antisera and the various standards used. Absence or low serum levels of one or more immunoglobulins may have three possible causes: (1) absence or decreased number of B cells in circulation of lymphoid tissue, (2) a defect in the immunoglobulin secretion by B cells, and (3) an increased rate of immunoglobulin catabolism. Tests that can be carried out to distinguish between the various possibilities involve the immunofluorescent staining of the membrane of the various lymphocytes to analyze the B-cell population in the circulation, as well as in the lymph nodes. In addition, one can look for the presence of germinal centers and plasma cells in the lymph nodes.

Tests for T-cell function. *The absolute lymphocyte count* in normal children usually is above 2000/mm^3 during the first 4 years of life. The lymphocyte count during maturation is an average of 2500 with a lower limit of 1000/mm^3. Normal infants should show a count greater than 1500 small lymphocytes per millimeter. *Delayed-type skin reactions* testing may employ five different antigens: *Trichophyton, Candida,* streptokinase-streptodornase, mumps, and purified protein derivative (PPD). Most normal persons show a positive response to one or more antigens. The most consistently positive antigen is *Candida,* which shows a positive delayed skin reaction in 80% to 95% of normal persons 7 months of age or older. If skin reactions to the aforementioned delayed-hypersensitivity antigens are negative, sensitivity tests to 2,4-dinitrochlorobenzene may be indicated. The *lymphocyte stimulation test* is an in vitro test useful in the diagnosis of thymic dysplasia in infants whose absolute lymphocyte count appears within the normal range. In this test a pure lymphocyte fraction obtained from peripheral blood is cultured with phytohemagglutinin (PHA). Lymphocytes from normal persons will show 50% or more conversion to blast forms, whereas cells from individuals with thymic abnormalities demonstrate little or no transformation of lymphocytes in culture. *Migration inhibitory factor* testing takes into account the principle that sensitized thymus-derived T lymphocytes in the presence of antigen release a number of factors, one of which inhibits the migration of macrophages from capillary tubes. Production of the migration inhibitory factor (MIF) is a good in vitro indicator of the presence of cell-mediated immunity. *Examination of circulating lymphocytes for T-cell markers* tests for surface receptor for sheep erythrocytes and provides a reliable marker for the identification of T cells. Erythrocyte rosette formation requires viable lymphocytes and has been shown to be dependent on a surface receptor. The percentage of peripheral blood lymphocytes that form E rosettes in normal adults varies between 65% and 78%. Antithymocyte serum, the antisera to T cells, has been developed by immunization of animals with human thymus cells and human or monkey thymus cell suspensions. If the absorbed antiserum is used in immunofluorescence tests, approximately 80% of peripheral blood lymphocytes are identified as T cells. Various studies have demonstrated a subpopulation of T cells with a surface receptor for the Fc portion of the IgG. This group of T cells with Fc receptors may represent T-helper cells. *Radiologic evidence* may be suggested in children by noting the presence of normal lymphoid tissue of thymus and pharynx. *Lymph node biopsy* may demonstrate a depletion of paracortical lymphoid cells, which indicates a T-cell defect.

Tests for B-cell function. The various tests for B-cell function could be presented as (1) tests for presence of immunoglobulins and existing antibodies to common antigens, and (2) tests for antibody formation following active immunization. The tests for presence of immunoglobulins and existing antibodies to common antigens include the following:

Schick test. If an individual has been previously immunized with diphtheria toxoid and his humoral immune system is normal, the Schick test will be negative. A positive Schick test in such cases is presumptive evidence of IgG deficiency.

A and B isohemagglutinins. Isohemagglutinins are present normally after about 1 year of age and are primarily of the IgM class. The absence of isohemagglutinins is presumptive evidence of IgM deficiency. The isoagglutinin titer in the first 2 years of life is low.

Immunoelectrophoresis. This test is used to determine qualitative levels of immunoglobulins IgG, IgM, and IgA. The sera of newborns show a normal absence of IgM and IgA.

Quantitative and immunoglobulin determinations. IgG concentration of 200 mg/dl is considered the lower adult threshold value. IgA deficiency shows less than 5 mg/dl of serum.

Quantitation of IgG subclasses. Patients with normal levels of immunoglobulins may have a history of recurrent pyogenic infection that is associated with selective IgG subclass deficiencies.

Rectal mucosal biopsy examination. A biopsy may be taken for routine histology and immunofluorescent localization of IgG, IgM, and IgA immunoglobulins. Infants over 1 month of age will have plasma cells in the lamina propria of the rectal mucosa. This is a good screening test for evidence of antibody production in suspected humoral immunodeficiency cases.

Circulating B lymphocytes for surface immunoglobulins. The presence of easily detectable surface immunoglobulin as determined by vital staining with immunofluorescent antisera of IgG heavy-chain determinants has been applied to identify B cells. The dominant surface Ig determinants on B cells in normal individuals are IgM and IgD. Many B cells carry both these determinants. The significance of the strong representation of IgD, besides its minor contribution to serum Ig, has suggested that it may be important in the clonal maturation of B cells or in triggering further events affecting B-cell response. The number of circulating B cells with easily detectable surface Ig in peripheral blood of normal adults has ranged from 8% to 15%. B cells have a surface receptor for the third component of complement and have been utilized as a means of detecting B cells in suspension. The most widely applied method demonstrates complement receptors using sheep erythrocytes sensitized with purified IgM antibodies and reacted with complement. These EAC cells can then be demonstrated to adhere to B lymphocytes to form rosettes through the complement surface receptor. Peripheral blood lymphocytes in normal individuals with EAC receptors also have surface Ig markers. Many B cells have receptors for the Fc portion of the IgG and may be identified by use of IgG-coated erythrocytes or fluorescent-tagged aggregated IgG. Such a receptor is also present on monocytes and some T cells. Since some B cells apparently lack Fc receptors, application of this technique as a lymphocyte marker probe is limited. The cell responsible for lymphoid cell–mediated antibody-dependent cytotoxicity has been shown to have Fc receptors without other identifying surface markers.

Tests for antibody formation following active immunization

Diphtheria, pertussis, and tetanus (DPT) vaccination. A standard dose is given weekly for 3 successive weeks. Following immunization with diphtheria toxoid, one can administer a Schick test. A positive Schick test is seen in agammaglobulinemia.

Active immunization with typhoid vaccine. Typhoid immunization can be given once a week for 3 weeks. Typhoid O and H agglutinins can be easily determined in the clinical laboratory. The anti-H titer after three injections will be 160 or greater, and patients with an antibody deficiency may have a titer of less than 1:5.

REFERENCES

1. American College of Chest Physicians, American Thoracic Society: Pulmonary terms and symbols, *Chest* 67:583, 1975.
2. Arnett FC et al: The American Rheumatism Association: 1987 revised criteria for the classification of rheumatoid arthritis, *Arthritis Rheum* 31:315, 1988.
3. Askenase PW: Effector and regulatory mechanisms in delayed-type hypersensitivity. In Middelton E Jr, Reed CE, Ellis E, editors: *Allergy: principles and practice,* ed 2, vol 1, St Louis, 1983, CV Mosby.
4. Back MK: Mediators of anaphylaxis and inflammation, *Annu Rev Microbiol* 36:371, 1982
5. Benacerraf B: Role of MHC gene products in immune regulation, *Science* 212:1229, 1981.
6. Bergsma D, editor: Immunologic deficiency diseases in man, *Birth Defects* 4:1968.
7. Biddison WE, Shae S: CD4 expression and function in HLA class II specific T cells, *Immunol Rev* 109:5, 1989.
8. Bierer BE et al: The biological roles of CD2, CD4, and CD8 in T-cell activation, *Annu Rev Immunol* 7:579, 1989.
9. Blomgren SF, Codemi JJ, Vaughn JH: Procainamide-induced lupus erythematosus: clinical and laboratory observations, *Am J Med* 52:338, 1972.
10. Brostoff J et al: *Clinical immunology,* London, 1991, Gower Medical.
11. Brostoff J et al: SLE and other connective tissue disorders, *Clin Immunol Immunopathol* 6:9, 1991.

12. Bruce CA et al: Quantitative inhalation bronchial challenge in ragweed hay fever patients: a comparison with ragweed-allergic asthmatics, *J Aller Clin Immunol* 56:33, 1975.
13. Bungaard M, deWeck AL: *Allergic reaction to drugs,* vol 63, Berlin, 1983, Springer-Verlag.
14. Burnet M: The clonal selection theory of acquired immunity, *Austr J Med NZ* 1957.
15. Carrao WM, Braman SS, Irwin RS: Chronic cough as the sole presenting manifestation of bronchial asthma, *N Engl J Med* 30:633, 1979.
16. Chandra RK: Immunodeficiency in undernutrition and overnutrition, *Nutr Rev* 39:225, 1981.
17. Chowdhury BA, Chandra RK: Prediction of the development of IgE-mediated atopic disorders and environmental engineering for their control, *Clin Rev Allergy* 7:1, 1989.
18. Cochran AJ: *Man, cancer and immunity,* New York, 1978, Academic Press.
19. Condemi JJ: The autoimmune diseases, *JAMA* 268:2882, 1992.
20. Cowan MD, Ammann AJ: Immunodeficiency associated with inherited metabolic disorders, *Clin Haematol* 10:139, 1981.
21. Dausset J, Svejgaard A, editors: *HLA and disease,* Baltimore, 1977, Williams & Wilkins.
22. Death due to chronic obstructive pulmonary disease and allied conditions, *MMWR* 35:507, 1986.
23. deWeck AL, Blumenthal MN, editors: HLA and allergy, *Monographs in Allergy,* vol 11, Basel, 1977, S. Karger.
24. Muller-Eberhard HJ: The membrane attack complex of complement, *Annu Rev Immunol* 108:151, 1986.
25. Muller-Eberhard HJ: Complement abnormalities in human disease. In Dixon FJ, Fisher DW, editors: *The biology of immunologic disease,* Saunderland, Mass, 1983, Sinauer Associates.
26. Fearson DT: Activation of the alternative complement pathway, *Crit Rev Immunol* 1:1, 1979.
27. Ferrone S, Curtoni ES, Gorini S, editors: *HLA antigens in clinical medicine and biology,* New York, 1979, Garland.
28. Fink JN: Hypersensitivity pneumonitis. In Lynch JP, Deremee RA, editors: *Immunologically mediated pulmonary diseases,* Philadelphia, 1991, JB Lippincott.
29. Fink JN: Hypersensitivity pneumonitis. In Lynch JP, DeRemee RA, editors: *Immunologically mediated pulmonary diseases,* Philadelphia, 1991, JB Lippincott.
30. Fox R et al: Sjogren's Syndrome: proposed criteria for classification, *Arthritis Rheum* 29:577, 1986.
31. Freedman SS: Skin testing for food sensitivity: its clinical significance, *Pediatr Clin North Am* 6:853, 1959.
32. Fye K, Sack K: Rheumatic disease. In Stites DP, Terr AI, editors: *Basic and clinical immunology,* Norwalk, Conn, 1991, Appleton & Lange.
33. Garovoy MR et al: Clinical transplantation. In Stites DP, Terr AI, editors: *Basic and clinical immunology,* Norwalk, Conn, 1991, Appleton & Lange.
34. Gell PGH, Bennacerat B: Studies on hypersensitivity. IV. The relationship between contact and delayed sensitivity: a study of the specificity of cellular immune reactions, *J Exp Med* 113:571, 1961.
35. Gerrard JW et al: Serum IgE levels in White and Metis communities in Saskatchewan, *Ann Allergy* 10, 1976.
36. Goldstein GB, Heiner DC: Clinical and immunological perspectives in food sensitivity, *L Allergy* 46:270, 1970.
37. Greenberger PA: Allergic bronchopulmonary aspergillosis. In Middleton E, Reed C, Ellis E, editors: *Allergy: principles and practices,* ed 3, St Louis, 1988, Mosby.
38. Halloran PF, Cockfield SM, Madrenas J: The molecular immunology of transplantation and graft rejection, *Immunol Allergy Clin North Am* 9:1, 1989.
39. Herberman RB, editor: *NK cells and other natural effector cells,* New York, 1982, Academic Press.
40. Hunder A, Bunch T: Treatment of rheumatoid arthritis, *Bull Rheum Dis* 32:1, 1982.
41. Inman RD, Day NK: Immunologic and clinical aspects of immune complex disease, *Am J Med* 70:1097, 1981.
42. Jaeger D et al: Latex-specific proteins causing immediate-type cutaneous, nasal, bronchial and systemic reactions, *J Allergy Clin Immunol* 89:759, 1992.
43. Janeway CA Jr et al: CD4+ T cells: specificity and function, *Immunol Rev* 100:39, 1988.
44. Kaliner M, Lemanske R: Rhinitis and asthma, *JAMA* 268:2807, 1992.
45. Kohler PF: Immune complexes and allergic diseases. In Middleton E Jr, Reed CE, Ellis E, editors: *Allergy: principles and practice,* ed 2, vol 1, St Louis, 1983, Mosby.
46. Marsh DG, Meyers DA, Bias WB: The epidemiology and genetics of atopic allergy, *N Engl J Med* 305:1551, 1981.
47. May CD, Block LA: A modern clinical approach to food hypersensitivity, *Allergy* 33:166, 1978.
48. McGhee JR, Mestecky J, editors: The secretory immune system, Proceedings of the Conference on the Secretory Immune System, May 4-7, 1982, *Ann NY Acad Sci* 409, 1982.
49. Mizel SB, editor: *Lymphokines in antibody and cytotoxic responses,* vol 6, *Lymphokines: a forum for immunoregulatory cell products,* New York, 1982, Academic Press.
50. Mullarkey MF: Eosinophilic nonallergic rhinitis, *J Allergy Clin Immunol* 82:941, 1988.
51. Oettgen HF: Immunologic aspects of cancer. In Dixon FJ, Fisher DW, editors: *The biology of immunologic disease,* Sunderland, Mass, 1983, Sinauer Associates.
52. Ogawa TH et al: IgE in atopic dermatitis, *Arch Dermatol* 103:575, 1971.
53. Oxelius VA et al: IgG subclass deficiency in selective IgA deficiency, *N Engl J Med* 305:1476, 1981.
54. Pahwa SG, Pahwa RN, Good RA: Heterogeneity of B lymphocyte differentiation in severe combined immunodeficiency disease, *J Clin Invest* 66:543, 1980.
55. Parker CW, Samter M, editors: *Hypersensitivity to drugs,* vol 1, London, 1972, Pergamon Press.
56. Pollat S et al: Epidemiology of acute asthma: IgE antibodies to common inhalant allergens as a risk factor for emergency room visits, *J Allergy Clin Immunol* 83:875, 1989.
57. Porter RR, Reid KBM: Activation of the complement system by antigen-antibody complexes: the classical pathway, *Adv Protein Chem* 33:1, 1979.
58. Rajka G: Prurigo Besnier (atopic dermatitis) with special reference to the role of allergic factors II. The evaluation of the results of skin cancer, *Acta Derm Venereol* (Stockh) 1961.
59. Reimer G: Autoantibodies in systemic sclerosis. In Le Roy EC, editor: *Rheumatic disease clinics of North America,* Philadelphia, 1991, WB Saunders.
60. Roitt I, Brostoff J, Mali D, editors: *Immunology,* St Louis, 1985, Mosby.
61. Rosenberg M et al: Clinical and immunological criteria for diagnosis of allergic bronchopulmonary aspergillosis, *Ann Intern Med* 1986: 405.
62. Sampson HA, McCaskill CC: Food hypersensitivity and atopic dermatitis: evaluation of 113 patients, *J Pediatr* 107:669, 1985.
63. Stobo JF: Autoimmune antireceptor diseases. In Dixon FJ, Fisher DW, editors: *The biology of immunologic disease,* Sunderland, Mass, 1983, Sinauer Associates.
64. Szentivanyi A, Szentivanyi J: Cellular and molecular foundations of immunity, immunologic inflammation and hypersensitivity: component parts and their relation to neurohumoral control mechanisms. In Sodeman WA, editor: *Sodeman's pathologic physiology: mechanisms of disease,* Philadelphia, 1985, WB Saunders.
65. Takafuji S, Suzuki S, Kiozumi K: Diesel exhaust particles inoculated by the intranasal route have an adjuvant activity for IgE production in mice, *J Allergy Clin Immunol* 79:639, 1987.
66. Talmage DW: Allergy and immunology, *Annu Rev Med* 3:239, 1957.
67. Townley RG, Dennis M, Itkin JM: Comparitive action of ocetyl-beta-

methacholine, histamine, and pollen antigens in subjects with hayfever and patients with bronchial asthma, *J Allergy* 36:121, 1965.
68. Townley RG, Hopp RJ: Inhalation methods for the study of airway responsiveness, *J Allergy Clin Immunol* 80:111, 1987.
69. Trentin JJ, editor: *Cross-reacting antigens and neoantigens* (*with implications for autoimmunity and cancer immunity*), Baltimore, 1967, Williams & Wilkins.
70. Twomey JJ, editor: *The pathophysiology of human immunologic disorders,* Baltimore, 1982, Urban & Schwarzenberg.
71. Van Oss CJ: Phagocytosis: an overview, *Methods Enzymol* 132:3, 1986.
72. Weigle WO: Analysis of autoimmunity through experimental models of thyroiditis and allergic encephalomyelitis, *Adv Immunol* 30:159, 1980.
73. Witting HJ et al: Age-related serum immunoglubulin E levels in healthy subjects and in patients with allergic disease, *J Allergy Clin Immunol* 66:305, 1980.
74. Yamamura Y, Kotani S, editors: Immunomodulation by microbial products and related synthetic compounds. Proceedings of an International Symposium, Osaka, Japan, 1981, Amsterdam, 1982, Excerpta Medica.
75. Zinkernegel RM, Doherty PC: Restriction of in vitro T-cell-mediated cytotoxicity in lymphocytic choriomeningitis within a syngeneic or semiallogeneic system, *Nature* 248:701, 1974.
76. Zmijewski CM: Immunologically mediated disease involving allogeneic antigens. In Bellanti JA, editor: *Immunology III,* Philadelphia, 1985, WB Saunders.

Part IV

SUSCEPTIBLE POPULATIONS AND SPECIAL PATIENT GROUPS

Chapter 28

GENERAL PRINCIPLES OF SUSCEPTIBILITY

Karen Reiser

Environmental factors influencing susceptibility
    Exposure to cigarette smoke
    Alcohol abuse
    Use of other drugs
    Nutritional status
    Physical activity
    Previous exposure history
Genetic factors influencing susceptibility
    Sex
    Genetic abnormalities
Miscellaneous factors affecting susceptibility
    Intercurrent diseases
    Psychophysiologic factors
    Age
Summary

For millennia it has been apparent that only some individuals in a given population become sick or die after exposure to a common environmental hazard. To what extent can we make predictions concerning the effects of environmental agents on individuals or groups? Determination of the exposure risk of an individual to a specific environmental agent involves analysis of the net influence of a large set of variables on the known effects of that agent. Some of these variables may enhance susceptibility, but others may diminish it. Not surprisingly, our present data base is not able to address all possible combinations of environmental hazards and susceptibility factors. Despite these difficulties, much progress has been made in our understanding of susceptibility. This chapter provides an overview of factors affecting susceptibility to environmental agents. Possible mechanisms are briefly discussed, as are techniques available for evaluating these factors.

There is little consensus over the most appropriate terminology to describe enhanced responsiveness to environmental agents. The terms *susceptible, hypersusceptible, high-risk, sensitive,* and *hypersensitive* have all been used more or less interchangeably to describe individuals who respond to toxic or carcinogenic substances at doses significantly lower than that to which the general population responds. In this chapter the term *susceptible* is used to refer to enhanced responsiveness regardless of cause.[1] There is also controversy over what constitutes a response that is significantly different from normal, because there is often little agreement on the normal values for a given parameter.[10,33]

Although there are many ways of categorizing the factors that contribute to susceptibility, most may be generally classified as either environmental or genetic. Environmental factors include attributes that are not innate and that are under at least partial control of the individual. These factors include such behavioral characteristics as smoking history and/or exposure to cigarette smoke, alcohol consumption, drug use, dietary habits, and level of physical activity. Occupational and nonoccupational exposures constitute another class of environmental factors. Genetic factors that affect susceptibility to environmental hazards comprise innate characteristics that are not (at least at present) capable of alteration by the individual. These factors include sex, ethnicity, and congenital genetic abnormalities; such abnormalities may be markers for susceptibility to a particular hazard or may be associated with overt disease. Other types of factors affecting susceptibility cannot be readily classified as either genetic or environmental. For example, some diseases that increase susceptibility to environmental hazards may result from a complex interaction between environmental and genetic factors in a given individual. Similarly, psychologic factors that affect susceptibility may represent variable mixtures of genetic and environmental influences. Finally, the age of the individual has been shown to significantly affect susceptibility independently of other factors.

Susceptibility seldom remains constant. An individual's susceptibility to environmental hazards may vary considerably during his or her lifetime as he or she grows and develops from a highly susceptible fetus to a mature, healthy adult; changes jobs; adopts various habits that enhance or impair his overall health; suffers intermittent illnesses or trauma; and develops chronic diseases in old age. Thus an individual's susceptibility profile may need to be reevaluated whenever there is concern about the potential adverse effects of environmental hazards.

ENVIRONMENTAL FACTORS INFLUENCING SUSCEPTIBILITY
Exposure to cigarette smoke

The relationship between smoking and susceptibility to environmental hazards has been the subject of extensive reviews; there is considerable evidence that smoking is associated with increased susceptibility to both nonneoplastic and neoplastic effects of other agents.[16,26,50] Many variables affect the degree to which smoking enhances susceptibility. Such variables include cumulative exposure to tobacco smoke; method of tobacco smoke exposure (pipe, cigar, cigarette); specific components present in tobacco smoke (including proprietary additives and pesticide residues); depth of inhalation; and, finally, individual susceptibility to tobacco smoke. Although smoking history as a susceptibility factor generally refers to active smoking by the individual, recent interest has focused on the role of passive smoking, or exposure to environmental tobacco smoke. The contribution of this indirect exposure to the development of chronic obstructive pulmonary disease (COPD) or to increased susceptibility to other pollutants remains controversial; recent reviews on this topic are available.[21,61] In addition, accurate histories concerning passive exposure to tobacco smoke in childhood may be difficult to obtain. Individual susceptibility to tobacco smoke also is difficult to evaluate unless the individual has a disease known to enhance susceptibility, such as alpha$_1$-antitrypsin deficiency or asthma; however, it is possible that eventually we may be able to predict susceptibility based on individual variability at the anatomic, physiologic, cellular, or molecular level.

There are many mechanisms by which smoking might enhance the effects of pollutants. For example, cigarette smoking is the major risk factor identified thus far for COPD, one of the leading causes of morbidity and mortality throughout the world.[62] If a smoker with impaired airflow from cigarette smoking is then exposed to environmental agents that also cause airway pathology, he or she is at greater risk for increased airway obstruction than is a nonsmoker; that is, the effects of cigarette smoke and the inhaled pollutants are additive. Because such agents are not confined to the workplace, including as they do smog, allergens, and dust and fumes from various hobbies, the smoker with impaired lung function may be considered to have increased susceptibility to a great many agents in his everyday environment. Even smokers with unimpaired lung function and no overt disease may have increased susceptibility to airborne pollutants, because cigarette smoke affects virtually all the cells in the lung. In the tracheal and bronchial epithelium, cigarette smoke causes cell necrosis and hyperplasia of the mucus-producing goblet cells; loss of cilia and disruption of alveolar macrophage function lead to impairment of the respiratory defense system. Any of these subclinical changes may affect distribution, retention, absorption, and clearance of inhaled pollutants.[26]

Cigarette smoke–enhanced susceptibility may be also be mediated by mechanisms other than clinical or subclinical lung damage. For example, smoking may transform inert chemicals into more toxic forms, as in the case of polymer-fume fever, in which the high combustion temperature of tobacco pyrolyzes certain fluorocarbon polymers.[66] Cigarette smoke may also serve as a delivery system for other toxic agents, primarily through inhalation but also through oral ingestion. This effect has been documented in the case of lead and most likely underlies the higher systemic toxicity of agents such as formaldehyde, boron trifluoride, organotin, methyl parathion, carbonyl, inorganic fluoride, and mercury in smokers than in nonsmokers.[59,61]

There is controversy concerning the mechanisms by which smoking enhances susceptibility to some environmental hazards.[26] For example, cigarette smoking appears to have a synergistic effect on the clinical symptoms of byssinosis; however, inconsistent results have been obtained concerning the effects of smoking on lung function in byssinosis.[3,24] It has been suggested that cotton dust and cigarette smoke interact in some as-yet-undetermined manner to cause a differential effect on clinical symptoms and pulmonary function under certain conditions. Similarly, studies of workers exposed to grain dust suggest that smoking may have a synergistic effect on symptoms such as wheezing and chest tightness but only an additive effect on changes in pulmonary function.[18] There is also controversy over whether the effects of smoking and asbestos exposure on radiographic changes and respiratory symptoms are additive or synergistic.[26]

There is both epidemiologic and laboratory evidence that tobacco smoke interacts with some environmental carcinogens to increase susceptibility to neoplastic disease synergistically rather than additively. For example, several studies have shown that smoking increases the risk of lung cancer due to asbestos exposure in a multiplicative, rather than an additive, fashion. Smoking does not affect the risk of developing mesothelioma, which is also associated with asbestos exposure.[44]

Data also suggest that smoking and alcohol exposure interact synergistically to increase the risk of development of cancer of the head and neck.[5] Controversy exists concerning the relationship between smoking, exposure to silica, and risk of lung cancer. Extensive reviews of large-scale epidemiologic studies and of animal data have failed to resolve the question.[25] Similarly, the effects of smoking on risk of development of lung cancer from radiation exposure are also controversial. Epidemiologic data, primarily studies of miners exposed to radon and radon daughters and of atomic bomb survivors, have provided evidence of both synergistic interactions and of additive effects. Results of animal studies also have been inconsistent.[16]

These conflicting results may be due in part to the extremely large number of variables involved in studies of the interaction between tobacco smoke exposure and exposure to other carcinogens. Variables related to smoking history have been described previously and may be difficult to measure quantitatively. Variables related to environmental exposures include assessment of cumulative exposure dose and route of exposure; even exposures that occurred long in the past may be implicated in carcinogenesis, because initiation of carcinogenesis by one agent need not occur contemporaneously with promotion by another. Further complicating the assessment of risk enhancement in smokers is that the interactions between tobacco smoke and most environmental hazards have yet to be studied. In theory there are many possible mechanisms by which tobacco smoke might enhance carcinogenesis of environmental agents, including altered absorption, distribution, excretion, and biotransformation; however, even for the few agents that have been extensively studied both epidemiologically and experimentally, there are few firm conclusions concerning the specific degree of risk enhancement by smoking.

Alcohol abuse

There is an extensive literature concerning the medical and social effects of alcohol abuse.[42,58] Alcohol use indirectly increases susceptibility to virtually any environmental hazard by impairing judgment and slowing reflexes, thus enhancing the likelihood that appropriate safety precautions may not be observed. Direct effects of alcohol use on susceptibility to other environmental agents have also been documented; interactions between alcohol and other drugs and chemicals have been recently reviewed.[11] Alcohol may enhance susceptibility to carcinogenic agents through several mechanisms, including increased cellular uptake of carcinogens, enhanced microsomal activity leading to more rapid metabolism of promutagens to mutagens, and promotion of carcinogenesis in cells already initiated by exposure to other environmental agents. The synergistic relationship between alcohol and smoking in the development of cancers of the head and neck has been extensively documented.[16,50]

Alcohol may also enhance susceptibility to nonneoplastic effects of environmental agents. There is evidence that toxicity of lead and pesticides is enhanced by alcohol ingestion. Hepatotoxicity associated with heavy alcohol use may also enhance susceptibility to other hepatotoxic agents. As in the case of smokers who have increased susceptibility to airborne pollutants even in the absence of functional pulmonary impairment, drinkers may be at increased risk from the effects of environmental hazards even if they have no clinically apparent liver disease. Subtle changes in hepatic function may result in decreased ability to metabolize toxins, leading to altered distribution, retention, and clearance of environmental agents and their metabolites. In addition, there is ample evidence that heavy alcohol use affects absorption, metabolism, and excretion of nutrients, many of which are directly implicated in susceptibility to various environmental agents, as described in detail later.[27]

Despite the many ways in which alcohol affects an individual's susceptibility, it may be extremely difficult to obtain an accurate assessment of this important factor. At present, there is no way of assessing cumulative alcohol exposure other than from the individual's own estimate of his intake, a notoriously inaccurate method. Although liver function tests may document overt hepatotoxicity, more subtle degrees of hepatic impairment are difficult to quantify, as is the corresponding enhancement of susceptibility to environmental agents.

Use of other drugs

Virtually any drug may alter an individual's susceptibility to environmental hazards through several possible mechanisms: organ system damage; altered absorption, metabolism, or excretion of exogenous agents; interaction with exogenous agents; and cross-sensitization of the individual.[56] There are many difficulties in the evaluation of the effects of drug use on susceptibility to pollutants, not the least of which is obtainment of an accurate history. Although an individual may provide reasonably detailed information concerning use of medically prescribed drugs, he or she may not be able to recall accurately amounts and types of over-the-counter medications, and he or she is unlikely to disclose details of recreational drug use. The context in which the information is obtained is likely to be a major determinant of its completeness and accuracy; very different histories may be obtained by a company physician performing a pre-employment examination, a trusted private physician, and an epidemiologist doing a field survey. Although current drug use can of course be assessed through use of drug screens, such an approach involves substantial ethical and legal implications. An additional problem in evaluation of the influence of drugs on susceptibility is the lack of an adequate data base; there are simply too many possible combinations of ingested drugs and exposure to exogenous environmental agents for it to be likely that information concerning all possible interactions will ever be available.

Nutritional status

The interrelationship between nutritional status and susceptibility to environmental hazards is also complex. Current evidence from both epidemiologic and experimental studies suggests that some dietary constituents directly affect susceptibility to various environmental agents.

A relationship between susceptibility to carcinogenesis and diet, especially intake of fat and vitamin A, has long been observed in animals. For example, vitamin A deficiency in animals has been associated with increased susceptibility to three different carcinogens in three different target organs: N-formamide–induced bladder cancer, aflatoxin B1–induced colon cancer, and 3-methylcholanthrene–induced lung tumors.[14] Similar relationships between diet and cancer in humans have more recently been suggested by epidemiologic studies that have shown an inverse relationship between vitamin A intake and cancer of the lung, oropharynx, esophagus, stomach, colon, and prostate.[14,69,70] It should be noted that the epidemiologic evidence regarding the relationship between vitamin A intake and risk of carcinogenesis is difficult to interpret, because vegetables, the main source of vitamin A, contain many compounds in addition to β-carotene that may also inhibit carcinogenesis, including various indoles, flavones, and phenols. In particular, indole-3-carbinole and benzylisothiocyanate, both of which are found in cruciferous plants, have been shown to inhibit development of tumors induced by benz[a]pyrene and 7,12-dimethylbenz[a]anthracene.[6]

Recent studies have, however, suggested that supplementation of the diet with β-carotene and vitamin A may reduce susceptibility to cancer induced by tobacco products. For example, studies on Filipino tobacco chewers, Inuit snuff dippers, and Indian tobacco or betel quid chewers have shown a significant reduction of genetic anomalies and oral leukoplakias in the oral mucosa in individuals receiving supplemental vitamin A and β-carotene.[57] One possible mechanism by which vitamin A affects susceptibility to carcinogens may involve its key role in normal differentiation of epithelial tissues: vitamin A deficiency has been associated with the development of squamous cell metaplasia, a precursor of carcinogenesis. β-Carotene, a precursor of vitamin A, may act as an electron scavenger of ultimate carcinogens or mutagens.[38]

In view of these studies suggesting an important role for vitamin A in carcinogenesis, there has been considerable interest in quantitative assessment of vitamin A status in human subjects. Because circulating levels of retinol (the hydrolyzed product of ingested vitamin A) are under strict homeostatic control, serum levels are affected only by extreme deficiency or excess in the diet. Nevertheless, because considerable individual variability exists in serum levels, circulating vitamin A levels were measured in several prospective studies examining factors influencing risk of cancer development. There was no correlation between serum retinol levels and the development of cancer.[6] Studies of cancer risk have also examined serum β-carotene levels. Several reports have suggested that there may be a relationship between serum β-carotene levels and the risk of development of several types of cancer.[28,55] At present, however, such assays cannot be used to evaluate an individual's susceptibility.

Other nutrients may also play a role in susceptibility to carcinogenesis induced by exogenous agents.[6,43] For example, vitamin C supplementation in animals has been shown to block the formation of bladder tumors induced with 3-hydroxyanthranilic acid.[47] In humans, there is evidence that vitamin C may have a protective effect against cancer of the esophagus, stomach, and cervix and has led to regression and/or decreased frequency of colonic polyps.[40] Some studies have suggested that vitamin E may exert a protective effect against carcinogens, but the evidence is not conclusive. Calcium has been observed to play a role in proliferation of colonic epithelium, and there is evidence that it exerts an antipromotional effect that protects against carcinogen-induced colon cancer. Finally, selenium compounds and sodium molybdate have been shown to protect against carcinogens in both animal studies and epidemiologic studies.[32,67]

Several nutrients have been observed to play a role in susceptibility to oxidant pollutants. This area is of considerable importance, because virtually all individuals are exposed at one time or another to such oxidant airborne pollutants as ozone and nitrogen dioxide, which are present in photochemical smog. The complex interrelationships between nutritional status, natural antioxidant defense mechanisms, and susceptibility to environmental oxidants have been the subject of recent reviews.[39,68] Most nutrients that influence susceptibility to oxidant pollutants do so through their role in antioxidant defense systems. For example, selenium is critical to the function of glutathione peroxidase, a metalloenzyme that protects cells from hydroperoxides by catalyzing the reduction of organic hydroperoxides formed from unsaturated fatty acids and the reduction of hydrogen peroxide formed from superoxide. Considerable experimental evidence suggests that animals deficient in selenium are more susceptible to oxidative damage as well as to carcinogenesis.[39] Studies of humans investigating the relationship between serum selenium levels and carcinogenesis have been inconclusive. It is likely that selenium concentration in hair and nails may be a more accurate reflection of long-term dietary intake; however, at present there are insufficient data to assess individual susceptibility based on these measurements. Vitamin E is another nutrient whose role in the body's natural antioxidant defense system in cell membranes has been studied extensively. Animal studies suggest that vitamin E deficiency is associated with increased susceptibility to oxidative damage; however, these experimental studies of deficiency cannot readily be used to assess the role of dietary vitamin E in human populations, because there is no evidence that human vitamin E deficiency exists in the United States. Furthermore, human studies demonstrating protective effects of vitamin E are limited and inconsistent. Similar difficulties exist in the assessment of the role of vitamin C in susceptibility to oxidant pollutants. There is no doubt it is an important antioxidant that scavenges free radicals; quenches lipid peroxidation; maintains sulfhydryl compounds, including glutathione in a reduced state; and may enhance the the antioxidant effects of vitamin E and selenium. However, we cannot yet extrapolate from animal studies to assess whether vitamin C supplementation beyond minimal requirements will decrease an individual's susceptibility to oxidant pollutants.

The effects of protein-calorie deficiency on susceptibility to environmental agents are even more complex and problematic than are the effects of deficiencies in specific nutrients.[45] Relatively few environmental agents have been rigorously investigated in malnourished humans or in experimental animals. This question is of considerable importance, given the large urban populations, particularly in Third World countries, that may be exposed over the long term to high levels of oxidant air pollutants. Several experimental studies in rats have specifically addressed the effects of malnutrition on susceptibility to airborne oxidant pollutants. Although protein deficiency and protein-calorie deficiency caused retardation in lung maturation and growth, there was no evidence that malnutrition in adult rats had any effect on lung injury due to oxidant exposure.[37] However, studies in neonatal and weanling rats suggested that there are critical periods of lung growth and development in which caloric deficiency may enhance the effects of oxidant exposure, resulting in irreversible lung damage. These studies suggest that malnourished children may constitute a susceptible subpopulation with regard to airborne oxidant pollutants.[39]

Overall, the effects of diet on susceptibility to environmental agents are difficult to assess, because of difficulties in patient recall regarding diet, lack of standardized methods for gathering such data, lack of standardized laboratory tests for measuring specific nutrients, and lack of a data base in which variabilities in diet are correlated with specific susceptibilities. At present it is unlikely that we can determine the influence of diet on an individual's susceptibility to a specific agent. Observations concerning dietary intake are more likely to be useful in the assessment of possible alterations in susceptibility in a subpopulation.

Physical activity

Level of physical activity may have both physiologic and psychologic effects that influence susceptibility to environmental hazards. For example, there is considerable evidence that exercise in the presence of airborne pollutants increases susceptibility; individuals included in this category include active children in urban environments and industrial workers with moderate-to-heavy levels of activity.[8,41] The total dose of any toxic particle or gas is determined by deposition and clearance, both of which may be influenced by exercise. In addition, switching to mouth breathing, which may occur in heavy exercise, profoundly alters both collection efficiency and distribution of the pollutant dose. Studies in both humans and animals have documented that exercising subjects sustain more damage from airborne pollutants than do sedentary controls; some of the agents studied have included organophosphorous insecticides, sulfur dioxide, and ozone. In addition to modification of the pulmonary dose by exercise, other factors associated with exercise may also affect susceptibility to a given pollutant. For example, increased pulmonary blood flow may alter the uptake of pollutant gases from the lungs. Biotransformation of pollutants, which usually occurs in the liver, may be decreased because hepatic blood flow declines during exercise. Hormonal alterations associated with exercise, especially changes in circulating levels of glucocorticoids, catecholamines, and endorphins, may alter responses to toxic gases and aerosols. Catecholamines may cause β-adrenergic–mediated bronchodilation, which in turn may alter distribution of inhaled pollutants as airway volume and airway resistance change. Other systemic responses to exercise include increased levels of circulating neutrophils and lymphocytes as well as variable alterations in eosinophils and basophils. Cellular function also is altered; it has been observed that phagocytic capacity of pulmonary macrophages is transiently suppressed. Other immune system alterations may also occur. Thus individuals who maintain high levels of physical activity in environments with airborne pollutants may be considered to be at risk for increased susceptibility to the effects of such pollutants, ranging from oxidative damage to perhaps increased risk of neoplasm, depending on the specific pollutants present. It is also possible that the physiologic changes induced by exercise may alter an individual's susceptibility to environmental hazards, even if the exercise is not performed in the presence of the environmental agent.

Exercise may also indirectly affect susceptibility to environmental agents. For example, to the extent that exercise decreases stress, a factor to be discussed in a later section, it is possible that susceptibility to certain types of environmental hazards is decreased by participation in a regular exercise program. Correlative behavior associated with an interest in physical fitness, such as attention to diet and decreased likelihood of smoking or excess drinking, also may contribute to decreased susceptibility.

Previous exposure history

Susceptibility to any environmental agent may be affected by an individual's previous exposure history. For example, exposure in the past to agents such as asbestos, tobacco smoke, or sensitizing drugs may profoundly affect an individual's response to specific environmental agents in the present. Assessment of the affects of previous exposure on susceptibility may require both a detailed history of previous exposures and specific tests to determine to what extent susceptibility has been affected. Several possible mechanisms may be responsible for altering susceptibility. First, susceptibility may be altered simply by increased body burden of a given environmental agent or its metabolites. For example, if the concentration of lead in the blood is greater than 50 µg/dL, the individual is precluded from further exposure to this agent.

Second, previous exposure to an environmental agent may enhance susceptibility by sensitizing the individual to that compound, either directly or by cross-sensitizion. Evaluations may consist of any of a series of tests designed to measure immune response, such as pulmonary function tests, radioallergosorbent tests, bronchial challenge tests, and skin tests.

Previous exposure leading to enhanced susceptibility to carcinogenic and mutagenic agents is often assessed through genetic monitoring. In contrast to genetic screening, which is discussed in a later section, genetic monitoring involves the periodic evaluation of individuals for evidence of genetic damage or alteration that may indicate enhanced susceptibility to specific agents or classes of agents. Genetic monitoring is often used to determine the presence of clastogenic effects (breakage or rearrangement of chromosomes) or mutagenic effects (heritable changes in deoxyribonucleic acid [DNA] in either germline or somatic cells). Extensive reviews of this topic are available.[1,60]

Cytogenetic techniques are generally used to evaluate chromosomal damage, which is most often caused by radiation, alkylating agents, or intercalating agents. Chromosomal aberrations may be analyzed by direct visualization of the chromosomes and by scoring of breakages and rearrangements. There is evidence that these aberrations may be associated with increased risk of disease. Elevations in the number of these aberrations have been found in lymphocytes of workers exposed to a variety of agents, including arsenic asbestos, benzene, lead, toluene, and vinyl chloride.[1] Chromosomal aberrations may also be assessed by measurement of the formation of micronuclei, which result from the exclusion of fragments from nuclei formed during mitosis. This assay is much less prone to observer error than are other cytogenetic assays. Increased levels of micronuclei have been observed in subjects exposed to ethylene oxide, styrene, and mixtures of petroleum hydrocarbons.

Sister chromatid exchange (SCE) has long been used as an indirect indicator of mutation. It can be a sensitive marker of DNA damage and repair. SCE occurs when apparently equivalent sections of the sister chromatids of the same chromosome are exchanged during cell divisions. SCEs that occur above the baseline rate may indicate exposure to DNA-damaging agents. They are most efficiently induced by agents that form adducts with DNA, distort DNA structure, or interfere with DNA precursor metabolism or repair. Generally SCEs are measured in peripheral blood lymphocytes; this test is easier and less costly than is evaluation of chromosomal aberrations. SCE measurement may be confounded by many variables, including cigarette smoking, alcohol ingestion, various drugs, and chemotherapy. Furthermore, frequency of SCEs may decrease with time after an acute exposure; thus the timing of the assay may be an additional variable in interpreting results.

Sperm cells are sometimes analyzed when the effects of environmental agents on the germline are of particular concern. Sperm count, morphology, motility, and karyotyping have all been used to evalute effects of environmental agents on sperm.[60] Abnormalities in sperm morphology have been associated with exposure to lead and carbaryl. Solvents such as ethylene glycol ethers, pesticides such as ethylene dibromide, metals such as mercury and arsenic, and alkylating agents such as ethylene oxide, have been shown to have spermatotoxic effects experimentally.[19]

Techniques for assessing mutagenicity at the molecular level are becoming available. Because most such assays are used predominantly as a research tool at present, these new methods are surveyed only briefly. A new, highly sensitive assay for mutagen exposure consists of analysis of T cells for evidence of mutation in the hypoxanthine–guanine phosphoribosyltransferase (HPRT) gene. At present it is unclear whether HPRT mutations directly presage carcinogenesis or are only a sentinel event. Several methods are now available for measurement of the formation of DNA adducts, which may be progenitors of genetic alterations. DNA adducts may be measured in virtually all body fluids as well as in tissue samples. At present there are insufficient data to correlate specific DNA adducts with specific toxic exposures, and measurement of adducts is not currently useful as a tool for evaluation of individual susceptibility. Determination of DNA repair activity in lymphocytes is another method used to measure exposure to genotoxic compounds. Quantification of DNA in individual cells also has been used to assess exposure to carcinogens. In one recent clinical study, workers exposed to bladder carcinogens were assayed with this technique; changes in DNA were observed in asymptomatic patients before clinical disease was confirmed by biopsy. Thus, at least in this instance, a genetic test was able to detect susceptible individuals, albeit after initiation of the disease but before its clinical manifestation. Similarly, assays for assessment of oncogene activity most likely will be useful in detection of cancer at a treatable stage rather than in identification of susceptible individuals before onset of the disease.[60]

For the most part, genetic monitoring cannot be used to predict health risks for an individual, although it may have predictive value for a group. Many difficulties exist in practical application of these tests, including ensuring consistency in test conditions, skill of technicians, appropriate timing of the test, use of an appropriate matched control population, and, finally, accurate interpretation. Excellent reviews of appropriate uses of genetic monitoring are available.[51,60]

GENETIC FACTORS INFLUENCING SUSCEPTIBILITY

Sex

The effects of sex on susceptibility to pollutants have been studied for only a few environmental agents, most notably airborne pollutants such as cigarette smoke and carbon monoxide.[2] Because sex affects many aspects of lung growth and development as well as structure and function, it is not surprising that there are sex-related differences in deposition of airborne pollutants and pulmonary response to such pollutants. Several epidemiologic studies of cigarette smoke have shown that, at the same exposure level, women are more resistant to lung damage than are men, as assessed by pulmonary function tests, the presence of chronic cough and sputum production, and the development of emphysema. For example, abnormalities of pulmonary function characteristic of small-airway dysfunction were observed in young male smokers but not in young female smokers, but abnormalities in large airways were observed in both men and women. The preferential dysfunction of small airways in men may presage the development of obstructive disease. Interestingly, the diffusion capacity for carbon monoxide was more affected in females than in males, suggesting increased parenchymal destruction.[49] Longitudinal studies have indicated that male smokers lose pulmonary function faster than do nonsmokers under age 45 but there was no difference in pulmonary function loss between female smokers and nonsmokers in this age range; however, in individuals older than age 45 the trend was reversed.[9]

The effects of sex on susceptibility to airborne pollutants may be influenced by other risk factors. For example, individuals who are heterozygous for α_1-antitrypsin deficiency, a genetic abnormality leading to early-onset emphysema, have an intermediate risk for development of lung disease. Some studies have shown that gender plays a role in determination of the likelihood of development of disease in smokers with this phenotype; however, other studies have not confirmed this finding and the issue remains controversial.

Sex differences in susceptibility to nonairborne environmental agents have been investigated for only a few compounds. For example, it has been shown that female rodents are far more susceptible than are males to the rare earth cerium but male rats are more susceptible to liver damage from rare earth chlorides.[35] Whether such sex-related differences in rodent response may be extrapolated to human workers is open to question.

Pregnancy constitutes a specifically sex-related susceptibility factor. Prenatal exposure to environmental hazards may put the fetus at risk for low birth weight, congenital abnormalities, developmental and behavioral disorders, and childhood cancer. There is a very large literature on the difficulties involved in evaluating safe exposure levels for pregnant workers. Unless specific studies have been done, it is extremely difficult to predict the dose received by a fetus based on maternal exposure.[2] Even when appropriate studies have been done in animals, extrapolation to humans is not always valid.

Genetic abnormalities

Genetic screening, in contrast to genetic monitoring, refers to the identification of individuals with specific genetic traits or disorders that may render them more susceptible to a given environmental agent. The concept that susceptible subpopulations might be defined by a single genetic trait has been of interest since the 1950s, when it was observed during the Korean conflict that certain soldiers taking primaquine developed hemolysis. This phenomenon was attributed to the fact that they were heterozygous for the glucose-6-phosphate deficiency (G6PD) gene. Investigators subsequently speculated that G6PD heterozygotes might also be hypersusceptible to other oxidant chemicals, such as aromatic nitro or amino compounds; by 1963 it was proposed that employees handling such chemicals be tested for G6PD before hiring. By the 1970s genetic screening was being used in the workplace to identify individuals with sickle cell trait and alpha$_1$-antitrypsin deficiency in addition to G6PD deficiency. Since then about 50 human genetic diseases that theoretically increase an individual's susceptibility to toxic or carcinogenic effects of environmental agents have been identified.[60] It should be emphasized that very few studies document that such risks exist clinically. Given that many genetic abnormalities are associated with specific ethnic groups, there is concern regarding possible discrimination against such groups. Genetic abnormalities of particular concern are discussed below.

G6PD deficiency is an X-linked disorder that occurs in about 10% of males and 1% of females of African and Mediterranean descent. Individuals are at risk for hemolytic episodes after exposure to primaquine, fava beans, vitamin K, and other compounds. On the basis of in vitro studies, exposure to any of a number of oxidant drugs and industrial chemicals, particularly aromatic amino and nitro compounds, could theoretically initiate a hemolytic episode; however, trinitrotoluene is the only agent for which excess risk has actually been documented in the workplace.[20]

Alpha$_1$-antitrypsin deficiency is a genetically caused abnormality in which the lungs are unable to inhibit adequately the activity of proteases released by resident lung cells, such as neutrophils and macrophages. The unopposed protease activity is associated with the development of panlobular emphysema. Serum immunoelectrophoresis is used to classify the protease inhibition (Pi) system; individuals with normal levels of the enzyme are designated as having the PiM phenotype. Homozygotes for the allele conferring deficiency are designated PiZZ. Homozygotes are likely to present early in life with lung disease. Difficulties have arisen in determining if heterozygotes with intermediate levels of enzyme constitute a susceptible population to certain airborne agents. Several clinical and epidemiologic studies have indicated that heterozygotes have a higher risk of developing lung disease in the absence of other exacerbating factors and that the risk is enhanced by smoking and exposure to grain dust.[23,31] Studies assessing susceptibility of heterozygotes to other specific airborne hazards are not available.

Sickle cell trait has been the subject of considerable controversy regarding whether it affects susceptibility to certain environmental conditions. It is a question of importance 7% to 13% of American blacks are heterozygous for the gene. Limited evidence suggests that heterozygotes are at increased risk for injury and death after vigorous exercise. It has been proposed that such individuals are also more susceptible to aromatic amino and nitro compounds, carbon monoxide, and cyanide; however, no conclusive experimental or epidemiologic evidence confirms that individuals with the trait are susceptible to specific environmental hazards.[34,60]

Thalassemia is a deficiency in hemoglobin production resulting in smaller erythrocytes. This autosomal recessive disease has both mild and severe forms. Ethnic groups at particular risk for having thalassemia include Americans of Italian and Greek descent (α-thalassemias) and blacks (β-thalassemia). There is limited evidence that β-thalassemic individuals are at increased risk after exposure to several chemicals, including benzene and lead; however, convincing data regarding other specific susceptibilities of these individuals are not available.[12]

Acetylation phenotype refers to the genetically determined rate at which the liver enzyme N-acetyltransferase detoxifies certain compounds through acetylation. At present, epidemiologic evidence suggests that slow acetylators are at increased risk for arylamine-induced bladder cancer; these findings also have been observed in animal models.[65]

MISCELLANEOUS FACTORS AFFECTING SUSCEPTIBILITY
Intercurrent diseases

Diseases that are not exclusively of genetic origin may also influence susceptibility to environmental agents. Mechanisms include damage to target organs as well as alterations in uptake, absorption, metabolism, and excretion of the environmental agents. This extensive topic is covered in Chapter 21, and specific examples of such diseases are provided.

Certain physiologic traits that are not usually considered diseases per se may also influence susceptibility. This category includes, for example, obesity, which increases susceptibility to certain hepatotoxins[29,30]; airway hyperreactivity; and atopy.[37,54]

Psychophysiologic factors

There is a large literature concerning the interaction between psychologic variables and susceptibility to disease. Various studies have suggested relationships between behavioral factors and cardiovascular disease, cancer, autoimmune diseases, and infections. This area of investigation, recently reviewed by Borysenko,[7] includes many diverse fields, making it particularly difficult to determine whether such variables can be used in a systematic way to assess susceptibility to environmental agents in either an individual or a subpopulation.

Both animal and human studies have shown that stress affects susceptibility to several types of disease.[64] A number of retrospective and prospective studies have shown a positive correlation between stress and risk of development of lung cancer. In several cases, psychosocial factors were better predictors of disease than were organic risk factors. Indeed, the best single predictor of malignancy was a significant loss in the previous 5 years. Recent studies investigating psychosocial factors, such as degree of support from social networks, strongly suggest that psychosocial variables indeed affect susceptibility to several diseases, including cancer.[13] Many studies of religious groups with strong social ties, such as the Mormons and Seventh-Day Adventists, have contributed to this data base; however, in these groups the effects of stringent dietary rules cannot be readily separated from the high degree of social support in such groups.[22,46] Interestingly, in recent studies of communities with few strictures regarding health habits, Bloom and colleagues[4] found that social support networks could in fact counteract the deleterious effects of excess drinking, smoking, obesity, and eating a diet high in animal fat. Overall, however, stress remains difficult to quantify, and differences among individuals, both innate and experiential, may result in very different responses to the same event.

Much current research is aimed at identifying physiologic variables that are directly correlated with stress and therefore could be used as biologic markers of stress. Studies in the past have focused on changes in hormonal levels and various measures of immunocompetence. Although some studies have shown that stress is associated with such immune function alterations as decreased natural killer cell activity and decreased mitogen response of T lymphocytes, at present there is no direct way of quantifying stress at the physiologic level. Thus the psychosocial history remains the best way of assessing this important susceptibility factor in an individual patient. Although it is not feasible to correlate stress in a given individual with susceptibility to specific environmental hazards, it is likely that universal, major life stressors, such as death of a spouse, render an individual more susceptible to virtually any environmental hazard.

Other psychologic variables that may represent varying combinations of innate and experiential factors also affect susceptibility to disease. There is a large literature on the relationship of depression to various diseases. For example, there is somewhat controversial epidemiologic evidence that depression is associated with increased risk of cancer and increased risk of death from cancer.[53] Possible mechanisms may include the known effects of depression on physiologic parameters such as immunocompetence, serum cortisol and catecholamine levels, and activity of microsomal enzymes. There is as yet no evidence that psychologic abnormalities are correlated with susceptibility to specific environmental hazards.

Chronobiologic stress constitutes a specific psychophysiologic variable that has received recent attention. There is an extensive literature concerning the psychologic and physiologic effects of shiftwork, particularly the effects of rotating shifts and other working conditions that disrupt normal circadian rhythms.[15,36] Recent investigations have focused on medical surveillance of such susceptible populations and possible interventional strategies.[17,48,52] Although there is little doubt that these factor contribute to stress, specific correlations with environmental agents have not been determined.

Age

Susceptibility to most environmental agents changes dramatically with age. The fetus, neonate, and child are all susceptible to many agents that have little effect on adults, but the physiologic changes that accompany normal aging also enhance susceptibility to many agents.

SUMMARY

In the design of a strategy for evaluation of susceptibility in an individual, there are few specific guidelines. Legal, ethical, financial, and pragmatic considerations preclude performance of every possible test for susceptibility on every patient. Thus the physician needs to clarify the purpose of the particular investigation and to understand the constraints pertaining to that investigation. The options of a company physician are quite different from those of a private consultant. Regardless of the particular circumstances of the investigation, the physician's obligation to the patient is to be thoroughly knowledgeable about all aspects of evaluating susceptibility and to use a great deal of common sense in performing such an evaluation.

REFERENCES

1. Ashford NA et al: *Monitoring the worker for exposure and disease,* Baltimore, 1990, Johns Hopkins University Press.
2. Beck BD, Weinstock S: Gender. In Brain JD et al, eds: *Variations in susceptibility to inhaled pollutants,* Baltimore, 1988, Johns Hopkins University Press.
3. Beck GJ et al: A prospective study of chronic lung disease in cotton textile workers, *Ann Intern Med* 97:645, 1980.
4. Bloom JR: Social support systems and cancer: a conceptual overview. In Cohen J, Cullen JG, Martin LR, eds: *Psychosocial aspects of cancer,* New York, 1982, Raven Press.
5. Blot WJ: Alcohol and cancer, *Cancer Res* 52:2119s, 1992.
6. Boone CW, Kelloff GJ, Malone WE: Identification of candidate cancer chemopreventive agents and their evaluation in animal models and human clinical trials: a review, *Cancer Res* 50:2, 1990.
7. Borysenko J: Psychophysiological variables. In Brain JD et al, eds: *Variations in susceptibility to inhaled pollutants,* Baltimore, 1988, Johns Hopkins University Press.
8. Brain JD et al: The effects of exercise on inhalation of particles and gases. In Brain JD et al, eds: *Variations in susceptibility to inhaled pollutants,* Baltimore, 1988, Johns Hopkins University Press.
9. Britt EJ et al: Sex differences in the decline of pulmonary function with age, *Chest* 80:79, 1981.
10. Brooks SM: Assessment of clinical changes in respiratory, cardiovascular, and other systems, *Ann Am Conf Gov Ind Hyg* 3:35, 1982.
11. Calabrese EJ: *Alcohol interactions with drugs and chemicals,* Chelsea, Mich, 1991, Lewis.
12. Carta PAM, Glacomina C: Occupational lead exposure, G6PD deficiency and beta-thalassemic trait, *Med Lav* 78:75, 1987.
13. Cohen J, Cullen JG, Martin LR, eds: *Psychosocial aspects of cancer,* New York, 1982, Raven Press.
14. Colditz GA, Stampfer MJ, Green LC: Diet. In Brain JD et al, eds: *Variations in susceptibility to inhaled pollutants,* Baltimore, 1988, Johns Hopkins University Press.
15. Colligan MJ, Rosa RR: Shiftwork effects on social and family life, *J Occup Med* 5:315, 1990.
16. Collins M, Schenker M: Susceptibility to neoplasia altered by tobacco smoke. In Brain JD et al, eds: *Variations in susceptibility to inhaled pollutants,* Baltimore, 1988, Johns Hopkins University Press.
17. Comperatore CA, Krueger GP: Circadian rhythm desynchronosis, jet lag, shift lag, and coping strategies, *J Occup Med* 5:323, 1990.
18. Cotton DJ et al: Effects of grain dust exposure and smoking on respiratory symptoms and lung function, *J Occup Med* 25:131, 1983.
19. Cullen MR, Cherniack MG, Rosenstock L: Occupational medicine, *N Engl J Med* 322:675, 1990.
20. Djerassi LS, Vitany L: Hemolytic episode in G6PD deficient workers exposed to TNT, *Br J Ind Med* 32:54, 1975.
21. Douville JA: *Active and passive smoking hazards in the workplace,* New York, 1990, Van Nostrand Reinhold.
22. Enstrom JE: Cancer mortality among Mormons in California during 1968-1975, *J Natl Cancer Inst* 65:1073, 1980.
23. Eriksson S, Lindell SE, Wiberg R: Effects of smoking and intermediate alpha 1-antitrypsin deficiency on lung function, *Eur J Respir Dis* 67:279, 1985.
24. Glindmeyer HW et al: Exposure-related declines in the lung function of cotton textile workers, *Am Rev Respir Dis* 144:675, 1991.
25. Goldsmith DF, Winn DM, Shy CM: *Silica, silicosis and cancer: controversy in internal medicine,* Philadelphia, 1985, Praeger.
26. Greaves IA, Schenker M: Tobacco smoking. In Brain JD et al, eds: *Variations in susceptibility to inhaled pollutants,* Baltimore, 1988, Johns Hopkins University Press.
27. Hall P, ed: *Alcoholic liver disease: pathobiology, epidemiology, and clinical aspects,* New York, 1985, Wiley.
28. Hennekens CH: A randomized trial of aspirin and beta-carotene among US physicians, *Prev Med* 14:165, 1985.
29. Hodgson M, van Thiel DH, Goodman-Klein B: Obesity and hepatotoxins as risk factors for fatty liver disease, *Br J Ind Med* 48:690, 1991.
30. Hodgson MJ et al: Liver injury tests in hazardous waste workers: the role of obesity, *J Occup Med* 31:238, 1989.
31. Horn SL, Tennet RK, Cockcroft DW: Pulmonary function in PIM and NZ grain workers, *Chest* 89:795, 1986.
32. Ip C: The chemopreventive role of selenium in carcinogenesis, *J Am Coll Toxicol* 5:7, 1986.
33. Janetos AC: Biological variability. In Brain JD et al, eds: *Variations in susceptibility to inhaled pollutants,* Baltimore, 1988, Johns Hopkins University Press.
34. Kark JA, Posey DM, Schumacher HR: Sickle cell trait as risk factor for sudden death in physical training, *N Engl J Med* 317:781, 1987.
35. Knight AL: The rare earths. In Zenz C, ed: *Occupational medicine,* Chicago, 1988, Year Book.
36. Knutsson A: Shiftwork and coronary heart disease, *Scand J Soc Med* 44(suppl):1, 1989.
37. Koren HS: The potential use of immunological markers in determining individuals susceptible to inhaled pollutants. In Utell MJ, Frank R, eds: *Susceptibility to inhaled pollutants,* Philadelphia, 1989, American Society for Testing and Materials.
38. Krinsky NI, Deneke SM: Interaction of oxygen and oxy-radicals with carotenoids, *J Natl Cancer Inst* 69:205, 1982.

39. Last JA: Nutritional status and oxidants. In Utell MJ, Frank R, eds: *Susceptibility to inhaled pollutants,* Philadelphia, 1989, American Society for Testing and Materials.
40. McKeown-Eysen G et al: A randomized trial of vitamin C and E in the prevention of recurrence of colorectal polyps, *Cancer Res* 48:4701, 1988.
41. Miller FJ, McDonnell WF, Gerrity TR: Exercise and regional dosimetry: an overview. In Utell MJ, Frank R, eds: *Susceptibility to inhaled pollutants,* Philadelphia, 1989, American Society for Testing and Materials.
42. Miller NS, ed: *Comprehensive handbook of drug and alcohol addiction,* New York, 1991, Marcel Dekker.
43. Moon T, Micozzi M, eds: *Nutrition and cancer prevention: the role of micronutrients,* New York, 1988, Marcel Dekker.
44. Muscat JE, Wynder EL: Cigarette smoking, asbestos exposure, and malignant mesothelioma, *Cancer Res* 51:2263, 1991.
45. Myers BA et al: Ozone exposure, food restriction and protein deficiency: changes in collagen and elastin in rodent lungs, *Toxicol Lett* 23:43, 1984.
46. Phillips RL et al: Mortality among California Seventh-Day Adventists for selected cancer sites, *J Natl Cancer Inst* 65:1097, 1980.
47. Pipkin GE: Inhibitory effect of L-ascorbate on tumor formation in urinary bladders implanted with 3-hydroxy-anthranilic acid, *Proc Soc Exp Biol Med* 131:522, 1979.
48. Rosa RR et al: Intervention factors for promoting adjustment to nightwork and shiftwork, *J Occup Med* 5:391, 1990.
49. Samet JM, Marbury MC, Spengler JD: Health effects and sources of indoor air pollution, part I, *Am Rev Respir Dis* 136:1486, 1987.
50. Saracci R: The interactions of tobacco smoking and other agents in cancer etiology, *Epidemiol Rev* 9:175, 1987.
51. Schulte PA: Methodologic issues in the use of biologic markers, *Am J Epidemiol* 126:1006, 1987.
52. Scott AJ, LaDou J: Shiftwork: effects on sleep and health with recommendations for medical surveillance and screening, *Occup Med* 5:273, 1990.
53. Shekelle RB et al: Psychological depression and 17-year risk of death from cancer, *Psychosom Med* 43:117, 1981.
54. Sheppard D: Mechanisms of airway hyperresponsiveness. In Utell MJ, Frank R, eds: *Susceptibility to inhaled pollutants,* Philadelphia, 1989, American Society for Testing and Materials.
55. Stahelin HB: Beta-carotene and cancer prevention: the Basel study, *Am J Clin Nutr* 53:265S, 1991.
56. Steinberg M: ACGIH TLVs and the sensitive worker, *Ann Am Conf Gov Ind Hyg* 3:77, 1982.
57. Stich HF et al: Remission of oral leukoplakias and micronuclei in tobacco/betel quid chewers treated with beta-carotene and with beta-carotene plus vitamin A, *Int J Cancer* 42:195, 1988.
58. Tabakoff B, Sutker PB, Randall CL eds: *Medical and social aspects of alcohol abuse,* New York, 1983, Plenum Press.
59. Tola S, Nordman CH: Smoking and blood lead concentrations in lead-exposed workers and an unexposed population, *Environ Res* 13:250, 1977.
60. US Congress Office of Technology Assessment: *Genetic monitoring and screening in the workplace,* OTA-BA-455, Washington, DC, 1990, US Government Printing Office.
61. US Department of Health and Human Services: *Smoking and health,* DHHS Pub No 79-50066, Washington, DC, 1979, US Government Printing Office.
62. US Department of Health and Human Services: *Chronic obstructive lung disease: summary of the health consequences of smoking: a report of the Surgeon General,* Washington, DC, 1984, US Government Printing Office.
63. US Department of Health and Human Services: *The health consequences of involuntary smoking: a report of the Surgeon General,* DHHS Pub No CDC 87-8398, Washington, DC, 1986.
64. van Dormolen M et al: The quest for interaction: studies on combined exposure, *Int Arch Occup Environ Health* 62:279, 1990.
65. Weber WW: Acetylation pharmacogenetics experimental models for human toxicity, *Fed Proc* 43:2332, 1984.
66. Wegman DH, Peters JM: Polymer-fume fever and cigarette smoking, *Ann Intern Med* 81:55, 1974.
67. Wei HJ, Luo XM, Yang SP: Effects of molybdenum and tungsten on mammary carcinogenesis, *J Natl Cancer Institute* 74:469, 1985.
68. Weinstock S, Beck BD: Age and nutrition. In Brain JD et al, eds: *Variations in susceptibility to inhaled pollutants,* Baltimore, 1988, Johns Hopkins University Press.
69. Ziegler RG: Vegetables, fruits and carotenoids and the risk of cancer, *Am J Clin Nutr* 53:251S, 1991.

Chapter 29

PREEXISTING CONDITIONS AND THE ELDERLY

Jessica Herzstein

Populations with preexisting conditions
    Chronic pulmonary disease
    Cardiovascular disease
    Diabetes
    Obesity
The elderly
    Neurotoxicants
    Respiratory toxins
    Carcinogen exposure
    Conclusion

The hazards of exposure to everyday chemical and physical agents in our environment are receiving increasing attention in our society. The broad spectrum of environmental exposures, their potential adverse effects, and the mechanisms of disease causation are not well understood for the most part. What has become clear however is that certain populations are more susceptible to potentially hazardous exposures than others. This differential susceptibility has been documented, for example, following urban smog alerts, nuclear warfare, and chemical contamination of water supplies, as well as worksite exposures to health hazards such as heavy metals, asbestos, pesticides, and solvents.

As research advances our understanding of exposure-related health effects, the issue of who is at increased risk for developing toxic and carcinogenic effects will come to the forefront in preventive health and in public policy. High-risk groups have long been recognized by EPA and OSHA in setting standards for "safe" exposure to potential hazards. However, the decisions about whom society wishes to protect and at what cost are still being addressed. Ethical conflicts are also apparent in discussing individual variation in susceptibility.[16] For example, are the risks attributed to the worker or to the hazardous working conditions? It is often easier to exclude individuals deemed to be at high risk rather than improve safety at the worksite.

Susceptibility can be viewed as a point on the continuum of normal human variation in response to environmental exposure. Hypersusceptible individuals experience an adverse effect at lower or shorter exposures than the general population. Adverse effects in a high-risk or hypersusceptible population are often indicative of some (future) risk for others who are similarly exposed. Thus the issue of safety for everyone is integral to defining risk and to protecting those at high risk from environmental toxins.

There are multiple causes of differential susceptibility, including age, genetic factors, preexisting conditions, and behavioral and life-style factors (including stress, tobacco and alcohol use, and nutritional status). Interactions between and among these factors may also affect susceptibility. Epidemiologic and animal data suggest that disease expression is modified by psychologic factors interacting with physiologic factors.

How are susceptible populations identified? Are the elderly (or some subgroup thereof) more likely than other populations to be adversely affected by ambient exposure to air pollutants? Are persons with preexisting lung or cardiovascular disease more likely to suffer ill effects after drinking water contaminated with hydrocarbon solvents? Which groups may be at particular risk if secondary smoke or formaldehyde off-gassing or pesticide residuals are present in indoor air? In each case how severe are the health effects experienced by susceptible persons? To estimate the exposure risk we must first know how host factors modify the exposure-disease relationship.

In this chapter the susceptibility of persons with preexisting conditions and the susceptibility of the elderly to environmental exposures are reviewed. Existing data on common exposures that may result in greater toxicity for these groups will be summarized. In many cases the data are preliminary or controversial. Indeed host-response differences are highly complex and have been incompletely studied. Studies of exposures in different populations are limited by many factors such as dose and duration of exposure, documentation of exposure, and the presence of confounding factors. Scientific data on low-level exposures and human toxicity are almost nonexistent. This, added to our very rudimentary knowledge of the mechanisms of chemical toxicity, means that no definitive answers can be offered for these important questions. The main objective here is to define the scientific basis for the role host factors play in response to specific environmental agents.

The influence of genetic and behavioral/life-style factors on susceptibility is presented in Chapter 28. The unique sensitivity of the fetus and child to a spectrum of environmental exposures is discussed in Chapters 31 and 33.

POPULATIONS WITH PREEXISTING CONDITIONS

Most workers are hired as healthy individuals. Over time, some of these workers will develop chronic health problems, work-related or otherwise. New legislation in the United States designed to prevent workplace discrimination against people with preexisting diseases (the Americans with Disabilities Act) may permit additional exposures for them unless the case can be made that diseased individuals are at greater risk of harm and should be excluded in certain cases. Nonworker populations also face potential risks from environmental exposures added to preexisting medical conditions. This has been best researched for those with chronic lung disease exposed to air pollutants.

Knowledge of the special risks of environmental exposures incurred by those with specific diseases is very limited. This will severely limit rational preventive practice, especially where the law requires that a worker be allowed to work unless sound data are available to recommend otherwise. The lack of scientific information also hampers physicians' ability to provide advice to their diseased patients concerning exposure to environmental stressors.

Chronic pulmonary disease

Groups of people with a spectrum of airway diseases appear to be at increased risk of adverse effects following airborne exposure to pollutants such as ozone, acid aerosols and particulates, and sulfur dioxide. Asthmatics have been the focus of this research, but the knowledge base in this field is limited. Some of the limitations include the methodology for measuring asthma severity and individual disease variability, estimation of inhaled dose, interaction of multiple exposures, and lack of nonasthmatic control groups.[8] Nonetheless, epidemiologic evidence suggests that asthmatics are at increased risk of experiencing a decline in respiratory function following certain inhaled environmental insults, including air pollutants.

Persons with asthma and airway hyperreactivity as well as atopic and allergic persons are potentially at increased risk for developing bronchoconstriction following exposure to air pollutants. Several types of investigation support this generalization. Controlled human exposures to low concentrations of sulfur dioxide have demonstrated that asthmatics experience bronchoconstriction at significantly lower concentrations than do nonasthmatics.[35] Asthma outbreaks in cities have also documented that asthmatics are more sensitive than the general population to acute increases in air pollution.[8] In Donora, Pennsylvania, in 1948, high levels of sulfur dioxide and particulates were trapped by a thermal inversion layer and 80% of persons with asthma experienced exacerbations.[11] Prospective epidemiologic studies are comparing the respiratory health of residents in a high-pollutant area with the health of persons residing in a low-pollutant area. In addition, animal models have demonstrated that inhaled pollutants such as ozone, sulfur dioxide, and nitrogen dioxide can enhance IgE production and asthma.[7]

Irritant gases, fumes, and particulates can precipitate respiratory symptoms in persons with asthma. This is a common mechanism of airway constriction in persons with underlying airway hyperreactivity. Vapors of volatile organic compounds, including common solvents such as toluene and formaldehyde, are often found in indoor air. Acute exposure of asthmatics to these irritant compounds may result in mild decrements in lung function and bronchial irritation.[19] Cigarette smoke is an irritant that may increase nonspecific bronchial reactivity in chronic smokers with normal lung function and perhaps in asthmatics. Low concentrations of irritants (such as sulfur dioxide) may cause bronchoconstriction in exercising asthmatics. People with atopy or allergy are more sensitive to the effects of some irritant inhaled pollutants (such as ozone), even if the individuals are asymptomatic.[6]

Another major mechanism of asthmatic responses to environmental exposures involves sensitization through synthesis of IgE (or IgG) antibodies. Occupational asthma caused by animal proteins or bacterial enzymes in the detergent industry is an example of IgE-mediated asthma. Atopic individuals are more likely than nonallergic persons to become sensitized to these high-molecular-weight substances. However, in other exposure settings (for example with polyurethane precursors or wood dust), there is no relationship between atopic status and the risk of hypersensitivity reactions.

Once an individual becomes asthmatic as a result of an environmental exposure, the bronchospasm can usually be triggered by a variety of nonspecific stimuli in the environment. A proportion of persons with new environmentally triggered asthma will have persistent airway hyperreactivity and respiratory symptoms for years after removal from the sensitizing agent.

Environmental tobacco smoke is a combination of irritant compounds that can induce symptoms of bronchospasm in a person with underlying airway disease. Environmental tobacco smoke has been shown to promote wheezing and increase airway reactivity in children.[20,39] Studies investigating the effects of passive cigarette smoke exposure on lung function in adult asthmatics have yielded contradictory results. There are some data to suggest that a subpopulation of asthmatics may be particularly sensitive to environmental tobacco smoke.[37]

Some of the major responses of atopics and asthmatics to common air contaminants that have been studied in controlled exposure and epidemiologic studies are presented in Table 29-1. There are many approaches and variables in the study of asthmatics as a susceptible group; this table presents data from some important exposure-effect studies but does not attempt to present a complete listing, nor does it detail the studies' strengths and weaknesses.

Clinical studies on nitrogen dioxide are limited, though some adult asthmatics may be in a reactive subgroup.[18,23] Some asthmatics failed to show increased sensitivity to these agents compared to nonasthmatics.[3,23]

Extensive clinical studies have been done on the health effects of ozone exposure, yet whether persons with asthma, COPD, angina pectoris, and allergic rhinitis are more likely to experience adverse effects remains unclear.[18] One study showed statistically significant differences in lung function response to ozone between asthmatics and nonasthmatics.[24] Recent data have documented a significant association between asthma visits to hospital emergency departments and ambient ozone concentrations.[12] The fact remains that ozone is a potent inducer of lung inflammation (as indicated by respiratory symptoms, increased airway responsiveness, and bronchoalveolar lavage and nasal lavage findings). In addition, clinical effects of ozone have been documented at very low exposure concentrations.[14] Despite clinical studies with variable results, it is reasonable to conclude that persons with underlying lung disease may be affected by ozone exposures below the current U.S. standards.[18]

Fine particulates are increasingly recognized as a potential source of serious adverse health effects[36] (see Table 28-1). They constitute a diverse mixture of pollutants, including arsenic, lead, sulfates, and carcinogens, and they are not covered by federal standards for ambient air quality. The fine particulates are capable of causing health effects at lower levels than other particulates (total suspended particulates, TSPs). Suspended sulfates, a major component of acid aerosols, have been related to respiratory tract infections and decreased lung function in children. Fine particulates are frequently deposited in the alveolae, and they may be carriers of toxic and carcinogenic vapors, even if the particulates themselves are inert. The particulates also interfere with the ciliary-mucosal filter system in the bronchial airways, thus promoting the potential toxicity of other inhaled toxins.[20]

Inhaled particulates have been associated with increased respiratory symptoms in asthmatics.[15,28] Increased hospitalization rates of those with asthma and COPD have been documented,[29,30] as has an increased relative risk of mortality for persons with COPD[33] following high particulate exposures.

Child asthmatics may be particularly susceptible to inhaled environmental exposures. Data from a 12-year follow-up in the Six City Study of air pollution have shown that exacerbations of symptoms in asthmatic children (but not pulmonary function levels) are associated with levels of exposure to particulates at or below the current ambient standards.[36] The occurrence of new cases of asthma did not appear to be related to ambient levels of pollutants. In contrast, children as a group do not have increased respiratory symptoms as pollutant exposures increase. The long-term consequences of modestly elevated ambient pollutant levels and increased symptom burden on asthmatic children are unknown at present.

Controlled exposure studies of adolescent asthmatics have shown increased sensitivity to inhaled sulfuric acid, a common atmospheric transformation product of sulfur dioxide, to a greater degree than adult asthmatic subjects have demonstrated.[18,22,23] In controlled exposure studies, exercising asthmatics appear to be an order of magnitude more sen-

Table 29-1. Environmental exposures and preexisting respiratory disease in adults

Clinical outcome	Exposure	Diseased population at risk?
Increased airway responsiveness	NO_2	Asthma
	O_3	Asthma
	SO_2	Asthma (with/without exercise)
	Sulfate aerosols	Asthma
Decreased lung function	VOCs	Asthma
	SO_2	Asthma
		Atopy (with exercise)
	Sulfate aerosols	Asthma
	O_3	Asthma (with exercise)
	NO_2	COPD
Increased respiratory symptoms	SO_2	Asthma
	Sulfate aerosols	Asthma
	Particulates	Asthma
	O_3	Asymptomatic allergic rhinitis
Increased mortality	Particulates	COPD
Increased hospitalization rates	Particulates	Asthma COPD

NO_2, Nitrogen oxides
O_3, Ozone
SO_2, Sulfur dioxide
VOCs, Volatile organic compounds
TSP, Total suspended particulates
COPD, Chronic obstructive pulmonary disease

sitive to inhaled sulfate aerosols than young adults.[18] The airway reactions have been detected with sulfur dioxide exposure levels below the mean ambient level, occur within 3 minutes of inhaling sulfur dioxide, and increase with exercise and exposure dose. Interestingly, persons with moderately severe COPD have not demonstrated significant symptoms or pulmonary function declines with sulfur dioxide exposure.[18]

The interactive effects of air pollutants may cause pulmonary toxicity that is not detected in single-exposure challenges. Very few studies have investigated the combined effects of pollutant exposures. Clinical aspects and potential mechanisms of the health effects of air pollutants and the significance for public policy have recently been reviewed.[5,18] Overall data suggest that a number of inhaled pollutants may affect pulmonary function and/or respiratory symptomatology of children and adult asthmatics.

Historic episodes of uncontrolled air pollution have demonstrated serious adverse health effects, particularly among those with preexisting respiratory diseases. In the London fog incident of 1952 the maximal 24-hour concentration of SO_2 soared to levels estimated at 10 times the current maximum permissible level. Among the 4000 excess deaths attributed to pollution, the majority were ascribed to bronchitis, pneumonia, tuberculosis, and other respiratory diseases.[26]

Chronic obstructive lung disease alters the structure and physiologic functioning of the lung, causing, for example, a loss of elastic recoil and a decrease in airway caliber with a resulting increase in resistance to flow. These changes affect both the deposition and clearance of inhaled particles. Particle deposition occurs more centrally because terminal air units are not accessible. More particles are deposited at sites of obstruction. Thus in diseased lungs inhaled toxins may exert more pronounced and varied effects compared to healthy lungs. For example, there are some data to suggest that persons with COPD experience significant decrements in pulmonary function as compared to elderly normals following acute NO_2 exposure.[27] Persons with COPD, particularly those with bronchoreactivity, are probably also at greater risk of developing symptoms (and possibly deteriorating lung function) from inhaled toxins than are persons without lung disease. Insufficient data preclude more specific conclusions about the risk of adverse effects following environmental exposures among persons with COPD.

Cardiovascular disease

Although there is epidemiologic evidence that patients with heart disease have increased susceptibility to inhaled pollutants, there are no controlled-exposure laboratory studies. In a small exercise study,[38] patients with coronary artery disease were exposed to high ambient ozone concentrations; no changes in pulmonary or cardiovascular function were detected. However, the authors caution that the limited exercise tolerance of these patients may have resulted in inhalation of low concentrations of ozone. Persons with cardiorespiratory disease that limits their exercise performance may thus have a protective mechanism restricting their total dose of inhaled pollutants.

Individuals with cardiovascular disease are considered to be at greatest risk for adverse effects from carbon monoxide exposure. Low levels of carbon monoxide can exacerbate myocardial ischemia during exercise.[1,25] This was confirmed in a multicenter study of patients with coronary artery disease.[2] Even small decreases in the oxygen-carrying capacity of blood in persons with coronary artery disease can produce myocardial ischemia because coronary blood flow cannot be augmented appropriately.

Persons with cardiomyopathies and cardiac dysrhythmias probably have an elevated risk for atrial and ventricular dysrhythmias following exposure to organic solvents, especially fluorinated ones.[17]

Diabetes

Diabetes mellitus is frequently complicated by symptoms and signs of peripheral neuropathy. A number of chemicals, including certain metals, solvents, gases, pesticides, and chemicals used in plastics, are known to be peripheral nervous system toxins. In theory there is reason to suspect that additive or perhaps synergistic toxicity could result when a diabetic is exposed to these toxins. Thus a diabetic may be more likely to develop peripheral neurotoxicity and the disease may be more extensive or more severe than in a nondiabetic following exposure to a neurotoxin. At the current time there are no epidemiologic data nor any accepted animal models that examine this theoretical possibility.

Obesity

Obesity may be associated with a reduction in lung volume.[31,32] The clinical picture of restrictive lung disease can be found in obese persons without intrinsic lung pathology. Since baseline pulmonary function is altered, obese persons might be at greater risk for development of further respiratory impairment following exposure to agents with respiratory toxicity. However, this has not been confirmed in human epidemiologic studies.

In addition, obese persons may be at risk for sudden increases in the concentration of lipophilic chemicals in the blood since these are largely stored in adipose tissue. Organochlorine pesticides, PCBs, and dioxins are some important examples. Higher amounts of lipophilic toxins accumulate in fat in an obese person than in a lean, athletic individual. The concentration of the toxin in the target organ is lowered by storage, and thus this toxin may manifest less toxicity in an obese than in a lean individual. However, when rapid mobilization of fat occurs, an obese person may have a greater increase in the concentration of the lipophilic chemical in the blood and therefore suffer acute toxic effects. This hypothesis has been studied and confirmed in animals exposed to organochlorine insecticides followed by starvation periods.[21] Clinical toxicity of this nature has not been proven in humans.

THE ELDERLY

The proportion of persons in our society who are age 65 or older is growing at a rapid rate. According to census projections, this proportion is increasing from 12% in 1986 to 22% in 2050.[13] Age is the most important determinant of incidence for most human diseases. Environmental exposures are known to be a factor in disease causation in the elderly, but to what extent these toxins account for morbidity or mortality in the elderly is not known.

A very large sector of society is placed at risk when exposures occur that may affect the extremes of age. The federal government has taken into account the susceptibilities of the very young in establishing national exposure standards, including drinking water and ambient air standards. However, while in theory the elderly may be highly susceptible to environmental exposures for a number of reasons (see Table 29-2), there is a paucity of research in this area and regulatory policies are virtually nonexistent.

The elderly are known to be more vulnerable than the rest of society to a number of stressors, including drugs, heat, and infections. However, studies on the health effects elderly populations experience following exposure to potentially hazardous acute or chronic environmental exposures have received very little attention in scientific research.

The current state of knowledge of geriatric responses to environmental exposures has been reviewed in Cooper[13] and Calabrese.[10] It has been suggested that since the elderly develop toxicity from drugs at lower doses than younger adults, the elderly may be more susceptible to toxic chemicals present in home, work, and outdoor environments.[10] Environmental agents (termed *gerontogens*) may also be capable of accelerating the onset and/or rate of progression of certain aging processes.[4]

The aging process is an important determinant of environmental exposure toxicity and susceptibility to lung disease. An elderly person may be at increased risk for adverse effects following an environmental exposure for a number of reasons.[13] Some proposed mechanisms underlying this susceptibility of the aged are listed in Table 28-2. For example, the cellular and biochemical responses to oxidant damage are age-dependent. Older animals are less protected from oxidant injury to the lung than are younger animals.[8] One hypothesis is that older cells are more susceptible than younger cells to oxidant stress (for example NO_2 and ozone) due to higher basal levels of peroxidation of lipid membranes in older cells. Decreased tissue antioxidants such as vitamin E may also contribute to the enhanced susceptibility to lung injury. Age-related decreases in pulmonary function, cough efficiency, mucociliary transport, and cell-mediated immunity are some changes that may affect susceptibility to other types of lung injury besides oxidant damage.[8]

Sensitivity to free radicals appears to be age-related.[10,13] Free radical stress may be more prevalent in the elderly, and the aging process may accumulate unrepaired damage caused by free radicals. The elderly have lower levels of superoxide dismutase, an important enzyme in antioxidant defense. These low levels may be a risk factor for oxidant pollutant toxicity; there is evidence that ozone and nitrogen dioxide cause pulmonary toxicity via free radicals. Xenobiotic-related effects such as carcinogenicity (such as carbon tetrachloride), hepatotoxicity (such as carbon tetrachloride and ethanol), nephrotoxicity (such as gentamicin), pulmonary fibrosis (such as bleomycin), and cardiotoxicity (such as adriamycin) are all age-related, and available evidence supports free radical mechanisms.[13]

The effect of a toxin may be enhanced in an elderly person by changes in tissue sensitivity and by changes in pharmacokinetics. Changes in absorption, distribution, metabolism, and excretion probably contribute. Research to date has focused on changes in hepatic metabolism with aging, but results have been contradictory. Despite the difficulty of assessing the potential for increased susceptibility of the elderly to xenobiotics, a number of agents have been identified that are more likely to cause adverse effects in older adults and/or the elderly. Various studies show higher rates of acute respiratory and neurologic toxicities, cancer, and other health effects compared with younger animals following exposure to a variety of chemicals.[10]

Further research is required before specific guidelines concerning the environmental susceptibility of aged individuals as a special subpopulation can be formulated.

Table 29-2. Sensitivity of the elderly to environmental toxins

Mechanism	Toxic effects
Changes in physiologic, biochemical, immune, and homeostatic parameters	Diminished inherent protective mechanisms Aging cells have an intrinsic sensitivity to certain toxins
Diminished functional reserve	A toxic dose is more likely to cause adverse effects
Decreased xenobiotic metabolism, increased production of toxic metabolites, less successful chromosome repair	Potentiation of the toxin's effects
Chronic	
Long exposure period to toxin and increasing life span	High total exposure dose Latency period exceeded and clinical toxicity apparent Interactions between chemicals (toxins and drugs) cause additional adverse effects

Neurotoxicants

The elderly are more susceptible to the adverse effects of pharmaceuticals than are younger individuals. Age can potentiate neurotoxicity associated with pharmaceuticals, as has been well demonstrated with the elderly's increased sensitivity to tardive dyskinesia after neuroleptic use and the rare occurrence of neuroleptic malignant syndrome in the elderly following administration of dopamine antagonists. These are examples of a senescent loss in neurons causing increased vulnerability to potential neurotoxicants. The age-related cell attrition causes reduced structural redundancy in the nervous system. Thus injury can occur without associated impairment until a threshold of viable cells is attained, at which point further damage causes more severe effects of longer duration than occurs in younger individuals.[13]

Aging can cause metabolic alterations, as well as changes in cell number, which may compound the neurotoxic effects of exposures. Carbon disulfide, acrylamide, lead, and the pesticides chlordecone, methylbromide, and DDT potentiate neurotoxicity in the elderly because they affect the catecholamine/indolamine "balance" that is already perturbed by aging. In addition, aging can result in reduced metabolism of toxic compounds and increased production of toxic metabolites.

Respiratory toxins

The aging process is an important determinant of susceptibility to lung disease, including toxic pulmonary effects. The association between exposure to ambient concentrations of air pollutants and a decline in lung function with age is controversial. Animal studies have shown an age-related sensitivity to the pulmonary toxicity of ozone and nitrogen dioxide.[13] In addition, nonspecific airway hyperresponsiveness increases with age, and therefore the elderly are potentially at increased risk for the irritant and bronchospastic effects of inhaled pollutants. In acute air pollution episodes such as those in Donora, Pennsylvania (1948), and in London (1952), the elderly had higher rates of illness and death. However, many of the elderly had preexisting disease.

Carcinogen exposure

The incidence of cancer increases markedly with age. This can be partially attributed to the fact that cumulative exposure to toxins is related to the development of cancer. For example, the longer duration of exposure accounts for the age-related increase in lung cancer in smokers. However, age also plays a direct role (in the form of tissue sensitivity or altered metabolism) in susceptibility to some environmentally induced cancers. Studies of people exposed to radiation from the bombs at Hiroshima and Nagasaki and from a single course of radiotherapy for ankylosing spondylitis reveal that the incidence of certain types of cancer (acute leukemia and lung cancer) was substantially higher in persons over 50 at the time of exposure, given the same exposure dose.[8,10]

The age-dependent susceptibility to carcinogens and other environmental toxins is not universal. Animal studies suggest that this depends on the chemical and the target organ.[8] Very limited human data exist except for ionizing radiation exposure.

CONCLUSION

Differential susceptibility to pollutant toxicity is a major area of concern in public health today. Persons with preexisting conditions, those at either end of the age spectrum, those with life-style habits that place them at higher risk, and those with genetically predetermined idiosyncrasy represent susceptible populations. Given the advances in science that allow greater understanding of the contributions of causative factors to disease, it is imperative that society address how information on disease risk and susceptibility is used. Which populations does society choose to protect, and which adverse affects are serious enough to merit regulatory attention? Further scientific investigation of the role host factors play in response to specific environmental agents is critical to future decision making in this area.

REFERENCES

1. Allred EN, Bleecker ER, Chaitman BR: Short-term effects of carbon monoxide exposure on the exercise performance of subjects with coronary artery disease, *N Engl J Med* 321:1426, 1989.
2. Allred EN et al: Acute effects of carbon monoxide exposure on individuals with coronary artery disease, Health Effects Institute, Research Report Number 25, 1989.
3. Angle CR: Indoor air pollutants, *Adv Pediatr* 35:239, 1988.
4. Baker SR, Rogul M, eds: *Environmental toxicity and the aging process,* New York, 1987, Alan R. Liss.
5. Balmes JR: Emerging issues in ambient air quality and respiratory health, *Probl Resp Care* 3:163, 1990.
6. Bascom R et al: Effect of ozone inhalation on the response to nasal challenge with antigen of allergic subjects, *Am Rev Respir Dis* 142:594, 1990.
7. Biagini RE et al: Ozone enhancement of platinum asthma in a private model, *Am Rev Respir Dis* 134:719, 1986.
8. Brain JD, Pikus AA, Greaves IA: Asthma and airway reactivity. In Brain JD et al, eds: *Variations in susceptibility to inhaled pollutants,* Baltimore, 1988, Johns Hopkins University Press.
9. Brain JD et al, eds: *Variations in susceptibility to inhaled pollutants,* Baltimore, 1988, Johns Hopkins University Press.
10. Calabrese EJ: *Age and susceptibility to toxic substances,* New York, 1986, Wiley.
11. Ciocco A, Thompson DJ: A follow-up on Donora ten years after: methodology and findings, *Am J Public Health* 51:155, 1961.
12. Cody RP et al: The effect of ozone associated with summertime photochemical smog on the frequency of asthma visits to hospital emergency departments, *Environ Res* 58:184, 1992.
13. Cooper RL, Goldman JM, Harbin TJ, eds: *Aging and environmental toxicology,* Baltimore, 1991, Johns Hopkins University Press.
14. Devlin RB et al: Exposure of humans to ambient levels of ozone for 6.6 hours causes cellular and biochemical changes in the lung, *Am J Respir Cell Mol Biol* 4:762, 1991.
15. Dockery DW et al: Effects of inhalable particles on respiratory health of children, *Am Rev Respir Dis* 139:587, 1989.
16. Draper E: *Risky business,* New York, 1991, Cambridge University Press.

17. Fine LJ, Rosenstock L: Cardiovascular disorders. In Cullen MR, Rosenstock L, eds. *Textbook of occupational and environmental medicine,* Philadelphia, 1994, WB Saunders.
18. Gong H Jr: Health effects of air pollution: a review of clinical studies, *Clin Chest Med* 13(2):201, 1992.
19. Harving H, Dahl R, Molhave L: Lung function and bronchial reactivity in asthmatics during exposure to volatile organic compounds, *Am Rev Respir Dis* 143:751, 1991.
20. Kane DN: *Environmental hazards to young children,* Phoenix, Ariz, 1985, Oryx Press.
21. Klaassen CD, Rozman K: Absorption, distribution and excretion of toxicants. In Amdur MO, Doull J, Klaassen CD, eds. *Toxicology: the basic science of poisons,* ed 4, New York, 1991, Pergamon.
22. Koenig JQ, Pierson WE, Horike M: The effects of inhaled sulfuric acid on pulmonary function in adolescent asthmatics, *Am Rev Respir Dis* 128:221, 1983.
23. Koenig JQ et al: The effects of ozone and nitrogen dioxide on pulmonary function in healthy and in asthmatic adolescents, *Am Rev Respir Dis* 136:1152, 1987.
24. Kreit JW et al: Ozone-induced changes in lung function and bronchial responsiveness in asthmatics, *J Appl Physiol* 66:217, 1989.
25. Lambert WE, Samet JM: The role of combustion products in building-associated illness, *Occupational Medicine: State of the Art Reviews* 4:4, 1989.
26. Logan WPD: Mortality in the London fog incident, *Lancet* 1:336, 1953.
27. Morrow PE et al: Pulmonary performance of elderly normal subjects and subjects with chronic obstructive pulmonary disease exposed to 0.3 ppm nitrogen dioxide, *Am Rev Respir Dis* 145:291, 1992.
28. Ostro B, Rothschild S: Air pollution and acute respiratory morbidity: an observational study of multiple pollutants, *Environ Res* 50:238, 1989.
29. Pope CA III: Respiratory disease associated with community air pollution and a steel mill, Utah Valley, *Am J Public Health* 79:623, 1989.
30. Pope CA III: Respiratory hospital admissions associated with PM_{10} pollution in Utah, Salt Lake, and Cache Valleys, *Arch Environ Health* 46:90, 1991.
31. Ray CS et al: Effects of obesity on respiratory function, *Am Rev Respir Dis* 128:501, 1983.
32. Rubinstein I et al: Airflow limitation in morbidly obese, nonsmoking men, *Ann Intern Med* 112(11):828, 1990.
33. Schwartz J, Dockery DW: Increased mortality in Philadelphia associated with daily air pollution concentrations, *Am Rev Respir Dis* 145:600, 1992.
34. Sheppard D et al: Exercise increases sulfur dioxide-induced bronchoconstriction in asthmatic subjects, *Am Rev Respir Dis* 123:486, 1981.
35. Sheppard D et al: Lower threshold and greater bronchomotor responsiveness of asthmatic subjects to sulfur dioxide, *Am Rev Respir Dis* 122:873, 1980.
36. Speizer FE: Asthma and persistent wheeze in the Harvard Six Cities Study, *Chest* 98:191S, 1990.
37. Stankus RP et al: Cigarette smoke-sensitive asthma: challenge studies, *J Allergy Clin Immunol* 82:331, 1988.
38. Superko HR, Adams WC, Daly PW: Effects of ozone inhalation during exercise in selected patients with heart disease, *Am J Med* 77:463, 1984.
39. Weitzman M et al: Maternal smoking and childhood asthma, *Pediatrics* 85:505, 1990.

Chapter 30

MULTIPLE CHEMICAL SENSITIVITY: CONTROVERSIES IN CLINICAL DIAGNOSIS AND MANAGEMENT

Robert Harrison

Epidemiology and case definitions
Etiology
    Psychiatric hypotheses
    Immunologic hypotheses
    Respiratory hypotheses
    Olfactory-limbic hypotheses
Clinical management
    History and physical examination
    Diagnostic tests
    Treatment

Over the past decade clinicians have been increasingly challenged by the individual with multiple complaints relating to low-level occupational or environmental exposures. Multiple central nervous system, musculoskeletal, gastrointestinal, and systemic symptoms are reported in relation to common environmental irritants such as perfumes, cigarette smoke, home or office furnishings, household cleaners, and a host of other petrochemical products. These symptoms occur with exposures well below the thresholds accepted by federal or state agencies as able to cause adverse effects in humans and may result in significant impairment with lost work time, complete job loss, or major alterations in social and family functions. Individuals may report the onset of initial symptoms following documented acute or chronic low-level occupational or environmental exposures, with persistent symptoms that are triggered by subsequent environmental irritants. Some individuals report these symptoms without obvious occupational or environmental etiology, but are concerned that *potential* exposure to environmental toxicants trigger or aggravate their symptoms. Often these individuals seek help from multiple healthcare providers who may have suggested a psychiatric etiology or treatment, obtained toxicologic or immunologic test batteries, or initiated a variety of empiric treatments. Worker's compensation or disability claims are often disputed, and employers often have difficulty accepting or accommodating clinician or patient requests for alternative work environments. As a result, frustration, anger, hostility, and suspicion may confront the clinician when significant impairment continues despite lengthy and expensive consultations.

Considerable controversy continues to surround the etiology, case definition, diagnosis, and treatment of individuals with this disorder.[10,38] The specialty of clinical ecology that emerged in the 1960s adopted theories of causation that differ from those of traditional allergy, immunology, and toxicology, thereby laying the basis for medical and legal disputes regarding legitimate or acceptable forms of treatment, medical or worker's compensation insurance reimbursement, and disability benefits. To guide the clinical evaluation of individuals with this disorder or respond to requests for epidemiologic investigation, the health care practitioner should be aware of these current controversies, including knowledge gaps and the need for further research.

EPIDEMIOLOGY AND CASE DEFINITIONS

Unfortunately there is no single term or universally accepted case definition for individuals with this disorder (Table 30-1). The term *environmental hypersensitivity* has been defined as a "chronic (that is, continuing for more than 3 months) multisystem disorder, usually involving symptoms of the central nervous system and at least one other system. Affected persons are frequently intolerant to some foods and react adversely to some chemicals and to environmental agents, singly or in combination, at levels generally tolerated by the majority. Affected persons have varying degrees of morbidity, from mild discomfort to total disability. On physical examination the patient is usually free from any abnormal objective findings. Improvement is associated with avoidance of suspected agents, and symptoms recur with re-exposure."[127] The term *environmental illness* has been described as an "acquired disease characterized by a series of symptoms caused and/or exacerbated by exposure to environmental agents. The symptoms involve multiple organs in the neurologic, endocrine, genitourinary, and immunologic systems."[62] The term *multiple chemical sensitivity* (MCS) has been defined as "an acquired disorder characterized by recurrent symptoms, referable to multiple organ systems, occurring in response to demonstrable exposure to many chemically unrelated compounds at doses far below those established in the general population to cause harmful effects. No single widely accepted test of physiologic function can be shown to correlate with symptoms."[35] Seven criteria were outlined in this definition:

1. The disorder is acquired in relation to some documentable environmental exposure(s), insult(s), or illness(es).
2. Symptoms involve more than one organ system.
3. Symptoms recur and abate in response to predictable stimuli.
4. Symptoms are elicited by exposures to chemicals of diverse structural classes and toxicologic modes of action.
5. Symptoms are elicited by exposures that are demonstrable (albeit of low level).
6. Exposures that elicit symptoms must be very low, by which is meant standard deviations below "average" exposures known to cause adverse human responses.
7. No single widely available test of organ function can explain symptoms.

By this definition patients with MCS are distinguished from those individuals with acute occupational diseases (for example, acute solvent intoxication, occupational asthma) and psychiatric disorders (for example, posttraumatic stress disorder, somatoform disorder, mass psychogenic illness). Other criteria have been proposed for MCS, including those based on a survey of occupational physicians, clinical ecologists, and internal medicine and otolaryngology specialists.[76] These criteria differ from those proposed by the National Research Council and the Agency for Toxic Substances and Disease Registry Working Groups (Table 30-2). In addition, an operational definition of multiple chemical sensitivity has been proposed based on the concept of "adaptations." With this operational definition, "the patient with multiple chemical sensitivities can be discovered by removal from the suspected offending agents and by re-

Table 30-1. Terms used to describe syndrome of symptoms in association with low-level occupational or irritant exposures

Environmental illness
Multiple chemical sensitivity
Chemical hypersensitivity
Universal allergy
Twentieth-century illness
Environmental allergy
Cerebral allergy
Chemically associated immune dysfunction

Table 30-2. Proposed case definitions for multiple chemical sensitivity

Cullen[35]	National Research Council[75a]	ATSDR[98]	Nethercott et al.[76]
Documentable environmental exposures	Symptoms elicited by low-level exposures	Change in health status	Symptoms reproducible with exposure
Symptoms in more than one organ system	Symptoms in more than one organ system	Symptoms triggered by multiple stimuli	Condition is chronic
Symptoms recur and abate to predictable stimuli	Symptoms and signs wax and wane with exposures	Symptoms for at least 6 months	Symptoms with low-level exposure
Symptoms elicited by diverse chemicals		Defined set of reported symptoms	Symptoms improve with avoidance
Symptoms elicited by demonstrable exposures		Symptoms in three or more organ systems	Responses to multiple substances
Symptoms elicited by very low exposures		Exclusion of other medical conditions	
No single test to explain symptoms			

challenge after an appropriate interval under strictly controlled environmental conditions. Causality is inferred by the clearing of symptoms with removal from the offending environment and recurrence of symptoms with specific challenge."[7,9] "Adaptation" refers to a sequence of stages (known as preadaptive, addictive, and postadaptive), along with stimulatory and withdrawal levels of reactions, by which an individual manifests symptoms as a result of cumulative environmental exposures.[84] A "stimulatory effect" from foods or chemicals is followed by "withdrawal" symptoms; eventually the individual becomes "addicted" or adapted to chronic environmental or food exposures. Clinical manifestations of adaptation are highly individualized and variable, with a broad range of gastrointestinal, cardiopulmonary, and central nervous system symptoms.[83] It is only by "withdrawing" the individual into an environment free from chemicals and food "incitants" that the illness can be "unmasked." Likewise a variety of intradermal and sublingual tests are used as diagnostic tools to provoke symptoms. These concepts were initially formulated in relation to food allergies, and then were extended to chemical exposures.[40,78,79] "Ecologic" or "environmental control" units have been established to provide chemical-free environments where these diagnostic and therapeutic techniques are employed.[80-82,110]

The field of clinical ecology emerged in the mid-1960s based on the proposal that chronic adverse reactions to low-level chemical or food exposures cause or exacerbate symptoms in susceptible individuals, and that changes in the frequency of and intervals between exposures can mask the clinical manifestations or alter the sensitivity to those substances.[14,24] Ecologic illness is defined as a "polysymptomatic, multisystem chronic disorder manifested by adverse reactions to environmental incitants, as they are modified by individual susceptibility in terms of specific adaptations. The excitants are present in air, water, drugs, and our habitats."[5] The controversy over these theories and clinical application has resulted in several reviews from professional medical organizations rejecting both the theoretical basis for ecologic illness as well as controversial diagnostic and treatment methods.[2-6,123] While recognizing that some individuals with MCS may have an organic basis for their disorders, a recent critique concluded that "no credible evidence exists at the present time that permits acceptance of MCS-related disorders or demonstrates the validity of treatments used by clinical ecology practitioners."[118] Other authors agree,[39,48,54,55] whereas others advocate for greater acceptance of the MCS patient and new, as yet untested theories.*

With the lack of a uniform case definition and the ongoing debate regarding the theories and practice of many practitioners of clinical ecology, it is not surprising that few epidemiologic data exist regarding this syndrome. No population-based data exist regarding the prevalence of MCS, or occupational or demographic characteristics of this syndrome. Four populations have been identified that may develop symptoms of MCS: industrial workers, occupants of "tight buildings" such as office workers and schoolchildren, residents of communities whose air or water is contaminated by chemicals, and individuals with unique, personal exposures to various chemicals in domestic indoor air, pesticides, drugs, and consumer products.[8] Other diagnostic subsets have been reported among individuals with solvent-associated psychoorganic syndrome, chemical headaches, and intolerance to solvents.[33] Records-based reports from an allergy practice, academic occupational medicine clinic, and environmental health center suggest that individuals with MCS are predominantly women in the 30- to 40-year age range, with a disproportionate number from service industries.[36,104,124] MCS patients in these reports tend to be of high socioeconomic status and had a diversity of both occupational and environmental exposures. The most common reported symptoms in one survey were headache, fatigue, confusion, shortness of breath, and arthralgias[104]; another survey found that previous psychologic difficulties (depression, anxiety, somatization, stress and stress-related functional illness) were prominent among MCS patients.[126]

Symptoms of MCS also resemble those of sick-building syndrome (SBS), a constellation of excessive work-related symptoms related to an indoor office environment (headache; eye, nose, and throat irritation; fatigue; dizziness) without an identifiable etiology.[52,75] Multiple chemical sensitivities has been reported to follow pesticide exposure among employees in a casino[34] and among several office workers following a large-scale outbreak of SBS.[130] Several symptoms included in the Centers for Disease Control case definition of chronic fatigue syndrome (CFS) (fatigue, confusion, memory loss, sleep difficulties, myalgias, headaches) are also common among individuals with MCS,[30] and affected individuals may be concerned about occupational or environmental etiologies for CFS. Aside from symptom overlap, there is currently no evidence linking CFS to occupational or environmental chemical exposures.

ETIOLOGY

Unfortunately the lack of a uniform case definition for individuals with MCS has hampered investigation of etiology, and the criteria for study eligibility have varied depending on the target population. Generally etiologic hypotheses have focused on either a primary psychiatric or physiologic etiology, with a central role of the immune and central nervous systems in the latter.[13,14,58] Individuals with thrombophlebitis, vasculitis, and cardiac disease have been reported in uncontrolled case series to have symptoms reproduced with specific chemical challenges, with symptom improvement following withdrawal in a chemical-free environment.[85-89] Signs and symptoms of chemical sensitivity have been assessed using low-dose chemical inhalant challenges and placebos in an environmental control

---

*References 31, 47, 49, 56, 68, 101.

unit,[94,95] but these studies have not been duplicated using more rigorous scientific methods, and they fail to shed any light on the mechanism by which symptoms are produced. No other carefully controlled inhalation challenge studies have been performed.

Psychiatric hypotheses

Individuals with MCS have been described as a medical subculture with a long history of preexisting psychologic symptoms and recurring physical complaints unsupported by objective physical findings, who search for physicians to confirm their own convictions regarding their symptoms, and who organize their life-style around their illness. In this view a society with a heightened awareness of toxic hazards, physicians with a ready explanation of symptoms based on physiologic theories, a favorable worker's compensation system, and medical, legal, and patient advocacy supports contribute to the emergence of MCS as a self-described medical disorder.[26] Other psychologic factors, such as the attribution of normal changes of aging to toxic exposure, traumatic neurosis, psychosis, work stress and conflicts, secondary gain from the sick role, and the need for vindication, also contribute to what has been described as a somatoform disorder.[27] Practitioners of clinical ecology become a last resort for many patients when traditional practitioners fail to explain the cause of bodily symptoms.[28] Symptom reports may be the result of a perceived toxic exposure, with a variety of perceptual biases and conscious or unconscious reporting biases determined in part by media influences, influence of other co-workers, monetary self-interest, and the forensic environment.[61]

The majority of patients with "twentieth century disease" in one case series were reported to have psychiatric conditions (psychoses, affective or anxiety disorders, or somatoform disorders—somatization, conversion, and hypochondriases), many with symptoms well before their diagnosis of environmentally related illness.[121] Some patients with persistent or recurrent medically unexplained symptoms may have an atypical posttraumatic stress disorder, where specific and recurrent somatic symptoms follow acute or chronic chemical exposures, and then subsequently experience symptoms repeatedly triggered by low-level environmental irritants.[107,108] Individuals with MCS may be a heterogeneous group of other psychiatric disorders, either causally related or secondary to MCS, with depression, anxiety, and a variety of somatoform disorders (hypochondriases, conversion disorder, somatization disorder).[109] Alternatively, prolonged physical symptoms and sensitivity to common environmental irritants have been described as a classical conditioned response[24] or an "odor-triggered panic attack."[113,114] Based on this view of MCS, specific cognitive and behavioral interventions such as systematic desensitization, relaxation techniques, self-hypnosis, or biofeedback have been suggested as treatment strategies.[24,109] Some MCS patients have been described as primarily ideational (obsessive/compulsive) in character, requiring a different psychotherapeutic approach focusing on the effect of physical symptoms on psychologic function, stress associated with physical and interpersonal isolation, or the frustration of multiple physician consultations.[103]

Neuropsychologic measures (EEG, scalp EMG, skin resistance) during relaxation in individuals who attribute medical and psychologic symptoms to chemical exposures ("universal reactors") have been compared with subjects with primary psychologic disorders and with a control group. "Universal reactors" did not differ from psychologic subjects, and both were significantly different from controls, suggesting that individuals with MCS may have primary emotional, anxiety, attentional, or personality disorders.[120] The "universal reactor" group also had a higher somatization score on a standard self-report symptom inventory, and a subset of these patients had a history of early childhood sexual abuse.[112] Others have argued that psychiatric and psychologic disorders may be a consequence, rather than a cause of MCS.[38]

Case-referent studies have compared subjects with MCS with age- and sex-matched controls using a variety of standardized psychologic interview schedules and self-administered symptom questionnaires. Case definitions and study populations have varied, but in general these studies suggest that psychologic disorders may explain some reported symptoms. Using the Diagnostic Interview Schedule, 26 subjects with a diagnosis by a clinical ecologist of environmental illness had a higher prevalence of affective disorders (particularly major depression), anxiety, and somatoform disorders compared with age- and sex-matched controls, and more environmental illness subjects met lifetime criteria for a major mental disorder.[22] In another study, 13 individuals who met a case definition for environmental illness among 36 individuals filing worker's compensation claims had a significantly greater prevalence of prior psychiatric morbidity (anxiety, depression, somatization trait) and significantly higher self-reported measures of somatization and hypochondriases.[115,116] The strongest predictor of environmental illness was a prior tendency toward somatization. In contrast, among 11 subjects referred to an academic occupational medicine clinic who met the case definition for MCS,[35] psychiatric evaluation did not suggest any premorbid psychiatric diagnosis or a premorbid tendency toward somatization.[42,43] Clinically significant psychiatric symptoms of depression and anxiety were present among most subjects, with a subset performing poorly on tests of verbal performance. In another prospective study 41 patients recruited from the practice of a community allergist with a reported diagnosis of chemical sensitivity were compared with 34 age- and sex-matched control patients from a university-based occupational musculoskeletal and back injury clinic.[116a] Cases of MCS reported a higher prevalence of current psychologic distress (depression, anxiety, somatization) and somatization symptoms preceding the onset of sensitivity symptoms; neuropsychologic performance did not differ when adjusted for level of psychologic distress. Regardless of whether psychiatric morbidity is the cause of or an outcome of MCS, it seems clear that psychologic distress is common in individuals with this disorder.[126a]

Immunologic hypotheses

Environmental and occupational chemical exposures may affect the immune system, with a variety of cellular and cell-mediated immunologic effects established in both animals and humans.* Xenobiotics may produce immunosuppression and alter host resistance in experimental animals following acute or subchronic exposure, and immunologic effects in humans have been reported in association with dusts (silica, asbestos), polyhalogenated aromatic hydrocarbons (dioxins, furans, polychlorinated biphenyls), pesticides, metals (lead, cadmium, arsenic, methyl mercury), and solvents.[67] Nonetheless, neither experimental immune dysfunction nor epidemiologic evidence of altered immunity have been well correlated with clinical disease.

Environmental illness has been postulated to be an immunologic disorder, with generalized immune dysregulation as a result of free radical generation and alkylation, structural alteration of antigens, or hapten/carrier reactions.[62] Chemicals are hypothesized to alter immune responses, triggering lymphokines leading to clinical symptoms of cell-mediated immune response.[96,97] Chemically sensitive patients are reported to have altered T and B lymphocyte counts, abnormal helper/suppressor ratios, and antibodies to a variety of chemicals.[51,92,93] Patients with building-related illness have been reported to have an abnormal antibody response and altered cellular immunity to formaldehyde,[128] although these findings have not been confirmed using controls and clinical correlation is absent.[32] MCS has also been hypothesized to be the result of an interaction between the immune and nervous systems.[70,71] In contrast, clinical case series of patients with environmental illness or MCS have found no consistent abnormalities in immunoglobulins, complement, lymphocytes, or B-cell or T-cell subsets.[59,124] A study of patients with MCS has found no evidence of increased autoantibodies, lymphocyte count, helper or suppressor cells, B or T cells, and TAl+ or interleukin-2+ cells when compared to control subjects.[116a] Based on available evidence to date, there is no convincing evidence that MCS is an immunologic disorder.[1,67,125]

Respiratory hypotheses

Because many individuals with MCS report a heightened sense of smell or develop symptoms at low levels of environmental irritant exposure, MCS has been hypothesized to represent an amplification of the nonspecific immune response to low-level irritants. Altered function of c-fibers, respiratory epithelium, or neuroepithelial interaction is postulated to result in increased symptom reporting correlated with physiologic abnormality.[11] A group of subjects with MCS was reported to have significantly higher nasal resistance and respiration rates,[41] and several patients with MCS were found with rhinolaryngoscopy to have marked cobblestoning of the posterior pharynx and/or base of the tongue.[72] The relevance of these findings to the etiology of MCS remains to be determined.

Olfactory-limbic hypotheses

Multiple chemical sensitivity has been postulated to be the result of environmental chemical exposure, with the triggering or perpetuation of affective and cognitive disorders as well as somatic dysfunction in vulnerable individuals via kindling mechanisms.[73,74] Kindling is a special type of time-dependent sensitization of olfactory-limbic neurons by drug or nondrug stimuli, with activation of neural structures such as the amygdala and hypothalamus.[16,17] In this model of MCS, sensitization to food or chemicals parallels the phenomenon of time-dependent sensitization from drugs or nondrug stressors, with heightened sensitivity to stimuli, gradual improvement following withdrawal, and reactivation of symptoms following reexposure. It has also been hypothesized that shy individuals may have hyperreactive limbic systems and may self-report greater symptoms of illness due to chemical exposures.[18] Further research is needed to determine whether the olfactory-limbic model may explain symptoms in patients with MCS.

CLINICAL MANAGEMENT
History and physical examination

A careful, thoughtful, and compassionate history is critical to the evaluation of the individual with multiorgan symptoms provoked by low-level chemical exposure. Although the etiology of MCS may be controversial, the patient may be suffering from disabling symptoms, frustrated with the lack of definitive answers from evaluating or treating practitioners, and sometimes desperately seeking advice and counsel regarding treatment. Approaching the history with the suspicion that the patient with MCS is suffering from a psychiatric disorder, is malingering, or is seeking monetary benefits is not helpful in establishing a therapeutic relationship. Acknowledgement of symptoms and the establishment of a trusting relationship should not necessarily be avoided because the etiology is uncertain or patient motivation is suspect.[44,64]

As with the evaluation of other occupational or environmental diseases, a history should be obtained of symptom onset in relationship to acute or chronic exposures. Particular attention should be paid to respiratory, dermal, neurologic, and systemic symptoms. Duration and severity of symptoms should be recorded, particularly in relationship to repeated exposures in the workplace or environment (for example, improvement away from work or on weekends/vacations, with worsening symptoms at work). An occupational history

---
*References 19, 21, 46, 65, 66, 122, 129, 131.

should be obtained, including past employment and exposure to chemicals, dusts, or fumes. Recent and past chemical exposures should be identified by product names or Material Safety Data Sheets, and any environmental monitoring data reviewed if available.[119]

The individual with MCS typically reports symptoms after exposure to common environmental irritants such as gasoline, perfumes, or household cleaners. Symptoms of headache, fatigue, lethargy, myalgias, and trouble concentrating may persist for hours to days or even weeks, with typical "reactions" reported after these common exposures. Often the individual with MCS will have already identified a variety of irritants that result in symptoms and will have initiated an avoidance regimen. Varying degrees of restrictions in social and work activities may be reported, including problems driving an automobile, grocery shopping, wearing certain types of clothing, or entering office buildings or other workplaces.

Individuals with MCS usually do not have concurrent presence of other obvious occupational or environmental diseases such as asthma or contact allergic dermatitis. However, a few patients may have underlying or concurrent hyperreactive airway disease and develop symptoms of chest tightness or shortness of breath on exposure to low-level environmental irritants. The physical examination is almost always normal in patients with MCS, but particular attention should be paid to examination of the lungs for the presence of wheezing that may indicate asthma.

Diagnostic tests

Several controversial techniques have been employed for the diagnosis of MCS, including provocation-neutralization testing, chemical and food challenges, immunologic testing, inhalant challenges, serologic testing for Epstein-Barr virus antibodies, autoantibodies, blood testing for organic hydrocarbon and pesticides, and hair testing for heavy metals.* Many of these tests have been extensively critiqued and found of no diagnostic utility.† There is no evidence linking MCS to past infection with the Epstein-Barr virus, and this test is therefore not useful and in fact often confuses the individual in its interpretation. Likewise, there is no confirmed association between MCS and levels of organic hydrocarbons or pesticides in blood or fatty tissue, and knowledge of minute residues of these chemicals may only serve to mislead and alarm the patient. Hair testing has no role in the diagnosis of patients with MCS.

Routine laboratory testing to rule out other medical conditions, or diagnostic tests (such as nonspecific airways challenge with methacholine or histamine) that are suggested by clinical complaints may be useful.[98] Neuropsychologic testing may be helpful for diagnostic purposes with a history of exposure to a known neurotoxin and symptoms suggestive of cognitive impairment. In the absence of other concurrent medical conditions suggested by history, physical examination, or routine lab testing, the diagnosis of MCS is usually made on the basis of history alone.

Treatment

A variety of controversial methods have been utilized for the treatment of MCS, including elimination or rotary diversified diets, vitamin therapy, antifungal and antiviral agents, thyroid hormone supplement, supplemental estrogen or testosterone, transfer factor, chemical detoxification through exercise and heat stress, intravenous gamma globulin, and intra- or subcutaneous neutralization.* A specially designed chemical-free environmental control unit has been advocated as an effective method to decrease blood pesticide levels and improve symptoms as well as intellectual and cognitive function.[20,90] These treatment methods have not been validated through carefully designed controlled trials, may have unwanted side effects, may serve to reinforce counterproductive behaviors, and are not recommended for the treatment of MCS.[5,6,23,126a] Nonetheless these methods offer hope of improvement to many individuals with MCS, and indeed some patients report symptom improvement over time. Many of these treatment methods are expensive and are rarely covered by health insurance. Patients should be advised that such treatments are controversial, have not been subject to controlled clinical trials, and are not recommended by most medical professional organizations.

Avoidance of those low-level environmental irritants that provoke symptoms is often already practiced by many patients, and many practitioners continue to recommend avoidance on an empirical basis, although most are reluctant to recommend specific changes in the home environment, work restrictions, or a trial away from work.[98] Elimination of exposures at home, workplace, or school through a variety of strategies (including room air filters) has been suggested.[132] Like other controversial treatment techniques, avoidance of low-level irritants has not been tested in controlled scientific studies. Indeed avoidance may reinforce the notion of disability and lead to further isolation, powerlessness, and discouragement.[117] Education regarding general principles of toxicology (for example, routes of exposure of toxic chemicals, routes of elimination) may be reassuring to the patient concerned about long-term storage of chemicals in the body and the fear of ongoing damage.[50]

Although it is not clear whether psychologic symptoms are the cause of MCS or simply accompany the diagnosis, specific cognitive and behavioral interventions may be useful in the treatment of MCS.[109,113,117,126a] Cognitive techniques or behavioral desensitization of the individual through relaxation techniques, breath-control exercises, and visualization or other hypnotic techniques have been suggested along with a structured plan to increase overall phys-

---

*References 45, 60, 63, 77, 93, 94, 111.
†References 2, 4-6, 48, 100, 123.

*References 25, 57, 63, 69, 102, 104, 106.

ical and social activity. Pharmacologic treatment targeted at specific symptoms suggestive of depression or anxiety, in conjunction with other behavioral techniques, may offer some relief.[117] Patients with MCS should be advised that, as with a chronic illness, treatment is not directed at a "cure," but rather at accommodation. Care should emphasize relief of symptoms and a return to an active work and home life.[53,64a,116a] These treatment strategies rely on the establishment of a treatment alliance between patient and clinician, without the judgment that MCS is purely a psychiatric illness. Regardless of the cause of MCS, it appears clear that psychologic symptoms play a prominent role in the syndrome. Until the cause of MCS is definitively identified, behavioral techniques aimed at the reduction of symptoms appear to be the most promising treatment approach.

REFERENCES

1. Albright JF, Goldstein RA: Is there evidence of an immunologic basis for multiple chemical sensitivity? *Toxicol Ind Health* 8:215, 1992.
2. American Academy of Allergy: American Academy of Allergy position statements: controversial techniques, *J Allergy Clin Immunol* 67:333, 1981.
3. American Academy of Allergy and Immunology: American Academy of Allergy and Immunology position statement: clinical ecology, *J Allergy Clin Immunol* 78:269, 1986.
4. American Academy of Allergy and Immunology: American Academy of Allergy and Immunology position statement: candidiases hypersensitivity syndrome, *J Allergy Clin Immunol* 78:269, 1986.
5. American College of Physicians: American College of Physicians position paper: clinical ecology, *Ann Intern Med* 111:168, 1989.
6. American Medical Association: Council on Scientific Affairs council report: clinical ecology, *JAMA* 268:3465, 1992.
7. Ashford NA, Miller CS: Chemical sensitivity: a report to the New Jersey State Department of Health, December 1989.
8. Ashford NA, Miller CS: *Chemical exposures: low levels and high stakes,* New York, 1991, Van Nostrand Reinhold.
9. Ashford NA, Miller CS: Case definitions for multiple chemical sensitivity. In *Multiple chemical sensitivities: addendum to biologic markers in toxicology,* Washington, D.C., 1992, National Research Council, National Academy Press.
10. Bascom R: Chemical hypersensitivity syndrome study, prepared at the request of the State of Maryland Department of the Environment, March 1989.
11. Bascom R: Multiple chemical sensitivity: a respiratory disorder? *Toxicol Ind Health* 8:221, 1992.
12. Bell IR: *Clinical ecology: a new medical approach to environmental illness,* Bolinas, Calif, 1982, Common Knowledge Press.
13. Bell IR, King DS: Psychological and physiological research relevant to clinical ecology: overview of the literature, *Clin Ecol* 1:15, 1982.
14. Bell IR: Environmental illness and health: the controversy and challenge of clinical ecology for mind-body health, advances, *Inst Advance Health* 4:45, 1987.
15. Bell IR et al: Depression and allergies: survey of a nonclinical population, *Psychother Psychosom* 55:24, 1991.
16. Bell IR, Miller CS, Schwartz GE: An olfactory-limbic model of multiple chemical sensitivity syndrome: possible relationships to kindling and affective spectrum disorders, *Biol Psych* 32:218, 1992.
17. Bell IR: Neuropsychiatric and biopsychosocial mechanisms in multiple chemical sensitivity: an olfactory-limbic system model. In *Multiple chemical sensitivities: addendum to biologic markers in toxicology,* National Research Council, Washington, DC, 1992, National Academy Press.
18. Bell IR et al: Self-reported illness from chemical odors in young adults without clinical syndromes or occupational exposures, *Arch Environ Health* 48:6, 1993.
19. Bellanti JA: Immunotoxicology: overview and future perspectives, *Ann Allergy* 66:465, 1991.
20. Bertschler J et al: Psychological components of environmental illness: factor analysis of changes during treatment, *Clin Ecol* 3:85, 1985.
21. Bigazzi P: Autoimmunity induced by chemicals, *Clin Toxicol* 26:125, 1988.
22. Black DW, Rathe A, Goldstein RB: Environmental illness: a controlled study of 26 subjects with "20th century disease," *JAMA* 264:3166, 1990.
23. Blonz ER: Is there an epidemic of chronic candidiasis in our midst? *JAMA* 256:3138, 1986.
24. Bolla-Wilson K, Wilson RJ, Bleecker ML: Conditioning of physical symptoms after neurotoxic exposures, *J Occup Med* 30:684, 1988.
25. Boyles JH: Chemical sensitivity, *Otolaryng Clin North Am* 18:787, 1985.
26. Brodsky CM: "Allergic to everything": a medical subculture, *Psychosomatics* 24:731, 1983a.
27. Brodsky CM: Psychological factors contributing to somatoform diseases attributed to the workplace, *J Occup Med* 25:459, 1983.
28. Brodsky CM: Multiple chemical sensitivities and other "environmental illness": a psychiatrist's view, *Occup Med* 2:695, 1987.
29. Broughton A, Thrasher JD, Madison R: Chronic health effects and immunological alterations associated with exposure to pesticides, *Comments Toxicol* 4:59, 1990.
30. Buchwald D et al: Chronic fatigue syndrome, *Toxicol Ind Health* 8:157, 1992.
31. Casanova-Roig R: Clinical ecology, multiple chemical sensitivity (M.C.S.): the debate, *Bol-Asoc Med PR* 83:553, 1991.
32. Chang CC, Gershwin ME: Perspectives on formaldehyde toxicity: separating facts from fantasy, *Regul Toxicol Pharmacol* 16:150, 1992.
33. Cone JE, Harrison RJ, Reiter R: Patients with multiple chemical sensitivities: clinical diagnostic subsets among an occupational health clinic population, *Occup Med* 2:721, 1987.
34. Cone JE, Salt TA: Acquired intolerance to solvents following pesticide/solvent exposure in a building: a new group of workers at risk for multiple chemical sensitivities? *Toxicol Ind Health* 8:29, 1992.
35. Cullen MR: The worker with multiple chemical sensitivities: an overview, *Occup Med* 2:655, 1987.
36. Cullen MR, Pace PE, Redlich CA: The experience of the Yale occupational and environmental medicine clinics with multiple chemical sensitivities, 1986-1991, *Toxicol Ind Health* 8:15, 1992.
37. Davidoff LL et al: Letter to the editor, *J Psychosom Res* 35:621, 1991.
38. Davidoff LL: Models of multiple chemical sensitivities (MCS) syndrome: using empirical data (especially interview data) to focus investigations, *Toxicol Ind Health* 8:229, 1992.
39. DeHart RL: Multiple chemical sensitivity—what is it? In *Multiple chemical sensitivities: addendum to biologic markers in toxicology,* Washington, D.C., 1992, National Research Council, National Academy Press.
40. Dickey LD: The food factor in disease: its history and documentation, *Clin Ecol* 1:65, 1982.
41. Doty RL et al: Olfactory sensitivity, nasal resistance, and autonomic function in patients with multiple chemical sensitivities, *Arch Otolarygol Head Neck Surg* 114:1422, 1988.
42. Fiedler N, Maccia C, Kipen H: Evaluation of chemically sensitive patients, *J Occup Med* 5:529, 1992.
43. Fiedler N, Kipen H: Neurobehavioral and psychosocial aspects of multiple chemical sensitivity. In *Multiple chemical sensitivities: addendum to Biologic Markers in Toxicology,* Washington, DC, 1992, National Research Council, National Academy Press.
44. Frumkin H: Care for "environmental illness," *Ann Intern Med* 111:542, 1989.
45. Galland L: Biochemical abnormalities in patients with multiple chemical sensitivities, *J Occup Med* 2:713, 1987.
46. Gleichmann E, Kimber I, Purchase IFH: Immunotoxicology: suppressive and stimulatory effects of drugs and environmental chemicals on the immune system, *Arch Toxicol* 63:257, 1989.

47. Green MA: "Allergic to everything": a 20th-century syndrome, *JAMA* 253:842, 1985.
48. Grieco MH: Controversial practices in allergy, *JAMA* 247:3106, 1982.
49. Harris C: Clinical ecology and the open mind, *Ann Intern Med* 111:690, 1989.
50. Hessl SM: Management of patients with multiple chemical sensitivities at occupational health clinics, *Occup Med* 2:779, 1987.
51. Heuser G, Wojdani A, Heuser S: Diagnostic markers of multiple chemical sensitivity. In *Multiple chemical sensitivities: addendum to biologic markers in toxicology,* Washington, D.C., 1992, National Research Council, National Academy Press.
52. Hodgson MJ: Clinical diagnosis and management of building-related illness and the sick building syndrome, *Occup Med* 4:593, 1989.
53. Jewett DL: Diagnosis and treatment of hypersensitivity syndrome, *Toxicol Ind Health* 8:111, 1992.
54. Kahn E, Letz G: Clinical ecology: environmental medicine or unsubstantiated theory? *Ann Intern Med* 111:104, 1989.
55. Kahn E, Letz G: Clinical ecology: environmental medicine or unsubstantiated theory? *J Allergy Clin Immunol* 85:437, 1990.
56. Kay AB: Alternative allergy and the General Medical Council, *Br Med J* 306:122, 1993.
57. Kilburn KH, Warsaw RH, Shields MG: Neurobehavioral dysfunction in firemen exposed to polychlorinated biphenyls (PCBs): possible improvement after detoxification, *Arch Environ Health* 44:345, 1989.
58. Kilburn KH: How should we think about chemically reactive patients? *Arch Environ Health* 48:4, 1993.
59. Kipen H et al: Immunologic evaluation of chemically sensitive patients, *Toxicol Ind Health* 8:1, 1992.
60. Laseter JL et al: Chlorinated hydrocarbon pesticides in environmentally sensitive patients, *Clin Ecol* 2:3, 1983.
61. Lees-Haley PR, Brown RS: Biases in perception and reporting following a perceived toxic exposure, *Percept Motor Skills* 75:531, 1992.
62. Levin AS, Byers VS: Environmental illness: a disorder of immune regulation, *Occup Med* 2:669, 1987.
63. Levin AS, Byers VS: Multiple chemical sensitivities: a practicing clinician's point of view—clinical and immunologic research findings, *Toxicol Ind Health* 8:95, 1992.
64. Lewis BM: Workers with multiple chemical sensitivities: psychosocial intervention, *J Occup Med* 2:791, 1987.
65. Luster MI et al: Development of a testing battery to assess chemical-induced immunotoxicity: National Toxicology Program's guidelines for immunotoxicity evaluation in mice, *Fundam Appl Toxicol* 10:1, 1988.
66. Luster MI et al: Pertubations of the immune system by xenobiotics, *Environ Health Persp* 81:157, 1989.
67. Luster MI, Bermolec DR, Rosenthal GJ: Immunotoxicology: review of current status, *Ann Allergy* 64:427, 1990.
68. McClellan RK: Biological interventions in the treatment of patients with multiple chemical sensitivities, *Occup Med* 2:755, 1987.
69. McClellan RK: Clinical ecology, *Ann Intern Med* 269:1634, 1993.
70. Meggs WJ: Multiple chemical sensitivities and the immune system, *Toxicol Ind Health* 8:203, 1992.
71. Meggs WJ: Immunological mechanisms of disease and the multiple chemical sensitivity syndrome. In *Multiple chemical sensitivities: addendum to biologic markers in toxicology,* Washington, D.C., 1992, National Research Council, National Academy Press.
72. Meggs WJ, Cleveland CH: Rhinolaryngoscopic examination of patients with the multiple chemical sensitivity syndrome, *Arch Environ Health* 48:14, 1993.
73. Miller CS: Possible models for multiple chemical sensitivity: conceptual issues and role of the limbic system, *Toxicol Ind Health* 8:181, 1992.
74. Miller CS, Ashford NA: Possible mechanisms for multiple chemical sensitivity: the limbic system and others. In *Multiple chemical sensitivities: addendum to biologic markers in toxicology,* Washington, DC, 1992, National Research Council, National Academy Press.
75. Morrow LA: Sick building syndrome and related workplace disorders, *Otolaryngol Head Neck Surg* 106:649, 1992.
75a. National Research Council Multiple Chemical Sensitivities: *Addendum to biologic markers in toxicology,* Washington, DC, 1992, National Academy Press.
76. Nethercott JR et al: Multiple chemical sensitivities syndrome: toward a working case definition, *Arch Environ Health* 48:19, 1993.
77. Pan Y, Johnson AR, Rea WJ: Aliphatic hydrocarbon solvents in chemically sensitive patients, *Clin Ecol* 5:126, 1988.
78. Randolph TG: Allergic-type reactions to indoor utility gas and oil fumes, *J Lab Clin Med* 44:913, 1954.
79. Randolph TG: Depressions caused by home exposures to gas and combustion products of gas, oil and coal, *J Lab Clin Med* 46:942, 1955.
80. Randolph TG: The ecologic unit, Part I, *Hosp Management* 97:45, 1964a.
81. Randolph TG: The ecologic unit, Part II, *Hosp Management* 97:47, 1964b.
82. Randolph TG: Ecologic orientation in medicine: comprehensive environmental control in diagnosis and therapy, *Ann Allergy* 23:7, 1965.
83. Randolph TG: Specific adaptation, *Ann Allergy* 40:333, 1978.
84. Randolph TG: Emergence of the speciality of clinical ecology, *Clin Ecol* 1:84, 1982.
85. Rea WJ: Environmentally triggered thrombophlebitis, *Ann Allergy* 37:101, 1976.
86. Rea WJ: Environmentally triggered small vessel vasculitis, *Ann Allergy* 38:245, 1977.
87. Rea WJ: Environmentally triggered cardiac disease, *Ann Allergy* 40:243, 1978.
88. Rea WJ et al: Food and chemical susceptibility after environmental chemical overexposures: case histories, *Ann Allergy* 41:101, 1978.
89. Rea WJ et al: Recurrent environmentally triggered thrombophlebitis: a five-year follow-up, *Ann Allergy* 47:338, 1981.
90. Rea WJ et al: Pesticides and brain-function changes in a controlled environment, *Clin Ecol* 2:145, 1984.
91. Rea WJ et al: T and B lymphocyte parameters measured in chemically sensitive patients and controls, *Clin Ecol* 4:11, 1986.
92. Rea WJ et al: T and B lymphocytes in chemically sensitive patients with toxic volatile organic hydrocarbons in their blood, *Clin Ecol* 5:171, 1987.
93. Rea WJ et al: Toxic volatile organic hydrocarbons in chemically sensitive patients, *Clin Ecol* 5:70, 1987b.
94. Rea WJ et al: Confirmation of chemical sensitivity by means of double-blind inhalant challenge of toxic volatile chemicals, *Clin Ecol* 6:113, 1988.
95. Rea WJ et al: Chemical sensitivity in physicians, *Clin Ecol* 6:135, 1988.
96. Rea WJ: Chemical hypersensitivity and the allergic response, *Ear Nose Throat J* 67:50, 1988.
97. Rea WJ et al: Considerations for the diagnosis of chemical sensitivity. In *Multiple chemical sensitivities: addendum to biologic markers in Toxicology,* Washington, D.C., 1992, National Research Council, National Academy Press.
98. Rest KM: Advancing the understanding of multiple chemical sensitivity (MCS): overview and recommendations from an AOEC workshop, *Toxicol Ind Health* 8:1, 1992.
99. Rest KM: A survey of AOEC physician practices and attitudes regarding multiple chemical sensitivity, *Toxicol Ind Health* 8:51, 1992.
100. Ritts RE: Clinical utility of immunologic tests, *Ann Intern Med* 96:779, 1982.
101. Roberts HJ: Clinicians and "clinical ecology," *J Fla Med Assoc* 77:533, 1990.
102. Root DE, Lionelli GT: Excretion of a lipophilic toxicant through the sebaceous glands: a case report, *J Toxicol Cut Ocular Toxicol* 6:13, 1987.
103. Rosenberg SJ et al: Personality styles of patients asserting environmental illness, *J Occup Med* 32:678, 1990.

104. Ross GH: History and clinical presentation of the chemically sensitive patient, *Toxicol Ind Health* 8:21, 1992.
105. Ross GH: Treatment options in multiple chemical sensitivity, *Toxicol Ind Health* 8:87, 1992.
106. Schnare DW, Robinson PC: Body burden reduction of PCBs, PBBs and chlorinated pesticides in human subjects, *Ambio* 13:378, 1984.
107. Schottenfeld RS, Cullen MR: Occupation-induced posttraumatic stress disorders, *Am J Psych* 142:198, 1985.
108. Schottenfeld RS, Cullen MR: Recognition of occupation-induced posttraumatic stress disorders, *J Occup Med* 28:365, 1986.
109. Schottenfeld RS: Workers with multiple chemical sensitivities: psychiatric approach to diagnosis and treatment, *Occup Med* 2:739, 1987.
110. Selner JC, Staudenmeyer H: The relationship of the environment and food to allergic and psychiatric illness. In Young S, Rubin J, eds: *Psychobiology of allergic disorders,* New York, 1985, Praeger.
111. Selner JC, Staudenmayer H: The practical approach to the evaluation of suspected environmental exposures: chemical intolerance, *Ann Allergy* 55:665, 1985.
112. Selner JC, Staudenmayer: Neurophysiological observations in patients presenting with environmental illness, *Toxicol Ind Health* 8:145, 1992.
113. Shusterman DJ, Dager SR: Prevention of psychological disability after occupational respiratory exposures, *Occup Med* 6:11, 1991.
114. Shusterman DJ: Critical review: the health significance of environmental odor pollution, *Arch Environ Health* 47:76, 1992.
115. Simon GE, Katon WJ, Sparks PJ: Allergic to life: psychological factors in environmental illness, *Am J Psych* 147:901, 1990.
116. Simon GE: Epidemic multiple chemical sensitivity in an industrial setting, *Toxicol Ind Health* 8:41, 1992.
116a. Simon G, Daniell W, Stockbridge H: Immunologic, psychological and neuropsychological factors in multiple chemical sensitivity: a controlled study, *Ann Int Med* 119:97, 1993.
117. Simon GE: Psychiatric treatments in multiple chemical sensitivity, *Toxicol Ind Health* 8:67, 1992.
118. Smith SJ, Loeb JM: Clinical ecology, *JAMA* 269:1635, 1993.
119. Sparer J: Environmental evaluation of workers with multiple chemical sensitivities: an industrial hygienist's view, *Occup Med* 2:705, 1987.
120. Staudenmeyer H, Selner JC: Neurophysiology during relaxation in generalized, universal "allergic" reactivity to the environment: a comparison study, *J Psychosom Res* 34:259, 1990.
121. Stewart DE, Raskin J: Psychiatric assessment of patients with "20th-century disease" ("total allergy syndrome"), *Can Med Assoc J* 133:1001, 1985.
122. Sullivan JB: Immunological alterations and chemical exposure, *Clin Toxicol* 27:311, 1989.
123. Task Force on Clinical Ecology, California Medical Association Scientific Board: Clinical ecology: a critical appraisal, *West J Med* 144:239, 1986.
124. Terr AI: Environmental illness: a clinical review of 50 cases, *Arch Intern Med* 146:145, 1986.
125. Terr AI: "Multiple chemical sensitivities:" immunologic critique of clinical ecologic theories and practice, *Occup Med* 2:683, 1987.
126. Terr AI: Clinical ecology in the workplace, *J Occup Med* 31:257, 1989.
126a. Terr AI: Multiple chemical sensitivities, 119:163, 1993.
127. Thomson GM et al: Report of the ad hoc committee on environmental hypersensitivity disorders, Provincial Court, Province of Ontario, Ontario, Canada, 1985.
128. Thrasher JD et al: Building-related illness and antibodies to albumin conjugates of formaldehyde, toluene diisocyanate and trimelletic anhydride, *Am J Ind Med* 15:187, 1989.
129. Vos J et al: Toxic effects of environmental chemicals on the immune system, *TiPs* 10:289, 1989.
130. Welch LS, Sokas R: Development of multiple chemical sensitivity after an outbreak of sick-building syndrome, *Toxicol Ind Health* 8:47, 1992.
131. Yoshida S, Golub MI, Gershwin ME: Immunological aspects of toxicology: premises not promises, *Regul Toxicol Pharmacol* 9:56, 1989.
132. Ziem GE: Multiple chemical sensitivity: treatment and follow-up with avoidance and control of chemical exposures, *Toxicol Ind Health* 8:73, 1992.

UNIQUE ISSUES AS THEY RELATE TO CHILDREN

Chapter 31

THE HAZARDS OF PESTICIDES TO CHILDREN

Richard J. Jackson

Pesticides as a hazard to children
What is a pesticide? A herbicide? A fungicide? An insecticide?
Sources and routes of pesticide exposure in children
Common pesticides and herbicides and their health effects
    Organophosphate insecticides
    Carbamate insecticides
    Organochlorine insecticides
    Pyrethrum and related compounds
    Chlorophenoxy herbicides
    Bipyridyl herbicides
Management of a poisoning

Children can be at great risk from pesticide exposures. Because of growth and development factors, some agents have greater toxic effects on children than on adults. In addition, children's exploratory behaviors and greater intake of air, water, and food can result in exposures higher than those to adults (see Chapter 10).

More than 800 active ingredients are registered or licensed as pesticides in the United States. These agents have effects through diverse toxicologic pathways.

PESTICIDES AS A HAZARD TO CHILDREN

Of the 10 million chemicals currently registered with the American Chemical Society, more than 15,000 are classified as pesticides. Pesticides, usually synthetic organic compounds, are used primarily by the agriculture industry in this country. Between 1964 and 1984, pesticide use increased in the United States from 540,000,000 lb to 1,080,000,000 lb per year (U.S. Environmental Protection Agency data), although use has remained relatively stable since that time.

Although environmental—and for some children, occupational—exposure to pesticides is the primary focus of this chapter, the most significant hazard to children remains the accidental ingestion. The most common cause of ingestion has been improper storage of pesticides, especially in food containers such as soft-drink bottles. The clinical management of such cases varies with the chemical ingested and is not the subject of this text.

Childhood death from pesticide exposure has declined significantly over the past three decades[11]; however, well over half of all pesticide exposures reported by this country's poison-control centers occur in children under the age of 6 years.

Pesticides are of particular concern in terms of child hazards because they are inherently toxic and because they are used in situations that intimately affect human activity: in food, in medications, on home and living-space structures. These uses can contaminate the air, water, and soil of human, animal, and plant habitats. Pesticides can pose significant occupational hazards, and can be deliberately or inadvertently brought into children's home environments.

Pesticide exposures and queries are the most frequent calls to poison-control centers. Although diagnosis in cases of ingestions may be straightforward, it can be extremely difficult with less dramatic environmental settings, because exposures can occur without parental awareness and can mimic more common childhood ailments. For example, the most common symptom of organophosphate ingestion is diarrhea.

Table 31-1. Pesticide classification by use

Pesticide class	Function
Insecticide	Kills insects
Herbicide	Kills weeds
Fungicide	Kills fungi
Rodenticide	Kills rodents
Nematicide	Kills nematodes
Bactericide	Kills bacteria
Acaricide	Kills spiders
Algicide	Kills algae
Miticide	Kills mites
Molluscacide	Kills snails and slugs (may include shellfish)
Avicide	Kills birds
Slimicide	Kills slime
Piscicide	Kills fish
Ovicide	Kills eggs
Chemical pesticides not bearing the *cide* suffix	
Disinfectant	Destroys or inactivates harmful microorganisms
Growth regulator	Stimulates or retards plant growth
Defoliant	Removes leaves
Desiccant	Speeds drying of plant
Repellent	Repels insects, mites, and birds
Attractant	Attracts insects
Chemosterilant	Sterilizes insects
Fumigant	Kills insects, bacteria, rodents, and other pests

From California Department of Health Services: *Pesticides: health aspects of exposure and issues surrounding their use,* Berkeley, Calif, 1988.

WHAT IS A PESTICIDE? A HERBICIDE? A FUNGICIDE? AN INSECTICIDE?

A pesticide is a chemical or biologic agent used to control or cause death to nonhuman organisms considered by humans to be pests (that is, inimical to human interest). The term encompasses many use categories, such as herbicides, fungicides, and insecticides (Table 31-1).

SOURCES AND ROUTES OF PESTICIDE EXPOSURE IN CHILDREN

Although the public may voice concern about low-dose environmental exposures to pesticides, the major hazards from pesticides result from ingestion episodes or from occupational exposure. The degree of exposure in these settings is far higher than in environmental settings. In manufacturing plants, workers may come in contact with highly concentrated technical-grade materials, and in formulation plants (where inert ingredients such as sticking agents are added to the technical-grade material), exposure may occur because engineering controls are often less strictly applied. Individuals who work in the storage or transportation of pesticides are of course at high risk for adverse effects of these chemicals. Agriculture exposures occur to mixers and loaders of the pesticides; to those applying the chemicals to crops; to flaggers, standing in the fields marking the rows for aerial dusting; and to fieldworkers and those involved in harvesting crops. Episodes of pesticide illness have occurred in workers involved in shipment of harvested crops, as in the case of cut flowers or when illegal or excessive use of pesticides has occurred.

Pesticide illnesses in working children have been identified. This illness is the result of the social reality that most farmworker families need two or more breadwinners and are usually paid for piecework. Lacking child care and being paid for the amount harvested, families frequently have children in the workplace. Large-scale picker poisonings not uncommonly include children.

Children are at risk from paraoccupational pesticide exposure when the clothing of their farmworker parents becomes contaminated and family garments are laundered together. Other such episodes of fouling of the nest occur when workers bring home industrial-strength chemicals for household problems such as roaches or head lice.

The general routes of pesticide exposure include oral ingestion—giving rise to systemic injury—and contact to the skin or eye. Dermal exposure can produce systemic effects as well as localized, irritant effects. Because pesticides are often applied as dusts, mists, sprays, or gases to permeate a given area more efficiently, aspiration or inhalation of a pesticide substance can theoretically reach the alveoli, where they are absorbed into the blood system via the pulmonary capillary bed.

COMMON PESTICIDES AND HERBICIDES AND THEIR HEALTH EFFECTS

Organophosphate insecticides

Toxicity. Of the thousands of different organophosphate compounds, fewer than 50 are used as insecticides, and only about 18 are used on food crops. Organophosphates exert their effects by phosphorylating the active site of the enzyme acetylcholinesterase and irreversibly inhibiting this enzyme. Some highly toxic organophosphates include ethyl-parathion (parathion), mevinphos (phosdrin), and methamidophos (Monitor). Organophosphates more likely to be seen in home or garden settings for children are malathion, diazinon, and dichlorvos (DDVP). The signs and symptoms of organophosphate poisoning result from the accumulation of acetylcholine at the nerve's receptor sites, leading to overstimulation of muscarinic receptors in the exocrine glands and smooth muscles. These events cause excessive salivation, tearing, urination, diarrhea, and constriction of the pupils (see box). Diagnosis of organophosphate poisoning is achieved with exposure history, cholinergic signs, and the patient's response to the antidote atropine.

Clinicians may find the mnemonic MUDDLES helpful in identifying a case of organophosphate or carbamate intoxication: M = miosis (often pinpoint pupils); U = urination (excessive and uncontrolled); D = diarrhea (especially with ingestions); D = disorientation; L = lacrimation; E = excitation (early—exhaustion and coma are late symptoms); S = salivation (excessive).

> **Signs and symptoms of cholinesterase-inhibitor poisoning (generally an organophosphate or carbamate)***
>
> General symptoms: Excitation; coma, if extreme; a chemical odor on the child or his or her clothing
> Vital signs: Bradycardia, hypotension, tachycardia if hypoxemic and agonal
> Head: Headache, mental confusion
> Eyes: Miosis, lacrimation, blurred vision
> Ears, nose, and throat: Rhinitis, salivation
> Chest: Difficulty breathing (bronchospasm and increased bronchial secretions)
> Heart: Bradycardia (vagal stimulation; may have tachycardia if hypoxic)
> Abdomen: Nausea, vomiting, and diarrhea
> Genitourinary system: Uncontrolled urination
> Extremities: Fasciculations
> Skin: Sweating

*No case presents with all of these symptoms.

Chronic effects. The most remarkable and serious long-term effect of organophosphate exposure has been noted only in adults. This effect, known as organophosphate-induced delayed polyneuropathy (OPIDN), is associated with ascending paralysis in the legs, sensory disturbances, weakness, and muscle fasciculation. Pesticides in current use are screened for these effects, and most chemicals with these significant OPIDN effects have been removed from commerce. The long-term effects of childhood intoxication with organophosphates and carbamates have not yet been adequately studied.

Carbamate insecticides

As with organophosphates, N-methyl carbamates exert their effects through the binding of the enzyme acetylcholinesterase, although this reaction is more readily reversible and the effects of exposure to carbamate insecticides usually abate within 6 to 8 hours. Although more short-lived in their effects than organophosphates, carbamates can be highly toxic. The most toxic of the carbamate insecticides is aldicarb (temik). Agents of lesser toxicity are methomyl (Lannate, Nudrin) and carbofuran (Furadan). An agent that may be more commonly seen in terms of home or backyard exposures to children is the chemical carbaryl, a chemical of relatively low acute toxicity.

Cholinergic symptoms may appear in a patient exposed to an unknown combination of organophosphate or carbamate compounds. Clinicians are advised to administer atropine and pralidoxime, because withholding pralidoxime can be fatal to the person actually exposed to an organophosphate insecticide.

Organochlorine insecticides

Toxicity. The organochlorine compounds are lipid-soluble, low-molecular-weight substances demonstrating a range of toxicities. Easily absorbed by inhalation or ingestion but not through the skin, the organochlorine insecticides are stored in body fat, which can influence their metabolic rate and excretion. Although not readily absorbed through the skin, the organochlorines appear difficult to remove by washing. Commonly available organochlorine pesticides include methoxychlor; lindane (gamma benzene hexachloride, or Kwell, the antilice and antiscabies treatment); and kelthane. Dichlorodiphenyltrichloroethane (DDT), the most notorious organochlorine insecticide, was banned from use in the United States in 1972, although it remains a contaminant of D.

Diagnosis. The organochlorine pesticides change the electrophysiologic and enzymatic properties of the cell membranes, producing abnormal nerve function that can manifest itself as seizures, such as those observed with DDT poisoning. Symptoms may begin insidiously and may include tremor, lack of muscle coordination, weakness, slurred speech, and changes in mental status. Children are often exposed to lindane as a treatment for head lice or scabies. The clinical signs of lindane poisoning are nausea, vomiting and central nervous system stimulation, such as a generalized seizure.

Treatment. The effects of organochlorine pesticide poisoning require symptom-specific therapy, such as intravenous anticonvulsants to halt a seizure. Some patients require endotracheal intubation or assisted ventilation. Low doses of dopamine are sometimes used to treat hypotension, if present, but epinephrine is not recommended, because some organochlorines may promote myocardial irritation.

Pyrethrum and related compounds

About six active pyrethrins are found in products that paralyze the insect nervous system, such as bug bombs and aerosol sprays. Pyrethrum, a natural product extracted from the chrysanthemum, may be combined with other chemical compounds to boost the toxicity of the product. Antilice shampoos such as Rid contain pyrethrins.

Toxicity. Because they are quickly metabolized by the mammalian liver, the pyrethrins have a low toxicity if ingested by children; however, allergic reactions in the form of a contact dermatitis can and do occur. Individuals chronically sensitized to these substances may suffer an anaphylactic episode consistent with histamine release, and symptoms can include tachycardia, pallor, fever, and sweating. Individuals with certain allergies may be prone to hypersensitivity reactions. Occasionally it is a cause of asthma.

Diagnosis. Pyrethrin exposure is often determined by the patient's history of recent exposure. Generalized allergic signs and symptoms often make diagnosis difficult.

Treatment. After decontamination and immediate removal of the offending substance, the patient's signs are treated directly. Antihistamines relieve any allergic reactions. Asthmatic reactions require more intensive treatment.

Chlorophenoxy herbicides

The chlorophenoxy herbicides are frequently used for deweeding because they block normal growth of grass and plants. Certain chlorophenoxy compounds appear to cause teratogenic effects in animals and are suspected to have similar effects in humans. Common products in this category include 2,4-dichlorophenoxyacetic acid (2,4-D), 2,4,5-trichlorophenoxypropionic acid (Silvex), and 4-chloro-2-methylphenoxyacetic acid (MCPA).

Toxicity. The toxicity of herbicides such as 2,4-D and related compounds remains low, usually appearing as local irritation after either ingestion or absorption through the skin. Inhalation exposure can lead to upper airway irritation. Other possible signs and symptoms of chlorophenoxy herbicide toxicity may include nausea, vomiting, spasms, and hypotonia, sometimes followed by tachycardia, seizures, fever, and coma.

Diagnosis. The diagnosis of chlorophenoxy herbicide poisoning is usually based on a history of exposure.

Treatment. After decontamination, patients should be observed for any further signs of illness and then treated accordingly. Intentional diuresis can hasten elimination of products such as 2,4-D and reduce symptoms.

Bipyridyl herbicides

The most well-known bipyridyl herbicides are paraquat and diquat, both nonselective plant-killing agents. The agriculture industry prefers these compounds because they become inactive on contact with the soil. Fatal or serious poisonings with bipyridyl herbicides have occurred after accidental or intentional ingestion in adults.

Toxicity. Paraquat or diquat can corrode the skin at high concentrations and can promote a delayed conjunctivitis and ulceration of the mouth and gastrointestinal tract if swallowed. Paraquat is associated with pulmonary toxicity, but diquat exposure appears to lead more readily to renal failures.

Diagnosis. Diagnosis of paraquat or diquat poisoning is confirmed by a quick urine test that determines the agent's presence if at a concentration of 1 ppm or higher. Common signs of paraquat exposure include vomiting, nausea, diarrhea, and erosions of the mucous membranes. Reduced urination may indicate renal failure. Hepatic and cardiac injury are often associated with exposure to these two herbicides.

Treatment. Death from bipyridyl herbicide poisoning occurs in approximately 60% of cases. No specific treatments are recommended other than immediate removal of the greatest amount of the compound, because the rate of failure is directly related to the amount of product ingested or absorbed. Gastric lavage using a clay or charcoal slurry may help some individuals. For patients with pulmonary complications, the prevention of respiratory failure remains the main goal. Patients with low plasma concentrations of the herbicide have a better chance for survival than do those with serum levels greater than 0.1 μg/mL. Because renal failure can occur rapidly after paraquat ingestion, the close monitoring of urine output is necessary. Dialysis is sometimes required in the optimal management of a patient with diquat poisoning.

Clinicians and pediatric health care providers can arrive at a diagnosis of pesticide-exposure poisoning by investigating the young patient's recent history of activity as related to exposure to insecticides, herbicides, and associated chemicals (see Table 31-2). More detail on the treatment of pesticide poisoning can be found in Chapter 23.

MANAGEMENT OF A POISONING

The clinical manifestation of pesticide poisoning can appear within minutes to hours to days of the actual exposure. An initial step in managing a pesticide-related poisoning is to assess the young patient's breathing status and oxygenation because most of the deaths associated with this type of poisoning result from the anoxia or respiratory failure. The

Table 31-2. Pesticides of potential concern with regard to children's environmental exposure

Agent	Chemical class	Common setting
Diazinon	Moderately toxic OP	Turf and garden, food uses, lanolin in breast creams
Oftanol	Highly toxic OP	Turf and lawn
Malathion	Low-toxicity OP	Home and garden, aerial bait (for example, versus Mediterranean fruit fly), food uses
Carbaryl	Low-toxicity carbamate	Garden and other sprays, food uses, pet flea powders
Fenthion	Moderately toxic OP	Flea bombs
Chlorpyrifos	Moderately toxic OP	Structural pest control, food uses, some paints
DDVP	Moderately toxic OP	Pest strips, pet flea dips and treatment
Pentachlorophenol	Moderately toxic phenolic	Wood treatment for decks and playground equipment
Diethyl-m-toluamide (DEET)		Insect repellant
Aldicarb	Highly toxic carbamate	Food residue, drinking water contaminant

OP, organophosphate.

clinician or attendant must ensure airway patency. Vital signs should be checked and supported if necessary.

Because carbamates, organophosphates, organochlorines, and paraquat can penetrate the skin, contaminated clothing should be removed and the patient should undergo a complete soap-and-water washing that includes the shampooing of the hair as well as thorough rinsing of the eyes and skin. The clinician should consult a poison-control center for appropriate advice on case management.

Clinical status in insecticide poisoning can change rapidly or deteriorate quickly. Details on the management of specific poisonings are available in the book *Recognition and Management of Pesticide Poisoning*.

An awareness of cumulative toxicity issues may aid the pediatric health care provider in advising patients. Many pesticides used on commonly ingested foods contain cholinesterase inhibitors, such as aldicarb found in potatoes and bananas. Because children ingest more fruit for their body size than adults, they are at an increased risk for overexposure to such substances. Cholinesterase inhibitors are heavily used in domestic insecticides and other pesticides and in agriculture and have contaminated drinking water in some locations (see Table 31-3). Because of their small body mass and proximity to ground level, children have a greater chance of exposure and ensuing toxic reactions to these chemicals.

Another aspect of pesticides in our environment is that parents especially worry about chronic toxicity effects. Of the more than 1400 active ingredients registered for pesticide use, 53 qualify as possible carcinogens and several have definite reproductive toxic effects. Pediatric health care providers can obtain updated information about toxic outcomes, legal ramifications, and government regulations from the sources listed later in the section Where to Get Help.

Health care providers can also advocate the use of other means to control pests. The dispersion of natural predators for pests, such as the release of ladybugs to control aphids, offers a safe alternative to spraying with malathion around a home with small children. The agriculture industry and universities are conducting research in biologic control methods, such as the release of sterile insects to decrease the pest population.

Case study 1: Respiratory arrest after pesticide exposure

An 11-day-old boy was brought to a San Francisco hospital in mid January because of cyanosis. In the waiting area, the infant suffered a respiratory arrest and was resuscitated but remained limp and unresponsive. A physical examination found pinpoint pupils and excess salivation. Because of suspected narcotic ingestion, the infant was treated with naloxone to no avail. His lungs were then mechanically ventilated for 16 hours.

The child's history was of a normal pregnancy and birth. At first, he had stayed with relatives because his parents' home had been treated with termite-and-roach spray on the day of his birth. After he was brought home, he developed vomiting after bottle feeding and became lethargic. Although the house continued to have a heavy odor of pesticides, his parents did not think that he had any direct exposure to the chemicals.

The treating medical team suspected organophosphate poisoning, which led to atropine treatment and an immediate increase in responsiveness. Blood chemistries showed a 50% depression in the infant's red blood cell cholinesterase concentrations, which supports the diagnosis of organophosphate poisoning. The local health department was notified of the diagnosis, and the parents' home was studied for chemical content.

The infant recovered steadily and left the hospital after 8 days. He and his parents moved into temporary housing while the health department investigated their home.

The California Department of Food and Agriculture found the pesticide chlorpyrifos on dish towels, surfaces used for food preparation, and the infant's clothing. Chloropyrifos is a long-term insecticide with a half-life of longer than 30 days indoors. Laws prohibit its use in food-preparation areas. The infant was most likely exposed to the pesticide through the skin and/or by mouth.

Case study 2: Aldicarb exposure through watermelon ingestion throughout several states

On July 13, 1985, the Oregon State Health Department contacted the California Environmental Protection Agency about three cases of people who had eaten watermelons from California and then developed headache, nausea, vomiting, diarrhea, excess salivation, blurred vision, and muscle fasciculation. An alerted San Francisco Poison Center reported three more cases of watermelon-related poisonings in adults, one of whom required resuscitation. On contact with six other California poison centers and 15 emergency departments, 30 additional cases of people who became extremely ill after ingesting watermelon were found. Oregon health officials analyzed the watermelon and did not find aldicarb itself, but its metabolic product known as aldicarb sulfoxide.

Table 31-3. Pesticides that have commonly contaminated drinking water

Pesticide	Effect
Soil fumigants	
Dibromochloropropane	Carcinogen, reproductive toxicant
Ethylene dibromide	Carcinogen, reproductive toxicant
Herbicides	
Alachlor	Carcinogen
Atrazine	Carcinogen

On receiving these results, the California Department of Health Services immediately banned the sale of watermelons on July 4. Aldicarb and its breakdown product, aldicarb sulfoxide, are extremely neurotoxic. The farm and agriculture industry cannot legally apply aldicarb to food crops because of its very high toxicity. This episode led to the destruction of $20 million to $25 million of fruit and to the establishment of a certification program for watermelons throughout the state.

REFERENCES

1. Berteau PE et al: Insecticide absorption from indoor surfaces: hazard assessment and regulatory requirements. In Wang RGM et al, eds: *Biological monitoring for pesticide exposure: measurement, estimation and risk reduction,* Washington, DC, 1989, American Chemical Society.
2. Borowitz SM: Prolonged organophosphate toxicity in a twenty-six-month-old child, *J Pediatr* 112:302-4, 1988.
3. California Department of Health Services: *Pesticides: health aspects of exposure and issues surrounding their use,* Berkeley, Calif, 1988.
4. Dunphy J et al: Pesticide poisoning in an infant: California, *MMWR* 29:1, 1980.
5. Edwards DL, Johnson CE: Insect-repellent-induced toxic encephalopathy in a child, *Clin Pharm* 6:496, 1987.
6. Fenske RA et al: Potential exposure and health risks of infants following indoor residential pesticide applications, *Am J Public Health* 80:689, 1990.
7. Garber M: Carbamate poisoning: the "other" insecticide, *Pediatrics* 79:734, 1987.
8. Goldman LR, Beller M, Jackson RJ: Aldicarb food poisonings in California: 1985-1988: toxicity estimates for humans, (in press).
9. Goldman LR et al: Acute symptoms in persons residing near a field treated with the soil fumigants methyl bromide and chloropicrin, *West J Med* 147:95, 1987.
10. Ladrigan PJ et al: Ethylene oxide: an overview of toxicologic and epidemiologic research, *Am J Ind Med* 6:103, 1984.
11. Mortensen ML: Management of acute childhood poisonings caused by selected insecticides and herbicides, *Pediatr Clin North Am* 33:421, 1986.
12. Moses M: Pesticide-related health problems and farmworkers, *AAOHN J* 37:115, 1989.
13. National Research Council, Committee on Scientific and Regulatory Issues Underlying Pesticide Use Patterns and Agricultural Innovation: *Regulating pesticides in food: the Delaney paradox,* Washington, DC, 1987, National Academy Press.
14. Ottesen EA et al: A controlled trial of ivermectin and diethycarbamazine in lymphatic filariasis, *N Engl J Med* 322:1113, 1990.
15. Prendergast T et al: Endrin poisoning associated with taquito ingestion: California, *MMWR* 38:345, 1989.
16. Rasmussen JE: Lindane: a prudent approach, *Arch Dermatol* 123:1008, 1987.
17. Romero P, Barnett PG, Midtling JE: Congenital anomalies associated with maternal exposure to oxydemeton-methyl, *Environ Res* 50:256, 1989.
18. Russell HH et al: Chemical contamination of California drinking water, *West J Med* 147:615, 1987.
19. Savage P, Scheidt B, Brockinton L: A cyanazine-birth defects link? *Chem Week* 136:11, 1985.
20. Schultz MW et al: Comparative study of 5% permethrin cream and 1% lindane lotion for the treatment of scabies, *Arch Dermatol* 126:167, 1990.
21. Zadikoff CM: Toxic encephalopathy associated with use of insect repellent, *J Pediatr* 95:140, 1979.
22. Zweiner RJ, Ginsburg CM: Organophosphate and carbamate poisoning in infants and children, *Pediatrics* 81:121, 1988.

SUGGESTED READINGS

Pesticide hazard assessment project: Harvester exposure monitoring field studies (1980-1986), vol 2, Government Reports Announcements and Index (GRA&I), 1988; Issue 14.

Committee on Scientific and Regulatory Issues Underlying Pesticide Use Patterns and Agricultural Innovation, Board on Agriculture, National Research Council: *Regulating pesticides in food: The Delaney paradox.* Washington, DC, 1987, National Academy Press.

Hayes W Jr: *Pesticides studied in man,* Baltimore, 1982, Williams & Wilkins.

Morgan DP: *Recognition and management of pesticide poisonings,* United States Environmental Protection Agency (EPA-540/9-80-005), ed 4, Washington, DC, 1989, United States Government Printing Office.

Poplyk J, ed: *Farm chemical handbook,* Willoughby, Oh, Meister (published annually).

Committee on Pesticides in the Diets of Infants and Children, National Research Council: *Pesticides in the diets of infants and children,* Washington, DC, 1993, National Academy Press.

Chapter 32

THE HAZARDS OF LEAD TO CHILDREN

Edward B. Hayes

Sources of lead
Health effects of lead
Clinical presentation
Diagnostic evaluation and laboratory testing
Patient management
Environmental interventions
Need for future research
Summary

Lead is a bluish gray metal found naturally in deposits in the earth's crust. It is soft and malleable, has a high density and a low melting point, is easy to cast, reacts electrochemically with sulfuric acid, and is chemically stable in water, air, and soil. From the beginnings of civilization through the industrial age, people have found lead to be useful in applications as diverse as sweetening wine, ballasting ships, glazing ceramics, powering automobiles, and painting children's cribs and bedroom walls. Because of lead's seemingly limitless usefulness in the daily activities of modern societies, people have come to live more intimately with lead than with almost any other known toxin.

Since before the turn of the twentieth century, physicians have been aware that high-dose exposure to lead can cause severe and sometimes fatal encephalopathy in children. A study published in 1943 indicated that children who recovered from this encephalopathy had long-term neurologic deficits. Over the past 10 years it has become increasingly evident that even low-dose lead exposure can cause subtle and long-lasting neurobehavioral deficits. The subtlety of lead's toxic effects and the intimacy with which we live with lead on a daily basis combine to make human lead exposure a vexing public health problem.

Public health efforts in the United States have succeeded in dramatically reducing the lead exposure of U.S. citizens over the past 20 years, largely by reducing the use of lead in gasoline. The geometric mean blood lead level of the U.S. population as a whole declined from more than 15 μg/dl in the 1970s to less than 5 μg/dl in the 1990s; however, subgroups of the population in this country continue to be exposed to high levels of lead in deteriorating household paint and in dust and soil in and around their homes. More than 30% of children tested in a major metropolitan lead-screening program in 1988 had blood lead levels greater than 14 μg/dl. The problem of balancing the need for affordable housing with the urgent need to reduce children's lead exposure is at the core of current public health approaches to further reductions in lead exposure in this country. Outside the United States, many countries have yet to control the use of lead in gasoline, an initial step in reducing the lead exposure of their citizens.

SOURCES OF LEAD

People may be exposed to lead from a variety of sources. Natural emissions, such as particulate lead emitted from active volcanoes, may contribute to the contamination of air, soil, and drinking water. Background levels of lead found naturally in surface soils are generally less than 50 ppm. The relative contribution of natural sources to total body lead burdens is smaller than that of various commercial sources. Workers in a wide range of occupations and industries may receive quite large doses of lead over long periods through occupational exposure. Specific industries and work activities that have been associated with occupational lead exposure include (but are not limited to) metal smelting, battery manufacturing and recycling, construction, automotive manufacture and repair, ceramics manufacture, work involving inorganic pigments, and work involving ammunitions and guns. A variety of hobbies are also associated with lead exposure. Workers that are occupationally exposed to lead may expose their families by bringing home lead dust on their clothing.

Populations that live in the vicinity of industrial facilities that release significant quantities of lead into the environment, such as smelters, may be exposed both by inhaling airborne lead and by ingesting lead deposited in the soil and dust of the surrounding area. In some countries, cottage industries for recycling and repairing lead batteries in and around homes may result in high concentrations of lead in the surrounding area, which may in turn cause fatal lead poisoning in exposed children.

With the extensive and increasing use of automobiles during this century, the use of lead in gasoline has been a major contributor to human lead exposure. Lead was first added to gasoline in the 1920s to increase the fuel's octane rating and to serve as an engine lubricant. In 1984 more than 30,000 tons of lead were emitted into the atmosphere from gasoline combustion in the United States alone. Lead emissions from the combustion of leaded gasoline contribute to human exposure, partly through inhalation but primarily by contaminating soil, dust, and food that are then ingested. The promotion of more fuel-efficient automobiles and regulations requiring the use of unleaded fuel have resulted in a decrease in airborne lead emissions from automobiles since the late 1970s. This has in turn resulted in dramatic declines in both air lead levels and blood lead levels in the United States. Leaded gasoline is still used in the United States in certain specialized vehicles, such as racing cars, and it continues to be the principal automobile fuel in many other countries.

The most important source of high-dose lead exposure for children is deteriorating lead-based paint. Lead had been added to paint since before the turn of the twentieth century to increase paint's durability. Many countries banned the use of leaded paint for household use in the early part of the century, but leaded paint was used extensively in the United States through the 1960s, and its use was not extensively regulated until 1978, when the Consumer Product Safety Commission required that all paint used on furniture, toys, and residential surfaces contain less than 0.06% lead by weight. In 1990 more than 50 million privately owned and occupied housing units in the United States were estimated to contain lead-based paint. Children living in homes with lead paint are at risk of high-dose lead exposure both from the ingestion of paint chips and from the more insidious long-term ingestion of leaded dust from deteriorated paint. Families may be inadvertently poisoned by renovations or remodeling projects that disrupt lead-painted surfaces and increase the amount of leaded dust in the household.

Lead can leach into household drinking water from plumbing systems that have lead pipes, copper pipes joined with lead solder, or brass fixtures that contain lead, especially if the water is hot or has a low pH or a low cation content (is ''soft''). Storage of drinking water in lead-lined water coolers also may result in high water lead levels. On the other hand, water with a high mineral content may coat the inner surface of leaded plumbing fixtures with deposits over time, thus reducing the leaching of lead into the drinking water.

In the past, food has been an important source of lead exposure. In 1982 the Food and Drug Administration estimated that a 2-year-old child in the United States ingested an average of 30 µg of lead per day in food. By the late 1980s the average dietary lead intake was reduced to an estimated 5 µg per day. This decreased lead contamination of food was attributed both to restrictions on the use of lead-soldered side-seam cans and to the decreased use of leaded gasoline. Lead-soldered cans have been virtually eliminated from the food industry in the United States.

Food grown in urban gardens may be contaminated by lead in the surrounding soil. The level of lead contamination is influenced by soil characteristics such as pH levels and the levels of other minerals as well as by the type of plant grown.

The glazes used on ceramics often contain lead. If the ceramics are improperly fired, lead may leach from the glaze into any food stored or cooked in the vessel. Acidic foods are particularly likely to leach lead, and children who consumed fruit juice stored in lead-glazed ceramic pitchers have acquired dangerously high blood lead levels. High levels of lead may also leach into acidic liquids stored in vessels made of leaded crystal.

Traditional remedies used in several cultures contain high levels of lead, and their use may result in childhood lead poisoning. Hispanic Americans may use *greta* or *azarcon* to treat or prevent a gastrointestinal condition in children called *empacho*. *Paylooah* is used by Southeast Asians to treat rash or fever, and *surma* or *kohl* may be used by Asian Indians and Arabs either as an eye cosmetic or to improve vision. Other names of lead-containing remedies include *bali goli, coral, ghazard, liga,* and *rueda*. Some individuals may be reluctant to report use of a traditional medicine because of concerns about the legality of such treatments or a lack of confidence in or understanding of Western medicine.

A seasonal pattern of childhood lead exposure has been noted in several studies, with blood lead levels tending to rise in the warmer months. This pattern was particularly noticeable in the past, when blood lead levels were higher. The number of children admitted to hospitals for lead poisoning increased during the summer months, and cases of lead encephalopathy were noted more frequently in summer than in winter. Several explanations have been proposed for the seasonal pattern, which was not consistently seen in all studies. Exposure from leaded gasoline was probably higher in summer months. Overall gasoline use in the United States tended to be higher in summer, and the concentration of lead in gasoline was increased in warmer months to compensate for decreased concentrations of more volatile ingredients. Other explanations include increased exposure to outdoor lead sources in warmer months, increased exposure to lead-paint dust in open window wells, the influences of rain on lead dust dispersion, and changes in the absorption of lead caused by the metabolic influences of sunlight on vitamin D. In the United States seasonal patterns of lead exposure may have become less noticeable as use of leaded gasoline has declined and blood lead levels overall have decreased.

Nutritional deficiencies, particularly of iron and calcium, may increase both lead absorption and children's susceptibility to the adverse effects of lead.

HEALTH EFFECTS OF LEAD

Clinically overt symptoms of lead toxicity are generally not seen until blood lead levels rise above 50 μg/dl. However, several prospective studies indicate that exposure to lead may impair children's neurobehavioral development at blood lead levels as low as 10 μg/dl. There is no known benefit of any amount of lead for normal development, and a safe lower threshold for lead exposure has not been identified. Studies on the neurobehavioral effects of low-level lead exposure indicate that for every increase of 10 μg/dl in children's blood lead levels, there tends to be a loss of between 2 to 6 intelligence-quotient (IQ) points on neurodevelopmental test scores. For someone with average development this loss is unlikely to be noticed, but shifting the population distribution of IQ scores down by several points would be expected to result in significant changes in the proportion of individuals at the extremely low and high ends of the distribution. If a population of children loses a few IQ points as a result of low-level lead exposure, the small decrease in mean IQ may reflect a substantial increase in the proportion of children with subnormal intellectual functioning as well as a decrease in the proportion with exceptionally high IQ scores.

At blood lead levels above 10 μg/dl a slight impairment of vitamin D metabolism and mild elevations of erythrocyte protoporphyrin (EP) levels may be seen. Nerve conduction velocity is impaired at blood lead levels above 20 μg/dl, and synthesis of hemoglobin is decreased at blood lead levels above 40 μg/dl. Frank anemia and other overt symptoms of lead toxicity, such as abdominal pain, constipation, and overt neurologic manifestations, are generally not seen until blood lead levels rise above 50 μg/dl. Blood lead levels of 70 μg/dl and higher may cause severe encephalopathy, and death may result from blood lead levels above 100 μg/dl; however, some individuals with blood lead levels well above 100 μg/dl may be asymptomatic.

In addition to the aforementioned effects, excess lead exposure appears to raise hearing thresholds and may impair normal growth in stature. Lead exposure has been associated with impaired renal function and hypertension in adults and also may adversely affect endocrine and reproductive function.

CLINICAL PRESENTATION

Because most children exposed to the damaging effects of lead are clinically asymptomatic, health care providers must rely on screening tests to determine whether a child has had excessive exposure to lead. Those few children who have symptoms may have abdominal pain, constipation, irritability, lethargy, headaches, nausea or vomiting, renal dysfunction, developmental delay, or a behavioral disorder. Children with acute encephalopathy due to lead poisoning may suffer from any or all of the following symptoms: vomiting, ataxia, incoordination, bizarre behavior, lethargy, seizures, and coma. Some children may simply present with a loss of recently acquired developmental skills. Any child with an elevated lead level who has overt symptoms should be managed as a medical emergency. (See later discussion.)

DIAGNOSTIC EVALUATION AND LABORATORY TESTING

The test of choice for determining an individual's exposure to lead is measurement of the venous blood lead level. Measurement of capillary blood lead levels may be used for screening, but because of the possibility of surface contamination of the skin by lead, a venous sample should be drawn for confirmation in any child with an elevated capillary blood lead level. With proper laboratory techniques, most proficient laboratories in the United States can accurately determine the lead level in a blood sample to within 4 μg/dl above and below the true value when the true value is less than 40 μg/dl and within 10% of the true value for higher blood lead levels. This measurement can usually be ascertained from a sample of less than 0.5 ml of blood. New instruments for more rapid measurement of blood lead levels that can be used at screening sites are currently under development.

In the past, children were screened for lead exposure by measuring serum erythrocyte-protoporphyrin (EP) levels, but because EP levels are normal in about 60% of children with blood lead levels above 15 μg/dl, measurement of EP is not an adequate test for low-level lead exposure; however, because EP levels generally take 2 weeks to rise, measurement of EP may provide an indication of the duration of lead exposure.

In general, blood lead measurements reflect an individual's exposure during the previous 1 to 3 months, although the rate of decline in blood lead levels may be influenced by the duration of previous exposure and by the total body burden of lead. Much of the long-term body burden of lead is stored in skeletal tissue. To ascertain cumulative lead exposure better, a few centers measure bone lead levels by using x-ray fluorescence. Although carefully collected hair and teeth samples may be used in studies for lead, neither provide as reliable a measure of current exposure as does the blood lead level.

Abdominal radiographs may be useful in identifying recent ingestion of paint chips or other objects containing lead. Radiographs of the long bones may provide an indication of the duration of lead exposure. Children who have been exposed to lead for longer periods of time tend to show lead lines, which are areas of increased mineralization or calcification. These lines are best recognized in the metaphyseal plate of the proximal fibula but may be seen in other bones as well.

Basophilic stippling of red blood cells is seen in some children with excessive lead exposure, but it is not a sufficiently consistent finding to be reliable as a screening test.

PATIENT MANAGEMENT

The underlying principle in the management of any patient with an elevated blood lead level is to ensure that his or her exposure to lead has been reduced or eliminated. In the United States, young children and occupationally exposed adults are at the highest risk of having elevated blood lead levels. For details on how to evaluate and manage occupationally exposed adults, refer to texts on occupational medicine. This section focuses on medical management of young children with elevated blood lead levels. Detailed, up-to-date guidelines for medical management may be found in the Centers for Disease Control (CDC) statement on lead, *Preventing Lead Poisoning in Young Children,* available directly from the CDC.

The CDC currently sets the blood lead level of concern at 10 µg/dl and recommends follow-up for individual children with blood lead levels of 15 µg/dl or higher. Parents of all children with blood lead levels of 10 µg/dl or above should be counseled on the sources of lead exposure and should be given simple recommendations on how to reduce their children's exposure. Lead-exposed children should receive adequate nutrition, particularly adequate amounts of iron and calcium. Careful follow-up and retesting of these children are needed to ensure that their blood lead levels do not increase. Specific recommendations for the frequency of retesting are available from the CDC.

Children with blood lead levels persistently at or above 15 µg/dl may benefit from an environmental inspection of their home to identify likely sources of lead exposure. If a specific source is found, it should be remediated or the child should be removed from the source. The child's blood lead level should then be monitored to ensure that the exposure has been curtailed.

Children with blood lead levels of 20 µg/dl or higher should be given a thorough medical evaluation with particular attention to the child's nutritional status, any history of pica, and a developmental and neurologic assessment. A thorough history of possible sources of lead exposure also should be obtained. The child's iron status should be assessed by measurement of serum ferritin or serum iron and total iron-binding capacity. Measurement of EP may provide an indication of the duration of lead exposure, because EP levels tend to increase about 2 weeks after significant lead exposure. A radiograph of the abdomen may identify paint chips or some other lead object, such as a fishing sinker, that has been ingested.

Children with blood lead levels above 24 µg/dl may require treatment with chelating agents to promote more rapid elimination of lead. Lead-chelating agents currently in use in the United States include edetate disodium calcium, dimercaprol, D-penicillamine, and succimer. Although chelation therapy has not been proven to improve or reverse the neurobehavioral effects of lead, the mortality from severe lead toxicity has been effectively reduced with proper chelation and intensive care. There are virtually no data to indicate that chelation of asymptomatic children with blood lead levels less than 40 µg/dl improves patient outcome, but many experts do administer chelating agents to such patients on the theoretical grounds that a more rapid lowering of the blood lead level may improve long-term outcome. Chelation therapy is not currently recommended for children with blood lead levels below 25 µg/dl.

Any child with symptomatic lead poisoning or a venous blood lead level of 70 µg/dl or higher should be admitted to a hospital with an intensive care unit and treated with appropriate chelating agents on an emergency basis.

The most important step in the management of any child with an elevated blood lead level is either to eliminate the source of his or her lead exposure or to remove the child from the lead source.

ENVIRONMENTAL INTERVENTIONS

Although most children exposed to lead are asymptomatic, they may eventually have adverse outcomes as a consequence of their lead exposure. There are essentially two public health approaches to lead poisoning prevention. The first and most important is primary prevention of lead toxicity by reducing the population's exposure to lead. This reduction can be accomplished by controlling lead emissions into the environment, reducing or eliminating the use of lead in any products that could result in increased human exposure, abating existing lead hazards such as deteriorated lead-based paint in housing and lead in soil and water, and educating the population about the sources of lead exposure and risks associated with such exposure. The second approach is to attempt to identify those groups at highest risk of an adverse outcome from lead exposure and to use blood lead testing to screen for and identify children who would benefit from interventions to reduce their exposure. Lead screening programs are useful both to identify groups of children at risk and to focus secondary prevention efforts on those children with the highest levels of lead exposure.

Because the most important effect of low-level lead exposure is impairment of neurobehavioral development, efforts to control lead exposure should be directed first toward children. Communities must identify the local sources of children's lead exposure and eliminate the exposure either by abating the source or blocking the pathway from source to child.

One of the most effective interventions to reduce human lead exposure in recent years has been the reduction of lead in gasoline. This reduction has contributed to dramatic declines in blood lead levels in the United States and could achieve similar results in many other countries of the world in which leaded gasoline is still extensively used. The use of more fuel-efficient automobiles has also contributed to the decrease in airborne lead emissions from combustion of leaded gasoline. The advantages to society of reducing the use of lead in gasoline have been supported by extensive cost-benefit analyses.

Perhaps the greatest challenge in reducing human lead exposure is presented by the extensive reservoir of lead-based paint in homes throughout the United States and in other countries. Ingestion of leaded paint chips may result in dangerously high, sometimes fatal lead exposure. Of less obvious but more widespread impact than the ingestion of paint chips is the daily exposure of children to dust and soil that has been contaminated by flaking or chalking leaded paint. Many children in the United States continue to be exposed to deteriorated lead-based paint in their homes, and some are at daily risk of severe lead poisoning. The Department of Housing and Urban Development estimated that in 1990, of more than 50 million homes in the United States that contained lead paint, close to 14 million had leaded paint in poor condition, and 3.8 million of them were homes of young children. In addition to their risk of ingesting paint chips or leaded dust from deteriorated painted surfaces, children may be exposed to poisonous levels of lead paint dust generated during renovation or remodeling of homes that contain lead paint.

In several studies researchers have attempted to evaluate the efficacy of environmental interventions to reduce children's exposure to lead-based paint, with varying results. From a retrospective review of the efficacy of limited lead-paint abatement conducted in St. Louis, researchers concluded that the interventions were more effective for children with blood lead levels above 35 μg/dl than for those with lower blood lead levels. The efficacy of lead paint abatement strategies such as replacing windows and doors that have lead-based paint, repairing deteriorated paint to a height of 5 feet, and replacing or covering any components that have lead-based paint and are subject to abrasion or friction is currently being studied prospectively, as are several other interventions designed to temporarily reduce lead-paint hazards. Current recommendations for management of lead hazards in the home include the careful removal or repair of deteriorated lead-based paint followed by thorough clean-up of lead-contaminated dust, regular wet mopping to reduce household dust, and avoidance of any activity that would generate lead paint dust or vapor, such as sanding or using heat to remove paint. In addition, all family members should be relocated from the dwelling whenever any remodeling, renovation, or lead paint abatement is taking place.

Given the extensive reservoirs of lead paint and lead-contaminated soil, the primary prevention of lead poisoning is particularly important and challenging. Lead poisoning prevention programs are searching for effective environmental intervention strategies in entire communities that will result in affordable housing without lead exposure hazards. If such strategies are successful, not only would the exposure of children living in those houses be prevented, so too would that of any children who might move into such homes in the future. The actual strategies for stabilizing or removing lead-based paint and reducing lead-contaminated dust economically and effectively, so that entire communities will be free of lead hazards, have not yet been clearly determined. Strategies for dealing with lead-contaminated soil also are being investigated.

The effect of educational programs to teach parents how to reduce their children's exposure to lead also requires further evaluation. Research is needed to determine the most effective strategies for communicating the risks of lead exposure and for encouraging individual action to reduce exposure.

Some communities have excessive amounts of lead in their water supplies. Adjustments in water pH and in the mineral content of water supplies may help reduce the leaching of lead from old municipal and household water pipes. When water may be contaminated by lead solder or plumbing within individual houses, flushing the pipes thoroughly before use and consuming water only from the cold-water tap may reduce the amounts of lead consumed in drinking water.

Legislative control of the use of lead in food production and packaging, regulation of the amounts of lead in public water supplies and emissions from industries, public education about the hazards of folk remedies that contain lead, and implementation of proper firing techniques or the use of lead-free glazes in the manufacture of ceramics are other interventions that may be effective in reducing children's lead exposure.

NEED FOR FUTURE RESEARCH

Efforts to prevent and eventually to eliminate lead toxicity require attention to a broad range of research questions. To pursue primary prevention in communities with extensive reservoirs of lead in older housing and surrounding soil, there is an urgent need to develop and test cost-effective strategies for remediating lead paint and leaded-soil hazards. In addition, strategies must be developed to determine which communities or housing units are most likely to pose a high risk of lead exposure to children. Investigations of the determinants of children's blood lead levels and the relative contributions of the various sources of lead in soil, dust, paint, water, and air are needed in different environmental settings and communities. The results of such studies would help focus intervention efforts where they are most needed and would assist in the development of health-based standards for lead concentration in various media. The efficacy of educational and nutritional interventions in reducing childhood lead exposure needs to be assessed.

The health effects of low-level lead exposure and of lead exposure among pregnant women and women who are breast-feeding their infants needs more extensive investigation. Well-controlled clinical trials of chelation therapy are needed to determine the efficacy of chelation in lowering children's blood lead levels, decreasing their brain exposure to lead, and, most important, improving their neurobehavioral outcome. Practical strategies for determining which children would benefit from chelation need to be developed on the basis of sound data on efficacy of treatment.

To make lead screening more useful and practical, research is needed to develop new and portable instruments to measure blood lead levels rapidly. The utility of methods to assess the total body burden of lead, such as x-ray fluorescence measurement of lead in bone, needs further evaluation.

SUMMARY

Lead is an environmental toxin that has gained widespread acceptance in society and has been ubiquitously used and applied in intimate proximity to people for many centuries. The health effects of lead are often subtle and insidious, but because lead impairs normal neurobehavioral development, widespread lead exposure may have substantial effects on the general well-being of large populations. Reductions in the use of lead in gasoline have contributed to substantial declines in human lead exposure. Children continue to be exposed to high levels of lead, primarily by living in housing with deteriorated lead paint. The goal of primary prevention of childhood lead poisoning by eliminating reservoirs of lead in paint, soil, and water presents a tremendous public health challenge for the coming decades.

SUGGESTED READINGS

Annest JL et al: Chronological trends in blood lead levels between 1976 and 1980, *N Engl J Med* 308:1373, 1983.

Aposhian HV, Aposhian MM: Meso-2, 3-dimercaptosuccinic acid: chemical, pharmacological and toxicological properties of an orally effective metal chelating agent, *Annu Rev Pharmacol Toxicol* 30:279, 1990.

Baghurst PA et al: Environmental exposure to lead and children's intelligence at the age of seven years: the Port Pirie cohort study, *N Engl J Med* 327:1279, 1992.

Baghurst PA et al: Determinants of blood lead concentrations to age 5 years in a birth cohort study of children living in the lead smelting city of Port Pirie and surrounding areas, *Arch Evniron Health* 47:203, 1992.

Bellinger DC, Stiles KM, Needleman HL: Low-level lead exposure, intelligence and academic achievement: a long-term follow-up study, *Pediatrics* 90:855, 1992.

Billick IH: Sources of lead in the environment. In Rutter M, Jones RR, eds: *Lead versus health,* Chichester, 1983, Wiley.

Billick IH, Curran AS, Shier DR: Analysis of pediatric blood lead levels in New York City for 1970-1976, *Environ Health Perspect* 31:183, 1979.

Billick IH, Curran AS, Shier DR: Relation of pediatric blood lead levels to lead in gasoline, *Environ Health Perspect* 34:213, 1980.

Blanksma LA et al: Incidence of high blood lead levels in Chicago children, *Pediatrics* 44:661, 1969.

Centers for Disease Control: Preventing lead poisoning in young children: a statement by the Centers for Disease Control, Washington, DC, 1991, US Department of Health and Human Services.

Centers for Disease Control: Preventing lead poisoning in young children: a statement by the Centers for Disease Control, Report no 99-2230, Atlanta, 1985.

Chisolm JJ Jr: The use of chelating agents in the treatment of acute and chronic lead intoxication in childhood, *J Pediatr* 73:1, 1968.

Chisolm JJ Jr: Management of increased lead absorption: illustrative cases. In Chisolm JJ Jr, O'Hara DM, eds: *Lead absorption in children: management, clinical, environmental aspects,* Baltimore, 1982, Urban and Schwarzenberg.

Chisolm JJ Jr, Mellits ED, Quaskey SA: The relationship between the level of lead absorption in children and the age, type, and condition of housing, *Environ Res* 38:31, 1985.

Chisolm JJ Jr: Evaluation of the potential role of chelating therapy in the treatment of low to moderate lead exposures, *Environ Health Perspect* 89:67, 1990.

Chisolm JJ Jr: Increased lead absorption and lead poisoning (plumbism). In Behrman RE, ed: *Nelson: Textbook of pediatrics,* ed 14, Philadelphia, 1992, WB Saunders.

Cory-Slechta DA, Weiss B, Cox C: Mobilization and redistribution of lead over the course of calcium disodium ethylenediamine tetraacetate chelation therapy, *J Pharmacol Exp Ther* 243:804, 1987.

Dietrich KN et al: The developmental consequences of low to moderate prenatal and postnatal lead exposure: intellectual attainment on the Cincinnati cohort lead study following school entry, *Neurotoxicol Teratol* 17:37, 1993.

Glotzer DE, Bauchner H: Management of childhood lead poisoning: a survey, *Pediatrics* 89:614, 1992.

Graziano JH, LoIacono NJ, Meyer P: Dose-response study of oral 2,3-dimercaptosuccinic acid in children with elevated blood lead concentrations, *J Pediatr* 113:751, 1988.

Graziano JH et al: Controlled study of meso-2-3-dimercaptosuccinic acid for the management of childhood lead intoxication, *J Pediatr* 120:133, 1992.

Hunter JM: The summer disease: an integrative model of the seasonality aspects of childhood lead poisoning, *Soc Sci Med* 11:691, 1977.

Jones RR: The contribution of lead in petrol to human lead intake. In Rutter M, Jones RR, eds: *Lead versus health,* Chichester, 1983, Wiley.

Kapoor SC et al: Influence of 2,3-dimercaptosuccinic acid on gastrointestinal lead absorption and whole-body lead retention, *Toxicol Appl Pharmacol* 97:525, 1989.

Markowitz ME, Rosen JF: Assessment of lead stores in children: validation of an 8-hour CaNa$_2$EDTA provocative test, *J Pediatr* 104:337, 1984.

Markowitz ME, Rosen JF: Need for the lead mobilization test in children with lead poisoning, *J Pediatr* 119:305, 1991.

Markowitz ME, Rosen JF, Bijur PE: Effects of iron deficiency on lead excretion in children with moderate lead intoxication, *J Pediatr* 116:360, 1990.

Marrero O et al: Seasonal patterns in children's blood-lead levels: a second peak in late winter, *Conn Med* 47:1, 1983.

McCusker J: Longitudinal changes in blood lead level in children and their relationship to season, age, and exposure to paint or plaster, *Am J Publ Health* 69:348, 1979.

Matte TD et al: Lead exposure among lead-acid battery workers in Jamaica, *Am J Ind Med* 16:167, 1989.

McElvaine MD et al: Evaluation of the erythrocyte protoporphyrin test as a screen for elevated blood lead levels, *J Pediatr* 119:548, 1991.

Mexico's experience, *Environ Sci Technol* 26:1702, 1992.

Mortensen ME, Walson PD: Chelation therapy for childhood lead poisoning: the changing scene in 1992, *Clin Pediatr (Phila)* (in press).

National Center for Health Statistics, Annest JL, Mahaffey K: *Blood lead levels for persons ages 6 months-74 years, United States, 1976-80,* Vital and Health Statistics, Series 11, No 233, Washington, DC, 1984, US Public Health Service.

Needleman HL et al: Deficits in psychologic and classroom performance of children with elevated dentine lead levels, *N Engl J Med* 300:689, 1979.

Osterloh J, Becker CE: Pharmacokinetics of CaNa$_2$EDTA and chelation of lead in renal failure, *Clin Pharmacol Ther* 40:686, 1986.

Perlstein MA, Attala R: Neurologic sequelae of plumbism in children, *Clin Pediatr (Phila)* 5:292, 1966.

Piomelli S et al: Blood lead concentrations in a remote Himalayan population, *Science* 210:1135, 1980.

Piomelli S et al: Management of childhood lead poisoning, *J Pediatr* 105:523, 1984.

Rabinowitz M et al: Environmental correlates of infant blood lead levels in Boston, *Environ Res* 38:96, 1985.

Rabinowitz M et al: Lead in umbilical blood, indoor air, tap water, and gasoline in Boston, *Arch Environ Health* 39:299, 1984.

Rabinowitz MB, Needleman HL: Temporal trends in the lead concentrations of umbilical cord blood, *Science* 216:1429, 1982.

Rabinowitz MB, Wetherill GW, Kopple JD: Magnitude of lead intake from respiration by normal man, *J Lab Clin Med* 90:238, 1977.

Romieu I et al: Vehicular traffic as a determinant of blood lead levels in children: a pilot study in Mexico City, *Arch Environ Health* 42:246, 1992.

Rosen JF et al: L-line x-ray fluorescence of cortical bone lead compared with the CaNa$_2$EDTA-treated lead-toxic children, *Environ Health Perspect* (in press).

Rutter M: Low level lead exposure: sources, effects, and implications. In Rutter M, Jones RR, eds: *Lead versus health,* Chichester, 1983, Wiley.

Schwartz J, Levin R: The risk of lead toxicity in homes with lead paint hazard, *Environ Res* 54:1, 1991.

Schwartz J, Pitcher H: The relationship between gasoline lead and blood lead in the United States, *J Official Statistics* 5:421, 1989.

Shannon M, Graef J, Lovejoy FH Jr: Efficacy and toxicity of D-penicillamine in low-level lead poisoning, *J Pediatr* 112:799, 1988.

US Department of Housing and Urban Development: *Comprehensive and workable plan for the abatement of lead-based paint in privately owned housing,* Report to Congress, 1990.

US Environmental Protection Agency: *Strategy for reducing lead exposures,* Washington, DC, 1991.

US Environmental Protection Agency: *Air quality criteria for lead,* vol 2, Research Triangle Park, NC, 1986.

von Schirnding Y et al: Blood lead levels in South African inner-city children, *Environ Health Perspect* 94:125, 1991.

Weinberger HL et al: An analysis of 248 initial mobilization tests performed on an ambulatory basis, *Am J Dis Child* 141:1266, 1987.

Chapter 33

THE HAZARDS OF AIR POLLUTION TO CHILDREN

Michael Lipsett

Background: susceptibility factors
    Differences in exposure
    Differences in pulmonary anatomy and physiology
    Increased susceptibility to infection
    Developmental susceptibility
    Conditions unique to or more common in childhood
Indoor pollutants
    Combustion products
    Building-related pollutants
Outdoor pollutants
    Ozone
    Particulate matter
Conclusions

BACKGROUND: SUSCEPTIBILITY FACTORS

Children represent the largest subpopulation susceptible to adverse effects of air pollution. During the past decade hundreds of published reports have documented the impact of both indoor and outdoor air pollutants on children. This chapter highlights the roles of some of the major indoor and outdoor air pollutants in the induction and exacerbation of disease in children. Though the principal site of impact is the respiratory tract, other systems may be affected as well.

Children are often considered a sensitive subpopulation because their bodies are still developing; therefore various organ systems, including the lungs, are more vulnerable to environmental insults than are those of adults. This generalization encompasses several facets of susceptibility, as described below.

Differences in exposure

By virtue of their shorter stature, children may experience greater exposure than adults to pollutants emitted close to the ground (such as automobile exhaust) or to those consisting of high-density gases or aerosols.[32] Older children and adolescents tend to spend more time than adults engaged in activities requiring vigorous physical exertion and an elevated ventilation rate, increasing the dose of pollutants to the lower respiratory tract.[74] This is of greater concern for exposure to outdoor than to indoor pollutants. In contrast, infants and young children spend a considerable amount of their indoor activities on the floor, where they will tend to receive greater exposure to some indoor pollutants. For example, treating carpets with pesticides can create a vertical concentration gradient, with the highest levels in infants' and toddlers' breathing zones.[21] Furthermore, infants' low mobility may subject them to aerosols generated by their parents, such as cooking fumes, cigarette smoke, and cleansers.

Finally, children spend much of their time in school, which may be a source of exposure to air contaminants. Radon and asbestos exposures may both be found in school environments, and various aeroallergens have been found at levels high enough to elicit symptoms in sensitized children with asthma.[52,86]

Differences in pulmonary anatomy and physiology

The relative contribution of the peripheral airways to total airway resistance appears to be greater in children age 5 and under than in older children and adults.[22] The narrow bronchioles of young children, particularly those with airway hyperresponsiveness, are more likely to become obstructed in response to environmental irritants than those of adults. In addition, because of their breathing patterns and pulmonary anatomy, small children are likely to inhale and retain greater quantities of air pollutants (particles) per unit body weight than adults. For any given level of activity, ventilation has been found to be related to body mass (plus a constant), so that a small person will inhale a greater quantity of air per unit mass. Phalen et al[60] used this relationship in a model incorporating airway dimensions measured in lung casts of people (aged 11 days to 21 years) to predict that particle deposition efficiency would be inversely related to body size (or age). This may tend to accentuate differences in exposure related to activity patterns.

Increased susceptibility to infection

Respiratory infections are the most common illness of childhood. Children have less acquired immunity than adults to a variety of respiratory pathogens, and experience more severe disease in response to certain organisms (for example, respiratory syncytial virus, parainfluenza virus, and *H influenzae*). A variety of air pollutants, particularly combustion products, increase the risk of pediatric respiratory infections, including those serious enough to require hospitalization. Sequelae of recurrent infection can include otitis media, bronchiectasis, induction and exacerbation of asthma, and possibly reduced lung growth.

Developmental susceptibility

Organ systems that develop postnatally, notably the nervous system and lungs, may be affected by childhood exposures. For example, the child's nervous system is markedly more sensitive than that of the adult to lead toxicity: childhood exposure to airborne lead may result in long-term and perhaps permanent effects on behavioral and cognitive development.[54] Historically, combustion of leaded gasoline was the largest single source of lead in blood in the United States, though this is no longer true because of the gradual elimination of this fuel.[2]

The neonate has the same number of generations of conducting airways as the adult, though there are structural differences that diminish with growth (such as a greater ratio of mucous glands in the epithelium, fewer respiratory bronchioles). While the overall airway structure is fully established by the seventeenth week of gestation, most alveoli ($\approx$85%) develop postnatally. The full-term infant has about 50 million alveoli, while the adult has approximately 300 million, though there is considerable variability.[89] Most of the adult complement of alveoli develop in early childhood (up to about age 2), though the number may increase to age 8 or beyond.[76] Alveolar multiplication coincides with postnatal increases in elastin and collagen, which contribute to the development of the mature lung's pressure-volume relationships and compliance.[89]

Environmental insults may impair normal lung growth and development and result in a lower peak lung capacity and possibly chronic lung disease in adulthood. High-level ozone exposure of young rats permanently decreases the number of respiratory bronchioles formed postnatally.[5] Childhood exposure to environmental tobacco smoke (ETS) and to polluted ambient air has both been associated with decreased lung development, as measured by pulmonary function tests.[16,17,81] The long-term implications of this phenomenon are unknown but may involve a premature decline of lung function into a range of clinical significance in some individuals.

Since cancer incidence increases exponentially with age during adulthood, exposure to airborne carcinogens during childhood can allow the cancer latency or induction period to elapse by middle age. Intense childhood exposure to ETS or to asbestos has been associated with lung cancer and mesothelioma, respectively, during adulthood.[33,34]

Conditions unique to or more common in childhood

The risk of certain conditions unique to childhood, such as sudden infant death syndrome (SIDS), is reportedly increased by exposure to ETS.[66] Some respiratory illnesses, such as asthma, are more common in childhood than in adulthood and can be exacerbated by exposure to both indoor (ETS and wood smoke) and outdoor pollutants (ozone and particles). Induction of childhood asthma has been linked to exposure to ETS and to indoor biologic aerosols (dust mite antigens).[75,81]

INDOOR POLLUTANTS

Time-activity studies indicate that children, especially younger children, spend about 85% of their time indoors, mostly at home.[8] Concentrations of many air contaminants have been found to be greater indoors than outside, due in part to energy conservation measures that reduce exchange rates of indoor and outdoor air.[59] The indoor environment itself is the source of most of the pollutants of health significance listed in Table 33-1, though some outdoor air pollutants can penetrate indoors in substantial quantities under certain circumstances. Many of the indoor pollutants are generated by daily human activities, others are the result of the physical chemistry of building materials or soil, and biologic aerosols represent the expansion of life into every available niche. The most important of the nonbiologic pollutants are described below.

Combustion products

Indoor combustion products include respirable particles, nitrogen oxides, carbon monoxide, various irritant gases (such as acrolein and formaldehyde), and numerous other respiratory toxicants. The principal sources include ETS (also known as passive) or secondhand smoke), emissions from cooking appliances and gas or kerosene heaters, and wood-burning devices (fireplaces and woodstoves). Of these, acute and chronic health effects of ETS have been the most extensively documented.[53,78,81] ETS is composed of

Table 33-1. Selected indoor pollutants of concern to children

Pollutant	Source	Potential health effects
Environmental tobacco smoke	Cigarettes, pipes, cigars	Respiratory infection (including bronchiolitis and pneumonia), otitis media, hearing loss, mucous membrane irritation, sudden infant death syndrome, decreased lung growth, chronic respiratory symptoms, induction and exacerbation of asthma, lung cancer, inflammatory bowel disease
Wood smoke	Fireplaces, wood stoves	Respiratory irritation, respiratory infections, otitis, exacerbation of asthma
Nitrogen oxides (NO, NO_2, HONO)	Unvented gas-burning appliances (stoves, heaters), wood-burning devices, kerosene heaters	Increased risk of respiratory infection, exacerbation of asthma
Carbon monoxide	Malfunctioning or unvented gas-burning appliances, cigarettes, wood-burning devices, automobile in attached garages, indoor use of hibachis or barbecues	Headaches, nausea, vomiting, impaired vision and incoordination, coma, death
Respirable particles	Cigarettes, wood-burning devices, cooking fumes, household cleansers and sprays, organic aerosols, house dust	Chronic respiratory symptoms, exacerbation of asthma, increased risk of respiratory irritation and infection
Formaldehyde	Pressed-wood furniture and wall paneling made of urea-formaldehyde resins (particle board, plywood, and fiberboard), cigarettes, wallpaper, permanent-press fabrics	Mucous membrane irritation, headaches, exacerbaton of asthma, respiratory cancer (chronic exposure in mobile homes)
Other VOCs (including benzene, tetrachloroethylene, styrene, methylene chloride)	Solvents, cleansers, adhesives, air fresheners, aerosol sprays, paint and paint strippers, dry-cleaned clothing, moth repellants, cooking fumes, pesticides	Mucous membrane irritation, headaches, neurological effects, potential cancer risk
Asbestos	Friable or otherwise damaged insulation or surfacing materials	Mesothelioma, lung cancer, benign pleural changes
Radon	Principally soil gas, but also construction materials, ground water	Lung cancer, leukemia?

4000 or more substances, including some respiratory irritants that are detectable at higher concentrations in sidestream smoke than in the smoke inhaled by the smoker.[53] The principal adverse effects of ETS reported in children include induction and exacerbation of asthma, increased risk (1.5- to twofold) of acute lower respiratory infection in infants and toddlers (particularly with maternal, but also with paternal, smoking), increased risk of otitis media and hearing loss, chronic respiratory symptoms (cough, wheezing, and excess phlegm), adverse effects on lung growth and development (as measured by pulmonary function tests), increasing severity of disease in children with cystic fibrosis, and increased risk of sudden infant death syndrome.* Children are also clearly vulnerable to irritation of the eyes and upper respiratory tract by ETS, which has been well described in adults.[6] A recent epidemiologic study suggests that intense exposure to ETS during childhood and adolescence approximately doubles the risk of lung cancer as an adult.[33] Nonsmoking adults living with smokers also have an approximately 30% increase in the risk of death from ischemic heart disease; whether this effect can also be caused by childhood exposures has not been investigated.[25]

Most of what is known about the adverse effects of wood smoke comes from studies of children living in homes equipped with wood-burning devices. Although the literature on wood smoke is relatively sparse, the adverse effects reported are, not surprisingly, similar to those associated with ETS. These include symptoms of chronic respiratory

---
*References 9-12, 19, 20, 53, 66, 78, 81.

irritation (wheezing without infection, frequent coughing), increased risk of hospitalization for pneumonia or bronchiolitis, otitis media, exacerbation of asthma, and increased risk of respiratory infection.[14,30,51,57]

Numerous studies have examined potential impacts of gas stove usage on the respiratory health of children, with mixed results. Though gas burns more completely than solid fuels, it produces respiratory irritants such as nitrogen dioxide and nitrous acid. A recent metaanalysis of 11 gas stove studies supports the existence of a link between gas stove use and respiratory illness in children.[28] The extensive documentation of the adverse effects of NO_2 on respiratory tract defenses supports the plausibility of a causal relationship between gas stove use and respiratory illness.[80] Epidemiologic studies of adult asthmatics link gas stove use with exacerbation of disease, which may occur in children with asthma as well.[43,58]

Carbon monoxide is a product of incomplete combustion of organic matter. Indoor sources include unvented or defective gas- or oil-burning appliances, cigarette smoke, wood combustion, entrainment of automobile exhaust from attached garages, ice resurfacing machines at skating rinks, and use of charcoal-burning hibachis or barbecues (used mainly by immigrants from Asia). An uncommon but potentially devastating childhood exposure can occur while riding in the back of pickup trucks with enclosed canopies, which can result in death or permanent neurologic damage.[26]

Building-related pollutants

Pollutants emitted from building materials or furniture may be related to both acute and chronic health effects in children. For example, volatile organic compounds (VOCs) emitted from carpet adhesives, particle board, and other construction materials, in an environment with inadequate ventilation, have been associated with a symptom complex called "sick building syndrome" (SBS—headaches, blocked or runny nose, dry eyes and throat, lethargy, difficulty concentrating). While SBS and other indoor-air-related health problems have usually been considered a problem in the workplace, these also occur in schools.[55] Formaldehyde, which may off-gas from particle furniture or building materials for years, is not only linked acutely with mucous membrane irritation, but is a recognized carcinogen as well. Long-term residence in mobile homes (which accumulate substantial quantities of formaldehyde) has been associated with an increased risk of nasopharyngeal malignancy.[84] Further discussion of indoor air pollution can be found in Chapter 37.

Radon and asbestos are two other indoor pollutants that also may pose long-term risks of cancer in adulthood from childhood exposures. Radon is a naturally occurring gas resulting from decay of uranium 238, which is nearly ubiquitous in soils. The gas enters buildings principally through apertures in floors and walls and tends to accumulate in basements and lower floors. Radon and its daughters ultimately decay to Pb^{206}, in the process emitting α- and β-particles. Its carcinogenic effect is probably mediated through α-particle bombardment of the respiratory epithelium. Estimates of lung cancer cases attributable to radon exposure in the United States range from about 10,000 to 20,000 cases per year, based on extrapolation from occupational studies of mortality in underground miners to the general population.[65] The magnitude of risk based on such extrapolations is controversial, especially since much of the risk is likely to be found in smokers. In some areas of the country, residential radon concentrations have been found to exceed current occupational exposure standards. Several recent epidemiologic studies also suggest that radon may be related to leukemia in children, though this has not yet been confirmed in case-control or cohort studies.[29] The U.S. Environmental Protection Agency and the Centers for Disease Control and Prevention have recommended universal testing for radon in homes, since test devices are inexpensive and remediation of elevated concentrations is relatively simple in most cases.[8]

Nonoccupational exposure to asbestos has been linked with respiratory cancer.[34] Adult urban dwellers carry a substantial asbestos fiber burden in their lungs. Autopsy evidence of asbestos fiber accumulation has been found in young children, including neonates and at least one stillborn.[27] The dynamics of childhood exposure to asbestos have not been extensively investigated, but potential sources include damaged asbestos-containing surfacing and insulation materials in schools or residences (or slipshod abatement of such materials), ambient air, contaminated play sand, improperly managed asbestos-containing waste, building demolition, and the use of asbestos-containing crushed rock on unpaved roads, among others. Children of asbestos workers run an increased risk of asbestos-related malignancy, due to "take-home" exposures.[34] The extent to which such risks would apply to low-level exposures occurring in schools or other buildings is controversial. However, any increased risk would be due to airborne fibers; asbestos-containing materials that are nonfriable and undamaged do not pose such risks. Failure to appreciate this relationship in the past has resulted in massive removal of asbestos in schools, even where the material was intact. On the other hand, where the potential for exposure is high—with friable or damaged asbestos—removal or encapsulation of the material is warranted.

OUTDOOR POLLUTANTS

In the United States regulation of outdoor air pollution has focused principally on six common or "criteria" pollutants: ozone, carbon monoxide, lead, nitrogen dioxide, sulfur dioxide, and particles. Industrial emissions of so-called "toxics," many of which are recognized carcinogens, will be increasingly controlled as the 1990 Clean Air Act amendments are implemented. Since the adoption of the Clean Air Act of 1970, concentrations of most of the criteria pollutants have decreased dramatically. For example, increasing use of unleaded gasoline has reduced airborne lead emissions in the United States by more than 90%, which has been accompanied by a dramatic decline in blood lead levels nationwide.[2,79] However, ambient concentrations of ozone and particles are still high enough in many areas to present hazards to children. Recent research indicates that acidic aerosols, for which there is no health-based standard, may also be associated with a variety of adverse respiratory effects. For a more complete description of the health impact of outdoor pollutants see Chapter 40.

Ozone

As an ambient air pollutant, ozone is formed by the action of solar radiation on nitrogen oxides and reactive hydrocarbons (both of which are emitted by motor vehicles and industrial sources); ozone levels therefore tend to be highest on warm, sunny days. Ozone concentrations typically peak in the afternoon, when children are likely to be outside playing. The causes and consequences of ground-level ozone air pollution are completely different from depletion of stratospheric ozone, which is due mainly to effects of man-made chlorofluorocarbons.

Exposure to ambient ozone has been consistently linked with acute and subacute effects in epidemiologic investigations and in controlled exposure studies in environmental chambers. For example, ozone causes cough, chest tightness, pain on inspiration, upper respiratory tract irritation, airway inflammation and hyperresponsiveness, increased bronchial epithelial permeability, and decrements in pulmonary function.* Nonrespiratory effects associated with ozone exposure include headache, nausea, malaise, and decreased ability to perform sustained exercise.[46,49] Epidemiologic studies link ozone exposure with exacerbations of asthma, as manifested by increased symptoms or hospitalizations.[67,77,88] Controlled chamber studies suggest, however, that low concentrations of ozone do not cause dramatic bronchoconstriction in adult asthmatic volunteers, although at higher concentrations asthmatics experience greater airway obstruction than do healthy study subjects.[37,42,44]

Healthy children experience decrements in pulmonary function of comparable magnitude to those observed in adults for an exposure to a given ozone concentration, but they do not report symptoms to the same extent.[3,4,48,70] While this may be an artifact of the experimental setting, it also suggests that children may not experience or recognize somatic signals to curtail exposure. Field studies suggest ozone effects on pulmonary function in children much greater than would be predicted from chamber studies.[70] Moreover, decreased peak flow in children has been reported to persist for up to a week following exposure to ozone concentrations lower than 0.2 ppm (the current stage 1 ''smog alert'' level), signaling the presence of damage to the respiratory tract.[15] Repeated exposures may result in persistent airway hyperresponsiveness.[91]

Controlled exposures of adults to low ozone concentrations (at and below the current federal standard of 0.12 ppm, 1-hour average) involving moderate levels of exercise for several hours have caused pulmonary function changes, respiratory symptoms, and dramatic increases in inflammatory markers in bronchoalveolar lavage fluid.[31,41] These findings are corroborated by animal studies indicating that repeated exposures to typical urban ozone concentrations produce centriacinar inflammation and small airway structural changes.[13] Such chronic inflammation also appears to occur in humans living in highly polluted areas: an autopsy study of the lungs of 107 youths (aged 14 to 25) who died of violent causes revealed a 75% prevalence of centriacinar inflammation and a 95% prevalence of chronic bronchitis.[69] At least one long-term epidemiologic study suggests that repeated exposure to photochemical smog (including ozone and particles) is associated with lower baselines and rates of growth of lung function.[16,17] However, whether repeated exposure to ozone is a cause of chronic lung disease in humans is still an open question.

Clinical and toxicologic evidence also demonstrates that ozone exposure can interact with other pollutants and biologic aerosols. Field studies indicate that exposures to complex mixtures of air pollutants may have synergistic acute effects on pulmonary function, and possibly on symptoms.[70,71] Even brief (1-hour) exposure to ozone ($\approx$ 0.12 ppm) can potentiate allergic asthmatic responses to aeroallergens or other pollutants.[38,50] There is, moreover, considerable experimental evidence in animals demonstrating that ozone can lower resistance to infection, facilitate sensitization and airway responses to airborne allergens, and act synergistically with airborne acidity to damage deep lung tissue.[24,56,87,90]

Particulate matter

Airborne particulate matter is a variable, complex mixture of solid and liquid particles from natural and synthetic sources, including numerous industries, motor vehicle exhaust, windblown dust, residential wood combustion, construction and demolition, agriculture, and other sources. Acidic aerosols are the result of combustion of sulfur-containing fossil fuels and of reactions of photochemical free radicals with nitrogen dioxide.

While it has long been recognized that very high levels of particulate matter cause respiratory injury, illness, and even death, epidemiologic studies of children and adults during the past few years suggest a significant impact of particles on respiratory health at concentrations far below the current federal standard (150 $\mu g/m^3$ of particles less than 10 μ in diameter, 24-hour average). Some of the pediatric outcomes correlated with ambient particle levels include acute occurrence of respiratory symptoms, hospital admissions for asthma and bronchitis, decrements in lung function, school

---
*References 31, 35, 36, 41, 46, 68.

absenteeism, and prevalence of chronic cough or chest illness.[18,61-64,85] Children with a history of lower respiratory symptoms are likely to be more susceptible to effects of particles.[18,61] Though the results of some studies are driven by winter particle levels and may therefore be subject to confounding by respiratory epidemics and low temperatures, strong associations with acidic and total suspended particles and ozone have also been identified in other seasons, including summer.[7,77] At present there is little toxicologic understanding of how low levels of particles could induce the various adverse effects identified (including mortality) in epidemiologic investigations. Acidic particles have been linked with small lung function decrements in adolescent asthmatics, with changes in tracheobronchial clearance and increased airway reactivity in controlled studies of normal subjects, but adverse effects have been observed in epidemiologic studies in the absence of significant acidity.[39,40,62,73,83]

CONCLUSIONS

Various factors related to size, physiologic maturity, and exposure patterns make children potentially more susceptible than adults to adverse effects of air pollution. Exposures during childhood may have long-lasting impacts on respiratory health. Indoor exposures of particular concern include combustion products (notably ETS) and some building-related pollutants (such as radon). Though concentrations of outdoor pollutants have decreased substantially since 1970, widespread exposures to ozone and particles continue to pose risks to pediatric health in North America.

REFERENCES

1. Adams WC: Effects of ozone exposure at ambient air pollution episode levels on exercise performance, *Sports Med* 4:395, 1987.
2. Annest JL et al: Chronological trend in blood lead levels for the US population ages 6 months–74 years, *N Engl J Med* 308:1373, 1983.
3. Avol EL et al: Respiratory effects of photochemical oxidant air pollution in exercising adolescents, *Am Rev Respir Dis* 132:619, 1985.
4. Avol EL et al: Short-term respiratory effects of photochemical oxidant exposure in exercising children, *J Air Pollut Control Assoc* 37:158, 1987.
5. Barr BC et al: Distal airway remodelling in rats chronically exposed to ozone, *Am Rev Respir Dis* 137:924, 1988.
6. Bascom R et al: Upper respiratory tract environmental tobacco smoke sensitivity, *Am Rev Respir Dis* 143:1304, 1991.
7. Bates DV, Sizto R: Air pollution and hospital admissions in southern Ontario: the acid summer haze effect, *Environ Res* 43:317, 1987.
8. California Air Resources Board: Study of children's activity patterns, Sacramento, Calif, Sept. 1991.
9. Campbell PW III et al: Association of poor clinical status and heavy exposure to tobacco smoke in patients with cystic fibrosis who are homozygous for the F508 deletion, *J Pediatr* 120:261, 1992.
10. Chen Y, Li WX, Yu S: Influence of passive smoking on admissions for respiratory illness in early childhood, *Br Med J (Clin Res Ed)* 293:303, 1986.
11. Chen Y et al: Chang-Ning epidemiological study of children's health: I. Passive smoking and children's respiratory disease, *Int J Epidemiol* 17:348, 1988.
12. Chilmonczyk BA et al: Association between exposure to environmental tobacco smoke and exacerbations of asthma in children, *N Engl J Med* 328:1665, 1993.
13. Crapo JD et al: Alterations in lung structure caused by inhalation of oxidants, *J Toxicol Environ Health* 13:301, 1984.
14. Daigler GE, Markello SJ, Cummings KM: The effect of indoor air pollutants on otitis media and asthma in children, *Laryngoscope* 101:293, 1991.
15. Dassen W et al: Decline in children's pulmonary function during an air pollution episode, *J Air Pollut Contr Assoc* 36:1223, 1986.
16. Detels R et al: The UCLA population studies of chronic obstructive lung disease. 9. Lung function changes associated with chronic exposure to photochemical oxidants; a cohort study among never-smokers, *Chest* 92:594, 1987.
17. Detels R et al: The UCLA population studies of CORD: X. A cohort study of changes in respiratory function associated with chronic exposure to SO_X, NO_X and hydrocarbons, *Am J Public Health* 81:350, 1991.
18. Dockery DW et al: Effects of inhalable particles on respiratory health of children, *Am Rev Respir Dis* 136:587, 1988.
19. Etzel RA, Pattishall EN, Haley NJ, Fletcher RH, Henderson FW: Passive smoking and middle ear effusion among children in day care, *Pediatrics* 90:228, 1992.
20. Evans D et al: The impact of passive smoking on emergency room visits of urban children with asthma, *Am Rev Respir Dis* 135:567, 1987.
21. Fenske RA et al: Potential exposure and health risks of infants following indoor residential pesticide applications, *Am J Public Health* 80:89, 1990.
22. Fraser RG et al: *Diagnosis of diseases of the chest,* ed 3, vol 1, Philadelphia, 1988, WB Saunders, pp 150-151.
23. Fujinaka LE et al: Respiratory bronchiolitis following long-term ozone exposure in bonnet monkeys: a morphometric study, *Exp Lung Res* 8:167, 1985.
24. Gardner DE: Oxidant-induced enhanced sensitivity to infection in animal models and their extrapolations to man, *J Toxicol Environ Health* 13:423, 1984.
25. Glantz SA, Parmley WW: Passive smoking and heart disease: epidemiology, physiology and biochemistry, *Circulation* 83:1, 1991.
26. Hampson NB, Norkool DM: Carbon monoxide poisoning in children riding in the back of pickup trucks, *JAMA* 267:538, 1992.
27. Haque AK et al: Asbestos in the lungs of children, *Ann NY Acad Sci* 643:419, 1991.
28. Hasselblad V, Eddy DM, Kotchner DJ: Synthesis of environmental evidence: nitrogen dioxide epidemiology studies, *J Air Waste Mgmt Assoc* 42:662, 1992.
29. Henshaw DL, Eatough JP, Richardson RB: Radon as a causative factor in induction of myeloid leukemia and other cancers, *Lancet* 335:1008, 1990.
30. Honicky RE, Osborne JS, Akpom CA: Symptoms of respiratory illness in young children and the use of wood-burning stoves for indoor heating, *Pediatrics* 75:587, 1985.
31. Horstman D et al: Ozone concentration and pulmonary response relationships for 6.6-hour exposures with five hours of moderate exercise to 0.08, 0.10 and 0.12 ppm, *Am Rev Resp Dis* 142:1158, 1990.
32. International Program on Chemical Safety, Commission of the European Communities: Environmental Health Criteria 59, *Principles for evaluating health risks from chemicals during infancy and early childhood: the need for a special approach,* Geneva, 1986, World Health Organization.
33. Janerich DT et al: Lung cancer and exposure to tobacco smoke in the household, *N Engl J Med* 323:632, 1990.
34. Joubert L, Seidman H, Selikoff IJ: Mortality experience of family contacts of asbestos factory workers, *Ann NY Acad Sci* 43:416, 1991.
35. Kehrl HR et al: Ozone exposure increases respiratory epithelial permeability in humans, *Am Rev Respir Dis* 135:1124, 1987.

36. Kinney PL, Ware JH, Spengler JD: Short-term pulmonary function change in association with ozone levels, *Am Rev Resp Dis* 139:56, 1989.
37. Koenig JG et al: Acute effects of 0.12 ppm ozone or 0.12 ppm nitrogen dioxide on pulmonary function in healthy and asthmatic adolescents, *Am Rev Respir Dis,* 132:648, 1985.
38. Koenig JQ et al: Prior exposure to ozone potentiates subsequent response to sulfur dioxide in adolescent asthmatic subjects, *Am Rev Respir Dis* 141:377, 1990.
39. Koenig JQ, Covert DS, Pierson WE: Effects of inhalation of acidic compounds on pulmonary function in allergic adolescent subjects, *Environ Health Perspect* 79:173, 1989.
40. Koenig JQ, Pierson WE, Horike M: The effects of inhaled sulfuric acid on pulmonary function in adolescent asthmatics, *Am Rev Respir Dis* 128:221, 1983.
41. Koren HS et al: Ozone-induced inflammation in the lower airways of human subjects, *Am Rev Resp Dis* 139:407, 1989.
42. Kreit JW et al: Ozone-induced changes in pulmonary function and bronchial responsiveness in asthmatics, *J Appl Physiol* 66:217, 1989.
43. Lebowitz MD, Collins L, Holberg CL: Time series analyses of respiratory responses to indoor and outdoor environmental phenomena, *Environ Res* 43:332, 1987.
44. Linn WS et al: Health effects of ozone exposure in asthmatics, *Am Rev Resp Dis,* 117:835, 1978.
45. Lioy PJ et al: Persistence of peak flow decrement in children following ozone exposures exceeding the National Ambient Air Quality Standard, *J Air Pollut Contr Assoc* 35:1068, 1985.
46. Lippmann M: Health effects of ozone: a critical review, *J Air Pollut Control Assoc* 39:672, 1989.
47. Martinez FD, Cline M, Burrows B: Increased incidence of asthma in children of smoking mothers, *Pediatrics* 89:21, 1992.
48. McDonnell WF et al: Respiratory responses of vigorously exercising children to 0.12 ppm ozone exposure, *Am Rev Respir Dis* 132:875, 1985.
49. McDonnell WF et al: Pulmonary effects of ozone exposure during exercise: dose-response characteristics, *J Appl Physiol* 54:1345, 1983.
50. Molfino NA et al: Effect of low concentrations of ozone on inhaled allergen responses in asthmatic subjects, *Lancet* 338:199, 1991.
51. Morris K et al: Wood-burning stoves and lower respiratory tract infection in American Indian children, *Am J Dis Child* 144:105, 1990.
52. Munir AKM et al: Allergens in school dust. 1. The amount of the major cat (Fel d I) and dog (Can f I) allergens in dust from Swedish schools is high enough to probably cause perennial symptoms in most children with asthma who are sensitized to cat and dog, *J Allergy Clin Immunol* 91:1067, 1993.
53. National Research Council: *Environmental tobacco smoke: measuring exposures and assessing health effects,* Washington, DC, 1986, National Academy Press.
54. National Research Council: *Measuring lead exposure in infants, children and other sensitive populations,* Washington, DC, 1993, National Academy Press.
55. Neuberger JS et al: Diminished air quality and health problems in a Kansas City, Kansas, elementary school, *J School Health* 61:439, 1991.
56. Osebold JW, Gershwin LJ, Zee YC: Studies on the enhancement of allergic lung sensitization by inhalation of ozone and sulfuric acid aerosol, *J Environ Pathol Toxicol* 3:221, 1988.
57. Ostro BD et al: Indoor air pollution and asthma; results from a panel study, *Am J Respir Crit Care Med* 149:1400, 1994.
58. Ostro BD et al: Asthmatic responses to airborne acid aerosols, *Am J Public Health* 81:694, 1991.
59. Pellizzari ED et al: The TEAM study: personal exposures to toxic substances in air, drinking water, and breath of 400 residents of New Jersey, North Carolina, and North Dakota, *Environ Res* 43:290, 1987.
60. Phalen RF et al: Postnatal enlargement of human tracheobronchial airways and implications for particle deposition, *Anat Rec* 212:368, 1985.
61. Pope CA, Dockery DW: Acute health effects of PM_{10} pollution on symptomatic and asymptomatic children, *Amer Rev Respir Dis* 145:1123, 1992.
62. Pope CA III et al: Respiratory health and PM_{10} pollution: a daily time series analysis, *Am Rev Respir Dis* 144:668, 1991.
63. Pope CA III: Respiratory disease associated with community air pollution and a steel mill, Utah Valley, *Am J Public Health* 79:623, 1989.
64. Ransom MR, Pope CA III: Elementary school absences and PM_{10} pollution in Utah Valley, *Environ Res* 58:204, 1992.
65. Samet JM: Indoor radon and lung cancer: estimating the risks, *West J Med* 156:25, 1992.
66. Schoendorf KC, Kiely JL: Relationship of sudden infant death syndrome to maternal smoking during and after pregnancy, *Pediatrics* 90:905, 1992.
67. Schoettlin CE, Landau E: Air pollution and asthmatic attacks in the Los Angeles area, *Pub Health Rep,* 76:545, 1961.
68. Seltzer J et al: O_3-induced change in bronchial reactivity to methacholine and airway inflammation in humans, *J Appl Physiol* 60:1321, 1986.
69. Sherwin RP, Richters V: Centriacinar region (CAR) disease in the lungs of young adults: a preliminary report. In Berglund RL, Lawson DR, McKee DJ, eds: *Tropospheric ozone and the environment,* Pittsburg, Pa, 1991, Air & Waste Management Association.
70. Spektor DM et al: Effects of ambient ozone on respiratory function in active, normal children, *Am Rev Respir Dis* 137:313, 1988.
71. Spektor DM et al: Effects of ambient ozone on respiratory function in healthy adults exercising outdoors, *Am Rev Respir Dis* 138:821, 1988.
72. Spektor DM et al: Effects of single- and multiday ozone exposures on respiratory function in active normal children, *Environ Res* 55:107, 1991.
73. Spektor DM, Yen BM, Lippmann M: Effect of concentration and cumulative exposure of inhaled sulfuric acid on tracheobronchial particle clearance in healthy humans, *Environ Health Perspect* 79:167, 1989.
74. Spier CE et al: Activity patterns in elementary and high school students exposed to oxidant pollution, *J Exposure Anal Environ Epidemiol* 2:227, 1992.
75. Sporik R, Platt-Mills TAE: Epidemiology of dust-mite-related disease, *Exp Appl Acarol* 16:141, 1992.
76. Thurlbeck WM: Growth, aging and adaptation. In Murray JF, Nadel JA, eds: *Textbook of respiratory medicine,* Philadelphia, 1988, WB Saunders, pp 37-46.
77. Thurston GD et al: A multi-year study of air pollution and respiratory hospital admissions in three New York state metropolitan areas; results for 1988 and 1989 summers, *J Exposure Anal Environ Epidemiol* 2:429, 1992.
78. U.S. Department of Health and Human Services: *The health consequences of involuntary smoking. A report of the Surgeon General,* PHS Publication No. CDC 87-8398, Washington, DC, 1986, U.S. Government Printing Office.
79. U.S. Environmental Protection Agency: *National air quality and emissions trends report, 1991,* publication no. 450-R92-001, Research Triangle Park, NC, 1992.
80. U.S. Environmental Protection Agency: Air quality criteria for oxides of nitrogen, 3 vols, publication no. EPA/600/8-91/049aA-cA, Research Triangle Park, NC, 1991.
81. U.S. Environmental Protection Agency: *Respiratory health effects of passive smoking: lung cancer and other disorders,* publication no. EPA/600/6-90/006F, Washington, DC, 1992.
82. U.S. Environmental Protection Agency, U.S. Department of Health and Human Services, U.S. Centers for Disease Control: *A citizen's guide to radon,* ed 2, publication no. 402-K92-001, Washington, DC, 1992, U.S. Government Printing Office.
83. Utell MJ, Morrow PE, Hyde RW: Airway reactivity to sulfate and sulfuric acid aerosols in normal and asthmatic subjects, *J Air Pollut Control Assoc,* 34:931, 1984.
84. Vaughan TL et al: Formaldehyde and cancers of the pharynx, sinus and nasal cavity: II. Residential exposures, *Int J Cancer* 38: 685, 1986.

85. Ware JH et al: Effects of sulfur oxides and suspended particles on respiratory health of preadolescent children, *Am Rev Respir Dis* 133:834, 1986.
86. Warner JA: Environmental allergen exposure in homes and schools, *Clin Exp Allergy* 22:1044, 1992.
87. Warren DL, Last JA: Synergistic interaction of ozone and respirable aerosols in rat lungs. III. Ozone and sulfuric acid aerosol, *Toxicol Appl Pharmacol* 88:203, 1987.
88. Whittemore AW, Korn EL: Asthma and air pollution in the Los Angeles area, *Am J Public Health,* 70:687, 1980.
89. Wohl MEB, Mead J: Age as a factor in respiratory disease. In Chernick V, Kendig EL, eds: *Kendig's disorders of the respiratory tract in children,* Philadelphia, 1990, WB Saunders, pp 175-182.
90. Yanai M, Ohrui T. Aikawa T: Ozone increases susceptibility to antigen inhalation in allergic dogs, *J Appl Physiol* 68:2267, 1990.
91. Zwick H et al: Effects of ozone on the respiratory health, allergic sensitization, and cellular immune system in children, *Am Rev Respir Dis* 144:1075, 1991.

Chapter 34

POISONING CAUSED BY HOUSEHOLD PRODUCTS

Ilene Anderson
Susan Kim

Nontoxic products
Personal hygiene products
Soaps and detergents
Bleach
Caustics
Hydrocarbons
Methanol
Ethylene glycol
Pesticides
Rodenticides
    Anticoagulants
    Strychnine

In a highly industrialized society, homes are filled with household products designed to make our lives easier and more pleasant. Given the ready availability of a vast array of products for home use, accidental or intentional poisoning by these agents seem almost inevitable. In 1993 over 1.8 million human poisoning exposures were reported to the poison control centers in the United States. Of these, 92% of the incidences occurred in the home. Children under the age of 5 were involved in about 60% of the cases. As a group, cleaning substances were cited as agents most frequently involved in human poisoning exposures. Cosmetics were the third most involved group.[47] Fortunately, the vast majority of these exposures are benign, producing little or no symptoms. However, some inappropriate exposures to products around the home carry a profound risk of serious morbidity and mortality.

When assessing the degree of danger posed by a poisoning exposure, getting a thorough and accurate history is of utmost importance. This cannot be emphasized enough. As is often stated, the dose makes the poison, so that a potentially toxic agent may not necessarily produce serious illness. Also, a product may be innocuous in one setting but highly dangerous in another; for example, ingestion of a mouthful of lighter fluid versus aspiration of the same amount produces markedly different outcomes. Getting an accurate history and recognizing the toxicity of the products involved will allow for appropriate treatment and, just as important, prevent overly aggressive interventions.

In this review of household products we discuss the toxicity of several groups of products commonly found around the home. They include the following: nontoxic products, personal hygiene products, soaps and detergents, bleach, caustics, hydrocarbons, methanol, ethylene glycol, pesticides, and rodenticides.

NONTOXIC PRODUCTS

The home contains many items that are considered nontoxic. Products classified as nontoxic possess no pharmacologic activity in the body in doses likely to be encountered. The items listed in the box are not expected to result in any significant harm upon ingestion. However, the taste or texture of the product may result in gagging or transient vomiting. Recognition of these items may avoid unwarranted mental stress as well as overtreatment of the patient. However, even nontoxic items may pose serious danger in some circumstances: for example, massive ingestions, pulmonary aspiration, choking hazard, foreign body obstruction, or ocular exposure. Proper management of these cases requires a thorough, reliable history. Most cases of nontoxic product ingestion may be managed by reassurance alone. A small

Air freshners	Fingernail polish	Putty
Aluminum foil	Floral preservatives	Rouge
Antiperspirants	Glow stick jewelry	Rust
Ashes, cigarette/fireplace/wood	Glue traps	Saccharin
Calamine lotion	Gypsum	Sheet rock
Candles	Hydrocortisone cream	Shoe polish
Caulk	Incense	Silica gel
Chalk	Indelible markers (without aniline dyes)	Silly Putty
Charcoal	Ink (without aniline dyes)	Simethicone
Charcoal briquettes	Etch-A-Sketch	Stamp pad ink
Cigarette filter tips (unsmoked)	Kitty litter	Soil
Clay	Latex paint	Spackle
Corticosteroids	Magic markers	Starch
Crayons	Make-up (foundation)	Styrofoam
Cyanoacrylate glues	Mascara	Sunscreen products
Chewing gum	Matches (<3 paper books)	Teething rings (fluid may have bacterial growth)
Deodorants	Mylar balloon	
Desiccants	Pencils (graphite)	Thermometers (mercury or phthlates/alcohol)
Disposable diapers	Photographs	
Erasers	Plaster	Water color paints
Felt-tip markers	Play-Doh	Zinc oxide ointment

amount of fluid may be offered to the patient to minimize any possible gastrointestinal upset.

PERSONAL HYGIENE PRODUCTS

A potpourri of personal hygiene products can be found in the typical American home. Many of these products are customarily left out on bathroom counters, allowing easy access to small children. These products are briefly discussed in Table 34-1, which focuses on the common formulations, toxicity following accidental exposures, and appropriate management. Unless otherwise stated, treatment usually entails administration of a small amount of fluid to minimize oral mucosa irritation. Ocular exposures require a 15-minute irrigation using cool or lukewarm tap water. Medical evaluation is indicated if the patient has persistent ocular complaints.

SOAPS AND DETERGENTS

Soaps are the salts of fatty acids produced from the addition of alkali to naturally occurring fats and oils. Detergents contain surface-active agents, or surfactants, which are designed to lower the surface tension of water, reducing the insoluble precipitates formed by soap and minerals in the water. Surfactants are divided into four categories based on their molecular charges: anionic, nonionic, cationic, and amphoteric.

Anionic and cationic surfactants contain negatively and positively charged ions, respectively. Examples of anionic surfactants, which are the most commonly used surfactants in commercial detergents, include alkyl sodium sulfate and sodium and lauryl sulfate. Most cationic surfactants are built upon a backbone of quaternary ammonium compounds, of which benzalkonium chloride is a common example. Both anionic and cationic surfactants possess irritant properties. Cationic surfactants, however, can cause caustic burns at higher concentrations (>10%).[74] Nonionic detergents are electrically neutral chains of sulfates, alcohols, or sulfonates. These produce less local irritation than anionic surfactants. Amphoteric surfactants, which contain both anionic and cationic moieties, are primarily used in industrial settings.

Anionic and nonionic surfactants are extensively used in products available in the home, including liquid and powder laundry detergents, dishwashing liquids, shampoos, and powdered cleansers. Some "heavy-duty" laundry detergents and most automatic dishwasher soaps contain builders to improve wetting and emulsifying properties. The most common builder was inorganic phosphates, until environmental concerns led to the use of other, more caustic salts, such as carbonates and silicates. These "low-phosphate" detergents are more likely to produce alkaline injury,[65] which will be discussed in detail in the next section. However, despite their alkaline nature, ingestion of liquid or powder automatic dishwasher detergents rarely results in burns.[41,79] Cationic detergents, many of which have bacteriostatic properties, are found in disinfectants, fabric softeners, and swimming pool algicides.

Ingestion of nonionic or anionic detergents typically produces self-limiting mucous membrane irritation. Immediate spontaneous emesis is common. Diarrhea and abdominal pain may also occur. Large ingestions may produce intractable vomiting, diarrhea, and hematemesis. Systemic toxicity is rare, except for cationic detergents. Very large ingestion of phosphate-containing products may produce hypocalcemia and tetany. Systemic absorption of cationic detergents

Table 34-1. Personal hygiene products

Product	General formulation	Comments
Artificial nail glue removers	Acetonitrile	Not commonly found in the home but rather at professional beauty salons. Cyanide is formed after ingestion. Death has been reported following small ingestions. Prompt medical evaluation is critical for all exposures.[14]
Baby powder	Talc	Aspiration pneumonitis if inhaled. Ingestion is nontoxic.
Baby wipes	Alcohol, lanolin	No effect expected due to the small amount available.
Bath oil beads	Oils, nonionic surfactants	Mild gastritis possible.
Betadine solution	Povidone-iodine 10% (1% available iodine)	Iodine toxicity is rare, with accidental ingestions due to poor gastrointestinal absorption.
Diaper pail deodorizers	Paradichlorobenzene	Gastritis possible.
Diaper rash creams/ointments	Lanolin, zinc oxide, petrolatum, cod liver oil	Possible laxative effect.
Hair conditioners	Cationic detergents	Nausea, vomiting, and rarely diarrhea may occur.
Hair dyes	Phenylenediamine may be present in brown or black hair dyes	Immediate or delayed ocular hypersensitivity reactions may produce conjunctival hyperemia, uveitis, and keratitis. Corneal necrosis has occurred. Dermatitis possible with skin exposure.[52]
Hair shampoos	Anionic nonionic surfactants	Nausea, vomiting, and rarely diarrhea may occur.
Hydrogen peroxide	Hydrogen peroxide	Common household formulation is 3%. Ingestion results in vomiting and burping. Higher concentrations (>20%) may be caustic.
Insect repellents	DEET (diethyltoluamide)	Sudden onset seizures.[71]
Lipstick	Waxes, oils	Diarrhea if more than one stick is ingested.
Nail polish	Toluene, xylene, acetone, phthalates	Toxicity is unlikely following ingestion, since the available amount of these solvents is small. Nausea and headache may accompany inhalation.
Nail polish remover	Ethyl acetate, acetone, isopropanol	Pediatric patients rarely ingest a toxic dose. Administer fluid and observe for 1 hour. If persistent vomiting or intoxication occurs, refer the patient to an emergency department.
Perfume, colognes, hairsprays, mouthwashes	Ethanol 15%-90%	Toxicity is rare following pediatric accidental ingestion. Administer juice; persistent vomiting or intoxication occurring within 1 hour warrants medical evaluation.
Rubbing alcohol	Isopropyl alcohol	Toxicity is rare following pediatric accidental ingestion. Administer fluid; persistent vomiting or intoxication occurring within 1 hour warrants medical evaluation.
Spermicides	Nonoxynol 9	Mild gastritis possible.
Sunscreen lotions	PABA, oils	Possible allergic reactions.
Toothpaste, tooth powders	Fluoride	Doses 3-5 mg fluoride/kg may result in gastritis. Administer calcium (Tums®). Doses greater than 5 mg/kg may result in cellular toxicity, and medical evaluation is indicated.

can cause restlessness, confusion, respiratory paralysis, and hypotension.[1]

In the vast majority of accidental poisonings with soaps and detergents, giving small amounts of water or milk to drink is adequate first aid. Emesis should not be induced. Gastric lavage should be performed for large intentional ingestions of cationic, corrosive, or phosphorus-containing detergents. For patients with persistent vomiting, dysphagia, or oropharyngeal burns suggestive of caustic injury, endoscopy may be needed.

BLEACH

Most household bleaches contain less than 5% sodium hypochlorite, which causes moderate mucosal irritation but usually not serious corrosive burns. Liquid bleach solutions are titrated to a moderately alkaline pH (10-12) to enhance stabilization of hypochlorite salts. Industrial bleaches or liquid chlorine mildew removers can contain much higher concentrations of sodium or calcium hypochlorites. "Bleach" also refers to other bleaching agents such as sodium perborate, sodium peroxide, and oxalic acids. Therefore, careful history taking, including the exact brand name, formulation, and ingredients, is essential.

Ingestion of household bleach produces rapid onset of nausea, vomiting, and less commonly diarrhea. For accidental ingestion of one to two mouthfuls of bleach, immediate oral dilution with milk or water is adequate. For large suicidal ingestions, gastric lavage should be considered, since untreated massive ingestions may lead to partial-thickness chemical burns and systemic hyperchloremic metabolic acidosis.[75]

Complaints about inhalation of bleach fumes are common, especially when bleach is mixed with other cleaners. Sodium hypochlorite fumes typically release small amounts of hypochlorous acid and chlorine gas, though the concentrations are too low to cause anything more than eye and throat irritation. However, mixing hypochlorite solution with acidic products, such as vinegar or toilet bowl cleaners, immediately liberates chlorine gas.[26] Similar problems result when a mildew remover and acid-containing products such as Shower Power or Lime Away are used together in the shower. Addition of ammonia to hypochlorite solutions creates chloramine gases, which form hydrochlorous acid and nascent oxygen upon contact with mucous membranes.

Exposure to chlorine or chloramine gases, especially in small, poorly ventilated rooms, can produce eye irritation, nausea, vomiting, coughing, hoarseness, wheezing, and stridor. The respiratory symptoms may progress to bronchitis, chemical pneumonitis, and rarely pulmonary edema.[64] Immediate cessation of exposure is of primary importance. In most cases respiratory symptoms resolve gradually without specific treatment. Some patients with persistent complaints have been considered to suffer from reactive airways dysfunction (RADs). Patients whose symptoms persist or worsen generally benefit from administration of humidified oxygen and/or inhaled bronchodilators.

CAUSTICS

A large number of chemicals produce corrosive effects. The discussion in this section is limited to those that can be broadly classified into acids or alkalies. Strongly caustic agents are readily available in the home for a variety of uses. For instance, toilet bowl cleaners, some drain cleaners, and automobile battery fluids contain high concentrations of hydrochloric or sulfuric acids. Muriatic acid, used in swimming pools, is 10% to 35% hydrochloric acid. Hydrofluoric acid is found in wire and spoke cleaners and rust removers.

Exceedingly strong alkali material is found in drain cleaners, which can be up to 100% sodium hydroxide. Automatic dishwasher detergents or low-phosphate laundry detergents contain alkali builders such as sodium metasilicate, sodium silicate, and sodium carbonate. Household ammonia contains ammonium hydroxide in concentrations ranging from 3% to 10%. Although rarely a problem, higher ranges can produce burns.[40]

Upon contact with tissues, acids cause an immediate coagulative-type necrosis with formation of scars (eschars) that tend to limit further damage. An exception is hydrofluoric acid, in which the fluoride ion, not the hydrogen, produces penetrating necrosis by combining with calcium and magnesium in tissues. Alkalis produce liquefaction necrosis by saponifying fats and proteins, which allows for continued penetration of deeper tissues and severe injury. Button batteries, the small disk-shaped batteries used in watches, calculators, and cameras, contain caustics such as sodium hydroxide, which can cause local corrosive injury.[48]

The extent of injury depends on several factors, such as the type of substance, volume, concentration, and contact time. In general, products with pH <2 or >12.5 are associated with tissue injury. The more concentrated the solution, the greater the probability of injury, regardless of other factors. And not surprisingly, the larger the volume and longer the contact time with tissues, the more severe and extensive the injury will be.

Ingestion of corrosives typically causes severe pain in the throat, chest, or abdomen, resulting in vomiting, drooling, and dysphasia. Upper airway obstruction may occur, manifest as aphonia, hoarseness, dyspnea, and stridor. Crystalline solid corrosives produce mainly throat and esophageal damage, whereas liquids are more likely to cause stomach and upper intestinal injury as well.[54,81] Perforation of the esophagus or stomach may occur, the risk being the greatest within the first 72 hours. Manifestations of perforation include severe chest or abdominal pain, hematemesis, tachycardia, shock, pancreatitis, or signs of peritonitis. Immediate surgery and extensive repair may be necessary. For stable patients with symptoms, endoscopy must be performed to determine the extent of injury. Whether or not asymptomatic patients need endoscopic exams is controversial.[15,19] Although esophageal or gastric burns are unlikely if the patient is completely asymptomatic, a small number of patients may have injury in the absence of oropharyngeal burns.[32] However, the extent of injury in these patients is likely to be limited. Deep or circumferential burns frequently lead to permanent scarring strictures and obstruction.

Systemic toxicity following caustic ingestions can be severe. With acid exposures, systemic acidosis, hemolysis, and shock may be seen.[13,70] Oxalic and hydrofluoric acids can cause life-threatening arrhythmias secondary to severe hypocalcemia. Hydrofluoric acid also produces hyperkalemia and hypomagnesemia, which contributes to the arrhythmogenic effects of the acid.[16] Systemic absorption of phenol (carbolic acid), which is used commonly as a disinfectant and chemical exfoliant, can cause seizures, coma, and arrhythmias.[49]

Treatment of ingested caustic depends greatly on the history, the nature of the caustic, and clinical findings. In general, giving one to two glasses of water or milk to drink is a safe and effect first aid. Careful administration of fluids orally helps to reduce contact time and increase dilution of the caustic. Emesis must not be induced, since vomiting reexposes tissues to the corrosive and increases the area of damage. Although controversial, gastric lavage following caustic ingestions may be beneficial, especially for liquids. Administration of activated charcoal should be avoided, since it may interfere with endoscopic exam. Endoscopy of symptomatic patients helps determine the extent of injury and identify those at risk of perforating. Although corticosteroids are thought to reduce the risk of stricture formation, the evidence is lacking, and routine use is discouraged.[2]

Dermal exposure to caustic materials requires initial copious irrigation with water. Specific treatment is not required except for hydrofluoric acid. Because the fluoride ion readily penetrates skin and causes deep-tissue destruction, topical application of calcium gluconate or magnesium sulfate helps bind the fluoride ion and limit the injury.[22] Hydrofluoric concentrations of <10% generally do not produce immediate pain but could still cause extensive tissue damage. Thus early recognition of potential injury and institution of appropriate therapy averts delayed complications. More severe injury may require subcutaneous injection or arterial perfusion of calcium gluconate.[3] Ocular exposures to caustics require immediate and profuse irrigation with water, and if readily available, saline; continuous irrigation for at least 15 minutes; and further treatment and examination in the emergency department.

HYDROCARBONS

There is a large number of household products that contain hydrocarbons, such as pine oil cleaners, furniture polishes, lubricants, lamp oils, gasoline, motor oil, turpentine, spot removers, fabric protectants, and paint thinner. Many household insecticides also contain hydrocarbon solvents. Hydrocarbons refer to organic compounds comprised of hydrogen and carbon atoms. Hydrocarbons have several classifications, including aliphatic (straight-chain), aromatic (containing a benzene ring), halogenated (containing a halogen, such as bromine, chlorine, or fluorine), and terpene (derived from pine).

Aliphatic hydrocarbons rarely result in systemic toxicity following accidental ingestion because of their poor gastrointestinal absorption. In contrast, aromatic, halogenated, and many other substituted hydrocarbons are more likely to result in systemic toxicity after acute ingestion. The acute oral dose for hydrocarbons and turpentine in humans remains unclear. Bratton et al[9] showed that gastric administration of 12 ml/kg of naphtha in animals did not produce any systemic toxicity. Erickson et al[23] reported an adult patient who received medical treatment after allegedly ingesting 250 to 500 ml of pine oil. Mild respiratory distress was the only complication.[23] However, aspiration of minute amounts may result in chemical pneumonitis.

Chemical pneumonitis is the most serious complication following ingestion of a hydrocarbon. Animal studies and roentgenographic findings indicate that the pulmonary complications are caused by aspiration of hydrocarbons, not by gastrointestinal absorption.[27,80] Hydrocarbons that pose the highest risk of aspiration possess low surface tension, low viscosity, and high volatility. These qualities enable the chemical to spread rapidly over pulmonary tissue and to penetrate deep into the distal airways.[80] Gasoline, kerosene, mineral seal oil, and naphtha pose a high aspiration risk. In contrast, mineral oil and motor oil have high viscosities and therefore pose a low aspiration risk.

If pulmonary aspiration occurs, the victim will usually experience immediate gagging, coughing, and choking. Over the next 6 hours tachypnea, dyspnea, chest pain/tightness, and possibly fever may develop. If the product has not been aspirated, the primary systems affected are the gastrointestinal tract and the central nervous system. Immediate burning of the throat, nausea, vomiting, abdominal discomfort, and burping is experienced following ingestion. These symptoms may persist for several days. Lethargy is the most common central nervous system effect, with a small percentage of patients developing coma and seizures.[61] Dermal exposure may result in chemical dermatitis. First- and second-degree burns have been reported after extended dermal exposure (more than 20 minutes) to kerosene.[56] Transient corneal irritation is generally the only effect following ocular exposure to hydrocarbons.

When hydrocarbons are inhaled in the vapor form, primarily for abuse, the principal complications involve the central nervous system and the myocardium.[63] Hydrocarbons sensitize the myocardium to endogenous catecholamines (epinephrine and norepineprine). Cardiac arrhythmias and sudden death have been reported following inhalation of gasoline fumes[4] and chlorinated hydrocarbons.[39]

Patients who are asymptomatic or who have initial symptoms that quickly resolve can be safely observed at home for symptoms of delayed pneumonitis.[50] Patients with symptoms consistent with aspiration (coughing, shortness of breath, chest tightness/pain) should be immediately referred to the emergency department. All patients who demonstrate signs of respiratory compromise should be admitted for observation and treatment. Supportive measures such as oxygen, bronchodilators, intubation, and PEEP should be instituted as needed.

The role of gastrointestinal decontamination is dependent on the type of hydrocarbon ingested. Hydrocarbons that are unlikely to result in systemic toxicity (gasoline, kerosene, naphtha, mineral spirits, and mineral seal oil) should not receive any gastrointestinal decontamination, which may increase the risk of aspiration.[46] In contrast, patients who have ingested hydrocarbons that are likely to result in systemic toxicity, such as halogenated hydrocarbons (trichloroethane, chlordane, carbon tetrachloride), aromatic hydrocarbons (toluene, xylene, benzene), or hydrocarbon pesticide mixtures (such as Diazinon) should receive gastric lavage and activated charcoal. Care should be taken to protect the airway. Ipecac syrup is generally contraindicated due to the risk of aspiration and sudden onset of coma and seizures.

Corticosteroids and prophylactic antibiotics have not been shown to be clinically efficacious in treating hydrocarbon-induced aspiration pneumonitis.[51,67]

METHANOL

Methanol is produced from the distillation of wood products; hence the name wood alcohol. Methanol is a common ingredient in windshield washing solutions, paint removers, "canned heat," duplicating fluids, and solvents. Since it is less expensive than ethanol but still results in an initial inebriation, it is sometimes used as an alcohol substitute by alcoholics. It is the metabolites of methanol (formaldehyde and formic acid) that are responsible for the delayed life-threatening symptoms of toxicity, not methanol itself (see Fig. 34-1). Methanol and ethanol compete for the enzyme alcohol dehydrogenase. The preference of this enzyme to

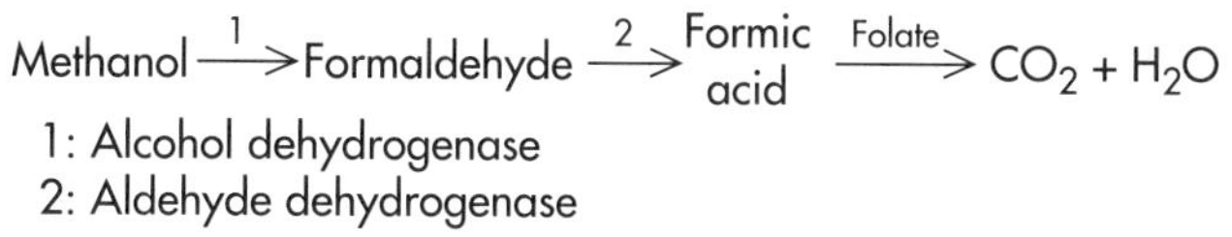

Methanol $\xrightarrow{1}$ Formaldehyde $\xrightarrow{2}$ Formic acid $\xrightarrow{\text{Folate}}$ $CO_2 + H_2O$

1: Alcohol dehydrogenase
2: Aldehyde dehydrogenase

Fig. 34-1. Methanol metabolism.

metabolize ethanol forms the basis for ethanol therapy in treatment.

Methanol is rapidly absorbed from the gastrointestinal tract, then slowly metabolized in the liver to formaldehyde and formic acid. Within 2 hours of ingestion, patients experience initial inebriation, and laboratory analysis will reveal an elevated osmolar gap. After a latency period of 12 to 24 hours, severe anion gap metabolic acidosis, visual disturbances, blindness, seizures, coma, and death may occur. Coingestion of ethanol will delay the onset of these symptoms even longer. The lethal dose of methanol has been estimated to range from 60 to 240 ml. Fatality has been reported following the ingestion of 15 ml of a 40% solution.[6] It is important to realize that just a few milliliters of 100% methanol may result in serious toxicity in a 10-kg child.

All significant ingestions of methanol should be referred to an emergency department for initial laboratory analysis and gastrointestinal decontamination procedures. Since stat methanol levels are rarely available, diagnosis is usually based on a history of the exposure, elevated osmolar and anion gaps, and clinical presentation. An osmolar gap as small as 5 to 10 mOsm/kg may indicate a toxic methanol level. Methanol serum levels greater than 20 mg/dl are considered toxic, and levels greater than 40 to 60 mg/dl may result in fatality if not aggressively treated. However, a methanol level of zero and a normal osmolar gap in a severely intoxicated patient does not rule out a serious intoxication, because all the methanol may have already been metabolized to formate.

Treatment consists of evaluation of the patient's risk, gastric lavage or ipecac syrup to minimize absorption, administration of ethanol to prevent the formation of toxic metabolites, administration of folate to promote the metabolism of formic acid to nontoxic metabolites,[57] and hemodialysis to remove methanol and its toxic metabolites from the serum.[30] Activated charcoal is ineffective in absorbing methanol from the gastrointestinal tract and may delay the absorption of orally administered ethanol.[58,78] Methanol serum levels greater than 20 mg/dl are considered toxic and indicate a need to institute folate and ethanol therapy. Symptoms of severe poisoning or methanol levels greater than 40 mg/dl indicate a need to institute hemodialysis as well.

ETHYLENE GLYCOL

Ethylene glycol is found in numerous commercial products but most commonly as the main ingredient in antifreeze. The sweet taste and euphoric effects contribute to ethylene glycol's role as an alcohol substitute by alcoholics, and as a

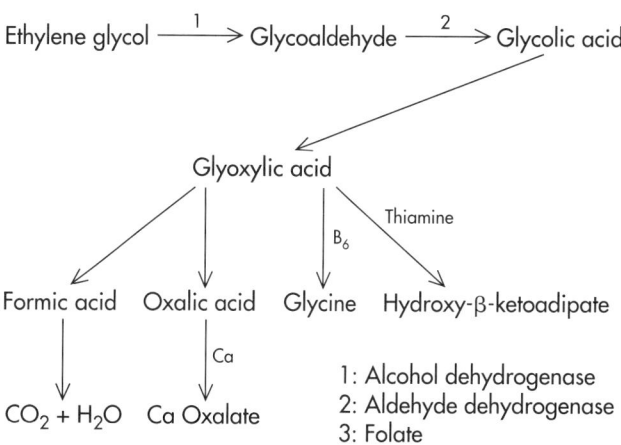

Fig. 34-2. Ethylene glycol metabolism.

culprit in pediatric and veterinary poisonings. The toxicity of ethylene glycol is very similar to methanol in that the metabolic products are more toxic than the parent compound (see Fig. 34-2). Glycolic,[37] glyoxylic, oxalic, formic, and lactic acids are responsible for the anion gap metabolic acidosis. Calcium oxalate crystals form when oxalic acid combines with calcium. These crystals deposit throughout the body, resulting in soft tissue destruction, hypocalcemia, and organ dysfunction. Like methanol, ethanol and ethylene glycol compete for the enzyme alcohol dehydrogenase. The preference of this enzyme for ethanol over ethylene glycol forms the basis for ethanol therapy in treatment.

Consumption of ethylene glycol results in initial inebriation and gastritis within the first 2 hours. After a latency period of 4 to 12 hours, hyperventilation, cardiac arrhythmias, renal dysfunction, coma, seizures, hypocalcemia, and metabolic anion gap acidosis may occur.[25] Coingestion of ethanol will further delay these symptoms. Renal failure is usually reversible but may require dialysis for 2 to 3 weeks. The estimated lethal dose of ethylene glycol is 1.5 ml/kg. Like methanol, it is important to remember that just a few milliliters of 95% ethylene glycol may result in serious toxicity in a 10-kg child.

All significant ingestions of ethylene glycol should be referred to an emergency department for initial laboratory analysis and gastrointestinal decontamination procedures. Since stat ethylene glycol levels are rarely available, diagnosis is usually based on a history of the exposure, elevated osmolar and anion gaps, presence of oxalate or hippurate crystals in the urine, and clinical presentation.[12] An osmolar gap greater than 10 mOsm/kg may indicate a toxic serum level of ethylene glycol. If antifreeze is the agent involved, then a Wood's lamp may be used to determine fluorescein presence in the urine. The absence of crystals or fluorescein in the urine does not rule out a significant ethylene glycol ingestion. Ethylene glycol serum levels > 20 to 50 mg/dl are usually associated with serious intoxication.

Treatment consists of gastric lavage or ipecac syrup to

minimize absorption, administration of ethanol to prevent the formation of toxic metabolites, administration of folate, thiamine, and pyridoxine (B_6)[28] to promote the metabolism of formic acid and glyoxylic acid to nontoxic metabolites, and hemodialysis to remove ethylene glycol and its toxic metabolites from the serum. Activated charcoal has not been shown to be efficacious in absorbing ethylene glycol, and it may delay the absorption of orally administered ethanol. Ethylene glycol levels greater than 20 mg/dl or symptoms of severe poisoning indicate a need to institute ethanol, folate, pyridoxine, thiamine, and hemodialysis.[60] Beware of rebound ethylene glycol levels after the completion of dialysis.

PESTICIDES

A wide variety of pesticides are available for home use. Some formulations are essentially nontoxic to humans whereas others are highly dangerous. This section is limited to agents classified as insecticides. The most commonly used insecticides for home or garden use can be divided into three groups: organophosphates, carbamates, and pyrethrins. Although most commercial brands of ant and roach killers contain less than 1% of the active insecticidal ingredients, some products for the garden are sold in concentrated forms that may be 50% or greater. These concentrated solutions present a significant poisoning hazard, since even a small accidental ingestion or inadvertent skin contact can result in serious toxicity. Ant baits or traps, which contain minute amounts of carbamates or organophosphates, almost never result in human poisoning.

Organophosphates and carbamates inactivate acetylcholinesterase enzymes by phosphorylation and carbamylation of the enzymes, respectively.[69] Organophosphates irreversibly bind acetylcholinesterases, and carbamates bind to them reversibly. Therefore initial signs and symptoms of toxicity from these insecticides are indistinguishable, although the duration of toxicity differs. By binding to acetylcholinesterases, these insecticides cause excessive accumulation of acetylcholine at muscarinic and nicotinic receptors and in the central nervous system.[35] Initial stimulation, then exhaustion, of the receptors produces a wide range of symptoms. Muscarinic (parasympathetic) manifestations include salivation, lacrimation, urination, and diarrhea (''SLUD''), along with vomiting, abdominal cramping, miosis, bradycardia, bronchorrhea, and bronchospasms. Nicotinic (ganglionic) effects include muscle fasciculation, tachycardia, and respiratory muscle paralysis. Among central nervous system effects are ataxia, seizures, and coma.[82]

The toxic doses needed to produce symptoms in man are crude estimations derived from animal data. Acutely toxic doses of pesticides are primarily determined by establishing the LD_{50} (dose needed to kill 50% of test animals) in a number of species, mainly rats and rabbits. Pesticides with LD_{50}s between 5 and 50 mg/kg are considered extremely toxic; between 50 and 5000 mg/kg they are moderately toxic. The following lists the LD_{50}s in rats of commonly used organophosphates and carbamates.[76]

ORGANOPHOSPHATES	mg/kg	CARBAMATES	mg/kg
Parathion	3	Aldicarb	0.9
Dichlorvos	25	Bendiocarb	34
Diazinon	66	Propopoxur	50
Malathion	2800	Carbaryl	500

Onset of symptoms after ingestion or inhalation is rapid, usually within the first 1 to 2 hours, and is often abrupt. Symptoms may be delayed for several hours following dermal exposure. Exceptions are very lipophilic organophosphates such as fenthion, which can have delayed onset of up to 5 days.[55] Respiratory paralysis left untreated can result in death quickly. Duration of toxicity varies widely, from a few hours for the more hydrophilic carbamates to up to several weeks to months for some lipophilic organophosphates.[7]

Treatment of organophosphate or carbamate exposure initially involves decontamination. Following dermal exposure, immediate removal of contaminated clothing and thorough washing of the affected area with soap and water are essential for reducing further absorption and for preventing secondary contamination of rescue personnel. For ingestions, syrup of ipecac *must not* be used, since loss of consciousness and seizures may occur concurrently with vomiting. Gastric lavage should be done for large ingestions. Since many insecticides are dissolved in hydrocarbon solvents, the airway needs to be protected to prevent aspiration, especially for lethargic or comatose patients. Activated charcoal should be given to help bind the toxins and decrease systemic absorption.

Antidotal treatment includes atropine and, for organophosphates, pralidoxime (2-PAM). Atropine reverses the muscarinic symptoms but does not affect nicotinic ones. Dosing is titrated to cessation of bronchorrhea or wheezing. Atropine often needs to be given repeatedly over the course of intoxication. For severe overdoses, cumulative doses of several grams are not uncommon.[29] Pralidoxime is a specific antidote that reverses organophosphate toxicity by reactivating phosphorylated cholinesterases and protecting the enzymes from further inhibition. Pralidoxime can dramatically reverse nicotinic symptoms such as muscle fasciculation and diaphragmatic weakness, and to a lesser degree, muscarinic effects. To be the most effective, pralidoxime needs to be given within the first 24 hours of the intoxication, before the cholinesterases are permanently ''aged'' by phosphorylation. However, therapy should not be withheld for those with delayed presentations if clinically appropriate. For adults, 1 to 2 gm of pralidoxime is given intravenously initially. The dose can be repeated every 4 to 6 hours as needed to treat recurrent symptoms.[72] For more serious overdoses requiring frequent dosing, continuous IV infusion of pralidoxime has been suggested.[24]

Use of pralidoxime for carbamate poisoning is controversial. Since carbamates reversibly bind to cholinesterases, "rescuing" the enzymes by using pralidoxime would not appear to be necessary. Some authors suggest that administration of pralidoxime for carbamate poisoning may be harmful, since it may worsen cholinesterase inhibition.[43] However, others have reported beneficial effects of pralidoxime following documented carbamate poisoning.[10,73] Since the initial presentations of organophosphate and carbamate toxicity are identical, pralidoxime probably should be used empirically when the identity of the intoxicant is unknown.

Pyrethrins are a class of insecticides derived from pyrethrum, the natural insecticide found in the chrysanthemum plant. Several synthetic pyrethrins, called pyrethroids, are used commercially, including allethrin, permethrin, and resmethrin. Pyrethrins are absorbed through the exoskeleton of arthropods and stimulate the nervous system. The mechanism of action is thought to involve delay in the closure of sodium channels of nerve cells, causing slow leakage of sodium at the end of depolarization. At high concentrations this effect is sufficiently large to depolarize the nerve membrane completely and block excitability. Paralysis and death follow.[62] Pyrethrins are usually formulated with piperonyl butoxide, which has little or no insecticidal activity but enhances the effects of pyrethrins by inhibiting pyrethrin's metabolism in arthropods.

Pyrethrins are widely used in the home as the active ingredients in flying insect killers, foggers, and pediculocides. Complaints after inhaling aerosolized insecticides are common. In nearly all cases, the symptoms, such as nausea, dizziness, headache, and coughing, are due to the solvents rather than the insecticides. The solvents, which typically comprise 80% to 90% of ready-to-use insecticide sprays and foggers, are primarily hydrocarbons and chlorinated hydrocarbons.

Although pyrethrins are potent mammalian neurotoxins, acute oral toxicity is low due to rapid hydrolysis of pyrethrins in the digestive tract and by liver microsomal esterases.[20] The oral LD_{50}s in rats range from several hundred or thousand mg/kg. However, natural pyrethrins are potent sensitizing agents, and susceptible individuals may exhibit allergic responses, including death. Reports of toxicity following ingestions are rare. A 21-year-old woman who ingested 30 ml of 2.5% (750 mg) of deltamethrin reportedly developed headache, muscle fasciculations, and seizures.[33] Accidental ingestion of pyrethrin-containing insecticides rarely requires aggressive treatment. Inhalational exposures can be treated simply by having the victim leave the area and breathe fresh air.

RODENTICIDES
Anticoagulants

The two most common rodenticides available for home use are the anticoagulants (both long- and short-acting) and strychnine. Examples of the long-acting anticoagulants (LAA) include brodifacoum, diphacinone, bromadiolone, chlorphacinone, and difenacoum. Brodifacoum is the most commonly utilized rodenticide today. Coumarin, a short-acting anticoagulant, is used less frequently as a rodenticide due to the growing numbers of resistant mice and rats. All of these agents exhibit their anticoagulant effect by preventing the activation of clotting factors II, VII, IX, and X via inhibition of vitamin K_1-2,3 epoxide reductase. Consequently, there is an accumulation of inactive clotting factor precursors resulting in anticoagulation.[44]

Chronic ingestion of coumarin is necessary for anticoagulation to occur. Doses as low as 0.2 mg/kg for 2 days have resulted in prolonged prothrombin times in children.[21] However, the long-acting anticoagulants such as brodifacoum require only a one-time ingestion to produce toxicity.[38] The minimum toxic dose of the LAA in humans is unknown. Adult cases resulting in anticoagulation involved large suicidal ingestions where the exact dose was difficult to obtain reliably. There is one case of a suicidal ingestion where a patient developed anticoagulation lasting 76 days after allegedly ingesting only 1 mg of brodifacoum.[17] Smolinske et al[66] reported eight pediatric patients with accidental LAA ingestions who developed slightly increased prothrombin times (1.04 to 1.44 times normal) without clinical symptoms of anticoagulation. Hemorrhage is the primary effect of these products following a significant ingestion. Manifestations include ecchymosis, gum and nasal bleeding, hemoptysis, hematuria, epistaxis, and melanotic stools.[77] Death has been reported after intracranial hemorrhage.[34,42]

The anticoagulant effect of both coumadin[18] and the long-acting anticoagulants are delayed 36 to 72 hours after ingestion.[66] However, their duration of action varies greatly. Coumadin's anticoagulant effect usually persists for only 4 to 5 days. In contrast, anticoagulation may persist for 2 to 8 months after a single ingestion of a long-acting anticoagulant.[36,45]

Diagnosis is determined by the history of ingestion, presence of clinical symptoms and elevation of the prothrombin time (PT), the partial thromboplastin time (PTT), and the International Normalized Ratio (INR). Since the onset of anticoagulation may be delayed, the prothrombin time should be monitored for a minimum of 48 hours after ingestion.

Treatment consists of gastrointestinal decontamination, Vitamin K_1, and fresh-frozen plasma. Small acute ingestions of coumarin or brodifacoum (<1 tsp of .005%) are not expected to result in toxicity, so treatment is rarely necessary. Induction of emesis with ipecac syrup may be used for children at home if initiated within 30 minutes of ingestion.[5,68] However, gut emptying should be avoided if the patient shows signs of active bleeding. Administer activated charcoal and cathartic to minimize absorption. Vitamin K_1 (phytonadione) is indicated if the patient has a prolonged prothrombin time or clinical symptoms of anticoagulation. Other forms of vitamin K such as vitamin K_3 (menadione) are ineffective. Vitamin K_1 should not be administered prophylactically in an asymptomatic patient because the prothrombin time may remain falsely normal for up to 5 days. Therefore, the required observation time of the patient will need to be lengthened from 2 to 5 days. Oral doses up to 400 mg a day have been required for anticoagulant reversal.[11] Lastly, fresh-frozen plasma is indicated for any patient showing signs of active bleeding.

Strychnine

Strychnine is an alkaloid prepared from the seed of the *Strychnos nux-vomica*. Today the only legitimate application of strychnine is as a rodenticide (primarily for gophers). The concentration available commercially is 0.5%, although higher concentrations are accessible to licensed pest control applicators. Strychnine is also utilized as an adulterant in illicit street drugs.

Strychnine competitively blocks the postsynaptic uptake of glycine, an inhibitory neurotransmitter, in the spinal cord and brainstem. Increased excitation occurs when normal glycine inhibition is disrupted.[53] Strychnine is rapidly absorbed from the gastrointestinal tract, resulting in symptoms within 15 to 30 minutes. Severe and often fatal intoxication may occur with very small doses. The toxic dose of strychnine is approximately 1.5 to 2 mg/kg.

The clinical presentation of strychnine is dramatic. Initially patients may experience apprehension, nausea, muscle twitching, and hyperreflexia. Mild intoxications may be restricted to these symptoms.[59] However, in cases of larger overdoses, life-threatening symptoms may progress rapidly. Tonic contractions, opisthotonus, and risus sardonicus in a patient who is awake is diagnostic of strychnine poisoning. Patients may eventually lose consciousness after reported tonic contractions. Auditory, visual, emotional, and cutaneous stimulation may trigger further tonic contractions.[8] The secondary complications include hyperthermia, rhabdomyolysis with renal failure, lactic acidosis, and permanent neurologic injury due to hypoxia.[31] In most cases of intoxication the acute life-threatening symptoms subside within 8 hours; however, hyperreflexia and muscle soreness may persist for up to a week.

All patients with a history of strychnine exposure should be immediately transported to the closest emergency department. Ipecac syrup is contraindicated because of the high risk of aspiration as well as the risk of triggering tonic contractions.

Treatment includes securing the patient's airway to ensure adequate ventilation; aggressive control of the tonic contractions with benzodiazepines (diazepam) and control of paralysis (neuromuscular blocker); gastrointestinal decontamination with activated charcoal and cathartic; and sodium bicarbonate to treat the acidosis and to minimize the risk of renal failure from myoglobinuria.

REFERENCES

1. Adelson L, Sunshine I: Fatal poisoning due to cationic detergent of the quaternary ammonium type, *Am J Clin Pathol* 22:656, 1952.
2. Anderson KD, Rouse TM, Randolph JG: A controlled trial of corticosteroids in children with corrosive injury of the esophagus, *N Engl J Med* 323:637, 1990.
3. Anderson WJ, Anderson JR: Hydrofluoric burns of the hand: mechanism of injury and treatment, *J Hand Surg* 13A:52, 1988.
4. Bass M: Death from sniffing gasoline, *N Engl J Med* 299:203, 1978.
5. Bennett DL et al: Long-acting anticoagulant ingestion: a prospective study, *Vet Hum Toxicol* 29:472, 1987.
6. Bennett IL et al: Acute methyl alcohol poisoning: a review based on experiences in an outbreak of 323 cases, *Med* 32:431, 1953.
7. Borowitz SM: Prolonged organophosphate toxicity in a twenty six month old child, *J Ped* 112:302, 1988.
8. Boyd RE et al: Strychnine poisoning, *Am J Med* 74:507, 1983.
9. Bratton I, Haddow JE: Ingestion of charcoal lighter fluid, *J Pediatr* 87:633, 1975.
10. Burgess JL, Bernstein JN, Hurlbut K: Aldicarb poisoning: a case of severe carbamate poisoning characterized by prolonged cholinesterase inhibition and improvement after pralidoxime administration, *Vet Hum Tox* 34:340, 1992.
11. Burucoa C, Mura P: Chlorophacinone intoxication: a biological and toxicological study, *Clin Toxicol* 27:79, 1989.
12. Cadnapaphornchai P et al: Ethylene glycol poisoning: diagnosis based on high osmolal and anion gaps and crystalluria, *Ann Emerg Med* 10:94, 1981.
13. Caravati EM: Metabolic abnormalities associated with phosphoric acid ingestion, *Ann Emerg Med* 16:904, 1987.
14. Caravati EM, Litovitz TL: Pediatric cyanide intoxication and death from an acetonitrile-containing cosmetic, *JAMA* 260:3470, 1988.
15. Cello JP, Fogel RP, Boland CR: Liquid caustic ingestion: spectrum of injury, *Arch Intern Med* 140:501, 1980.
16. Chan KM, Svancarek WP, Creer M: Fatality due to acute hydrofluoric acid exposure, *Clin Toxicol* 25:333, 1987.
17. Chen TW, Deng JF: A brodifacoum intoxication case of mouthful amount, *Vet Hum Toxicol* 28:488, 1986.
18. Coumadin. *Physician's desk reference*, ed 47, 1993.
19. Crain EF, Gershel JC, Mezey AP: Caustic ingestions: symptoms as predictors of esophageal injury, *AJDC* 138:863, 1984.
20. Dorman DV, Beasley VR: Neurotoxicology of pyrethrin and the pyrethroid insecticides, *Vet Hum Toxicol* 33:238, 1991.
21. Doyle JJ et al: Anticoagulation with sodium warfarin in children: effect of a loading regimen, *J Pediatr* 113:1095, 1988.
22. El Saddi MS et al: Hydrofluoric acid dermal exposure, *Vet Hum Toxicol* 31:243, 1989.
23. Erickson T et al: Pine oil cleaners in prison, *Ann of Emerg Med* 19:158, 1990.
24. Farrar HC, Wells TG, Kearns GL: Use of continuous infusion of pralidoxime for treatment of organophosphate poisoning in children, *J Ped* 116:658, 1990.
25. Frommer P, Ayus JC: Acute ethylene glycol intoxication, *Am J Nephrol* 2:1, 1982.
26. Gapany-Gapanavicius M et al: Pneumomediastinum—a complication of chlorine exposure from mixing household cleaning agents, *JAMA* 248:345, 1982.
27. Gerarde HW: Toxicological studies on hydrocarbons: V. Kerosene, *Toxic Appl Pharmacol* 1:462, 1959.
28. Gibbs DA, Watts RWE: The action of pyridoxine in primary hyperoxaluria, *Clin Sci* 38:277, 1970.
29. Golsousidis H, Kokkas V: Use of 19,590 mg of atropine during 24 days of treatment, after a case of unusually severe parathion poisoning, *Human Toxicol* 4:339, 1985.
30. Gonda A, Gault H, Churchill D, Hollomby D: Hemodialysis for the methanol intoxication, *Am J Med* 64:749, 1978.
31. Gordon AM, Richards DW: Strychnine intoxication, *JACEP* 8:520, 1979.
32. Gorman RI et al: Initial symptoms as predictors of esophageal injury in alkaline corrosive ingestions, *Am J Emerg Med* 10:189, 1992.

33. He F, Wang S, Lin L et al: Clinical manifestations and diagnosis of acute pyrethroid poisoning, *Arch Toxicol* 63:54, 1989.
34. Helmuth RA et al: Fatal ingestion of a brodifacoum-containing rodenticide, *Lab Med* 25, 1989.
35. Hodgson MJ, Parkinson DK: Diagnosis of organophosphate intoxication, *N Engl J Med* 313:329, 1985.
36. Hoffman RS et al: Evaluation of coagulation factor abnormalities in long-acting anticoagulant overdose, *Clin Toxicol* 26:233, 1988.
37. Jacobsen D et al: Glycolate causes the acidosis in ethylene glycol poisoning and is effectively removed by hemodialysis, *Acta Med Scand* 216:409, 1984.
38. Katona B, Wason S: Superwarfarin poisoning, *J Emerg Med* 7:627, 1989.
39. King GS, Smialek JE, Troutman WG: Sudden death in adolescents resulting from the inhalation of typewriter correction fluid, *JAMA* 253:1604, 1985.
40. Klein J, Olson KR, McKinney HE: Caustic injury from household ammonia, *Am J Emerg Med* 3:320, 1985.
41. Krenzelok EP: Liquid automatic dishwashing detergents: a profile of toxicity, *Ann Emerg Med* 18:60, 1989.
42. Kruse JA, Carlson RW: Fatal rodenticide poisoning with brodifacoum, *Ann Emerg Med* 21:331, 1992.
43. Kurtz PH: Pralidoxime in the treatment of carbamate intoxication, *Am J Emerg Med* 8:68, 1990.
44. Leck JB, Park BK: A comparative study of the effects of warfarin and brodifacoum on the relationship between vitamin K1 metabolism and clotting factor activity in warfarin-susceptible and warfarin-resistant rats, *Biochem Pharmacol* 30:123, 1981.
45. Lipton RA, Klass EM: Human ingestion of a "superwarfarin" rodenticide resulting in a prolonged anticoagulant effect, *JAMA* 252:3004, 1984.
46. Litovitz T, Greene AE: Health implications of petroleum distillate ingestion, *Occup Med: State of the Art Review* 3:555.
47. Litovitz TL et al: 1992 Annual Report of the American Association of Poison Control Centers Toxic Exposure Surveillance System, pending publication, 1993.
48. Litovitz T, Schmilz BF: Ingestion of cylindrical and button batteries: an analysis of 2382 cases, *Pediatrics* 89:747, 1992.
49. Lober CW: Chemexfoliation-indications and cautions, *J Am Acad Dermatol* 17:109, 1987.
50. Machado B, Cross K, Snodgrass WR: Accidental hydrocarbon ingestion cases telephoned to a regional poison center, *Ann Emerg Med* 17:804, 1988.
51. Marks MI, Chicoine L, Legere G: Adrenocorticosteroid treatment of hydrocarbon pneumonia in children—a cooperative study, *J Pediatr* 81:366, 1972.
52. McCally AW, Farmer AG, Loomis EC: Corneal ulceration following use of lash-lure, *JAMA* 101:1560, 1933.
53. McGuigan MA: Strychnine, *Clin Toxicol Rev* 6:1, 1983.
54. Meredith JW, Kon ND, Thompson JN: Management of injuries from liquid lye ingestion, *J Traum* 28:1173, 1988.
55. Merrill DG, Mihn FG: Prolonged toxicity of organophosphate poisoning, *Crit Care Med* 10:550, 1982.
56. Mosconi G et al: Kerosene "burns": a new case, *Contact Dermatitis* 19:314, 1988.
57. National Institutes of Health: Use of folate analogue in treatment of methyl alcohol toxic reactions is studies, *JAMA* 242:1961, 1979.
58. North DS, Thompson JD, Peterson CD: Effect of activated charcoal on ethanol blood levels in dogs, *Am J Hosp Pharm* 37:864, 1981.
59. O'Callaghan WG, Joyce N, Counihan HE: Unusual strychnine poisoning and its treatment: report of eight cases, *Br Med J* 285:478, 1982.
60. Peterson CD et al: Ethylene glycol poisoning: pharmacokinetics during therapy with ethanol and hemodialysis, *N Engl J Med* 304:21, 1981.
61. Press E et al: Report of the subcommittee on accidental poisoning: cooperative kerosene poisoning study, *Pediatrics* 29:648, 1962.
62. Ray DE: Pesticides derived from plants and other organisms. In Hayes WJ, Laws ER, eds: *Handbook of pesticide toxicology,* San Diego, 1991, Academic Press.
63. Reinhardt CF, Mullin LS, Maxfield ME: Epinephrine-induced cardiac arrhythmia potential of some common industrial solvents, *J Occup Med* 15:953, 1973.
64. Reisz GR, Gammon RS: Toxic pneumonitis from mixing household cleaners, *Chest* 89:49, 1986.
65. Simonowitz D, Lee JF, Block GE: Corrosive injury to the stomach and esophagus by nonphosphate detergents: an experimental study, *Am J Surg* 123:652, 1972.
66. Smolinske SC, Scherger DL, Kearns PS et al: Superwarfarin poisoning in children: a prospective study, *Pediatrics* 84:490, 1989.
67. Steele RW, Conklin RH, Mark HM: Corticosteroids and antibiotics for the treatment of fulminant hydrocarbon aspiration, *JAMA* 219:1434, 1972.
68. Sullivan MP et al: Long-acting anticoagulant rodenticides: an evaluation of 88 cases, *Vet Hum Toxicol* 31:361, 1989.
69. Tafuri J, Roberts J: Organophosphate poisoning, *Ann Emerg Med* 16:193, 1987.
70. Teixeira F, Morgan J, Kikeri D et al: Hemolysis following 80% acetic acid ingestion, *Vet Human Toxicol* 34:340, 1992.
71. Tenenbein M: Severe toxic reactions and death following the ingestion of diethyltoluamide-containing insect repellents, *JAMA* 258:1509, 1987.
72. Thompson DR et al: Therapeutic dosing of pralidoxime chloride, *Drug Intell Clin Pharm* 21:590, 1987.
73. Tsao TC-Y et al: Respiratory failure of acute organophosphate and carbamate poisoning, *Chest* 98:631, 1990.
74. Van Berkel M, de Wolff FA: Survival after acute benzalkonium chloride poisoning, *Human Toxicol* 7:191, 1988.
75. Ward MJ, Routledge PA: Hypernatremia and hyperchloremic acidosis after bleach ingestion, *Human Toxicol* 7:37, 1988.
76. Ware GW: Toxicity and hazards of pesticides. In *The pesticide book,* Fresno, Calif, 1989, Thomas.
77. Weitzel JN et al: Surreptitious ingestion of a long-acting vitamin K antagonist/rodenticide, brodifacoum: clinical and metabolic studies of three cases, *Blood* 76:2555, 1990.
78. Whalen JE: Inadequate removal of methanol and formate using the sorbent based regeneration hemodialysis delivery system, *Clin Nephrol* 11:318, 1979.
79. Winter ML, Ellis MD: Automatic dishwashing detergents: their pH, ingredients and a retrospective look, *Vet Hum Toxicol* 28:536, 1986.
80. Wolfe BM, Brodeur AE, Shields JB: The role of gastrointestinal absorption of kerosene in producing pneumonitis in dogs, *J Pediat* 76:867, 1970.
81. Zargar SA et al: Ingestion of corrosive acids: spectrum of injury to upper gastrointestinal tract and natural history, *Gastroenterology* 97:702, 1989.
82. Zwiener RJ, Ginsburg CM: Organophosphate and carbamate poisoning in infants and children, *Pediatrics* 81:121, 1988.

Chapter 35

WORK-RELATED INJURIES AND EXPOSURES IN CHILDREN AND ADOLESCENTS

Susan Pollack

Overview
Pediatric occupational fatalities
Agricultural fatalities and injuries
Occupational injury
Occupational exposure
Public health issues

OVERVIEW

More than 4 million adolescents are legally employed in the United States today.[8] The 12-year-old delivering newspapers, the 14-year-old stocking supermarket shelves, and the 16-year-old serving fast food or pumping gas all may be legally employed. In addition, a large number of children and adolescents are employed under conditions that violate wage, hour, and/or safety regulations. Among 1106 high school students with work experience surveyed in 1988, 24% had been asked to work "off the books."[9] Illegal employment of children and adolescents occurs in industries ranging from agriculture and construction to leather manufacturing and home assembly of radar detectors.

Exposure of working minors to hazardous substances and dangerous machinery is prohibited under the federal Fair Labor Standards Act (FLSA) of 1938. Child labor laws in some states are even more stringent in their regulation. The existence of such legislation has led to the general impression that the health and safety of American youth are adequately protected in this century. Although little is known about occupational exposures and resulting illness among working adolescents, analysis of work-related fatalities and injuries among employed adolescents under the age of 18 suggests otherwise.

> A 16-year-old boy was brought by his mother to an adolescent clinic in a northeastern city during the winter of 1992 with complaints of fatigue, headache, and dizziness. Further history revealed that he was running a thriving T-shirt business, which made a major contribution to the family's finances. He used an airbrush to paint the designs with solvent-based paints, working in his room for several hours a day after school with the windows tightly closed. He then slept in his room for approximately 6 hours a night. Neither the patient nor his family was willing to consider closing the T-shirt business. The cost of a commercial spray booth was prohibitive, but they agreed to move production from his bedroom to another room.

With thanks to Leslie Sanders, M.D., Adolescent Medicine, Children's Hospital of Pittsburgh, for sharing the case.

PEDIATRIC OCCUPATIONAL FATALITIES

The Occupational Safety and Health Administration (OSHA) investigated 104 occupational fatalities to minors occurring from 1984 through 1987.[8] Almost one third of these deaths (30%) involved industrial vehicles and equipment; electrocution accounted for 17% and falls 11%. Citations for safety violations were issued by OSHA in 70% of the fatalities. Forty-three (41%) of the deaths occurred while adolescents were engaged in work specifically prohibited by FLSA. In a review of these cases, Suruda and Halperin[18] found 14 deaths (13%) in children aged 15 and under. These cases actually underestimate the true number and spectrum of adolescent work-related fatalities, because

OSHA concentrates on the 25% of deaths that occur in construction and manufacturing industries and does not investigate agriculture, mining, federal employees, homicides, or transportation accidents.

In contrast, the National Traumatic Occupational Fatality (NTOF) data base consists of all deaths for which the "injury at work" box on death certificates was checked "yes." Although OSHA investigated 47 fatalities among minors under the age of 18 during 1984 and 1985, there were 111 deaths among 16- and 17-year-olds recorded by NTOF during the same period. These findings led the National Institute for Occupational Safety and Health (NIOSH) to estimate that there are at least 100 work-related deaths among children under 18 in the United States every year.[18]

Castillo et al[6a] from NIOSH reviewed 670 occupational fatalities among 16- and 17-year-olds recorded in NTOF from 1980 to 1989. Death occurred at an average annual rate of 5.11/100,000 full-time-equivalent workers. Motor vehicle (24%) and machinery injuries (17%), electrocution (13%), and homicide (7%) were leading causes of death, with 92% involving males. Poisoning accounted for 3% of deaths. Fourteen youths who died were employed in mining, which is specifically prohibited for those under age 18. The authors concluded that employed 16- and 17-year-olds were at greater risk than adult workers for occupational death by electrocution, suffocation, drowning, poisoning, and natural and environmental factors.

In a study of North Carolina adolescent occupational fatalities, Dunn and Runyan[8a,8b] found that 90% were male, and the youngest victim was 11 years old. Homicide was the leading occupational killer of adolescent females, as it is for adult women. More than 50% of fatalities involved a motor vehicle. Many of these were tractors, as field or farm accounted for 27% of the injury locations. Employment in activities that appeared to violate the Fair Labor Standards Act characterized 86% of fatalities in workers under age 18.

AGRICULTURAL FATALITIES AND INJURIES

In a study of agriculture, Rivara[16] found that nearly 300 children and adolescents die each year from farm injuries and 23,500 suffer nonfatal trauma.[4] The fatality rate increases with age; the rate for 15- to 19-year-old boys is double that of young children and 26 times that for girls. More than half of those injured die before reaching a hospital. Farm machinery is the most common cause of fatal injury, with tractors accounting for half of the machinery-related deaths, followed by farm wagons, combines, and forklifts. In a review of tractor fatalities in Wisconsin, Karlson and Noren[12] found that 29% of farm-work fatalities between 1971 and 1975 occurred among male farm residents under the age of 19. Cogbill et al[7] echoed Rivara's concern about prehospital deaths in agricultural injuries and found a bimodal distribution of pediatric farm injuries, with peaks occurring at ages 4 and 14. All 13- to 18-year-olds were working at the time of their injury.[17] A similar bimodal peak was noted by Swanson et al[19] in a review of injuries to rural Minnesota adolescents. Among the 88 adolescents injured, one third were definitely working at the time of injury, and an additional 20 may have been working.

In a study of agricultural occupational injuries among minors in the state of Washington, 36% of workers' compensation claims for children under 14 and 17% of claims filed by 14- or 15-year-old adolescents were related to farm work.[10] Although 16% of all claims filed by minors were for serious injuries, 26% of farm worker claims involved serious injuries.

A review by Belville et al[2] of workers' compensation awards to 14- to 17-year-olds in the state of New York from 1980 through 1987 supports the important role that agriculture plays in occupational injury of minors, despite the relatively few adolescents employed in that industry. Half the deaths among 14-year-olds involved work with agricultural machinery, and by the age of 17 agriculture is the most hazardous industry in which to work for adolescents, as it is for adults. In addition to machinery, chemical exposures and large animals can be hazards.

OCCUPATIONAL INJURY

In the state of New York, more than 1000 minors received workers' compensation awards each year for injuries incurred at work.[2] There were 35 known deaths during that time. Every year more than 400 adolescents sustained a work-related injury resulting in some degree of permanent disability. The lowest injury award rates were found among 14- and 15-year-olds (8.2 and 8.3 per 10,000, respectively), but for 17-year-olds rates were 46.8 per 10,000. Boys were injured three times as often as were girls, despite their employment in equal numbers. Manufacturing (newspaper delivery) and agriculture were the industrial sectors with the two highest overall rates of injury awards (49.0 and 46.2 per 10,000, respectively). Newspaper delivery accounted for 50% of deaths among 14-year-olds and all deaths to those under 14. The trade sector had the third-highest injury rate, 33.2/10,000. Because almost half of all working adolescents were employed in the trade sector, it accounted for almost 56% of all compensated adolescent injury awards.

A similar 1-year study of compensated injuries to employed Connecticut youth revealed that most injuries were lacerations and occurred in grocery stores.[1] An intervention to lessen these injuries is currently being carried out by medical personnel, a major grocery-store chain, and the manufacturer of a new blade for opening boxes.

Work-related injuries severe enough to result in death, although undercounted, are probably more likely to be recognized than are injuries requiring only outpatient treatment. Brooks, Davis, and Gallagher[4] reviewed work-related injuries to 14- to 17-year-olds in Massachusetts collected through the Statewide Childhood Injury Prevention Program from 1979 through 1982. During this time 8662 injuries with a known location were treated in emergency departments.

Of these, 1152 occurred at work. Both the number and the proportion of occupational injuries increased with age: among 14-year-olds, 2.5% of all injuries with a known location were work related, but among 17-year-olds, approximately 26% were work related. In contrast, only 17% were related to sports.

OCCUPATIONAL EXPOSURE

Illegal employment of minors has implications for occupational injuries and illness, because wage-and-hour violations frequently are accompanied by health-and-safety violations. One of the most egregious examples of occupational exposure includes application of solvents by hand in New York City belt shops in which children also work and that have been fined repeatedly for violation of child labor laws.[13] Another example is pesticide exposure of working (and nonworking) migrant farm workers' children.

In a 1989-1990 survey of 50 adolescent Mexican-American migrant farm workers,[2] (4%) were found to have mixed and loaded pesticides.[14] Neither of these boys had either training in pesticide handling or protective equipment. Forty-eight percent of the workers reported having worked in fields still wet after application of pesticides, despite federal reentry times that are calculated to ensure that workers are not exposed. Forty-two percent had been sprayed while working in the fields, either directly by plane or tractor or indirectly by wind-borne spray drift. One boy had been sprayed while eating his lunch. Although documented acute pesticide poisoning has been rare among this group, the consequences of long-term exposures to chemicals that may have reproductive or carcinogenic effects after long latency periods are unknown.

The exposures of this group of working migrant farm worker children in the state of New York are similar to conditions found in other areas of the country, including Virginia, Maine, Michigan, Washington, and California. The importance of these exposures from a public health standpoint lies in the potential for acute poisoning of mass numbers of people similar to that seen in the November 1989 episode in Ruskin, Florida, in which 112 workers were poisoned and required medical care.[6,20] Men, women (including two who were pregnant), and adolescents were sent to work in a cauliflower field less than 12 hours after the field had been sprayed with Phosdrin, a potent organophosphate. (This brief reentry time was in violation of both federally mandated minimal reentry times of 48 hours and the manufacturer's recommendations for proper use of the chemical but is not an uncommon practice.) The presence of an unusually heavy dew that morning led to workers' rapidly becoming soaked with pesticide-laden water. Within a few hours the first of them became ill and went to the Ruskin Migrant and Community Health Center. Ultimately, 84 workers were treated there, 50 people received care in emergency departments at five different hospitals, and 13 people were hospitalized, at least one of them requiring intensive care for life-threatening illness.

Another group of adolescents who potentially have occupational exposures are those involved in work-study, vocational-technical, or school-to-work programs. Many work-study and vocational-technical programs have exemptions from the hazard restrictions that are normally imposed on working teenagers by the FLSA. These exemptions are based on the assumption that work is occurring under supervised conditions in safe environments, but such is not always the case. Thus adolescents employed in work-study or vocational-technical settings may have a number of exposures. For example, adults in automotive shops in which radiator repair work is done are known to be at risk for elevated lead levels. It may be inferred that youth working on radiators in small automotive shops have a similar lead risk, but no survey of adolescent auto repair workers has ever been undertaken. In the United States, learning-disabled and mentally handicapped youth tend to be preferentially funneled into vocational-technical programs. The implications of this funneling for health and safety are significant but have not been investigated by either the pediatric or the occupational medicine communities. Curricula for vocational-technical programs do include modules on safety but have little or no information on potentially hazardous exposures. Some vocational-technical programs have the benefit of a long-term school nurse, who may be familiar with the machinery and substances used in the school and who may perform inspections at the start of each school year. There are other programs in which increased interaction between educators, the medical community, and the occupational health community would be advantageous both for improving the safety and health of the children and for maximizing this opportunity to teach new workers about occupational safety and health in ways that provide a foundation for their entire working future.

Although conditions of work may be somewhat different in the United States, a survey of adolescents in apprenticeship programs in Switzerland revealed a number of work-related health complaints that may also be relevant in the United States.[11] Among 1198 apprentices surveyed by Holtz and Boillat,[11] 119 reported problems with solvents, other chemical exposures, dust, smoke, and noise. Thirty-eight youths had sought medical care for work-related exposures. Injuries requiring medical care were incurred by an additional 191 adolescents, mostly during their first year as apprentices, and an additional 46% reported near accidents. Injuries were most commonly related to cuts, foreign bodies and toxic splashes in the eyes, electric shocks, and falls. Meat cutters and butchers had the highest frequency of injuries, a point of particular interest given recent discussions and in the United States about whether to permit adolescents to work with delicatessen slicers, which is currently prohibited under hazard restrictions of the FLSA. Swiss firms with fewer than 20 employees were more likely to be associated with both near injuries and injuries necessitating medical care than were larger firms. A feeling of intoxication related to solvent exposure was reported by 47% of floor layers and 32% of painters, yet 46%

of floor layers reported that required personal protective equipment was unavailable to them.

Bremberg and Nilsson[3] reported occupation-specific health complaints identified by Swedish trade-school students. They included cough and breathing difficulties from indoor dust in construction and headache and nausea among mechanics working in poorly ventilated automotive shops.

In one of the only American studies to investigate occupational illness specifically in adolescents, Broste et al[5] followed up audiometric examination results on 872 high-school vocational agriculture students for 3 years. Students who were involved in farm work had a higher prevalence of high-frequency, early noise-induced hearing loss than did their peers who were not actively involved in farm work. This study has led to an intervention program to supply hearing-protection equipment.

PUBLIC HEALTH ISSUES

There is at present a dearth of knowledge specifically addressing occupational exposures for teenagers, although extrapolation of what we know about adult occupational hazards and adolescent occupations provides a starting point. Heat exposure in farm and lawn work; pulmonary exposures from dusts, grain, and ammonia in animal barns and in mines; formaldehyde and dye exposure in the garment industry; solvents in paint and automotive shops; and asbestos and lead in building abatement all are potential health issues for adolescents as they are for adults.[15]

Some aspects of adolescence may lead to more age-specific risks, such as outdoor jobs with prolonged sun exposure in a population that often uses photosensitizing medication for acne. Of special concern may be early exposure to substances that may have cumulative toxicities or have long latency periods of carcinogenic effects. Benzene exposure among teenagers who work at service stations is an example of such an exposure. Although adolescents have mature physiologic systems, they are in a period of rapid growth, and it is unclear what implications this growth may have when coupled with chemical exposures. Any chemical exposure with effects on the endocrine system also might be of special concern. Perhaps more important, the employment of adolescents in some of the dirtiest and most hazardous work, which continues to take place illegally, places them at potential risk for incurring exposures to substances that may be health hazards. Although the normal risk-taking behavior of adolescents is well known, adolescents wish to be responsible adults and good employees may actually lead to some of the greatest risk taking in the workplace and places them in a particularly vulnerable position to be exploited in hazardous tasks. An adolescent who is asked to work with a delicatessen slicer, to use a large piece of machinery with difficult-to-reach pedals, or to apply pesticides may not know that each activity is legally prohibited for safety reasons, but even if he or she does know, there may be great reluctance to challenge a supervisor and to appear unable or unwilling to do the job.

In summary, it is important that the employment of adolescents continue to be regulated in ways that adequately protect their health and safety, that we educate adolescents about occupational health and safety issues both before they begin to be employed and as they enter the work force, and that we also educate their parents about work and its potential hazards as well as benefits. Health professionals need to be educated that occupational illness and injury is an important part of adolescent health care. More research is needed to investigate exposures and effects. Enforcement of protective laws is important for public health. Last, great potential benefit might result from more interaction among educators, pediatricians, and occupational and environmental health professionals, and it is hoped that this chapter may contribute to that end.

REFERENCES

1. Banco L, Lapidus G, Braddock M: Work-related injury among Connecticut minors, *Pediatrics* 89:957, 1992.
2. Belville R et al: Occupational injuries among working adolescents in New York State, *JAMA* 269:2754, 1993.
3. Bremberg S, Nilsson A: A model for prevention of future working place injuries by means of involving and preparing students at trade schools. Presented at the First World Conference on Accident and Injury Prevention, Stockholm, Sweden, September 17-21, 1989.
4. Brooks DR, Davis L, Gallagher SS: Work-related injury among Massachusetts children: a study based on emergency department data, *Am J Ind Med* 24:313, 1993.
5. Broste SK et al: Hearing loss among high school farm students, *Am J Public Health* 79:619, 1989.
6. Brown J: Florida's largest pesticide poisoning occurs in Ruskin, *Health Beat,* Winter 1989.
6a. Castillo DN, Landen DL, Layne LA: Occupational injury and deaths of 16- to 17-year-olds in the United States, *Am J Public Health,* 84:646, 1994.
7. Cogbill TH, Busch HM, Stiers GR: Farm accidents in children, *Pediatrics* 76:562, 1985.
8. Corban T: *Current trends in youth employment,* Albany, 1988, Division of Research and Statistics, New York State Department of Labor.
8a. Dunn KA, Runyan CW: Deaths at work among children and adolescents, *AJDC* 147:1044, 1993.
9. Durski L: Child labor law survey of teenagers. In *Child labor law review: report to New York State Commissioner of Labor.* Albany, 1988, Intradepartmental Task Force on Child Labor.
10. Heyer HJ, et al: Occupational injuries among minors doing farm work in Washington State: 1986-1989, *Am J Public Health* 82:557, 1992.
11. Holtz JF, Boillat M-A: Health and health related problems in a cohort of apprentices in Switzerland, *J Soc Occup Med* 41:23, 1991.
12. Karlson T, Noren J: Farm tractor fatalities: the failure of voluntary safety standards, *Am J Public Health* 69:146, 1979.
13. Pollack S: Personal observation.
14. Pollack S: Unpublished data.
15. Pollack SH, Landrigan PJ, Mallino DL: Child labor in 1990: prevalence and health hazards, *Annu Rev Public Health* 11:359, 1990.
16. Rivara FP: Fatal and nonfatal farm injuries to children and adolescents in the United States, *Pediatrics* 76:567, 1985.
17. Stiers G: Personal communication.
18. Suruda A, Halperin W: Work-related deaths in children, *Am J Ind Med* 19:739, 1991.
19. Swanson JA et al: Accidental farm injuries in children, *Am J Dis Child* 141:1276, 1987.
20. Tarrant C: Balm, Florida pesticide poisoning chronology, *Tampa Tribune,* South Bay Bureau (chronology provided by the Ruskin Migrant and Community Health Center).

Chapter 36

ENVIRONMENTAL HEALTH IN MINORITY COMMUNITIES

Lynette Benson

Conceptual problems
Methodologic problems
Conclusion

CONCEPTUAL PROBLEMS

Characterization of environmental health risk tends to be based either on extrapolation from animal studies or on epidemiologic studies of white middle- and upper-class individuals. Extrapolation of adverse health effects in humans from animal studies is at best risky and at worst misleading. Populations chosen for epidemiologic study have tended to be those with the resources to investigate toxic exposures and their connection with adverse health effects. According to recent investigations, however, these are the populations least likely to live in enclaves of toxic waste.[3]

Recent research has shown that environmental health risk is inequitably distributed across the United States, with minority, low-income, and other disadvantaged populations bearing the brunt of increasing exposure to environmental toxicants and suffering increased morbidity and mortality.[4] Toxic waste facilities, for example, are often located in communities with high percentages of poor, elderly, young, and minority residents.[3] A 1983 U.S. General Accounting Office report found that race was by far the most significant factor associated with the location of commercial hazardous-waste landfills. Air pollution levels in inner-city neighborhoods can be as much as five times greater than in suburban areas, contributing to increased rates of asthma, emphysema, lung cancer, and other pulmonary disorders in these populations.[3]

Assumptions about exposure in these communities based on the attitudes, beliefs, and behaviors of the white middle class may prove to be highly inaccurate. For example, if we find that Asian residents of a community are more likely to grow vegetables for their own consumption than are other community residents, it changes their exposure to environmental toxicants in significant ways. They may be involved in moderately strenuous exercise outdoors for longer periods than are other residents, which would increase their inhalation of airborne toxicants. Pesticide application is less rigorously monitored. Foods consumed from the garden may contain higher or lower levels of toxic chemicals and heavy metals than do those purchased at a supermarket. Toxicants may enter the food chain at this point from contaminated water, air, or soil. The recognition that part of the study population engages in subsistence gardening may cause investigators to take soil samples when previously they had not expected that this might be a significant route of exposure.

The priority placed on agents that have the highest toxicity to the greatest number of people have left pockets of ignorance about populations that are unusually susceptible or that may be exposed simultaneously to multiple agents.[19] The result of this emphasis is that the special needs of individual communities are rarely considered as the basis for the identification or analysis of potential impact of environmental degradation.[12] Although many community organizations have been able to hire independent consultants or researchers to conduct health studies,[7,9] mobilization of such resources is often difficult for members of minority populations.[3] Racial and ethnic minorities, the economically disadvantaged, the elderly, and the differently abled often constitute atomized and peripheral segments of society. Their diversity makes them difficult to integrate into models based on the white middle class. These are the populations that most frequently have to bear the brunt of society's errors and whose participation and consent in the decision-making process are least likely to be sought.[6,18]

Traditional approaches to risk assessment and management tend to ignore the sociocultural context of environmental hazards. Experts divide the subject of risk into the categories of risk perception, encompassing inaccurate characterizations of risk by the public, and actual risk, involving quantitative measurements and statistical analysis, which creates an adversarial atmosphere. This pits technical against experiential evaluations of risk[1,17] and exacerbates existing conflicts based on perceptions (of both the community and the researchers) based on class, race, sex, or other demographic or cultural categories. The quantitative approach discounts the public's perception of risk and disenfranchises those most likely to face the consequences of an increasingly hazardous environment. On the other hand a purely qualitative assessment can frequently result in overestimation of a risk that is insignificant to human health in the face of more critical environmental health challenges.[20] To invest our limited resources in areas in which they will have optimal impact and to empower minority communities, it is necessary to focus on the intersection of minority communities. It is also necessary to focus on the intersection of minority community concerns about and scientific evaluations of environmental health risks.

One of the dilemmas involved in the mitigation of environmental health hazards in minority and economically disadvantaged populations is that these communities tend to be the very ones that most desperately need the economic development often associated with environmental conditions leading to adverse health effects. Traditionally, community consent has been inferred from the participation of the community in the economic benefits that are typically alleged to accrue to it from accepting (voluntarily or involuntarily) increased environmental risk.[20] This trade-off of jobs, an increased tax base, or other economic incentives for increased health risk from toxic exposures has been termed *job blackmail* or *environmental blackmail*[14] because it often creates a coercive atmosphere in which the choice is between adverse economic or adverse health effects. Once a locally undesirable land use (LULU) is located in a community, the location of subsequent LULUs is seen to have a lesser impact in that community than in a so-called virgin community,[3] making the creation of toxic enclaves almost inevitable. Current siting policies indicate that such enclaves are populated largely by the poor and minorities. Given our limited knowledge about interactions between multiple contaminants and toxicants, the impact of such policies has unknown but potentially disastrous effects on human health, especially on the health of our most vulnerable populations. In addition, the economic benefits of industrialization may accrue disproportionately to populations other than those assuming the burden of risk.[2,3] Clearly, for any attempt to improve conditions in target communities to be effective, economic development and environmental health objectives must be integrated.

There is a perception that minorities and other disadvantaged groups are less concerned about their environment than are mainstream middle- and upper-class populations. In one study, however, women, minorities, and persons of lower socioeconomic status exhibited greater concern over the dangers of technology, including such hazards as contaminated water, pesticides, air pollution, and cancer-causing chemicals.[16] Green and Isely[11] found that, despite dispersed settlement, lack of formal education, and transportation difficulties, a poor rural community was eager to participate in the construction of "a simple technology in response to a felt need." When there is ambivalence about project objectives on the part of the target population, as is often the case with minority populations, the importance of respect of traditional patterns of leadership and community organization is central to achievement of optimal participation. Knowledge of such patterns and the use of such knowledge in promoting community participation may be the deciding factors in achievement of a successful outcome.[11,13]

It is vital to the development of effective environmental health policy that the priorities of concerned poor and minority communities be examined and included in research objectives. The myth of the "concern and action gap"[22] may be related to disadvantaged groups framing their environmental concerns in a civil-rights, rather than a mainstream environmental, context. Mistrust of the environmental movement is engendered in economically and politically disenfranchised people when they see use of environmental reforms to direct social and economic resources away from the problems of the poor toward priorities of the affluent.[3] Recent research shows that underprivileged people are struggling to gain control over their environment through instrumental action aimed at establishment of environmental equity and fairer redistribution of environmental risk. The Congressional Black Caucus, for example, has the most consistently environmentally conscious voting record in Congress. Minorities and disadvantaged populations have begun to organize, both locally and nationally, to assert their rights to live in a healthy environment.[3]

It is critical to explore both intracommunity and intragroup diversity as well as the more obvious intergroup distinctions. This exploration is important because traditional methods used in environmental health tend to treat the exposed community as a monolith. Even those who recognize intracommunity diversity by developing analytical categories based on race, class, or other variables tend to ignore intragroup diversity that may affect the distribution of environmentally induced disease. One of the most important sources of intragroup diversity in health is sex. Other demographic categories tend to homogenize ethnicity and race in ways that do not reflect their complexity. For example, a Haitian immigrant and an African American have significant cultural differences, including language, diet, education, and access to health care. These factors may be more significant in estimation of some exposures and in creation of models of environmental health than that both individuals have black skin.

METHODOLOGIC PROBLEMS

Psychometric investigation has often been used to characterize public reactions to and perceptions of environmental health risk.[8,10,15] Although such investigations have been very useful in attracting attention to and measuring less tangible effects of environmental risks, they have serious limitations in the study of environmental risk in minority populations. Most of this research either is based on white middle-class communities or does not explicitly treat demographic factors such as race and ethnicity as independent variables. Research emphasizing the use of such traditional tools as personality inventories, structured questionnaires, and Likert scales is limited to the investigation of variables defined by the researcher. Researchers tend to be white, male, and upper- or middle-class and thus may miss variables that could be very important to populations with other cultural backgrounds.[5] One solution to this problem is to increase the use of ethnographic methods for qualitative data collection in environmental health research. Ethnographic methods of data analysis are data driven, meaning that coding categories are derived from data collected in open-ended interviews. These methods work to increase the validity of the findings by ensuring that all relevant categories are included.

Estimation of exposure is another problem of environmental health research in culturally diverse communities. Exposure is often measured in terms of a single toxicant and a single pathway. The complexity of human exposure to environmental hazards places serious limitations on the utility of this approach for approximation of actual exposures. Total human exposure is a function of the routes, magnitude, duration, and frequency of exposure.[19] Assumptions based on the lives and activities of the community of academic investigators may result in inaccurate estimations of exposure for populations with other sociocultural backgrounds. Ethnographic methods such as participant observation and life histories, in addition to such traditional instrumental measurements as ambient concentrations and body burdens, can provide more accurate, reliable, and generalizable data on total human exposure in minority populations.

Analysis of environmental health risk in minority communities is complicated by the problem of obtaining a large-enough sample size for valid inferences to be made.[1,23] Once again ethnographic methods may be useful in the evaluation of environmental health in minority communities. Such methods have long been used to collect data with extremely high internal validity among very small populations. A synthesis of data collection and analysis at regional, community, and subcommunity levels could increase the overall validity and reliability of the data. Data gathered on exposure and endpoints in a minority community, placed into a regional context, could facilitate the quantification of environmental health inequity in minority populations.

A systematic approach to characterization and quantification of environmental health risk in minority populations has eluded the grasp of researchers for many reasons. The problem of environmental health in toxic enclaves whose residents do not conform to the assumptions of largely middle-class white investigators is a complex one, involving social, political, economic, and cultural forces as well as the more obvious behavioral, clinical, and toxicologic factors. The lack of an interdisciplinary approach has resulted in research in which essential pieces of information are missing. Minority populations are often difficult for mainstream academic investigators to reach and interview effectively. The solution is to incorporate community residents into all phases of environmental health research, transferring instrumental, analytic, and problem-solving skills to community members through formal and informal training and education.[21]

CONCLUSION

There is currently no method for measuring the degree to which political, social, and economic factors have affected the environmental health risks of minority populations. The political powerlessness of such populations not only has targeted them for toxic exposure but keeps their problems from receiving top priority from agencies faced with complaints from more vocal and influential communities. Development of methods for measurement, analysis, communication, and management of environmental health risks and hazards in racially, ethnically, and culturally diverse communities depend on the ability of clinicians, environmental scientists, epidemiologists, and social scientists to work together in developing a new, more culturally sensitive paradigm for estimation of environmental health risk in minority populations.

REFERENCES

1. Brown P: Popular epidemiology and toxic waste contamination: lay and professional ways of knowing, *J Health Soc Behav* 33:267, 1992.
2. Brown S: Quantitative risk assessment of environmental hazards, *Annu Rev Public Health* 6:247, 1985.
3. Bullard R: *Dumping in Dixie: race, class, and environmental quality,* Boulder, Colo, 1990, Westview Press.
4. Button G: Class, ethnicity, race, and toxic waste disposal. Paper presented at the annual meeting of the American Anthropology Association, Chicago, November 22, 1991.
5. Curtis SA: Cultural relativism and risk-assessment strategies for federal projects, *Human Organization* 51:65, 1992.
6. Douglas M, Wildavsky A: *Risk and culture: an essay on the selection of technological and environmental dangers,* Berkeley, Calif, University of California Press.
7. Edelstein M: *Contaminated communities: the social and psychological impacts of residential toxic exposure,* Boulder, Colo, 1988, Westview Press.

8. Fischhoff B, Slovik P, Lichtenstein S: *Managing technical hazards: research needs and opportunities,* Boulder, Colo, 1977, University of Colorado Press.
9. Freudenberg N: *Not in our backyards! Community action for health and the environment,* New York, 1984, Monthly Review Press.
10. Gatchel R, Newberry B: Psychophysiological effects of toxic chemical contamination exposure: a community field study, *J of App Soc Psychol* 21:1961, 1991.
11. Green EC, Isely RB: Significance of settlement pattern for community participation in health, *Human Organization* 47:158, 1988.
12. Gregory, R, Keeney R, von Winterfeldt D: Adapting the environmental impact statement process to inform decision makers, *J Policy Anal and Manag* 11:58, 1992.
13. Hanks LM, Hanks JR: Diphtheria immunization in a Thai community. In Paul BD, ed: *Health culture and community,* New York, 1955, Russell Sage Foundation.
14. Kazis R, Grossman R: *Fear at work: job blackmail, labor, and the environment,* New York, 1983, Pilgrim Press.
15. Markowitz JS, Gutterman EM, Link BG: Self-reported physical and psychological effects following a malathion pesticide incident, *J Occup Med* 28:377, 1986.
16. Pilisuk M, Acredolo C: Fear of technological hazards: one concern or many? *Social Behavior* 3:17, 1988.
17. Plough S, Krimsky A: The emergence of risk communication studies: social and political context, *Science, Technology and Human Values* 12:4, 1987.
18. Rayner S, Cantor R: How fair is safe enough? The cultural approach to societal technology choice, *Risk Anal* 7:3, 1987.
19. Sexton K et al: Estimating human exposures to environmental pollutants: availability and utility of existing databases, *Arch Environ Health* 47:398, 1992.
20. Shrader-Frechette KS: *Risk and rationality: philosophical foundations for populist reforms,* Berkeley, Calif, 1991, University of California Press.
21. Swan SH, Robins JM: Comment, *J Am Stat Assoc* 81:604, 1986.
22. Taylor E: Blacks and the environment: toward an explanation of the concern and action gap between blacks and whites. *Environ Behav* 21:175, 1989.
23. US Public Health Services, Department of Health and Human Services: *Healthy people 2000: national health promotion and disease prevention objectives,* DHHS Pub No (PHS)91-50212, Washington, DC, 1991, US Government Printing Office.

Part V

SPECIFIC ENVIRONMENTAL EXPOSURE SOURCES

Chapter 37

INDOOR AIR POLLUTION

Enrique Fernandez-Caldas
Roger W. Fox
Ira S. Richards
Timothy C. Varney
Stuart M. Brooks

Potential health issues
Terminology
What are the solutions to the problem?
Sources of indoor exposures
    Outdoor sources
    Building factors
    Human activities
    Economic factors
Examples of indoor air pollutants
    Indoor allergens
Human factors influencing responses to indoor air pollutants
    Host susceptibility
Health issues
    Volatile chemicals
    Ventilation rates
    Biologic agents
Environmental tobacco smoke
Approach to the problem
    Multifactorial problem
    Assessing the building
    What is not known
Specific control procedures
    Procedures for specific pollutants
    Room air-cleaning devices
Philosophic approach to sick building syndrome
    Whose fault is it anyway?
    Possible procedure to follow
Conclusion

Construction and architectural modifications were introduced in the 1970s as a result of the worldwide energy crisis, because approximately one third of the energy consumed was used in the heating and cooling of indoor air. The approach was to add insulation and reduce building ventilation to conserve fuel. Older buildings became better insulated, and newer buildings became tighter thermal envelopes, with less fresh air infiltrating the structure. Windows were dispensed with and replaced by mechanically controlled ventilation in most new office buildings. Other types of building changes incorporated were prefabricated exterior sections mounted on steel frames; inoperable windows; a heating, ventilation, and air-conditioning system (HVAC) with combined intake and exhaust located on the roof; greater use of organic-emitting building materials and furnishings; tight construction of homes; less maintenance of buildings because they had become so complex; and changes in formulation of cleaning agents used to clean buildings' interiors.[80,81,83,94] As a result of all these changes, many buildings became havens for building-related health complaints.

POTENTIAL HEALTH ISSUES

It soon became clear that indoor air pollution may develop in the tight, energy-efficient home or building with poor ventilation and air-exchange rates or when the air-handling system is contaminated with microorganisms (Table 37-1). Although many investigations of workplace environments clearly documented the role of occupational air pollutants in causing adverse health complaints and disease, the initial observations of poor air quality and health complaints from nonindustrial indoor settings (for example, offices in commercial, institutional, and public buildings; residences; and vehicles) were not readily accepted by

Table 37-1. Average fresh air exchange rates for various indoor situations

Location	Air exchange rate per hour
Automobile with windows open	5 to 50
Jet airplane	4 to 7
Conventional home	1 to 2
Tight home	About 0.5
Supertight home	0.1 to 0.3
Mobile or prefabricated home	About 1 per 24 hours

Table 37-2. Average hours spent in locations for adults*

Location	Employed men	Employed women	Housewives
Home	13.4 (56%)	15.4 (64%)	20.5 (85%)
Work	6.7 (28%)	5.2 (22%)	— (0%)
In transit	1.6 (7%)	1.3 (5%)	1.0 (4%)
Outside	0.7 (3%)	0.3 (1%)	0.4 (2%)
In other structures	1.6 (7%)	1.8 (7%)	2.1 (9%)

*Data based on studies of 44 U.S. cities, 1972.

scientists, governmental agencies, and the public as being important. Furthermore, the precise health significance resulting from a prolonged exposure in a so-called tight or sick building is controversial. An important issue is whether a prolonged exposure to poor indoor air quality can lead to a permanent condition or whether the complaints are simply an inconvenience, with no identifiable illness produced at any time. There is a legitimate concern about potential health effects of indoor air pollution, because the concentrations of some pollutants may reach levels higher than outdoor concentrations and may in some instances exceed the national standard for such exposures outdoors. People residing in urban areas spend more than 90% of their time indoors, with the home being where people spend as much as 70% of their time (Table 37-2). Furthermore, individuals considered to be the most susceptible (the young, the elderly, and the infirm) spend the greatest amount of time indoors.[92]

TERMINOLOGY

The adverse health complaints that appeared to be associated with the indoor air contamination have been given such designations as *sick building syndrome, tight building syndrome,* and *building-related illness.* Precise designations have been provided by investigators.[80,81] The term *building-related illness* has been reserved for specific medical conditions of known origin that usually are discerned by objective physical signs and laboratory findings. Such illnesses include more serious conditions such as asthma, hypersensitivity pneumonia, and respiratory infections (for example, Legionnaires' disease). In contrast to sick building syndrome, building-related illnesses are often traceable to a specific contaminant source, such as mold infestation and microbial growth in cooling towers, air handling systems, and water-damaged furnishings. Building-related asthma is a more serious aftermath of a building-related illness and was reported to occur among 512 Denver office workers; the prevalence of new-onset asthma or exacerbation of preexisting asthma was 4.9 times greater among the affected population.[35]

WHAT ARE THE SOLUTIONS TO THE PROBLEM?

Not enough attention has been given to the methods available for the prevention and control of poor indoor air quality problems, which are often expensive and time consuming to introduce. Each indoor environment is unique, and the air quality may vary from room to room; however, practical measures to detect poor air quality and methods to implement proper environmental control can be developed. Perhaps it is an oversimplification to state that the goals to achieve in environmental control of poor indoor air quality are to identify, remove, isolate, and/or replace the source of the pollution. It is clear that the problem is more complicated, that certain host factors may make some people more susceptible, and that psychologic, economic, and anthropologic factors are involved in many instances. Source control of indoor air pollution may not be easily achieved, and corrective measures may be costly, especially when they involve a home rather than an office building. For example, the removal of a domestic pet from the home of a cat-allergic individual has emotional barriers that make implementation difficult or impossible. Removal of carpeting and furniture containing house dust mite or cat allergens to which an individual is allergic may be impractical and costly. Major expenses may be incurred when installation or modification of ventilation systems or air conditioning units is required. Furthermore, building owners, managers, or homeowners must be convinced that the modification and expenditure are essential and that a substantial health benefit will follow. Medical advice should be obtained to determine the relative role of the indoor environment on the patient's medical problem. Other contributing factors, such as allergic sensitivities, other occupational exposure, cigarette smoking, psychosocial factors, and other medically related problems, must be evaluated. Furthermore, lack of insight into the effects of indoor air quality on a person's health may result in needless continuation of chronic medications or the worsening of symptoms.

SOURCES OF INDOOR EXPOSURES

The type and concentration of an indoor air pollutant are influenced by its sources of generation (both outdoors and indoors) and the rate of removal from the environment.[80,81,92] Indoor sources include the building and its furnishings as well as the indoor sources generated by human activities. An individual's actual exposure to indoor air pollutants depends on the concentration of the pollutants in question and the time the person spends in the environment. Chapter 2 discusses various aspects of the concept of total human personal exposure. A number of excellent reviews on indoor air pollution provide additional information.* The characteristics of indoor air pollution may be influenced by building sources, interior furnishing sources, and/or human activities sources.[92] An exposure may be influenced by the way it is generated (such as by combustion); by the type of pollutant group present (for example, volatile organic compounds [VOCs], fibers); and by location, rate, or pattern of emissions. The chemical attributes of any indoor chemical exposure are important and include chemical type and reactivity, irritation capacity, chemical bioactivity, concentration or dose, and potential synergism with other accompanying chemicals. Some building materials, furnishings, and household products release pollutants continually, and other sources are related to activities carried out in the home or office and release pollutants intermittently. The latter activities include cigarette smoking, house cleaning, and maintenance activities. The major indoor air pollutants are listed in the box at left, and Table 37-3 summarizes some important types of sources of indoor air pollution.

*References 25, 80, 81, 92-94, 103, 104.

Outdoor sources

The concentrations of ozone, sulfate, aerosols, sulfur dioxide, and metals (such as lead and vanadium) are lower indoors than outdoors, with levels ranging between 20% and 80% of the outdoor concentrations [92]; respirable-sized particles (that is, outdoor aerosols) also can penetrate the indoor environment. Radon in the home, also considered an indoor pollutant, originates from the earth and rocks beneath the home, well water, and some building materials. Radon enters the home through cracks in concrete walls and floors and floor drains and becomes a problem when it is trapped in buildings.[79] Exposure to radon produces no immediate symptoms, but it has been suggested that environmental radon exposure poses a substantial risk to the general popu-

---

Major indoor air pollutants

Respirable particles
Oxides of nitrogen
Carbon monoxide
Carbon dioxide
Biologic agents and indoor allergens
Formaldehyde
Radon and radon daughters
VOCs and semivolatile organic compounds
Asbestos fibers

Table 37-3 Types and sources of indoor air pollution

Respirable particles	Nitrogen dioxide	VOCs	Semivolatile organic compounds	Infectious and allergic causes	Carbon monoxide
Fireplaces	Gas ranges	Plasticizers	Pesticides	Dust mites	Gas ranges
Space heaters	Pilot lights	Oils	Transformer fluid	Cockroaches	Pilot lights
Coal stoves	Space heaters	Solvents	Termiticides	Bacteria	Space heaters
Wood stoves	Gasoline engines	Mothballs	Wood combustion	Fungi	Gasoline engines
Tobacco smoke	Outside air	Cleaning fluids	Tobacco smoke	Viruses	Outside air
Outside air	Hockey rinks	Glues	Kerosene	Pollen	Hockey rinks
Attached facilities		Photocopiers	Wood preservative		Tobacco smoke
Occupant activities		Personal-care products	Fungicide		Gas furnaces
		Resins			Attached garage
		Gasoline			
		Formaldehyde			
		UF foam			
		Glues			
		Fiberboard			
		Pressed board			
		Plywood			
		Particle board			
		Carpet backing			
		Fabrics			

lation and is responsible for approximately 10% of all new cases of lung cancer in the United States.[99] Smokers are at higher risk of developing radon-induced lung cancer; however, the significance of radon as a major health issue continues to be controversial, and there is much scientific uncertainty about the quantitative risk for lung cancer and data on the most accurate exposure projection for the population at large. The estimated national average is estimated to be 1.5 pCi/L, but levels as high as 200 pCi/L, and occasionally even 800 pCi/L, have been detected in some homes.[79] The National Council on Radiation Protection action level is 8 pCi/L. The Environmental Protection Agency (EPA) recommends that home owners take action to reduce the level of radon if it exceeds 4 pCi/L of air as an annual average concentration.[99]

Building factors

Building factors include proceedings essential to building operations and processes, unique working conditions of the people employed in the building, building maintenance practices, engineering characteristics, lighting, temperature, humidity, and fresh air ventilation. Concrete, stone, plywood, particle board, insulation, fire retardants, adhesives, and paints can emit pollutants to the indoor air. There may be off-gassing from building materials, which is greater in newly constructed buildings and may continue for several months.[90] Radon may be emitted from building materials such as cinder block, aggregate, and building stone, and particle board and plywood (made from formaldehyde-containing resin bonding agents) can release formaldehyde vapors.[92,93] Deteriorating or displaced asbestos and asbestos-containing products (such as ceiling and vinyl floor tile, pipe insulation, ceiling plaster, spackling compounds, concrete, and acoustic and thermal insulating materials), which were formerly used extensively in homes, office buildings, and schools, can release asbestos fibers into the air. Recent surveys by the EPA have documented very low fiber counts in public buildings and schools, with fiber counts averaging between 0.0002 and 0.00008 fibers per cm^3, depending on the building tested. Because of the low fiber counts and because asbestos removal often generates higher fiber levels, the EPA has published new recommendations that encourage management in place and worker protection.[100] Interior furnishings, such as wall-to-wall carpeting glued to the floor with adhesives, draperies of synthetic materials, and furniture constructed with particle board, can release VOCs of a variety of types. Other emissions include organic dusts and fibrous glass particles from deteriorating foam cushions and curtains; VOCs are emitted from plastic- and fabric-covered room dividers. In offices, photocopying machines may emit ozone and VOCs, small refrigerators may leak chlorodifluoromethane (Freon), blueprint machines may release ammonia, and photographic equipment may release acetic acid.[92]

Human activities

Cooking, heating, smoking, and hobbies can lead to indoor air pollution (Table 37-4). Other etiologic factors include the use of home office equipment, home care, room deodorizers, furniture polish, disinfectants, carpet shampoos, aerosol sprays, cosmetics, moth crystals, fabric-care products, pesticides, cleaning products, and personal and other household products are sources of indoor air pollutants (see box). The indoor use of fuel for heating and cooking can lead to a build-up in the indoor air of carbon monoxide (CO), carbon dioxide (CO_2), sulfur dioxide, nitrogen oxides, and a variety of VOCs, especially in homes with unvented appliances. One of the most important types of indoor pollution is from tobacco smoke, which contributes to levels of respirable particles, nicotine, polycyclic aromatic hydrocarbons, CO, acrolein, nitrogen dioxide (NO_2), N-nitrosodimethylamine, acetone, and benzene.*

Economic factors

Economic factors could conceivably influence prevalence of symptomatology by increasing the use of a product that causes an exposure. A rush job may require increased office

---

*References 80, 81, 92-94, 103.

Table 37-4. Exposures related to human activities

Origin of personal exposure	Pollutant
Unvented combustion	CO, NO_2, particles
Solvents, paints, glues, sprays	VOCs
Grinding and abrasion	Dusts
Furnishings and building materials	Formaldehyde, VOCs, solvents
Soil gas	Radon, biocides, organics
Insects	Dust mites
Pets	Dander
Water leaks and standing water	Mold, *Legionella*
Tobacco smoke	CO, particles
People	CO_2, body odors
Computers and copiers	Ozone, particles
Garages and loading docks	CO, particles, VOCs
Wall insulation	Asbestos, fiberglass

CO, carbon monoxide; NO_2, nitrogen dioxide, CO_2, carbon monoxide.

Indoor allergens

Domestic mites
Furry pets (cats, dogs, rabbits, gerbils, mice, rats, hamsters, guinea pigs, and others)
Birds
Insects (cockroaches, fleas)
Molds (outdoor and indoor molds)
Molds and bacteria in air-conditioning units

personnel activity, with production and duplication of many reports on copying machines and laser printers. There may be increased psychologic stress because of employee discontent. Finally, economic factors may preclude an employer from properly maintaining or modifying a building.

EXAMPLES OF INDOOR AIR POLLUTANTS

Respirable particles evolve from fireplaces, wood and coal stoves, unvented kerosene heaters, and environmental tobacco smoke. Concentrations exceeding 500 µg/m³ have been detected in bars, meetings, and waiting rooms; between 100 and 500 µg/m³, in smoking sections of airplanes; and between 10 and 100 µg/m³ in homes. The EPA's 24-hour outdoor ambient air standard is 265 µg/m³, whereas 75 µg/m³ is the annual outdoor ambient air standard. There are no indoor standards for respirable particles. The principal health complaints reported to be caused by respirable particles include eye, nose, and throat irritation; respiratory infections and bronchitis; headaches; and lung cancer. Tobacco smoke is the primary contributor to respirable particles. There has been concern that the concomitant inhalation of respirable particles and a toxic gas or carcinogen may lead to the adsorption of the gas or carcinogen to the large surface area of the particle, leading to a longer lung retention time, greater concentration of the toxic agent, and thus more of a likelihood of an adverse event.

Combustion products such as oxides of nitrogen (nitric oxide [NO], NO_2), CO, and CO_2 may be present in indoor environments. The usual sources of NO and NO_2 are gas ranges and pilot lights, kerosene and gas stoves and heaters, gasoline engines, some gas furnaces, environmental tobacco smoke, and the outside air. A normal range for homes with gas stoves is 25 to 75 parts per billion (ppb). Peak values in kitchens with gas stoves or kerosene gas heaters reach 100 to 500 ppb. The World Health Organization safety standard is 160 ppb for 1-hour maximal exposure. Irritation of the eyes, nose, and throat is the principal health effect of exposure to NO_2. Inhalation of NO_2 may cause impairment on lung function tests and an increased risk of respiratory infections in children.

Tobacco smoke, pilot lights, gas ranges, unvented kerosene and gas heaters, wood stoves, and gasoline engines are important sources of CO. At low levels, inhalation of CO fatigues healthy people and provokes chest pain in people with ischemic heart disease. Higher concentrations impair vision, disturb coordination, and provoke headaches, dizziness, confusion, and nausea. Inhalation of high concentrations of CO can be fatal. The average level in homes without gas stoves ranges between 0.5 and 5 ppm.

Human breath unvented kerosene and gas heaters, tobacco smoke, and the outside air are important indoor sources of CO_2. Its concentration in the outdoor air varies from 320 to 400 ppm. Concentrations of 2000 to 5000 ppm can be measured in crowded and inadequately ventilated indoor environments. A CO_2 concentration below 1000 ppm usually indicates an adequate fresh air supply.

VOCs and semivolatile organic compounds are emitted from household products such as paints, paint strippers, aerosol sprays, and some art supplies (Table 37-5). The most common health effects of exposure to these compounds are eye, nose, and throat irritation; headaches; loss of coordination; nausea; and, in more severe cases, potential damage to the liver, kidneys, and central nervous system. VOCs may also transiently increase the degree of airway reactivity. There are hundreds of different types of VOCs, among them benzene, chloroform, trichloroethane, and formaldehyde. The EPA has identified more than 500 different VOCs in surveys of public buildings.[90] The indoor level of VOCs is several times higher than that outdoors, and in some cases it can be several orders of magnitude higher, especially after use of paint stripper.

Pesticides, fungicides, herbicides, and the combustion of wood, tobacco, or kerosene are important sources of semivolatile organic compounds. These compounds include chlorinated hydrocarbons and polycyclic compounds. Only limited data are available, and no indoor standards have been established.

Formaldehyde is a VOC present in urea formaldehyde foam insulations (UFFI), glues, fiberboard, pressed board, plywood, particle board, carpet backing, and fabrics. Formaldehyde concentrations vary from 0.1 to 0.8 ppm in houses with UFFI. In mobile homes, the average concentration is 0.5 ppm. Concentrations higher than 1 ppm have been detected in a few houses and mobile homes. Exposure to high concentrations of formaldehyde can cause irritation of the eyes and throat, nausea, and difficulty in breathing. Several states have adopted a concentration of 0.2 to 0.5 ppm as a safety standard.

Table 37-5. Some examples and sources of VOCs and semivolatile organic chemicals

Chemical	Example of source of exposure
Benzene	Automobile exhaust
Chloroform	Showers
Methylene chloride	Paint strippers
1,1,1-Trichloroethane	Office machine cleaning fluids
Trichloroethylene	Cosmetics, nail polish remover
Carbon tetrachloride	Strong cleaning solutions
Toluene	Paints
Xylene	Adhesives
Terpenes	Deodorizers
Limonenes	Fabric softener
Chlorpyrifos	Insecticide
Chlordane	Termiticide
Polyaromatic hydrocarbons	Burning wood
Polychlorinated biphenyls	Leaking transformers
Perchlorethylene	Dry cleaning

Indoor allergens

Indoor allergens are the variety of allergens that occur within human dwellings and are found in most home environments. Immunochemical methods have been developed to identify and estimate their concentrations in the air and in settled dust.* Indoor allergens are products of living organisms such as cats, dogs, and other pets as well as insects, molds, bacteria, and mites. Almost half of the homes in the United States contain a cat, a dog, or other furry pet. Homes have been carpeted, heated, cooled, and/or humidified to make them energy efficient, which has provided an ideal habitat for dust mites, cockroaches and other insects, and mold and bacteria in air-conditioning ducts. All play a role in potential sensitization of home dwellers, in particular, those with an atopic background. House dust is the main source of indoor allergens and is composed of a variety of inorganic and organic compounds, including fibers, mold spores, pollen grains, insects, insect feces, mammalian dander, mites, and mite feces. It is estimated that 40% to 80% of all asthmatics are sensitized to one or more of the house dust allergens[61]; high specific immunoglobulin E (IgE) titers to mite, cat, and cockroach allergens are highly prevalent among asthmatic individuals treated in emergency departments in the southeastern United States.[18,26,67,68]

The association between exposure to some allergens and symptoms may be obvious, especially with cats and other mammalian species; however, the association between exposure to house dust and symptoms is not as clear. Even so, many house dust–allergic individuals with perennial allergic rhinitis and or asthma note exacerbation of symptoms when exposed to house dust. Exacerbation of atopic dermatitis (eczema) has also been associated with contact with house dust. The World Health Organization has recognized house dust mite allergy as a universal health problem.[62]

Pets are an important source of respiratory allergens. Cats are the most common source, but other pets, such as dogs, mice, rats, guinea pigs, gerbils, rabbits, and hamsters, also can be troublesome. Bird proteins cause hypersensitivity pneumonitis, which commonly affects pigeon breeders. Occasionally parakeets, budgerigars, and canaries can cause similar problems as well as respiratory allergies.

Molds also are an important source of allergens, but much additional information is necessary to determine the importance of mold allergens in the home environment. Infectious agents such as viruses and bacteria also are present in the indoor environment. Endotoxins, a part of the outer membrane of gram-negative bacteria, are potent proinflammatory substances that may play an important role in the clinical manifestations of a respiratory disease.[49,50]

House dust and storage mites are the main sources of dust-derived allergens. Mite allergens are present in mite bodies, secreta, and excreta. It has been demonstrated that mite feces are an important source of allergens and that 95% of the allergen accumulated in mite cultures is derived from fecal particles.[97] The family Pyroglyphidae consists of 47 species in 17 genera. Most live in nests of birds and small mammals, but 11 species in 5 different genera are found in house and mattress dust; of them, *Dermatophagoides pteronyssinus, Dermatophagoides farinae,* and *Euroglyphus maynei* are the most important. Significant progress in the understanding of mite biology and immunochemistry has been made in recent years. House dust mite allergy is recognized as an important clinical problem in many areas of the world, and positive skin tests and bronchial reactivity to mite extracts can be detected in most asthmatic individuals. Mites feed on human and animal skin scales and can be found in carpets, on floors, in mattresses, and in overstuffed furniture. Optimal conditions for growth are 22°C to 26°C and 75% relative humidity, and the cycle can be lengthened or shortened with lower or higher temperatures and humidity. Mites need high humidity to survive (70% to 80% relative humidity) and cannot live where the relative humidity is less than 50%. *D. farinae* appears to survive better in dryer climates than does *D. pteronyssinus.* Altitude also affects their survival, because of the effects of altitude on temperature and humidity. In Switzerland and France, above 1200 m, the numbers and species of mites decrease, most likely because of the lower temperature and absolute humidity.[82,95,102] Asthmatic persons with mite allergy who have been transferred to a high altitude have improved their asthmatic state[102]; however, such improvement does not occur in mountainous regions of the Andes, such as Peru and Colombia, where high humidity promotes mite growth and sensitization at high altitudes.[82]

Storage mites inhabit stored food products and hay and require abundant food and high humidity for survival. The most common species belong to the genera *Tyrophagus, Glycyphagus, Acarus, Lepidoglyphus, Chortoglyphus, Carpoglyphus, Aleuroglyphus,* and *Tarsonemus.* These mites, usually found in stored grain, barns, hay, and straw, have also been identified in house dust. Allergic rhinitis, contact dermatitis, urticaria, and asthma have been associated with storage mites. Another mite species that seems to be of clinical importance is *Blomia tropicalis,* a domestic mite commonly found in tropical and subtropical environments. Its allergenicity has been demonstrated by skin tests, radioallergosorbent assay (RAST), and RAST inhibition.[3,23]

Purified allergens from mites have been prepared, with the first mite allergen to be purified being *Der p* I from *D. pteronyssinus,* which is secreted into its alimentary canal. It is a heat-labile glycoprotein with physicochemical properties similar to *Der f* I, the major allergen from *D. farinae* and a homologous allergen produced by *D. microceras* (*Der m* I).

---

*References 7, 23, 45, 66, 69, 85, 96.

These allergens, which are cysteine proteinases of the papain superfamily and occur in high concentrations in mite feces, are removed rapidly by elution from fecal particles and have been described as group I mite allergens.[61] They have an approximate molecular weight of 24 kd, multiple isoallergenic forms (isoelectric point to range 4.7 to 7.1), and a similar N-terminal amino acid sequence. Purification of second allergens from *D. pteronyssinus* (*Der p* II) and *D. farinae* (*Der f* II) also has been accomplished. These allergens (group II mite allergens) have an identical molecular weight (15 kd) and are more concentrated in mite bodies than in mite feces extracts. A third allergen from *D. farinae*, *Der f* III, has been purified. *Der f* III has a molecular weight of approximately 30 kd and a chemical structure very similar to that of trypsin.[36] Group IV mite allergens with a molecular weight of approximately 60 kd and a chemical nature very similar to amylase have been described[42] (see Table 37-3).

Cats are very potent sensitizers; 9% to 41% of asthmatic individuals have a positive skin test reaction to cat allergens. The major allergen in cat extract, *Fel d* I, has been isolated and characterized immunochemically; it is found in large quantities in cat pelt and saliva and sebaceous glands of cat skin. Voided urine but not urine obtained by bladder puncture contains *Fel d* I.[2,59] Several groups of investigators have also developed monoclonal antibodies against *Fel d* I and demonstrated that very high concentrations of *Fel d* I can accumulate in house dust.[7,15] Other allergens have also been identified in cat extracts, but their clinical significance and physicochemical characteristics have not been established.

Dog allergy is not as common as allergy to other mammals; however, 5% to 30% of allergic individuals have positive results of skin tests with dog extracts. Dog allergens are present in saliva, epidermal scales, serum, and urine. An important dog allergen has been purified from an extract of dog hair and dander. This allergen, *Can d* I, has a molecular weight of 25 kd and is present in large concentrations in saliva.[16,84] In IgE binding experiments, *Can d* I accounted for approximately 25% of the allergenic activity of dog hair and dander extracts, and approximately 70% of dog-allergic individuals reacted to this allergen. Dog saliva is a very strong source of *Can d* I; dog urine and feces contain very little *Can d* I.

Insects may also cause allergy. Cockroach hypersensitivity, increasingly recognized as a cause of allergic diseases, especially asthma, is now established as responsible for problems among allergic individuals living in cockroach-infested environments, particularly in dilapidated inner-city dwellings. IgE-mediated allergic response to cockroach allergens among urban patients with asthma has been documented.[37] Cockroaches belong to the class insecta, order *Orthoptera*; there are more than 3500 members of the family Blattidae, which contains the most common cockroaches: German cockroach (*Blatella germanica*), American cockroach (*Periplaneta americana*), Asian cockroach (*Blatella orientalis*), Australian cockroach (*Periplaneta australasiae*), and brown-banded cockroach (*Supella supelledium*). An important allergen from each of two cockroaches of major domiciliary importance, the American and the German, has been isolated. These cross-reactive allergens, *Per a* I and *Bla g* I, have molecular weights of approximately 25 kd and have been used to develop assays to determine exposure to cockroach allergens.[84-86] Two allergens from the German cockroach have been isolated and characterized with use of monoclonal antibodies.[69] These monoclonal antibodies have been used to determine cockroach allergen concentrations in the indoor environment and to establish the sources of cockroach allergens.[69]

Other biologic pollutants include infectious agents such as paramyxovirus (measles), influenza virus, *Mycobacterium* (tuberculosis), and some upper respiratory viruses that are transmitted through the air.[6] Various thermophilic and mesophilic actinomycetes, including *Mycropolyspora faeni*, *Thermoactinomyces vulgaris*, *Thermoactinomyces sachari*, and *T. candidus*, may be present in home central air-conditioning systems, farming environments, and contaminated humidification systems and may cause outbreaks of hypersensitivity pneumonitis. Actinomycetes are members of the order Eubacteriales, although they have the morphology of fungi and are often mistaken for and identified as such.[44] They grow best in decaying organic matter such as hay and bagasse at high temperatures (37°C to 60°C) and relative humidities (above 80%). The encapsulated yeast *Cryptococcus neoformans* is commonly associated with pigeon droppings in attics and lofts and above ceilings in office buildings and homes.

Proteins derived from feathers, serum, and excrement of several avian species have been shown to produce hypersensitivity pneumonitis. Pigeon-breeder's disease, duck fever, and turkey-handler's disease have been associated with exposure to avian antigens. Toxic and irritant agents such as bacterial endotoxins can also cause building-related illness. They have been isolated from humidifier reservoirs contaminated with *Pseudomonas* and *Flavobacterium* species. Symptoms related to exposure to high levels of endotoxins consist of fever, chills, chest tightness, and difficult breathing. Airborne endotoxin levels in the range of 0.13 to 0.39 $\mu g/m^3$ have been measured and were associated with bacterial levels of $100/m^3$. Bacteria also produce other pyrogenic toxins, which include gram-positive exotoxins and enterotoxins.[6]

HUMAN FACTORS INFLUENCING RESPONSES TO INDOOR AIR POLLUTANTS

A number of human factors influence an individual's response to an indoor air pollutant.

Genetic factors may be influential in increasing the risk of development of an irritant response, although there is minimal knowledge concerning this issue. Such genetic factors as individual differences in clearance rates and bronchial and nasal anatomy, among other factors, may be important. The site at which antigen or environmental particles come into contact with responding tissue may be an important determinant of the nature and severity of the conjunctival, nasal, or bronchial responses. The number of mast cells is greatest in the terminal bronchioles, and more peripheral distribution of an inhaled pollutant may have more serious consequences. The site of deposition of inhaled particles depends on the anatomic and physiologic status of the airways. In the presence of increased bronchial tone and narrowing, the airway radius decreases and deposition occurs more by impaction. The net effect is a more central deposition of inhaled material. As bronchial constriction subsides, the particles can reach more peripheral airways. The normal pulmonary defenses may be impaired by environmental pollutants indigenous to the building, including cigarette smoke, biologic agents, chemicals, and dust. This situation may in turn impair particle clearance, possibly leading to longer persistence of a particulate within the lung.

Environmental tobacco smoke (ETS) may increase the risk of susceptible individuals to adverse health effects from indoor air pollution. A hypothetical mechanism to explain the connection between cigarette smoking and allergic sensitization is that the inhalation of cigarette smoke produces an injury to the bronchial epithelium.[54] Possibly as a result of widening of the tight junctions between epithelial cells, the epithelial injury could enhance bronchial epithelial permeability and lead to increased penetration of antigen through the epithelial layer, thus presumably increasing the possibility of an immunologic response. Passive tobacco smoke is one of the most important serious type of exposures related to indoor air pollution and is discussed later.

Host susceptibility

Host factors, including atopy and preexisting respiratory illness, are important in determining whether an individual will show a more acute response to ETS.[11,89] Normally, small immediate changes in results of lung function testing may occur after exposure to environmental tobacco smoke.[91] It appears that groups of susceptible persons are at an increased risk for developing asthma from indoor air pollution.[35] The contention assumes that a susceptible person may have preexisting but asymptomatic, nonspecific airway hyperresponsiveness, which is a more common event than was previously suspected, especially among children and adolescents. The hypothesis that there may be a sensitive or susceptible subpopulation in the general population has been considered by others,[10] and human exposure studies document that some persons are more sensitive to low levels of irritants.[17] Although a prolonged low-level exposure to irritant gas produces some airway inflammation in normal persons, a similar exposure in asthmatics and atopic persons leads to an exaggerated response.[4,54] Persons with nonspecific airway hyperresponsiveness respond more adversely to irritant exposures. Airway epithelial damage can be present in asthmatic subjects (and atopic persons) who display minimal symptoms and who require little or no medication. Bronchial mucosa–mast cell degranulation and mediator release occur continuously in atopic asthmatic subjects. The constellation of changes results in a segment of the population who may be more susceptible to irritant-induced airway injury and with the potential to develop asthma or other respiratory effects.

HEALTH ISSUES

The most widely used designation of sick building syndrome concerns alleged health effects resulting from poor indoor air quality in nonresidential and nonindustrial buildings. The usual complaints are nonspecific and afflict the eyes, skin, and upper airways but also include symptoms of headache and fatigue. The symptoms are generally not traceable to a specific substance but are usually attributable to exposures to a combination of substances or to an individual's increased susceptibility (for example, due to atopy or preexisting asthma) to lower concentrations of contaminants.[83] In most cases, the symptoms are reversible, disappear, or are dissipated once the individual leaves the building.

The term *building-related illness* has been reserved for specific medical conditions of known cause that usually are discerned by objective physical signs and laboratory findings. Such illnesses include more serious conditions, such as asthma, hypersensitivity pneumonia, and respiratory infections (for example, Legionnaires' disease). Fig. 37-1 presents potential building-related illnesses. In contrast to sick building syndrome, building-related illnesses are often traceable to a specific contaminant source, such as mold infestation and microbial growth in cooling towers, air handling systems, and water-damaged furnishings. New-onset asthma has been discerned as a building-related health issue.[35]

The magnitude of the sick building syndrome has not been well determined, but an accumulating body of data now suggests that it represents a very serious health problem. The EPA estimates that at any one time, 10 to 25 million people in 800,000 to 1.2 million commercial buildings in the United States have symptoms typical of the sick building syndrome. This situation translates into an economic impact of billions of dollars, reduced productivity of workers, and increased absences from work.

Volatile chemicals

Careful human laboratory investigations have documented a variety of respiratory, olfactory, and neurobehavioral effects from VOCs.[36,39,60] Norback and associates[57] performed exposure assessments for VOCs, formaldehyde, and 15 common hydrocarbons. Tobacco smoking, self-reported exposure to static electricity, and total indoor hydrocarbon

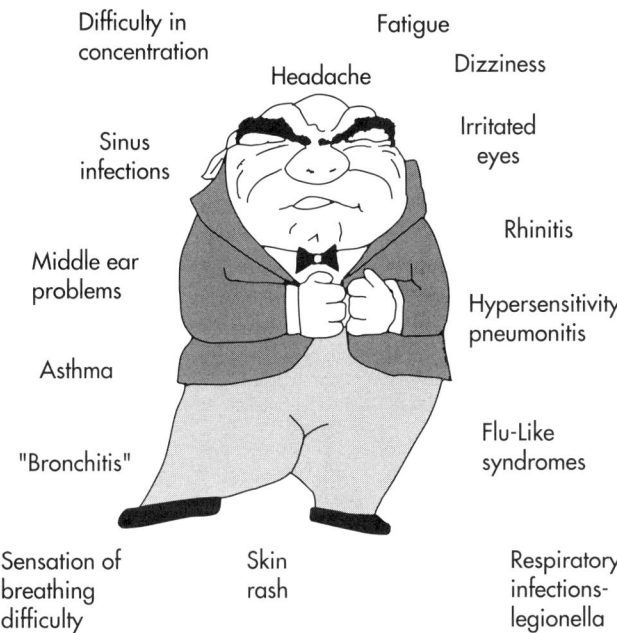

Fig. 37-1. Some building-related illnesses including asthma, hypersensitivity pneumonia, and respiratory infections (e.g., Legionnaires disease). The most common complaints related to a sick building syndrome are mucous membrane and upper airway irritation symptoms. Less discerning complaints may include skin rash, dizziness, difficulty in concentrating, and sensation of difficulty in breathing.

concentration (ranging between 0.05 and 1.38 mg/m^3) correlated with symptoms; however, the personal factor that most strongly correlated with symptoms was "symptoms of hyperreactivity in situations outside the sick building" (that is, bronchial hyperreactivity). It is clear that persons with atopy or documented bronchial hyperresponsiveness seem more sensitive to low levels of indoor VOCs. Harving et al[33] examined the effects of a 90-minute exposure to low concentrations (2.5 to 25 mg/m^3) of a mixture of 22 volatile organic solvents (such as n-hexane, n-nonane, cyclohexane, 3-xylene, ethylbenzene, isopropanol, n-butanone, and ethoxyethylacetate) on the lower airways of 11 atopic persons (with hyperresponsiveness to histamine) under controlled conditions in a climatic chamber.[33] The decline in forced expiratory volume in 1 second with a 25-mg/m^3 exposure was most pronounced for those persons with the greatest degree of airway hyperresponsiveness to histamine.

Reports have shown important relationships among indoor concentrations of volatile hydrocarbons, work at terminals, video display static electricity, and psychosocial factors and the development of complaints of sick building syndrome.[58] The role of psychological factors per se cannot justifiably explain symptoms associated with indoor air pollution or a sick building syndrome, although working in a contaminated environment appears to have deleterious psychological consequences for some persons.[5,75] Environmental exposures during childhood, exposure to fresh paint, the presence of preschool children at home, childhood exposure to maternal tobacco smoke, and exposures from urban outdoor environment also need to be taken into consideration. It is important to realize that preventive measures intended to reduce the prevalence of sick building syndrome should not focus exclusively on specific types of pollutants but also should take other possible exposures and personal factors into account.

Ventilation rates

Building ventilation has been shown to be influential in causing symptoms.[1] An investigation of the effects of changing the supply of outdoor air in four office buildings on symptoms reported by workers and their perception of the indoor environment was undertaken by Menzies and colleagues.[48] The supply of outdoor air averaged 7% and 32% in the ventilation system and 30 and 64 ft^3/min per person in the work site at the lower and higher ventilation levels, respectively. Increases in the supply of outdoor air did not appear to affect the workers' perception of their office environment or their reporting of symptoms, because the changes in the supply of outdoor air were not associated with changes in the participant's rating of the office environment or in symptom frequency. Information from six epidemiologic studies focused on buildings not designated as sick buildings and revealed that sealed buildings with air conditioning are consistently associated with an increased prevalence of work-related headache, lethargy, and upper-respiratory and mucous-membrane symptoms, but mechanical ventilation without air conditioning is not so associated.[47] In fact, air-conditioned buildings with water-based humidification may be associated with a higher prevalence of symptoms than are buildings with steam humidification, which may indicate a greater risk is associated with biologic aerosols from water within the ventilation system. It is important to point out some confounding factors of air-conditioned buildings: on average they tend to be newer and to contain fluorescent lighting; inner offices distant from windows, without natural light; open-plan office layout; and newer synthetic materials with high-absorption surface area (carpets, cloth-covered partitions, and the like capable of accumulating and releasing physical, chemical, and biologic contaminants).

Biologic agents

Increased respiratory complaints (and other symptoms) among children and adults are associated with the presence of home dampness and molds, suggesting that biologic agents may be responsible for some of the symptoms reported in sick building syndrome.[12] Harrison et al[32] also concluded that biologic agents seemed important in some cases of sick building syndrome. In the home environment, allergens are especially prevalent and were discussed previously.

ENVIRONMENTAL TOBACCO SMOKE

ETS is known to contain more than 400 constituents, including over 40 carcinogens and numerous respiratory irritants. Beginning in the 1970s, a large body of data has consistently demonstrated adverse effects, including cancer, from ETS exposure. The earliest studies of ETS exposure focused on respiratory health outcomes.[101] Several studies have shown that ETS increases the risk of lower respiratory tract infections in infants and children. The EPA has estimated that between 150,000 and 300,000 cases of lower respiratory tract infections in infants and young children below the age of 18 months can be attributed to ETS exposure annually. ETS also is associated with irritation of the upper respiratory tract and with small but statistically significant reductions in pulmonary function in children. Several studies have observed a consistent association between ETS exposure and fluid in the middle ear, and the effects persist after control for other risk factors.

Smoking by the mother or maternal caregiver is the exposure variable most strongly associated with the asthmatic state in children. Maternal smoking is an important predictor of wheezing-associated morbidity during childhood,[46] and maternal smoking holds the greatest risk for recurrent wheezing before the age of 18 months.[3] The EPA estimates that each year ETS may exacerbate asthmatic symptoms in as many as 1 million children under the age of 18 years. The role of atopy and susceptibility to irritant exposures seems important.[20] Because maternal smoking in the households of asthmatic children is all too common, reduction of this potentially important risk factor should be the target of practitioners and health educators working with the families of asthmatic children. Studies directed at helping develop policy and intervention strategies for ETS smoke have been addressed.[21,22,76,109]

In adults ETS causes small changes in pulmonary function in nonsmokers and may lead to increased respiratory complaints, including cough, phlegm production, and chest discomfort.

In 1981 two epidemiologic investigations revealed a significantly increased risk of lung cancer among nonsmoking wives of cigarette smokers. Since then, more than 30 epidemiologic studies in eight countries have addressed lung cancer risk from ETS exposure in nonsmokers. These investigations, employing a variety of study designs and comprising more than 3000 lung cancer cases, consistently demonstrate an increased risk of lung cancer from ETS exposure. In studies that considered different levels of ETS exposure, a majority observed a dose-response relationship. Taken with the demonstration of carcinogen in ETS and biologic markers of ETS exposure in nonsmokers, the evidence meets causal criteria for ETS as a carcinogen. The EPA has classified ETS as a known human carcinogen and estimates that it is responsible for approximately 3000 lung cancer deaths annually in U.S. nonsmokers.

It has become apparent to industry that it was more expensive to hire a cigarette smoker than a nonsmoker. It costs a company about $700 per year for each employed smoker.[41] A more discomforting estimate was a $4611 annual cost per smoker.[106] Smokers have between 50% and 100% greater rates (depending on the amount of smoking) of hospitalizations.[41,73] Absenteeism and general illness may be 50% higher in smokers than in nonsmokers,[41] and about 45% more work days are estimated to be lost per person per year because of smoking.[111] An estimated 77 million to 80 million work days are lost because of smoking.[41] The economic cost, which includes the cost of work lost, reduction of company productivity and profit, and increased morbidity and mortality, was estimated at $53.7 billion in 1984.[73]

Smokers are said to have more adverse life-style behavior patterns, including more automobile accidents and moving violations and more likely use of illicit drugs, alcohol consumption, and arrests for drunk driving. Current smokers have 75% more motor vehicle accidents than do nonsmokers[24]; however, there are no differences in the rates between ex-smokers and nonsmokers. This suggests that factors relating specifically to current smoking may play a role in accidents. There are several possible mechanisms to explain this observation. Distraction due to cigarette manipulation at a critical moment could result in a collision. Drug use may be important because smokers are reported to be about twice as likely as nonsmokers to use illicit drugs.[28] Alcohol consumption may be a factor in smokers. Finally, body burden of CO and nicotine from smoking could affect driving ability.

The adverse health effects of ETS include cardiac disease.[72,88,107] ETS is associated with a 30% increased risk of death from heart disease, and there seems to be an apparent dose-response effect.[27] The number of estimated deaths from heart disease may be as much as 10 times more than the estimated number of lung cancer deaths. The mechanism may relate to an effect on platelet function and damage to arterial endothelium. Exposure to passive smoke impairs the cardiac performance of both survivors of myocardial infarctions and healthy volunteers. In a smoking environment, survivors of infarction show statistically higher postexercise plasma CO and lower expired breath CO levels than do healthy persons, possibly reflecting silent cardiac failure, impaired cardiac hemodynamics, and alterations in ventilation-perfusion ratios.[43]

APPROACH TO THE PROBLEM
Multifactorial problem

The practitioner and health professional should be aware that, contrary to popular opinion, indoor air quality and building-related health complaints are much more complicated than high CO_2 levels in the building and occupants' complaints of headaches. If there is a defining aspect to this phenomenon, it is that causation is in every sense of the term multifactorial.

Assessing the building

From a practical standpoint, the technical aspect of the problem can be reduced to the following elements: (1) poor building setting and design; (2) poor and/or inadequate HVAC system design, including reduced fresh air intake; (3) inadequate maintenance and cleaning of HVAC systems and other building components; (4) contamination of the indoor environment by chemical and biologic agents; (5) long-term exposure of building occupants to multiple contaminants at low concentrations; (6) difficulty in relating symptoms and/or health complaints to a causative agent; (7) confusion regarding sampling, analyses, and problem definition; and (8) failure to realize that a problem exists and the employer or building owner's failure to respond in a timely manner. Given these considerations, a systematic approach to the elucidation and resolution of the problem is necessary. One approach is summarized in Fig. 37-2, taken from an EPA publication that presents an approach in flowchart format.

Initial inspection and survey. Making a walk-through survey of the problem area and obtaining an assessment of the health and symptom history are essential first elements. The walk-through survey can include a consultant such as a professional engineer or industrial hygienist who is familiar with inspection procedures necessary for building-related problems. The physician or health professional can be instrumental in organizing and/or interpreting the results from a questionnaire administered to all building occupants. Conducting the health and symptoms history provides an important window to temporal and spatial clinical patterns of exposure that are often overlooked. This clinical information becomes increasingly important as the size and complexity of the building enlarge and hence the population at risk increases. A review of the health symptoms history assists greatly in identification of the most appropriate course of medical intervention and may also be of value in the design of area sampling and analyses. Although many of the symptoms associated with sick building situations involve irritation (such as burning of eyes, scratchy throat, nasal discharge, or stuffiness), some health complaints are more significant and need to be addressed.

HVAC system evaluation. During the course of the building survey, particular attention must be directed at the HVAC system, its operation, and its state of maintenance. The evaluation of the HVAC system is the most important parameter to inspect, and frequently a deficiency in the system is the cause of the indoor air-quality problem. It is important to remember that HVAC systems not only provide ventilation functions but also could serve to transport airborne contaminants to virtually every area receiving airflow. During the course of this process, the HVAC system and all

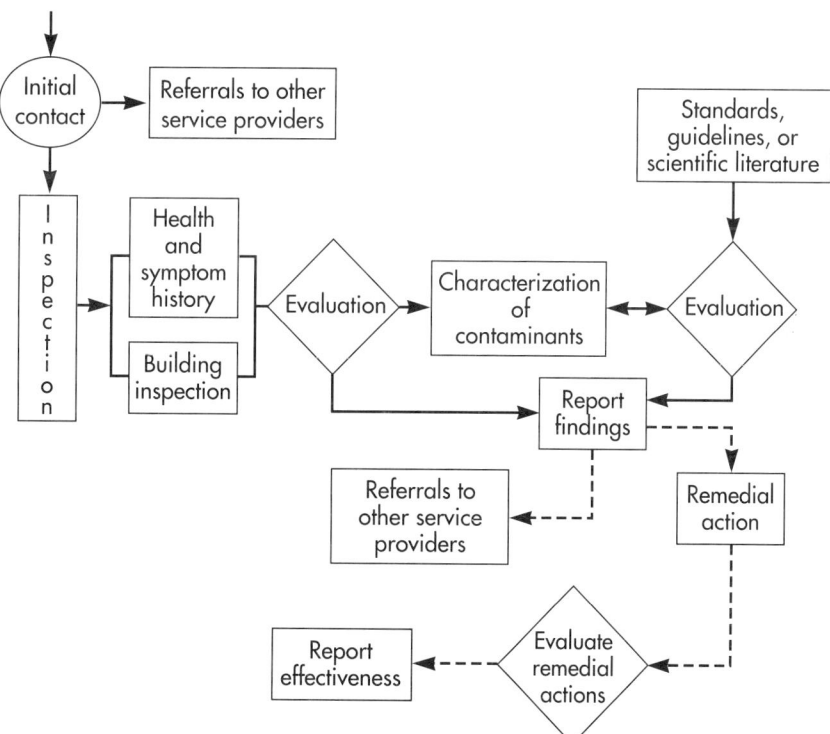

Fig. 37-2. Flow chart taken from an Environmental Protection Agency publication presents an investigation strategy for indoor quality problems (see text).

of its components also become contaminated. Although the HVAC system deserves careful attention, inspections of HVAC systems are often incomplete or oversimplified. The following are common HVAC system shortcomings: (1) There are inadequate fresh-air ventilation rates, marked by excessive CO_2 levels (from occupant-expired breath CO_2 build-up) above 1000 ppm and the build-up of other contaminants in the breathing space, usually because there is no (or less than 5%) fresh-air intake occurring and a total dependence on recirculated air. (2) Fresh-air intake is placed near a contaminated source and/or favors the entry of exhaust air. (3) Dirty fresh-air intake is clogged with particulates and growths of algae, fungi, and bacteria. (4) There is inadequate air filtering, and the filters used to clean the air are bypassed or there has been a failure to change dirty filters. (5) There are dirty cooling coils and condensate pans, dirty supply and return grills, and/or dirty supply fans and ducts, which consequently promote the growth of undesired fungi, bacteria, insects, and protozoa. (6) There is an inadequate control of temperature and humidity, promoting biologic amplification and occupant discomfort.

Sampling and analyses. Once the requirements of the building inspection and the health and symptoms survey have been satisfied, attention may be directed to sampling and analyses, which require consultation and the service of a professional qualified to perform this task. A certified industrial hygienist or professional building engineer is appropriate, but the professional's experience in the area and qualifications should be examined. Sampling and analyses may consist of air, environmental, and surface wipes and bulk material that may include rugs, ceiling tiles, insulation, particulate debris, and other materials. Sampling may consist of short- or long-term protocols varying from grab or instantaneous sampling to intervals spanning 24 hours or longer. Sampling may focus on area-wide collecting or personal air sampling pumps placed on individuals in the building during the course of daily activities.

Which contaminants are found in the indoor environment depend on the building use and location, but some common types and sources of contaminants are: CO, CO_2, oxides of nitrogen and sulfur, ozone, VOCs, and particulates from industrial and vehicular emissions; (2) VOCs from paints, solvents, fuels, carpets, furnishings, pressed woods, cleaning solutions, and plumbing systems; (3) pesticides applied inside and around the outside of buildings; (4) heavy and toxic metals from deteriorating HVAC systems, pesticide applications, paints, printing inks, and nearby combustion sources; (5) radon from natural sources and building materials; (6) asbestos from insulation, coatings, plasters, tiles, mastics, wallboards, shingles, and pipe wraps; and (7) biologic agents from contaminated HVAC systems, rodents, birds, bats, medical waste, leaking sewer systems, water-damaged carpets and ceiling tiles, animal cages, terrariums, and potted plants.

In the indoor setting, sampling and analyses often result in the discovery of diverse chemical contaminants at very low levels, generally in the parts-per-billion range. Biologic agents, on the other hand, may be found to range in excess of 10^6 colony-forming units per cubic meter (CFUs/m^3) or 10^7 CFUs/g of bulk sample. Irrespective of these findings, there is a need to follow through on some form of exposure-risk assessment for individuals occupying the area or areas of concern. Fig. 37-3 presents a general outline of how this process might be approached.

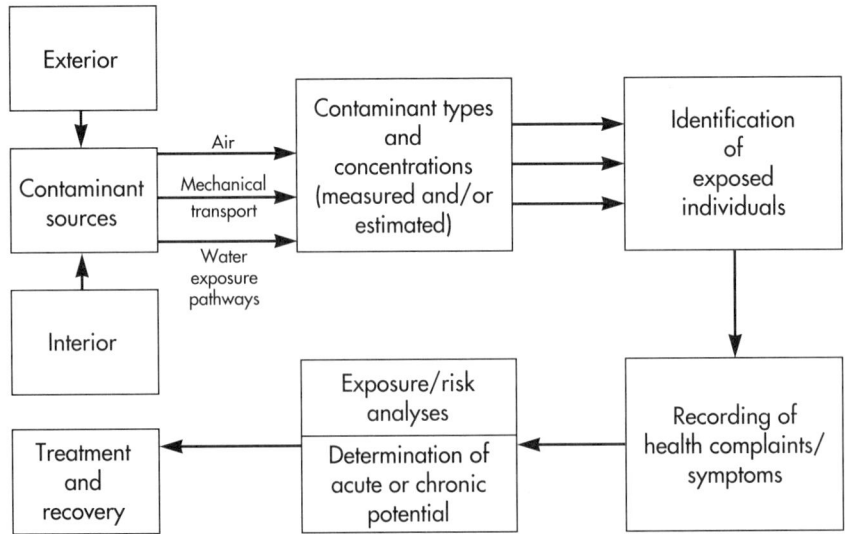

Fig. 37-3. General outline of an exposure-risk assessment for individuals occupying the area(s) of poor indoor air quality.

What is not known

Indoor environments must be viewed as finite systems, and consequently their ability to handle contaminants and to provide a healthy and comfortable environment is limited. For the most part, indoor environments that have been permitted to become contaminant sinks gradually worsen with time as their HVAC systems become more contaminated and decline in efficiency. Reversal of this trend requires a concerted effort to develop more effective educational and information distribution programs at the federal, state, and local levels. Irrespective of increased indoor air quality awareness and growing scientific inquiry, several important aspects require further explanation. The following is by no means an exhaustive list but does identify common and recurring problems and deficiencies associated with indoor air quality and building-related health complaints. In essence, these aspects constitute important research needs: (1) better understanding of the effect of long-term low-concentration exposures to multiple chemical contaminants in indoor settings; (2) better understanding of the effect of long-term exposure to multiple biologic contaminants not historically recognized as pathogenic; (3) better understanding of indoor contaminant transport dynamics in both temporal and spatial contexts for gases, particulates, aerosols, and biologic agents; (4) design of analytic and diagnostic protocols geared to the identification of causation in relation to specific health complaints; (5) refinement of contaminant sampling and analytic protocols for low-concentration, multiple-contaminant indoor environments; (6) refinement of HVAC systems design to achieve a higher level of health maintenance and occupant comfort, particularly when laboratories and the housing of animals are part of the building-use scenario; (7) development and selection of interior design materials with low potential for release of VOCs and growth of biologic agents; and (8) reevaluation of the indoor use of pesticides in terms of chemistry, concentrations, and frequency of application.

SPECIFIC CONTROL PROCEDURES

There are three basic strategies to improve indoor air quality. These strategies include source control, ventilation improvements, and the use of air cleaners.

Procedures for specific pollutants

Combustion products. The principal step to reduce exposure to respirable particles consists of not smoking and discouraging others from smoking in the home, venting all furnaces to the outdoors, and having a trained professional inspect, clean, and tune up central heating systems annually. Important steps to reduce exposure to NO, NO_2, and CO consist of keeping all gas appliances properly adjusted and isolating the garage from the rest of the home. A high concentration of CO_2 in the indoor environment is a consequence of inadequate fresh air intake. An increase in the fresh-air intake rate significantly decreases the concentration of CO_2. A CO_2 value below 1000 ppm is considered acceptable. A sufficient fresh-air mixture to the recirculated air is at least 10%.

Radon. There are several steps to reduce exposure to radon in a home. The general recommendations consist of testing the indoor air for radon and getting professional advice before planning and carrying out radon-reducing measures. Cracks and other openings in the basement floor should be sealed. Crawl spaces should be ventilated, and subslab ventilation should be installed. Radon-contaminated water should be treated by aeration or filtration through granulated activated charcoal.

VOCs. VOCs should be used in well-ventilated areas. Insecticides and pesticides should be applied only in the recommended quantities and should not be stored indoors. Formaldehyde concentrations in homes with UFFI decline by 50% every 2 to 3 years. Average concentrations in older homes without UFFI are below 0.1 ppm. Concentrations greater than 0.3 ppm can be detected in homes with large amounts of pressed-wood products. These products should be replaced with plywood-containing phenolic resins if possible. Other palliative measurements consist of increasing ventilation, sealing off the sources of VOCs, and using dehumidifiers and air conditioners.

Asbestos. Professional help should be requested when the presence of asbestos is suspected or its removal is planned. An increase in ventilation does not result in adequate protection.

House dust and storage mites. House dust and storage mite allergens commonly exacerbate symptoms in people with asthma, allergic rhinitis, or eczema. Environmental control measures to reduce symptoms in mite-allergic individuals have been contradictory. Some mite-allergic patients have shown an improvement in asthma symptoms and decreased bronchial hyperreactivity after their removal from mite-infested environments.[63,105] Successful studies on dust avoidance have used rigid avoidance measures in bedrooms, including removal of carpets, covering of mattresses, and regular washing of bedding in hot water. Other studies have found that high concentrations of mite allergens are present in sofas and carpets outside the bedroom, and allergen levels remain high in some sites for several months after the humidity falls.[64] Therefore, house dust mite control should include all the rooms of the home. A successful mite control should combine the killing of mites and the removal, immobilization, or denaturation of mite allergens. At present, the reduction of dust mite allergen level required to achieve clinical improvement has not been determined. The box on page 432 provides some environmental control measures for house dust.

Several methods to kill mites have been proposed. They include the use of acaricides, the control of microfungi on which mites depend for predigestion of their food, and phys-

> **Environmental control measures for house dust**
>
> Replace feather pillows with Dacron (washable) pillows, and wash regularly.
> Vacuum mattress, base of the bed, carpet, and sofa.
> Encase mattress and boxspring in a plastic enclosure, and damp dust regularly.
> Remove objects that collect dust from the bedroom.
> Wash pillow cases, sheets, mattress pad, and blankets in hot water ($\geq 130°F$), and vacuum around the bed regularly.
> Keep fur-bearing pets out of the home. If a fur-bearing animal has resided in the home a 3% tannic acid solution should be used.
> Air conditioners, air-filtration devices, and dehumidifiers may also be beneficial. Relative humidity should be maintained at or below 50%.
> If these measures are not effective, use acaricides on mattresses, carpets, and sofas.

ical methods such as heating, freezing, and drying. The use of acaricides presents a potential problem of toxicity to humans and pets and damage to household contents. Several chemicals are currently in use. Pirimifos-methyl (Actelic, Imperial Chemical Industries, U.K.), a mosquito insecticide with acaricidal activity, is currently used to protect grain against storage mites.[53] A compound of benzoic acid esters combined with acrylate polymers is an effective acaricide and is currently employed as a household acaricide in Europe and the United States (Acarosan, Fisons, N.Y.).[38] A benzyl tannate complex solution (Allersearch DMS, Australia), a combination of an acaricide and an allergen-reducing agent, is currently being marketed in Australia.[30] A study demonstrated the acaricidal effect of pure caffeine. Caffeine-treated *D. pteronyssinus* cultures showed a significant decrease in mite numbers and in mite allergen after 2 months.[74]

Fungicides such as a 10% application of natamycin resulted in a 40% mortality in a population of *D. pteronyssinus* after 2 weeks.[77] Results of clinical trials on the efficacy of Tymasil (natamycin) to control house dust mites and mite-induced asthmatic symptoms are contradictory.[9,70,78] Mites can grow on animal proteolytic substrates as well as on substrates of vegetal glucidic origin. It also appears that the development of mites is conditioned by the lipid and vitamin B content of the culture medium.[77] The presence of *Aspergillus glaucus* and *Aspergillus restrictus, Eurotium amstelodami,* and especially *Aspergillus penicilloides* in the culture medium actively stimulates the development of *D. pteronyssinus*. These molds predigest the food medium, especially the lipids, and facilitate the absorption of food by the mites.

The weekly washing of bed linens is of benefit to patients if the temperature of the washing water destroys mites (at least 130°F). Warm or cold water does not kill mites, and washing living mites out of a fabric is difficult. Bleach also kills house dust mites. Electric blankets also are effective in reducing relative humidity and the concentration of house dust mites in the surface of mattresses.[14,55]

Liquid nitrogen has been successfully used to control mite populations.[8] Dorward et al[19] demonstrated a 95% reduction of live mites after 8 weeks in liquid nitrogen–treated mattresses of 10 asthmatics, compared with a 19% reduction in the control group. The treated group had a significant improvement in symptom scores and results of lung function tests.

Humidity is a major factor limiting the abundance of house dust mites. They are able to absorb water vapor from unsaturated air until the absolute indoor humidity reaches 7 to 8 g/m^3 (equivalent to approximately 50% relative humidity at 20°C). At lower humidities, they dehydrate and die. Korsgaard[40] observed that a relative humidity above 60% in the house prevents sufficient reduction of mites to be clinically useful. Because mite-allergic patients improved markedly in a controlled environment such as a hospital, where the relative humidity is 40% to 50%, patients should be advised to control the relative humidity in their homes. Low humidity (below 50%) also prevents mold and bacteria growth. Inadequate ventilation, a consequence of energy saving, also seems to be an important risk factor for house dust mite sensitization in temperate regions.[110]

A reduction in the exposure to mite allergens can also be achieved by removal of mite allergens by vacuuming, damp cleaning, denaturing mite allergens, and encasing mattresses and pillows. Attempts to remove mites from furniture by vacuuming are generally unsuccessful because the mites attach themselves to the fibers. Vacuum cleaning removes surface dust and fecal pellets that otherwise become airborne, but inadequate suction and a leaking bag temporarily increase the concentration of house dust mite aeroallergens.[98] Mite allergens become airborne during cleaning activities, and they have been detected in large (10 µm) and in small (less than 5 µm) particles, the latter of which can readily enter the small airways of the lung.[65,96] Therefore, masks should be used by mite-allergic individuals during housecleaning activities.

Air filtration removes only airborne allergens and can have a significant impact on allergen exposure only when low amounts of allergen become aerosolized. Most indoor allergens only become airborne during cleaning activities.

A 3% tannic acid solution (Allergy Control Products Inc., Conn.) is used in the United States to denature mite allergens in house dust.[29,50]

Encasing mattresses, pillows, and blankets in plastic covers also is an important strategy in avoidance of mite allergens.

Furry pets. Fur-bearing pets to which family members are allergic should not be allowed in the home. This measure may not be altogether effective, because mammalian allergens can be transported on clothing of individuals who come in contact with such animals. Studies have demonstrated that there is a variability in cat allergen shedding and that male cats shed more allergen than do female cats.[108] These results are consistent with the observation that some cats provoke more symptoms than do others. Washing cats weekly is effective in reducing cat allergen concentrations in homes.[13] Cat allergens can remain airborne for extended periods,[13] which could explain why cat-allergic individuals experience allergic symptoms on immediate exposure to the presence of a cat. Therefore, benefits from removal of the cat from the home may not become apparent for a long time because of the large reservoir of animal allergens in settled dust.[112] A 3% tannic acid solution is effective in reducing cat allergen concentrations by denaturing cat allergens and can be used in such cases.[52] Most environmental control work with fur-bearing animals has been done with cats; however, it is suspected that such information is applicable to gerbils, guinea pigs, dogs, hamsters, and other furry pets.

Insects and other biologic agents. Regular thorough cleaning of the home and pest control for cockroaches are the ideal methods for controlling these insects and their allergens in the home.

The long-term treatment of patients with hypersensitivity pneumonitis depends on the recognition and elimination of exposure to the causative agent and its source. The elimination of the antigen from the patient's environment helps control the disease and prevents sensitization in other exposed individuals. Reducing the indoor humidity with a dehumidifier and cleaning with a 5% bleach solution significantly reduce the amount of mold and bacteria in homes. The effect of cleaning air ducts on clinical symptoms has not been studied in a controlled manner.

Room air-cleaning devices

Removal or modification of a contaminant source and environmental control measures are necessary to correct identified indoor air-quality problems. Removal or reduction of the airborne pollutants can be accomplished by increasing natural ventilation, improving mechanical ventilation systems, and by employing room air-cleaning devices (RACDs). The latter can be incorporated into the central air-conditioning system, or a portable unit can be placed in a specific room. Three types of air cleaners are currently used: those that include simple panel filters, pleated extended surface filters, or high-efficiency particular air filters; electronic devices that incorporate electrostatic precipitators or negative ion generators; and those that use absorbents such as activated charcoal.

The long-term effectiveness of air cleaners in removing pollutants from the air is a function of the efficiency of the filtration device and the amount of air passing through the device. For example, portable RACDs vary widely in cost, filtration efficiency, and clean-air delivery rates. It must be emphasized that it is a simplistic approach to the complex issue of poor indoor air quality from any source to use an RACD as the only approach for removing the causative airborne impurities.

There are several obstacles that prevent a given RACD from reducing the concentration of air pollutants. Large quantities of house dust mite and animal dander allergens can be isolated in mattresses, pillows, sofas, and carpeting. Inhalation of these allergens occurs with close contact with the source, such as sleeping on a mite-infested pillow. These allergens, especially mite allergens, are transiently airborne, and RACDs cannot remove the sequestered causative allergens. The filtering or precipitating capacity of a given RACD may not permit removal of an overwhelmingly large quantity of allergens or pollutants. Many RACDs are not designed to remove gaseous pollutants.

An ad hoc committee of the American Academy of Allergy and Immunology reported on the types, performances, and the clinical effectiveness of RACDs.[56] The last two recommendations of their report were (1) the role of indoor RACDs is not defined (with regard to health issues) but their use without appropriate environmental control is not sensible and (2) there is clearly a need for studies of RACDs that monitor effects on aeroallergen levels, symptoms, and objective criteria, for example, results of pulmonary function testing (in asthmatics), under suitable, controlled conditions. Data from controlled investigations have yet to substantiate and ensure medical efficacy. Although published clinical studies on RACDs have shown some benefits for some individuals, the data generated are insufficient to permit selection of an RACD for use in a specific indoor environment or for a specific individual.[71] The efficacy of RACDs depends on many clinical factors and uncontrolled variables (type of residence, air quality, allergen concentrations, ventilation systems, environmental control efforts, patient's sensitivities, and severity of symptoms). RACDs have a wide range of performances, requiring the establishment of a uniform, national standard performance test to compare their air-cleaning capacities. The American Home Appliance Manufacturers have developed performance standards for their RACDs as home appliances. They issue a consumer buying guide that informs the consumer about the amount (in cubic feet) of air cleaned by their RACDs, which allows comparative evaluation of their various units. Tests of air cleaning efficiency are performed separately with cigarette smoke, Arizona road dust, and paper-mulberry pollen to provide a wide spectrum of particle sizes.[56]

Carefully controlled, well-executed multicenter double-blind studies must be performed to quantify before-and-after of RACDs on air concentrations of aeroallergens and pollutants and their influence on the clinical status of matched subjects. The decision to use an air cleaner in an attempt at environmental control of a possible indoor air quality problem is left to the individual consumer. The EPA and medical specialty groups have not publicly endorsed the use of these devices in homes or nonindustrial workplaces as effective medical treatment. Additional scientific and clinical research is required to establish medical performance standards for RACDs. RACDs are only an adjunctive method or ancillary piece of equipment that, in combination with other environmental control methods, could improve poor indoor air quality.

PHILOSOPHIC APPROACH TO SICK BUILDING SYNDROME
Whose fault is it anyway?

It has been reiterated by many experts in the field that building-related problems are difficult to resolve and seem to continue for inordinate periods, often in the face of a "pollution problem" that would be expected to be easily solvable, at least from an engineering perspective; however, the chronology and circumstances of events that surround a sick building event often lead to an adversarial state between employees and employer. It is clear that indoor air contaminants can cause diseases and health issues and are a matter of concern. Nevertheless, the issue of critical importance is the status of the relationship between the employees or occupants and the manager or employer or building owner; at issue is whether there is employee discontent, anger, and job dissatisfaction. In the final analysis, a sick building pollution problem is no different than any other work-related problem; however, the resolution of the problem requires the employer's full attention, high priority, and positive attitude. What most employers do not realize is that a building-related air pollution problem often becomes a personnel issue. In this context, it is the administrative and leadership skill of a manager to expedite and solve this work-related problem in a prompt, effective, and convincing manner that is likely the single most conclusive way to resolve the problem.

Each party (employees and employer or manager) looks at the indoor pollution issue differently. The employee may perceive it as a serious health issue and quite differently from the manager's view. Because of this perception, the employees must not be made to think that they are victims nor made to feel ill-advised because they complained of symptoms. It is important to mention that affected workers can generally accept events that are not predictable or are not controllable (such as hurricanes, tornadoes). It becomes an unacceptable situation to most present-day employees when they think that they have been made unhealthy or sick because of a circumstance in the building in which they work or are in a health-related situation that seems to be out of their control and that no one promptly resolves the problem. The workers become frustrated because they must remain in the sick building because they must work to maintain an income. The employees views the sick building as being the responsibility of the employer or manager or some other person or organization. Employees develop anger when they interpret management's inactions as a cover-up or when information concerning their health is not freely exchanged. Of course, the employer may be more concerned with legal issues and future lawsuits against the company or filing of workers' compensation claims that will raise the workers compensation insurance; the employer is often reluctant to provide information to employees about building-related issues, especially if the cause was a failure of proper maintenance or a decision by management to save money and reduce energy costs. This lack of communication and different perspectives lead the employee to view the employer or manager as the "bad guy," who is incompetent or insensitive to the health issues of the employee.

Clearly the most important failures of management are not to accept their responsibility for resolving the building-related problem, not to communicate important information adequately, and not to address the concerns and complaints of the employee sufficiently in a prompt and effective manner. In a confrontational or adversarial milieu, the resolution of a sick-building problem becomes more difficult because, in this type of setting, it no longer represents a health issue but rather has evolved into an employer-employee issue. Thus the resolution of the sick building problem now becomes more time consuming and consequently more costly. It is important to emphasize that once a sick building situation is identified, its complexity is a management issue and its resolution depends directly on the effectiveness and competence of an administrator to resolve a personnel problem!

To work out the problem and bring it to a close, administrators (or supervisors) must recognize five important A's when dealing with a sick building situation—attitude, attention, adversary, acceptance, and acknowledgment: (1) Have a sensitive and compassionate attitude; (2) pay attention to the problem promptly and give it a high priority; (3) avoid an adversarial situation; (4) accept responsibility for resolution of the problem and project a demeanor of trying to solve the problem promptly; and (5) acknowledge information and communicate with all interested parties; present a trustful relationship with employees by not hiding information and by communicating results, progress, and other issues effectively and promptly. Once the work-related problem is dealt with in this way, resolution becomes less difficult.

Possible procedure to follow

It is essential that expert help be obtained and a building evaluation be completed in the manner discussed in previous sections. Additionally, employee issues need addressing. It is suggested that management communicate a written plan of action for handling possible future occurrences and how the present problem will be handled. It is important to develop an approach that is proactive and preventive. By proactive it is meant that a program of surveillance and case finding be initiated, and by preventive it is means that future problems are to be identified at an early time before there are serious consequences. The plan requires designation of the party responsible for building maintenance and the type of building inspection and care that will be provided in the future. In other words, if a problem occurs in the future, where does the buck stop? Periodic review of absenteeism of employees by the personnel director (or designee) may be one way to identify future health problems early, when preventive actions can be introduced. Persons believing the building is causing a health problem should not be discouraged from medical evaluation and should be referred to a practitioner knowledgeable about indoor air quality problems. The employer can organize or direct the facility's safety committee to address the issue in meetings. Educational materials and information can be made available to employees as part of the right-to-know legal requirements in the state.

CONCLUSION

There is a legitimate concern about potential health effects of indoor air pollution, for a variety of reasons. Persons spend most of their times indoors. The adverse health complaints may be associated with contamination of various types of indoor pollutants. Each indoor environment is unique, and the air quality may vary from room to room; however, practical measures to detect poor air quality and methods to implement proper environmental control can be developed. As an oversimplification, the requirement to achieve environmental control of poor indoor air quality is to identify, remove, isolate, and/or replace the source of the pollutant. Source control of indoor air pollution may not be easily achieved, and corrective measures may be costly. Building owners, managers, or home owners must be convinced that the modification and expenditure are essential and that not only will a substantial health benefit follow but failure of resolution will lead to employee dissatisfaction and inefficiency. Medical advice from physicians and nurses should be obtained to determine the relative role of the indoor environment in the patient's medical problem. Other contributing factors, such as allergic sensitivies, other occupational exposure, cigarette smoking, psychosocial factors, and other medically related problems, must be evaluated. Lack of insight into the effects of poor indoor air quality on a person's health may result in needless continuation of medication use or the worsening of symptoms and in some cases to unnecessary legal involvement.

REFERENCES

1. Abbritti G et al: High prevalence of sick building syndrome in a new air-conditioned building in Italy, *Arch Environ Health* 47:16, 1992.
2. Anderson M, Baer H, Ohman JJ: A comparative study of the allergens of cat urine, serum, saliva and pelt, *J Allergy Clin Immunol* 76:563, 1985.
3. Arruda L et al: Exposure and sensitization to dust mite allergens among asthmatic children in São Paulo, Brazil. *Clin Exp Allergy* 21:433, 1991.
4. Bascom R et al: Effect of ozone inhalation on the response to nasal challenge with antigen of allergic subjects, *Am Rev Respir Dis* 142:594, 1990.
5. Bauer R, Grieve K, Besch E: The role of psychological factors in the report of building-related symptoms in sick building syndrome, *J Consult Clin Psychol* 60:213, 1992.
6. Burge H: Bioaerosols: prevalence and health effects in the indoor environment, *J Allergy Clin Immunol* 86:687, 1990.
7. Chapman M et al: Monoclonal antibodies to the major feline allergen Fel d I. II. single-step affinity purification of Fel d I N-terminal sequence analysis, and development of a sensitive two-site immunoassay to assess Fel d I exposure, *J Immunol* 140:812, 1988.
8. Colloff M: Use of liquid nitrogen in the control of house dust mite populations, *Clin Allergy* 16:41, 1986.
9. Colloff M, Lever R, McSharry C: A controlled trial of house dust mite eradication using natamycin in homes of patients with atopic dermatitis: effect on clinical status and mite populations, *Br J Dermatol* 121:199, 1989.
10. Committee for Study of Aldehydes: *Formaldehyde and other aldehydes,* 1981, Board on Toxicology and Environmental Health Hazards, National Academy of Science, Washington, DC.
11. Cummings K et al: Variations in sensitivity to environmental tobacco smoke among adult non-smokers, *Int J Epidemiol* 20:121, 1991.
12. Dales R, Burnett R, Zwanenburg H: Adverse health effects among adults exposed to home dampness and molds, *Am Rev Respir Dis* 143:505, 1991.
13. De Blay F et al: Airborne cat allergen (Fel d I): environmental control with the cat in situ, *Am Rev Respir Dis* 143:1334, 1991.
14. De Boer R: The control of house dust mite allergens in rugs, *J Allergy Clin Immunol* 86:808, 1990.
15. de Groot H et al: Monoclonal antibodies to the major feline allergen Fel d I: serologic and biologic activity of affinity purified Fel d I and of Fel d I–depleted extract, *J Allergy Clin Immunol* 82:778, 1988.
16. de Groot H et al: Affinity purification of a major and a minor allergen from dog extract: serologic activity of affinity-purified Can f I and of Can f I depleted extract, *J Allergy Clin Immunol* 87:1056, 1991.
17. Devlin R et al: Exposure of humans to ambient levels of ozone for 6.6 hours causes cellular and biochemical changes in the lung, *Am J Respir Mol Biol* 4:72, 1991.
18. Di Nicolo R et al: Allergen-specific IgE levels in children presenting to the emergency room with acute asthma, *J Allergy Clin Immunol* 87:234, 1991.
19. Dorward A et al: Effect of house dust mite avoidance measures on adult atopic asthma, *Thorax* 43:98, 1988.
20. Ehrlich R et al: Childhood asthma and passive smoking: urinary continue as a meslces of exposure, 145:594, 1992.
21. Emmons K et al: Exposure to environmental tobacco smoke in naturalistic setting, *Am J Public Health* 82:24, 1992.
22. Erwin S et al: A smoke-free environment, *J Psychosoc Nurs Ment Health Serv* 29:12, 1991.
23. Fernández-Caldas E et al: House dust mite in Florida: mite survey in households of mite-sensitive individuals in Tampa, Florida, *Allergy Proc* 11:263, 1990.
24. Gabel H, Colley-Niemeyer B: Smoking in a public health agency: its relationship to sick leave and other life-styles behavior, *South Med J* 83:13, 1990.
25. Gammage R, Kaye S: *Indoor air and human health.* Chelsea, Mich, 1985, Lewis.
26. Gelber L et al: Serum IgE antibodies and allergen exposure as risk factors for acute asthma, *J Allergy Clin Immunol* 85:193, 1990.
27. Glantz S, Parmley W: Passive smoking and heart disease: epidemiology, physiology and biochemistry: Clinical Progress Series, *Circulation* 83:1, 1991.
28. Goode E: Cigarette smoking and drug use on college campus, *Int J Addict* 7:133, 1972.
29. Green W: Abolition of allergens by tannic acid, *Lancet* 2:160, 1984.
30. Green W et al: Reduction of house dust mites and mite allergens: effect of spraying carpets and blankets with Allersearch DMS, an acaricide combined with an allergen reducing agent, *Clin Exp Allergy* 19:203, 1989.
31. Halken S et al: Recurrent wheezing in relation to environmental risk factors in infancy, *Allergy* 467:507, 1991.

32. Harrison J et al: An investigation of the relationship between microbial and particulate indoor air pollution and the sick building syndrome, *Respir Med* 86:225, 1992.
33. Harving H, Dahl R, Molhave L: Lung function and bronchial reactivity in asthmatics during exposure to volatile organic compounds, *Am Rev Respir Dis* 143:751, 1991.
34. Heymann P et al: Antigenic and structural analysis of group II allergens (Der f II and Der p II) from house dust mites (*Dermatophagoides* spp), *J Allergy Clin Immunol* 83:1055, 1989.
35. Hoffman R et al: Building-related asthma in Denver office workers, *Am J Public Health* 83:89, 1993.
36. Hudnell H et al: Exposure of humans to a volatile organic mixture. II. Sensory, *Arch Environ Health* 47:31, 1992.
37. Kang B: Cockroach allergy, *Clin Rev Allergy* 8:87, 1990.
38. Kniest F et al: Clinical evaluation of a double-blind dust-mite avoidance trial with mite-allergic rhinitic patients, *Clin Exp Allergy* 21:39, 1991.
39. Koren H et al: Exposure of humans to a volatile organic mixture. III. Inflammatory response, *Arch Environ Health* 47:39, 1992.
40. Korsgaard J: House-dust mites and absolute indoor humidity, *Allergy* 38:85, 1983.
41. Kristein M: Economic issues in prevention, *Prev Med* 6:252, 1977.
42. Lake F et al: House dust mite–derived amylase: allergenicity and physicochemical characterization, *J Allergy Clin Immunol* 87:1035, 1991.
43. Leone A et al: Indoor passive smoking: its effect on cardiac performance, *Int J Cardiol* 33:24, 1991.
44. López M, Salvaggio J: Hypersensitivity pneumonitis. In Murray J, Nadel J, eds: *Textbook of respiratory medicine,* Philadelphia, 1988, WB Saunders.
45. Luczynska C et al: Airborne concentrations and particle size distribution of allergen derived from domestic cats *(Felis domesticus),* *Am Rev Respir Dis* 141:361, 1990.
46. McConnochie K, Roghmann K: Wheezing at 8 and 13 years: changing importance of bronchiolitis and passive smoking, *Pediatr Pulmonol* 6:138, 1989.
47. Mendell M, Smith A: Consistent pattern of elevated symptoms in air-conditioned office buildings: a reanalysis of epidemiologic studies, *Am J Public Health* 80:1193, 1990.
48. Menzies R et al: The effect of varying levels of outdoor-air supply on the symptoms of sick building syndrome, *N Engl J Med* 328:821, 1993.
49. Michel O, Duchateau J, Sergysels R: Effect of inhaled endotoxin on bronchial reactivity in asthmatic and normal subjects, *J Appl Physiol* 66:1059, 1989.
50. Michel O et al: Domestic endotoxin exposure and clinical severity of asthma, *Clin Exp Allergy* 21:441, 1991.
51. Miller J et al: Effect of tannic acid spray on dust-mite antigen levels in carpets, *J Allergy Clin Immunol* 83:262, 1989.
52. Miller J et al: Effect of tannic acid spray on cat allergen levels in carpets, *J Allergy Clin Immunol* 85:226, 1990.
53. Mitchell E et al: Reduction of house dust mite allergen levels in the home: use of the acaricide, pirimiphos methyl, *Clin Allergy* 15:235, 1985.
54. Molfino N et al: Effect of low concentrations of ozone on inhaled allergen responses in asthmatic subjects, *Lancet* 338:199, 1991.
55. Mosbech H, Korsgaard J, Lind P: Control of house dust mites by electrical heating blankets, *J Allergy Clin Immunol* 81:706, 1988.
56. Nelson H et al: Recommendations for the use of residential air-cleaning devices in the treatment of allergic respiratory diseases, *J Allergy Clin Immunol* 82:661, 1988.
57. Norback D, Michael I, Widstrom J: Indoor air quality and personal factors related to the sick building syndrome, *Scand J Work Environ Health* 16:121, 1990.
58. Norback D et al: Environmental, occupational, and personal factors related to the prevalence of sick building syndrome in the general population, *Br J Ind Med* 48:451, 1991.
59. Ohman J, Lowell F, Bloch K: Allergens of mammalian origin. III. Properties of a major feline allergen, *J Immunol* 113:1668, 1974.
60. Otto D et al: Exposure of humans to a volatile organic mixture. I. Behavioral assessment. *Arch Environ Health* 47:23, 1992.
61. Platts-Mills T, Chapman M: Dust mites: immunology, allergic disease and environmental control, *J Allergy Immunol* 80:755, 1987.
62. Platts-Mills T, de Weck A: Dust mite allergens and asthma: a worldwide problem. *J Allergy Clin Immunol* 83:416, 1989.
63. Platts-Mills T et al: Reduction in bronchial hyperreactivity during prolonged allergen avoidance, *Lancet* 69:220, 1982.
64. Platts-Mills T et al: Seasonal variation in dust mite and grass pollen allergens in dust from the houses of patients with asthma, *J Allergy Clin Immunol* 79:781, 1986.
65. Platts-Mills T et al: Airborne allergens associated with asthma: particle sizes carrying dust mite and rat allergens measured with a cascade impactor, *J Allergy Clin Immunol* 77:850, 1986.
66. Platts-Mills T et al: Measurements of airborne allergen using immunoassays. In Solomon W, ed: *Airborne allergens (Immunology and allergy)*, Philadelphia, 1989, WB Saunders.
67. Pollart S et al: Epidemiology of emergency room asthma in northern California: association with IgE antibody to ryegrass pollen, *J Allergy Clin Immunol* 82:224, 1988.
68. Pollart S et al: Epidemiology of acute asthma: IgE antibodies to common inhalant allergens as a risk factor for emergency room visits, *J Allergy Clin Immunol* 83:875, 1989.
69. Pollart S et al: Environmental exposure to cockroach allergens: analysis with monoclonal-based enzyme immunoassays, *J Allergy Clin Immunol* 87:505, 1991.
70. Reiser J et al: House-dust mite allergen levels and an antimite mattress spray (natamycin) in the treatment of childhood asthma, *Clin Exp Allergy* 20:561, 1990.
71. Reisman R et al: A double blind study of the effectiveness of a high-efficiency particulate air (HEPA) filter in the treatment of patients with perennial allergic rhinitis and asthma, *J Allergy Clin Immunol* 85:1050, 1990.
72. *Report to the Surgeon General: the health consequences of involuntary smoking,* Washington, DC, 1986, US Department of Health and Human Services.
73. Rice P et al: The economic cost of the health effects of smoking, 1984, *Milbank Mem Fund Q* 64:489, 1986.
74. Russel D et al: Caffeine: a natural acaricide, *J Allergy Clin Immunol* 87:107, 1991.
75. Ryan C, Morrow L: Dysfunctional building or dysfunctional people: an examination of the sick building syndrome and allied disorders, *Clin Psychol* 60:220, 1992.
76. Ryan J et al: Occupational risks associated with cigarette smoking: a prospective study, *Am J Public Health* 82:29, 1992.
77. Saint Georges-Gridelet D: Mise au point d'une stratégie de contrôle de l'acarien des poussières *(Dermatophagoides pteronyssinus)* par utilization d'un fongicide, *Acta Oecol Appl* 2:117, 1981.
78. Sakaguchi M et al: Measurement of allergens associated with dust mite allergy. II. Concentrations of airborne mite allergens (Der I and Der II) in the house, *Int Arch Allergy Appl Immunol* 90:189, 1989.
79. Samet J, Spengler J: Indoor air pollution. In Rom W, ed: *Environmental and occupational medicine,* Boston, 1992, Little, Brown.
80. Samet J, Marbury M, Spengler J: Health effects and sources of indoor air pollution, part I, *Am Rev Respir Dis* 136:1486, 1987.
81. Samet J, Marbury M, Spengler J: Health effects and sources of indoor air pollution, part II, *Am Rev Respir Dis* 137:221, 1988.
82. Sánchez Medina M et al: Prevalence of specific IgE to 5 different mite species in Bogotá, Colombia, *J Allergy Clin Immunol* 85:185, 1990.

83. Scannel G: *Occupational exposure to indoor air pollutants: request for information,* Washington, DC, 1991, OSHA.
84. Schou C, Løwenstein J: Purification and characterization of the important dog allergen Can f I (Ag 13), *J Allergy Clin Immunol* 85:170, 1990.
85. Schou C, et al: Environmental assay for cockroach allergen, *J Allergy Clin Immunol* 87:828, 1991.
86. Schou C et al: Identification and purification of an important cross-reactive allergen from American *(Periplaneta americana)* and German *(Blatella germanica)* cockroach, *J Allergy Clin Immunol* 86:935, 1990.
87. Reference deleted in proofs.
88. Schwartz J et al: Passive smoking, air pollution and acute respiratory symptoms in a diary study of student nurses, *Am Rev Respir Dis* 141:62, 1990.
89. Sexner S et al: Tobacco use: selection, stress or culture? *J Occup Med* 33:1035, 1991.
90. Sheldon L et al: *Indoor air quality in public buildings,* Washington, DC, 1988, Environmental Protection Agency.
91. Shephard R: Respiratory irritation from environmental tobacco smoke, *Arch Environ Health* 47:123, 1992.
92. Spengler J: Outdoor and indoor air pollution. In Tarcher A, ed: *Principles and practice of environmental medicine,* New York, 1992, Plenum.
93. Spengler J, Sexton K: Indoor air pollution: a public health perspective, *Science* 221:9, 1983.
94. Spengler J et al: Indoor air pollution (special issue), *Environ Int* 8:3, 1982.
95. Spieksma F, Spieksma-Boezeman M: High altitude and house dust mites, *Br Med J* 1:82, 1971.
96. Swanson M, Agarwal M, Reed C: An immunochemical approach to indoor aeroallergen quantitation with a new volumetric air sampler: studies with mite, roach, cat, mouse, and guinea pig antigens, *J Allergy Clin Immunol* 76:724, 1985.
97. Tovey E, Chapman M, Platts-Mills T: Mite faeces are a major source of house dust allergens, *Nature* 289:592, 1981.
98. Trudeau W et al: Mite aeroallergen concentrations before, during and after vacuum cleaning, *J Allergy Clin Immunol* 83:264, 1989.
99. U.S. Environmental Protection Agency: *A citizen's guide to radon: what it is and what to do about it,* Washington, DC, 1986, Government Printing Office.
100. U.S. Environmental Protection Agency: *Managing asbestos in place: a building owner's guide to operations and maintenance programs for asbestos-containing material,* Washington, DC, 1990, Office of Pesticides and Toxic Substances.
101. U.S. Environmental Protection Agency: *Respiratory health effects of passive smoking: lung cancer and other disorders,* NIH Pub No 93-3605, Washington, DC, 1993, US Department of Health and Human Services.
102. Vervloet D et al: Altitude and house dust mites, *J Allergy Clin Immunol* 69:290, 1982.
103. Wadden R, Scheff P: *Indoor air pollution,* New York, 1983, Wiley-Interscience.
104. Wallace L, Pellizzari E, Gordon S: Organic chemicals in indoor air: a review of human exposure studies and indoor air quality studies. In Gammage R, Kaye S, eds: *Indoor air and human health,* Chelsea, Mich, 1985, Lewis.
105. Walshaw M, Evans C: Allergen avoidance in house dust mite sensitive adult asthma, *Q J Med* 58:199, 1986.
106. Weis W: Can you afford to hire smokers? *Personnel Administrator* 26:71, 1981.
107. Weiss S: What are the health effects of passive smoking? *J Respir Dis* 9:46, 1988.
108. Wentz P, Swanson M, Reed C: Variability of cat allergen shedding, *J Allergy Clin Immunol* 85:94, 1990.
109. White J et al: Respiratory illness in nonsmokers chronically exposed to tobacco smoke in the work place, *Chest* 100:39, 1991.
110. Wickman M et al: House dust mite sensitization in children and residential characteristics in a temperate region, *J Allergy Clin Immunol* 88:89, 1991.
111. Wilson R: Cigarette smoking, disability days, and respiratory conditions, *J Occup Med* 15:236, 1973.
112. Wood R et al: The effect of cat removal on Fel d I content in household dust samples, *J Allergy Clin Immunol* 85:328, 1990.

Chapter 38

ASBESTOS EXPOSURE IN BUILDINGS

Michael Gochfeld

What is asbestos
Asbestos in commerce
Chronology of knowledge about asbestos hazards
Asbestos in the environment
Exposure
    Uptake, absorption, and distribution in the body
    Fiber content of lung and pathology
Secondary asbestos exposure
Measuring asbestos
Asbestos-related diseases
    Asbestosis
    Pleural plaques or pleural asbestosis
    Lung cancer
    Pathogenesis of cancer
    Mesothelioma
    Intestinal tract cancers
    Immunologic effects
    Medical surveillance
    Epidemiology
    Smoking and asbestos disease
    Fiber types and pathogenesis
    Risk from asbestos in indoor air
    Asbestos in the home
    Asbestos as a hazardous waste
Preventing exposure to asbestos
    Standards governing asbestos exposure
    Working safely with asbestos
    Managing asbestos
    Magnitude of the problem
    Abatement decisions
    Asbestos removal
    Risk communication and asbestos exposure
    For further information

Asbestos has emerged as one of the most complex, alarming, costly, and tragic environmental health problems.

There is a huge primary, secondary, and popular literature on asbestos, dealing with its sources, commercial uses, toxicity, exposure, risk, removal, and disposal.[1] Probably more has been written about the health hazards of asbestos than about any other environmental toxicant, with the possible exception of lead. Nonetheless, its mechanisms of action are probably unique, and there remain many gaps in our knowledge of the pathogenesis of and risk factors for asbestos-induced disease.

Asbestos continues to be a significant occupational hazard, with a whole new workforce, abatement workers, now potentially exposed. Moreover, because of the long latency, exposure occurring 30 or more years ago continues to exact its toll on the former workforce. But a major concern today is with long-term low-level exposure from asbestos mainly as an indoor air pollutant.[95] A growing number of studies of such populations exist,[135] but for the most part it is necessary to make extrapolation from studies on occupational asbestos exposure, disease, and risk.

The economic issues involved in asbestos are staggering. Although most uses are banned in the United States and most other developed nations, there continues to be extensive use of asbestos products in Japan and in the developing nations. Market concerns have fueled the controversy over just how dangerous asbestos is, and asbestos companies have invested heavily in studies aimed at demonstrating that some kinds of asbestos can be used safely. The potential legal liability of asbestos product manufacturers is enormous as well, with more than 200,000 pending legal tort cases in the United States and an average of 50 new cases filed daily.[21] Outstanding claims for asbestos-related disease caused Johns Manville to seek bankruptcy protection,[18] and affected workers have yet to receive compensation.[21]

Table 38-1. The five forms of asbestos fiber, their relative use in construction, and their role in lung cancer and mesothelioma*

Name	Classification	Color name	Use in construction	Lung cancer	Mesothelioma	Metal content
Chrysotile	Serpentine	White	Very frequent	+++	+++	Mg, Fe
Amosite	Amphibole	Brown	Frequent	++	+++	Mg, Fe
Tremolite	Amphibole	—	Infrequent	++	++	Ca, Mg, Fe
Crocidolite	Amphibole	Blue	Scarce	++	++++	Na, Fe
Anthophyllite	Amphibole	Gray	Scarce	++?	++?	Mg, Fe

*Only the fibrous forms of these minerals are named "asbestos."
+, plus marks indicate attributable causation; the more marks the stronger the causation.

WHAT IS ASBESTOS

Asbestos refers to a family of fibrous minerals that are hydrated silicates of magnesium and iron. *Fiber* is a generic term referring to a particulate that is at least three times as long as thick. Table 38-1 lists the types of asbestos and some of their properties.[35] There are two subdivisions of asbestos, the serpentine group containing only chrysotile, and the amphibole group containing several minerals. Chrysotile consists of bundles of curly fibrils, whereas the amphiboles tend to be more straight and rigid.[123] The formula for chrysotile is

$$(Mg,Fe)_6(OH)_8Si_4O_{10}$$

For the amphiboles the generic formula is

$$(Cation)_x(OH)_2Si_8O_{22}$$

There are many other nonfibrous silicates that do not have the same hazardous properties as asbestos, and conversely, fibrous zeolites, which are nonasbestos silicates, cause some of the same cancers as asbestos,[168] heightening the emphasis on understanding the relationship between fibrous properties and pathogenesis.

ASBESTOS IN COMMERCE

Asbestos rock occurs in many parts of the world, but most of it is mined in Quebec, South Africa, Russia, and Brazil. The coarse rock is crushed and then milled to yield fibers that are then split into finer fibers that can be woven into textiles or used to impregnate plastics, cement, and other material. The processed asbestos is then fabricated into a wide variety of materials that have been used in consumer products such as cigarette filters, wine filters, hair dryers, brake linings, vinyl floor tiles, and cement pipe, and in construction materials as shown in Table 38-2.[114]

The fire-resistant properties of asbestos have been known for millennia. In Roman times it was woven into cloth, and even then bladder membranes were used as respirators to protect the slaves who wove the fabric.[21] However, it was not until the 1870s, fairly late in the industrial revolution, that asbestos came into widespread commercial use. Its magical properties included resistance to fire, chemicals, and friction; these same properties, however, account for its unique toxicity.

In the early 1900s asbestos was used to insulate boilers (including in steam locomotives) and as insulation around heating pipes. Later it came into use as thermal insulation in buildings, although most of this market was subsumed by fiberglass. After the end of World War II many building codes, particularly for schools, required the use of asbestos for fireproofing. At least 95% of the asbestos used in the United States was chrysotile, but amosite was an important constituent of thermal insulation and soundproofing material, much of which was friable and therefore particularly hazardous.

CHRONOLOGY OF KNOWLEDGE ABOUT ASBESTOS HAZARDS

The box on the following page is a synoptic, chronologic history of knowledge related to the health effects of asbestos. Reports of pulmonary disease were published shortly after asbestos came into widespread use.[21] Respiratory and wasting disease were recognized in Europe and Great Britain by 1898 and were attributed to inhalation of the dust. By 1918 the fibrous lung disease associated with asbestos was well known, although the term *asbestosis* was not coined until 1927.[30] In 1918 insurance companies, recognizing the in-

Table 38-2. Uses of asbestos*

Uses of asbestos	% of total asbestos used	% that is chrysotile
Asbestos-cement pipe	15	57
Flooring	20	99+
Friction products	21	~100
Roofing	3	~100
Sheeting	5	~100
Coating and papers	10	~100
Packings and gaskets	5	99
Thermal insulation	<0.1	95
Electric insulation	<0.1	~100
Other	25	—

*From report by the U.S. Bureau of Mines, 1983.[20]
~, nearly 100%.

Chronologic history of knowledge of the hazards of asbestos

1897 First report of pulmonary problems associated with dust[21]

1902 Oliver's *Dangerous Trades* mentions asbestos weaving as an age-old occupational hazard[21]

1907 Murray's report to British parliament is first description of asbestosis, a fatal case with fibrosis[21]

1906-1910 Reports on multiple asbestos-related deaths from France, Italy, Britain[21]

1912 Beattie produces lung fibrosis in animals inhaling asbestos[21]

1914 Fahr [Germany] gives pathologic description of lung scarring[21]

1918 Hoffman of Prudential reported that 9 of 13 asbestos workers insured by Prudential died before age 45. Documented that insurance companies denied life insurance to asbestos workers[78]

1918 Pancoast reports x-ray abnormalities in asbestos workers[137]

1924 Cooke [Britain] case report of worker with TB and asbestosis in *British Medical Journal*[29]

1925 Pancoast [U.S.] reports radiographic evidence of asbestos[138]

1927 Cooke uses term "pulmonary asbestosis"[30]

1927 McDonald uses term "asbestos bodies"[21]

1927 First U.S. compensation award to an asbestos victim for occupational lung disease[21]

1927-1928 *JAMA* carries abstracts and editorials reporting evidence of asbestosis[21]

1930 Johns Manville reviews recent literature on asbestosis[21]

1930 Merewether publishes an epidemiologic survey of asbestos of 374 workers, finding about 30% with asbestosis. He reports a 5-year latency between exposure and disease. Report includes measurement of dust counts in factory air.[113]

1930 First U.S. case of asbestosis published[118]

1930 Workmen's Compensation Act in Britain extended to cover asbestosis[21]

1930 Labor journal *The Asbestos Worker* [U.S.] reports hazards[21]

1930 Metropolitan Life Insurance study [published 1935] of 126 asbestos workers showed 50% with definite asbestosis[21]

1931 Sparks reports on progression of disease after termination of exposure[164]

1930-1935 Period of rapid growth of medical literature on asbestosis

1935 Asbestos manufacturers discourage publication of negative health information in their trade journal[21]

1933 Gloyne's report of lung cancer in cases of asbestosis[21]

1935 Lynch reports lung cancer with asbestosis in United States[105]

1935-1940 Eight papers document increased lung cancer rates in about 17% of asbestosis victims[21]

1938 Exposed mice (81%) developed cancer in industry-supported study at Saranac Laboratory [results never published][21]

1942 Hueper's book on *Occupational Tumors* reports evidence of increased cancer risk[82]

1942 Holleb & Angrist report lung cancer in insulation workers[79]

1943 Germany lists asbestosis and lung cancer combination as compensable[21]

1943 Saccone & Coblentz review world literature with no connection mentioned with asbestos[21]

1943 Pleural disease reported in tremolite talc millers in New York[162]

1947 Mallory's case of mesothelioma had had asbestos exposure, but association was not made

1950 Cartier [Quebec] reports two cases of pleura mesothelioma[21]

1951 Stoll & Angrist describe lung cancer in insulation worker and argue that it is compensable[167]

1952 Behrens [Germany] summarizes 509 published autopsied cases of asbestosis victims; 14% had lung cancer[21]

1953 Doll's epidemiologic study confirmed high rate of lung cancer[39] in asbestos workers

1953 Weiss reports two mesotheliomas among 31 autopsied asbestosis victims[21]

1954 Breslow's study linked asbestos work with lung cancer[17]

1955 Doll's study of asbestos textile workers showed lung cancer (SMR = 1375)[40]

1955 Bonser et al. reported four peritoneal cancers with asbestosis[21]

1956 Pleural asbestosis recognized as common finding[63]

1957-1963 Resurgence of case reports of lung cancer and asbestos[21]

1959 Cecil & Loeb textbook of medicine mentions cancer and asbestos[22]

1950-1960 Industry and government express skepticism over carcinogenicity[21]

1960 Wagner [South Africa] reports 33 mesothelioma cases, including some with only community exposure[171]

1963 Wagner reports on 120 cases, more than half of which had only community exposure[21]

1963 Lanza [U.S.], in his book *Pneumoconioses*, doubts that asbestos is carcinogenic[96]

1963 Mancuso publishes epidemiologic study showing excess of lung cancer and five cases of peritoneal mesothelioma[109]

1964 Selikoff reports first epidemiologic study of insulation workers with 20+ years of exposure showing excess lung cancer, intestinal cancer, and mesothelioma and shortened life[154]

1965 New York Academy of Science Symposium on Biological Effects of Asbestos[131]

1965 London study shows several mesotheliomas in community residents and household contacts[130]

1968 Observation of synergism between smoking and lung cancer[155]

1972 New York City bans sprayed-on asbestos[94]

1973 EPA bans sprayed on asbestos[94]

1979 Selikoff publishes excess risks of kidney, larynx, pharynx, and oral cavity cancer[156]

1979 New York Academy of Science publishes an asbestos symposium

1986 Asbestos School Hazard Abatement Act (AHERA) passed

1990 Asbestos School Hazard Abatement Act Reauthorization Accreditation requirements extended to contractors working in public or commercial buildings

1991 New York Academy of Science Symposium: The Third Wave of Asbestos Disease[95]

1992 Fifth district vacates part of EPA ban

creased risk, stopped selling life insurance to asbestos workers.

From 1935 to 1955 there were more than two dozen reports of lung cancer occurring in asbestos-exposed workers or asbestosis victims. There was remarkable consistency among these studies, most of which reported that 13% to 18% of the subjects had lung cancer.[21] By 1987 most uses of asbestos were banned in the United States and many other nations, although a recent court order has upset part of the ban on a legal technicality, creating the mistaken impression that the United States no longer considers asbestos so hazardous. Asbestos use has declined drastically in the United States and has stabilized worldwide, although it is still in widespread use in Japan and in many developing nations.

ASBESTOS IN THE ENVIRONMENT

Asbestos is neither water-soluble nor volatile, so that the form of concern is microscopic fibers. The fibers may dissolve slowly over time, but they are not broken down by bacteria and they do not move readily through the soil. Bioaccumulation in plants and animals is not a problem. The smallest fibers are very light and may remain "entrained" in the air for many hours, but sooner or later they settle onto surfaces. Natural weathering of rocks can release asbestos into the air and water, but by far the major source is anthropogenic from the many different industrial and commercial uses of asbestos and from uncontrolled waste sites.

The ambient air level in rural areas is below 3 fibers/m^3 or 3×10^6 fibers per cc. In urban areas the levels reach 300 fibers/m^3, while near asbestos mines or factories it can exceed 2000 fibers/m^3.[1] With the elimination of asbestos from brake linings in the United States, the urban ambient should decline. The OSHA Permissible Exposure Limit for Asbestos is 0.1 fibers/cc, about 1000 times higher than the highest level in the urban background.

EXPOSURE

For asbestos fibers to cause disease they must gain access to the body. They do not pass through the intact skin, so their main entry routes are by inhalation or ingestion of contaminated air or water. Community exposure can come from a variety of facilities, including mines, mills, and factories that manufacture asbestos products, from demolition of buildings, and from improperly controlled hazardous waste sites. Indoor air and household exposure can come from a variety of asbestos-containing building materials (ACBM), particularly sprayed-on asbestos and asbestos insulation around boilers and pipes, and from consumer products. Air and water are the main media of contamination, but contaminated soil can be ingested or can generate airborne asbestos in the form of dust, and in some cases food may be contaminated as well. Table 38-3 summarizes the main pathways for nonoccupational exposure.

Air: Most knowledge of asbestos exposure comes from occupational exposure to workplace air usually measured as fibers/cc and summarized in terms of the fiber/cc-year for various epidemiologic studies. However, other important temporal features include age at onset of exposure, latency since first exposure, and duration of exposure. The cumulative or lifetime fiber dose appears to correlate well with lung cancer data, but age at onset and duration are more important than total fiber exposure for mesothelioma risk.[125] A study of lung cancer in South African asbestos miners showed that both duration of exposure and latency since first exposure were significant contributors to lung cancer risk for those exposed to crocidolite, but for amosite exposure only duration of exposure was important,[163] and there was a

Table 38-3. Exposure matrix for nonoccupational asbestos contact*

	Inhalation	Ingestion	Dermal
Air	++++ Disturbance of intact material or dust; renovations & demolition brake linings	++ Deposition on food in school or on surface water used for drinking	0
Water	0 (Asbestos is not volatile)	++++ Water may contain natural asbestos or may extract it from asbestos-cement pipe	0
Soil	+++ Dust may stir up asbestos in soil or on HW sites	+ Children may eat about 50-100 mg/soil but occasionally more	0
Food	0	Negligible Occasionally through deposition on food (no food chain concentration)	0
Dust	Can be stirred up and either breathed in or ingested		

*Environmental and Occupational Health Sciences Institute.
0, route unimportant; ++++, route very important

significant risk of asbestosis for workers exposed to only 2 to 5 fibers/cc-year.[163]

Water: Asbestos in drinking water can be derived from (1) natural geophysical processes such as the erosion of asbestos-containing deposits, (2) asbestos waste, and (3) leaching of fibers from asbestos-cement piping. The water supply of Duluth, Minnesota, was found to be contaminated by asbestos from industrial debris.[27] An EPA[53] study of asbestos in drinking water in 365 cities found that 55% had undetectable or negligible asbestos fiber, while 20% had >1 million and 11% had more than 10 million fibers/cc.[117]

Asbestos-cement pipe: Originally developed to be resistant to deterioration, asbestos cement piping (ACP) is widely used in North America and is being increasingly used in the developing nations. Most of the asbestos in ACP is chrysotile, but some pipe contains crocidolite. An industry survey in the mid-1970s estimated that 38% of U.S. cities had ACP,[32] and at that time about 65 million people were receiving water through such pipes.[124] From engineering and cost perspectives there are significant advantages to ACP over metal piping; however, research in the laboratory and the field shows that asbestos can be released from ACP,[33] particularly by soft water with relatively low pH (so-called aggressive water).

A Connecticut study of 149 public water supplies (mostly with soft water) revealed asbestos fiber counts as high as 700,000 fibers/L and an estimate that in 16% of towns with the most aggressive water, asbestos concentrations might reach 10 million fibers/L. By contrast a study in Michigan, where water was generally hard, revealed negligible fiber release.[69] The Safe Drinking Water Committee of the National Research Council[124] explored ACP in depth, but did not conclude whether ACP is safe for use.

Uptake, absorption, and distribution in the body

For airborne asbestos the largest fibers are filtered out in the nose and the upper airway, while the smallest impact on the bifurcations of the alveolar ducts. The mucociliary escalator carries some of the fibers upward so that they are expectorated or swallowed. In addition, some fibers are ingested directly, particularly if people eat or drink where there is asbestos exposure or if water contains asbestos. Ingested or swallowed asbestos fibers can be absorbed from the GI tract and can be detected in the urine.[28] Fibers in the lung attract macrophages and stimulate fibrosis (see below).

Once the fibers reach the alveoli or the intestinal mucosa, they are not readily absorbed into the bloodstream. Thus their main effects are probably at the site of deposition. Most fibers that enter the intestinal tract are excreted directly, although some enter the mucosal cells, and a few penetrate the intestinal tract and enter the bloodstream, lymphatics, or even abdominal cavity.

Asbestos bodies. Asbestos fibers ingested by macrophages may become coated by a mucopolysaccharide in an iron-rich matrix that assumes a dumbbell-like shape known as an asbestos body (AB). Although only about 1% of fibers become coated, these ABs are readily detectable under the light microscope by their shape and golden color and can be quantified as an index of asbestos exposure.[169] The coating appears to play a role in detoxifying the fibers, and amphibole fibers are more likely to be coated than chrysotile fibers. There is a rough correlation between exposure, extent of fibrosis, and the pulmonary burden of coated and uncoated asbestos fibers.[23] Pathologic examination of lung tissue of the general population reveals fewer than 500 ABs/g of lung tissue (dry weight), but persons with pleural plaques may have 20,000 AB/g, and those with asbestosis often have more than 1,000,000 AB/g.

Fiber content of lung and pathology

There have been many studies of the fiber burden of the lung in connection with asbestosis, pleural disease, and mesothelioma. The results are too complicated to review here. There is often a poor correlation between the mass of asbestos fibers and the extent of fibrosis, but some studies show a dose-response relationship with fiber counts. Once compromised by fibrosis, the lung may accumulate fibers that, although not primarily responsible for disease, may remain to be counted at autopsy. Chrysotile fibers are cleared from lung tissue more quickly than amphibole fibers. This may be due in part to dissolution and in part to migration. Most of the fibers found near the pleura are chrysotile fibers.

SECONDARY ASBESTOS EXPOSURE

Indirect exposure to asbestos, like secondhand tobacco smoke, causes disease. Selikoff found asbestos-related disease in family members of insulation workers from dust brought home on the workers' clothing.[5] Li[99] reported mesothelioma in the otherwise unexposed wife and daughter of an insulation worker (exposed mainly to chrysotile), and household contacts of workers developed mesothelioma.[107,171] Kilburn et al[91] reported that 11% of wives and 4% of children of shipyard workers had radiologic evidence of asbestosis and were therefore at increased risk of future mesothelioma and lung cancer. Indeed among 115 deaths of household contacts of asbestos workers there were 38% cancer deaths, including 10% lung cancer deaths and 3% mesothelioma deaths,[89] that is about half the risk faced by the workers themselves. Community exposure has also resulted in mesothelioma.[16,130,171]

MEASURING ASBESTOS

Asbestos can be analyzed in air, water, wipe samples of dust, or "bulk" samples of solid material (Table 38-4). Standard air samples are collected on a filter paper and fibers greater than 5 μm long are counted with a phase contrast microscope.[52] An experienced laboratory is essential, and EPA proficiency testing showed that many laboratories performed poorly. Alternative approaches include both scanning (SEM) and transmission (TEM) electron microscopy and x-ray diffraction.

Table 38-4. Units used for reporting results of asbestos analysis*

Workplace air	Fibers/cc mg/m^3
School or nonworkplace air	Fibers/m^3
School or nonworkplace air (includes asbestos and nonasbestos material under TEM)	Structures/cc (s/cc)
Bulk samples	Percentage by weight
Concentration in water	Millions of fibers/L (MFL)
Lung tissues	Fibers/g (wet or dry weight)
Epidemiology dose reconstruction	Million particles/cubic ft year (mppcf-yr) or (mpcf)
Lifetime exposure	Total fibers; mfcc-yr

*Environmental and Occupational Health Sciences Institute.

ASBESTOS-RELATED DISEASES

There are several long-term studies of asbestos-exposed workers, including the Quebec miners and millers,[107] textile workers,[37,38,106] asbestos-cement workers,[84] and insulation workers.[156,159] Much of the critical epidemiologic research that resulted in banning asbestos uses was performed by the late Irving J. Selikoff, MD, and his colleagues at Mt. Sinai Medical School in New York. Selikoff, already well known for his research in tuberculosis, followed a cohort of 17,800 insulation workers for many years, documenting their causes of death. Four classes of disease (Table 38-5) were elevated in this cohort. About 10% of the cohort died of asbestosis, 20% of lung cancer, 8% of mesothelioma, and 8% of intestinal cancers, making this undoubtedly the most hazardous profession known. There have been many other epidemiologic studies that tend to verify most of the findings, albeit with varying degrees of risk, in many different types of asbestos exposure. The conditions were covered in Chapter 23.

Asbestosis

Asbestosis is a restrictive fibrotic lung disease, one of the pneumoconioses.[157] It is mainly a disease of occupational exposure; for example, 86% of shipyard workers had asbestosis.[158] The severity of the lung reaction is correlated with the exposure level, usually measured in fiber $\times$ years of exposure. Asbestosis is usually detected after 10 years of exposure, but long-term exposure is not essential for developing asbestosis,[153] and it can even occur in household contacts.[4,91] It can be caused by any of the types of asbestos fiber.[36,133,159]

Diagnostic criteria for asbestosis. The classical picture of asbestosis includes a history of significant asbestos exposure, x-ray evidence of fibrosis (at least ILO category 1/1 with irregular opacities and pleural changes), reduced FVC ($<$ 80% predicted value), end inspiratory rales, and reduced diffusing capacity ($<$ 80% predicted value). Clubbing occurs in advanced cases with hypoxia, but is otherwise seldom seen and is not required for diagnosis. Diagnosis can be confirmed by demonstrating asbestos bodies in biopsies or bronchoalveolar lavage or by gallium-67 lung scans, but with a good history such aggressive approaches are not required.

The primary means of diagnosing asbestosis is with a so-called B-reading of the posteroanterior (PA) chest radiograph based on internationally accepted guidelines published by the International Labour Office for x-ray diagnosis of the pneumoconioses.[86] Some of the reporting criteria are listed in Table 38-6, and more detailed illustrations are provided

Table 38-5. Mortality causes among 17,800 asbestos workers[156,159]

	Standardized Mortality Ratio (SMR) (1991)		
	1979	Death cert. 1991	Best evidence 1991
All cause mortality	146	143	143
Total cancer mortality	400	279	301
Lung cancer	436	375	435
Gastrointestinal cancer	140	139	139
Noninfectious lung disease		321	350
All other causes		93	84
Laryngeal cancer	171		
Oral cancers	220		
		Actual deaths recorded (too rare to calculate SMR)	
Pleural mesothelioma		89	173
Peritoneal mesothelioma		92	285
Asbestosis		201	427

All values significantly elevated (or reduced) at the .001 level.

Table 38-6. ILO scoring system for profusion of parenchymal fibrosis[86]*

0/- 0/0	No fibrosis
0/1	Minimal changes, not enough for category 1
1/0 1/1 1/2	Slight profusion
2/1 2/2 2/3	Intermediate profusion
3/2 3/3 3/-	Great profusion
p	Round infiltrates $<$1.5 mm
q	Round infiltrates 1.5-3 mm
r	Round infiltrates $>$ 3 mm
s	Irregular infiltrates ca $<$1.5 mm
t	Irregular infiltrates ca 1.5-3 mm
i	Irregular infiltrates ca 3-10 mm
A,B,C	Large opacities

Note: All results are referenced against a standard set of x-rays used for training and scoring. The report form also includes entries for film quality, site and extent of pleural abnormalities, locations of lesions, and abnormalities unrelated to dust disease. For example, a 2/1 reading indicates a category 2 profusion, but the reader seriously considered category 1 before deciding on 2. This allows for classification of intermediate profusion.

*By permission of Environmental and Occupational Health Sciences Institute; adapted from ILO 1980.[86]

by Merchant and Schwartz.[112] B-readers are trained in reading x-rays specifically to detect subtle changes according to these criteria. Although originally designed for epidemiologic purposes, this grading system has proven useful for clinical and compensation purposes as well.[44] In the United States B-readers are certified by NIOSH. Radiologists who are not B-readers very often miss asbestosis, but occasionally they overdiagnose it as well.[77,143]

Although there is great variability in radiographic diagnosis,[44] most cases of parenchymal asbestosis are detectable on a typical PA view, but 19% of cases were detected only on a lateral.[76] Kipen et al[92] caution that a chest x-ray is not infallible, since 18% of workers with autopsy-proven parenchymal fibrosis had "negative" chest x-rays indeed, 11% of those with "severe fibrosis" at autopsy were read as negative. Traditional CT scans can be useful in assessing pleural disease, but were not advantageous for pulmonary asbestosis.[13] However, high-resolution CT augments the detection and interpretation of both parenchymal and pleural disease,[104] and new phosphor-based digital radiography offers promise as well.[67]

Clinical features of asbestosis. Asbestosis can be graded from I (peribronchiolar fibrosis with asbestos bodies) to IV (honeycombing). Even mild cases reveal a reduction in forced vital capacity (FVC), total lung capacity, and diffusing capacity. With advanced disease, persons have exertional dyspnea and reduced arterial oxygen saturation. FVC may be more sensitive than x-ray in detecting asbestosis,[12] and some studies show a correlation between the two.[115,146,148] Even asbestos workers with normal chest x-rays had an average FVCs only 88% of predicted.[115]

Pathogenesis. After depositing in or near the alveoli, fibers may remain in place, be slowly dissolved, or migrate directly through tissue, or via the bloodstream or lymphatics. Fibers elicit a complement-mediated chemotaxis, attracting macrophages, and within an hour of experimental exposure, macrophages engulf the fibers.[97] Short fibers may be successfully phagocytized, while longer fibers only partially surrounded may distort and damage the macrophage. Macrophages secrete a growth factor that is a chemoattractant and a strong stimulant of fibroblast mitosis,[97] resulting in a great proliferation of fibrous tissue immediately around the fiber. There is also a positive feedback, for as fibrosis progresses, the percentage of fibers retained in the lung increases.[103] See Chapter 14 for further details.

The activated macrophages may also play a role in upregulating proto-oncogenes,[74] which in turn may increase cell responsiveness to growth factors also secreted by the macrophages, increasing the likelihood of malignant transformation.[68] There is also a release of active oxygen species, free radicals that may in turn damage cell membranes through lipid peroxidation.[122] Cellular proliferation can be demonstrated by the uptake of tritiated thymidine by macrophage and alveolar epithelial cells exposed to chrysotile.[126]

Pleural plaques or pleural asbestosis

Diffuse pleural thickening and pleural plaques are characteristic of asbestos exposure and can occur at levels insufficient to produce x-ray-positive fibrosis. Increasingly they are referred to as "pleural asbestosis." A study of 12,000 sheet metal workers showed a prevalence of pleural disease ranging from 10% (for those with 20 to 24 years since onset) to 22% (for those with 40+ years), whereas parenchymal disease was detected in less than 10%.[173] However, pleural thickening can be detected in schoolteachers and maintenance workers exposed to much lower levels of asbestos in public buildings.

Plaques begin with thickening of the pleura, mainly over the diaphragm and in the costophrenic angle, but may become confluent over much of the lung and can develop calcifications. The distinction between pleural thickening and pleural fat is facilitated by use of high-resolution CT scanning.[104] Pleural thickening and plaques are probably the first x-ray evidence of asbestos exposure.

There is a 50% increased detection with the use of oblique films in addition to PA and lateral,[10] although interobserver reliability is lower.[142]

Significance of pleural plaques. Until recently most clinicians assumed that plaques were an incidental marker of asbestos exposure and did not have pathologic consequences, and there is still debate over whether plaques represent a physiologic defect associated with spirometric abnormalities, a predictor of increased cancer risk, or perhaps even a precursor of mesothelioma. Studies of workers with pleural plaques have found two- to threefold increased risk of mesothelioma and lung cancer.[60,61] Pleural plaques also exert an independent effect on lung function,* with a decline of 5% to 10%.[148]

Lung cancer

Lung cancer is the largest killer of asbestos workers in some studies,[153,156,158,159] and it has been recognized as a hazard since the 1930s (see box on p. 440). Asbestosis is a risk factor for cancer. Amphibole-exposed workers with slight and with moderate to pronounced asbestosis experienced lung cancer SMRs of 416 and 562, respectively, while those with no radiographic opacities had an SMR < 100.[163] However, in animal studies, lung cancer can occur at levels that do not cause fibrosis,[141] although with chrysotile, at least, cancers are most likely to arise in the lobes with fibrosis.[34] The causal relationship between asbestos exposure and lung cancer was recognized in part because of the evidence of asbestosis in the lungs of cancer victims,[40,41] raising the question of whether asbestosis is a necessary precursor[83] or simply an indicator of exposure. The process of inflammation may be a "promotor" of lung cancer in victims of asbestosis. Thus asbestos fibers could initiate DNA damage

---
*References 9, 59, 88, 102, 151.

and the concomitant inflammation could promote the development of cancer.

Pathogenesis of cancer

It is not clear how asbestos causes cancer. Its role as an initiator (direct damage to DNA or chromosomes) has been challenged,[125] but there is recent evidence to support it. There is also a promoting role, perhaps related to the inflammatory response generated by the fibers. One early hypothesis was that polyaromatic hydrocarbons and other initiators adsorbed to the asbestos fiber, which serves mainly as a vehicle, and that the smoother surfaces of glass fibers made them less active in this role.[45,120]

Mesothelioma

Primary cancer of the pleura or peritoneal membrane is a very rare condition (incidence less than 1/100,000 per year) in people who have not been exposed to asbestos and related fibrous silicates. The first mesothelioma case in an asbestos worker was reported in 1943. Wagner et al[171] described 33 cases from in and around a South African crocidolite mine; 5% of deaths among crocidolite workers were mesotheliomas. Selikoff et al[156] estimated that 8% of deaths among insulation workers exposed mainly to chrysotile were mesotheliomas.

Clinical picture. Mesothelioma often presents with a pleural effusion and/or chest pain, dyspnea, and weight loss. In some cohorts peritoneal tumors predominate. Many mesotheliomas have been misdiagnosed as lung cancer, because nosology emphasizes site rather than histology. The histologic picture resembles fibrosarcoma. In addition to location and cytologic features, mesothelioma can be distinguished from adenocarcinoma by the presence of certain biomarkers (for example, cytokeratin) and the absence of others (for example, CEA, Leu MI).

In most cases (at least 85%) of malignant mesothelioma, a history of asbestos exposure can be identified. The risk is not augmented by cigarette smoking. Although all fiber types can cause mesothelioma, crocidolite seems to be the worst offender. Mesothelioma rates were similar in two Quebec townships, despite a sevenfold difference in tremolite contamination of the chrysotile, leading him to conclude that chrysotile caused mesothelioma in humans.[147]

Both pleural and peritoneal mesotheliomas are caused by asbestos exposure, and in these cases pleural tissue has high concentrations of asbestos fibers, particularly chrysotile.[93] The mode of transfer from lung or intestine to the pleura or peritoneum can be either lymphogenous, hematogenous, or direct penetration, and this is no doubt influenced by the fiber morphology and perhaps chemistry.

In insulation workers, where more than 50% of mesotheliomas were peritoneal, there has been a decline in peritoneal but not in pleural mesotheliomas.[159] In contrast, only 5% of mesotheliomas in Italian railroad machinists were peritoneal.[108]

Intestinal tract cancers

Several studies provide evidence of excess rates of intestinal cancer in asbestos-exposed workers.[6,49,128,159,172] Other studies do not find this. Some studies show slight increase in GI cancers in populations exposed to asbestos in drinking water,[26,81,90] and a National Toxicology Program lifetime feeding study with chrysotile produced GI cancers in male rats.[127]

Since fibers are readily swallowed or directly ingested and since fibers can be demonstrated in the GI tract, there is no question that the mucosa is exposed to asbestos. Nonetheless alternative explanations offered for the increased risk include misdiagnosis, diet, and alcohol.[42,43] The Agency for Toxic Substances and Disease Registry (1993) concludes that although ''none of these lines of evidence are entirely convincing ... it seems only prudent to consider increased risk of gastrointestinal cancer an effect of concern.'' The evidence from multiple positive studies shows clearly that asbestos causes GI cancer.

Immunologic effects

Several studies have identified alterations in cell-mediated immunity,[116] but although this may influence susceptibility to complications of advanced disease, the immunologic changes do not seem to be necessary for the development of either asbestosis or cancer, although impairment of immunosurveillance of abnormal cells may contribute.

Medical surveillance

Workers with past or current exposure to asbestos, such as asbestos-abatement workers, are required to have periodic medical evaluations. Such examinations can have important benefits for those with exposure and a substantial risk of future disease. For example, Selikoff et al[158] found five previously undetected lung cancers among 286 shipyard workers screened. Judging by the 86% with radiologic evidence of asbestosis, this was certainly a high-risk cohort.

Epidemiology

There have been many epidemiologic studies of asbestos that have used various approaches to overcome the lack of adequate exposure information or other sources of potential bias; studies based on union records have tended to find steeper dose-response curves than those based on social security or company records.[47] Recognizing the limitations of death certificate studies, particularly where underdiagnosis of a disease may be part of the hypothesis, Selikoff and associates developed a ''best evidence'' approach to diagnosis.[156,160] They reviewed medical records of decedents, including x-rays and biopsy and autopsy results to cross-validate death certificate diagnoses, and they reported SMRs based on both death certificates and ''best evidence.''[160] Using this approach, Selikoff et al[156] reported the SMRs shown in Table 37-5. They concluded that of all the deaths in this cohort exposed to chrysotile, there was a 31% excess of cancer mortality and a 9% excess of asbestosis. In other words, 40% of the people who died died because of their asbestos exposure.

Quebec miners showed an SMR of 161 for lung cancer, and asbestosis was elevated in both the miners and the surrounding community.[107] Other studies of chrysotile-exposed workers showed lung cancer SMRs of 214,[140] 221, and 237,[48] and one study reported a higher SMR for mixed chrysotile-crocidolite exposure[75] than for chrysotile alone. Dement et al[38] reported an overall SMR of 135 but an SMR of 728 for workers with 20 or more years of exposure. Conversely an epidemiologic study of an asbestos workforce that did not have elevated air levels of asbestos reported no excess of lung cancer.[129]

Dose-response curves. Epidemiologic data on asbestos allows one to demonstrate dose-response relationships. In general the relative risk in a large cohort is a nearly linear function of the cumulative fiber-years of exposure. A fiber-year is obtained by multiplying the estimated exposure (fibers/cc) times the number of years over which such an exposure occurred. Since in most cases there are no actual measurements, one must use a dose-reconstruction approach, based on existing data for a particular plant and/or process, using the worker's history or company records to determine the duration of work in a particular job title or building.

In studies of Quebec miners, however, the dose-response curves are not linear and the slope is much flatter[107] than the slope derived from textile workers.[37] Doll and Peto[43] showed that the incidence of mesothelioma increases in proportion to the intensity of exposure, the duration of exposure, and the third power of the number of years since exposure began.

The data from Selikoff and Seidman[159] show that the SMR for lung cancer continues to rise for cohorts until they have been followed for 35 to 39 years from onset of exposure (SMR 511). There was very little excess detected in men followed for only 15 years from onset of exposure, although individual cases with only 10-year latency have been reported.[101]

Latency. The long latency period between onset of exposure and diagnosis of cancer poses a challenge to epidemiologists trying to elucidate their causes. Mesothelioma is among those tumors with the longest latency periods, and only its rarity and relative uniqueness to asbestos exposure allowed it to be identified as an asbestos-related disease. For 94 mesothelioma cases in London dockworkers, only 15 occurred within 30 years of first exposure, and 7 occurred more than 60 years later. The peak latencies were between 30 and 50 years.[14,161] For pleural mesothelioma the peak is at 45 to 49 years from onset, when it reaches 513 cases/100,000, almost 5000 times the background rate. A similar trend was observed for peritoneal mesothelioma and for asbestosis.[159]

Smoking and asbestos disease

Cigarette smoking interacts synergistically with asbestos exposure to cause lung cancer. It does not seem to be implicated in mesothelioma, and there are conflicting studies regarding a role in asbestosis. In 1968 Selikoff et al[155] made the alarming discovery for 283 asbestos workers who smoked that they had a ninety-twofold increased risk of dying of lung cancer compared with men who had neither exposure. Further study of this cohort showed that asbestos workers have 5 times the risk of developing lung cancers as controls, while smoking confers an elevenfold increased risk compared with nonsmokers. Insulation workers who smoked had a fifty-threefold greater risk of lung cancer than those who had neither smoking nor asbestos exposure.[156] This is remarkably close to the 55 predicted by a truly multiplicative or synergistic interaction, and this represents the best example of true synergism between two environmental exposures. Smoking cessation is therefore the main preventive strategy available to asbestos-exposed individuals.

Smoking also increases or accelerates asbestosis,[15] perhaps because of interference with fiber clearance. Smokers were much less likely than nonsmokers to have normal chest x-rays and averaged about 5% lower FVCs than nonsmokers, a significant finding since about 80% of the cohort had smoked.[115] Moreover, impairment began about 10 years earlier in smokers.[31] However, some studies found no relationship between smoking history and asbestos mortality.[100]

Fiber types and pathogenesis

A fiber is defined as being three times as long as its diameter, and the effective or aerodynamic diameter is three times the actual diameter.[103] Thus fibers broader than 3μm do not reach the alveoli. Conversely, the smallest fibers with diameter <0.1 μm are likely to remain airborne and to be exhaled with the subsequent breath; longer fibers are more likely to be retained within the lung.[103]

Stanton proposed that fibers less than 0.5 μm in diameter and more than 5 μm long have greater pathogenic potency,[165,166] while Harington[71] believed that for mesothelioma the most carcinogenic fibers had diameters <.05 μm and length <3 μm. The relationship between fiber size, aspect (shape), and carcinogenicity is certainly not simple, and the fiber size distribution of the different types of asbestos does not coincide with the epidemiologic data. In some studies of chrysotile[24] and amosite[25] fibrosis has been negatively correlated with the fiber size distribution. For example, reference samples of crocidolite and Canadian chrysotile have only 3% of fibers >5 μm long, while amosite and Rhodesian chrysotile have 6% of fibers >5 μm,[144] yet the former are more pathogenic.

Some writers have argued that chrysotile is less hazardous than the amphiboles,[111,121] and this viewpoint has serious economic consequences as well as health implications.[119] The American Conference of Governmental Industrial Hygienists[3] distinguishes different hazard levels by setting a threshold limit value (TLV) for crocidolite of 0.2 fibers/cc, for amosite of 0.5 fibers/cc, and for chrysotile and other amphiboles of 2 fibers/cc. However, OSHA and EPA do not distinguish, reflecting their conclusion that chrysotile is no less hazardous than the other fiber types. It has long been known that all types of asbestos fibers can cause fibrosis, lung cancer, and mesothelioma in animals,[1,80] and tumor incidence is similar for chrysotile exposure and amphibole exposure.[170]

The arguments that chrysotile is somehow "safer" and that Canadian chrysotile was not carcinogenic are not new, and were rebutted in the pages of *Science*,[145] and by the International Agency for Research on Cancer in 1977[85] with the words, "Uncontrolled exposure to chrysotile asbestos . . . has the potential for serious human disease. Reassurance is unwarranted. . . ."[85] The debate has recently heightened as the asbestos industry seeks to expand world markets for chrysotile and argues that chrysotile has low carcinogenic potential and can be used "safely." The International Program on Chemical Safety (IPCS), a branch of the World Health Organization, whose decisions will have significant impacts on international trade treaties, is reexamining its position on chrysotile, hearing claims from certain governments and industries that wish to expand the worldwide use of chrysotile.

Pathogenicity of chrysotile. Chrysotile was the main exposure for the most completely studied cohort of asbestos workers, Selikoff's insulation workers.[159] This cohort experienced dramatic excess of certain cancers. Mossman and colleagues[119] have advanced what has come to be called the "amphibole" hypothesis, namely that the diseases attributed to chrysotile are really due to tremolite or other amphibole contaminants. This is a subject of heated debate. Several authors have criticized the amphibole hypothesis on the following grounds: (1) The mesothelioma rates in two Quebec cities where chrysotile was mined were similar, despite the fact that the percent of tremolite contamination varied sevenfold.[147] (2) Since the amphibole represented only 1% of the asbestos present, its potency would have to be more than 100 times greater than that of chrysotile in order for it to be the predominant contributor. (3) The Tremolite fiber present in the lung now would be positively correlated with the total fiber exposure and therefore with the chrysotile exposure, which took place many years earlier. (4) tremolite fibers are generally shorter than the size identified by Stanton as "optimal."[166] (5) There is no practical way to eliminate the tremolite from the asbestos.[94]

Fiber burden in lungs. Examining data on the Quebec chrysotile miners, Mossman et al[119] point to the correlation between risk of mesothelioma and the lung content of tremolite as evidence in favor of the amphibole hypothesis and against the carcinogenicity of chrysotile. Beginning in the mid-1980s many studies have appeared investigating the persistence of asbestos fibers in the lung and their movement from the lung parenchyma to the pleura and other tissues.

The results are conflicting, but some studies show that chrysotile is cleared from the parenchyma and shows a much higher tendency to concentrate in the pleura than does amosite.[93] Baker[8] cautions that such fiber burden studies are limited by potential biases.

Epidemiologic evidence. Dement[37,38] has followed a cohort of textile workers who used almost exclusively Quebec chrysotile. Three studies of textile workers exposed to chrysotile show uniformly steep dose-response curves when the relative risk is plotted against fiber counts, while the comparable curve for chrysotile miners is much more gradual. He cautions against generalizing from the miner data or concluding that chrysotile is not a lung carcinogen, and suggests that the greater carcinogen rates among textile workers may reflect exposure to longer and thinner and more potent fibers.[37] Except for miners there is a 0.5% to 4.3% risk for every year of exposure to 1 f/cc[133] regardless of fiber type. Hughes and Weill[83,84] concluded that a mixed exposure to chrysotile plus crocidolite was somewhat more potent at producing mesothelioma in humans, but that chrysotile was just as potent as crocidolite in causing lung cancer. Mesothelioma rates were similar in cohorts that were exposed to 97% chrysotile, 60% chrysotile, and 100% amosite. It appears that crocidolite is more potent in causing mesothelioma, but chrysotile is equivalent to amosite, and both are more potent than tremolite in causing mesothelioma.

In addition there is substantial animal data. Wagner et al[170] demonstrated that chrysotile, whether from Canada or Rhodesia, was more potent than any amphibole in producing lung cancer, particularly adenocarcinomas in rodents. Moreover, the Canadian chrysotile (which contains 1% tremolite) was just as potent as pure crocidolite, tremolite, or amosite in causing mesothelioma. Therefore the cancer rates could not be due to the tremolite contaminant alone.

In vitro evidence. Cytotoxicity is related at least in part due to fiber morphology and, for example, nonfibrous serpentine is not cytotoxic.[62] Chrysotile is more cytotoxic than crocidolite.[122] Experiments using short (<2 μm) and long (>10 μm) fibers of chrysotile and crocidolite showed that the former were taken up by epithelial cells, while the latter were partially phagocytized with a release of superoxide anion radicals.[122] In some studies chrysotile proved to be a complete carcinogen,[73] not requiring an additional promotor.

Mineral oil hypothesis. Another hypothesis, the so-called mineral oil hypothesis argues that the apparent carcinogenicity of chrysotile should be blamed on the mineral oil applied to it in the textile industry. However, Dement[37] tested this hypothesis and found that mineral oil exposure did not contribute appreciably to the lung cancer rates in a cohort of asbestos textile workers, and mineral oil is also used the same way in the cotton textile industry where no excess of lung cancer is seen.

Conclusions on chrysotile carcinogenesis. Nicholson[133] concludes that "both human and animal data demonstrate that chrysotile asbestos is as potent a carcinogen to the lung as any other variety of asbestos.'' Based on in vitro studies, animal studies, and epidemiologic studies, Harington[72] and Rom[147] concluded that chrysotile is a significant human carcinogen. Doll[42] concluded that chrysotile is just as likely to cause lung cancer as amphiboles. Hughes, Weill, and Hammad reported that chrysotile causes lung cancer.[84] Doll and Peto[43] concluded that there is no point in blaming tremolite unless the tremolite can be removed from the chrysotile. Thus chrysotile must be considered as much a human carcinogen as the amphiboles, and although it may be less potent than crocidolite in causing mesothelioma, its greater potency as a lung carcinogen must be emphasized since lung cancer is a much more common cause of death in asbestos workers. There are no grounds for complacency regarding chrysotile. Experience at trying to protect workers in the highly regulated asbestos abatement industry suggests that although it is theoretically possible to work safely with any hazardous material, it will never be practical to work safely with asbestos.

Risk from asbestos in indoor air

In the late 1970s the nation's attention was riveted on the potential for widespread exposure from asbestos-containing materials (ACBM) in public buildings. No longer was asbestos a problem of mines, factories, and shipyards. Asbestos was present in many school buildings and offices, and there might be nonoccupational exposures (schoolchildren, office workers, shoppers) as well as occupational exposure (custodial staff, remediation workers.) (Table 38-7)[134]

In 1984 the National Research Council Committee on Non-occupational Health risks of Asbestiform Fibers published an extensive report,[125] including a quantitative risk assessment assuming an ambient air level of .0004 fibers/cc of air, about 1/250 of the workplace PEL. A lifetime exposure at this level corresponded to a mesothelioma risk of nine in a million. The risk of lung cancer would range from 64 per million for male smokers to 3 per million for female nonsmokers. Aroesty and Wolf[7] pointed out an error in the NRC[125] calculations, determining a lifetime background risk of mesothelioma of 800/million coupled with a school-acquired risk of 399 per million. The comparable risk for exposure to .0004 fibers/cc and .002 fibers/cc for lung cancer ranged from 14 (female nonsmoker at low dose) to 1459 per million (for male smoker at high dose).

Mossman and Gee[121] argued that nonoccupational exposure to asbestos was not a hazard, but ignored several studies that showed asbestos disease among household contacts of asbestos workers and community residents near asbestos mines and factories. In addition, several studies have shown that occupants of buildings containing ACBM do develop asbestos-related diseases. These include asbestosis[11,98,135] and mesothelioma[4] among maintenance workers, and asbestosis[64] and mesothelioma[101] among schoolteachers.

Asbestos in the home

Asbestos is widespread in private homes constructed prior to 1978, mainly around hot water pipes and furnace boilers, and as asbestos cement used around furnace fittings. Although asbestos-cement sheeting, a grayish-white, brittle, thin, boardlike material, is easily recognizable, there are many asbestos-containing products that cannot be recognized without testing. The gaskets around the doors on furnaces and coal or wood-burning stoves often contain asbestos, and these should be replaced before they become severely worn. Asbestos-impregnated paper products were widely used as pipe insulation, although most insulation installed after 1980 is asbestos free. Drywall patching material and spackle produced before 1978 often contained asbestos, as did textured paint. Asbestos siding, vinyl asbestos floor tiling, and roofing felt with asbestos were also widely used. None of these materials routinely release asbestos fiber unless they become friable due to water damage, or unless there is manipulation such as drilling, cutting, or removal. Some states have produced a model document for homeowners.[50]

Asbestos as a hazardous waste

Asbestos materials were frequently removed and discarded during building renovations and demolition (see Table 38-7). When repairing pipes and replacing damaged insulation, plumbers frequently discarded soggy and fragmented asbestos on the floor, where dust accumulated over many years, exposing subsequent generations of maintenance workers.[66] Many landfills received construction debris, and some have piles of uncontained asbestos. Since 1980 only certain landfills are approved to receive asbestos waste, and this must be properly double-bagged and labelled according to EPA specifications.

PREVENTING EXPOSURE TO ASBESTOS

In the United States the Environmental Protection Agency (EPA) is the main agency responsible for regulating uses, transportation, releases, and disposal of asbestos. Permits for building renovation and demolition require a site assessment for asbestos and a plan for safe prior removal and disposal. The EPA regulates the sites that can accept and dispose of asbestos safely.

Table 38-7. EPA survey of asbestos in buildings[57]

	Buildings	% of Friable	% of Type	Million sq feet
Total with friable asbestos	733,000	100	20	1200
Residential apartment buildings	208,000	28	59	
Private nonresidential	511,000	70	16	
Federal government	14,000	2	35	
School survey	35,000		35	169

For drinking water there is a substantial gap between the ambient water quality guideline of .0003 fibers/L proposed by the EPA[54] and the Minimum Contaminant Level Guideline of 7 million fibers/L.[58] The latter would allow a typical adult to consume 14 million fibers in a typical day. However, most drinking water supplies contain well under 1 million f/L.

The EPA banned most uses of asbestos and required a 10-year phaseout. However, a federal court reversed the ban, except for procedures and products already banned prior to 1987. Nonetheless, because of insurance and liability considerations, most asbestos use in the United States has terminated.

Standards governing asbestos exposure

In 1971 the OSHA permissible exposure limit (PEL) was 5 fibers (longer than 5 μm) per cc, based on an 8-hour time-weighted average, which would allow a person to inhale 100 million fibers a day. This was lowered to 2 f/cc in 1976, which was deemed sufficient to prevent asbestosis but not to prevent cancer,[139] and it was lowered to 0.2 f/cc in 1986 and to 0.1 f/cc in 1994. In 1986 OSHA issued a companion standard to regulate asbestos exposure in the construction industry to control removal, encapsulation, renovation, maintenance, insulation, spill cleanup, transportation, disposal, and storage of asbestos. The National Emission Standards for Hazardous Air Pollutants (NESHAP) require that asbestos emissions be controlled with the best available control technology (BACT).[51]

Working safely with asbestos

For people who must work with asbestos, for example in abatement, heavy emphasis is placed on protecting the worker with proper equipment and training. The asbestos industry argues[119,121] that it is possible to work safely with asbestos, while at the same time it decries the removal of asbestos from buildings because of the great cost. Paradoxically, the great cost arises in large part because of the need to remove it safely—the training and protection of abatement workers and building occupants. If, as the industry itself argues, the cost of asbestos abatement is prohibitive, it is not likely that such costly safeguards will be part of everyday operations, particularly in the developing world, where worker protection is generally primitive.

Managing asbestos

Asbestos Hazard Emergency Response Act (AHERA). In 1986 Congress passed AHERA, which required local school districts to evaluate their facilities for the presence and condition of asbestos and to develop a management plan. EPA estimated a cost of about $7000 per school building, and established a $74 million school aid program that was terminated in 1993.[56,57] It also required the EPA to develop regulations for asbestos response by school districts and conduct a nationwide study to determine the extent of danger to human health. The box below and the one on the next page identifies some key requirements in the EPA regulations developed under AHERA.

Magnitude of the problem

Asbestos-containing materials are widespread in public buildings such as schools.[134] Under AHERA New York State determined that there were over 250 million square feet of asbestos in school buildings, of which about 9% was either friable or deteriorated, and a New York City survey showed that 67% of buildings had asbestos, and 13% of these had deteriorated asbestos.[94] A systematic survey of Vermont schools found 75% with asbestos and 40% with asbestos in student-occupied areas; significantly, in prior self-assessments by school districts, only 10% of such schools had been identified.[134] A Boston school survey cited by Oliver[135] found 43% of schools with ACBM requiring prompt corrective action, 13% where asbestos was present but intact, and only 11% with no asbestos. The EPA's report to the U.S. Congress[57] estimated 733,000 buildings containing friable asbestos, but most of this was in pipe and boiler insulation, which poses a more isolated and manageable problem (see box on the following page).

Removal costs are astronomical, estimated at over $14 million for one school alone.[46] Alternatively, some schools use a quick-and-dirty removal method that is cheaper and more hazardous. One district spent $180,000 to remove 100,000 square feet of asbestos; a photograph clearly illustrates an improperly protected worker using improper tech-

---

Provisions of the AHERA requirements for local education agencies[56]

By Dec. 14, 1987, each LEA* must

Select and train a "designate person" responsible for all activities

Use accredited personnel to design and carry out response actions

Train maintenance staff

Post warning labels where asbestos has been identified

Abide by maintenance requirements when asbestos may be disturbed

Transport and dispose of asbestos waste safely

Maintain records necessary to verify compliance

By Oct. 12, 1988, each LEA must

Complete initial inspection to locate all asbestos-containing building materials (ACBM)

Develop and submit an asbestos management plan based on inspection

By July 9, 1989, each LEA must

Begin implementation of management plan

*Local Educational Agency (e.g., Board of Education).

nique.[110] The overall estimate for asbestos abatement in the United States is as high as $150 billion.[121]

Abatement decisions

Beginning in 1979 the EPA[52] developed guidelines for managing ACBM and criteria for determining whether to remove it or manage it in place. Remarkably, these have withstood the test of time and the appearance of new remediation techniques.[65] It is generally agreed that ACBM that is not releasing fibers is not a health threat, but the public and insurers do not always accept this, and do not want to overlook future hazards should the ACBM become unstable. The decision over whether to remove, encapsulate, enclose, or observe asbestos depends on the type and condition of the material and the potential for human exposure. Alternative views range from "Removal should be avoided if possible"[111] to "All ACBM must come out of buildings when they are demolished; the issue is when, not whether to spend the money."[135] New Jersey has argued for a more middle-of-the-road position.[65]

Any form of management entails costs and health risks, but well-established guidelines exist for reaching decisions. The quick-and-dirty removal or out-of-sight, out-of-mind approaches are untenable. The following factors enter into the decision process (see box below).

Friable versus cementitious. This describes the form of ACBM at the time of application. Some is hard and plaster-like while other is soft and cottony. The latter is "friable," tending to pull apart and to separate from its support when disturbed. Friable material is soft and compressible. Friable asbestos used for thermal insulation contains a high proportion of amosite, while the cottony spray surfacing used for soundproofing or fireproofing contained chrysotile or amosite and occasionally even crocidolite. The cementitious materials contained mainly chrysotile with about 1% tremolite.[133] Friability per se may constitute grounds for removal when the ACBM can be directly contacted by building occupants. Cement-like ACBM will release fiber when damaged or when cut, but not under normal circumstances.

Condition. Either friable or cementitious asbestos may become damaged by building activities, or most often by water. Plaster-like material, becoming water-sodden, may separate and partially disintegrate, and begin to release fibers as it dries. In this condition it behaves like "friable" asbestos, but the term "friable" is not synonymous with "damaged."

Accessibility. Particularly in schools where children may brush up against or damage the ACBM, this is grounds for abatement. Vandalism by school occupants frequently results in the gouging or scarification of ceilings in hallways and classrooms (personal observations in New Jersey high schools). Repair work by maintenance workers also releases fibers. But even the normal wear-and-tear and vibration of an occupied building can jar loose fibers from friable or damaged ACBM or can stir up asbestos-containing dust from various surfaces.

Measurement of air levels. Air sampling is not an acceptable criterion for deciding whether to remove asbestos, and air level measurements are neither required nor appropriate for making decisions regarding abatement,[132] although a high air level may prompt more immediate actions.[65] Often there is no difference in air levels of asbestos in buildings with no ACBM, with intact ACBM, and with damaged ACBM, although air levels average about 10 times higher than outside urban ambient levels.[19,57] Sawyer et al.[149] showed that fiber counts could be undetectable, even in the presence of grossly visible settled asbestos dust subject to being stirred up and breathed in. Elevated air levels are likely to be episodic due to disturbance of dust by maintenance or custodial workers or by building occupants, which can increase air levels above the occupational PEL.[150] Therefore the arguments by Mossman et al.[119] that indoor air levels are very low reflect the inadequacy of air analysis as a decision tool, rather than a low level of risk. Air analysis is important during abatement activities, however.

Abatement versus observation and management. Friable, deteriorating, or highly accessible ACBM to which building occupants are exposed should be removed. Otherwise damaged material can be encapsulated or enclosed if it

---

Asbestos management program

Analysis

Verify presence or absence of asbestos in building materials
Take bulk samples and analyze if necessary

Inspection

Is the asbestos friable?
What is its condition: intact, deteriorated, severely damaged?
What is the distribution of friability or damage?
Is it accessible to people?
What are the target populations?
How can exposure occur?

Operations and management (O&M) program

Categorize all asbestos with regard to potential exposure
Make decision—manage in place, remediate, remove
Asbestos removal or abatement plan
O & M plan (inspection, containment, medical monitoring, training)

Notification

Written report to all occupants

Abatement

Certified contractors
Contract embodies health and safety provisions
Follow EPA guidelines for asbestos containment
Air monitoring during removal
Postremoval assessment

is localized and there is no regular opportunity for exposure. Intact, stable ACBM can be left in place and managed under an observation and management (O & M) program. However, an O & M program is not cheap, and it is "not a trivial matter that can be relegated to building custodians."[87]

Asbestos removal

If removal were only costly, it would be easier to deal with, but the process of removal is likely to greatly increase the levels of airborne fibers, at least temporarily, and thereby jeopardizes the health of removal workers as well as other building occupants. Any asbestos abatement or removal project should conform to the EPA's guidance documents.[52,56,150] It is important that contracts for removal specify the health and safety requirements, and that on-site enforcement of the specifications be made by an independent industrial hygienist. The contractors and workers must be highly motivated and trained to follow the guidelines.[149]

Removal of asbestos without wetting produces fiber counts regularly in excess of 30 f/cc and sometimes greater than 100 f/cc. Therefore, wet procedures are required, and the use of amended water, containing a surfactant to penetrate the asbestos, lowers the count to about 1 f/cc, in well-controlled removals, while outside the containment area fiber counts averaged 0.1 f/cc.[149] The EPA requires both personal monitoring and air sampling during removal procedures. Air levels measured in the breathing zone of removal workers averaged 50% higher than the area samples.[149] More worrisome, however, is the fact that air level measurements obtained by removal contractors themselves averaged one-quarter the levels measured by experienced, independent industrial hygienists.[149] Self-policing by contractors is therefore inadequate.

Risk communication and asbestos exposure

Although the public is rightfully concerned about asbestos, it is important to emphasize that as with any hazardous material there must be actual exposure and the material must actually enter the body to cause harm. In view of concern over exposure of schoolchildren, the American Academy of Pediatrics studied asbestos exposure and drafted a statement:

> Pediatricians can provide careful, reasoned and influential advice. . . . they need to understand and communicate the basis of the long-term health concerns and the available corrective options. The goal should be to promote effective prevention. . . . remedial options range from complete removal of asbestos or the establishment of physical barriers . . . to simply, an ongoing maintenance and inspection program for asbestos materials that are not an immediate hazard. . . . Sloppy removal and cleanup procedures by inadequate contractors will do more harm than good because they will increase the exposure and hazard to students.[2]

This continues to be sound advice.[65]

Asbestos-containing materials must be identified and their condition must be monitored. Any renovation involving such material must be done to prevent dissemination of asbestos fiber. Any evidence of damage to the material requires further assessment. If ACBM is either friable or damaged and may release fiber into an area occupied by people, abatement is required. This may involve removal or some intermediate action such as encapsulation or enclosure. Only contractors with asbestos certification should perform the abatement work. Building occupants must be notified at each step of the way. Neither alarm nor complacency are warranted.

For further information

The Toxicologic Profile on Asbestos by ATSDR[1] provides an extensive review of the epidemiologic and experimental literature on asbestos. Several groups serve victims of asbestos exposure, including the following:

White Lung Association
P.O. Box 1483
Baltimore, Md 21203

Asbestos Victims Special Fund Trust
1500 Walnut Street, Mezzanine Level
Philadelphia, PA 19102

REFERENCES

1. Agency for Toxic Substances and Disease Registry: *Toxicological profile for asbestos,* Atlanta, 1993, Centers for Disease Control.
2. American Academy of Pediatrics: Asbestos exposure in schools, *Pediatrics* 79:301, 1987.
3. American Conference of Governmental Industrial Hygienists: *Threshold limit values and biological exposure indices for 1992-1993,* Cincinnati, 1992.
4. Anderson HA et al: Mesothelioma among employees with likely contact with in-place asbestos-containing building materials, *Ann NY Acad Sci* 643:550, 1991.
5. Anderson HA et al: Asbestosis among household contacts of asbestos factory workers, *Ann NY Acad Sci* 330:397, 1979.
6. Armstrong et al: Mortality in miners and millers of crocidolite in Western Australia, *Br J Ind Med* 45:5, 1988.
7. Aroesty J, Wolf K: Risk from exposure to asbestos, *Science* 234:923, 1986.
8. Baker DB: Limitations in drawing etiologic inferences based on measurement of asbestos fibers from lung tissue, *Ann NY Acad Sci* 643:61, 1991.
9. Baker EL, Dagg T, Greene RE: Respiratory illness in the construction trades. I. The significance of asbestos-associated pleural disease among sheet metal workers, *J Occup Med* 27:483, 1985.
10. Baker EL, Greene R: Incremental value of oblique chest radiographs in the diagnosis of asbestos-induced pleural disease, *Am J Industr Med* 3:17, 1982.
11. Balmes JR, Daponte A, Cone JE: Asbestos-related disease in custodial and building maintenance workers from a large municipal school district, *Ann NY Acad Sci* 643:540, 1991.
12. Becklake MR: Asbestos-related diseases of the lung and other organs: their epidemiology and implications for clinical practice, *Am Rev Respir Dis* 114:187, 1976.
13. Begin R et al: Radiographic assessment of pleuropulmonary disease in asbestos workers: posteroanterior, four view films, and computed tomograms of the thorax, *Br J Ind Med* 41:373, 1984.
14. Bianchi C et al: Asbestos-related mesothelioma in Monfalcone, Italy, *Am J Ind Med* 24:149, 1993.
15. Blanc P: Cigarette smoking, asbestos, and parenchymal opacities revisited, *Ann NY Acad Sci* 643:133, 1991.
16. Bohlig H et al: Epidemiology of malignant mesothelioma in Hamburg: a preliminary report, *Environ Res* 3:365, 1970.

17. Breslow L et al: Occupations and smoking as factors in lung cancer, *Am J Public Health* 44:171, 1954.
18. Brodeur P: *Outrageous misconduct: the asbestos industry on trial,* New York, 1985, Pantheon.
19. Burdett GJ, Jaffrey S: Airborne asbestos concentrations in buildings, *Ann Occup Hyg* 30:185, 1986.
20. Bureau of Mines: *Asbestos: minerals yearbook 1982,* Washington, DC, 1983, U.S. Department of Interior.
21. Castleman BI: *Asbestos: medical and legal aspects,* ed 3, Englewood Cliffs, NJ, 1990, Prentice Hall Law & Business.
22. Cecil RL, Loeb RF: *A textbook of medicine,* ed 10, Philadelphia, 1959, WB Saunders.
23. Churg A: Fiber counting and analysis in the diagnosis of asbestos-related disease, *Human Pathol* 13:381, 1982.
24. Churg A et al: Mineralogic correlates of fibrosis in chrysotile miners and millers, *Am Rev Respir Dis* 139:891, 1989.
25. Churg A et al: Mineralogic parameters related to amosite asbestos-induced fibrosis in humans, *Am Rev Respir Dis* 142:1331, 1990.
26. Conforti PM et al: Asbestos in drinking water and cancer in the San Francisco Bay area: 1969-1974 incidence, *J Chronic Dis* 34:211, 1981.
27. Cook PM, Glass GE, Tucker JH: Asbestiform amphibole minerals: determination and measurement of high concentrations in municipal water supplies, *Science* 185:853, 1974.
28. Cook PM, Olson GF: Ingested mineral fibers: elimination in human urine, *Science* 204:195, 1979.
29. Cooke WE: Fibrosis of the lungs due to the inhalation of asbestos dust, *Br Med J* 2:147, 1924.
30. Cooke WE: Pulmonary asbestosis, *Br Med J* 2:1024, 1927.
31. Cotes JE, Chinn DJ: Is respiratory function diminished? *Ann NY Acad Sci* 643:149, 1991.
32. Craun GF, Millette JRL: Exposure to asbestos fibers in water distribution systems. Proceeding of the American Water Works Association, ninety-seventh annual conference, Denver, 1977.
33. Dangel RA: *Study of corrosion products in the Seattle Water Department Tolt Distribution System,* Cincinnati, 1975, U.S. Environmental Protection Agency, EPA 670/2/75-036.
34. Davis JM, Cowie HA: The relationship between fibrosis and cancer in experimental animals exposed to asbestos and other fibers, *Environ Health Perspect* 88:305, 1990.
35. Deer WA, Howie RA, Zussman J: *An introduction to the rock-forming minerals,* London, 1966, Longman.
36. de Klerk NH et al: Radiographic abnormalities and mortality in subjects with exposure to crocidolite, *Br J Ind Med* 50:902, 1993.
37. Dement JM: Carcinogenicity of chrysotile asbestos: evidence from cohort studies, *Ann NY Acad Sci* 643:15, 1991.
38. Dement JM et al: Estimates of dose-response for respiratory cancer among chrysotile asbestos textile workers, *Ann Occup Hyg* 26:869, 1983.
39. Doll R: Bronchial carcinoma: incidence & aetiology, *Br Med J* 2:521, 1953.
40. Doll R: Mortality from lung cancer in asbestos workers, *Br J Ind Med* 12:81, 1955.
41. Doll R: Etiology of lung cancer, *Adv Cancer Res* 3:1, 1955.
42. Doll R: Mineral fibers in the non-occupational environment. In Bignon J, Peto R, Saracci R, eds: *Non-occupational exposure to mineral fibers,* Lyon, France, 1989, IARC Scientific.
43. Doll R, Peto J: Effects on health of exposure to asbestos. Report to the Health and Safety Commission, London, 1985, Her Majesty's Stationery Office.
44. Ducatman AM: Variability in interpretation of radiographs for asbestosis abnormalities: problems and solutions, *Ann NY Acad Sci* 643:108, 1991.
45. Eastman A, Mossman BT, Bresnick E: The influence of asbestos on the uptake of benzo[a]pyrene and DNA alkylation in hamster tracheal epithelial cells, *Cancer Res* 43:1251, 1983.
46. Eng L: McAteer cost overruns triple, *San Francisco Examiner,* June 23, 1988.
47. Enterline PE: Pitfalls in epidemiological research: an examination of the asbestos literature, *J Occup Med* 18:150, 1976.
48. Enterline PE, Hartley J, Henderson V: Asbestos and cancer: a cohort followed up to death, *Br J Ind Med* 44:396, 1987.
49. Enterline PE, Henderson VL: Type of asbestos and respiratory cancer in the asbestos industry, *Arch Environ Health* 27:312, 1973.
50. Environmental and Occupational Health Information Program: *A guide to asbestos in the home for New Jersey residents,* Trenton, 1989, New Jersey Dept. Health.
51. Environmental Protection Agency: *National emission standard for hazardous air pollutants: amendments to asbestos standard,* 40 CFR Fed Reg 43(118) 26372, June 19, 1978.
52. Environmental Protection Agency: *Asbestos containing materials in school buildings: a guidance document, Part 1,* Washington, DC, 1979, Office of Toxic Substances.
53. Environmental Protection Agency: *Interim primary drinking water regulations. Amendments,* Fed Reg 44:42246-42259, July 19, 1979.
54. Environmental Protection Agency: *Ambient water quality guidance document,* EPA 440/5-80-022, Washington, DC, 1980.
55. Environmental Protection Agency: *Airborne asbestos health assessment update,* EPA 600/8-84-003F, Washington, DC, 1986.
56. Environmental Protection Agency: *Asbestos-in-schools: a guide to new federal requirements for local education agencies,* Washington, DC, 1988, Office of Toxic Substances.
57. Environmental Protection Agency: *EPA study of asbestos-containing materials in public buildings: a report to congress,* Washington, DC, 1988.
58. Environmental Protection Agency: Part II, *Federal Register* 56:3526-3528, 1991.
59. Ernst P, Bourbeau J, Becklake MR: Pleural abnormality as a cause of impairment and disability, *Ann NY Acad Sci* 643:157, 1991.
60. Finklestein MM, Vingilis JJ: Radiographic abnormalities among asbestos-cement workers: an exposure-response study, *Am Rev Respir Dis* 129:17, 1984.
61. Fletcher DE: A mortality study of shipyard workers with pleural plaques, *Br J Ind Med* 29:142, 1972.
62. Frank AL et al: Biological activity in vitro of chrysotile compared to its quarried parent rock (platy serpentine), *J Exp Pathol Toxicol* 2:1041, 1979.
63. Frost J, Georg J, Moller FP: Asbestosis with pleural calcification among insulation workers, *Dan Med Bull* 3:202, 1956.
64. Gochfeld M, Glazner L: *Report on the Cherry Hill School District: asbestos exposure in school teachers,* Trenton, 1979, New Jersey Dept. Health.
65. Gochfeld M et al: *Asbestos in New Jersey's institutions of higher education: an assessment of risk with recommendations,* Piscataway, NJ, 1990, Environmental and Occupational Health Sciences Institute.
66. Gochfeld M, Patel D: *Preliminary report on asbestos exposure in maintenance workers at state institutions,* Trenton, 1979, New Jersey Dept. Health.
67. Greene R, Schaefer CM, Oliver LC: Improved detection of asbestos-related pleural plaques with digital radiography, *Ann NY Acad Sci* 643:90, 1991.
68. Guillemin B et al: Role of peptide growth factors in asbestos-related human lung cancer, *Ann NY Acad Sci* 643:245, 1991.
69. Hallenbeck WH et al: Is chrysotile asbestos released from asbestos-cement pipe into drinking water? *J Am Water Works Assoc* 70:97, 1978.
70. Hammond EC, Selikoff IJ, Seidman H: Asbestos exposure, cigarette smoking and death rates, *Ann NY Acad Sci* 33:473, 1979.
71. Harington JS: Fiber carcinogenesis: epidemiologic observations and the Stanton hypothesis, *J Natl Cancer Inst* 67:977, 1981.
72. Harington JS: The carcinogenicity of chrysotile asbestos, *Ann NY Acad Sci* 643:465, 1991.

73. Hei TK et al: Chrysotile fiber is a strong mutagen in mammalian cells, *Cancer Res* 52:6305, 1992.
74. Heintz H et al: Chrysotile induces protooncogenes, *Proc Natl Acad Sci* 90:3299, 1993.
75. Henderson VL, Enterline PE: Asbestos exposure: factors associated with excess cancer and respiratory disease mortality, *Ann NY Acad Sci* 330:117, 1979.
76. Hillerdal G: Short report: value of the lateral view in diagnosing pleural plaques, *Arch Environ Health* 41:391, 1986.
77. Hilt B et al: Chest radiographs in subjects with asbestos-related abnormalities: comparison between ILO categorizations and clinical reading, *Am J Ind Med* 21:855, 1992.
78. Hoffman FL: *Mortality from respiratory diseases in the dusty trades [inorganic dusts],* Bureau of Labor Statistics Report No. 231:172-180, 1918.
79. Holleb HB, Angrist AA: Bronchogenic carcinoma in association with pulmonary asbestosis, *Am J Pathol* 18:123, 1942.
80. Holt PF, Mills J, Young DK: Experimental asbestosis in the guinea pig, *J Pathol Bacteriol* 92:185, 1966.
81. Howe HL et al: Cancer incidence following exposure to drinking water with asbestos leachate, *Public Health Reports* 104:251, 1989.
82. Hueper WC: *Occupational tumors and allied diseases,* Springfield, Ill, 1942, Charles C Thomas.
83. Hughes JM, Weill H: Asbestos exposure: quantitative assessment of risk, *Am Rev Respir Dis* 133:5, 1986.
84. Hughes JM, Weill H, Hammad YY: Mortality of workers employed in two asbestos cement manufacturing plants, *Br J Ind Med* 44:161, 1987.
85. International Agency for Research on Cancer: *Monographs on the evaluation of carcinogenic risk of chemicals to humans,* vol 14, Lyon, France, 1977, Asbestos.
86. International Labour Office (ILO): *Guidelines for the use of ILO international classification of radiographs of pneumoconioses,* revised edition, Occup Safety & Health Series No 22, Geneva, 1980.
87. Irwig HG et al: Asbestos in place: a building management perspective, *Ann NY Acad Sci* 643:589, 1991.
88. Jarvholm B, Sanden A: Pleural plaques and respiratory function, *Am J Ind Med* 10:419, 1986.
89. Joubert I, Seidman H, Selikoff IJ: Mortality experience of family contacts of asbestos factory workers, *Ann NY Acad Sci* 643:416, 1991.
90. Kanarek MS et al: Asbestos in drinking water and cancer incidence in the San Francisco Bay area, *Am J Epidemiol* 112:54, 1980.
91. Kilburn KH et al: Asbestos disease in family contacts of shipyard workers, *Am J Publ Health* 75:615, 1985.
92. Kipen HM et al: Pulmonary fibrosis in asbestos insulation workers with lung cancer: a radiological and histopathological evaluation, *Br J Ind Med* 44:96, 1987.
93. Kohyama N, Suzuki Y: Analysis of asbestos fibers in lung parenchyma, pleural plaques, and mesothelioma tissues of North American insulation workers, *Ann NY Acad Sci* 643:27, 1991.
94. Landrigan PJ: A population of children at risk of exposure to asbestos in place, *Ann NY Acad Sci* 643:283, 1991.
95. Landrigan PJ, Kazemi H: The third wave of asbestos disease: exposure to asbestos in place, *Ann NY Acad Sci* 643:1, 1991.
96. Lanza AJ: *The pneumoconioses,* New York, 1963, Grune & Stratton.
97. Lasky JA, Bonner JC, Brody AR: The pathogbiology of asbestos-induced lung disease: a proposed role for macrophage-derived growth factors, *Ann NY Acad Sci* 643:239, 1991.
98. Levin SM, Selikoff IJ: Radiological abnormalities and asbestos exposure among custodians of the New York City Board of Education, *Ann NY Acad Sci* 643:530, 1991.
99. Li FP et al: Familial mesothelioma after intense asbestos exposure at home, *JAMA* 240:46, 1978.
100. Liddell FDK, McDonald JC: Radiological findings as predictors of mortality in Quebec asbestos workers, *Br J Ind Med* 37:257, 1980.
101. Lilienfeld DE: Asbestos-associated pleural meosthelioma in school teachers: a discussion of four cases, *Ann NY Acad Sci* 643:454, 1991.
102. Lilis R et al: The effect of asbestos-induced pleural fibrosis on pulmonary function: quantitative evaluation, *Ann NY Acad Sci* 643:162, 1991.
103. Lippmann M: Asbestos and other mineral fibers. In Lippmann M, ed: *Environmental toxicants,* New York, 1992, Van Nostrand Reinhold.
104. Lynch DA, Gamsu G, Aberle DR: Conventional and high resolution computed tomography in the diagnosis of asbestos-related diseases, *Radiographics* 1989:523, 1989.
105. Lynch KM, Smith WA: Pulmonary asbestosis. III: Carcinoma of the lung in asbestos-silicosis, *Am J Cancer* 24:56, 1935.
106. McDonald AD et al: Dust exposure and mortality in an American factory using chrysotile, amosite and crocidolite in mainly textile manufacture, *Br J Ind Med* 39:368, 1983.
107. McDonald JC et al: Dust exposure and mortality in chrysotile mining 1910-75, *Br J Ind Med* 37:11, 1980.
108. Maltoni C, Pinto C, Mobiglia A: Mesotheliomas due to asbestos used in railroads in Italy, *Ann NY Acad Sci* 643:347, 1991.
109. Mancuso TF, Coulter EJ: Methodology in industrial health studies, *Arch Environ Health* 6:210, 1963.
110. Maske M: Montclair State ends dorm peril: college removes asbestos ceiling hazard, *Star Ledger,* Newark, NJ, Aug. 10, 1977.
111. Massey DG, Fournier-Massey G: Asbestos removal from buildings: a review, *Hawaii Med J* 46:153, 1987.
112. Merchant JA, Schwartz DAL: Chest radiography for assessment of the pneumoconioses. In Rom W, ed: *Environmental and occupational medicine,* ed 2, Boston, 1992, Little, Brown.
113. Merewether ERA: The occurrence of pulmonary fibrosis and other pulmonary affections in asbestos workers, *J Ind Hyg* 12:198, 1930.
114. Michaels L, Chissick SS, eds: *Asbestos: properties, applications, and hazards,* New York, 1979, J Wiley.
115. Miller AG: Application of pulmonary function tests to the evaluation of asbestosis, *Ann NY Acad Sci* 643:145, 1991.
116. Miller LG, Sparrow D, Ginns LC: Asbestos exposure correlates with alterations in circulating T-cell subsets, *Clin Exp Immunol* 51:110, 1983.
117. Millette JR, Clark PJ, Pansing MF: *Exposure to asbestos from drinking water in the United States,* EPA 600/1-79-028, Washington, DC, 1979, U.S. Environmental Protection Agency.
118. Mills RG: Pulmonary asabestosis: report of a case, *Minn Med* 13:495, 1930.
119. Mossman BT et al: Asbestos: scientific developments and implications for public policy, *Science* 247:294, 1990.
120. Mossman BT et al: The effects of crocidolite and chrysotile asbestos on cellular uptake, metabolism and DNA after exposure of hamster tracheal epithelial cells to benzo(a)pyrene, *Environ Health Perspect* 51:331, 1983.
121. Mossman BT, Gee JBL: Asbestos-related diseases, *N Engl J Med* 320:1721, 1989.
122. Mossman BT, Landesman JM: Importance of oxygen-free radicals in asbestos-induced injury to airway epithelial cells, *Chest* 83(suppl):50, 1983.
123. National Research Council: *Drinking water and health,* Washington, DC, 1977, National Academy Press.
124. National Research Council: *Drinking water and health,* vol 4, Washington, DC, 1982, National Academy Press.
125. National Research Council: *Asbestiform fibers—nonoccupational health risks,* Washington, DC, 1984, National Academy Press.
126. National Research Council: *Biologic markers in pulmonary toxicology,* Washington, DC, 1989, National Academy Press.
127. National Toxicology Program: *Toxicology and carcinogenesis studies of chrysotile asbestos in F344/N rats (feed studies),* Research Triangle Park, NC, 1985, National Institute for Environmental Health Sciences.
128. Newhouse ML, Berry G: Patterns of mortality in asbestos factory workers in London, *Ann NY Acad Sci* 330:53, 1979.

129. Newhouse ML, Sullivan KR: A mortality study of workers manufacturing friction materials 1941-86, *Br J Ind Med* 46:176, 1989.
130. Newhouse ML, Thompson H: Mesothelioma of pleura and peritoneum following exposure to asbestos in the London area, *Br J Ind Med* 22:261, 1965.
131. New York Academy of Science: Biological effects of asbestos, *Ann NY Acad Science,* vol 136, New York, 1965, The Academy.
132. Nicholson WJ: *Airborne asbestos health assessment update,* EPA/600/8-84/003F, Washington, DC, 1986, U.S. Environmental Protection Agency.
133. Nicholson WJ: Comparative dose-response relationships of asbestos fiber types: magnitudes and uncertainties, *Ann NY Acad Sci* 643:74, 1991.
134. Novick LF et al: Asbestos in Vermont schools: findings of a statewide on-site investigation, *Am J Public Health* 71:744, 1981.
135. Oliver LC: Asbestos in public buildings. In Rom WN, ed: *Environmental and occupational medicine,* Boston, 1993, Little, Brown.
136. Oliver LC, Sprince NL, Greene R: Asbestos-related abnormalities in maintenance personnel, *Ann NY Acad Sci* 643:521, 1991.
137. Pancoast HK, Miller TG, Landis RM: A roentgenologic study of the effects of dust inhalatin upon the lungs, *Am J Roentgenol* 5:129, 1918.
138. Pancoast HK, Pendergrass EP: A review of our present knowledge of pneumoconiosis, based upon roentgenologic studies with notes on the pathology of the condition, *Am J Roentgenol* 14:381, 1925.
139. Peto J: Dose-response relationships for asbestos-related disease: implications of hygiene standards, *Ann NY Acad Sci* 33:195, 1979.
140. Peto J et al: Relationship of mortality to measures of environmental asbestos pollution in an asbestos textile factory, *Ann Occup Hyg* 29:305, 1985.
141. Reeves AL, Puro HE, Smith RG: Inhalation carcinogenesis from various forms of asbestos, *Environ Res* 8:178, 1974.
142. Reger RB et al: The detection of thoracic abnormalities using posterior-anterior (PA) vs PA and oblique chest roentgenograms, *Chest* 81:290, 1982.
143. Reger RB et al: Cases of alleged asbestos-related disease: a radiologic re-evaluation, *J Occup Med* 32:1088, 1990.
144. Rendall REG: The data sheets on the chemical and physical properties of the UICC standard reference samples. In Shapiro HA, ed: *Pneumoconioses,* Oxford, 1970, Oxford University Press.
145. Rohl AN, Langer AM, Selikoff IJ: Chrysotile asbestos: effects of human exposure, *Science* 198:1202, 1977.
146. Rom WN: Accelerated loss of lung function and alveolitis in a longitudinal study of non-smoking individuals with occupational exposure to asbestos, *Am J Ind Med* 21:835, 1992.
147. Rom WN: Asbestos-related diseases. In Rom WN, ed: *Environmental and occupational medicine,* Boston, 1993, Little, Brown.
148. Rosenstock L et al: The relation among pulmonary function, chest roentgenogrphic abnormalities and smoking status in an asbestos-exposed cohort, *Am Rev Respir Dis* 138:272, 1988.
149. Sawyer RN, Rohl AN, Langer AM: Airborne fiber control in buildings during asbestos material removal by amended water methodology, *Environ Res* 36:46, 1985.
150. Sawyer RN, Spooner CM: *Sprayed asbestos-containing materials in buildings: a guidance document,* Washington, DC, 1978, U.S. Environmental Protection Agency.
151. Schwartz DA: The clinical relevance of asbestos-induced pleural fibrosis, *Ann NY Acad Sci* 643:169, 1991.
152. Seidman H, Selikoff IJ, Gelb SK: Mortality experience of amosite asbestos factory workers: dose-response relationships 5 to 40 years after onset of short-term work exposure, *Am J Ind Med* 10:479, 1986.
153. Seidman H, Selikoff IJ, Hammond EC: Short-term asbestos work exposure and long-term observation, *Ann NY Acad Sci* 330:61, 1979.
154. Selikoff IJ, Hammond EC, Churg J: Asbestos exposure and neoplasia, *JAMA* 188:22, 1964.
155. Selikoff IJ, Hammond EC, Churg J: Asbestos exposure, smoking and neoplasia, *JAMA* 204:104, 1968.
156. Selikoff IJ, Hammond EC, Seidman H: Mortality experience of insulation workers in the United States and Canada, 1943-1976, *Ann NY Acad Sci* 330:91, 1979.
157. Selikoff IJ, Lee DHK: *Asbestos and disease,* New York, 1978, Academic Press.
158. Selikoff IJ, Nicholson WJ, Lilis R: Radiological evidence of asbestos disease among ship repair workers, *Am J Ind Med* 1:9, 1980.
159. Selikoff IJ, Seidman H: Asbestos-associated deaths among insulation workers in the United States and Canada, 1967-1987, *Ann NY Acad Sci* 643:1, 1991.
160. Selikoff IJ, Seidman H: Use of death certificates in epidemiological studies, including occupational hazards: variations in discordance of different asbestos-associated diseases on best evidence ascertainment, *Am J Ind Med* 22:481, 1992.
161. Sheers G, Coles R: Mesothelioma risks in a naval dockyard, *Arch Environ Health* 35:276, 1980.
162. Siegel W, Smith AR, Greenburg L: The dust hazard in tremolite talc mining including roentgenological findings in talc workers, *Am J Roentgen Radium Ther* 49:11, 1943.
163. Sluis-Cremer GK: Asbestos disease at low exposures after long residence times, *Ann NY Acad Sci* 643:182, 1991.
164. Sparks JV: Pulmonary asbestosis, *Radiology* 17:1249, 1931.
165. Stanton MF et al: Carcinogenicity of fibrous glass: Pleural response in the rat in relation to fiber dimension, *J Natl Cancer Inst* 58:587, 1977.
166. Stanton MF et al: Relation of particle dimension to carcinogenicity in amphibole asbestoses and other fibrous minerals, *J Natl Cancer Inst* 67:965, 1981.
167. Stoll R, Bass R, Angrist AA: Asbestosis associated with bronchogenic carcinoma, *Arch Intern Med* 88:831, 1951.
168. Suzuki Y: Carcinogenic and fibrogenic effects of zeolites: preliminary observations, *Environ Res* 27:433, 1982.
169. Suzuki Y, Churg JL: Structure and development of the asbestos body, *Am J Pathol* 55:79, 1969.
170. Wagner JC et al: The effects of the inhalation of asbestos in rats, *Br J Cancer* 29:252, 1974.
171. Wagner JC, Sleggs CA, Marchand P: Diffuse pleural mesothelioma and asbestos exposure in the northwestern Cape Province, *Br J Ind Med* 17:260, 1960.
172. Weiss W: Asbestos and colorectal cancer, *Gastroenterology* 99:876, 1990.
173. Welch LS, Michaels D, Zoloth S: Asbestos-related disease among sheet-metal workers, *Ann NY Acad Sci* 643:287, 1991.

Chapter 39

MAN-MADE MINERAL FIBERS

Stuart M. Brooks

Exposures to MMVF
Features of fiber toxicity
    Fiber size and distribution
    Fiber type and concentration
    Fiber durability and solubility
    Fiber chemical composition
    Fiber surface properties
Potential human health effects
Human mortality studies of MMVF
Animal inhalation studies
    Fibrous glass
    Mineral wool
    RCF
    Potassium titanate and potassium octatitanate
    Silicon carbide
    Carbon fiber
    Aramid fibers
Conclusion

Although man-made fibers have long been used in industry and construction, their use has accelerated in the past decade with the phasing out of asbestos from many uses. Synthetic vitreous fibers (MMVF)—mineral wool, glass fiber, and ceramic fiber—are used as insulation products replacing asbestos in many commercial situations. Mineral wool is slag wool and rock wool. Production occurs by melting and fiberizing iron ore furnace slag or melting and fiberizing naturally occurring basaltic rock or siliceous limestone. Glass fiber includes glass wool, continuous glass filament, and special-purpose glass fiber. Glass wool, often used synonymously with *glass fiber*, is frequently used in home insulation. Glass fiber is manufactured into glass from the raw material silicon dioxide with varying amounts of intermediate oxides or stabilizers such as aluminum, titanium, and zinc; there are also modifiers, or fluxes, such as sodium, potassium, calcium, barium, lithium, and magnesium.

Refractory ceramic fibers (RCF) are characterized by their ability to resist temperatures as high as 2600°F. Ceramic fibers are produced from kaolin clay, alumina-silica, or alumina-silica-zirconia. The physical characteristics of ceramic fibers can be changed by modifying the amount of stabilizers and fluxes. RCF constitutes only about 1% or 2% of worldwide MMVF production. An important use of RCF is for the lining of furnaces and kilns. When RCF are heated to temperatures above 1800°F, they undergo partial conversion to cristobalite (or crystalline silica-like).

The average diameter of RCF is in the range of 1.0 to 5.0 μm. Most glass wool fibers have diameters between 1 and 15 μm, depending on their intended end use specifications. Early production processes produced a greater range of diameters of fibers, between 1 and 40 μm. Special-purpose glass fiber is less than 3 mm in diameter (by flame attenuation process), with a range between 0.05 and 7 μm. Continuous glass filament ranges between 3 and 25 μm, depending on the end use. The slag wool production process produces discontinuous fibers with diameters ranging between 3.5 and 7 μm.

EXPOSURES TO MMVF

In the occupational setting the concentration of airborne fiber depends on the average diameter of the fiber under process and the fiberizing process. To compare the magnitude of exposures in the industry, let us assume that the average concentration of glass fiber in the outdoor ambient air is 0.00001 to 0.0001 fiber/cm^3. A summary of average occupational exposure levels of MMVF would be as follows: special-purpose glass fiber and ceramic fiber, 0.1 to 1.0 fibers/cm^3; mineral wool, 0.01 to 0.01 fibers/cm^3; continuous glass filament, 0.001 to 0.01 fibers/cm^3.[8,41] The smaller the average diameter of fiber under production, the greater the airborne concentration of respirable-size fiber.

In 1977 the National Institute for Occupational Safety and Health (NIOSH) recommended an occupational standard for exposure to fiberglass of 3 fibers/cm^3 as a time-weighted average. This standard was applied to other MMVF with diameters less than or equal to 3.5 μm and length greater than or equal to 10 μm. On the other hand, the Occupational Safety and Health Administration (OSHA) has assigned a permissible exposure limit (PEL) for MMVF under its dust standard as 5 mg/m^3 for respirable dust and 15 mg/m^3 for total dust. NIOSH's recommended standard and OSHA's PEL are assigned under the Air Contaminants Standard for the construction, maritime, and agricultural industries and are currently under review, and a new standard will be recommended. This new standard will apply to general industry and most likely will be below or at 1 fiber/cm^3. European standards also are considered. The recommended standard for MMVF in the United Kingdom is 2 fibers/cm^3; in Sweden, it is 1 fiber/cm^3; and in Australia it is 0.5 fiber/cm^3.

FEATURES OF FIBER TOXICITY

The major concern about MMVF relates to its fibrous forms and possible production of consequences similar to that of asbestos, which causes pulmonary fibrosis, bronchogenic carcinoma, mesothelioma, and possibly other types of cancers.

Fiber size and distribution

Much of the relevant research on fiber toxicity has been conducted on asbestos fibers. Although it is clear that the fiber concentration in the lung is a paramount factor in disease development, other aspects of lung fiber content, including fiber distribution and fiber size, are important. Research by Stanton and co-workers[74-76] showed that direct implantation of fibers of similar size into the pleura of rats produced mesotheliomas. A multitude of investigations have addressed various aspects of fiber toxicity; important characteristics of fibers that influence toxicity are fiber size and distribution, fiber type and concentration, fiber durability and solubility, fiber chemical makeup, and fiber surface properties. Fiber size and geometry determine fiber entry and intrapulmonary distribution within the host. An essential determinant of lung deposition is the aerodynamic diameter.[77] Fibers with an aerodynamic diameter of less than 12 μm are not likely to reach the respiratory region in humans; fibers of an aerodynamic diameter of less than 6 μm are not likely to reach the respiratory units of rodents.[69] The Stanton-Pott hypothesis suggests that fibers longer than 8 μm and thinner than 0.25 μm have high carcinogenicity potential. Most ceramic fibers are thicker than the Stanton fibers but theoretically could achieve the critical Stanton fiber size during lung clearance. Although both aspects of size (length and diameter) are important, the diameter of the fiber appears to be of greater significance in relation to initial deposition and translocation within the lung and the extension to the pleural and peritoneal surfaces. The length of the fiber has an impact on the ability of the lungs to clear the fiber once it is deposited within the lung respiratory tissue; longer fibers are cleared less effectively than are shorter fibers.[26] In general, on a one-to-one basis, long fibers appear to be more fibrogenic, and long, high-aspect (length-to-width ratio) fibers are more dangerous with regard to production of mesotheliomas than are short- or low-aspect fibers.[1,2,16,76,81]

In vivo studies using radiolabeled glass fibers with similar diameters (geometric mean diameter of 1.5 μm) but different lengths (5- or 60-μm length) were examined.[7] There was little difference in clearance time between the long (half-life of 35 days) and short (half-life of 38.5 days) glass fibers at 19 weeks after instillation; however, the short fibers were apparently successfully phagocytosed by alveolar macrophages and cleared to the lymph nodes, but the long fibers were not. The long fibers produced a foreign-body granulomatous response in the lungs. On the other hand, Morgan and associates[52] concluded that longer glass fibers were more soluble than were shorter ones. Examining glass fibers of the same diameter (1.5 μm), the investigators found that 90% of 5-μm fibers were cleared from the lung during the 12-month period but 80% of 10-μm fibers were cleared. Neither the 60-μm or 30-μm fibers were cleared to any extent during the same period.

Investigations on rock wool found no significant change in the geometric mean diameter of instilled rock wool fibers in rat lungs.[49] When observed after 6 months, the fibers were noted to have become thinner at their ends than in their middle and that slow dissolution occurred.

The importance of fiber distribution is emphasized by the anatomic distribution of certain asbestos-related diseases, such as asbestosis, in which a peripheral lower lobe severity is noted. The fibrosis is greatest in the portion of the parenchyma served by short airways with few branches[14]; however, examination of lung tissue does not divulge a gradient of deposition whereby the lower lung has a greater deposition of fibers than has the upper lung.[47,50] The fiber distribution seems to be influenced by the fiber type. For example, when lungs of deceased workers are examined, chrysotile fibers are always found in the pleura, but amphiboles cannot be detected.

Fiber type and concentration

Much of the information pertaining to fiber differences comes from studies conducted on asbestos. There is a dose relationship between asbestos fiber burden and the type of disease present.[14] The pleura seems more sensitive to amphibole exposure than the parenchyma, both for benign and for malignant changes. As opposed to the amphiboles, in which mesothelioma appears at much lower lung burdens than does asbestosis, in chrysotile exposure both mesothelioma and asbestosis appear with approximately the same burden, which is extraordinarily high. In general and in comparison with the general population, asbestosis is seen with a very high lung burden, and the grade of asbestosis (that is, the amount of scarring) is proportional to the asbestos burden.

Fiber durability and solubility

Although their dimensions influence the entry and deposition of fibers in the lungs, the critical basis for the accumulation of a lung burden of fibers is durability and dissolution potential of fibers.[26] In the case of asbestos, the more durable amphiboles accumulate in the lungs in quantities that correlate with cumulative exposure but the less durable chrysotile does not.[53,54] Comparable data on MMVF are not available. The mechanism of clearance of inhaled particles from the lungs involves mucociliary transport, translocation to lymph nodes by alveolar macrophages, and dissolution by extracellular fluid. It is likely that the fibers are attacked by fluids normally present in the lung that cause fragmentation to shorter fibers, which are biologically less active and are more readily removed from the lungs by clearance mechanisms or total dissolution.[6,51]

An important fiber property is solubility, which influences the lung residence time and clearance rate.[41,90] Studies of asbestos fibers show that chrysotile is more soluble than crocidolite.[3] In general, amphibole fibers are very resistant to dissolution and consequently reside in lung tissue for prolonged periods of time.[17,78] The dissolution rate of MMVF depends on the chemical composition and there are differences among fiber types by several orders of magnitude.[33] Other factors that seem influential are the rigidity of fibers, their surface properties, and fiber-end architecture (such as smooth, grainy, or spiculed edges).[39,40] The in vitro solubility of MMVF varies over a wide range and depends on the composition of the fibers.[38] In summary, glass wool is the least durable, followed by rock and slag wool, and ceramic fibers are the most durable.* Special-purpose glass fibers can demonstrate increased durability when alterations in the type and amount of stabilizers and fluxes are made.

Fiber chemical composition

An important feature of the chemical nature of the fiber is its ability to induce a biologic effect and interact with cell constituents, including deoxyribonucleic acid (DNA). The chemical make-up of a fiber may relate to its influence on solubility of the fiber. Investigations have studied in vitro determination of dissolution rates by using a constant flow of physiologic Gamble's solution.[41] One protocol examined change in fiber properties after leaching had occurred for 180 days. Parameters examined included total specimen weight, surface area, and surface morphology. When fibrous glass (borosilicate fibers) is compared with chrysotile asbestos, more silica is dissolved from the borosilicate fibers (36% to 90%) than from the asbestos fibers (1%). The solubility rate of the borosilicate fibers was determined to be 650 to 17,000 times greater than that of chrysotile asbestos. The solubility change in surface area of the borosilicate fibers can be confirmed by scanning electron microscopy, showing surface distortions from the leaching process, with pitting, cracking, breaking, and segmentation of the fibers.

Fiber surface properties

Substantial data suggest that fiber surface charge is an important determinant of fiber cytotoxicity.[9] For asbestos there are interactions between the asbestos fiber and the cell surface. Charge-mediated effects occur with positively charged fibers such as chrysotile asbestos. Another type of interaction is reported to occur with amphibole or glassy fibers and is mediated by fibronectin, which first binds to the fiber. The bound protein then attaches to receptors on the cell surface. Toxicity may also be associated with fiber surface area available for interaction.[19]

The fiber surface properties may be modified by in vivo host factors. Serum factors can augment the cytotoxic potential of fibers by increasing the interaction of the fibers with the epithelial cell membrane and vacuoles within the cell. Damage to alveolar epithelial cells may be due to neutrophils activated by stimuli induced by fibers.[32] Toxicity is enhanced by an increased intracellular oxidant stress, for example, iron in amosite asbestos. Serum-altered toxic effects of asbestos may be reduced by chelation of the iron in asbestos fibers or by augmentation of intracellular antioxidant lung defenses.

A great deal of information has been gleaned from studies of quartz, which has the ability to damage cell membranes and this mechanism may be important in the effects of MMVF. The surface of the quartz crystal interacts with cell membranes (such as alveolar macrophage membranes; and epithelial cells) and causes cell membrane damage; this alteration leads to inflammation and resultant fibrosis. Lysis of red blood cells has been used as an indicator of biologic activity and cell membrane damage.[56] Silica crystals coated with the proton-acceptor polymer polyvinyl pyridine-N-oxide (PVPNO) loses its ability to lyse red blood cells. Possibly, PVPNO forms a coating of several hundred angstroms thick that rendered the negatively charged SiO^- groups inaccessible for interaction with cell membranes. Alternatively, red blood cell lysis may be due to negative surface charge from the ionized silanol groups (SiO^-) on the quartz surface.[60] The coating of the (SiO^-) groups with a strong Lewis acid (such as $AlCl_3$ or $FeCl_3$) causes the quartz to lose its ability to lyse red blood cells, even though the surface SiOH groups were available for hydrogen bonding.

---
*References 6, 8, 24, 31, 33, 35, 40, 48.

In another study using chrysotile asbestos, toxicity (as determined by hemolysis test and P38 cytotoxicity assay) was reduced by dyeing (chelating) it with suitable dyestuffs that form colored lakes or chelates with magnesium.[44] The study by Nolan et al[59] effectively used the in vitro membranolytic activity (red blood cell hemolysis) test to investigate the differences in toxicity of various palygorskite and sepiolite clays. The test was also used by Wallace and associates[83] to demonstrate the protective influences of lung surfactant.

Another theory considers the role of spatial arrangement of oxygen atoms on the crystal structure in the formation of molecular contacts (such as hydrogen bonding or electrostatic) during crystal-cell interactions. The distribution of oxygen atoms on the crystal surface is considered important in defining a molecular surface topology that is supportive of crystal-cell interactions. Quartz surfaces modified with selected organosilanes also alter the ability to lyse red blood cells and resultant pulmonary inflammation and fibrosis.

There may be possible alteration of the effective biological activity (e.g., lysis of red blood cells and pulmonary inflammation and fibrosis) of quartz crystals by chemical modifications of its crystalline surface. Quartz surfaces can be modified with selected organosilanes to examine the biologic activity when different surfaces are presented to red blood cells or are instilled into the lungs of mice and resultant pulmonary inflammation and fibrosis are judged.[85] Organosilanes were considered ideal for this purpose because they covalently attach to quartz surfaces and have known structures that allow relatively easy determination of the exact crystal surface structure and surface properties. The results of the study support that the electrostatic interaction is more important than hydrogen bonding. The Q-amine (N-trimethoxysilylpropyl-N,N,N-trimethylammonium chloride) surface-substituted crystal had significantly higher biologic activity than that of the P-amine (3-aminopropyltriethoxysilane) surface-substituted crystal despite the ability of the NH_2 groups of the P-amine–modified crystal to hydrogen bond. Similar processes may be important in other types of dust diseases, such as asbestosis.[21]

POTENTIAL HUMAN HEALTH EFFECTS

A number of animal and in vitro investigations have addressed the problem of carcinognesis.* The morbidity studies for fibrous glass and rock wool show no substantial nonmalignant pulmonary disease among workers exposed to the fibers over many years. There is no evidence for interstitial fibrosis; however, the prevalence of pleural changes as noted on chest radiographs seems to be increased in this population. Respiratory morbidity studies measuring pulmonary symptoms, lung function tests, and chest roentgenographic changes have essentially not shown any adverse health trends in glass-fiber or rock- and slag-wool manufacturing facilities.* Workers involved with manufacturing RCF are currently being observed in a longitudinal morbidity study.[41] There is a 3.4% prevalence of pleural changes, with more than 90% classified as pleural plaques. Of 70 employees with more than 20 years of employment, eight (11.3%) had pleural changes. No interstitial changes were noted. In comparison, the prevalence of pleural thickening in glass-fiber and mineral-wool manufacturing workers was 1.8%.[84] The prevalence of pleural thickening in a non–dust-exposed blue-collar population has been reported to be 0.21% in men and 0.2% in women.[11,67]

HUMAN MORTALITY STUDIES OF MMVF

Previous mortality studies in the United States and Europe, encompassing more than 17,000 glass-fiber manufacturing workers and 25,000 production-plant workers, have not demonstrated a significant increase in mortality from malignant respiratory disease[41]; however, a recent examination showed a small but significant increase in respiratory cancer in workers in glass-wool plants (standard morbidity ratio [SMR] 113.5) and for mineral-wool plants (SMR 134.2). The excess respiratory cancer mortality ratio in mineral-wool workers with 20 years or more since first employment was limited to the slag-wool manufacturing facilities.[18,43] The European study of 25,000 mineral wool and glass fiber manufacturing workers reported an increase SMR of 152 for workers with 30 or more years of employment.[41] A weak association between exposure between exposure and lung cancer was noted for 2500 Canadian workers exposed to glass wool.[70]

ANIMAL INHALATION STUDIES
Fibrous glass

Chronic inhalation studies performed with use of fibrous glass have failed to induce tumors in the animal models investigated (guinea pig in one, hamster in two, and rats in seven).† In two parallel rat studies using JM100 fibrous glass exposure of 10 mg/m³ for 12 months, there was no significant increase in lung tumors during the lifetime of the animals; an exposure to a similar concentration of chrysotile asbestos caused a significant increase in lung tumors.[45,80] The study by Smith et al[72] reported no observed tumors in rats and hamsters after inhalation of 3 to 12 mg/m³ of several different compositions of fibrous glass. Currently, additional multidose studies are under way at Research and Consulting Company (RCC) in Geneva.[26]

Mineral wool

Three chronic inhalation studies using mineral wool also have not shown tumors.[34,72,80] Studies by Wagner et al[80] and LeBouffant et al[35] reported no tumors in rats over their lifetime breathing rock wool, but 25% and 19% incidences of

---

*References 4, 20, 30, 46, 58, 61, 65, 66, 68, 79, 82, 87, 88.

*References 41, 42, 57, 71, 84, 89.
†References 23, 26, 34, 36, 45, 55, 72, 80.

tumors were noted in the two studies in which chrysotile asbestos was inhaled.[73,74] A study by Smith et al[72] used hamsters and rats exposed to 10 mg/m³ of mineral wool (slag wool) for 24 months. Tumor incidence in the control group exposed to short crocidolite asbestos was not increased. Additional dose-response studies have been conducted for two different compositions of mineral wool at RCC.[26]

RCF

At least three long-term inhalation studies have been performed with RCF. Results of investigations have been published.* Davis et al[15] exposed 48 rats to RCF (dose of fibers longer than 5 μm long, 95 fibers/cm³) by inhalation for 7 hours per day, 5 days per week, for 224 days. Sacrifice of animals at the end of the study revealed an average of 5% pulmonary fibrosis, and eight rats were found to have developed pulmonary tumors, with three of the animals demonstrating lung carcinomas; there was one peritoneal mesothelioma. Smith et al[72] exposed hamsters and rats to RCF at 200 fibers/cm³ for 6 hours per day, 5 days per week, for 24 months. The rats showed no tumors and little pulmonary fibrosis. In hamsters there was one mesothelioma in 50 animals, but no fibrosis was observed. In a third study, four different types of RCF special-size fibers (average 1 μm diameter and 20 μm long) were aerosolized for 6 hours per day, 5 days per week, to the maximum tolerated dose (MTD) (30 mg/m³, about 200 to 250 fibers/cm³).[25] Hamsters were exposed to only kaolin RCF. Positive controls (chrysotile asbestos) and negative controls (filtered air) were included. Early results report lung fibrosis beginning at 9 months and the development of mesothelioma in 36 of 102 hamsters (35%) exposed to RCF.[25,26]

Potassium titanate and potassium octatitanate

Pulmonary responses to respirable potassium titanate and potassium octatitanate (Fybex) fibers in rats, hamsters, and guinea pigs were compared with those to amosite asbestos.[36] Unlike amosite fibers, potassium titanate caused no tumors but Fybex produced three mesotheliomas in hamsters and several lung tumors in rats with exposure at concentrations of 80 and 370 mg/m³, respectively. The investigation points out the problem of species susceptibility and differences. The hamster was the more susceptible to Fybex for lung fibrosis than was the guinea pig but less susceptible than was the rat, but Fybex caused more pleural fibrosis in hamsters than in rats or guinea pigs.

Silicon carbide

Subchronic inhalation studies performed in rats have been published.[12,13] Histologic findings in the rats studied included adenomatous hyperplasia of the lung, subpleural inflammation, mild visceral pleural fibrosis, and visceral and parietal pleural hyperplasia. The rats (50 males and 50 females) were exposed for 6 hours per day, 5 days per week, for 13 weeks to silicon carbide fibers (4.5 μm diameter, 0.2 μm long) at average concentrations of 3.93, 10.7, and 60.5 mg/m³ (630, 1740, and 7276 fibers/cm³); the positive control was crocidolite asbestos (1.5 μm wide, 0.2 μm long) at 1298 fibers/cm³, and the negative control was filtered air. In vivo studies on sheep also reveal interstitial lung changes.[5] The animal studies lend support to human epidemiologic investigations showing pulmonary effects.[22,62,64,73]

Carbon fiber

Two short-term and one subchronic inhalation study of carbon fiber have been determined to be inadequate because of the extremely low concentrations used and the short duration of exposure and observation.[26-28,63]

Aramid fibers

Ultrafine para-aramid fibers were shown to cause a low level of lung fibrosis at the three highest concentrations used.[37] A dose-related increase in lung carcinomas was noted in female rats exposed to the highest dose level. An in vitro study confirmed the toxicity of aramid fibers.[86]

CONCLUSION

Human morbidity studies on populations with exposures to fibrous glass and rock wool show no substantial respiratory disease among workers exposed to the fibers over many years, but the prevalence of pleural changes as noted on chest radiographs may be increased among ceramic workers. The data suggests that significant environmental exposures are unlikely outside of the workplace. Human cancer risks do not seem to be an important issue for glass fibers. The cancer risks associated with occupational exposures to glass wool and mineral wool also seem small but are mainly an issue among workers with longer duration of exposures. Therefore these types of fibers are not likely to be a problem for the consumer or in the home environment. The carcinogenic potential of ceramic fibers is still being investigated, but data to date suggest that there may be some carcinogenic potential to certain types of ceramic fibers. Taking this finding into account, it is not likely that the quantity and quality of nonoccupational exposures would put consumers at substantial risk; however, careful investigations on this type of fiber must continue.

REFERENCES

1. Adamson I, Bowden D: Response of mouse lung to crocidolite asbestos I. Minimal fibrotic reaction to short fibers, *J Pathol* 152:99, 1987.
2. Adamson I, Bowden D: Response of mouse lung to crocidolite asbestos: II. Pulmonary fibrosis after long fibers, *J Pathol* 152:109, 1987.
3. Abraham J, Smith C, Mossman B: Chrysotile and crocidolite asbestos pulmonary fiber concentration and dimensions after inhalation and clearance in Fischer 344 rats, *Ann Occup Hyg* 32:203, 1988.
4. Barrett J: Role of chromosomal mutations in asbestos-induced cell transformation. In Harris C, Lechner J, Brinkley B, eds: *Cellular and molecular aspects of fiber carcinogenesis,* ed 1, Plainview, NY, 1991, Cold Spring Harbor Laboratory Press.

---
*References 10, 15, 25, 26, 29, 72.

5. Begin R et al: Carborundum pneumoconiosis. In Mossman B, Begin R, eds: *Effects of mineral dusts on cells,* Berlin, 1989, Springer-Verlag.
6. Bellman B et al: Persistence of man-made mineral fibres (MMMF) and asbestos in rat lungs, *Ann Occup Hyg* 31:693, 1987.
7. Bernstein D, Drew R, Kuschner M: Experimental approaches for exposure to sized glass fibers, *Environ Health Perspect* 34:47, 1980.
8. Bernstein D et al: Pathogenicity of MMMF and the contrast with natural fibers. In Guthe T, ed: *Biological effects of man made mineral fibres: proceedings of a WHO/IARC conference in association with JEMRB and TIMA, Copenhagen, April 20-22, 1982,* 1984, World Health Organization, Geneva.
9. Brown R et al: Factors affecting the interaction of asbestos fibers with mammalian cells, *Ann Occup Hyg* 35:25, 1991.
10. Bunn W et al: Manmade mineral fibers. In *Medical toxicology of hazardous materials,* Baltimore, 1991, Williams & Wilkins.
11. Castellan R, Anderson W, Peterson M: Prevalence of radiographic appearance of pneumoconiosis in an unexposed blue collar population, *Am Rev Respir Dis* 131:684, 1985.
12. Chamberlain W: Subchronic (39 week) inhalation toxicity study of silicon carbide fibers in rats, Washington, DC, 1985, US Environmental Protection Agency.
13. Chamberlain W: Subchronic (39 week) inhalation toxicity study of silicon carbide fibers in rats, Washington, DC, 1987, US Environmental Protection Agency.
14. Churg A: Mineral analysis of lung parenchyma. In Crystal R, West J, eds: *The lung: scientific foundation,* ed 1, vol 2, New York, 1991, Raven Press.
15. Davis J et al: The pathogenic effects of fibrous ceramic aluminum silicate glass administered to rats by inhalation or peritonea injection. In Guthe T, ed: *Biological effects of man-made mineral fibres: proceedings of a WHO/IARC conference in association with JEMRB and TIMA,* Copenhagen, April 20-22, 1982, 1984, World Health Organization.
16. Davis J et al: The pathogenicity of long versus short fibre samples of amosite asbestos administered to rats by inhalation and intraperitoneal injection, *Br J Exp Pathol* 67:415, 1986.
17. Du Toit R: An estimate of the rate at which crocidolite asbestos fibres are cleared from the lung, *Ann Occup Hyg* 35:433, 1991.
18. Enterline P: Carcinogenic effects of man-made vitreous fibers, *Annu Rev Public Health* 12:459, 1991.
19. Finch G et al: Influence of physiochemical properties of beryllium and nickel compounds on cultured cell toxicity. In Mossman B, Begin R, eds: *Effects of mineral dusts on cells,* Berlin, 1989, Springer-Verlag.
20. Fischer A: Induction of sister chromatid exchanges by fibrous dusts alone and in combination with other xenobiotics in Chinese hamster cells. In Mossman B, Begin R, eds: *Effects of mineral dusts on cells,* Berlin, 1989, Springer-Verlag.
21. Gallagher J, George G, Brody A: Sialic acid mediates the initial binding of positively charged inorganic particles to alveolar macrophage membranes, *Am Rev Respir Dis* 135:1345, 1987.
22. Gauthier J, Ghezzo H, Martin R: Pneumoconiosis following carborundum (silicon carbide) exposure, *Am Rev Respir Dis* 131:191, 1985.
23. Gross P: The effects of glasswool fiber dust on the lung of animals, Washington, DC, 1976, HEW.
24. Hammad Y: Deposition and elimination of MMMF. In Guthe T, ed: *Biological effects of man made mineral fibres: proceedings of a WHO/IARC conference in association with JEMRB and TIMA. Copenhagen, April 20-22, 1982,* 1984, World Health Organization.
25. Hesterberg T et al: Chronic inhalation toxicity and oncogenicity study of refractory ceramic fibers in Fischer 344 rats, *Toxicologists* 11:85, 1991.
26. Hesterberg T et al: Use of animal models to study man-made fiber carcinogenesis. In Harris C, Lechner J, Brinkley B, eds: *Cellular and molecular aspects of fiber carcinogenesis,* ed 1, Plainview, NY, 1991, Cold Spring Harbor Laboratory Press.
27. Holt P: Submicron carbon dust in guinea pigs, *Environ Res* 28:434, 1982.
28. Holt P, Horne M: Dust from carbon fibre, *Environ Res* 17:276, 1978.
29. Imamura T et al: Evaluation of pulmonary functions during chronic inhalation studies with refractory ceramic fibers (RCF) and an experimental fiber in rats, *Toxicologists* 10:7, 1990.
30. Jaurand M-C et al: Neoplastic transformation of rodent cells. In Harris C, Lechner J, Brinkley B, eds: *Cellular and molecular aspects of fiber carcinogenesis,* ed 1, Plainview, NY, 1991, Cold Spring Harbor Laboratory Press.
31. Johnson N, Griffiths D, Hill R: Size distribution following long-term inhalation of MMMF. In Guthe T, ed: *Biological effects of man made mineral fibres: proceedings of a WHO/IARC conference in association with JEMRB and TIMA, Copenhagen, Arpil 20-22, 1982,* 1984, World Health Organization.
32. Kamp D et al: Serum promotes asbestos-induced injury to human pulmonary epithelial cells, *J Lab Clin Med* 116:289, 1990.
33. Law B, Bunn W, Hesterberg T: Solubility of polymeric organic fibers and manmade vitreous fibers in Gambles solution, *Inhalation Toxicology* 2:321, 1990.
34. Le Bouffant L et al: Distribution of inhaled MMMF in the rat lung: Long-term effects. In Guthe T, ed: *Biological effects of man made mineral fibres: proceedings of a WHO/IRAC conference in association with JEMRB and TIMA, Copenhagen, April 20-22, 1982,* 1984, World Health Organization.
35. LeBouffant L et al: Experimental studies on long-term effects of inhaled MMMF on the lungs of rats, *Ann Occup Hyg* 31:765, 1987.
36. Lee K et al: Comparative pulmonary responses to inhaled inorganic fibers with asbestos and fiberglass, *Environ Res* 24:167, 1981.
37. Lee K et al: Lung response to ultrafine Kevlar aramid synthic fibrils following 2-year inhalation exposure in rats, *Fundam Appl Toxicol* 11:1, 1988.
38. Leineweber J: Solubility of fibres in vitro and in vivo. In Guthe T, ed: *Biological effects of man made mineral fibres: proceedings of a WHO/IARC conference in association with JEMRB and TIMA, Copenhagen, April 20-22, 1982,* 1984, World Health Organization.
39. Lippman M: Review: asbestos exposure indicies, *Environ Res* 46:86, 1988.
40. Lippman M: Man-made mineral fibers (MMMF): human exposures and health risk assessment, *Toxicol Ind Health* 6:225, 1990.
41. Lockey J, Weise N: Health effects of synthetic vitreous fibers, *Clin Chest Med* 13:329, 1992.
42. Malmberg P et al: Pulmonary function in workers of a mineral rock fiber plant. In Guthe T, ed: *Biological effects of man made mineral fibres: proceedings of a WHO/IARC conference in association with JEMRB and TIMA, Copenhagen, April 20-22, 1982,* 1984, World Health Organization.
43. Marsh G et al: Mortality among a cohort of US man-made mineral fiber workers: 1985 follow-up, *J Occup Med* 32:594, 1990.
44. Martin M et al: Toxicity of chrysotile asbestos through surface modification with chelating agents. In Mossman B, Begin R, eds: *Effects of mineral dusts on cells,* Berlin, 1989, Springer-Verlag.
45. McConnell E, Wagner J, Skidmore J: A comparative study of the fibrogenic and carcinogenic effects of UICC Canadian chrysotile B asbestos and glass microfibre (JM 100). In Guthe T, ed: *Biological effects of man made mineral fibres: proceedings of a WHO/IARC conference in association with JEMRB and TIMA, Copenhagen, April 20-22, 1982,* 1984, World Health Organization.
46. Molloy C et al: Oncogenes and signal transduction in malignancy. In Harris C, Lechner J, Brinkley B, eds: *Cellular and molecular aspects of fiber carcinogenesis,* ed 1, Plainview, NY, 1991, Cold Spring Harbor Laboratory Press.
47. Morgan A, Holmes A: Distribution and characteristics of amphobile asbestos fibres measured with light microscope, in the left lung of an insulation worker, *Br J Ind Med* 40:45, 1983.

48. Morgan A, Holmes A: The deposition of MMMF in the respiratory tract of the rat, their subsequent clearance, solubility in vivo and protein coating. In Guthe T, ed: *Biological effects of man made mineral fibres: proceedings of a WHO/IARC conference in association with JEMRB and TIMA, Copenhagen, April 20-22, 1982,* 1984, World Health Organization.
49. Morgan A, Holmes A: Solubility of rockwool fibers in vivo and the formation of pseudo-asbestos bodies, *Ann Occup Hyg* 28:307, 1984.
50. Morgan A, Holmes A: The distribution and characteristics of asbestos fibers in the lungs of Finnish anthophyllite mine-workers, *Environ Res* 33:62, 1984.
51. Morgan A, Holmes A: Solubility of asbestos and manmade mineral fibers in vitro and in vivo: its significance in lung disease, *Environ Res* 39:475, 1986.
52. Morgan A, Holmes A, Davison W: Clearance of sized glass fibres from the rat lung and their solubility in vivo, *Ann Occup Hyg* 25:317, 1982.
53. Mossman B, Light W, Wei E: Asbestos: mechanisms of toxicity and carcinogenicity in the respiratory tract, *Annu Rev Pharmacol Toxicol* 23:595, 1983.
54. Mossman B et al: Scientific developments and implications for public policy, *Science* 247:294, 1990.
55. Muhle H et al: Inhalation and injection experiments in rats to test the carcinogenicity of MMMF, *Ann Occup Hyg* 31:755, 1987.
56. Nash T, Allison A, Harrington J: Physiochemical properties of silica in relation to its toxicity, *Nature* 210:259, 1966.
57. Nasr A et al: The prevalence of radiographic abnormalities in the chests of fiber glass workers, *J Occup Med* 13:371-376, 1971.
58. Nettersheim P et al: In vitro analysis of multistage carcinogenesis, *Environ Health Perspect* 75:71, 1987.
59. Nolan R, Langer A, Herson G: Membranolytic activity and morphological characterization of palygorskite and sepiolite. In Mossman B, Begin R, eds: *Effects of mineral dusts on cells,* Berlin, 1989, Springer-Verlag.
60. Nolan R et al: Quartz hemolysis as related to its surface functionalities, *Environ Res* 26:503, 1981.
61. O'Connell T, Rheinwald J: Biology of normal, malignant, and oncogene-transfected human mesothelial cells in culture. In Harris C, Lechner J, Brinkley B, eds: *Cellular and molecular aspects of fiber carcinogenesis,* ed 1, Plainview, NY, 1991, Cold Spring Harbor Laboratory Press.
62. Osterman JW et al: Work related decrement in pulmonary function in silicon carbide production workers, *Br J Ind Med* 46:708, 1989.
63. Owen P et al: Sub-chronic inhalation toxicology of carbon fibers, *J Occup Med* 28:373, 1986.
64. Peters J et al: Pulmonary effects of exposure to silicon carbide manufacturing, *Br J Ind Med* 41:109, 1984.
65. Pfeifer A et al: Control of growth and squamous differentiation in normal human bronchial epithelial cells by chemical and biological modifiers and transferred genes, *Environ Health Perspect* 80:209, 1989.
66. Reider C, Sluder G, Brinkley B: Some possible routes for asbestos-induced aneuploidy during mitosis in vertebrate cells. In Harris C, Lechner J, Brinkley B, eds: *Cellular and molecular aspects of fiber carcinogenesis,* ed 1, Plainview, NY, 1991, Cold Spring Harbor Laboratory Press.
67. Rogan W et al: US prevalence of occupational pleural thickening: a look at chest x-rays from the first national health and nurtrition examination survey, *Am J Epidemiol* 126:893, 1987.
68. Rom W: Activated alveolar macrophages from individuals with asbestosis release peptide growth factors. In Harris C, Lechner J, Brinkley B, eds: *Cellular and molecular aspects of fiber carcinogenesis,* ed 1, Plainview, NY, 1991, Cold Spring Harbor Laboratory Press.
69. Schlessinger R: Comparative deposition of inhaled aerosols in experimental animals and humans: a review, *J Toxicol Environ Health* 15:197, 1987.
70. Shannon H et al: Mortality experience of Ontario glass fiber workers: extended follow-up, *Ann Occup Hyg* 31:657, 1987.
71. Skuric Z, Stahuljak-Beritic D: Occupational exposure and ventilatory function changes in rock wool workers. In Guthe T, ed: *Biological effects of man made mineral fibres: proceedings of a WHO/IARC conference in association with JEMRB and TIMA, Copenhagen, April 20-22, 1982,* 1984, World Health Organization.
72. Smith D et al: Long-term health effects in hamsters and rats exposed chronically to man-made vitreous fibers, *Ann Occup Hyg* 31:731, 1987.
73. Smith T et al: Respiratory exposures associated with silicon carbide production: estimation of cumulative exposure for an epidemiologic study, *Br J Ind Med* 41:100, 1984.
74. Stanton M, Wrench C: Mechanism of mesothelioma induction with asbestos and fibrous glass, *J Natl Cancer Inst* 48:797, 1972.
75. Stanton M et al: Carcinogenicity of fibrous glass: pleural response in the rat in relation to fiber dimensions, *J Natl Cancer Inst* 58:587, 1977.
76. Stanton M, et al: Relationship of particle dimension to carcinogenicity in amphibole asbestos and other fibrous minerals, *J Natl Cancer Inst* 67:965, 1981.
77. Stober W: Dynamic shape factors of nonspherical aerosol particles. In Mercer TEA, ed: *Assessment of airborne particles,* Springfield, Ill, 1972, Charles C Thomas.
78. Timbrell V: Deposition and retention of fibres in the human lung, *Ann Occup Hyg* 26:347, 1982.
79. Van der Meeren A et al: Production of growth factors by rat pleural mesothelial cells in vivo and in vitro transformed by chrysotile fibers. In Mossman B, Begin R, eds: *Effects of mineral dusts on cells,* Berlin, 1989, Springer-Verlag.
80. Wagner J et al: Animal experiments with MMM(V)F—Effects of inhalation and intrapleural inoculation in rats. In Guthe T, ed: *Biological effects of man-made mineral fibres: proceedings of a WHO/IARC conference in association with JEMRB and TIMA, Copenhagen, April 20-22, 1982,* 1984, World Health Organization.
81. Wagner J et al: Biologic effects of tremolite, *Br J Cancer* 45:352, 1982.
82. Walker V et al: Expression of fms-related oncogene in carcinogen-induced neoplastic epithelial cells, *Proc Natl Acad Sci* 84:1804, 1987.
83. Wallace W et al: Mineral surface-specific differences in the adsorption and enzymatic removal of surfactant and their correlation with cytotoxicity. In Mossman B, Begin R, eds: *Effects of mineral dusts on cells,* Berlin, 1989, Springer-Verlag.
84. Weill H et al: Respiratory health effects in workers exposed to man-made vitreous fibers, *Am Rev Respir Dis* 128:104, 1983.
85. Weissner J et al: The effects of chemical modification of quartz surface on particulate-induced pulmonary inflammation and fibrosis in the mouse, *Am Rev Respir Dis* 141:111, 1990.
86. Wheeler C, Garner C: The effect of aramid and metaphosphate fibers on macrophage viability and function. In Mossman B, Begin R, eds: *Effects of mineral dusts on cells,* Berlin, 1989, Springer-Verlag.
87. Wilson V et al: Chemical carcinogen-induced decreases in genomic 5-methyloxycytidine content of normal human bronchial epithelial cells, *Proc Natl Acad Sci USA* 84:3298, 1987.
88. Wilson V et al: Genomic 5-methyldeoxycytidine decreases associated with the induction of squamous differentiation in cultured normaal human bronchial epithelial cells, *Carcinogenesis* 9:2155, 1988.
89. Wright G: Airborne fibrous glass particles: chest roentgenograms of persons with prolonged exposures, *Arch Environ Health* 16:175, 1968.
90. Yamato H et al: Determinant factors for clearance of ceramic fibres, *Br J Ind Med* 49:182, 1992.

Chapter 40

AIR POLLUTION IN THE OUTDOOR ENVIRONMENT

Mark J. Utell
Jonathan M. Samet

Sources and classification
Personal exposure to air pollution
Sources of information on ambient air quality
Principles of inhalation injury
Health effects of specific outdoor pollutants
    Sulfur oxides, particulate matter, and acid aerosols
    Ozone
    Nitrogen oxides
    CO
    Lead
Susceptible populations
    Clinical studies of asthmatics and patients with COPD
    Clinical studies of patients with heart disease
Control strategies
    Patient-oriented strategies
    Community-oriented strategies

Outdoor air pollution has long been associated with clinically significant adverse health effects. Dramatic episodes of fatalities associated with outdoor air pollution occurred at Donora, Pennsylvania, in 1948 and in London in 1952, providing clear evidence that pollutants in outdoor air can cause deaths. Although clinicians may become involved in the evaluation and treatment of patients with acute, severe, and potentially fatal effects of toxic exposures, the clinician is more typically concerned with outdoor pollutants as a cause of respiratory morbidity. Patients often turn to their physicians for advice concerning possible harmful consequences of air pollution and steps that may be taken to minimize any adverse effects. Physicians may also be viewed as the community's experts on the consequences of air pollution; pulmonary physicians are often regarded as having special expertise in this regard. Thus the scope of physician involvement with air pollution is broad, ranging from issues arising in the care of the individual patient to public health concerns.

This chapter addresses the broad sources of pollution in outdoor air and introduces the concept of total personal exposure to air pollutants. The health effects of the principal outdoor air pollutants are then reviewed, as are the effects of pollutant exposure on persons with asthma and chronic obstructive pulmonary disease (COPD) as well as individuals with coronary artery disease. Finally, approaches to controlling adverse effects of air pollution exposure are addressed.

SOURCES AND CLASSIFICATION

Myriad pollutants, both man-made and natural, can be detected in outdoor air. Some naturally occurring pollutants in outdoor air are well documented to cause or exacerbate pulmonary diseases, for example, pollens and fungi. More attention has been focused, however, on the effects of man-made pollutants, which may reach potentially hazardous levels in urban areas or near point sources, such as power plants or manufacturing facilities; some man-made pollutants, for example, acid aerosols and photochemical smog, now contaminate broad regions of the United States and other countries.

In the United States, the principal outdoor pollutants are generally classified within the framework provided by the Environmental Protection Agency (EPA), which identifies

Table 40-1. Criteria pollutants: NAAQS and principal health effects

Pollutant	Primary standards*	Average time	Health effects
Ozone	0.12 ppm (235 µg/m³)	1 hr	Decrements in lung function, possibly chronic lung disease
PM_{10}†	50 µg/m³	Annual (arithmetic mean)	Chronic respiratory disease, altered lung function in children
	150 µg/m³	24 hr	
SO_2	0.03 ppm (80 µg/m³)	Annual (arithmetic mean)	Exacerbation of asthma
	0.14 ppm (365 µg/m³)	24 hr	
NO_2	0.053 ppm (100 µg/m³)	Annual (arithmetic mean)	Increased respiratory infections, risk of acute lung disease
Carbon monoxide	9 ppm (10 mg/m³)	8 hr	Aggravation of coronary artery disease
	35 ppm (40 mg/m³)	1 hr	
Lead	1.5 µg/m³	Quarterly average	Developmental effects on children

*Standard to protect against adverse health effects.
†Particulate matter with a diameter of 10 µm or less.

two sets of pollutants, criteria pollutants (Table 40-1) and hazardous pollutants. The criteria pollutants include primarily combustion-related pollutants (sulfur dioxide [SO_2], nitrogen dioxide [NO_2], carbon monoxide [CO], and particles), the secondary pollutant ozone, and lead. The hazardous pollutants are predominantly carcinogens, such as asbestos; the sources are diverse but principally include industries and waste products.

These two groups of pollutants are regulated through different mechanisms. For the criteria pollutants, National Primary Ambient Air Quality Standards (NAAQS) are set after extensive review of all relevant evidence; the standards must afford protection to the entire population, including those with heightened susceptibility, and must offer an adequate margin of safety. The hazardous pollutants are predominantly carcinogens, such as asbestos and radionuclides, and standards for maximal concentrations also are intended to provide a margin of safety. The Clean Air Act includes mechanisms for achieving levels within the standards and for enforcement. Despite federal standards for ambient air quality, levels in excess are common in many areas of the country, particularly for ozone.

The goal of achieving a set level of air quality should afford protection to most people; however, particular combinations of susceptibility and exposure might still produce clinically relevant effects in some persons at pollutant levels below the standards.

PERSONAL EXPOSURE TO AIR POLLUTION

In developed countries the patterns of time of use and activity put children and adults in diverse indoor and outdoor environments throughout the day, each environment possibly having its own unique set of air contaminants.[17] Perhaps because of the distinct sources contaminating outdoor air and indoor air and the separate regulatory mechanisms for outdoor air, the workplace, and the home, the health effects of air pollution have often been addressed separately for outdoor and indoor air.

However, the concept of total personal exposure is more relevant for health; personal exposure to air pollution represents the time-weighted average of pollutant concentrations in microenvironments, environments having relatively homogeneous air quality, where time is spent.[26] Thus for an office worker, relevant microenvironments might include home, office, car, outdoors at home, outdoors at work, and a movie theater. For some pollutants, for example, ozone or acid aerosols, outdoor environments make the predominant contribution to total personal exposure; for others, such as radon and formaldehyde, indoor locations are most important. In considering the health consequences of air pollution, the physician should recognize that outdoor air is only one potential vector for pollution exposure.[17]

SOURCES OF INFORMATION ON AMBIENT AIR QUALITY

Achieving a full understanding of the health effects of any air pollutant is a daunting task. The relevant literature potentially includes information on sources and concentrations and complementary data from toxicologic investigations, human exposures, and epidemiologic studies. Each approach has specific strengths and weaknesses in evaluation of the impact of pollutants on human health.

Epidemiologic studies involve examination of the relation between exposure and health effects in the community setting, typically in large populations.[6] Respiratory effects are usually assessed by questionnaire and tests of pulmonary function that can be used in the field setting, most often spirometry. Inherent methodologic problems may limit the results of epidemiologic studies. Accurate estimation of exposure to a pollutant is typically difficult, and many outdoor pollutants of concern occur as components of complex mixtures. Confounding factors, including environmental agents other than the pollutant of concern and factors determining the susceptibility of subjects, may further limit interpretation of epidemiologic studies.

Controlled human exposures, involving short-term inhalation of pollutants by small groups of subjects in the laboratory, allow strict control of the experimental subject and the environment. The limitations of use of environmental exposure chambers rest on ethical and practical considerations. The safety of volunteer subjects is a primary concern, so long-term exposures cannot be performed and the investigator is limited to examining mild, acute, and reversible effects. Exposures to pollutants are usually for short durations, such as a few hours, and at low concentrations. The results of controlled human exposures cannot be extrapolated to chronic effects. Clinical studies have proved quite effective, however, in determining threshold concentrations of individual pollutants that may cause specific health effects; susceptible populations have often been the focus of clinical studies.

Animal studies provide the opportunity to evaluate pathogenetic mechanisms of injury by pollutants. Carefully performed exposure-response data can be collected with use of a wide array of biologic parameters in multiple species; however, the use of data from animal exposures introduces uncertainty through the need for extrapolation from an animal model to human health effects. Differences in respiratory tract morphology, regional deposition of pollutants within the lung, and interspecies differences in biologic and physiologic sensitivity to given concentrations of pollutants contribute to the uncertainty of this extrapolation.

Information on air pollution from these investigative approaches is published in a broad array of journals and technical reports. The criteria documents prepared by the EPA offer lengthy reviews that are periodically updated, but even these summary reports are potentially overwhelming in size and scope. The American Thoracic Society has periodically prepared summary statements for health professionals on the health effects of ambient air pollution.

PRINCIPLES OF INHALATION INJURY

Atmospheric pollutants exist in both gaseous and particulate forms. In relating clinical diseases to specific exposures the clinician should recognize that penetration into and retention within the respiratory tract of toxic gases can vary widely, depending on the physical properties of the gas (such as its solubility), the concentration of the gas in the inspired air, the rate and depth of ventilation, and the extent to which the material is reactive.[33] Gases that are highly water soluble, such as SO_2, are almost completely extracted by the nose and pharynx of resting healthy subjects during brief exposures. In contrast, the removal of less water-soluble gases, such as NO_2 and ozone, is much less complete, and thus these gases penetrate deeper into the respiratory tract.[16,23] CO is poorly soluble in water and is not removed in the upper airways. On reaching the lung CO diffuses across the alveolar-capillary membrane and binds avidly to hemoglobin in the blood.

Penetration of gases into the deep lung, and thus the total dose to the airway target can be greatly enhanced by exercise. Not only does exercise increase the dose directly by increasing minute ventilation but also, because many people switch from nasal to oral breathing during moderate-to-heavy exercise, the more efficient uptake by the nasal passages is bypassed.

Pollutants in particulate form are usually found in nature as aerosols. These small liquid droplets or solid particles are dispersed in the atmosphere with sufficient stability to remain in suspension. Examples of common aerosols are sulfuric acid mists, sulfate salts, and nitrate salts. Although deposition of inhaled particles depends on many factors, including the aerodynamic properties of the particle (primarily size), airway anatomy, and breathing pattern, several generalizations can be made. Particles larger than 10 μm are effectively filtered out of the nose and nasopharynx. These relatively large particles tend to deposit rapidly because of impaction against surfaces and gravitational forces. Particles trapped in the nose and nasopharynx are cleared in nasal secretions, coughed out, or swallowed. Particles less than 10 μm in aerodynamic diameter may be deposited in the tracheobronchial tree; deposition in the lung's alveoli is maximal for particles of 1 to 2 μm in diameter. Particles smaller than 0.5 μm are carried by diffusion to the alveolar level, where they collide with gas molecules by brownian movement and are impacted on alveolar surfaces. Removal of particles from the upper airways is efficient and occurs within hours; this rapid clearance contrasts with clearance from the deep lung by alveolar macrophages, which may require days to months.

The mechanisms by which inhaled gases and particles injure the lung are diverse and not yet fully understood. Oxidant gases—ozone and NO_2—cause inflammation of the respiratory epithelium, presumably through the production of toxic oxidant species and release of potent mediators. SO_2 also is an irritant gas. The response to particles varies with the chemical nature of the particles. Acidic compounds on particles may dissolve into tissue fluids and induce an inflammatory response. Organic materials on particles may also produce inflammation or act as initiators or promoters of cancer.

HEALTH EFFECTS OF SPECIFIC OUTDOOR POLLUTANTS

About 102 million people in the United States lived in counties that exceeded one air quality standard during 1987: by pollutant, the numbers include ozone, 88.6 million; CO, 29.4 million; particulate matter, 21.5 million; NO_2, 7.5 million; and SO_2, 1.6 million. Although the pollutants are considered on an individual basis in the following section, it should be reemphasized that exposure is often difficult to characterize, because a mixture of pollutants is often involved. This chapter does not address the health effects of the hazardous pollutants because of the large number of agents of concern.

Sulfur oxides, particulate matter, and acid aerosols

Sulfur oxides are produced by combustion of fuels containing sulfur, such as coal from the eastern United States and crude petroleum. In the past, scientific research and regulatory concern in relation to the sulfur oxides was directed primarily at the health effects of SO_2.[2] Particulate matter was considered separately. Particles in the air have numerous natural and man-made sources, including the same combustion processes that also produce SO_2 and another group of oxidant gases, the nitrogen oxides. The chemical composition of particles is complex and highly variable, but along with the size of the particle, it is a major determinant of toxicity in the respiratory tract.

Asthmatics are particularly susceptible to SO_2, responding to exposure in chamber with increased airways resistance and reduced level of lung function.[27] With hyperventilation, which increases the dose delivered to the respiratory tract, some asthmatics are adversely affected at levels common in ambient air and well below those that might occur transiently with direct exposure to the plume from a power plant or factory.

The adverse effects of particles depend on chemical composition, for example, presence of trace metals and hydrocarbons, and on size, which determines the site of deposition within the respiratory tract. Inflammation with symptoms and reduction of lung function in normal persons, asthmatics, and persons with COPD is of concern, as is carcinogenesis. New epidemiologic findings suggest that the present NAAQS for particulate matter may not be protecting against adverse health effects with the adequate margin of safety mandated by the Clean Air Act. Some of these new findings include positive associations between mortality rates and levels of particulate matter in a number of U.S. cities* and between respiratory morbidity and pollution with particulate matter with a diameter of 10 μm or less in the Utah Valley, the site of a steel mill.[19-21] The new mortality findings are remarkable for the demonstration of an apparent adverse effect of particulate-matter pollution in concentration ranges under currently allowable levels; however, the toxicologic mechanism by which inhaled particulate matter could lead to cardiopulmonary morbidity and mortality has yet to be established[34] and could temper the interpretation of data.

New data suggest that large numbers of persons in the United States and other industrialized countries are exposed to acid aerosols arising from combustion pollutants.[4,31] Tall stacks release SO_2, NO_2, and particles high into the atmosphere, where transformations yield acid particles containing sulfate and nitrate species. This problem of acid aerosols predominantly affects the central eastern United States and Canada, but point sources can produce local problems. Epidemiologic data indicate associations of acid aerosol levels with mortality and respiratory symptoms in children.[22] Asthmatics also appear sensitive to acid aerosols.[14,35] The evidence on acid aerosols and health was recently reviewed by a committee of the American Thoracic Society.[4] Persons considered to be at greatest risk were those working outdoors and thus highly exposed and persons with increased airways responsiveness or asthma. Health effects of concern included increased respiratory symptoms and decreased lung function.

Ozone

Photochemical pollution is a complex oxidant mixture produced by the action of sunlight on vehicle exhaust. Through a series of photochemical reactions involving hydrocarbons and nitrogen oxides, various oxidant pollutants are produced, including ozone, which serves as an index for this type of pollution. Photochemical pollution was first recognized about 40 years ago in southern California, where the combination of sunlight and heavy vehicle travel promotes its formation. Ozone has now become a problem in many other locations, including other western cities with similarly sprawling growth and in the eastern United States during the summertime.

The toxicology of ozone has been extensively investigated.[16] Low-level exposures cause damage to the small airways of experimental animals; the demonstration of subtle fibrosis in one animal model raises concern about permanent structural alteration.[16] Volunteers exposed to ozone at concentrations in the range of the present standard, often present during pollution episodes, have transient reductions of lung function; normal subjects have a range of responsiveness that is broad but repeatable for individuals. More recently, evidence of an inflammatory response and biochemical changes in bronchoalveolar lavage fluid have been detected 18 hours after an exposure to ozone at a level below the current standard. Taken together, the progressive decrements in pulmonary mechanics during exposure and the persistent biochemical changes many hours after cessation of exposure indicate the potential for chronic effects from repeated inhalation. Surprisingly, asthmatics have not been shown to have increased susceptibility to ozone in clinical studies. The evidence of short-term effects of ozone exposure on the lung function of normal volunteers has raised concern about possible long-term effects of living in southern California and other locations with sustained photochemical pollution. Relevant epidemiologic data are suggestive of chronic effects of ozone, but these data are not definitive.[16]

Nitrogen oxides

Nitrogen oxides, like sulfur oxides, are produced by combustion processes and contribute to the formation of acid aerosols. NO_2 is regulated by the EPA as a criteria pollutant, although most of the population's exposure in the United States reflects indoor exposure from gas stoves and space heaters. NO_2 is an oxidant gas that can penetrate to the small airways and alveoli of the lung. Toxicologic evidence suggests that NO_2 exposure can impair lung defenses against

---
*References 7-9, 12, 21, 25.

respiratory pathogens and cause airways inflammation, with associated effects on lung function and respiratory symptoms.[23] The epidemiologic evidence remains inconclusive, largely because of methodologic problems arising in attempts to separate the effects of NO_2 from those of other pollutants. A recent metaanalysis using data from 11 studies found that a long-term increase in NO_2 exposure of approximately 15 ppb, consistent with the presence of a gas stove in the home, is associated with a 20% increase in the risk of respiratory illness in children.[11] On the other hand, a large study of children under the age of 2 years in Albuquerque found no association between indoor NO_2 exposure and respiratory illness.[24] Similarly, recent controlled clinical studies provide inconsistent findings on the effects of low-level NO_2 on lung function of asthmatics.[23] The conflicting results are probably related to differences in subject selection and exposure protocols. Individuals with COPD may represent a group with increased susceptibility to short-term NO_2, but further study of this issue is needed.

CO

CO, another criteria pollutant, binds to hemoglobin to form carboxyhemoglobin (COHb) and reduces the capacity of the blood to deliver oxygen to the tissues. At high levels CO can cause severe neurologic damage and even death in normal persons. At lower levels normal persons may have reduced oxygen uptake during exercise. Recent evidence indicates that controlled CO exposure to patients with stable coronary artery disease can induce earlier subjective and objective evidence of myocardial ischemia at venous COHb levels as low as 2% to 4%.[1] Such data are relevant to the urban environment, where individuals may be exposed to sufficient air pollution to raise blood COHb levels to this range. Furthermore, moderate exercise results in even greater CO loading. Thus for patients with coronary disease exposure to CO can exacerbate myocardial ischemia. In addition, at a COHb level of 6%, patients with coronary artery disease have an increased frequency of arrhythmias.[30] On a practical level physicians should advise patients with exertional myocardial ischemia that personal exposure to CO is potentially modifiable. Persons with COPD and fetuses also may be susceptible to CO. The EPA has recently required areas that are not in compliance with the CO standard to add methyl tertiary-butyl ether, as an oxygenate, to gasoline to enhance oxidative combustion.

Lead

The population may be exposed to lead through many environmental media, including ambient air. Fortunately, in the United States the importance of ambient air as a source of population exposure to lead has diminished with the removal of lead from gasoline. Children are particularly vulnerable to lead exposure. Even levels previously considered safe have been associated with adverse neurologic effects.[18]

SUSCEPTIBLE POPULATIONS

The legislative history of the Clean Air Act mandated that primary NAAQS were to be set low enough to protect the health of all susceptible groups[5,32] (Table 40-2) within the population, with the exception of those requiring life-support systems, namely, patients in intensive care units and newborn infants in nurseries. Only two diseases, asthma and emphysema, were specifically identified in the Clean Air Act as associated with increased susceptibility. Controlled clinical studies have identified asthmatics as susceptible to SO_2, sulfuric acid aerosols, and perhaps NO_2, whereas individuals with COPD may be more responsive to nitrogen dioxide. Rather surprisingly, asthmatics and healthy volunteers have demonstrated nearly equivalent responses in terms of pulmonary decrements to ozone.

Clinical studies of asthmatics and patients with COPD

Controlled laboratory studies of volunteers have attempted to identify specific effects of individual pollutants as assessed primarily by pulmonary mechanics. Such studies often examine groups thought to be at high risk from pollutants, such as asthmatics, individuals with COPD, and normal subjects who undergo periods of heavy exercise.

The most striking effect of acute exposure to SO_2 at concentrations at or below 1.0 ppm is the induction of bronchoconstriction in asthmatics after exposures lasting only 5 minutes. In contrast, inhalation of concentrations of SO_2 in excess of 5 ppm causes only small decrements in airway function in normal subjects. Lung function responses to SO_2

Table 40-2. Populations considered susceptible to air pollution

Population	Potential mechanism	Consequences
Asthmatics	Increased airways responsiveness	Increased risk for exacerbation of respiratory symptoms
Cigarette smokers	Impaired defense and clearance, lung injury	Increased damage through synergism
Elderly	Impaired respiratory defenses, reduced functional reserve	Increased risk for respiratory infection, increased risk for clinically significant effects on function
Infants	Immature defense mechanisms of the lung	Increased risk for respiratory infection
Persons with CHD	Impaired myocardial oxygenation	Increased risk for myocardial ischemia
Persons with COPD	Reduced level of lung function	Increased risk for clinically significant effects on function

CHD, coronary heart disease.

in asthmatics are greater when SO_2 exposure is accompanied by increased ventilation, usually stimulated by exercise.[28] SO_2-induced bronchoconstriction can be exacerbated by breathing cold air and/or dry air and oral breathing instead of nasal breathing. The SO_2 bronchoconstrictor response can be reduced or inhibited in asthmatics by anticholinergic agents such as atropine, mast-cell stabilizers such as cromolyn,[27] and β-agonist bronchodilators such as metaproterenol.[15]

Inhalation of acidic aerosols generally produces little alteration of pulmonary function in normal subjects even at the workplace permissible exposure limit of 1 mg/m^3. As with SO_2, asthmatic subjects have been found to be susceptible to the effects of acidic aerosol exposure, although different laboratories have found differing threshold exposure concentrations. Adult asthmatics exposed to 450 and 1000 μ/m^3 H_2SO_4 aerosols demonstrated decrements in specific airway conductance.[35] Adolescent asthmatics appear to be more sensitive to the effect of acidic aerosols than are adult asthmatics. Functional decrements have been observed in adolescents at levels as low as 70 $\mu g/m^3$, a level occasionally experienced in outdoor air.[14] The apparent difference in sensitivity of adult and adolescent asthmatics may also be due to differences in aerosol sizes or exposure protocols, but adolescent asthmatics respond to concentrations of H_2SO_4 aerosols at exposures an order of magnitude lower than that to which normal subjects respond. In these studies,[14] young asthmatics showed functional decrements at exposure levels near peak outdoor levels in the northeastern United States. Field studies in summer camps of both normal and asthmatic children reported decrements in pulmonary function during pollution episodes that included increased levels of acidic aerosols,[22] reinforcing concern that children and adolescents may be particularly susceptible to effects of acidic atmospheres.

Although several controlled human studies have found asthmatics to be responsive to low levels of NO_2, the findings have not been consistent.[23] The conflicting results among these several studies are probably related to the differences in subject selection and exposure protocols. Individuals with COPD may represent a group with increased susceptibility to short-term NO_2 exposure, but further study of the issue is needed.

Consonant with the provisions of the Clean Air Act and its legislative history, a group that appears to be at potential risk from exposure to ozone is the subgroup of the general population characterized as having preexisting respiratory disease; however, in the case of asthmatics, emerging data from controlled studies indicate no greater responsiveness to ozone in mild asthmatics than in normal, healthy populations. Pretreatment of healthy volunteers with β-adrenergic agents prior to ozone exposure and exercise has not prevented bronchoconstriction, whereas pretreatment with atropine or indomethacin reduced the decrement in lung function.[16] Because exercise greatly potentiates the response to ozone, the best strategy is to avoid outdoor exercise during periods of high-ozone pollution.

Clinical studies of patients with heart disease

Individuals with coronary heart disease have also been identified as a group at risk from elevated air pollution levels. In the presence of coronary artery disease there is limited ability to increase coronary blood flow in response to increased myocardial oxygen consumption during exercise. When myocardial blood flow is not sufficient to meet oxygen demand, the myocardium becomes ischemic, resulting in angina pectoris of electrocardiographic changes, or both. Several recent studies conducted at various COHb levels have investigated the effects of CO exposure on exercise capacity and on the occurrence of myocardial ischemia.[1,13,29] All three studies reported a decrease, or results were consistent with a decrease, in the time to the occurrence of myocardial ischemia in persons with coronary artery disease during exercise after CO exposure. The lowest CO dose to produce a decrease in time to the onset of angina was observed at 2% COHb.[1] In this study, there was a mean 4.2% decrease in the time to angina and a mean 5.1% decrease in the time to electrocardiographic changes indicative of myocardial ischemia at 2% COHb, compared with control (air exposure) days, and there were greater effects at 3.9% COHb. The clinical studies have shown a significant dose-response relationship for the individual differences in time to the onset of electrocardiographic changes at increasing COHb levels. In addition, at a COHb level of 6%, patients with coronary artery disease have an increased frequency of arrhythmias.[30] It is interesting that adverse effects have not been observed in animal studies at COHb levels as low as those for which effects have been observed in humans.

CONTROL STRATEGIES
Patient-oriented strategies

Approaches for limiting the health risks of breathing polluted ambient air have received little investigation. Present understanding of the determinants of exposure suggests that modifying time-activity patterns to limit time outside during episodes of air pollution represents the most effective strategy. The levels of some reactive pollutants tend to be lower indoors than outdoors. Ozone levels in buildings are lower than outdoor levels but can be driven upward by increases in the rate of exchange of indoor with outdoor air. Fine acid aerosols can penetrate indoors, but neutralization by ammonia produced by occupants, pets, and household products may reduce concentrations. Other types of particles in outdoor air may also enter indoor air. Nevertheless, health care providers can reasonably advise patients to stay indoors during pollution episodes. Vigorous exercise outdoors, which increases the dose of pollution delivered to the respiratory tract, also should be avoided at such times.

Susceptible patients should be counseled about the nature and degree of their susceptibility. The use of medication should follow the usual clinical indications, and therapeutic regimens should not be adjusted because of the occurrence of a pollution episode without evidence of an adverse effect on symptoms or function. In the laboratory, inhalation of cromolyn sodium and bronchodilating agents may block the response to some pollutants, but use of these drugs solely because of exposure to air pollution cannot be advised.

Respiratory protective equipment has been developed for use in the workplace to minimize exposure to toxic gases and particles. Many of these devices, particularly those likely to be most effective, add to the work of breathing and are not well tolerated by persons with respiratory disease. Under most circumstances, health care providers should not suggest respiratory protection as a method for reducing the risks of ambient air pollution. Similarly, air cleaners have not been shown to have health benefits.

Community-oriented strategies

Frequently communities become concerned about the impact of particular local sources, perhaps a power plant or manufacturing facility. Concern about the health risks may quickly lead to controversy and litigation. Thus understanding the health risks posed by local sources may be difficult and may require skills in community health, epidemiology, and toxicology.[10] Local physicians may become involved through concerns about the health of their patients or as advocates for the community's environment of the polluting facility. Most often the dimensions of such complex problems exceed the skills of local physicians. Nevertheless, involvement may be appropriate but guidance should be obtained from appropriate public health and environmental agencies.

The interplay of factors that must be manipulated to prevent environmentally induced disease is complex, but standards are considered to be objective indicators of successful preventive measures or strategies. In 1976 the EPA proposed cautionary statements for public reporting of outdoor air quality, the Pollutant Standards Index for criteria pollutants. The actions taken when alert levels are reached or expected to be reached include the issuance of health advisories (or cautionary statements) to the public. The EPA's advice is intended to be applied by local air pollution agencies in preparation of daily air quality summaries that are disseminated to the media. Although the cautionary statements require some revisions, especially as related to ozone exposures, useful guidelines are offered for the physician and public health officials.

REFERENCES

1. Alfred EN et al: Short-term effects of carbon monoxide exposure on the exercise performance of subjects with coronary artery disease, *N Engl J Med* 321:1426, 1989.
2. American Thoracic Society: Health effects of air pollution, *ATS News* 6:1, 1978.
3. American Thoracic Society: Environmental controls and lung disease, *Am Rev Respir Dis* 142:915, 1990.
4. American Thoracic Society: Health effects of atmospheric acids and their precursors, *Am Rev Respir Dis* 144:464, 1991.
5. Brain JD et al: *Variations in susceptibility to inhaled pollutants: identification, mechanisms, and policy implications,* Baltimore, 1988, Johns Hopkins University Press.
6. Committee on the Epidemiology of Air Pollutants, Board on Toxicology and Environmental Health Hazards, Commission on Life Sciences, National Research Council: *Epidemiology and air pollution,* Washington, DC, 1985, National Academy Press.
7. Dockery DW, Schwartz K, Spengler JD: Air pollution and daily mortality: associations with particulates and acid aerosols, *Environ Res* 59:362, 1992.
8. Dockery DW et al: An association between air pollution and mortality in six U.S. cities, *N Engl J Med* 329:1753, 1993.
9. Fairley D: The relationship of daily mortality to suspended particulates in Santa Clara county, 1980-1986, *Environ Health Perspect* 89:159, 1990.
10. Goldstein BD, Gochfeld M: Role of the physician in environmental medicine, *Med Clin North Am* 74:245, 1990.
11. Hasselblad V, Kotchmar DJ, Eddy DM: Synthesis of environmental evidence: nitrogen dioxide epidemiology studies, *J Air Waste Manage Assoc* 42:662, 1992.
12. Kinney PL, Özkaynak H: Associations of daily mortality and air pollution in Los Angeles county, *Environ Res* 54:99, 1991.
13. Kleinman MT et al: Effects of short-term exposure to carbon monoxide in subjects with coronary artery disease, *Arch Environ Health* 44:361, 1989.
14. Koenig JQ, Covert DS, Pierson WE: Effects of inhalation of acidic compounds on pulmonary function in allergic adolescent subjects, *Environ Health Perspect* 79:173, 1989.
15. Linn WS et al: Effect of metaproterenol sulfate on mild asthmatics' response to sulfur dioxide exposure and exercise, *Arch Environ Health* 43:399, 1988.
16. Lippmann M: Health effects of ozone: a critical review, *Air Pollution Control Assoc* 39:672, 1989.
17. National Research Council, Committee on Advances in Assessing Human Exposure to Airborne Pollutants: *Human exposure assessment for airborne pollutants, advances and opportunities,* Washington, DC, 1991, National Academy Press.
18. Needleman HL, Gatsaris CA: Low-level lead exposure and the IQ of children: a meta-analysis of modern studies, *JAMA* 263:673, 1990.
19. Pope CA III: Respiratory disease associated with community air pollution and a steel mill, Utah Valley, *Am J Public Health* 79:623, 1989.
20. Pope CA III: Respiratory hospital admissions associated with PM_{10} pollution in Utah, Salt Lake, and Cache Valleys, *Arch Environ Health* 46:90, 1991.
21. Pope CA III, Dockery DW: Acute health effects of PM_{10} pollution on symptomatic and asymptomatic children, *Am Rev Respir Dis* 145:1123, 1992.
22. Raizenne ME et al: Acute lung function responses to ambient acid aerosol exposures in children, *Environ Health Perspect* 79:179, 1989.
23. Samet JM, Utell MJ: The risk of nitrogen dioxide: what have we learned from epidemiological and clinical studies?, *Toxicol Ind Health* 6:247, 1990.
24. Samet JM et al: *Nitrogen dioxide and respiratory illness in children,* Health Effects Institute Research Report No 58, Montpelier, Vt, 1983, Capital City Press.
25. Schwartz J, Dockery DW: Increased mortality in Philadelphia associated with daily air pollution concentrations, *Am Rev Respir Dis* 145:600, 1992.
26. Sexton K, Ryan PB: Assessment of human exposure to air pollution: methods, measurements, and models. In Watson AY, Bates RR, Kennedy D, eds: *Air pollution, the automobile, and public health,* Washington, DC, 1988, National Academy Press.
27. Sheppard D: Mechanisms of airway responses to inhaled sulfur dioxide. In Loke J, ed: *Lung biology in health and disease,* vol 34, New York, 1988, Marcel Dekker.

28. Sheppard D et al: Exercise increases sulphur dioxide–induced bronchoconstriction in asthmatic subjects, *Am Rev Respir Dis* 123:486, 1981.
29. Sheps DS et al: Lack of effect of low levels of carboxyhemoglobin on cardiovascular function in patients with ischemic heart disease, *Arch Environ Health* 42:108, 1987.
30. Sheps DS et al: Production of arrhythmias by elevated carboxyhemoglobin in patients with coronary artery disease, *Ann Intern Med* 113:343, 1990.
31. Spengler JD, Brauer M, Koutrakis P: Acid air and health, *Environ Sci Technol* 24:946, 1990.
32. Utell MJ, Frank R, eds: *Susceptibility to inhaled pollutants,* Philadelphia, 1989, American Society for Testing and Materials.
33. Utell MJ, Samet JM: Environmentally mediated disorders of the respiratory tract, *Med Clin North Am* 74:291, 1990.
34. Utell MJ, Samet JM: Particulate air pollution and health, *Am Rev Respir Dis* 147:1334, 1993.
35. Utell MJ et al: Airway responses to sulfate and sulfuric acid aerosols in asthmatics, *Am Rev Respir Dis* 128:444, 1983.

Chapter 41

FIRE AND PYROLYSIS PRODUCTS

Michael Gochfeld

Firefighting: unique hazards and exposures
Exposure to fire products
Specific toxic agents
    Carbon monoxide
    Oxides of nitrogen
    Hydrogen chloride
    Hydrogen cyanide
    Benzene
    Phenol
    Formaldehyde
    Phosgene
    Acrolein
    Polychlorinated biphenyls
    Chlorinated polyaromatics
    Radiation
    Metal and polymer fumes
Health effects in fire victims
    Smoke inhalation
    Heat stress and cardiovascular events
Chronic disease risks for firefighters
    Respiratory disease
    Cancer
Emergency evaluation and care of fire victims
FEMA/USFA algorithm for smoke inhalation injuries

Fires in both natural and man-altered environments are common and devastating occurrences. In addition to the severe property damage that they cause, fires are a major source of illness, injury, and death for firefighters (both volunteer and salaried) and the public. Aside from the acute injurious effects of fire, clinicians must be alert to the pathophysiologic changes associated with exposure to heat and smoke and to the chronic sequelae, both physical and psychologic. Most of the information available on health effects of fires involves firefighters, but many of the principles apply equally to other victims exposed to fire and smoke.

Emergency treatment of firefighters can be complicated, and guidelines for emergency room treatment have been published by the Federal Emergency Management Agency[12] and the New Jersey Department of Health.[15] In addition to the management of burns and trauma, it is necessary to evaluate firefighters for all acute systemic effects of exposure to smoke, heat, or toxic substances; recognize toxic effects that may be obscured by more serious traumatic effects; be alert for delayed consequences; and recognize acute and chronic exposure and health effects due to toxic chemicals found in smoke.

FIREFIGHTING: UNIQUE HAZARDS AND EXPOSURES

Firefighters are at increased risk of chronic respiratory and other systemic disease, because they have recurrent exposure to fire and pyrolysis products. Contrary to some popular accounts, firefighters are usually reluctant to visit emergency rooms and seek medical attention. In many cases they believe that their employment may be jeopardized if they are found to have medical conditions.

Clinicians are likely to take the obvious dangers of firefighting for granted without recognizing that it is a mentally and physically demanding occupation.[7,23–26] Burns, falls, and crushing injuries are commonplace, but the impact of smoke and toxic pollutants in smoke complicates both the immediate treatment and any follow-up. Clinicians must understand the fire environment, the potential constituents of smoke, and the tasks of the firefighter to make decisions on admission, treatment, referral, follow-up, and return-to-work clearance.

Even though firefighters are selected on the basis of physical fitness, they experience increased rates of mortality due to myocardial infarctions,[21] which in some jurisdictions (such as the city of New York) are automatically considered work-related regardless of where or when they occur (presumption of work-relatedness). Moreover, chronic medical conditions such as cardiovascular disease, respiratory impairment, increased predisposition to various forms of cancer, noise-induced hearing loss, and anxiety regarding prior exposures present problems for firefighters.[39]

Several organizations have reported statistics on injuries among firefighters, among them the International Association of Fire Fighters,[19,21] the National Fire Protection Association,[54] and the Federal Emergency Management Administration (FEMA) of the US Department of Commerce.[11] Overall the injury rate for firefighters is about 42 per 100 worker-years,[19] and fatalities run about 80 per 100,000 worker-years.[54] The injury rate is 1.5 times as high as for mining and the mortality rate is twice as high as in police work.[39]

Of 2 million people treated annually for burns, about 10,000 civilians and firefighters die, mainly because of inhalation of toxic and irritating products of combustion.[4] Figs. 41-1 and 41-2 provide breakdowns of 31,403 nonfatal injuries[19] and 113 fatalities.[54] Musculoskeletal injuries accounted for 35% and inhalation for 11% of the injuries, and myocardial infarction accounted for 39% and smoke inhalation for 22% of fatalities. About two thirds of the injuries and fatalities occur at the scene of the fire.[54]

Major urban areas have paid, full-time fire companies, but rural areas and small towns are likely to be served by volunteer companies. A paid company is likely to respond to more than three alarms per day, whereas volunteers may respond to three per week.[39] Volunteers outnumber paid firefighters (for example, by 10 to 1 in New Jersey[39]) but the proportion varies from state to state.

There are three phases to firefighting: (1) rescue, (2) extinguishment (what most people consider firefighting), and (3) overhaul (the search for smoldering materials that might reignite). Although burns and smoke inhalation are most severe during the first two phases, the overhaul phase may be the most hazardous for inhalation of toxics. At this stage firefighters are likely to remove their protective gear and search through the rubble for persistent fires while surrounded by smoldering and smoking debris releasing various toxic gases.

About 30% of fires are primarily structural. Fig. 41-3 shows the distribution of fire types causing injuries. Most

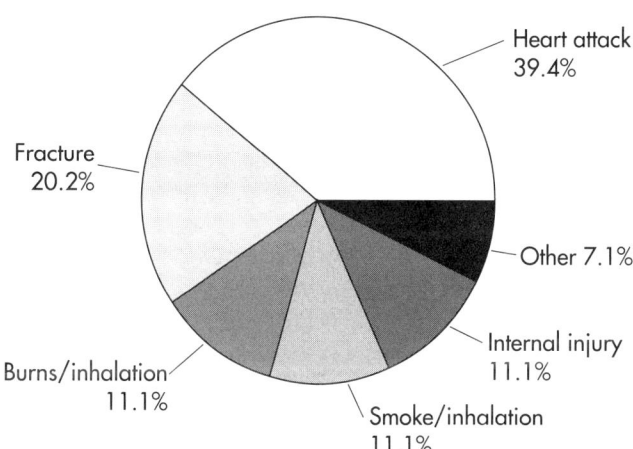

Figure 41-2. Breakdown of causes of death for 113 firefighter fatalities. (From Washburn AE, Harlow DW, Horn S: United States fire fighter deaths in the line of duty during 1979: National Fire Protection Association, *Fire Command* 47:30, 1980.)

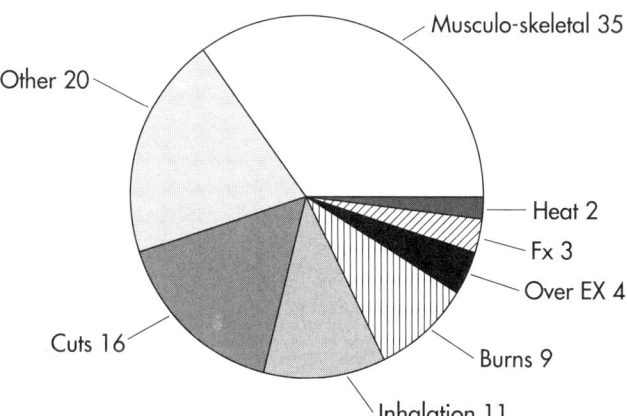

Figure 41-1. Breakdown of 31,403 nonfatal injuries among firefighters. Numbers are percentages adding to 100%. Fx = Fracture. Over EX = Overexertion injuries. (From International Association of Fire Fighters: *Annual death and injury survey,* Washington, DC, 1980, the Association.)

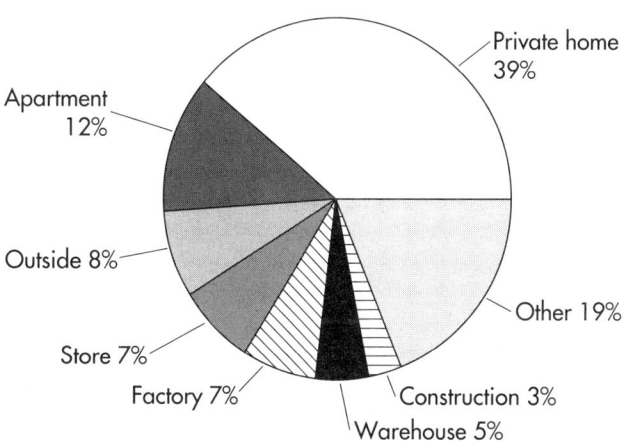

Figure 41-3. Types of fires causing injuries to firefighters. (From Federal Emergency Management Agency: *Highlights of fire in the United States,* Washington, DC, 1980, US Department of Commerce.)

firefighters are injured at fires in private homes or apartments (51%), and factories and warehouses account for 12% of injuries[11]; however, on a per-fire basis, factory fires were the most hazardous (7 injuries per 100 fires), and residential fires were the least hazardous (3.6 injuries per 100 fires[11]).

There have been major advances in the design of firefighting equipment; however, not all companies have access to modern equipment, and paradoxically suburban volunteer companies are more likely to have newer protective equipment than are urban paid companies. In addition, for major fires that require more than one shift on duty, there is often not enough protective gear for all participants at the scene.

Because the fire scene is likely to be hypoxic, firefighters, particularly those entering a burning building, should always wear a self-contained breathing apparatus (SCBA). Respirators of the cartridge or gas-mask type do not provide oxygen, and their chemical-protective properties may be overwhelmed after a short time. SCBA tanks generally provide air for only about a half hour, and for large fires requiring many hours to extinguish, it may not always be feasible to refill tanks quickly enough, so a company may sometimes run out of air.

EXPOSURE TO FIRE PRODUCTS

Combustion is a complex process involving high-temperature oxidation, during which many chemical reactions can occur. Pyrolysis (incomplete combustion) of wood releases many simple and complex organic compounds, including lignin. With the introduction of many new construction and finishing products including plastics, there are many new pyrolysis products, including cyanide (from nitriles) and chlorine (for example, from polyvinyl chloride plastics). They are highly toxic and can also react with other organics to produce new toxic and irritant chemicals. Incomplete combustion and firefighting water also may produce highly acidic aerosols.[8,47]

Very hot fires (temperatures above 1400°C) may cause complete combustion, but under most fire conditions combustion is incomplete, and many toxic products are released from smoldering or partially controlled fires. During the overhaul phase many toxic pyrolysis products have been identified,[16,17,22] and this phase may be a source of significant exposure, because protective clothing is often removed at this time.

Many chemicals are produced in a fire, whether it is a burning cigarette yielding thousands of different substances, some of which are human carcinogens,[57] or mixtures of wood, paper, and plastics found in homes. In general, however, only about a dozen are present at high concentrations.[39]

Combustion products vary dramatically with the objects burning, the conditions of temperature, oxygen availability, and substances used to fight the fire. Carbon monoxide, nitrogen dioxide, sulfur dioxide, cyanide, hydrogen chloride, phosgene, acrolein, formaldehyde, other aldehydes and organic acids, benzene, chlorine, and ammonia are among the common toxic pollutants released during fires.

Knowledge of the materials undergoing combustion helps predict the toxic products that will be formed in the fire and the chemical changes that can continue to occur in the atmosphere. Ultimately, exposure is determined by the concentration reaching the person, the volume of air breathed in, and the bioavailability of the toxin (see Chapter 4). Exposure and absorption depend on whether the material is released as vapor or a smoke or is carried by steam, liquid droplets, or ash. Ingestion and dermal absorption may contribute to exposure in some cases.

Industrial hygiene measurements of contaminants have been reported for some fires.[3,16,50] Table 41-1 shows the proportion of fires that produced levels of selected agents that were above the Occupational Safety and Health Administration (OSHA) short-term exposure limits (STELs) or above levels considered immediately dangerous to life and health (IDLH).[38] It is apparent that at most fire sites the concentration of toxic air contaminants is below these levels, and in most cases firefighters are adequately protected; however, because several of the contaminants (such as respiratory irritants) have the same effects, their concentrations (as a percentage of their respective PELs) may be added to provide a more meaningful picture of site contamination. Also, about 5% of fires produce very high exposures. Because firefighters respond to hundreds of alarms each year, they will certainly find themselves in some life-threatening toxic situations. For the community, the main problem is short-term exposure, because any given member of the public should be exposed to fires only rarely.

SPECIFIC TOXIC AGENTS

Several of the more hazardous and common combustion products are discussed in detail herein; others are considered in other chapters.

Carbon monoxide

Carbon monoxide is always present at fires. The main symptoms of carbon monoxide poisoning are dizziness, headache, nausea, weakness, and tachypnea, followed, at

Table 41-1. Percentage of fires that produced air contamination levels above the ACGIH short-term exposure limit (STEL) and above the NIOSH immediately-dangerous-to-life-and-health (IDLH) levels

	Percentage with values above STEL	Percentage dangerous above IDLH
Carbon monoxide	18	5
Hydrogen chloride	30	2
Acrolein	57	4

From New Jersey State Department of Health: *Firefighting in New Jersey: hazards and methods of control,* Trenton, 1982, *ACGIH,* American Conference of Governmental Industrial Hygienists.

higher amounts, by loss of consciousness, coma, convulsions, and death. Neurobehavioral changes, such as prolonged reaction time and interference with cognitive functions, can be detected with exposure levels as low as 50 ppm.[28] The standard monitoring is measurement of the carboxyhemoglobin (HbCO) level in blood, which is less than 1% in nonsmokers, although smokers may have transient levels approaching 10%. Certain chemicals such as methylene chloride (present in paint strippers) may confound the situation, raising HbCO to dangerous levels.[29] After a fire, most firefighters have HbCO levels above 10%.[22] This exposure can be serious in persons with cardiovascular disease, because angina has been reported to occur after 90 minutes' exposure to 50 ppm.[43]

Subacute and long-term exposure to carbon monoxide may accelerate atherosclerosis and increases the risk of arrhythmias (even as much as 2 weeks after exposure). Acute myonecrosis has been associated with carbon monoxide poisoning.[18]

In a normal person HbCO levels below 20% are not associated with symptoms. At HbCO levels between 20% and 40% headache, nausea, vomiting, and neurobehavioral changes occur. At 40% to 60% visual and general impairment occur and consciousness diminishes, and a 70% HbCO level is likely to be fatal. Patients with an elevated HbCO level are likely to have an elevated or at least normal arterial partial pressure of oxygen (PaO_2) but reduced arterial saturation of oxygen (SaO_2). There is controversy about the role of hyperbaric oxygen treatment of persons with serious carbon monoxide poisoning. Prompt treatment may prevent nervous system damage. Morbidity and duration of hospitalization can be reduced with administration of 100% oxygen at 2 atm, which facilitates dissociation of HbCO and forces oxygen into tissues, relieving the hypoxemia.

Oxides of nitrogen

Oxides of nitrogen, a family of compounds including nitrogen dioxide and nitrous oxide among others, are released on combustion of organic compounds, many of which contain nitrogen (amines, amides). Nitrogen dioxide, the most serious offender, is irritating to the eyes and throat and can yield nitric acid when dissolved in the liquid on the mucous membranes. Some oxides of nitrogen may change the hemoglobin to methemoglobin, which also interferes with oxygen transport. Severe exposure to nitrogen dioxide produces irritation of the lower airway, leading to pulmonary edema. Nitrogen dioxide concentrations are likely to be highest in basement fires involving electrical lines and equipment. Concentrations of 25 to 50 ppm for 1 hour cause severe respiratory irritation, chest pain, and, possibly, pulmonary edema.[39]

Hydrogen chloride

With the dramatic increase in the use of polyvinyl chloride materials in construction, there has been an increase in exposure to hydrogen chloride gas, which is generated from the pyrolysis of polyvinyl chloride. In addition to burning eyes and throat, the vapors may produce edema of the glottis, acute bronchitis, pulmonary edema, and death. Exposure to levels of 10 to 50 ppm is very irritating, and most individuals can detect exposure to 5 ppm.[43]

Hydrogen cyanide

Pyrolysis of asphalt, wool, acrylonitrile, urethane, nylon, and other plastics that contain urethane cross-linkages may yield hydrogen cyanide. Exposure and illness from burning acrylonitrile have been documented after several major fires.[33,35]

Sublethal exposure to cyanide may produce weakness, headache, nausea, vomiting, confusion, and other symptoms of central nervous system toxicity, including coma. Cyanide gas is only mildly irritating to the eyes and throat. Several hours of exposure in the 20- to 40-ppm range may cause symptoms, and only 30 minutes' exposure to 135 ppm or 10 minutes' exposure to 180 ppm may be fatal.[43]

Treatment with sodium nitrite or amyl nitrite converts hemoglobin to methemoglobin, which then binds cyanide as cyanmethemoglobin, thereby competitively inhibiting its toxic effects. This treatment is followed immediately by administration of intravenous aqueous sodium thiosulfate, which reacts with cyanide to form thiocyanate, which is excreted in urine.

Benzene

At high concentrations benzene is a central nervous system depressant, but at fires relatively low concentrations are encountered, and the main concern is whether recurrent exposure is sufficient to cause leukemia. OSHA has established a PEL for benzene of 1 ppm averaged over an 8-hour working day. A New Jersey Department of Health study[39] found that benzene was present in most fires, often at levels exceeding 1 ppm.[39] Firefighters are thus exposed to a level close to or above the PEL of 1 ppm, but this exposure is not usually sustained for an entire day. Epidemiologic studies have shown that firefighters are at an increased risk of leukemia, but it is not known whether it is due specifically to their benzene exposure.

Phenol

Phenolic resins are commonly present in construction materials because of their chemical inertness, but on decomposition they release phenol, which is highly corrosive to any tissue. Severe respiratory burns, hypoxemia, and shock may ensue.

Formaldehyde

Many construction materials contain formaldehyde or substances that form formaldehyde on combustion. These materials include phenolic resins present in plywood and laminates. This colorless gas has a characteristic odor and is highly irritating to eyes and mucous membranes. Individuals vary greatly in their sensitivity to formaldehyde. This gas is so irritating that persons usually cannot inhale high concentrations without choking. Coughing, shortness of breath, and pulmonary edema may occur if the person cannot escape. Formaldehyde is an animal carcinogen and is considered a probable human carcinogen.[32]

Phosgene

Phosgene, a highly reactive compound, is widely used in industry as a raw material for chemical syntheses, for example, in the production of aniline dyes, and it is also well known as a chemical warfare agent; however, it is also commonly formed from pyrolysis of chlorinated compounds. It does not have an unpleasant odor and is not immediately irritating; therefore it readily enters the respiratory tract without causing choking and reaches the lower airway, where it dissolves and forms hydrochloric acid in the smaller bronchi and alveoli, inducing severe irritation. The most characteristic problem is the delayed pulmonary edema, which can be fatal. If death from pulmonary edema is averted, care must still be taken to avoid pneumonia.

Acrolein

Combustion of propylene, a common plastic, releases acrolein, which is severely irritating to eyes and the respiratory tract even at concentrations as low as 0.25 ppm. The OSHA PEL is 0.1 ppm, and the IDLH is 5 ppm.[38] Acrolein has a pungent odor and is so irritating that although upper-airway irritation occurs, there are rarely lower-airway effects. Prolonged exposure can cause dermal burns and dermatitis. Exposure to 1 ppm becomes intolerable and can produce pulmonary edema. Acrolein was found in 69% of fire-atmosphere samples.[50]

Polychlorinated biphenyls

Although production and most uses of polychlorinated biphenyls (PCBs) were terminated before 1980, these persistent chlorinated hydrocarbons were widely used, particularly in electrical equipment, and are still present in old transformers and capacitors and in the environment. Although they are acutely toxic at high doses, it is their subacute and chronic effects on the skin and nervous system as well as their carcinogenic properties and effects on reproductive health that are of concern. Firefighters accumulate PCBs with age and length of service, presumably as a result of small, recurrent exposures.[32] The main source of exposure is to firefighters and building occupants when fires have involved electrical transformers. Serum PCB concentrations can be used to document recent exposure to PCBs (see Chapter 52).

Chlorinated polyaromatics

Compounds such as dioxins and furans can be formed by the combustion of wood, paper, and plastic materials in typical structural fires. The modern household provides a complex mix of chemicals in the kitchen, basement, and garage. In many cases, however, firefighters have an additional exposure risk from fighting fires at industrial facilities, transport spills, chemical warehouses, and chemical dump sites, where there may be high level exposure to some esoteric toxic compounds. Much of the dioxin and furan emissions from fires involve the higher chlorinated compounds (hepta- and octachlor compounds) rather than the more toxic tetrachlor compounds such as 2,3,7,8-tetrachlorodiberzo 20-p-dioxin.

Radiation

Fires at nuclear facilities or in laboratories that handle radioactive material may lead to exposure or contamination of firefighters or their gear. Emergency personnel should have advance information and an emergency plan regarding any nuclear facilities in their catchment area.[52] Decontamination of the clothing of a victim is important, both for his or her own sake and to prevent exposure of emergency personnel handling the victim.

Metal and polymer fumes

A special combustion problem arises when certain metal compounds (such as paint pigments) or polytetrafluoroethylene compounds burn. A person who inhales the fumes of these compounds may develop chest tightness and cough, as well as a flulike syndrome of fever, chills, and rapid pulse. The disease has a delayed onset and usually resolves spontaneously within 2 days.

HEALTH EFFECTS IN FIRE VICTIMS

Table 41-2 lists the kinds of damage commonly associated with fires. Acute effects include burns, trauma, smoke inhalation, and cardiovascular stress. Subacute and long-term effects may involve multiple organ systems.

Smoke inhalation

Smoke inhalation can lead to hypoxemia by interfering with either air movement in the upper airway or gas exchange in the lower airway. The pathophysiologic effects of smoke depend on the presence and concentrations of particular substances in the smoke, the temperature of the inhaled air, and the duration of exposure.[6] There are both direct respiratory and systemic effects from substances absorbed into the blood. The main toxic agent is carbon monoxide, present in all fires, and carbon monoxide poisoning must be considered in all cases of smoke inhalation.

The face, mouth, and throat are subject to thermal injury, but even hot air cools rapidly in the upper respiratory tract, preventing thermal burns to the lung parenchyma; however, inhalation of steam causes lower-airway burns. Moreover, hot particulates that evade defense mechanisms may cause microscopic burns in the bronchioles and alveoli.

Thermal and chemical burns of the upper airway may cause swelling of the pharynx, larynx, and trachea, with potentially lethal results. Bronchospasm due to chemical irritation may complicate the picture. Soluble gases such as

Table 41-2. Types of acute injury due to fire exposure

Acute	Chronic
Burns (superficial, deep, internal)	Chronic cardiovascular disease
Thermal	Chronic respiratory disease
Chemical	Noise-induced hearing loss
Dermal reactions to toxicants	Posttraumatic stress disorder
Eye irritation and burns	Cancer
Smoke inhalation: direct and toxic	
Cardiovascular strain	
Musculoskeletal trauma	
Heat stress	
Neuropsychiatric effects	
Posttraumatic stress disorder	
Renal damage due to myoglobinemia	
Stresses inherent in shift work	

Data from New Jersey State Department of Health: *Firefighting in New Jersey: hazards and methods of control,* Trenton, 1982, and International Association of Fire Fighters: *1982 annual death and injury survey,* Washington, DC, 1983, The Association.

hydrogen chloride and sulfur dioxide dissolve mainly in the moisture on the mucous membrane surface of the upper airway, whereas phosgene and nitrogen oxides reach the terminal bronchi and cause severe irritation and pulmonary edema.

Subacute phase. The period between 12 hours and 7 days after exposure is a subacute phase that requires especial vigilance in persons who have had significant exposure to smoke. Respiratory and kidney disease may evolve during this period and are dangerous because the patient may have been discharged from the emergency department in apparently good health.

Chronic phase. Respiratory injury may persist for weeks or months after a particularly serious exposure and can be documented by both restrictive and obstructive changes on spirometry.[42,51] Firefighters frequently experience such symptoms as frequent or prolonged headaches, black-sputum production, chronic cough, nausea, and vomiting.[5,45]

Heat stress and cardiovascular events

Firefighters are vulnerable to myocardial infarction through a combination of exposures and high levels of carbon monoxide, which combine to increase the demand for cardiac output and oxygen delivery and interfere with oxygen transport and release.[26] The major heat stress syndromes associated with protective gear include heat stroke, heat exhaustion, heat cramps, and related events.[10]

In addition to the delayed acute and subacute respiratory illnesses associated with firefighting, cardiac disease may manifest itself during the subacute period. Ischemic changes, conduction abnormalities, arrhythmias, and myocarditis may become manifest during this period.[49]

CHRONIC DISEASE RISKS FOR FIREFIGHTERS
Respiratory disease

Respiratory symptoms in a firefighter may reflect cumulative irritant exposures rather than simply the effects of the most recent fire[31,34]; however, there are not good data distinguishing acute disease after individual fires from chronic disease after recurrent exposures.[34] Bronchitis, emphysema, and pneumonitis are more common among firefighters than in the general population.[1,42,46] Personnel who fought the Chemical Control fire in Elizabeth, New Jersey, in 1980 experienced a high incidence of radiographic and spirometric abnormalities and corresponding symptoms[30] that persisted for several years. This finding also was true for firefighters fighting an acrylonitrile fire.[35]

Cancer

Firefighters' cancer rates are higher than those of the general population.[20] They are regularly exposed to carcinogens such as vinyl chloride, asbestos, benzene, and polycyclic aromatic hydrocarbons at real and simulated fires; however, they have elevated risks of brain, colon, rectal, skin, and male breast cancer but not of angiosarcoma, mesothelioma, and lung cancer. They do have an elevated leukemia risk, perhaps related to benzene exposure.[13,26] In addition, firefighters are exposed to diesel emission,[14] which are suspected to have carcinogenic properties.[37] Elevated respiratory cancers among a group of firefighters who fought a chemical waste fire in 1978 were attributed to career exposures[36] rather than to that fire.

EMERGENCY EVALUATION AND CARE OF FIRE VICTIMS

Emergency treatment begins in the field. As soon as possible, the history of the fire exposure should be determined, including the type of fire, substances burning, duration of exposure, and other factors influencing exposure, such as enclosed spaces or use of respiratory protection. A rapid physical assessment should determine the functional status of the upper airway, lungs, and cardiovascular system. With toxic exposures, other organ systems, particularly the central nervous system and kidney, may be affected.

Chemical exposure may contaminate the victim's clothing, resulting in continued exposure to both the victim and emergency personnel. The victim's clothing should be removed before he or she is brought into the emergency room. Some hospitals maintain decontamination rooms in which to remove the clothing and wash the victim, which are most applicable to firefighters after a fire at a chemical facility or chemical waste site. Decontamination procedures should not jeopardize the victim.[2,40,48]

Oxygen administration often begins during transportation. Arterial blood gas and carboxyhemoglobin levels are routinely obtained, but thiocyanate levels are seldom measured. Calculation of SaO_2 should not be made from the PaO_2, because there must be correction for HbCO. Blood gas levels form the basis for decision making in the FEMA protocol. A wide alveolar-arteriolar gradient may denote significant lung damage requiring further evaluation (that is, with xenon lung scans) or treatment (for example, with steroids or bronchodilators). Hyperbaric oxygen treatment is sometimes required. In the acute phase a chest radiograph is likely to be normal, even in the presence of symptoms, but it may be an important baseline in the event of pulmonary edema, consolidation, or atelectasis.

Personnel taking a history from the firefighter or another person should inquire about the respiratory-protection history, both for the recent event and in general. Knowledge of whether a firefighter was adequately protected can influence evaluation of his or her risk.[15]

Clinicians tend to have little idea of the importance of vigilance for delayed effects in fire victims,[15] and often, because symptoms improve after administration of 100% oxygen, the patient is discharged without adequate evaluation. Life-threatening laryngeal or pulmonary edema from inhaled toxins may not be evident until 8 to 24 hours after the exposure.[9] Once supportive treatment, usually including oxygen administration, is established, clinicians must be alert to these possibilities.

Eye damage is frequent, ranging from conjunctival reddening to, rarely, retrobulbar neuritis and cortical blindness. The retina may show characteristically flame-shaped hemorrhages due to carbon monoxide poisoning.[49] A rare but serious complication is myonecrosis due to carbon monoxide poisoning.[18] It can be recognized by muscle tenderness, diminished strength, and altered creatine kinase levels in serum, with presence of an mm band.

An electrocardiogram is recommended to evaluate possibly cardiotoxic effects of carbon monoxide and other volatile compounds. Enzyme measurement for cardiac damage should be considered in all victims presenting with more than minor complaints; however, most deaths from acute carbon monoxide poisoning are mainly due to arrhythmias. The ischemia of the ventricle secondary to carbon monoxide poisoning can be superimposed on underlying coronary artery disease. As a result, papillary muscle dysfunction, mitral valve prolapse, and aberrant motion of the ventricular wall may occur. Electrocardiographic changes include T-wave abnormalities, ST-segment ischemic changes, atrial flutter, atrial fibrillation, premature ventricular contractions, and conduction disturbances.[49]

Continuous cardiac monitoring throughout the observation period is indicated. Carbon monoxide binds to myoglobin as well as to hemoglobin and, in fact, is released more slowly. A potential rebound increase in HbCO may follow treatment with oxygen. Moreover, there is a preferential binding to cardiac myoglobin, thereby further compromising oxygen delivery to the myocardium.[49]

Although there is a substantial literature on treatment of thermal burns, there is less information on chemical burns. Chemical burns may involve the skin, eye, mucous membranes, and lungs. Prompt treatment should include[53] removal of chemical-soaked clothing to avoid continued exposure to chemicals, adequate water lavage, discernment of exposed area (distinguished from suntan), and diagnosis of gas injuries.[27,44,49,56]

FEMA/USFA ALGORITHM FOR SMOKE INHALATION INJURIES

The Federal Emergency Management Agency's Fire Administration (FEMA/USFA[12]) provides an algorithm (Table 41-3), developed by the American College of Emergency Physicians, to assist the emergency physician in the evaluation and treatment of smoke-inhalation victims.[12] It relies on clinical findings (from history and physical examination) and laboratory investigation (arterial blood gases) to divide patients into three groups: minimal exposure (probable discharge), moderate exposure (observation and evaluation), and severe exposure (probable admission).

The history provides information on the type of fire, presence of synthetic materials or hazardous chemicals, use or misuse of personal protective gear, and combustion of synthetic materials or chemicals. If arterial blood gas measurements show a partial pressure of oxygen (PO_2) above 70, a partial pressure of carbon dioxide (PCO_2) between 35 and 45, or a pH between 7.35 and 7.45, continued support and observation are indicated while HbCO measurement results are pending. If HbCO is below 5%, the patient should be considered for discharge. If HbCO is between 5% and 10%, continued support and observation with administration of 100% oxygen and a second HbCO determination in 2 hours are suggested. If the HbCO level is then below 5%, discharge is considered. No further ancillary testing is performed in this group.

If history and clinical findings indicate moderate exposure, the observation and support period is longer and diagnostic studies are more extensive than in the minimal-exposure group. Increased respiratory effort, reflected by dyspnea, use of accessory muscles of respiration, hoarseness, or wheezes on physical examination, mandate the use of supplemental oxygen. Measurement of arterial blood gases and of HbCO level and baseline chest radiography are performed. Blood gas results showing a PO_2 below 70, PCO_2 below 30, and pH above 7.35 classify the patient as one who may soon improve and be discharged or may worsen and require admission. If a firefighter is kept in the hospital for observation, the physician should also be vigilant for delayed presentation of pulmonary edema and laryngeal or tracheal edema.

HbCO levels between 10% and 20% also place the patient in the moderate-exposure category. Oxygen therapy should

Table 41-3. FEMA algorithm for emergency evaluation of persons exposed to fires and smoke

Observation of chief complaint				
Asymptomatic		Moderate dyspnea		Hypoventilation apnea
Consider oxygen		Oxygen		100% oxygen and respiratory support
Physical examination				
Consider arterial blood gases		Do arterial blood gas and carboxyhemoglobin		Do arterial blood gas and carboxyhemoglobin
PE normal		PE→hoarseness/wheezes		Cyanosis, ronchi, rales
Provide any other necessary support		Continue oxygen		100% oxygen and respiratory support
Observe		Chest x-ray		Chest x-ray
Results of arterial blood gases				
PO_2 <70		PO_2 <70		PO_2 <60
PCO_2 35–45		PCO_2 <30		PCO_2 <45
pH 7.35–7.45		pH <7.35		pH <7.35
Support and observe		Continue oxygen		100% oxygen and respiratory support
		Await HbCO and x-ray		Evaluate acidosis
Carboxyhemoglobin				
HbCo <5%	HbCo 5%–10%	HbCO 10%–20%	HbCO > 20%–40%	HbCO > 40%
Support and observe	Oxygen	100% oxygen	100% oxygen	Consider hyperbaric oxygen
Observe	Repeat HbCO	Repeat HbCO	Repeat HbCO	Repeat HbCO
Discharge when stable				
Chest x-ray results				
	Normal	Abnormal	Pulmonary edema	Pulmonary edema and persistent acidosis
	Discharge when stable	Continue support	100% oxygen PEEP	Consider CN kit
		Reevaluate	Admit	Admit

From Gochfeld M, Szenics J: *Guidelines for the emergency management of firefighters,* Trenton, 1992, New Jersey Department of Health.
PE, physical examination; *PEEP,* positive end-expiratory pressure; *CN,* Cyanide. HbCO Carboxyhemoglobin.

be administered, and HbCO measurement repeated in 2 hours. Continued elevation of the HbCO level calls for maintenance of support and possible admission. A second chest radiograph may be helpful in this regard, because developing pulmonary edema may interfere with clearance of carbon monoxide. Individuals with severe exposure as denoted by history, physical examination, and laboratory findings are strong candidates for hospital admission. Physical findings such as cyanosis, rhonchi, and rales, and arterial blood gas measurements showing a PO_2 below 60, PCO_2 above 45, pH below 7.35, or HbCO above 20% argue strongly for such respiratory support. If HbCO exceeds 40%, hyperbaric oxygen therapy should be considered to prevent permanent neurologic damage.[41,55,56] Patients whose chest radiographs show pulmonary edema should be considered for positive end-expiratory pressure treatment.

Patients who fall into the moderate or severe exposure categories are likely to experience abnormalities of multiple organ systems; hence, early attention to renal function, hydration status, potential for development of stress ulceration of the gastrointestinal tract, and so on is indicated.

REFERENCES

1. Brandt-Rauf PW et al: Health hazards of firefighters: exposure assessment, *Br J Ind Med,*
2. Bronstein A, Currance P: *Emergency care for hazardous materials exposure,* St Louis, 1988, CV Mosby.
3. Burgess WA, Treitman RD, Gold A: Air contaminants in structural firefighting, NFPCA Grant 7X008, Boston, 1979, National Fire Prevention and Control Administration.
4. Cohen MA, Guzzardi LI: Inhalation of products of combustion, *Ann Emerg Med* 12:628, 1983.
5. Cook C, Cone M: Deadly smoke, *Santa Ana (Calif) Register* December, 1983.
6. Crapo RO: Smoke-inhalation injuries, *JAMA* 246:1694, 1981.
7. Davis PO et al: Relationship between simulated fire fighting tasks and physical performance measures, *Med Sci Sports Exerc* 14:65, 1982.
8. Dyer RF, Esch VH: Hydrogen chloride toxicity in fires, *JAMA* 235:393, 1976.
9. Edlich RF: Early respiratory insufficiency in the burn patient, *Current Concepts in Trauma Care.* Spring 1979, pp 15-18
10. Favata E, Buckler G, Gochfeld M: Heat stress in hazardous waste workers: evaluation and prevention, *State-of-the-Art Reviews in Occupational Medicine* 5:79, 1990.
11. Federal Emergency Management Agency: *Highlights of fire in the United States,* Washington, DC, 1980, US Department of Commerce, Federal Emergency Management Agency, US Fire Administration.

12. Federal Emergency Management Agency: *The medical management of victims of smoke and toxic gas inhalation,* FA-79, Washington, DC, 1988, US Chamber of Commerce, Federal Emergency Management Agency, US Fire Administration.
13. Feuer E, Rosenman K: Mortality in police and fire-fighters in New Jersey, *Am J Ind Med* 9:517.
14. Froines JR et al: Exposure of firefighters to diesel emissions in fire stations, *Am Ind Hyg Assoc J* 48:202, 1987.
15. Gochfeld M, Szenics J: *Guidelines for the emergency management of firefighters,* Trenton, 1992, New Jersey Department of Health.
16. Gold A, Burgess WA, Clougherty EV: Exposure of firefighters to toxic air contaminants, *Am Ind Hyg Assoc J* 39:534, 1978.
17. Grand AF, Kaplan HL, Lee GH III: Investigation of combustion atmosphere in real building fires: final report to Society of the Plastics Industry, New York, and US Fire Administration, 1981.
18. Herman GD: Myonecrosis in carbon monoxide poisoning, *Vet Hum Toxicol* 20:28, 1988.
19. International Association of Fire Fighters: *Annual death and injury survey,* Washington, DC, 1980, The Association.
20. International Association of Fire Fighters Department of Health: *Occupational cancer and the firefighter,* Washington, DC, 1982, The Association.
21. International Association of Fire Fighters: *1982 annual death and injury survey,* Washington, DC, 1983, The Association.
22. Ives JM, Hughes E, Taylor JK: Toxic atmospheres associated with real fire situations, NVS 10-807, 1972. Washington, DC, US Department of Commerce, National Bureau of Standards. US Department of Commerce, National Bureau of Standards.
23. Kilbom A: Physical work capacity of firemen with special reference to demands during firefighting, *Scand J Work Environ Health* 6:48, 1980.
24. Lemon PW, Hermiston RT: The human energy cost of fire fighting, *J Occup Med* 19:558, 1977.
25. Manning JE, Griggs TR: Heart rate in fire fighters using light and heavy breathing equipment: simulated near-maximal exertion in response to multiple work load conditions, *J Occup Med* 25:215, 1983.
26. Melius JM: Fire fighters. In Zenz C, ed: *Occupational medicine,* ed 2, Chicago, Ill, 1988, Year Book.
27. Mills J, ed: *Current emergency diagnosis and treatment,* Los Altos, Calif, 1983, Lange.
28. National Academy of Science: *Carbon Monoxide,* Washinton, DC, 1977, Committee on Medical and Biological Effects of Environmental Pollutants, National Academy of Science.
29. National Institute for Occupational Safety and Health: *Occupational diseases: a guide to their recognition,* Washington, DC, 1977.
30. National Institute for Occupational Safety and Health: *Health hazard evaluation report: chemical control facility, Elizabeth, New Jersey,* HETA 80-118. 1980.
31. National Institute for Occupational Safety and Health: *Health hazard evaluation report: Federated Fire Fighters of Nevada,* HETA 81-137-990, 1981, Cincinnati.
32. National Institute for Occupational Safety and Health: *Formaldehyde evidence of carcinogenicity,* Current Intelligence Bulletin 34, 1981.
33. National Institute for Occupational Safety and Health: *Health hazard evaluation report: International Association of Firefighters, New Jersey,* HETA 82-319-1569, 1982, Cincinnati.
34. National Institute for Occupational Safety and Health: *Health hazard evaluation report: Fire Department, Houston, Texas,* HETA 82-114-1097, 1982, Cincinnati.
35. National Institute for Occupational Safety and Health: *Health hazard evaluation report: Fire Department, Stamford, Connecticut,* HETA 83-157-1373, 1983.
36. National Institute for Occupational Safety and Health: *Health hazard evaluation report: Chester Fire Department, Chester, Pennsylvania,* HETA 83-360-1495, 1984.
37. National Institute for Occupational Safety and Health: *Carcinogenic effects of exposure to diesel exhaust,* Current Intelligence Bulletin 50, Atlanta, 1988.
38. National Institute for Occupational Safety and Health, Occupational Safety and Health Administration: *Pocket guide to chemical hazards,* Washington, DC, 1980, US Government Printing Office.
39. New Jersey Department of Health: *Firefighting in New Jersey: hazards and methods of control,* Trenton, 1982.
40. Papanek P Jr: *Hazardous materials medical management protocols,* Los Angeles, 1989, California Emergency Medical Services Authority and the Toxics Epidemiology Program, Los Angeles County Department of Health Services.
41. Peirce EC et al: A registry for carbon monoxide poisoning in New York city, *J Toxicol Clin Toxicol* 26:419, 1988.
42. Peters JM et al: Chronic effect of firefighting on pulmonary function, *N Engl J Med* 291:1320, 1974.
43. Proctor NH, Hughes JP: *Chemical hazards of the workplace,* Philadelphia. 1978, JB Lippincott.
44. Rosen P, ed: *Emergency medicine: concepts and clinical practice,* St Louis, 1983, Mosby.
45. Rubin P: Careers in ashes. Phoenix *New Times.* 1988.
46. Sidor R, Peters JM: Firefighting and pulmonary function, *Am Rev Respir Dis* 109:249, 1974.
47. Stutz DR et al: *Hazardous materials injuries: a handbook for prehospital care,* Beltsville, Md, 1982, Bradford Communications.
48. Terrill JB et al: Toxic gases from fires, *Science* 200:1343, 1978.
49. Tintinalli JE, ed: *Emergency medicine: a comprehensive study guide,* ed 2, New York, 1988, McGraw-Hill.
50. Treitman RD, Burgess WA, Gold A: Air contaminants encountered by firefighters, *Am Ind Hyg Assoc J* 41:796, 1980.
51. Unger KM et al: Smoke inhalation in firemen, *Thorax* 35:838, 1980.
52. US Department of Energy: *Firemen: emergency handling of radiation accident cases,* DOE/EV-0023, Washington, DC, 1979.
53. Walt AJ: *Early care of the injured patient,* ed 3, Philadelphia, 1982, WB Saunders.
54. Washburn AE, Harlow DW, Horn S: United States fire fighter deaths in the line of duty during 1979: National Fire Protection Association, *Fire Command* 47:30, 1980.
55. Welch GW et al: The use of steroids in inhalation injury, *Surg Gynecol Obstet* 45:539, 1977.
56. Wilkins EW, ed: *Emergency medicine: scientific foundations and current practice,* ed 3, Baltimore, 1989, Williams & Wilkins.
57. Wynder EL, Hoffmann D: Tobacco and health: a societal challenge, *N Engl J Med* 300:894, 1979.

Chapter 42

WATER POLLUTION

Joseph P. Brown
Richard J. Jackson

Regulatory programs and standards
The water standard development process
Technical issues
    Noncancer versus cancer endpoints
    Multiroute exposures for volatile organics
    Risk-management issues
    Perspective
Toxicants in water
    Arsenic
    Radon
    Asbestos-cement pipe
    Nitrate and nitrite
    Chloroform and disinfection by-products

Contamination of drinking water with toxic chemicals has become widely recognized as a public health concern since the discovery of 1,2-dibromo-3-chloropropane (DBCP) in drinking water in California's Central Valley and solvents in water in New Jersey in 1979. Increased monitoring since then has shown that many other pesticides and industrial chemicals can be detected in drinking water. Contaminants of drinking water also include naturally occurring substances such as asbestos, arsenic, selenium, and radionuclides such as radium, radon, and uranium. Disinfection by-products, formed when chlorine reacts with trace organics in water, including chloroform, other trihalomethanes, and haloacetic acids, are also of concern. Public water systems and commercially bottled and vended water must meet the same state and federal standards with regard to toxic contaminants, and California has taken measures to prevent future water pollution problems through a variety of new statutes, regulations, and programs.

The vulnerability of the groundwater to chemical contamination with pesticides was most dramatically revealed by the 1979 discovery of DBCP in the Central Valley of California. Like other soil fumigants, DBCP was injected into the soil to kill nematodes. Since 1955 about 1.4 million kg (3 million lb) DBCP was applied annually in California before its use was suspended in 1977 after findings of sterility and reduced sperm counts in male workers at a Central Valley formulating plant.

In California approximately 2500 wells were found to be contaminated with DBCP; more than half of these wells were made unusable as drinking-water sources, because DBCP concentrations exceeded the state health advisory guideline (action level) of 1 part per billion (ppb). The state promulgated a more stringent enforcement level (maximum contaminant level [MCL]) of 0.2 ppb, which was subsequently supported by a federal primary standard at the same level. Several Central Valley water utilities have introduced specialized water treatment to meet this new standard. Recently, the city of Sanger settled an important lawsuit with a number of DBCP manufacturers under which the latter will pay for a portion of the water-treatment costs. It has been estimated that more than 200,000 people are exposed to DBCP levels between 0.05 and 0.2 ppb. DBCP has also been found in wells in Arizona, South Carolina, Maryland, and Hawaii. Its widespread occurrence and persistence in groundwater (one study estimates its half-life in soil at 141 years[7]) underscore the need for pollution prevention rather than cleanup. A similar story involved aldicarb (Temik) contamination of groundwater on Long Island, New York.

Monitoring for pesticides and industrial chemicals in drinking water has greatly increased in California since 1979. The California State Water Resources Control Board has verified 441 cases of groundwater contamination by 54 different pesticides in 28 counties, not including the DBCP cases.[13] Many of these incidents may have come from spills or improper disposal of pesticides rather than from agricultural use.

The results from the sampling of approximately 3000 wells of large public water systems for organic contaminants under California's AB1803 program show that 18.3% of the wells had some contamination and 5.6% exceeded one or more state standards.[8] About 41% of the contaminated wells were in Los Angeles County, which indicates that industrial sources such as leaking storage tanks, improper holding ponds, leaking sewers, and even parking-lot runoff are significant sources of contaminants.

A subsequent sampling of approximately 4500 small water system wells between 1985 and 1989 revealed that 7.9% showed some contamination, with 3.1% exceeding one of the state MCLs and 2.1% exceeding one of the state's action levels.[9] Of some 263 chemicals analyzed, 46 were found to contaminate small public water system wells. The most frequent contaminants were DBCP, perchlorethylene (PCE), and chloroform. DBCP was the most common contaminant, found in 11% of 1082 wells sampled.

Finally, the 1992 Well Inventory Database, covering the years 1986 through 1992, reports on 260,693 analyses of well water from 17,713 wells taken during 251 separate groundwater monitoring surveys under California's AB2021 (Pesticide Contamination Prevention Act). Sixty-eight pesticides were detected and 36 confirmed in 3697 wells in 44 counties.[11] Twenty-five pesticides (see box) were found in concentrations in excess of MCLs or other standards such as state action levels or U.S. Environmental Protection Agency (EPA) lifetime health advisories.

In 1978 the New Jersey Department of Environmental Protection published a report on its groundwater survey of 500 wells.[6] Overall water quality exceeded the federal drinking water standards, but almost all wells contained traces of organics; pesticides were detected mainly in agricultural areas, and organic chemicals, mainly in industrialized urban areas. Statewide, 6% of wells exceeded the standards for one or more chemicals.

Asbestos from asbestos-cement pipe has also been a concern; however, an epidemiologic study in Connecticut did not find a relationship between the use of asbestos-cement pipe and the occurrence of intestinal cancer.[24]

REGULATORY PROGRAMS AND STANDARDS

The history of federal legislation protecting water dates to the Rivers and Harbors Act of 1899, prohibiting the discharge of refuse into navigable waterways. It was followed by the Federal Water Pollution Control Act of 1948, which with subsequent amendments became the Clean Water Act. The Clean Water Act is one of the major enabling laws for the U.S. EPA, requiring it to ensure compliance with permit programs and authorizing it to inspect and monitor facilities and to seek both civil and criminal penalties. Central to the act is the prohibition against discharge of any pollutant into a navigable waterway without a permit. The act covers point sources, such as sewage-treatment facilities and factories, and the handling of dredged material from adjacent waters. Many specific provisions of the act differentially affect existing and proposed facilities, imposing harsher standards on the latter. A major breakthrough was the requirement that industries discharging pollutants to a publicly owned treatment works must provide pretreatment to minimize water degradation at the point of ultimate discharge.

The thrust of the Safe Drinking Water Act of 1974 is quite different. It aimed at ensuring that public water supplies were safe and that valuable aquifers are protected. This act protects not only surface waters but also groundwater, regulating underground discharge of contaminants. During the Reagan administration the EPA repeatedly needed to provide evidence to the Office of Management and Budget that federal protection of drinking water quality was required.

Under the authority of the Safe Drinking Water Act (PL 93-523), the EPA has had national authority since 1974 over drinking water quality and the regulation of public drinking-water systems, but states may create and administer their own safe drinking-water programs if they meet minimal EPA standards. The California Safe Drinking Water Act states that water delivered by public water systems in the state shall "be at all times pure, wholesome, and potable."[12]

To ensure drinking water quality, the EPA or the states set standards for contaminants in drinking water, called MCLs. These standards were set to protect public health while taking into account the economic costs and technologic feasibility of treatment or removal of the contaminants. MCLs are divided into two categories: primary, for chemicals that have adverse health effects, and secondary, for those that have mainly undesirable aesthetic effects, that is, in the taste, odor, and appearance of the water. MCLs are legally enforceable standards. The EPA has established relatively few MCLs in the past. Until the mid 1980s, primary MCLs covered only 10 inorganic and 7 organic chemicals

---

Pesticides detected in well water at excessive concentrations[11]

Alachlor	Dieldrin
Aldicarb	Dinoseb
Aldicarb sulfone	Endothall
Aldicarb sulfoxide	EDB
Aldrin	1,1,2,2,-TCA
Atrazine	Heptachlor
Ethylene dichloride	Lindane
Bentazon	Molinate
Chlordane	Naphthalene
1,2-D	Simazine
DBCP	Telone
DDD	Toxaphene
Diazinon	

and radionuclides. Because of delays at the federal level and unique water contamination issues in California, the California Department of Health Services (CDHS) has set 36 MCLs for California over the past 4 to 6 years. Since 1991 the EPA has remarkably increased the number of standards issued, currently at 86. The states are required to adopt federal standards, set more stringent state standards, or obtain an exemption based on low vulnerability of state water systems to a particular pesticide or other contaminant.

When contaminants without MCLs are detected in drinking-water supplies, the EPA and some states develop nonenforceable health advisory guidelines (called action levels in California). The guidelines help distinguish between hazardous and nonhazardous exposures and prompt water utilities to notify customers and to take corrective measures when action levels are exceeded. Although public notification of action-level excesses formerly were voluntary, the CDHS now requires large water suppliers to notify customers whenever action levels or MCLs are exceeded. California legislation (AB 1803) requires water suppliers to monitor wells for all chemicals that are used in the area of the aquifer rather than just for chemicals with MCLs, as was previously required. The California Office of Environmental Health Hazard Assessment (OEHHA) also develops action levels for new contaminants detected in drinking water systems and evaluates health effects of contaminants found in private wells.

Chemicals recently evaluated in this regard include Freon 12, methyl *tert*-butyl ether, methyl chloride, tetrachloroterephthalate, metam sodium, and methyl isothiocyanate. In 1989 the California legislature passed the Safe Drinking Water Act of 1989 (AB21). This bill revamps the state's drinking-water program and most significantly provides for the active improvement of drinking-water quality. In addition to requiring periodic review of MCLs, the law requires the establishment of recommended public health levels (RPHLs), which are wholly health-based standards analagous to the EPA's maximum contamination level goals (MCLGs) and the state's action levels. In addition to meeting MCLs for chemical contaminants, water suppliers with more than 10,000 service connections are required to improve water quality to the RPHL or reporting values if economically and technically feasible.

THE WATER STANDARD DEVELOPMENT PROCESS

The development of California RPHL/MCL standards parallels the federal process; beginning with an in-depth review and analysis of the best available data on the toxicology, metabolism, human exposure, and related information. The work is conducted by OEHHA staff, in-house consultants, and contractors in the state's university system and federal national laboratories. Staff of the University of California, Davis, and the Lawrence Livermore National Laboratory have been involved with about one third of the health risk assessments conducted during the past few years. Comprehensive risk assessment documents on individual chemicals that are produced through contract are subjected to two external peer reviews by independent experts. On the basis of peer-review contracted or internally generated risk assessments, the OEHHA staff prepares a summary document that includes a rationale for and calculation of a water concentration at which no adverse health effects are expected. Previously, this was a concentration known internally as a proposed maximum contaminant level, but in future it will be called an RPHL.

The CDHS Office of Drinking Water staff performs a technical-feasibility and economic analysis based on the OEHHA document and prepares a regulatory document proposing an MCL and RPHL. The regulatory document is released for public comment, and a public hearing is held. DHS/OEHHA staff respond to public comments and revise the regulation and numerical values as necessary. The Office of Administrative Law reviews the statutory authority, format, completeness of responses to comments, and other issues as necessary. If all is in order, the regulation is sent to the secretary of state for promulgation. The new MCL (and RPHL) values would appear in subsequent versions of Title 22, California Code of Regulations (Article 4, Section 64435). The process can take 1.5 to 3 years to complete. Recent proposals within OEHHA to enhance peer review of all scientific and regulatory products may affect this process.

TECHNICAL ISSUES
Noncancer versus cancer endpoints

To establish standards, toxicologists consider the data on acute and chronic effects, neurotoxicity, teratogenicity, mutagenicity, and carcinogenicity. With noncarcinogenic contaminants, scientists often recommend that the standard be set at a level 100, 1000, or even 10,000 times below the no-observed-adverse-effect level (NOAEL) determined from experiments in animals. These values are called safety factors or uncertainty factors (see Chapter 3). These uncertainty factors reflect differences in toxic response between animal species and humans and differences in individual susceptibility in humans. It may be increased when there are inadequacies in the available toxicologic data, such as when the NOAEL has not been determined or when the study is too brief to detect long-term effects. Exceeding an RPHL or action level indicates an encroachment into the margin of safety but does not necessarily indicate an endangerment of public health.

Because of the nature of the carcinogenic process, however, NOAELs are generally nonexistent. Carcinogenesis is believed in most cases to involve the interaction of a carcinogen with deoxyibonucleic acid (DNA) or other target marcomolecules, and cancer can ensue from this interaction even within a single cell.[23,43] Regulatory agencies therefore generally consider carcinogenesis to be essentially a nonthreshold process.

Mathematical models (such as the linearized multistage model) are used to assess cancer risks. Because only 50 or fewer treated animals per dose are usually used in cancer bioassay experiments, the doses must be high enough to produce statistically meaningful results but not so great as to produce serious adverse effects other than tumors. From the data points at the high experimental doses, a curve is extrapolated downward to estimate the effects that would occur at the very low doses found in environmental exposures. Use of high doses to determine effect of chemicals that normally exist at very low levels in the environment is scientifically controversial but, when challenged, has usually been confirmed as representing prudent public health policy.

Whenever feasible, MCL standards and action levels for carcinogens are established as acceptable, or de minimis, risk. The EPA has established the upper limits of acceptable risks between one additional case of cancer in a population of 10,000 to one in 1 million (10^{-4} to 10^{-6}) over a 70-year lifetime.[33] Similarly, the OEHHA considers lifetime extra risks at the one-in-a-million level or below to be negligible. The risk level is intended to be health conservative because it involves involuntary risk. Public health officials believe that although society willingly accepts much higher voluntary risks, it will not tolerate similar risks for someone else's economic benefit.

One risk assessment study of the drinking water in 25 cities has noted that contaminants in drinking water are usually present in mixtures and that the aggregate risks from these mixtures in most of the cities studied "are comparable to other risks that society puts up with but tries to control."[18] In drinking water found to have a high aggregate risk, such as 2.5 persons per 1000, most of the risk was due to the presence of the by-products of chlorination. (See discussion of trihalomethanes below.)

Multiroute exposures for volatile organics

Human exposure to volatile compounds in water can occur by routes other than direct ingestion. They include inhalation of contaminants transferred to the air from showers, baths, toilets, dishwashers, washing machines, and stoves and dermal absorption of contaminants while washing, bathing, and showering.[40]

Showering, for example, creates an aerosol and allows volatile compounds to vaporize into the confined space, resulting in inhalation. A New Jersey community had benzene levels in drinking water as high as 1.5 ppm, resulting in sufficient airborne contamination to produce a cancer risk estimate of 1 in 1000 excess cases.[1]

McKone[31] employed a three-compartment model to simulate the 24-hour concentration profile within showers, bathrooms, and the remaining household volumes of a typical dwelling. The model was used to estimate factors for seven compounds: chloroform, ethylene dibromide, dibromochloropropane, methyl chloroform, perchloethylene, trichloroethylene (TCE), and carbon tetrachloride. Exposure estimates for these compounds indicate that indoor inhalation exposures attributable to contaminated tap water can be between 1.5 and 6.0 (0.8 to 4 for DBCP) times the exposure from ingestion of 2 L/day tap water by a 70-kg adult. More than half of the daily inhalation exposure is projected to occur in the shower stall, with an additional one third in the bathroom. In the case of chloroform exposure via showering, Jo et al.[27,28] have recently shown by breath analysis that a single 10-minute shower resulted in exposure equivalent to drinking 1.4 L water with the same chloroform concentration. These results are in fair agreement with McKone's estimates.

The dermal absorption of VOCs in connection with tap-water exposure has been investigated by Brown et al.[4] On the basis of published skin absorption rates and Fick's law, they determined permeability constants for ethyl benzene, styrene, toluene, and xylene; calculated doses for nine different exposure situations; and compared them to oral doses. They found that skin absorption contributed from 29% to 91% of total dose, averaging 64%. The calculated permeability constants ranged from 0.0006 $L/cm^2/hr$ for stryene to 0.001 $L/cm^2/hr$ for ethylbenzene and toluene (not measured). The 0.001-$L/cm^2/hr$ value has been used as a default assumption in several risk assessments of water pollutants. Recently Bogen et al.[2] measured percutaneous absorption from dilute aqueous solutions of carbon-14–labeled TLE, chloroform, and PCE in sedated, immersed hairless guinea pigs. The permeability constants obtained were approximately 0.0008 $L/cm^2/hr$ for chloroform, 0.001 $L/cm^2/hr$ for TCE, and 0.003 $L/cm^2/hr$ for PCE. These values are quite close to earlier estimates.

Risk-management issues

Cost and technical feasibility are major limitations in control of cancer-causing pollutants at desirable levels. For example, the individual extra lifetime cancer risk due to DBCP exposure at the current MCL of 0.2 ppb is more than 1 in 10,000. The cost of reducing cancer risk further would cost more than $2 million per additional cancer case avoided. Federal and state regulatory actions to control environmental carcinogens usually cost $1 million to $2 million or less per theoretical cancer case avoided. New statutes are designed to push technology so that lower levels of pollutants may be detected and cost-effectively removed when feasible, but this process will take many years to achieve wholly satisfactory results.

Perspective

Drinking-water standards are not set as limits for pollution, that is, as permits for contamination to the stated level. Drinking-water MCLs indicate when contamination levels in drinking water have reached such an unacceptable level that alternate water sources should be considered or the water should be treated further to protect human health. RPHLs and action levels, although health based, do not reflect environmental bioaccumulation in plants and animals, the fate and toxicity of chemical degradation products, or human exposure to the interaction of complex chemical mixtures in various media. Because these standards are developed for individual chemicals, they are not suitable clean-up numbers for mixtures of pollutants, for example, in hazardous waste sites, where other sources of exposure may be significant.

Recently the EPA's Office of Water has issued a public education fact sheet calling attention to threats to drinking-water quality, including new or expanded industrial, commercial, or residential construction; road repairs; pesticides; fertilizers; landfills; and leaking underground storage tanks.[20] Although it calls attention to potential pollution of private drinking wells, it is important to realize that public or commercial water providers also may have contaminated sources.

TOXICANTS IN WATER
Arsenic

Arsenic is found naturally in the environment in both organic and inorganic forms. Arsenate (As +5) is the principal form of inorganic arsenic found in drinking water. Some arsenite (As +3) also is found in drinking water, and these inorganic forms of arsenic are more acutely toxic than organic arsenic compounds. Arsenite is thought to be the principal toxicant in cancer induction, although the mechanism of action is unknown.

Since 1985 new human epidemiologic studies on arsenic have provided persuasive evidence that arsenic in drinking water not only causes skin cancer, which has been known for many years, but also can cause liver and lung cancer and increases the risk of bladder, kidney, and nasal-cavity cancers in both sexes and prostate cancer in males.[15,16] Smith et al,[36,37] in a recent analysis of the human data, estimated that the cancer potency of arsenic, based on skin cancer, was $5.3 \times 10^{-3}/\mu/kg/day$. At a 10^{-6} or negligible lifetime risk this is equivalent to drinking 2 L/day water at 6.2 parts per trillion (0.0062 ppb). Assuming linearity of response, the risk at 50 ppb is about 1%. Comparable risks were estimated for other tumor sites, ranging from 0.2/1000 (liver cancer in males) to 17.2/1000 (lung cancer in females) at 2-L/day intake at the current MCL at 50 µ/L (50 ppb). The sum of all internal tumor sites gives risks of 18.8/1000 and 34.6/1000 for males and females, respectively, and an average risk of 26.8/1000.[35]

At 50 ppb, the lifetime cancer risk of arsenic exposure via drinking water is approximately 1% to 2%, a risk comparable to radon exposure or secondhand cigarette smoke. Most public water systems in California have less than 25 ppb arsenic in their drinking water, and only 15 water systems in six counties have arsenic concentrations above the 50-ppb MCL. These water systems have been unable to meet the arsenic water standard by closing highly contaminated wells and blending water from various wells. Some public water suppliers have installed treatment facilities to reduce arsenic levels to comply with the federal standard, and additional treatment is required to meet more stringent future standards. The reevaluation of arsenic using newly available data on internal cancers will result in a lowering of the federal MCL, closer to the 2-ppb limit of detection. At this level, as many as 300 water systems in California and 13,000 nationally would be noncompliant. OEHHA has already proposed a significantly lower RPHL for inorganic arsenic in drinking water.[5]

Radon

In the indoor environment, exposure to radon can occur by the direct ingestion of drinking water or, more significantly, via inhalation after radon has volatilized from tap water or has seeped into living spaces from soil and bedrock located directly beneath the house's foundation.

The EPA has estimated the relative lung cancer risk from radon from epidemiologic data obtained from groups of smoking underground metal ore miners to be $4.9 \times 10^{-7}/pCi/L_w$ and $1.5 \times 10^{-7}/pCi/L_w$, via the inhalation and ingestion routes, respectively.[41] In 1991 the EPA proposed an MCLG of 0 and an MCL of 300 pCi/L_w for radon and classified it as a group A human carcinogen. Cancer risk from radon shows a strong multiplicative effect with cigarette smoking. The EPA based its 300-pCi/L_w MCL on risk to an average population somewhat between former smokers and light smokers. Risks to nonsmokers are only 20% of the average population risk.[41] The EPA is probably overestimating the risks of lung cancer due to radon exposure in the general population, because smoking is on the decline in many areas.

At present radon in homes is estimated to account for as many as 40,000 lung cancer deaths annually, but only 1% to 5% of the deaths are attributed to radon in drinking water.[33] Although the EPA is required under the 1986 amendments to the Safe Drinking Water Act to regulate radon and other radionuclides in drinking water, it was not given any legal authority to regulate the much higher risk of radon in indoor air. Water utilities are concerned that the proposed regulation, which will be very expensive to implement, reduces only a minor portion of the overall risks from radon exposure whereas the main risk from radon in homes remains unregulated; however, ingested radon alone represents a higher cancer risk than that of many other regulated organic contaminants in drinking water.

In California radon contamination in groundwater is found in wells adjacent to radon rock formations of granite, sandstone, or feldspar, which commonly occur in the San Joaquin Valley. On the basis of aquifer geology, the greatest potential of radon occurrences in groundwater (1,000 to 10,000 pCi/L_w) are in the counties of Alpine, Amador, Calaveras, El Dorado, Fresno, Kern, Madera, Mariposa, Riverside, San Diego, Tulare, and Tuolumne.[42] Overall, the coastal areas of California contain few locations with elevated radon contamination of groundwater. It is estimated that in California, more than 7000 large and small water systems wells are noncompliant with the proposed 300-pCi/l_w radon rule.[42] At 1000 pCi/L_w, only about 1700 wells (13%) would be noncompliant.

Asbestos-cement pipe

Asbestos-cement was first used for water distribution systems in Europe in the early 1900s, and its use has become widespread. The addition of asbestos fibers to the portland cement mixture was designed to provide a strong, durable conduit, particularly one tolerant of high pressure. Asbestos-cement pipe was first used in the United States in 1930, and an estimated 65 million people may receive water through asbestos-cement pipe. Because it does not rust, asbestos-cement was considered beneficial; however, subsequent research has demonstrated that under certain so-called aggressive water conditions, the calcium carbonate of the cement is dissolved and asbestos fiber may be released. Depending on the manufacturer, asbestos fiber may make up to 10% to 70% of asbestos-cement pipe. Water with a low pH, a low calcium level, and a low level of dissolved solids tends to be aggressive.[37]

Metals in water, such as iron and zinc, can coat the pipe and prevent water from reacting with the cement. Studies in Connecticut revealed that 19 of 149 water samples contained asbestos fibers, from 10,000 fibers/L to 700,000 fibers/L[17]; however, an epidemiologic study in Connecticut did not find a relationship between the use of asbestos-cement pipe and the occurrence of intestinal cancer.[24]

Nitrate and nitrite

Nitrate is a common groundwater contaminant found in many agricultural areas in California. Nitrate is found in groundwater as a result of contamination with nitrogenous fertilizers or organic wastes from humans or animals. The principal health concern for excessive nitrate levels in drinking water is the development of methemoglobinemia in infants. After ingestion, nitrate is converted to nitrite in the gut of the infant. The absorbed nitrite reacts with hemoglobin in the blood, forming methemoglobin, which significantly reduces the oxygen-carrying capacity of the blood, giving rise to a so-called blue baby syndrome. More detailed environmental and toxicologic assessment of nitrate can be obtained from other publications.[21,34]

According to the CDHS more public water supply wells in California have been closed because of violations of the nitrate standard than for any other contaminant or class of contaminants.[38] Monitoring of water supply wells (drinking and irrigation wells) and public drinking water wells for nitrate showed that approximately 10% were found to have levels exceeding the drinking water standard of 10 mg/L nitrate (measured as nitrogen, NO_3-N). Contaminated wells are found in the coastal counties Orange, Los Angeles, San Diego, Ventura, Monterey, Santa Clara, and Contra Costa and in the agricultural zone of the Central Valley stretching from Kern County to Sacramento County. Because the margin of safety of the 10-mg/L standard is slim or nonexistent for infants under 6 months of age, well owners with nitrate problems and infants are strongly advised to use bottled water for infant drinking and formula preparation.

Chloroform and disinfection by-products

One of the great public health breakthroughs was the use of halogens to purify water. Chlorination has been practiced throughout the world, and the incidence of gastrointestinal disease rapidly declines as purification is accomplished; however, use of chlorine products for disinfection relies on the release and killing power of free chlorine, which in turn is free to react with various organic compounds present in the water, producing chlorinated hydrocarbons, many of which are possible or probable human carcinogens.

The National Research Council published an entire volume devoted to disinfection, comparing chlorination with other approaches, including use of activated charcoal and ozonation. Most chemical additives react to produce some unwanted and unhealthful by-products, such as the trihalomethanes. The introduction of a water clarification scheme involving coagulation, sedimentation, and filtration can remove some of the organic precursors with which chlorine reacts. Similarly, granular activated charcoal as the last step in the disinfection process removes many toxic chemicals, including the trihalomethanes.[36]

The primary public health concern with respect to chloroform and other disinfection by-products in drinking water is chronic toxicity, particularly cancer. A number of human epidemiologic studies have identified an association between human consumption of chlorinated drinking water and cancer incidence*; however, after reviewing these and many other data the International Agency for Research on Cancer (IARC) concluded that chlorinated drinking water is ''not classifiable'' (group 3) with respect to human or animal carcinogencity.[26] More recently, results of metanalysis of pooled data from 10 studies on cancer incidence and chlorinated water exposure suggested that as many as 18% of 45,000 cases of rectal cancer and 9% of the annual 51,600 cases of bladder cancer may be attributed to consumption of chlorinated water.[32] Thus the epidemiologic picture with respect to human cancer and chlorinated water is still uncertain.

The trihalomethane chloroform is frequently found in finished drinking water. It is readily absorbed after ingestion, inhalation, or dermal exposure and is distributed to all tissues, particularly those with a high lipid content. Chloroform

---

*References 10, 14, 22, 25, 30, 48.

is primarily metabolized to phosgene, which may undergo spontaneous hydrolysis to CO_2 and HCl, or it may react with cellular constituents. Other reactive metabolites such as free radicals may be produced under reductive conditions. Chloroform's ability to cause liver and kidney toxicity depends on its metabolism. Radiolabeled chloroform metabolites have been found to bind to cellular proteins and lipids and, to a lesser extent, to DNA.[10]

Mutagenicity tests of chloroform in bacteria and fungi have largely been negative. A few positive results have been reported for sister chromatic exchange in cultured human lymphocytes and mouse bone marrow cells and in the micronucleus test in mouse bone marrow. Chloroform is a mitotic poison in an invertebrate test system. Although the preponderance of results of genetic toxicity tests on chloroform have been negative to date (for example, results of only 7 of 59 tests were positive or weakly positive in the EPA/IARC Genetic Activity Profile Database), it is not possible to exclude a genotoxic mechanism in the observed carcinogenicity of chloroform in animal bioassays. Chloroform is carcinogenic in rodents, producing liver tumors in both sexes of mice, kidney tubular epithelial tumors in male rats, and chloangiocarcinomas in rats.[10] The quantitative risk estimation conducted by CDHS[10] included data from four studies in experimental animals: National Cancer Institute (NCI)[35]; Jorgenson et al[29]; Roe[34]; and Tumasonis.[39] Cancer potency estimates by the linearized multistage model (Global 86) were made from these studies, based on applied and metabolized (pharmocokinetic) doses. The oral potency values ranged from 4.7×10^{-3} to 0.167 $(mg/kg/day)^{-1}$ for metabolized doses and from 4.3×10^{-3} to 0.14 $(mg/kg/day)^{-1}$ for applied doses.[10] The CDHS scientists who reviewed these study data and potency values concluded that the studies by the NCI and Jorgenson et al were the more reliable and that the four potency values (metabolized and applied) for renal tubular adenoma and carcinoma in male rats from these studies should be combined with geometric mean of the potency values for the Roe and Tumasonis studies (renal adenoma or hypernephroma in male mice and hepatic cholangiocarcinomas in male and female rats, respectively). The arithmetic mean of these six values (three metabolized dose and three applied dose estimates) gave the best estimate of the oral potency, or slope factor: 0.031 $(mg/kg/day)^{-1}$.[10] Based on this potency, a negligible-risk water concentration for 2-L/d ingestion would be about 1.0 ppb. The EPA's estimate of negligible risk based solely on data from the study by Jorgenson et al[29] data is 6.0 ppb.

Recently published bioassay data from Dunnick and Melnick[19] for male rat kidney tumors induced by chloroform administered in oil gavage[35] similarly indicate an average slope factor of 0.028/mg/kg/day.

The cancer potency for the trihalomethane bromodichloromethane (BDCM, $CHBrCl_2$) was calculated based on a National Toxicology Program (NTP) animal bioassay. In this study, 50 $B_6C_3F_1$ mice or F344/N rats of each sex were treated with BDCM in corn oil by gavage 5 days per week for 102 weeks. Treatment-related increases of tumor were observed in the large intestine and kidney in rats and in the kidneys and liver in mice.

In rats tumor incidence of adenomatous polyps or adenocarcinomas in the large intestine were 0/50, 13/50, and 45/50 in males and 0/46, 0/50, and 12/47 in females at doses of 0, 50, or 100 mg/kg/day (time-weighted average [TWA] doses 0, 35.7, or 71.4 mg/kg/day), respectively. The incidences of tubular cell adenoma or adenocarcinoma in the kidney were 0/50, 1/50, and 13/50 in males and 0/50, 1/50, and 15/50 in females at doses of 0, 50, or 100 mg/kg/day, respectively.

In mice, tumors were observed in the kidney in males and in the liver in females. The incidences of kidney tubular cell adenomas or adenocarcinomas were 1/49, 2/50, and 9/50 at 1, 25, and 50 mg/kg/day (TWA doses 0, 17.9 or 35.7 mg/kg/day) respectively. The incidences of liver hepatocellular adenoma or carcinoma were 3/50, 18/48, and 29/50 at 0, 75, and 150 mg/kg/day (TWA doses 0, 53.6, or 107.1 mg/kg/day), respectively.

Because tumors in the large intestine are rare in F344/N rats, tumor incidences of adenomatous polyps or adenocarcinomas in male rats were used for the calculation of a BDCM cancer potency. With use of the linearized multistage model, the upper-bound animal cancer potency was calculated to be 2.85×10^{-2} $(mg/kg/day)^{-1}$, which was rounded off to 0.03 $(mg/kg/day)^{-1}$. A negligible-risk water concentration based on a 70-kg adult drinking 2 L water per day can be calculated as 0.9 ppb, which could be rounded to 1.0 ppb.

The cancer potency of chlordibromomethane (CDBM, $CHBr_2Cl$) was calculated based on an NTP animal bioassay.[38] In this study, 50 $B_6C_3F_1$ mice or F344/N rats of each sex were treated with CDBM in corn oil by gavage 5 days per week for 104 weeks. No increase of tumors were observed in the rats, but liver tumors were observed in the mice.

The incidences of hepatocellular carcinomas were 10/50, 9/50, and 19/50 in male mice and 4/50, 6/50, and 8/50 in female mice, at doses of 0, 50, or 100 mg/kg/day (TWA doses 0, 35.7, or 71.4 mg/kg/day), respectively. The male and female mice in the low-dose group were accidentally overdosed at week 58. Thirty-five male mice were killed in week 58 to 59, but female mice were not affected. Tumor incidences of the male mice thus was considered by NTP to be inadequate for analysis. With use of tumor incidences in female mice and the linear multistage model, the slope factor was calculated to be 3×10^{-3} $(mg/kg/day)^{-1}$. With use of surface area scaling for interspecies extrapolation, the human slope factor is 0.04 $(mg/kg/day)^{-1}$. At 2-L/day consumption a negligible-risk water concentration of 0.7 ppb can be calculated.

The cancer potency of bromoform (BF, $CHBr_3$) was calculated on the basis of a NTP animal bioassay. In this study,

50 $B_6C_3F_1$ mice and F344/N rats of each sex were treated with BF in corn oil by gavage 5 days per week for 103 weeks. BF was not carcinogenic in the mice, but treatment-related increases of large intestine neoplasma were observed in the rats.

Tumor incidences of adenomatous polyps or adenocarcinomas in the large intestine were 0/50, 0/50, and 3/50 in male rats and 0/50, 1/50, and 8/50 in female rats at doses of 0, 100, or 200 mg/kg/day (TWA doses 0, 71.4, or 142.8 mg/kg/day), respectively. With use of tumor incidence in female rats and the linear multistage model, the animal slope factor was calculated to be 1.15×10^{-3} (mg/kg/day)$^{-1}$. A negligible-risk water concentration of 4 ppb can be calculated.

The present federal MCL for trihalomethanes in finished drinking water is 100 ppb for the sum of all four trihalomethanes compounds. This standard is currently under review by the EPA in a negotiated rule-making process designed to produce a new standard acceptable to all interests. In addition to the trihalomethanes, the process also is evaluating the need for standards on other disinfectants and by-products, including dichloroacetic and trichloroacetic acids, chloral hydrate, bromate, chlorite and chlorate, chlorine dioxide, chloramine, and chlorine. Significantly, a primary standard for source water organic matter (total organic carbon) also is being considered. Because most problems with residual disinfectant by-products result from chlorination of water high in organic matter, it may represent the most cost-effective control measure in many cases.

REFERENCES

1. Bishop BL, Rosenman KD, Patel DB: *An exposure-risk assessment for benzene in shower air,* Trenton, 1984, New Jersey Department of Health.
2. Bogen KT, Colston BW, Machicao LK: Dermal absorption of dilute aqueous chloroform, trichloroethylene, and tetrachloroethylene in hairless guinea pigs, *Fundam Appl Toxicol* 18:30, 1992.
3. Brenniman GR et al: Case-control study of cancer deaths in Illinois communities served by chlorinated or nonchlorinated water. In Jolly R et al, eds: *Water chlorination: environmental impact and health effects,* vol 3, Ann Arbor, 1980, Ann Arbor Science Publishers.
4. Brown HS, Bishop DR, Rowan CA: The role of skin absorption as a route of exposure for volatile organic compounds (VOCs) in drinking water, *Am J Public Health* 74:479, 1984.
5. Brown JP, Fan AM: *Arsenic: recommended public health level for drinking water* (Draft Document), Berkeley, Calif, 1992, Office of Environmental Health Hazard Assessment, California Environmental Protection Agency.
6. Burke TA, Tucker RK: *A preliminary report on the findings of the State Groundwater Monitoring Project,* Trenton, 1978, New Jersey Department of Environmental Protection.
7. Burlison NE, Lee LA, Roseblatt DH: Kinetics and products of hydrolysis of 1,2-dibromochloropropane, *Environ Sci Technol* 16:627, 1982.
8. California Department of Health Services: *Organic chemical contamination of large public water systems in California,* Sacramento, 1986.
9. California Department of Health Services: *Organic chemical contamination of small public water systems in California,* Sacramento, 1990.
10. California Department of Health Services: *Health effects of chloroform,* Berkeley, 1990, Hazard Identification and Risk Assessment Branch, Air Toxicology and Epidemiology Section.
11. California Department of Pesticide Regulation: *Sampling for pesticide residues in California well water: 1992 well inventory data base, Cumulative Report 1986-1992,* Sacramento, 1992.
12. California Safe Drinking Water Act of 1986, California Health and Safety Code, div 5, pt 1, chap 7 s4010.
13. California State Water Resources Control Board: *Water quality and pesticides: a California risk assessment program,* vol 1, Sacramento, 1984.
14. Cantor RP et al: Association of cancer mortality with halomethanes in drinking water, *J Natl Cancer Inst* 61:979, 1978.
15. Chen CJ, Wang CJ: Ecological correlation between arsenic level in well water and age-adjusted mortality from malignant neoplasms, *Cancer Res* 5:5470, 1990.
16. Chen CJ et al: A retrospective study of malignant neoplasms of bladder, lung and liver in Blackfoot disease endemic area in Taiwan, *Br J Cancer* 53:399, 1986.
17. Craun GF, Millette JR: Exposure to asbestos fibers in water distribution systems. In Proceedings of the 97th Annual American Water Works Association, Denver, Col, 1977.
18. Crouch EAC, Wilson R, Zeise L: The risks of drinking water, *Water Resource Res* 19:1359, 1983.
19. Dunnick JK, Melnick RC: Assessment of the carcinogenic potential of chlorinated water: experimental studies of chlorine, chloramine and trihalomethane, *J Natl Cancer Inst* 85:817, 1993.
20. Environmental Protection Agency: Ground water protection: a citizen's action checklist, Public Education Fact Sheet Series, Office of Water, U.S. Environmental Protection Agency, EPA 810-F-92-002, 1992.
21. Fan AM, Willhite CC, Book SA: Evaluation of nitrate drinking water standard with specific references to methemoglobinemia and reproductive toxicity, *Reg Toxicol Pharmacol* 7:135, 1987.
22. Gottlieb MS, Carr JK, Morris DT: Cancer and drinking water in Louisiana: colon and rectum, *Int Epidemiol* 10:117, 1981.
23. *Guidelines for chemical carcinogen risk assessment and their scientific rationale, California Department of Health Services,* Berkeley, 1986, pC-10.
24. Harrington JM et al: An investigation of the use of asbestos cement pipe for public water supply and the incidence of gastrointestinal cancer in Connecticut, 1935-1973. *Am J Epidemiol* 107:96, 1978.
25. Hogan MD et al: Association between chloroform levels in finished drinking water supplies and various site-specific cancer mortality rates, *J Environ Pathol Toxicol* 2:873, 1979.
26. International Agency for Research on Cancer: Chlorinated drinking-water; chlorination by-products; some other halogenated compounds; cobalt and cobalt compounds, In *IARC Monogr Eval Carcinogenic Risks Hum 1991,* vol 52, Lyon, 1991, IARC.
27. Jo WK, Weisel CP, Lioy PJ: Routes of chloroform exposure and body burden from showering with chlorinated tap water, *Risk Anal* 16:575, 1990.
28. Jo WK, Weisel CP, Lioy PJ: Chloroform exposure and the health risk associated with multiple uses of chlorinated tap water, *Risk Anal* 10:581, 1990.
29. Jorgenson TA et al: Carcinogenicity of chloroform in drinking water to male Osborne-Mendel rats and female B6C3F1 mice, *Fund Appl Toxicol* 5:760, 1985.
30. Lynch CF et al: Chlorinated drinking water and bladder cancer: effect of misclassification on risk estimates, *Arch Environ Health* 44:252, 1989.
31. McKone TC: Human exposure to volatile organic compounds in household tap water: the indoor inhalation pathway, *Environ Sci Technol* 21:1194, 1987.
32. Morris RD et al: Chlorination, chlorination by-products and cancer: a meta-analysis, *Am J Public Health* 82:955, 1992.
33. National Academy of Sciences: *Health effects of exposure to low levels of ionizing radiation,* BEIR V, Washington, DC, 1990, National Academy Press.

34. National Academy of Sciences: *Nitrates: an environmental assessment,* Washington, DC, 1978, NAS.
35. National Cancer Institute: *Report on carcinogenesis bioassay of chloroform,* National Cancer Institute Carcinogenesis Program, Bethesda, 1976, The Institute.
36. National Research Council Drinking Water and Health, vol 2, Safe Drinking Water Committee, Washington, DC, 1980, National Academy Press.
37. National Research Council Drinking Water and Health, vol 4, Safe Drinking Water Committee, Washington, DC, 1982, National Academy Press.
38. National Toxicology Program: *Toxicology and carcinogenesis studies of chlorodibromomethane in F344/N rats and $B_6C_3F_1$ mice (gavage studies),* NTP TR 282, US Department of Health and Human Services, Public Health Service, National Institutes of Health, 1985.
39. National Toxicology Program: *Toxicology and carcinogenesis studies of bromodichloromethane in F344/N Rats and $B_6C_3F_1$ mice (gavage studies),* NTP TR 321. US Department of Health and Human Services.
40. National Toxicology Program: *Toxicology and carcinogenesis studies of tribromomethane in F344/N rats and $B_6C_3F_1$ mice (gavage studies),* NTP TR 350. US Department of Health and Human Services.
41. Roe, FJC et al: Safety evaluation of chloroform. I. Long-term studies in mice, *Pathol Toxicol* 21:799, 1979.
42. Sakajii, RH: *Radon in California's groundwater: a Water Quality Survey Assessment.* Office of Drinking Water, California Department of Health Services, Berkeley, Oct. 1991.
43. Smith AH et al: Cancer risks from arsenic, *Environ Health Perspect* 97:259, 1992.
44. Smith AH et al: *Health risk assessment for arsenic,* Berkeley, Calif, 1990, University of California Press.
45. Tumasonis CF et al: Lifetime toxicity of chloroform and bromodichloromethane when administered over a lifetime in rats, *Ecotox Environ Saf* 9:233, 1985.
46. U.S. Environmental Protection Agency: *National Drinking Water Regulations. Radionuclides. Proposed rules, Federal Register* 33050, 1991.
47. Young TR et al: Epidemiologic study of drinking water chlorination and Wisconsin female cancer mortality, *J Natl Cancer Inst* 67:191, 1991.

Chapter 43

FOOD: ITS QUALITY AND ROLE AS A PATHWAY OF EXPOSURE

James Craner

Diet as a vector of contaminants
Heavy metals
   Routes of metal contamination of foods
   Dietary sources of toxic heavy metals
   Arsenic
Organics
   Polychlorinated biphenyls (PCBs)
   Polybrominated biphenyls (PBBs)
   Polychlorinated dibenzodioxins (PCDDs)
Pesticides
   Measurement of residues
   Regulatory issues
   Consumer choices: alternatives or reassurance?
   Clinical evaluation for pesticides
Food preparation and cooking
Food additives
   Regulation
   Color additives
   Food preservatives
   Ethylene dibromide
   Fat and sugar substitutes
   Food additives and hyperactivity in children
   Summary of relative risks of food additives
Packaging
   Food storage principles and safety issues
   Plastics
   Metals
   Paper
Nutrition and factory farming
   Animal health products
   Entry of animal drugs into human food supply
Food irradiation
   Process history and development
   Purpose
   Description of irradiation process
   Toxicologic aspects
   Regulation
   Public concerns/barriers to widespread acceptance
Genetic engineering
   Scope
   Safety concerns and regulation
Conclusion

The tremendous growth in agricultural output in industrialized nations since the end of World War II has produced a food supply that potentially offers the widest availability, highest quality, and greatest safety. However, while the use of pesticides, food preservatives, packaging, and methods of monoculture agriculture and intensive animal "farming" have all contributed to the success of the food industry, they also introduce certain risks. Consumers have become so accustomed to having access to fresh, safe, affordable, perfect-appearing food year-round that they unrealistically have come to expect food to be risk-free (see box).[82]

Over the same period the dramatic rise of chemical manufacturing has exponentially increased various forms of pollution, which directly affects the safety of the food supply, and food is one of the major environmental media to which we are exposed. In many documented cases, human and ecological damage, some of it irreversible, has occurred as a result of pollution induced food contamination. As scientific and epidemiologic information accumulates, our society is questioning to what degree these technologies and by-products contribute to the steadily rising incidence rates of certain

Proximate and ultimate sources of food contamination

Proximate sources

Agriculture, mariculture, livestock
  -Bioaccumulation or other contamination of raw ingredients
  -Pesticide residues
  -Agricultural waste runoff
Food processing
  -Cooking utensils
  -Manufacturing equipment/conditions
  -Food additives
Packaging and storage
  -Aluminum
  -Plastics

Ultimate sources

Agriculture, mariculture
  -Pesticides
  -Fertilizers
  -Drugs/other chemicals
Industrial waste
Sludge/sewage treatment
Mining

---

cancers, chronic disease, birth defects, and other health problems for which the etiology is not well understood. New food processing technologies, such as genetic engineering and food irradiation, are thus being scrutinized intensely by the public and by regulatory officials and lawmakers.

A tremendous amount of research has been published in many areas of medicine and food science on both intentional and unintentional contaminants in food. This chapter summarizes the most important clinical topics of food safety as they relate to environmental medicine. It provides the clinician with a base of information to answer cogently and credibly such commonly asked questions from individual patients or groups as "Should I eat organic food?" or "Will plastic containers, or pesticides, or food irradiation, increase my risk of cancer?" Traditional food-related public health issues of microbes and diseases, basic nutrition, and drinking water quality are not covered here. (The subject of natural anticarcinogens and carcinogens in food is covered in Chapter 44.)

Clinicians find it difficult to advise patients about the potential health risks of various environmental exposures, including food quality and contamination. Consumers receive conflicting messages about health and food safety from many sources with divergent agendas. The media, consumers, and public interest organizations have increased public awareness of the potential adverse effects of environmental contamination in food, but their information may not be sufficiently objective or comprehensive for individual consumers to make informed choices. The industries that produce and distribute food products have a vested economic interest in ensuring that their products are safe, yet their credibility continues to be challenged by sporadic episodes of food contamination, questions of food safety, and sometimes questionable advertising practices. Caught in between are the government regulatory agencies who are responsible for enforcing in the food industry the laws that protect public health and the environment. The public tends to list pesticide residues in food as the main problem, followed by hormone residues, food irradiation, and food additives and preservatives.[46,82]

The diet in industrialized nations has changed drastically in the past 100 years and is associated with a significant shift in the patterns of disease. Infectious diseases and nutritional deficiencies, which accounted for most of the mortality and shorter life expectancy until the end of World War II, have been supplanted by the implementation of public sanitation measures, the rise of an abundant food supply, and the discovery of vitamins and antibiotics. Coronary artery disease, certain major cancers, stroke, hypertension, obesity, diabetes, diverticulosis, and several other chronic diseases caused by or strongly associated with a high-fat, animal-based diet (plus other unhealthy life-style behaviors, such as cigarette smoking, lack of exercise, and excessive alcohol consumption) have become the principal causes of morbidity and mortality in Western nations.[44] Modern medical practice is oriented toward *treating the symptoms* of these life-style–induced, *preventable* diseases. Although ample medical evidence points to *voluntary,* unhealthy behaviors as the leading risk factor for these major diseases, the public often perceives risk from *uncontrollable* factors, such as pesticide residues or food additives, to be greater.

The challenge to the general physician is to respond to patients' concerns about pollutant exposure in an organized fashion, to ascertain if the exposure really exists, to recognize and estimate other potential routes of exposure, to perform appropriate diagnostic testing and interpret the results in light of the data limitations, and to communicate risks (or absence of risks) effectively.

Physicians should also report potential exposures to local and/or state public health and environmental agencies for follow-up investigation and possible epidemiologic evaluation and should refer cases to appropriately qualified professionals in medicine and other fields for technical support and recommendations for intervention.

DIET AS A VECTOR OF CONTAMINANTS

Detecting and addressing sources of environmentally induced food contamination by heavy metals, as well as organic and inorganic pollutants, chemicals, and pesticides, often require interdisciplinary efforts by professionals from various fields, including agricultural scientists, soil and hydrology engineers and chemists, toxicologists, epidemiologists, and environmental medicine physicians. Physicians need to appreciate that low-level dietary exposures to certain chemicals and metals may not result in the same pathophysiologic manifestations as acute or chronic higher-dose occupational exposures (which typically occur through respiratory and/or dermal routes).

HEAVY METALS

Heavy metal contamination of foods has been a public health problem since humans first began to mine and utilize metals. Certain metals that are essential trace elements, for example, chromium and selenium, are toxic to humans and other living organisms at high concentrations. Some metals (such as lead, cadmium, and mercury) have no beneficial biologic function.

Indeed metals may be present and measurable in body tissues without posing any clinically significant harm. In other situations biologic measurements for certain metals may be inadequate or difficult to interpret, yet if a history of exposure and appropriate correlation with symptoms exists, there may be sufficient justification for medical intervention. For many metals, however, the human health implications of low-level, subclinical exposures remain unknown.

This section will provide an overview of several environmentally important toxic metals that enter the food supply (see box). Mercury contamination of fish is explored in depth to underline the complexity that characterizes the chemistry, multiple routes of exposure, metabolism, biologic monitoring, assessment of health effects, and rationale for medical interventions. Detailed discussions of the rationale for specific biologic monitoring and other diagnostic studies for exposure or toxicity from particular metals can be found in the references cited herein.

Routes of metal contamination of foods

Toxic metals are introduced into the environment and subsequently the food or water supply by two major man-made routes: accumulation from point sources of pollution (for example, sewage treatment plants, industrial discharge pipes, leaching from municipal landfills) and nonpoint sources (for example, farmland irrigation and fertilzer, sewage sludge applied as fertilizer, other fertilizer applications, incinerator fly ash.) Subsequent bioamplification through the food chain is important. Some plants are able to accumulate certain elements to high concentrations; for example, certain wild legumes in the Great Plains region of the United States accumulate selenium to levels that are toxic to cattle that graze on these plants.[73] Most plants, however, cannot take up heavy metals in their root systems because these metals damage or kill the plants. The use of municipal sewage sludge as fertilizer for topsoil is an increasingly common practice (for example, New York City sludge shipped to farmers in Texas; see sludge section of Chapter 45) that can introduce high levels of certain metals into the soil, such as boron (from laundry detergent preparations), and lead, cadmium, and mercury discharged from residential and indus-

---

Heavy metals and synthetic organic compounds: Summary of health effects (with examples of human contamination epidemics)

Heavy metals
MERCURY (Hg) (Minimata Disease)
Acute symptoms: Nonspecific paresthesias, anorexia, nausea, diarrhea, irritability, sleep disturbances, personality changes
Long-term health effects: Bilateral constriction of vision, ataxia, tremors, dementia, teratogenic effects, especially psychomotor retardation and other congenital neurologic deformities
Acceptable limits: 30 µg/day (1 ppm in fish)
Clinically significant levels: 200 µg/L
LEAD (Pb)
Acute symptoms: Abdominal colic, constipation, mental confusion, personality changes
Long-term health effects: Arthralgias, neurobehavioral changes, impotence
Measurement: µg/L (water); ppm (air)
Clinically significant levels: >40 µg/dl (blood); >10 µg/dl (pediatric)
CADMIUM (Cd)
Acute symptoms: Bone pain, stress fractures (Itai-Itai disease)
Long-term health effects: Kidney and lung disorders
Safe weekly intake: 0.5 mg
Clinically significant levels: >5 µg/L (blood); >1 µg/g creatinine (urine)

Synthetic organic compounds
POLYCHLORINATED BIPHENYLS (PCBS)
(Araclor, Monsanto: 1930-1977)
Acute symptoms: Chloracne, hyperpigmentation, sensory and motor disturbances, elevated liver enzymes (Yusho disease)
Long-term health effects (possible): Increased risk of hepatic microsomal enzyme induction, increased estrogenic activity, liver cancer, in vitro immunosuppression
Measurement: parts per billion (ppb)
POLYBROMINATED BIPHENYLS (PBBS)
(Firemaster; Nutrimaster)
Acute symptoms: None known
Long-term health effects (possible): Liver function abnormalities, immunosuppression
POLYCHLORINATED DIBENZODIOXINS (CDDs)
(2,3,7,8-TCDD "Dioxin"; 2,4,5-T; 2,4-D; Pentachlorophenol)
Acute symptoms: ??
Long-term health effects: Not known; suspected carcinogen
Measurement: Parts per trillion (ppt)
Average adjusted body burden in fat: 22 ppt

---

trial sources into municipal sewage systems. Synthetic fertilizers may also contain high concentrations of cadmium and lead. Other metals are used as pesticides and include copper sulfate (on grapes and as an algicide), arsenic salts, and organic mercury. However, these uses have been declining as episodes of toxic exposures have increasingly occurred in farmworkers, the general population, and sensitive ecosystems.

Food processing and cooking are other potential contributors to metal contamination of food. Perhaps the most infamous example occurred in ancient Rome, where chronic lead poisoning was caused by leaching of the metal from glazed pottery vessels used to stored wine. Even today, wine stored in leaded glass crystal takes up lead from glass. Stainless steel used in food processing equipment may leach small quantities of copper, nickel, iron, and chromium; the extent of migration depends on the food being processed, temperature, pH, contact time, and especially the grade and quality of the steel. Cast-iron skillets transfer small amounts of iron to food, but not in toxic quantities. While leaching of some metals may go unnoticed in the food, other metals directly affect the color, taste (such as nickel rapidly induces rancidity of fats and spoiling), texture, and/or shelf life, making contamination more obvious.

Dietary sources of toxic heavy metals

Mercury (Hg) contamination of foods represents a significant source of environmental pollution that directly affects human health. Several large-scale human disasters, resulting in many deaths and incapacitating disease, have resulted from mercury contamination of food supplies. Man-made water pollution affecting fish represents the largest source of human mercury exposure from the food supply and ultimately from the environment.[98] In the sediment of lake and sea bottoms metallic mercury and mercuric salts undergo aerobic and anaerobic methylation by microorganisms to form methylmercury cation, CH_3Hg^+. Methylmercury is rapidly absorbed by other aquatic microorganisms and gradually bioaccumulates in the food chain.[67] Fish may also concentrate methylmercury directly from aqueous intake through their gills.[89]

The muscles of large predator fish such as tuna, shark, halibut, and freshwater pike have been found to accumulate organic mercury to levels 3000 to 10,000 times the concentration found in water. Larger, older fish tend to have higher levels of methylmercury in their muscles. Methylmercury's half-life in fish is roughly 2 years, due to slow excretion and continuous absorption. Levels greater than 1.2 mg/kg have been reported in shark, swordfish, pike, tuna (Mediterranean), walleye, and bass.[98] Species such as tuna from polluted waters may contain as much as 10 mg/kg methylmercury in their muscles, in comparison with 0.2 to 1.0 mg/kg typically measured in fish from unpolluted waters, and 0.1 to 0.2 mg/kg is typically found in terrestrial animals (with higher concentrations in organ meats). Industrial water pollution from pulp mills that utilize mercury as a catalyst in the chlorine-bleaching process can cause concentrations of mercury in bottom sediment to increase thirtyfold, though this may not necessarily be reflected in mercury tissue levels of locally caught fish.[67] Chloralkali factories that discharge untreated waste into local waters have also been documented as significant contributors to the mercury burden in fish in Sweden and Canada, while in Australia and New Zealand natural deposits of mercury-laden sediment have been largely responsible.[73] The mercury content (mostly in inorganic form) of vegetables, cereals, and dairy products is typically low (5 to 10 μg/kg), though uptake by plants of mercury can be increased by addition of sewage sludge fertilizer that contains high levels of inorganic mercury.

Humans' absorption of methylmercury from the intestine is highly efficient. Methylmercury enters the bloodstream, where it binds to erythrocytes and then becomes distributed to other tissues. The brain has a particularly high affinity for methylmercury, accumulating it up to six times the concentration of any other tissue.[73] Methylmercury is the most biologically toxic form of mercury to many life forms, particularly mammals, because of its high avidity for sulfhydryl groups of proteins, which disrupts the tertiary structure and function of the proteins. The half-life of methylmercury in humans, approximately 70 days, is relatively long but varies among individuals. Since the primary route of excretion is biliary, urinary mercury is not suitable for monitoring dietary exposure, although it is used to monitor short-term occupational exposures to elemental and ionic forms of mercury. Blood mercury levels (HgB) correlate reasonably well with recent (i.e., within a few days) exposure and total body mercury burden. Dietary intake of 10 to 20 grams/day of fish (the average amount consumed in the United States) significantly affects HgB, and accounts for most of the ''background'' HgB levels of up to 5 μg/L.[98] Since methylmercury is eventually metabolized in the body to mercuric cation, it is slowly excreted in the urine, accounting for ''background'' urine levels in the population. Carefully collected hair mercury levels are a useful measure of past cumulative intake for exposed populations.[66,70] Paresthesias of the extremities and around the tongue and lips are typically the first symptom of methylmercury toxicity, but they may occur only after a significant amount of subclinical, irreversible organ damage has occurred. No biologic markers have been developed to measure early signs of neurologic damage at a potentially reversible stage.

The toxic effects of dietary methylmercury exposure were dramatized by the epidemic known as Minamata disease. Over several years in the mid-1950s in the small villages surrounding Minamata Bay in Japan, over 100 people and many animals, notably cats, developed a debilitating, unusual neurologic disease. Over 50 fatalities were recorded, as well as a significantly increased incidence of congenital neurologic deformities (cerebral palsy, mental retardation). By 1956 epidemiologic studies identified fish caught from the bay as the vector of disease, and an acetaldehyde manufacturing plant discharging effluent into the bay as the source of the fish contamination.[90] Not until 1963, however, was methylmercury identified as the causal agent. Many people continued to consume contaminated fish and develop disease in the interval, despite government advisories, as the pollution continued unabated. Fish and shellfish in the bay had levels as high as 29 mg/kg of methylmercury in their tissues.[73] A similar episode occurred in the 1960s in the coastal village of Niigata, Japan, where industrial water pollution also went unchecked. These episodes were among the first to demonstrate the role of environmental metabolism (inorganic to organic mercury) and bioaccumulation (with methymercury nontoxic to fish but toxic to humans, and cats, when concentrated in the food supply) of a pollutant-causing human health damage.

Several episodes of organomercury poisoning from contaminated grain have occurred. The largest episodes occurred in Iraq in 1960 and again in 1971 when people consumed bread made from grains intended for use as seed that had been treated with phenylmercury fungicide.[7] In the latter episode, over 6000 people were hospitalized for organomercury toxicity; 459 died, and many babies suffered congenital neurotoxicity. Farmers who processed the grain were aware that it had been treated with a potentially poisonous compound, but they wrongly assumed that a superficial washing (which removed the warning dye) and testing for safety by observing no immediate ill effects in farm animals ensured that it was safe. Grain treated with organomercury fungicide fed to pigs resulted in human poisonings after human consumption of the contaminated pork. As a result of these poisonings, organomercury fungicides have been largely replaced by other chemical classes of fungicides in most developed nations.

The disasters due to acute toxicity from high levels of mercury contamination in fish prompted concern in many nations about the long-term toxicity of lower concentrations of methylmercury consumed in the food supply, especially from the regular consumption of fish and other seafood. Extrapolation of human toxicity data from the Japanese and Iraqi poisonings, plus toxicokinetic studies on human volunteers using radiolabeled mercury, has led to estimates that the lowest blood mercury level (HgB) associated with the earliest signs of organomercury toxicity and paresthesias is approximately 200 μg/L, which corresponds to a minimum daily intake of 300 μg of methylmercury in the diet.[89] Paresthesias, often the first symptom seen in methylmercury poisoning, are rather nonspecific unless there is a history of mercury exposure. A complaint of paresthesia should not prompt an evaluation for mercury intoxication before other much more likely causes (e.g., medications, inflammatory diseases, other toxins, and nutritional deficiencies) are reasonably evaluated and excluded. Other nonspecific complaints of organomercury toxicity may include nausea, diarrhea, anorexia, irritability, sleep disturbances, and personality changes. Symptoms of chronic exposure to methylmercury include bilateral constriction of vision (such as tunnel vision), ataxia, tremors, and dementia. There is no firm understanding of the variability of individual responses to methylmercury, including subclinical effects from very low exposures.

Recognizing the limitations in these estimates and incorporating an uncertainty factor of 10 because of extrapolating to low-dose, dietary exposure, the Joint FAO/WHO Expert Committee on Food Additives in 1972 established a "tolerable" weekly intake of total mercury of 0.3 mg, of which no more than 0.2 mg should be methylmercury. This translates to allowable methylmercury consumption of approximately 33 μg/day.[89] In the United States, the FDA set a corresponding "acceptable daily intake" of 0.3 mg, with an "action level" of 1.0 ppm mercury in fish in 1987. Other nations have comparable limits.

Numerous studies have been conducted to estimate potential exposure to humans from eating fish. Fish consumption has been found to be a major predictor of blood mercury levels. For some cultures, fish represents a major percentage of the daily protein intake. In one such nation, Sweden, some families were found to consume fish containing 0.3 to 7 mg/kg mercury, with HgB levels as high as 60 μg/L, but no detectable symptoms or signs of neurotoxicity were observed.[89] Market basket studies in the United States show that the average American consumes approximately 18 grams/day of fish, with tuna the most common species eaten.[76] In estimating risks from fish the U.S. EPA considers 165 grams/day as high average consumption[91]; however, Puerto Rican fishermen consumed an average of 284 grams/day[13] to 370 grams/day.[14] Data from the FDA in 1979 show the highest mean level of mercury is found in swordfish. Based on worst-case scenarios of individuals consuming the most contaminated species of fish on a regular basis at amounts two standard deviations above the mean, the daily intake of mercury would still fall below 0.2 mg/day. In a British population of 942 individuals whose mean fish consumption per capita was 50 grams/day, largely of fish from estuaries with high mercury levels due to industrial pollution, the average HgB was 8.8 μg/L.[83] Thus, even the individuals in the upper 0.1 to 0.2% of a population who consume the largest quantity of fish on a regular basis appear to be below the estimated minimum risk level for (methyl)mercury toxicity, while the remainder of the population, particularly in the United States, is substantially below this threshold.

Fetotoxicity: Of special concern is the vulnerability of the fetal nervous system to the toxic effects of methylmercury transferred across the placenta. Fetotoxic effects may occur even when the mother is asymptomatic.[73] Epidemiologic data from Japan and Iraq indicated that exposures occurred prenatally and through breast milk. Fetal blood concentrations may exceed those in maternal blood.[45] Clarkson[18] found that elevated maternal hair mercury levels during pregnancy predicted an increased probability of adverse effects, particularly psychomotor retardation, in the offspring. Studies in New Zealand of children whose mothers had high fish consumption during pregnancy also suggest that mental development and school performance may be adversely affected by prenatal methymercury exposure.[42]

Although governmental agencies in the United States and other nations have issued advisories or placed outright bans on the consumption of certain fish because of mercury or other chemicals, there is a tendency for certain sectors of the public, particularly fishermen, to ignore these posted warnings.[15] In the United States most states analyze fish and shellfish caught within their waters as part of their environmental monitoring programs as required under section 304 of the Clean Water Act (1987). This program helps to identify polluted waters and point sources of toxic discharges, and to develop discharge control strategies.[91] The EPA, FDA, and state and local governments may vary in their methods of risk assessment (e.g., extrapolation of animal data, estimates of consumption of locally caught fish) and risk management, which may tend to make some agencies appear more conservative in their approach than others.

In summary, our understanding of the toxic effects of low-level exposures to dietary mercury continues to evolve, particularly for high-risk populations such as pregnant women and young children. Reducing this risk depends on implementation of and industrial compliance with state and federal regulations designed to minimize the sources of metal pollution. It is possible that the dietary recommendations frequently espoused by cardiologists, dieticians, and other health professionals to increase fish consumption because of its putatively beneficial effect on lipid profiles and cardiovascular disease risk[3] may increase health risks from certain environmental contaminants.

Lead (Pb) is present in trace quantities in many foods (see Table 43-1), leading to an average U.S. daily consumption of 0.3 mg from food plus 0.1 mg from water and air. This is consistent with the WHO estimate of 0.2 to 0.3 mg worldwide.[96] Intestinal lead absorption is approximately 10% in adults and 50% in children.[1] In special cases there may be excessive dietary lead intake, for example, where local industrial pollution has contaminated fish, resulting in elevated blood lead levels in fish eaters.[50] As in Roman times, lead poisoning occasionally occurs from wine and spirits prepared in home distilleries using piping and vessels containing lead. Beer is the major dietary source of lead for adult Germans and Australians, where per capita consumption of this alcoholic beverage is relatively high.[6,50]

Lead-glazed earthenware remains a problem today, particularly in pottery imported from countries where lead-based glazes are still popular and legal.[27] Tinned copper cooking vessels used in restaurants and homes contain as much as 0.2% lead.

Individuals who consume wild game animals killed with lead shot are potentially exposed, but a far greater source of exposure for the U.S. general population comes from the 15 billion lead shot each year that miss their target and end up in surface water and vegetation. Lead bioaccumulates in animals that consume the contaminated plants and water.[73] However, only humans who rely on hunting for a significant amount of their food are likely to develop lead poisoning. Finally, the major source of ingested lead in children comes from eating leaded paint chips. While this is not a dietary exposure per se, it represents a significant public health problem regarding lead exposure.

Symptoms in adults consistent with acute lead poisoning (abdominal colic, new-onset constipation, mental confusion or personality changes, peripheral muscle weakness) or chronic poisoning (more insidious onset of symptoms, notably neurobehavioral changes, arthralgias, impotence) should be evaluated through an appropriate history, including occupation, hobbies, and diet; physical examination (mostly to rule out more likely organic diagnoses); and appropriate tests, including blood lead level (PbB), zinc protoporphrin (ZPP), and a peripheral blood smear. In adults, a PbB above 40 ug/dl is consistent with the clinical diagnosis of lead poisoning; however, the range of individual responses varies widely, depending on the source and time course of exposure and the patient's baseline health status. For chronic exposures an elevated ZPP may be the only significant effect, particularly because neurobehavioral symptoms may be vague and the diagnosis may thus not be entertained. In children, there is epidemiologic evidence that exposure to lead at levels previously considered safe may be associated with neurobehavioral deficits that persist into early adulthood,[61] and food may occasionally contribute to elevated PbB.

In general, investigation of food and/or water sources for lead exposure should be undertaken only if clinical suspicion is high. Attention to proper analytical methodology and epidemiologic assessment (i.e., investigating other potentially exposed individuals or groups, and comparing them with controls) is vital to ensuring accurate, clinically meaningful results. Symptoms from foodborne lead poisoning are rarely life-threatening (in contrast to some occupational exposures) and are usually treated by identifying and removing or remediating the source of the exposure, and following the patient clinically with serial blood tests as necessary.

Cadmium (Cd) has many industrial uses and is widespread as an environmental contaminant capable of producing kidney and lung disease with high exposure.[10] Itai-Itai

Table 43-1. Typical concentrations of lead in food derived from Environmental Protection Agency data

Food	Concentration (ng/g)
Dairy products	3-83
Meat, fish, poultry	2-159
Grain and cereal	2-136
Vegetables	5-649
Fruit and fruit juices	5-223
Oils, fats, shortenings	8-28
Sugar	6-73
Beverages (μg/L)	2-41

(literally "ouch ouch") disease, characterized by bone pain, was first recognized in Japan in the 1960s, resulting from cadmium-laden mining wastes discharged into waters used to irrigate rice fields. Villagers, particularly postmenopausal women, developed severe osteomalacia, manifested by painful fractures in the vertebrae and femurs, as a result of cadmium-induced proximal renal tubular disease with calcium wasting. Genetic and dietary conditions also likely contributed to the development of this epidemic.

Cadmium normally occurs in low concentrations in foods. Estimates of average daily ingestion in Canada range from 7 to 34 μg (mean 13.8 μg), with significantly higher exposures through inhalation by cigarette smokers (0.5 to 2.0 μg Cd absorbed/pack). The highest content is typically found in animal products such as poultry, beef, and shrimp.[22] Cadmium levels in organ meats are closely correlated with cadmium content of animal feeds. Fish and other seafood from bodies of water polluted with cadmium have been found to have cadmium concentrations of 0.05 to 3.66 mg/kg in the United States, and can account for as much as one-half of daily dietary cadmium intake. Sewage sludge used as fertilizer can also contribute to cadmium uptake by crops and animals. Water is typically a small contributor (<1 μg/l) unless cadmium is leached from zinc-plated (galvanized) pipes and cisterns;[73] soft drinks dispensed from vending machines with cadmium-plated storage tanks can contain 100 to 1000 times the amount of cadmium found in untainted drinking water. Galvanized iron pots are coated with zinc that contains low traces of (1% to 2%) cadmium, which can leach into weakly acidic foods and liquids. The WHO/FAO has established a "safe" weekly intake of approximately 0.5 mg. Acute toxicity from cadmium ingestion, manifested as severe gastrointestinal symptoms and acute renal failure, was seen when cadmium-plated cooking utensils were used many years ago, but is rarely seen now that this practice has been abandoned.[10]

Aluminum (Al) is widely used in containers for cooking and packaging and is also a key ingredient in baking powder, many commercial antacid preparations and in antiperspirants. The average daily amount of aluminum ingested by adults is 12 to 14 mg.[69] Based on the FDA Total Diet Study (1984), the leading sources of aluminum in the American diet are processed cheese (American cheese is highest with 411 mg/kg) and flour products such as biscuits (16.3) and flour tortillas (129), which are prepared with aluminum-based baking powder. Certain teas, herbs, and spices are naturally high in aluminum as well. In contrast, water is not an important contributor to dietary aluminum intake unless aluminum sulfate (alum) has been added to water supplies as a coagulant.[73]

Cooking utensils and containers made from aluminum represent a major use for this metal, but also remain controversial because of concerns that they contribute significantly to the aluminum content of foods and beverages. Aluminum cooking or storage surfaces can release aluminum into some foods, particularly acidic foods or liquids, but in one experiment the aluminum concentration of potatoes cooked in an aluminum pan was no different than in a glass pan.[69] Aluminum concentration in tomatoes, however, increased 100-fold and in cabbage 300-fold after they were cooked in aluminum cookware, while no changes were observed when they were cooked in glassware. Storage of food in aluminum foil, as well as cooking or reheating in foil, also resulted in increased aluminum concentrations. Levels in acidic beverages such as fresh orange juice and tomato juice have been observed to increase from 1.3 mg/kg to 12.4 mg/kg after storage in an aluminum container for several hours.[69] Aluminum concentration can reach 5 to 10 mg/L without affecting the flavor of beer or soda. Resins and other alloying metals may be used with aluminum containers to improve corrosion resistance.[73]

Though migration of aluminum from cookware or packaging is evident, the clinical significance of dietary aluminum exposure remains unclear. Intestinal absorption varies but is generally less than 10%. Aluminum citrate is readily absorbed; aluminum phosphate is poorly absorbed. Normally functioning kidneys efficiently excrete the small amount of aluminum absorbed each day, resulting in neutral aluminum balance.[73] However, when aluminum is introduced into the body other than orally—e.g., through dialysis, total parenteral nutrition, and perhaps dermally or inhaled through antiperspirants—the body burden increases and toxicity can occur. The use of aluminum-containing water in the dialysate of chronic renal failure patients is thought to contribute to the development of dialysis dementia in those patients for whom dialysis cannot sufficiently excrete the excess aluminum. Such patients are also advised to avoid aluminum-containing preparations for binding phosphate (which builds up to toxic levels in patients with renal failure) for the same reason. There are no reliable biologic monitoring tests for chronic, low-level aluminum exposure. Blood aluminum levels are not an appropriate indicator of elevated body burden or chronic exposure.

Among a number of putative effects attributed to chronic aluminum ingestion over the past 100 years since its use in cookware, the most controversial is its association with Alzheimer's disease. Although elevated levels of aluminum have been found in brain tissue of autopsy specimens of Alzheimer patients, the metal's role in causation, if any, has not been proved.[69] Elimination of aluminum cookware on this basis does not appear warranted, but is certainly feasible given the many alternatives. If an individual wishes to reduce aluminum exposure, he should know that processed cheeses and breads and possibly antiperspirants appear to be the sources of greatest potential exposure.

Tin (Sn) alloys have been used in cooking and utensils for hundreds of years with generally safe results. While studies of dietary tin intake have focused on exposure from canned goods, another and more toxic hazard is organotin compounds. Dibutyltin salts used as stabilizers in PVC wrapping films and trialkyl- and triaryltin compounds used as biocides are potential contaminants in a wide range of foods. Of particular concern is tributyltin (TBT), which is widely used in paints as an antifouling agent on most recreational and commercial boats and ships. Extremely high residues have been found in Sydney (Australia) harbor and the Georges River estuary, where oysters have been found to contain up to 500 times greater concentration of TBT than oysters from unpolluted waters.[8] Similar contamination has been found in British waters. The use of TBT has been banned in certain types of paints used on boats in several parts of Australia. There is little toxicological information on dietary organotin compounds. With high-level, chronic industrial exposures these compounds are potent neurotoxins.

Radioactive metals, most notably strontium 90, iodine 131, and cesium 137, are dispersed into the environment by radioactive fallout from nuclear tests, malfunctioning power plants, and natural volcanic eruptions. Fallout settles in soil, where it is taken up by plants. Strontium (in the same periodic column as potassium) is especially taken up by grains and grass.[73] As a result, the largest dietary source of radioactivity is milk and dairy products, in which radioactive metals are concentrated. The contribution of these sources to dietary radioactivity intakes is many orders of magnitude more important than naturally occurring isotopes of biologically active elements, such as potassium (^{40}K) and carbon (^{14}C). Pollution from nuclear fission reactors into local bodies of water can also result in high concentrations of ^{137}Cs in fish and edible seaweed, as has been observed in the Irish Sea.[65] The release of radioactive elements from the Chernobyl nuclear reactor in the Ukraine in 1986 resulted in contamination of soil, water, vegetation, and animals over wide areas of Europe and Asia. Measured levels of radioactivity led to restrictions on the sale and consumption of a wide variety of foodstuffs throughout Europe and Russia. The long-term implications of these sources of dietary radioactivity for human health await further study.

Arsenic

For most people ingestion of food (particularly seafood) is the main pathway for exposure to arsenic with an average exposure of 46 μg/day.[2] The main use of arsenic is as a biocide, with an emphasis on wood preservation. The background level in food is below 150 ppb. Fatal ingestion of arsenic can be accidental or can occur as homicide or suicide. High-level exposure to arsenic occurred with the medicinal ingestion of Fowler's solution (1% potassium arsenite) used to treat syphilis. Arsenic occurs mainly as the inorganic ions As^{+3} or As^{+5}. Most studies of oral arsenic poisoning refer to inorganic forms of arsenic, usually As^{+3}, and most of the organic arsenical compounds are considered to have relatively low toxicity.[2]

Arsenic occurs in grain, meats, and seafood, with levels in the latter averaging up to 5 ppm, but occasionally reaching 170 ppm.[56] This is mostly organic arsenic, but in some cases food may contain substantial amounts of the more toxic inorganic compounds.[2]

ORGANICS

Synthetic organic chemicals represent a significant source of contamination for the food supply. The likelihood of uptake by plants and animals is influenced by many toxicologic, soil, and biotic factors, for example, sunlight, the chemistry of soil water, and microbial activity. Biomagnification through the food chain is important for some chemicals; however, only a few organic chemicals have been noted to significantly enter the human food chain and/or cause human illness (see the box on p. 490). Many others persist in the environment and may cause damage to other species and ecosystems. This section will discuss a few of the better-studied organic pollutants that affect the food supply and their ramifications for human health. Other organic pollutants that more directly affect drinking water supplies are discussed in the chapter on water.

Polychlorinated biphenyls (PCBs)

PCBs were manufactured in the United States by Monsanto under the trade name Araclor between 1930 and the mid-1970s. Foreign manufacturers also produced PCBs under various trade names. During that period over 1 billion pounds were produced. All PCB isomers are lipophilic and hydrophobic and have low electrical conductivity and high heat capacities.[80] By the 1970s, as a result of industrial accidents, regular leakages from products in service, and leaching from landfills into waterways, PCBs were found to be ubiquitous in the environment. Episodes of acute human toxicity and concern about potential human health and ecological effects from this persistent substance led to the banning of production in the United States by the EPA in 1977. Production and/or active use in other parts of the world continues today.

The problem of bioaccumulation of PCBs in fish was first noticed when large groups of fish-eating birds died in the U.K. in 1969. Studies of PCBs in fish in the upper Hudson River (New York) revealed levels of 5 ppm and higher by the mid-1970s, while levels in Great Lakes fish ranged from 3 to 12 ppm.[20] The highest levels were found in larger, older fish. Biomagnification of PCBs in fish was extensive: in Hudson River water, concentrations were 0.3 to 3.0 ppb; in river-bottom sediment, <13 ppm; and in fish, 5 to 20 ppm.[80] Because of their environmental persistence, PCBs remain detectable today in the sediment of lakes and streams, though in lower concentrations than 20 years ago. In places where PCB levels in fish exceeded these tolerances, fishing was banned.

Human exposure to PCBs through the food supply has also occurred as a direct result of hundreds of documented industrial accidents.[77] The most striking episode, the Yusho incident, occurred in Japan in 1968 when over 1000 people developed symptoms of chloracne, hyperpigmentation of the skin, sensory and motor disturbances (visual dysfunction, weakness, numbness, headaches), and elevations in liver enzymes due to consumption of cooking rice oil ("yusho") contaminated with PCB and dibenzofurans that leaked from a heat exchanger in the food processing plant. The frequency and severity of symptoms were found to be proportional to blood PCB levels.[20]

A number of PCB contamination episodes have involved contamination of animal feed with PCB-tainted feed, with resultant high PCB levels detected in animal products such as milk, chicken, and beef that were consumed by humans. For example, in 1978-1979, at a feedlot in Kansas where a contaminate oil-based insecticide was regularly applied to decrease fleas and other surface parasites, hundreds of animals developed a severe neurologic disorder and gastrointestinal hemorrhaging that resulted in the deaths of over 50 animals.

Fish and seafood are potential sources of dietary PCBs. Cooking produces a 20% reduction in PCB levels in crab claws, and removal of the hepatopancreas before cooking greatly reduced PCB residues. PCBs were recovered from boiling cooking water. Puerto Rican fisherman who stewed whole fish had significantly higher potential exposure to PCBs and other lipophilic contaminants than those who ate fried fillets.[13]

While the acute toxicity in animals and humans is well known, the chronic health effects of PCB exposure are not. Chronic feeding studies performed on laboratory animals revealed significant reproductive effects in certain species at low dietary concentrations (2.5 ppm), and PCBs induce hepatic microsomal enzymes and have some estrogenic activity in vitro. They also cause immunosuppression and liver cancer.[80] For studying the risk of cancer, the FDA utilized high-dose feeding studies on laboratory animals to develop a tolerance level of 5 ppm in fish, which was later decreased to 2 ppm. Tolerances for other foods are lower. As in all its other risk assessments, the FDA assumed worst-case scenarios for exposure, concentration, and potency that may have overestimated the carcinogenicity risk by orders of magnitude.[53] In humans blood and adipose levels of PCBs are measurable in ppb concentrations. However, from studies of populations with documented low-level dietary exposure to (and concomitantly elevated tissue levels of) PCBs over many years through high fish consumption, no adverse health effects (including cancer) have yet been documented. However, epidemiologic studies must extend for many more years before any definitive conclusions can be made about PCB toxicity to humans.

Polybrominated biphenyls (PBBs)

Chemically related to PCBs, PBBs were manufactured as flame-retardant materials for use in plastic electronic and automotive parts. In late 1973 Michigan chemical company, which manufacturered PBBs along with other products, accidentally substituted PBB "Firemaster" into a similarly named formulation, "Nutrimaster," used for animal feed. Only after several months, when cattle and pigs with PBB levels from 4000 to 13,500 ppm, who consumed the feed became ill, was the accident discovered.[80] The tainted beef, poultry, and dairy products were consumed by thousands of people before the cause was discovered 9 months later. Widespread consumption of the contaminated foods occurred throughout Michigan and neighboring states. Although the affected animals and animal products were quarantined and destroyed, a long-term prospective study conducted by the Michigan Department of Public Health revealed that PBB residues remained present in the blood of 71% of the "exposed" group 5 years after the contamination occurred. In the southern peninsula of Michigan, 98% of nursing mothers had PBB in their breast milk, as did 43% in the northern pensinsula.[62] Though PBBs have been found to have a number of toxic effects in laboratory animals, no acute health effects were observed in the most highly exposed groups (families living on affected farms, who had higher blood PBB levels) when compared with controls.[20] While there is some suggestion of increased frequency of liver function abnormalities and immunosuppression in this group, no significant adverse chronic health effects have been observed. Follow-up data of this cohort through this decade may better elucidate the nature of the chronic health effects of this past exposure.

Polychlorinated dibenzodioxins (PCDDs)

This class of compounds, of which 2,3,7,8-TCDD ("dioxin") is the most toxic, is a by-product of the production of chlorinated phenol herbicides and fungicides (such as 2,4,5-T; 2,4-D; pentachlorophenol) and of refuse incineration. Dioxin has been implicated as a cause of ill health in soldiers exposed to Agent Orange during the Vietnam War. PCDDs and the related compounds, polychlorinated dibenzofurans (PCDFs), have also been found in soil around power plants and municipal waste incinerators.[80] Like PCBs and PBBs, PCDDs and PCDFs are highly lipophilic and chemically stable, with the ability to biomagnify in the food chain. They have been identified in all animal food products, and the average body burden (fat concentration) of total PCDDs in Americans, adjusted relative to 2,3,7,8-TCDD's potency, is 22 parts per *trillion*,[16] of which 5 ppt is contributed by 2,3,7,8 TCDD itself.

FOOD PREPARATION AND COOKING

The manner in which food is prepared and cooked can significantly alter exposure to contaminants. Trimming of fat from meat and removal of the hepatopancreas or green gland of crabs[101] are mechanical ways of eliminating pollutants that accumulate in these tissues. Fishermen who stewed whole fish rather than frying fillets were exposed to higher levels of mercury[13] while boiling rather than steaming eliminated PCBs from crabs.[101] The high temperatures of cooking and baking can drive off volatile compounds from tissues, reducing the amount ingested, but potentially increasing the amount inhaled if the kitchen is not well ventilated. Cooking reduced PCB levels in crab flesh by 20%.[101]

Some toxic substances are generated during the cooking process. Carcinogenic PAHs such as benzo[a]pyrene are produced from meat fat during grilling,[93] and the amount varies with the cooking method. Hamburger cooked over an open flame had high levels of this carcinogen, while microwaving produced negligible concentrations.[21]

PESTICIDES

Pesticide residues on food remain the major food safety concern of American consumers. While over four-fifths of consumers surveyed by the Food Marketing Institute in 1989 felt confident that the food supply is safe, this level dropped to 67% after the Alar incident (discussed below) in 1990.[79] These concerns have been addressed in thousands of scientific studies, and continue to consume much attention at the regulatory level. This section will focus on the evidence for health effects of chronic exposure to residues on food, regulatory efforts and problems, and implications for individual consumers and patients. In the United States, pesticide use is regulated by the EPA under the Federal Insecticide, Fungicide and Rodenticide Act (FIFRA). Residues on animal feed are regulated by the FDA and the U.S. Department of Agriculture (USDA).

In 1993 the National Research Council published a report entitled *Pesticides in the Diets of Infants and Children.*[59] The report concluded that diet is an important source of pesticide exposure. The study found differences in susceptibility and how children and adults process pesticides. But small children have much greater exposure to pesticide-bearing foods, putting them at greater risk of chronic effects.

Measurement of residues

The FDA is responsible for monitoring and enforcing of the tolerances established by the EPA for pesticide residues on raw commodity foods traded in interstate commerce in the United States. The USDA is responsible for inspecting residues in meat, poultry, and raw egg products. Over 600 active pesticides (not including propellant and diluent carrier compounds) are registered for use on food crops. Of these, 350 account for 98% and 150 account for greater than 80% of the total amount used in U.S. agriculture.[9] Between 1983 and 1986, the FDA analyzed pesticides in 27,700 food samples. In 60% of the samples, *no* residues were detected (versus 55% in 1978 to 1982).[99] Only 3% of produce sampled exceeded FDA standards, mostly because no tolerances had yet been established for newer agents or metabolites. A slightly higher percentage (5%) of violations were found in imported foods, principally from Mexico, the largest exporter of food to the United States. The percentage of imported samples having no detectable residues was 45% to 49%.[99] Data from the leading agricultural states, however, indicate the highest frequency of elevated pesticide levels are in cheese and egg products, tropical fruits, and waxy green vegetables.[9]

Organochlorine pesticides (many of them banned in the 1970s) were the major substances found in bottom-feeding, freshwater fish, particularly from the Great Lakes. In samples of domestic and imported chocolate, and especially in commercial cocoa preparations used for food processing, residues of lindane, aldrin, and dieldrin (all banned organochlorine insecticides) have been detected, though usually below their respective tolerance levels.[68] In a study of the nine major fruit and vegetable crops grown in New Jersey (lettuce, green peppers, white potatoes, snap beans, spinach, sweet corn, tomatoes, apples, and peaches) obtained from farms and from supermarkets in the state, none had residues of 26 priority pesticides (15 of them suspected carcinogens) above EPA tolerance limits,[51] and 76% of the samples had no detectable levels of residues.

While pesticide residues are infrequently detected in processed foods, when they are found they are usually in lower concentrations than in the raw product.[17] Washing, peeling, and cooking tend to remove residues via mechanical action, chemical degradation, and hydrolysis. There are some exceptions, however, such as ethylene-*bis*-dithiocarbamate (EBDC), a carbamate fungicide and class B2 carcinogen, which often resists washing and peeling and, upon heating, is transformed into ethylenethiourea (ETU), the principal toxic metabolite.[17,99] Food processors must follow strict standards under the National Food Protection Act (1960) to monitor and report pesticide residues on the raw products they receive, and to restrict the types and amounts of pesticides used on raw crops. In 1985 of 20,310 processed food products, 93% had no detectable pesticide residues.[17]

Another method of estimating human exposure used by the FDA is the Total Diet Study (TDS), initiated in the 1950s. This approach utilizes consumer market-basket surveys conducted each year in different regions of the nation. These "typical" diets, including processed foods, are prepared in experimental kitchens and then analyzed for over 100 potential pesticide residues. Levels of detectable pesticides are quantified at concentrations 5 to 10 times below tolerance levels.[49] This type of study more realistically reflects actual consumer exposure than monitoring of field crops and processed food. In 1989 the FDA took 19,000 samples of TDS foods (44% domestic, 56% imported). Data from 1988 reveal that *no* residues were found in 60% and 62% of domestic and imported foods, respectively, while less than 1% of each were over tolerance levels.[49] The TDS results through the end of the 1980s indicate that dietary intakes of pesticides in typical American diets are *less than 1%* of the acceptable daily intake (ADI) established by FAO

Table 43-2. Agencies and regulations dealing with food

Agencies

Agency	Function
World Health Organization (WHO)	Sets acceptable daily intakes (ADI) for toxic substances
Food and Agriculture Organization (FAO)	Research
Food and Drug Administration	Sets acceptable limits of exposure in United States
	Research
	Issues fines and injunctions, closes plants, blocks sale of hazardous imports for all food *except* poultry, meat, and raw eggs
U.S. Department of Agriculture (USDA)	Inspects poultry, meat, and raw eggs
International Food Biotechnology Council (IFBC)	Develops comprehensive criteria and procedures to evaluate safety of food (plants microorganisms) produced through genetic engineering
Joint Expert Committee on Irradiated Foods (JECIF)	Research policy on food irradiation

Regulations

Federal Food, Drug, and Cosmetic Act (FDCA), 1938	Sets maximum allowable residue metabolite concentrations in food for all registered pesticides
Food Additives Amendment, 1954 (Delaney Clause)	Prohibits EPA approval of any additive, including pesticides, shown to be carcinogenic
National Food Protection Act, 1960	All food processors must monitor and report pesticide residues on raw materials

and WHO. For environmentally persistent agents like dieldrin, consumption has declined to 5% of that in 1970. In summary, food monitoring at the state and federal levels indicates that pesticide residues fall well below the established tolerance levels.[9]

Regulatory issues

While residue monitoring and toxicologic studies comprise the framework of health risk assessment for human consumption of pesticide residues, inherent conflicts arise in the way in which these data are interpreted, and in particular how risk is regulated (Table 43-2). At the center of this conflict is the Federal Food, Drug, and Cosmetic Act (FFDCA, 1954). Under section 408 of the Act, the EPA is required to establish for each registered pesticide a "tolerance" or maximum allowable residue level in raw agricultural commodities that affords reasonable protection of the public health. Tolerances are established primarily for enforcement purposes (i.e., to monitor for misapplication) rather than for direct public health protection.[5] By stipulating "tolerable" residue levels, the Act explicitly recognizes that certain minimum health and environmental risks are "acceptable" in return for the benefits pesticides provide in assuring "an adequate, wholesome, and economical food supply."[57] Pesticide residues that concentrate in *processed* food above the tolerance level set for their parent raw commodities are regulated as *food additives* under section 409. Unlike section 408, section 409 requires that these residues must be proven "completely safe" for consumption, with no recognition of a tolerable, acceptable risk. Specifically, the Delaney Clause in section 409 prohibits EPA approval of any food additive, including pesticide residues, that has been shown to be "carcinogenic"—which the EPA defines as substances that produce benign and/or malignant tumors in humans or laboratory animals.[57]

This inherent conflict within the law, dubbed "the Delaney paradox," raises major questions about the regulatory agencies' ability to implement policies that both protect public health and enhance food safety and availability.[57] The EPA is required under FIFRA to reassess and approve or reject by 1997 those pesticides registered prior to 1984. Under the regulatory framework of FDCA and FIFRA, the EPA's policy has been to revoke the use of pesticides in processed food that exceed their tolerance levels under section 409, *and* to deny granting a section 408 tolerance for residues in the raw, parent crop. While this policy has been consistently applied to new pesticides and new uses of existing agents, this has not been the case with regard to the hundreds of pesticides that were registered before newer toxicologic assays, sophisticated analytical exposure monitoring methods, and mathematical dose-response models were incorporated into the risk assessment process.[9] As discussed earlier, the EPA's database on toxicologic properties and exposure for many agents is limited and outdated for most agents that were approved by now-outdated standards. When these older agents are tested by contemporary standards, many are considered to be (suspected) carcinogens. Moreover, as more information on concentrated residues in processed foods becomes available, many more pesticides may fall under the purview of the Delaney Clause.

First, the EPA assumes all exposures occur at the highest allowable level—the tolerance level—even though the average residue levels are less than 30% of tolerance for most crops, and only a low percentage of crops or processed foods are found to have residues that exceed the tolerance limit. Second, the EPA assumes that each agent is applied to 100% of the crops for which it is registered.[9] The calculation of a pesticide's carcinogenic potency ("Q*") can also vary by several orders of magnitude (see Chapter 3). Testing is done at high doses in animals—often orders of magnitude above those to which humans are exposed—to allow detection of potential "weak" carcinogens. Of the 28 currently registered compounds considered most important for cancer risk assessment by the National Research Council's (NRC) Board on Agriculture, 10 of them account for 80% to 90% of the total potential cancer risk. Although only processed foods are covered by the Delaney Clause, nearly half of the estimated dietary carcinogenic risk, based on EPA calculations, is from foods that remain unprocessed, that is, fruits, vegetables, meat, cow's milk, and poultry products.[57]

The EPA thus faces many dilemmas in deciding how to reconcile its mandate from the Delaney Clause with the need for timely, accurate regulatory action on hundreds of pesticides. Each pesticide typically takes several years of testing and analysis before a risk estimate is derived. A number of regulatory scenarios have been proposed by NRC to address this problem. Currently, the EPA favors relaxing the Delaney provision as it applies to processed food by replacing the zero-risk criterion with a "negligible" (or "acceptable") risk increase of 1×10^{-6}.[78] The establishment and enforcement of tolerance levels does not necessarily ensure long-term safety, and therefore measuring only the percentage of residue samples that exceed tolerance levels may not be as meaningful in terms of protecting public health. Yet given the high percentage of residue samples that are well under the established tolerances for most foods, it is also unclear whether lowering these levels will actually reduce health risks from chronic exposure. Scientists, physicians, policymakers, and the public still have not reached a consensus on what level of risk (of cancer or other diseases) is "acceptable."

One example of the wide uncertainty in the risk assessment process, for a noncancer end point, is the series of three outbreaks between 1985 and 1988 in California involving over 1000 people who developed food poisoning caused by the carbamate insecticide aldicarb (Temik), applied to watermelons and cucumbers.[31] Illnesses involved symptoms of cholinesterase inhibition, including nausea, vomiting, diarrhea, abdominal pain, dizziness, confusion, weakness, and blurred vision. No deaths were reported. Aldicarb, which was not registered for use on these crops, breaks down rapidly into a number of metabolites in plants and in the soil; these are absorbed systemically, the metabolite aldicarb sulfoxide (ASO) being the principal toxic agent. A study performed on 12 human volunteers in 1971 before the insecticide was registered by the newly established EPA suggested a Lowest Observed Effect Level (subclinical cholinesterase depression) in humans of 0.025 mg/kg (ppm). Measurements of ASO residues by FDA and California laboratories on the contaminated fruits and vegetables in 1985 to 1988 ranged from the limit of detection (0.2 ppm) up to 4.7 ppm. Based on estimates of the amounts consumed by affected individuals over several days, ASO dose intake ranged from 0.003 to 0.006 mg/kg. These results suggested that aldicarb is significantly more toxic than the initial studies indicated.

Alar: The problems with regulating based only on cancer risk are best demonstrated by the 1989 uproar over daminozide (Alar), a chemical growth regulator used since the 1960s by apple growers to improve the crop's yield, appearance, and storage characteristics.[75] Research conducted at the Eppley Institute for Research in Cancer (Omaha, NE) beginning in 1973 found that a metabolite of Alar, unsymmetrical 1,1-dimethylhydrazine (UDMH), caused various tumors of lung, kidney, liver, and blood vessels in mice. Alar contains approximately 1% UDMH, and this content is increased to approximately 5% by heat processing used in the production of apple juice and applesauce. In addition, approximately 1% of Alar is metabolized to UDMH in the human liver. As a result, EPA ordered a "special review" of this new toxicologic data. However, only after several years of lobbying by Alar's manufacturer, Uniroyal Chemical Co., and subsequent lawsuits by the Natural Resources Defense Council (NRDC), a public interest organization, did the review occur. The Eppley studies were reviewed by a panel of specially appointed academic experts who found significant methodologic issues—in particular, the very high doses of Alar used on the animals—which cast some doubt on the validity of the studies. The EPA ruled in January 1986 that insufficient evidence was present to cancel Alar's registration. The EPA then directed Uniroyal to perform residue analysis and animal feeding studies. The results of Uniroyal's studies several years later all showed no increase in tumor incidence in mice or rats for either Alar or UDMH, even at the maximum tolerated doses, $35,000 \times$ the highest estimated daily intake of UDMH for children regularly consuming apple juice and applesauce (the theoretically most highly exposed human population). The higher doses necessary to produce more tumors also caused most of the mice to die prematurely of other toxic effects.

The EPA used the above toxicity threshold to extrapolate human risk, and estimated (worst-case) that human exposure would produce an additional 45 cancers per million people, an unacceptable risk. The EPA announced in 1989 that it would ban the use of Alar on apples after July 1990. Simultaneously, in a report published by NRDC entitled "Intolerable Risk: Pesticides in Our Children's Food,"[60] NRDC estimated an even higher lifetime cancer risk, 240 lifetime cancers per million children. Both the EPA and NRDC estimated children's consumption of processed apple products based entirely on USDA consumer surveys. A more recent study[59] confirms that children have higher pesticide exposure than adults because of their diet.

Consumer choices: alternatives or reassurance?

Given the many uncertainties in regulatory and scientific assessment of health risks from pesticide residues, the public's difficulty with understanding or accepting risk, and our agricultural industry's intensive dependence on pesticides, some consumers and farmers have reacted by shifting to organically grown foods (no pesticides or synthetic fertilizers). Certified organic produce typically costs more money (largely because of smaller economies of scale), sometimes has a less uniform, "perfect" appearance, and may lack the year-round availability of conventionally grown foods, all of which limit its appeal to most of the population. At the same time, people who buy organic produce with the belief that it will protect their health may continue to follow unhealthy lifestyle and dietary choices (in particular, a low-fiber, high-fat diet centered around animal foods), which present far greater risks for short- and long-term adverse health effects.

Clinical evaluation for pesticides

While isolated cases of pesticide-related, acute illnesses have occurred (such as from exposure to aldicarb), there is no evidence that chronic exposure to pesticide residues in food is responsible for many of the diseases and ill-defined symptoms (chronic fatigue syndrome, environmental allergies) that currently defy etiologic explanation. Far more pesticide-related poisonings occur in industrial manufacturing, agricultural application, and inappropriate application of pesticides by homeowners and gardeners. Physicians should evaluate patients who seek to blame pesticides for their ills with an appropriate dietary and occupational/environmental history, and provide an objective assessment and information in a manner that enables the patient to decide whether his/her explanation is really valid. If a significant foodborne exposure is suspected, referral to a qualified occupational/environmental medicine physician is warranted. Blood pesticide residue ''screens'' are rarely a useful diagnostic test in the absence of a positive exposure history.

FOOD ADDITIVES

The addition of chemical preservatives, coloring agents, and other substances to foods (including beverages) has been practiced since ancient times. The principal benefits are to improve the taste, attractiveness, and convenience of preparation of foods; to increase storage life; to prevent or retard microbial contamination and spoilage; and in some cases, to provide nutrient fortification. All of these measures result in reduced costs and increased availability of many foods. Largely as a result of urbanization of much of the population and the demand for fresh fruits and vegetables year-round, produce in the United States travels an average distance of 1500 miles from farm to market. Consumer demand for these advantages and the resultant market response has created the impetus for the development of hundreds of commercial food additives serving a variety of functions. While a surprising number of the naturally derived colorants and preservatives used for hundreds of years remain in commercial use, most of the additives intentionally added to foods (i.e., direct additives) today are synthetically manufactured. Substances can also enter food as a result of microbial contamination, pollution, packaging, cooking, processing, and other treatments (indirect additives).

This section will briefly summarize the health hazards of some of the more controversial classes of direct additives and review the laws designed to regulate them. Indirect additives such as pollutants, packaging, and food irradiation are covered in other sections. The topic of food additives has been intensively studied, and a number of comprehensive, detailed reviews are available.[54,81,100]

Regulation

All food additives are regulated by the FDA under the Federal Food, Drug, and Cosmetic Act (FFDCA, 1938). This law was intended to prohibit food, processing methods, and packaging that are potentially hazardous to human health from entering the marketplace.[25] FDA has jurisdiction over all foods except raw meat, poultry, and eggs, which are under the jurisdiction of the U.S. Department of Agriculture (USDA). The Food Additives Amendment (Delancy Clause, 1954) to FFDCA specifically gave the FDA authority over this class of agents, as well as indirect additives, including pesticide residues, animal drug residues, certain animal products, and food irradiation. The amendment also established a regulatory framework that shifted to the manufacturer the burden of demonstrating scientific proof of the safety of each new additive to the FDA for consideration for approval. This amendment also included the Delaney Clause, which prohibits FDA approval of any additive in *processed* foods that has been found to cause cancer in humans or (laboratory) animals. (The controversies surrounding the implementation of the Delaney Clause have been discussed under **Pesticides**.)

The FDA process of evaluating and approving a food additive for safety is complex and often requires several years. The FDA requires data not only on toxicity, carcinogenicity, mutagenicity, and teratogenicity (largely from animal feeding studies) but also the manufacturing process, chemical composition, and specific intended uses and concentrations expected in these foods or beverages.[81] To ensure uniformity and purity of food additives, the FDA requires every manufacturer to meet the production and quality specifications of the Food Chemical Codex, developed by the National Academy of Sciences, and to follow the Good Manufacturing Practice (GMP) criteria, which specify the types of raw materials, processing, and packaging allowable in producing each approved food additive substance. The FDA's monitoring programs enforce the allowable concentration (tolerance level) established for each additive that is necessary to achieve its intended effect. Approximately 700 substances (e.g., colorants, preservatives) that were approved for use before 1954, and which have been deemed safe by food science experts based on scientific studies and extensive commercial experience, are classified as ''generally recognized as safe'' (GRAS) and are exempted from pre-market safety approval.[100] Each of these substances also has a defined tolerance that is enforced.

Problems with the ranking of carcinogenic hazards—the risk assessment process—are myriad. Criticisms include the high levels of uncertainty produced by extrapolation from high-dose rodent studies to lower-level human dietary exposures; the lack of sound data on the mechanism of cancer induction and thus the appropriate dose-response curve(s); the question of how much weight should be given to negative data; and the public health effects of regulating known tumor promoters (such as dietary fat in vegetable oils), as opposed to genotoxic initiators (identified by animal and in vitro tests). Interspecies differences are highlighted by the finding that 226 of the 392 chemicals (natural and synthetic) tested positive for carcinogenicity in either rats or mice, but many were not positive in both species. Despite limitations, animal tests remain important sources of data on human carcinogens.

Color additives

Food colorants have long been used to add aesthetic qualities to foods. Natural spices such as turmeric (yellow), paprika (red), and saffron (orange) are examples of colorants still used today, largely for their flavoring properties. The late 1800s saw the synthesis of organic chemical dyes, initially as derivatives from coal tar. Today seven (water-soluble) food dyes are fully approved by FDA as ''FD&C colors'' for certain applications in food, based on extensive safety testing.[12] In addition, a number of ''FD&C lakes'' (dyes attached to an aluminum hydrate or calcium moiety in order to make them water-insoluble) are approved. The National Research Council estimates that less than 4 grams of synthetic colors are consumed per capita per year in the United States. Natural colorants, such as the spices listed above, are exempt from the certification process. All approved color additives must be identified on food labels and must meet the tolerance levels established under GMP. The FDA considers toxicity as well as estimated exposure in establishing levels that provide ''reasonable certainty that no harm will result from the intended use of the color additive'' (21 CFR, Section 70.3(i), (1989). The Delaney Clause is strictly applied to food colorants; 63 agents have been removed from the market as a result.[100]

Food preservatives

Nitrates and nitrites: These compounds, found naturally in many foods but best known as preservatives in cured meats, can react with oxygen through metabolism in the body, or through certain cooking methods, to form *N*-nitroso compounds (NOCs, chemical structure R—N=N—O). Two major categories of NOCs have been discovered: *N*-nitrosamines, which tend to be formed in foods during cooking and then ingested; and *N*-nitrosamides, which are mostly formed in the digestive tract. Risk for stomach cancer is associated with high exogenous nitrate exposure, but is inversely associated with intake of foods high in vitamin C, a potent antioxidant. Achlorhydria, in which gastric nitrite levels are elevated, also increases gastric cancer risk. Both classes of nitros compounds contain many proven mutagens that induce tumors in laboratory animals at numerous sites, depending on the R-group.[36] Nitroso compounds exert their mutagenicity through metabolism to an electrophile, carbonium ion (R_2CH^+), which readily alkylates DNA bases. Acutely, nitrites (directly ingested or metabolized from nitrate) can induce methemoglobinemia, particularly in neonates, when ingested in high concentrations.[94]

The largest source of exposure to preformed nitrosamines is through tobacco (parts per thousand). Vegetables, particularly celery, lettuce, cabbage, and spinach, account for the largest percentage of total daily ingestion of nitrates, but this source of nitrosamines (via internal metabolism) is small compared to cigarette smoke or chewing tobacco.[36] Moreover, many of the same green, leafy vegetables contain vitamin C and other antioxidants that inhibit the NOC formation reaction. Drinking water is typically low in nitrates, except when contaminated by agricultural fertilizer runoff.[94] Fermented foods contain moderate amounts of nitrates and nitrites. The largest dietary exposures, however, come from two man-made sources: nitrate and nitrite additives used to stabilize the colors and inhibit oxidation in cured meats, such as bacon, and from grilling and smoking of meats and fish, in which proteins, urea, guanidine, creatinine, and other endogenous amines are oxidized in the presence of nitrogen to form nitroso compounds. Total dietary nitrate/nitrite ingestion in the United States is typically <1 μg/day.[36] However, in certain societies such as parts of Japan where smoked fish and preserved meats as well as fermented foods are consumed in large quantities, dietary exposure to nitrates, nitrites, and preformed NOCs is much higher (smoking prevalence is also high). This epidemiologic association may explain why the risk of stomach cancer is significantly higher in Japan than in the United States and other Western nations.

BHA and BHT: At the levels allowable in food (0.02% of fat or oil content), two of the most commonly used antioxidants in fats and fatty foods, BHA (2- 3-tert-butyl-4-hydroxyanisole) and BHT (3,5-di-tert-butyl-4-hydroxytoluene), exhibit few adverse effects in laboratory animals or humans.[81] Occasional cases of urticaria and other allergic reactions have been reported.[32] Weak carcinogenic effects in rodents have been observed at chronic ingestions only at much higher concentrations.[23] The FDA regulates these two compounds and related preservatives that have been in use for decades as GRAS, as long as they are used within their assigned allowable concentrations. Amounts consumed by Americans are well under the established ADI.

Sulfites: Sulfiting agents (sulfur dioxide, sodium sulfite, and sodium and potassium salts of bisulfite and metabisulfite, collectively referred to as ''sulfites'') have been used for centuries to control browning of fruits and vegetables, to limit microbial and mold growth in wine and fruits, and to inhibit oxidation reactions. Their fate in food depends upon the nature of the food product, the type and degree of food processing, and storage conditions.[100] In most foods sulfites are oxidized to harmless sulfates and excreted in the urine, or to sulfur dioxide, which volatilizes out of food. In a few foods such as lettuce, sulfites remain unreacted and therefore bioavailable. Americans typically consume 6 mg/day (more for heavy wine or beer drinkers), in comparison with the ADI of 50 mg (for a 70-kg man).

The most familiar adverse health effect associated with sulfites are allergic reactions, manifested as asthma exacerbation, contact dermatitis, and rarely anaphylaxis. Fewer than 1% of mild to moderate asthmatics are sensitive, but up to 8.4% of severe asthmatics may be affected.[94] The highest exposures to dietary sulfites have occurred in raw vegetables and dried fruits at restaurant salad bars; as a result of the low-probability but potentially fatal reaction from this source of sulfites, the use of sulfites for this purpose has been prohibited by the FDA. Sulfites have been shown to reduce the content of certain B vitamins, particularly thiamine, in certain foods.[71] Overall, however, this class of preservatives has shown little systemic toxicity or carcinogenicity in laboratory animals. The validity of extrapolation of these results to humans is limited by differences in metabolism, as rodents have 10 to 20 times the level of the detoxifying enzyme, sulfite oxidase, as humans.[94] Nevertheless, both humans and rodents have an enzymatic capacity that far exceeds the dosages regularly encountered in average American diets.

Ethylene dibromide

EDB is a potent biocide used as a gas to fumigate stored grain and other foodstuffs. Although volatile, EDB residues can persist on food and remain present in flour. Since EDB is a potent alkylating agent and a carcinogen, its presence in food products was alarming, and in 1983 several states required food companies to withdraw contaminated foods such as cake mixes from grocery shelves. The magnitude of risk was low, overall, but children who consumed large quantities of baked goods would have experienced an unacceptable cancer risk.

Fat and sugar substitutes

Saccharin and cyclamate are two of the better-known synthetic sugar substitutes that have been labeled as suspected carcinogens; one (cyclamate) was banned, while the other (saccharin) remains on the market. Aspartame has been successfully marketed, with few adverse effects. The reader is referred to one of the comprehensive references cited in this section for a review of the history of these compounds. With the public increasing its demand for low-fat, low-calorie foods, but reluctant to alter their diets toward foods naturally low in fat, food processors are also focusing on developing starch- and protein-based fat substitutes.[88] Most of the products introduced to date are natural starches, such as carageenan, a seaweed extract, which is added to ground beef to reduce the fat content. Safety testing of each of these new products will take many years; some, such as Procter and Gamble's Olestra, an indigestible glucose polyester with fatty acid linkages, have been approved by FDA, only to fail to gain market acceptance. The cost to food manufacturers for development, safety testing, and the approval process is substantial.

Food additives and hyperactivity in children

This controversy, beyond the scope of this chapter, dates back to 1973, when Benjamin Feingold reported that more than half of the children he examined with behavioral or learning disorders had adverse reactions to food additives but improved on the "Feingold diet," which eliminated synthetic preservatives and food colors.[38] There have been positive and negative studies of this and other dietary and environmental modifications, some of which showed dramatic reduction of hyperactivity in young boys.[40]

Summary of relative risks of food additives

The public perception of risk from food additives appears to be partly related to the complex chemical names of additives used in trace quantities in foods and the perception of involuntary exposure to man-made chemicals. Yet 95% of the total amount of direct additives that consumers ingest have long records of safe use.[100] The regulatory and public preoccupation with carcinogenicity detracts from attention to broader changes in the food choices of the typical American diet that would have far greater impact on protecting public health. Public recognition that the regulatory process ensures a reasonably safe, but not completely risk-free food supply is necessary to balance the extensive testing that is required to appropriately permit additives that are safe for human consumption.

PACKAGING

Food packaging plays an important role in enabling the food supply to have the variety, storage life, nutritional integrity, safety, and resultant economy that is enjoyed by consumers. Packaging has evolved into a science as well as a major part of the food industry. Yet excessive packaging contributes in a major way to product costs, resource waste, and solid waste disposal problems. Today, plastics, metals and alloys, paper, and ceramics, and combinations thereof (for example, aseptic juice cartons) are the mainstay of packaging materials. Maintaining the integrity of the packaging material under various conditions (heating, transport, freezing) is important not only for protecting the contents of the package but also for ensuring that the material does not interact with or contaminate the food. Increasing concerns about the effect of these materials on food safety have prompted in-depth studies and risk assessments. This section will briefly discuss some of the major issues of food packaging's effects on foods. Migration of lead, aluminum, and tin from containers into food has been discussed in part in the section on heavy metals.

Food storage principles and safety issues

The stability of food is influenced largely by the amount of light, oxygen (O_2) content, and moisture, as well as its own chemical and physical composition.[33] Through appropriate packaging as well as proper handling and processing methods, these factors can be controlled, thus minimizing the oxidation of fats, vitamin degradation, and other enzymatic and nonenzymatic reactions that may alter the taste, appearance, and nutritional value of the food.

Whether these substances represent a significant health risk depends on their concentration, their interaction with other molecules in the foodstuff (particularly vitamins and minerals) that may diminish (or enhance) their toxicity (such as vitamin E or selenium acting as antioxidants), and the body's ability to metabolize and detoxify them. To place the significance of these substances in proper perspective, they should be considered in comparison with the toxins and mutagens produced by traditional cooking methods and with "natural carcinogens" found in foods considered important for good health (e.g., vegetables).[4,44]

In assessing dietary exposure to packaging residues and regulating human risks, the use of sensitive analytical methodologies is crucial for meaningful health risk assessment and regulation.[41] Analytical technology has improved substantially in the past 30 years, lowering detection limits by orders of magnitude, that is, from parts per million to parts per billion and lower. Because of the difficulties in accurately analyzing many actual foodstuffs for trace quantities of migrant plastic compounds (and other residues such as metals and organic pollutants), the FDA uses food "simulants" (water/alcohol mixtures, 3% acetic acid, vegetable oils) at different storage temperatures to test packaging materials for chemical migration.[30] Estimated consumption of residues is also monitored by population-wide dietary surveys and individual food-recall studies, as well as from packaging industry sales data.[41]

In the United States the FDA regulates food packaging as a "food additive," requiring premarket safety approval (unless considered GRAS) before the material is allowed to enter into commercial usage. FDA compares the estimated consumer exposure (often taken as the upper bound of the confidence interval for the estimated consumption for each residue) with an estimated "acceptable daily intake" (ADI) derived by extrapolation of the "no observable adverse effect level" (NOAEL) from animal toxicity studies. Approval is granted if the estimated human exposure is less than the ADI. In the case of proven or suspected carcinogens, the FDA has allowed residues at "tolerance" levels that pose "negligible risk" of additional cancers (1×10^{-6}). As for regulation of other additives, this approach has received substantial criticism because of its conflict with the Delaney Clause and its overreliance on quantitative risk assessment methods that involve uncertainties. Less stringent regulation is utilized by the USDA in its jurisdiction over meat and poultry products.[25] There is very little epidemiologic data on the health effects from chronic exposure to approved packaging polymers, metals, or additives.

Plastics

As the number of plastic compounds used in packaging and storage materials has increased exponentially in the past 20 years, migration of potentially toxic, low-molecular-weight moieties from plastic polymer packaging materials has become a major safety and food quality issue. Numerous chemical materials have the potential to migrate from plastic into food.[30] While the various heat and light stabilizers, antioxidants, plasticizers, and other processing aids are required for proper functioning of the packaging material, residual monomers and oligomers of plastic polymers are not. Some materials may migrate independently of the food contents of the package, while others migrate ("leaching") depending on the acidity, temperature, and other properties of the food.[25] Certain packaging aids, such as antifogging, antistatic, and slip agents, are designed to work at the surface of the material, thereby remaining in regular contact with both the package and the food contents.[41]

Many studies have been conducted to assess the degree of migration of plastic monomers into food and the potential risk to humans who consume them over time. At concentrations in food of greater than 10 ppb, styrene may impart a noticeable taste to foods.[55] Studies of styrene monomer in milk and other dairy products of varying fat content, stored for 19 to 56 days in polystyrene (PS) containers, revealed styrene monomer concentrations of 17 to 77 ppb (except for sour cream, which contained 242 ppb).[30] In margarine stored in PS tubs, styrene monomer was less than the minimum detection limit (MDL) of 25 ppb. Similarly low results have been obtained in food simulation studies. Benzene residues (a starting material in PS production) have not been found (detection limit 0.35 ppb) in samples of boiling water contained in PS foam cups for 1 hour, though trace amounts (0.56 ppb) of benzene were measured in the cup itself.[30] These levels fall far below the FDA's allowable limit of 0.5% (500 ppm) for styrene in fatty foods and 1% in water-based foods or liquids.[55]

The case with vinyl chloride monomer (VCM), the building block of polyvinyl chloride (PVC), is not as straightforward. PVC film is used for food wrappers, as a liner in soda bottle-caps, in semirigid form for meat blister packs, and in a rigid form for liquor and oil bottles. In 1973 VCM was detected at 20 ppm in liquor and at lower levels in various foods. At that time, VCM had been confirmed as an animal and human carcinogen (hepatic angiosarcoma). As a result, the FDA banned PVC for use in packaging that involved food contact.[41] The plastics industry responded by changing its PVC manufacturing techniques, which resulted in drastically lower VCM residue levels. For example, VCM levels in oils, concentrated fruit drinks, and margarine went from >200 ppb to <5 ppb, and levels in liquor declined to 1 ppm. The overall estimated daily intake thus decreased from 1.3 to 0.1 µg/day/person.[41] As a result, the FDA's restriction was withdrawn, and new VCM residue limits were set at 50 ppb. FDA established an ADI (25 ng/day) of this carcinogen as a level that posed a "negligible risk" to human health. This decision was again in conflict with the Delaney Clause.

A situation similar to that of VCM occurred with acrylonitrile (AN) monomer. AN has widespread use (as a copolymer of butadiene and styrene) in containers for margarine, dairy products, vegetable oils, and carbonated beverages. This monomer, has produced increased frequencies of various tumors in animals when administered at high levels. Trace amounts (0.24 to 0.35 ppm) were detected in some food products in 1974.[30] After the FDA withdrawal of approval for use of AN, manufacturing changes lowered residues to a point that appeared to pose negligible carcinogenic risk. Other compounds, such as plasticizers (such as dioctyl phthalate) and adhesives (2,4-toluenediamine), are examples of suspected carcinogens now undergoing regulatory evaluation.

Metals

Containers made from metals such as tin, steel, and aluminum are utilized for their ability to resist physical impacts and corrosion and to preserve food for extended lengths of time under variable external conditions. However, migration of metals into food at very slow rates is known to occur.

When they were introduced 150 years ago, "tin cans" (steel cans with an inner layer of tinplate), leached significant amounts of tin into food. Since 1950 the percentage of metallic tin used in tinplate has been halved.[52,73] Organic resin lacquers (synthetic or natural) have also been applied to coat the inner tinplate layer to provide a further barrier to tin corrosion. As a result of these protective measures, tin corrosion is extremely slow.

Soldering of the seams, tops, and bottoms of rolled steel cans represents a significant source of migration of tin and, more importantly, lead. Solder contains 2% tin and 98% lead, though higher percentages of tin have been introduced primarily to decrease lead migration into food.[52] Studies of canned versus fresh tomato purees and orange juice have shown that the canned foods contained slightly higher concentrations of lead.[64] The differences were on the order of 0.1 ppb, which is clinically insignificant for adults but which may be significant for baby foods. Indeed, some countries have banned the use of lead solder in baby food containers, shifting instead to completely welded or cemented cans.[52] Less acidic foods may not produce as marked an effect on metal migration.

Other types of storage containers can introduce heavy metals, including lead, into food. As discussed earlier, ceramic vessels can be glazed with pigments containing various metals, including lead, cadmium, and chromium. The porous nature of these vessels and the relative instability of the glazing (especially when not fired at sufficiently high temperatures) can produce significant leaching of these metals into food over short periods of time. Cases of lead poisoning from liquids stored in ceramic pitchers have been reported. Recently, as a result of legislation passed in California, American manufacturers of china have agreed to reduce the lead content of their products by 50%, and to warn consumers of the hazard.[27] Many imported and handmade ceramics still contain high levels of lead, however. Colored enamel coating on commercial casserole dishes and saucepans can also be a source of these metals. Lead has been found in food stored in polyethylene bread wrappers turned inside-out and used as lunch bags.[95] Polyethylene bags contain 25 grams/kg lead from printing inks and plastic stabilizers.[73] The role of aluminum in storage containers is discussed in the section on heavy metals.

Paper

Relatively little has been written about food contamination from paper products other than metals leaching from decorative printing inks from wrappers to feed. Recently publicized concerns include the migration of dioxin (2,3,7,8-TCDD) from bleached paperboard cartons into milk and juices, and the leaching of lead from bread bags into food.[95]

NUTRITION AND FACTORY FARMING

The average American adult consumes 112 pounds of beef, plus more than 50 pounds of chicken, pork, and fish each year, in addition to large quantities of dairy and egg products. In the United States animal products account for approximately 65% of the dietary protein.[62] Many chronic diseases in the United States and other affluent nations are caused by or strongly associated with this high-cholesterol, high-saturated-fat, low-fiber diet. The American public has responded to somewhat conflicting health messages from the USDA, health organizations, medical professional organizations, and food industries by consuming less "red meat" products but eating much more poultry, fish, oils, and dairy products (particularly high-fat cheeses). The net result over the past 10 years has been little change in the overall fat content of the American diet, and minimal if any improvement in the incidence rate of the major dietary diseases.[92] Much of the demand for animal products is generated by advertising from the beef, poultry, pork, and dairy industries, which represent economically powerful constituencies. While the American consumer is accustomed to purchasing animal products in neatly packaged wrappers and containers at the supermarket, the intensive methods employed to bring billions of pounds of animal products to market—factory farming—are carefully hidden from the view of consumers, including physicians and other health providers. This section will attempt to highlight some of the important aspects of this topic.

Animal health products

One major result of the intensely stressful, confining, and, to most first-time observers, inhumane conditions under which animals are raised for human consumption is widespread internal and external bacterial and other microbial contamination. Animal foods account for nearly 58% of foodborne microbial illness in the United States, most of which is due to improper sanitation during processing, inadequate refrigeration, or improper cooking methods that allow these microbes to flourish.[46] To counter these infectious disease problems and to improve efficiency in the growth of the animals, antibiotics, pesticides, hormones, vaccines, and feed additives are used. Nearly 80% of all chickens, pigs, and dairy and beef cattle are fed antibiotics.[48] Antibiotics such as tetracyclines have been used as broad-spectrum antimicrobial agents as well as anabolic growth promoters for many years, but have declined in use as a result of concerns about toxic human exposures (possible idiosyncratic aplastic anemia). Many narrow-spectrum antibiotics and antimicrobials used to alter the bacterial content of cows' rumen (stomach) to reduce intestinal disease, however, are not sold for use in humans. Other growth stimulants given to cattle and other animals include anabolic steroid implants (in the ear), synthetic progesterones, and arsenic-based compounds. The use of these compounds results in decreased production costs that save the consumer approximately 9% in the cost of beef.[62]

Entry of animal drugs into human food supply

Potential adverse human health effects from consumption of animal products tainted with animal drugs ranks high on the list of consumers' food hazard concerns. The relatively few overt episodes of meat, dairy, or egg contamination from animal drugs have resulted from incorrect (or illegal) applications, or insufficient allowance of ''withdrawal time'' between administration and slaughter/milking/laying.[62] The development of allergies or hypersensitivity reactions in humans to animal antibiotics, especially penicillins, sulfa compounds, and tetracyclines, has been minimal. Finally, the concentrations of synthetic progesterones and anabolic steroids found in animal tissues and milk are far lower in concentration and potency than corresponding endogenous hormones in humans, and certainly many orders of magnitude lower than in women ingesting oral contraceptives.[62] The use of a new product of biotechnology, bovine somatotropin hormone, to raise cows' milk output even higher has stimulated recent debate because of its potential to enter into milk and produce adverse endocrinologic effects on children. While some consumers believe that eating ''organically'' bred beef, chicken, or eggs will be more heathful, most of the significant health hazards posed by these animal foods appears to come from the excessive amounts of fat and protein, the lack of fiber or starch, and toxic substances produced by cooking them, rather than from pesticide or drug residues.

FOOD IRRADIATION

Irradiation of certain foods as a method of preservation and protection from microbial contamination has been promoted as a food processing technology for many years, yet it remains controversial. Its inability to gain acceptance as a viable commercial enterprise in the United States is largely due to a public perception of adverse health risks. However, as other food preservation and processing technologies, most notably pesticides, come under increasing regulation, the health and economic benefits of food irradiation become more visible. Accurate information about the benefits and potential risks of this technology is essential both to appropriate regulation of the industry and to physicians who are asked to address safety concerns of individuals and groups of patients.

Process history and development

Treating various foods with ionizing radiation was first introduced in Britain in 1905 as a method of food preservation. Intensive research into improving methods of producing gamma radiation began in the 1940s in the United States. By the late 1950s ^{60}Co (cobalt) had been introduced and tested for its preservative effects as well as its toxicologic properties on food sources.[24] In 1957 selected spices were treated commercially with irradiation in Germany, and in 1960 the U.S. Army began to regularly irradiate meat for use in military rations. In 1964 the Food and Agricultural Organization (FAO) of the World Health Organization (WHO) and the International Atomic Energy Agency (IAEA) formed the Joint Expert Committee on Irradiated Foods (JECIF). This international body of experts from numerous disciplines representing numerous public and private interests initiated extensive toxicologic (animal feeding) studies, short-term screening tests, and chemical analyses of irradiated foods.[26] By 1980, based on hundreds of studies conducted during the 1970s, JECIF concluded that ''irradiation of any food commodity up to an average dose of 10 kGy (kilogray—see definition below) presents no toxicological hazard.''[97]

Purpose

Irradiation offers several potential benefits in terms of the safety, nutritional adequacy, and cost of certain foods. Most obviously, its application can decrease or in some cases prevent food spoilage via destruction of certain pathogenic organisms. Though irradiation can preserve the freshness of certain foods beyond their existing shelf life, it cannot hide the effects of food spoilage or natural degradation; this is a common misperception. With these benefits should come decreased costs and increased quality to the consumer. In theory the selected use of irradiation as a food preservation technique could lead to a reduction in the use of chemical pesticides, fumigants, and preservatives, as well as energy savings from reduced refrigeration requirements. In reality, irradiation is mostly used in conjunction with these other methods.

Description of irradiation process

Several sources of ionizing radiation have been approved for use in food treatment. The most commonly used source is ^{60}Co, which emits (high energy) gamma rays. Use of ^{137}Cs (cesium) has been curtailed by its limited supply, higher cost, lesser penetrating power, and difficulty with reprocessing. The other major commercial source of gamma irradiation is the electron accelerator, which has been in use since the 1950s for sterilization of medical equipment, generation of x-rays for medical therapy, and other applications. The energy absorbed by a particular foodstuff per unit time is measured in Grays (Gy), in which 1 Gy represents 1 Joule/kilogram of food. Formerly this absorbed dose was measured in rads (where 100 rads equals 1 Gy). Food, either packaged or raw, is placed on a conveyer belt that moves through an enclosed concrete structure in which it is exposed to energy from the radiation source for a specified length of time. The treated food receives only energy, not radioactivity. Thus the actual amount of radiation given off by the ^{60}Co source (measured in curies) is important only in ensuring that a sufficient amount of energy is emitted. Determination of the specific dosage of irradiation required for each foodstuff incorporates the type of food involved (fruit, animal product, solid versus liquid), its density, conveyer speed, and type of packaging. The effective dose must also account for natural heterogeneities in the content of each foodstuff. Chemical dosimeters are used to measure the absorbed energy dose and depth of penetration of the energy beam. Tolerances for the ratio of maximum to minimum depth are established for each foodstuff, with a goal of overall average dose reaching >50% absorption established by JECIF.

The primary goal of food irradiation is destruction of microorganisms that produce food spoilage and/or human disease. The dose of radiation required to damage DNA in microorganisms or insects does not significantly alter the composition of other macromolecules in the food (enzymes, nucleoproteins, lipids, carbohydrates). There are several reasons for this phenomenon: (1) the DNA in microorganisms represents a relatively large target, with only one copy per cell, in comparison to many times greater concentrations of smaller macromolecules found in foodstuffs; (2) DNA is far more sensitive to radiation energy than enzymes, nucleoproteins, lipids, and other potentially susceptible macromolecules in the foodstuff; and (3) DNA in the cells of the foodstuff is no longer actively replicating, unlike that in live contaminant microorganisms and insects. Thus a dose of 0.1 kGy will damage 2.8% of the DNA in bacterial cells, which will be lethal to a significant percentage of the irradiated cells, whereas the same dose will damage only 0.14% of the enzymes and 0.005% of the amino acids, which will have essentially no measureable impact on food quality.[72] With far less DNA than insects, bacteria are less radiosensitive than insects, and therefore require larger doses of irradiation to achieve destruction. Very high dosages (25 to 45 kGy) of radiation can completely, permanently sterilize the foodstuff (radappertization). Lower dosages (2 to 8 kGy) will reliably reduce the number of viable, non–spore-forming bacteria to minimally detectable levels (radicidation) or acceptably low levels necessary to prevent spoilage for a limited period of time (radurization, 0.4 to 10 kGy).[24] Thus food irradiation rarely is intended to ''sterilize'' food in the same way that medical equipment needs to be sterilized, since minimal levels of bacteria are safe in food and persist with all other present methods of food preservation.

Food irradiation dosages have been approved by the JE-CIF for up to 10 kGy, at which level no observable effect on the quality of the foodstuff or production of toxic by-products has been observed. Most major bacterial food pathogens (*Salmonella, Campylobacter, Bacillus cereus, Staphylococcus aureus,* molds, and yeasts) are reliably destroyed in foods at dosages under 10 kGy. More resistant organisms, such as *Clostridium botulinum,* are reduced in number at these dosages and also become less resistant to heat, pH, and salt.[24] Proper food handling and packaging practices are clearly the most essential measures to prevent the growth of these potential pathogens. Pathogenic viruses, which can normally survive under 12 hours in slaughtered animals intended for human consumption, are typically only partially inactivated at dosages of <10 kGy, and conventional cooking methods are still required for thorough inactivation. Finally, parasites such as *Entamoeba* and *Toxoplasma* are readily killed at relatively lower doses of irradiation, around 0.25 kGy.

Toxicologic aspects

The energy absorbed by the foodstuff from the radiation source leads to the formation of ions and short-lived free radicals in the target food compound. These particles, particularly the latter, undergo secondary reactions to form *radiolytic* compounds, many of which are chemically stable. The major radiolytic products are formed by reactions with water, the most abundant compound in all foods. The products include reactive intermediates such as hydroxyl radical, hydrogen atom, and hydrogen peroxide.[24] Foods highest in water content (fruits and vegetables) yield the highest amounts of radiolytic products. The oxygen content of the food and its immediate environment (packaging) also influence the degree of oxidation and formation of reactive peroxyl radicals ($\cdot RO_2$). While the commercially maximum irradiation dose of 10 kGy produces approximately 300 mg of radiolytic products per kilogram of food, this is far less in amount, but similar in content, to that produced by traditional cooking methods, such as frying or boiling.[34] Indeed, in numerous analytical studies of irradiated foodstuffs, only a very small fraction of energy-induced by-products have been found to be unique to the irradiation process. Free radicals are generated in all processes that result in energy absorption (such as heating, pasteurizing), regardless of the energy source, and the chain-reaction by-products are determined largely by the type of food, temperature, and competing chemical reactions. Most experimental studies of food irradiation chemistry have been conducted on simplified solutions of glucose, amino acids, and other basic components of human foods. Since the extent of by-product formation increases with aqueous dilution, this laboratory method does not reflect the realistic situation in whole foods, where hundreds or thousands of substances are naturally present in each foodstuff and may interact with the principal macromolecules.

Irradiation of certain foods, most notably processed

foods, can be done safely inside packaging. Proper packaging is essential to prevent microbial contamination, water loss, and degradation. In extensive testing most plastic, glass, and metal food packaging materials show minimal degradation at doses up to 10 kGy.[24] Certain plastic films and some paper (cardboard) packaging can be weakened at higher doses. To date, commercial experience has not seen packaging as a significant problem in terms of quality or toxicity.

Regulation

Currently the FDA regulates food irradiation as an *additive*, not as a process. Section 201(s) of the Food, Drug, and Cosmetic Act (1958) specifically addresses irradiation and certain processing and packaging applications as "substances" that are expected to become a component of food or which may affect the characteristic of the food.[24] The standards of safety are regulated under several subsections of section 409, and depend upon the probable amount of consumption and cumulative health effects (in humans or laboratory animals). This approach presents an inherently paradoxical obstacle to commercial viability, since estimating probable consumption or cumulative effects is based on the industry's limited commercial experience in the United States. Clearly, these regulations were intended for intentional chemical food additives. In 1986 the FDA finally ruled that doses of up to 1 kGy were permissible for growth and maturation inhibition of certain fruits; disinfestation of arthropod pests in spices, herbs, and dry enzyme preparations; and treatment of pig carcasses for *Trichinella*. To date these are the only current usages of food irradiation in the United States, though only 0.5% of all spices sold in the United States are irradiated.[74] The FDA requires that irradiated food be labeled "irradiated" at the wholesale and retail levels, though processed foods containing an irradiated ingredient need not be identified. Virtually every major nation has established its own list of foods that may be irradiated, and the doses and purposes, many of them broader than that of the United States.

Numerous problems emerge when applying food additive safety testing methods to irradiation of foodstuffs. As discussed earlier, only minute amounts of numerous radiolytic products are produced, all of them common to other traditional cooking and processing methods. Studies of animals fed 100% irradiated diets, and of mice fed extremely high-fat, nonphysiologic diets irradiated up to 800 times the accepted maximum commercial dose, have shown no increases in toxic end points.[24] Regulation of irradiation as a *process* would undoubtedly abet its regulatory evaluation. Well-designed studies of whole foodstuffs irradiated at commercial doses (under 10 kGy) and kept stored under normal conditions have repeatedly shown no mutagenic effects.[26]

Human volunteer studies in China, including over 400 participants consuming irradiated foods for 7 to 15 weeks, revealed no differences in chromosomal abnormalities versus controls. No acute adverse health effects were seen. The only human study that has suggested genotoxicity found an increase in polyploidy in the lymphocytes of five malnourished Indian children who consumed irradiated wheat immediately after it had been treated with 0.75 kGy, compared with no polyploidy observed in children who consumed wheat that had been irradiated and then stored for 12 weeks.[11] However, numerous caveats limit the validity of the study. For example, (1) only group data was provided; (2) extremely small numbers of subjects were involved; (3) there was a relatively high background rate of polyploidy (0.8 to 1.8%); (4) the mode of preparation of the wheat (fried, cooked, raw) was not described; (5) no other clinically significant chromosomal abnormalities (breaks, gaps, deletions) were observed between the cases and controls; and (6) animal studies failed to confirm this singular finding. Numerous attempts to repeat these studies in India and in other nations have failed to reveal similar findings. As a result, the Indian government in 1976 concluded that polyploidy is not related to wheat irradiation.

In 1983 a worldwide standard covering irradiated foods was adopted by the Codex Alimentarius Commission, which represents the FAO and WHO. Based on the findings of the JECIF from 1969 to 1980, it concluded that "irradiation of any food commodity" up to a dose of 10 kGy "presents no toxicological hazard" and therefore requires no further testing.[19]

Public concerns/barriers to widespread acceptance

Despite the lack of evidence pointing to health and environmental hazards of food irradiation, the industry has gained very limited commercial acceptance in the United States. Other industrialized nations, including Japan, the Netherlands, and France, irradiate grains, potatoes, onions, and other products in large-scale facilities. In addition, adverse environmental and occupational experience with chemical pesticides has made irradiation a more attractive alternative in these other nations. Yet as of 1990 the total amount of food irradiated worldwide was only 0.5 million tons.[37]

A major public perception and marketing barrier is the false belief that the irradiation process makes food radioactive. Much opposition comes from consumers' false belief that *anything* treated with radiation is unsafe.[74] As explained, this is entirely untrue; the food is exposed to energy emitted by a radioactive source, but does not come in contact with the radioactive source. All food contains trace amounts of natural isotopes (^{14}C, ^{40}K, ^{3}H) such that minute amounts of radioactivity are consumed each day. The same irradiation process is applied to sterilize medical supplies and cosmetics, which the public does not question. Much of this misperception comes from a lack of public education about radiation, confusion about the difference between nuclear power and irradiation, and the publicity that has been given to serious nuclear energy accidents like Chernobyl that resulted in real contamination of food with radioactive particles. Companies engaged in commercial food irradiation are regulated as closely, if not more so, than any others in the food processing industry. The public must also recognize the potential benefits of replacing or reducing current methods of food preservation, for example, using ethylene oxide and ethylene dibromide—both highly toxic and with potential long-term health effects—to preserve stored grains, fruits, and nuts, with applications of low doses (0.2 to 0.7 kGy) of irradiation.[24] Similarly, potatoes now treated with chemical sprout inhibitors, some of which are banned in some countries, or kept for long periods in refrigerators (high cost), could be comparably preserved for 1 year in cool (15° C), unrefrigerated storage with 0.15 kGy of irradiation. Irradiation will not reverse improper handling techniques that result in cuts and bruises, which in turn allow entry of rot-causing organisms. Irradiation is not known to increase the toxicity of pesticides, chemical additive residues, or food packaging.[29]

In summary, decades of scientific scrutiny have shown food irradiation to be a safe, effective method of food preservation. New analytical methods, such as thermoluminescence measurement and electron spin resonance, may allow identification of unique radiolytic products, which to date have not been found. While no accurate method presently exists to distinguish food that has been irradiated, labeling requirements must convey health—and environmental—benefits and risks to consumers based on scientific information available. Irradiation is unlikely to replace well-established, cost-effective preservation methods, but rather will be used selectively.

GENETIC ENGINEERING

Genetic engineering involves the manipulation of genes between organisms, and holds out the promise of providing new beneficial strains of crops, supplementing more classical breeding approaches.[39] The use of genetic manipulation techniques such as recombinant DNA and cell fusion allows genetic material to be specifically transferred between almost any pair of organisms, and in many cases, to allow the specific expression of a transferred gene(s) into the new host organism. With this advanced technology, however, comes numerous ethical, environmental, and human safety concerns. The focus of this section will be on human health issues, discussed in the context of a few examples of genetically engineering food products currently being developed and/or marketed for public consumption.

Scope

It is unlikely that genetic engineering will altogether replace conventional plant breeding. Only a few species are capable of being genetically engineered, and most of the current "successes" involve the expression of a single gene for a single purpose, for example, disease resistance or delayed ripening. Many traits involve the complex interaction of numerous genes and modifying proteins that cannot be manipulated with present technologies. The primary purpose of agricultural genetic engineering is to speed up the process of selective breeding to enhance crop yields, diversity, and positive attributes (taste, appearance, shelf life), and through direct manipulation of specific genes allow stable replication of the desired gene/trait in offspring during conventional plant (or animal) breeding.[39] Numerous applications exist for this type of technology. At present, plant foods are the primary commercial goal. Resistance to insect pests, such as in tomatoes, has been successfully enhanced by introduction of the BT protein gene of the bacterium *Bacillus thuringiensis*. The advantages of this selective introduction of a "natural" insect control over conventional chemical insecticides are obvious: only the insects that eat the plant are affected, and the toxin is limited to the plant. Therefore the toxin does not become widespread in the environment where, like pesticide agents, it can affect other plants, nontarget insects, and mammals, including humans.

The controversial "ice minus" case involved the "release" of plants containing a genetically engineered freeze-resistant gene. The researchers failed to realize that the public was concerned more with the failure of the process to investigate environmental and health effects than with the actual risks. Therefore no amount of risk assessment could quell the concerns.[43]

Another direction of genetic engineering is improving shelf life and storage of foods. Numerous food, chemical, and pharmaceutical companies, for example, have developed genetic engineering methods to improve the quality of major market-fresh crops like tomatoes. Thus the use of genetic engineering can significantly improve the taste and texture of market tomatoes by allowing them to "naturally" vine-ripen, reducing spoilage losses, and at the same time reduce the energy (refrigeration) and handling costs. Processing ripe tomatoes for tomato paste and puree may also be improved as heat processing becomes unnecessary. Calgene and its competitors' tomatoes are just being introduced into the U.S. market at the time of this writing.

A more controversial area is the development of herbicide-tolerant plants. While herbicide tolerance could facilitate herbicide control of weeds that compete with the desired crop, it is altogether possible that this approach will foster excessive use of herbicides. Another questionable application is the modification of the nutritional composition of plant materials, for example, increasing the methionine or lysine content of corn or soy meal for cows and pigs. One may argue that consumption of these animal products is inherently unhealthy, economically costly, and environmentally destructive, and that better use could go to feeding these foods directly to people. Finally, and perhaps most objectionable, is research aimed at genetically altering mammals. In response to the high-fat, animal-centered American diet and its resultant diseases (coronary disease, certain cancers, obesity, stroke), numerous bodies, including the U.S. Department of Agriculture and the National Research Council, have recommended that "part of the solution to the high-fat American diet may be to put farm animals on a diet of their own" by genetically engineering the animals in addition to existing methods of selective breeding and altering the composition of their feed.[87] Included in this arena is the administration of bovine somatotropin (BST) produced by recombinant DNA technology to increase muscle content and decrease fat content of cows and their milk. This development conflicts with recommendations for the public to reduce animal protein consumption in favor of plant foods. This major consumer shift motivated by health concerns also benefits the environment and is less costly, since plant protein is produced with 10× greater efficiency on the same amount of land (see Chapter 61). This is particularly important when one considers that the average American diet has not changed significantly—still 36% of calories of fat—from 1976-1980 to 1990, despite widespread promotion of the health benefits of a lower fat diet.[92]

Safety concerns and regulation

Genetic engineering of foods raises safety concerns not only for individual consumers but also for our society as a result of the introduction of genetically altered organisms into the environment. In 1988 the International Food Biotechnology Council (IFBC), composed of experts from academia and industry (food, biotechnology), was established to develop comprehensive criteria and procedures to evaluate the safety of foods and food ingredients produced through genetically modified plants and microorganisms.[47] (The council did not consider genetically modified animals or ecologic implications of the technology.) The final report, issued in 1990, incorporated extensive reviews by government agencies in 13 nations, public interest organizations, academicians, and industrial scientific organizations. The IFBC concluded that no additional regulatory measures beyond those currently required by the FDA and USDA are needed for genetically modified plant products. The council established three major criteria for regulation: knowledge of the genetic background and procedures for genetic modification; composition of food products (nutrients and toxicants); and pertinent toxicologic data.

For regulation of genetically engineered microorganisms, the FDA has jurisdiction regarding health concerns. The FDA assesses whether the microbe itself ends up in the food product, whether some aspect of the vector or the expression product for which the DNA codes (for example, an enzyme) is unsafe for use in food, and whether the microbe is free of other extraneously introduced DNA that could code for a toxic product.[47]

The public in all nations is anxious about genetically engineered foods. There are broad ethical and social concerns that may override safety issues about individual foods, such as the genetically altered tomato. The American public's general lack of scientific sophistication, coupled with media attention to potential adverse effects, overemphasizes many potential risks while ignoring others.

CONCLUSION

Although there is some scientific basis for many of the concerns voiced regarding food quality, in most cases the fears appear exaggerated. Although episodes of metal and pesticide poisoning have been attributed to contaminated food, such events are infrequent. "For the majority of consumers, the perception of benefit or risk appears to be more important than scientific justifications. Thus the concept of zero tolerance in the case of hazardous substances appeals to many consumers who cannot understand why there should be any amount of a potentially harmful substance in a food."[63]

REFERENCES

1. Agency for Toxic Substances & Disease Registry (ATSDR): *Toxicological profile for lead,* Atlanta, 1992, Agency for Toxic Substances and Disease Registry.
2. Agency for Toxic Substances & Disease Registry (ATSDR): *Toxicological profile for arsenic,* Atlantic, 1992, Agency for Toxic Substances and disease registry.
3. American Heart Association/National Heart, Lung, and Blood Institute: *Dietary treatment of hypercholesterolemia,* Dallas, 1988, American Heart Association.
4. Ames BN, Magaw R, Gold LS: Ranking possible carcinogenic hazards, *Science* 236:271, 1987.
5. Archibald SO, Winter CK: Pesticides in our food: assessing the risks. In Winter CK, Seiber JN, Nuckton CF, eds: *Chemicals in the human food chain,* New York, 1990, Van Nostrand-Reinhold.
6. Australian Academy of Science: *Health and the environment in Australia,* Canberra, 1981, Australian Academy of Science.
7. Bakir F et al: Methyl mercury poisoning in Iraq, *Science* 181:230, 1973.
8. Batley GE et al: Accumulation of tributyltin by the Sydney rock oyster, *Saccostrea commercialis, Australian J Mar Freshwater Res* 40:49, 1989.
9. Benbrook CM: What we know, don't know, and need to know about pesticide residues in food. In Tweedy BG et al, eds: *Pesticide residues and food safety: a harvest of viewpoints,* Symposium Series 446, Washington, DC, 1991, American Chemical Society.
10. Bernard A, Lauwerys R: Cadmium in human population, *Experientia* 40:143, 1984.
11. Bhaskaram C, Sadasivan G: Effects of feeding irradiated wheat to malnourished children, *Am J Clin Nutr* 28:130, 1975.
12. Borzelleca JF, Hallagan JB: Safety and regulatory status of food, drug, and cosmetic color additives. In Finley JW, Robinson SF, Armstrong DJ, eds: *Food Safety Assessment,* Washington DC, 1992, American Chemical Society.
13. Burger J, Gochfeld M: Fishing a Superfund site: dissonance and risk perception of environmental hazards by fishermen in Puerto Rico, *Risk Analysis* 11(2):269, 1991.
14. Burger J, Cooper K, Gochfeld M: Exposure assessment for heavy metal ingestion from a sport fish in Puerto Rico: estimating risk for local fishermen, *J Toxicol Environ Health* 36:355, 1992.
15. Burger J, Staine K, Gochfeld M: Fishing in contaminated waters: knowledge and risk perception of hazards by fishermen in New York City, *J Toxicol Environ Health* 39:95, 1993.
16. Byard JL: The toxicological significance of 2,3,7,8-tetrachlorodibenzo-p-dioxin and related compounds in human adipose tissue, *J Toxicol Environ Health,* 22(4):381, 1987.

17. Chin HB: The effect of processing on residues in foods: the food processing industry's residue database. In Tweedy BG et al, eds: *Pesticide residues and food safety: a harvest of viewpoints,* Symposium Series 446, Washington, DC, 1991, American Chemical Society.
18. Clarkson TW: Human health risks from methylmercury in fish, *Environ Toxicol Chem* 9:957, 1990.
19. Codex Alimentarius Commission: *The microbiological safety of irradiated foods,* Rome, 1983.
20. Cordle F, Kolbye AC: Environmental contaminants in food. In Hathcock JN, ed: *Nutritional toxicology,* New York, 1982, Academic Press.
21. Creighton PJ, Greenberg A, Lioy PJ: The effect of cooking methodology on benzo(a)pyrene exposure from "home-cooked" bacon and hamburgers and "fast-food chain" hamburgers, *J Exposure Anal Environ Epid* 2:27, 1992.
22. Dabeka RW, McKenzie AD, LaCroix GMA: Dietary intakes of lead, cadmium, arsenic and fluoride by Canadian adults: a 24-hour duplicate diet study, *Food Addit Contam* 4:89, 1987.
23. Daniel JW: Phenolic antioxidants. In Walker R, Quatrruci E, eds: *Nutritional and toxicological aspects of food processing: Proceedings of an international symposium, Rome, April 14-16, 1987,* New York, 1988, Taylor & Francis.
24. Diehl JF: *Safety of irradiated foods,* New York, 1990, Marcel Dekker.
25. Downes TW: Practical and theoretical considerations in migration. In Gray JI, Harte BR, Miltz J, eds: *Food product-package compatibility: proceedings of a seminar, July, 1986,* Lancaster, Pa, 1987, Technomic.
26. Elias PS: Wholesomeness of irradiated food. In Walker R, Quatrruci E, eds: *Nutritional and toxicological aspects of food processing: Proceedings of an international symposium, Rome, April 14-16, 1987,* New York, 1988, Taylor & Francis.
27. Environmental Defense Fund (EDF): China makers agree to cut lead 50%, *EDF letter* 24(2):1, 1993.
28. Environmental Protection Agency (EPA): *Air quality criteria for lead,* Cincinnati, Ohio.
29. Food and Drug Administration (FDA): Irradiation in the production, processing, and handling of food: final rule, Federal Register 54:13376, 1986.
30. Giacin JR, Brzozowski A: Analytical measurements of package components from unintentional migrants. In Gray JI, Harte BR, Miltz J, eds: *Food product-package compatibility: proceedings of a seminar, July, 1986,* Lancaster, Pa, 1987, Technomic.
31. Goldman LR, Beller M, Jackson RJ: Aldicarb food poisonings in California, 1985-88: toxicity estimates for humans, *Arch Environ Health* 45(3):141, 1990.
32. Goodman DL et al: Chronic urticaria exacerbated by the antioxidant food preservatives BHA and BHT, *J Allergy Clin Immunol* 86:570, 1990.
33. Gray JI, Harte BE: An overview of food component interaction during processing and storage. In Gray JI, Harte BR, Miltz J, eds: *Food product-package compatibility: proceedings of a seminar, July, 1986,* Lancaster, Pa, 1987, Technomic.
34. Griffith G: Irradiated foods: new technology, old debate, *Trends Food Sci Tech* 3(3):251, 1992 (editorial).
35. Gruenwendel DW: Industrial and environmental chemicals in the human food chain. I. Inorganic chemicals. In Winter CK, Seiber JN, Nuckton CF, eds: *Chemicals in the human food chain,* New York, 1990, Van Nostrand-Reinhold.
36. Hotchkiss JH et al: Nitrate, nitrite, and N-nitroso compounds: food safety and biological implications. In Finley JW, Robinson SF, Armstrong DJ, eds: *Food safety assessment,* Washington DC, 1992, American Chemical Society.
37. International Consultative Group on Food Irradiation: *Facts about food irradiation,* Vienna, Austria, 1991, FAO/WHO/IAEA.
38. Joneja JV, Bielory L: *Understanding allergy, sensitivity, immunity: a comprehensive guide,* New Brunswick, NJ, 1990, Rutgers University Press.
39. Jones JL: Genetic engineering of crops: its relevance to the food industry, *Trends Food Sci Technol* 3:54, 1992.
40. Kaplan B et al: Dietary replacement in preschool-aged hyperactive boys, *Pediatrics* 83:7, 1989.
41. Kirkpatrick DC, Ripley RA, Pelletier MA: Food packaging materials: health implications. In Hathcock JN, ed: *Nutritional toxicology,* vol 3, New York, 1989, Academic Press.
42. Kjellstrom T et al: *Physical and mental development of children with prenatal exposure to mercury from fish,* Report 3080, Solna, Sweden, 1986, National Swedish Environmental Protection Board.
43. Krimsky S, Plough A: *Environmental hazards: communicating risks as a social process,* Dover, Mass, 1988, Auburn House.
44. LaChance P: Diet-health relationship. In Finley JW, Robinson SF, Armstrong DJ, eds: *Food safety assessment,* Washington DC, 1992, American Chemical Society.
45. Lansdown ABG: Teratogenicity and reduced fertility resulting from factors present in food. In Conning DM, Lansdown ADG, eds: *Toxic hazards in food,* New York, 1983, Raven Press.
46. Lechowich RV: Current concerns in food safety. In Finley JW, Robinson SF, Armstrong DJ, eds: *Food safety assessment,* Washington DC, 1992, American Chemical Society.
47. Lindemann J: Biotechologies and food: a summary of major issues regarding safety assurance, *Regul Toxicol Pharmacol* 12:96, 1990.
48. Livingston RC: Antibiotic residues in animal-derived food, *J Assoc Anal Chem* 68:966, 1985.
49. Lombardo P, Yess NJ: The FDA program on pesticide residues in food. In Tweedy BG et al, eds: *Pesticide residues and food safety: a harvest of viewpoints,* Symposium Series 446, Washington, DC, 1991, American Chemical Society.
50. Louekari K, Salminen S: Intake of heavy metals from foods in Finland, West Germany, and Japan, *Food Addit Contam,* 3:355, 1986.
51. Louis JB et al: Pesticide residues measured in fruits and vegetables. In Weigmann DL, ed: *Pesticides in the next decade: the challenges ahead,* Proceedings of the Third National Research Conference on Pesticides, Blacksburg, Va, 1991, Virginia Water Resources Research Center.
52. Mannheim C: Interaction between metal cans and food products. In Gray JI, Harte BR, Miltz J, eds: *Food product-package compatibility: proceedings of a seminar, July, 1986,* Lancaster, Pa, 1987, Technomic.
53. Maxim LD, Harrington L: A review of the Food and Drug Administration risk analysis for polychlorinated biphenyls in fish, *Regul Toxicol Pharmacol* 4:192, 1984.
54. Miller SA: Food additives and contaminants. In Amdur MO, Doull J, Klaassen CD, eds: *Casarett and Doull's toxicology,* ed 4, New York, 1991, Pergamon.
55. Miltz J: Migration of low molecular weight species from packaging materials: theoretical and practical considerations. In Gray JI, Harte BR, Miltz J, eds: *Food product-package compatibility: proceedings of a seminar, July, 1986,* Lancaster, Pa, 1987, Technomic.
56. National Research Council: *Arsenic,* Washington, DC, 1977, National Academy of Sciences.
57. National Research Council, Committee on scientific and regulatory issues underlying pesticide use patterns and agricultural innovation, and Board on Agriculture: *Regulating pesticides in food: the Delaney paradox,* Washington, DC, 1987, National Academy Press.
58. NRC: *Dolphins and the Tuna Industry,* Washington, DC, 1992, National Research Council.
59. National Research Council; *Pesticides in the diet of infants and children,* Washington, DC, 1993, National Academy Press.
60. Natural Resources Defense Council (NRDC): *Intolerable risk: pesticides in our children's food,* New York, 1989.
61. Needleman HL et al: The long-term effects of exposure to low doses of lead in childhood: an 11-year follow-up report, *N Engl J Med* 322:83, 1990.

62. Norman BB, Edmondson AJ: Sources of chemicals in animal products. In Winter CK, Seiber JN, Nuckton CF, eds: *Chemicals in the human food chain,* New York, 1990, Van Nostrand-Reinhold.
63. O'Brien J: Genetic engineering: a rough ride ahead? *Food Sci Technol* 3:53, 1992 (editorial).
64. Oduoza CF: Studies of food value and contaminants in canned foods, *Food Chem* 44:9, 1992.
65. O'Flaherty T: Reducing the risk to human health from radioactivity in the food chain. In *Proceedings of the conference on pure food production: implications of residues and contaminants,* Dublin, 1988, The Agricultural Institute.
66. Oskarssen A, Ohlin B, Ohlander E-M, Albanus L: Mercury levels in hair from people eating large quantities of Swedish freshwater fish, *Food Addit Contam* 7:555, 1990.
67. Paasivirta J et al: Food chain enrichment of organochlorine compounds and mercury in clean and polluted lakes of Finland, *Chemosphere* 12:239, 1993.
68. Pastoni F et al: Organochlorine residues in imported foodstuffs. In Walker R, Quatrruci E, eds: *Nutritional and toxicological aspects of food processing: Proceedings of an international symposium, Rome, April 14-16, 1987,* New York, 1988, Taylor & Francis.
69. Pennington JAT: Aluminum content of foods and diets, *Food Addit Contam* 5:161, 1987.
70. Phelps RW, Clarkson TW, Kershaw TG, Wheatley B: Interrelationships of blood and hair mercury concentrations in a North American population exposed to methylmercury, *Arch Environ Health* 35(3):161, 1980.
71. Pizzoferrato L, Quattrucci E, DiLullo G: Antinutritional effects of sulfites in foods. In Walker R, Quatrruci E, eds: *Nutritional and toxicological aspects of food processing: Proceedings of an international symposium, Rome, April 14-16, 1987,* New York, 1988, Taylor & Francis.
72. Pollard EC: Phenomenology of radiation effects on microorganisms. In Diethelm L et al, eds: *Handbook of medical radiology,* vol 2, New York, 1966, Springer.
73. Reilly C: *Metal contamination of food,* ed 2, London, 1990, Applied Science Publishers.
74. Rogan A, Glaros G: Food irradiation: the process and implications for dieticians, *J Amer Diet Assoc* 88:833, 1988.
75. Rosen JD: Much ado about Alar, *Issues Sci Tech* 85, 1990.
76. Safina, C: Bluefin tuna in the West Atlantic: negligent management and the making of an endangered species. Conserv Biology 7:229-238, 1993.
77. Sawhney BL, Hankin L: Polychlorinated biphenyls in food: a review, *J Food Prot* 48:442, 1985.
78. Schneider K: EPA plans to seek loosening of a law on food pesticides, *New York Times,* Feb 2, 1993, p 1.
79. Scroggins CD: Consumer attitudes toward the use of pesticides and food safety. In Tweedy BG et al, eds: *Pesticide residues and food safety: a harvest of viewpoints,* Symposium Series 446, Washington, DC, 1991, American Chemical Society.
80. Seiber J: Industrial and environmental chemicals in the human food chain. II. Organic chemicals. In Winter CK, Seiber JN, Nuckton CF, eds: *Chemicals in the human food chain,* New York, 1990, Van Nostrand-Reinhold.
81. Senti FR: Food additives and contaminants. In Shills ME, Young VR, eds: *Modern nutrition in health and disease,* ed 7, Philadelphia, 1988, Lea & Febiger.
82. Shank FR, Carson KL: What is safe food? In Finley JW, Robinson SF, Armstrong DJ, editors: *Food safety assessment,* Washington, DC, 1992, American Chemical Society.
83. Sherlock JC et al: Duplication diet study on mercury intake by fish consumers in the United Kingdom, *Arch Environ Health* 37(5):271, 1982.
84. Sherlock JC, Smart GA: Tin in foods and the diet, *Food Addit Contam* 1:271, 1984.
85. Shubat P: *Health risk assessment for the consumption of sport fish contaminated with mercury, PCB, and TCDD,* Minnesota Dept. of Health, Jan., 1991, Minneapolis, Minn.
86. Stoewsand GS: Trace metal problems with industrial waste materials applied to vegetable producing soils. In Graham HD, ed: *The safety of foods,* ed 2, Westport, Conn, 1980, AVI Publishing.
87. Sun M: Designing food by engineering animals, *Science* 240:136, 1988.
88. Thayer AM: Food additives, *Chem Eng News* 26-44, June 15, 1992.
89. Tollefson L, Cordle F: Methylmercury in fish: a review of residue levels, fish consumption and regulatory action in the United States, *Environ Health Perspect* 68:203, 1986.
90. Tsuchiya K: The discovery of the causal agent of Minamata disease, *Am J Ind Med* 21:275, 1992.
91. US Environmental Protection Agency (EPA): *Assessing human health risks from chemically contaminated fish and shellfish: a guidance manual,* Washington, DC, Sept. 1989.
92. US Public Health Service: *A Public Health Service progress report on Healthy People 2000: nutrition,* Washington, DC, 1992, US Dept. of Health and Human Services.
93. Waldman JM et al: Analysis of human exposure to benzo(a)pyrene via inhalation and food ingestion in the Total Human Environmental Exposure Study (THEES), *J Exposure Anal Environ Epid* 1:193, 1991.
94. Walker R: Toxicological aspects of food preservatives. In Walker R, Quatrruci E, eds: *Nutritional and toxicological aspects of food processing: Proceedings of an international symposium, Rome, April 14-16, 1987,* New York, 1988, Taylor & Francis.
95. Weisel C, Demak M, Marcus S, Goldstein BD: Soft plastic bread packaging: lead content and reuse by families, *Am J Public Health* 81:756, 1991.
96. World Health Organization (WHO): *Environmental health criteria 3: lead,* Geneva, 1976.
97. World Health Organization (WHO): *Wholesomeness of irradiated foods,* Technical Report Series 659, Geneva, 1981.
98. World Health Organization (WHO): *Environmental health criteria 101,* Geneva, 1990.
99. Yess NJ, Houston MG, Gunderson EL: Food and Drug Administration pesticide residue monitoring of foods: 1983-1986, *J Assoc Off Anal Chem* 74:273, 1991.
100. York GK, Gruenwendel SHO: Food additives in the human food chain. In Winter CK, Seiber JN, Nuckton CF, eds: *Chemicals in the human food chain,* New York, 1990, Van Nostrand-Reinhold.
101. Zabik ME, Harte JB, Zabik MJ: Effects of preparation and cooking on PCB distributions in blue crabs. NJ Dept Environ Prot Energy, Research Project Summary, 1992.

Chapter 44

NATURAL CARCINOGENS AND ANTICARCINOGENS IN THE DIET

Randy L. Shuler
Jeffrey D. Laskin

Diet has been found to be one of the leading contributors to the development of human cancers. Carcinogenic compounds occur in foods of many kinds, particularly in those of plant origin. Foods also contain a large variety of compounds that help protect the body against the harmful effects of carcinogenic compounds. A *carcinogen* is any substance that can initiate the development of cancer. Many carcinogens arise through metabolic activation of an exogenous compound in the liver or a sensitive tissue.[16,17] Any factor that can enhance the development of previously damaged cells into cancerous cells is often referred to as a *tumor promoter*. Tumor promoters are not necessarily carcinogenic by themselves. Compounds that block or suppress these effects are considered to be *anticarcinogens* or *antitumor promoters*. Genetic and environmental influences excluded, the possibility of the development of human cancers from carcinogenic agents found in the diet may depend on the critical balance of carcinogens and anticarcinogens that are consumed and metabolized.

Foods contain numerous naturally occurring carcinogens. Several examples of these are listed in Table 44-1.[2] Aflatoxin, one of the most potent carcinogens known, is present in mold-contaminated foods such as cheese, corn, fruits, and nuts. The chlorogenic acid present in coffee is not only a natural mutagen but also an antinitrosating agent, thereby acting as both a carcinogen and an anticarcinogen. Many hydrazine carcinogens act by producing reactive oxygen species, and nitrates are involved in the formation of nitrosamines and other nitroso compounds. When activated by sunlight, the psoralens damage deoxyribonucleic acid (DNA) directly and also produce oxygen radicals. Quercetin has been found to be genotoxic in a number of experimental systems.[9] It is easy to visualize the potential for widespread tumorigenesis that could result solely from eating food, were there not mechanisms to counteract the effects of these dietary carcinogens.

The process of cooking foods also has been found to generate many carcinogenic compounds. Several examples provide a perspective on the different types of reactions occurring in cooked foods.[2] The caramelization of sucrose by slow heating leads to the formation of hydroxymethylfuraldehyde. Heterocyclic aromatic amines are formed by the Maillard-Browning reaction when meats are cooked.[6,13,17] Heating serine and threonine residues gives rise to acrylamide cross-linkages in proteins. Unsaturated fatty acids and cholesterols in fat are easily oxidized to mutagens and carcinogens by heating. The products of this rancidity reaction include fatty acid and cholesterol hydroperoxides and epoxides, endoperoxides, enols and other aldehydes, and alkoxy and hydroperoxy radicals.[2]

Anticarcinogens can be classified into three groups based on their mechanism of action. The first group are compounds that prevent the formation of carcinogens from precursors. Some examples include ascorbic acid (vitamin C) and α-tocopherol (vitamin E). The second group is composed of compounds that prevent carcinogenic substances from reaching or reacting with critical target sites in the tissue and are termed *blocking agents*. Blocking can occur by prevent-

Table 44-1. Dietary sources of carcinogens

Food source	Carcinogen
Beets, spinach	Nitrates
Celery, parsley, limes	Psoralens
Coffee	Chlorogenic acid
Food molds	Aflatoxin
Fruits, vegetables	Quercetin
Mushrooms	Hydrazines

Table 44-2. Common dietary sources of anticarcinogens

Food source	Anticarcinogen
Allium species (garlic, onions, leeks, and shallots)	Organosulfur compounds
Beans and seeds	Protease inhibitors
Citrus fruit oils	Terpenes
Cruciferous vegetables	Indoles, isothiocyanates, dithiolethiones
Green tea	Epigallocatechin

Table 44-3. Anticarcinogenic blocking agents and suppressing agents found in foods

Blocking agents	Suppressing agents
β-Carotene	β-Carotene
Curcumin	D-limonene
Flavones	Protease inhibitors
Indoles	Retinoids
Organosulfides	Selenium
Tannins	Vitamin A

ing the metabolic activation of carcinogens, by increasing detoxification, or by trapping reactive carcinogenic species. Many blocking agents acting against tumor promoters do so by preventing oxygen radical formation or trapping those that are formed.[19] The third group is the suppressing agents, which act by suppressing the development of neoplasia in cells previously exposed to carcinogens.[19]

Table 44-2 provides a brief list of several common sources of dietary anticarcinogenic compounds.[19] The anticarcinogens are further broken down into either blocking agents or suppressing agents in Table 44-3.[19] The mechanisms of action of these anticarcinogens are many and varied. Some of the dietary antioxidants are mentioned herein. Vitamins C[3] and E[12] and β-carotene shield lipid membranes from oxidative damage.[20] Dietary glutathione is effective against both oxidative and alkylating carcinogens and is an effective anticarcinogen against aflatoxin.[2] Selenium protects against lipid peroxidation by activating glutathione peroxidase, which destroys hydrogen peroxide and lipid hydroperoxides.[8]

The beneficial properties of dietary fiber also deserve mention. It has been well established that dietary fiber increases that transit time of foods through the digestive system. Wheat bran and cellulose, in particular, have a protective effect against the development of cancers of the colon, because of their low fermentability.[1,5] The products of fermentation of fibers such as pectin and guar are acetate, propionate, and butyrate (short-chain fatty acids). The physiologic consequences arising from these fermentation products are decreased colonic pH, decreased dilution potential, and increased cell proliferation, all factors that may lead to cancer of the colon.[10,11]

There has been much recent emphasis on the beneficial properties of food extracts such as green tea. Polyphenolic extracts of green tea have been shown to inhibit several different types of cancers.[4,14,18] Some of the components of green tea are epigallocatechin, flavonols, and catechin, which possess potent antioxidant activity. Curcumin, flavones, and tannins are protective against carcinogens through inhibition of the arachidonic acid cascade, prevention of oxidative damage, or modulation of hormonal responses.[19] The broad group of organosulfides increases the activity of hepatic phase II enzymes and induces glutathione S-transferase activity. Similarly, indoles also stimulate glutathione S-transferase activity.[19]

Other anticarcinogens act via different mechanisms. D-Limonene and the other terpenes induce hepatic phase I and phase II detoxification enzymes and cytochrome P-450 enzymes.[7] Ornithine decarboxylase activity is induced by the retinoids. Vitamin A deficiency leads to increased DNA synthesis and mitotic activity in epithelial cells.[16] These are but a few of the ways in which the anticarcinogens neutralize the effects of carcinogenic agents.

CONCLUSION

Carcinogens in the foods that are eaten are probably the most important risk factors that human populations encounter.[15] A major focus for prevention of cancer has been directed toward understanding dietary carcinogens and anticarcinogens. There is certainly a wide variety of both carcinogens and anticarcinogens in the foods we consume. The delicate balance between these harmful and beneficial agents is maintained better in some individuals than in others. Some develop cancer, but others do not. There should be error on the side of precaution with attempts to consume more foods containing anticarcinogens to improve the chance that cancer does not develop.

REFERENCES

1. Alberts DS et al: Effects of dietary wheat bran on rectal epithelial cell proliferation in patients with resection for colorectal cancers, *J Natl Cancer Inst* 82:1280, 1990.
2. Ames BN: Dietary carcinogens and anticarcinogens: oxygen radicals and degenerative diseases, *Science* 221:1256, 1983.

3. Chen LH, Boissonneault GA, Glauert HP: Vitamin C, vitamin E and cancer, *Anticancer Res* 8:739, 1988.
4. Conney AH et al: Inhibitory effect of green tea on tumorigenesis and tumor growth in mouse skin. In Huang M-T, Ho C-T, Lee CY, eds: *Phenolic compounds in food and their effects on health. II. Antioxidants and cancer prevention,* Washington, DC, 1992, American Chemical Society.
5. DeCosse JJ, Miller HH, Lesser ML: Effect of wheat fiber and vitamins C and E on rectal polyps in patients with familial adenomatous polyposis, *J Natl Cancer Inst* 81:1290, 1989.
6. Felton JS, Knize MG: New mutagens from cooked food. In Pariza MW et al, eds: *Mutagens and carcinogens in the diet,* New York, 1990, Wiley-Liss.
7. Gould MN: Chemoprevention and treatment of experimental mammary cancers by limonene, *Proc Am Assoc Cancer Res* 32:474, 1991.
8. Hocman G: Chemoprevention of cancer: selenium, *Int J Biochem* 20:123, 1988.
9. Huang M-T, Ferraro T: Phenolic compounds in food and cancer prevention. In Huang M-T, Ho C-T, Lee CY, eds: *Phenolic compounds in food and their effects on health. II. Antioxidants and cancer prevention,* Washington, DC, 1992, American Chemical Society.
10. Jacobs LR: Fiber and colon cancer, *Gastroenterol Clin North Am* 17:747, 1988.
11. Jenkins DJ et al: Starchy foods, type of fiber, and cancer risk, *Prev Med* 16:545, 1987.
12. Knekt P: Role of vitamin E in the prophylaxis of cancer, *Ann Med* 23:3, 1991.
13. Larsen JC et al: New mutagens from cooked food. In Pariza MW et al, eds: *Mutagens and carcinogens in the diet,* New York, 1990, Wiley-Liss.
14. Laskin JD et al: Inhibitory effect of a green tea polyphenol fraction on 12-*O*-tetradecanoylphorbol-13-acetate-induced hydrogen peroxide formation in mouse epidermis. In Huang, M-T, Ho C-T, Lee CY, eds: *Phenolic compounds in food and their effects on health. II. Antioxidants and cancer prevention,* Washington, DC, 1992, American Chemical Society.
15. Newberne PM, Conner MW: Dietary modifiers of cancer, *Prog Clin Biol Res* 259:105, 1988.
16. Shils ME: Nutrition and diet in cancer. In Shils ME, Young VR, eds: *Modern nutrition in health and disease,* ed 7, Philadelphia, 1988, Lea & Febiger.
17. Sugimura T, Wakabayashi K: Mutagens and carcinogens in food. In Pariza MW et al, eds: *Mutagens and carcinogens in the diet,* New York, 1990, Wiley-Liss.
18. Wang ZY et al: Inhibition of nitrosamine-induced tumorigenesis by green tea and black tea. In Huang M-T, Ho C-T, Lee CY, eds: *Phenolic compounds in food and their effects on health. II. Antioxidants and cancer prevention,* Washington DC, 1992, American Chemical Society.
19. Wattenberg LW: Chemoprevention of cancer by naturally occurring and synthetic compounds. In Wattenberg L et al, eds: *Cancer chemoprevention,* Boca Raton, Fla, 1992, CRC Press.
20. Weisburger JH: Nutritional approach to cancer prevention with emphasis on vitamins, antioxidants, and carotenoids, *Am J Clin Nutr* 53(suppl):26S, 1991.

Chapter 45

SOIL: SOURCES, DYNAMICS, AND ROUTES OF EXPOSURE

Michael Gochfeld

Exposure to soil contaminants
Types or classes of soil
Physical and chemical properties of soil
Soil profiles
Aquifers
Hardpans and laterites
Sediments
Sources of contamination of soil and groundwater
    Natural contaminants in soil
    Industrial waste
    Leachate from landfills
    Landfills and soil and water pollution
    Sludge disposal
Leachate treatment
Soils and siting
Soil percolation tests
Environmental fate and transport
Soil and sewage
Bioavailability
Plant uptake of contaminants from soil
Contaminants in soil
    Naturally occurring metals
    Petroleum hydrocarbons
    Chlorinated polyaromatics: dioxins and polychlorinated biphenyls
Soil as a source of human exposure
    Direct contact with soil
    Airborne contamination from soil
    Water contamination from soil
    Contamination of food
Methods for evaluating soil contamination
    Soil sampling
    Priority pollutant scan
    Analytic techniques
Conclusion

The soil that underlies forests, fields, factories, and towns is the repository of critical nutrients that support agriculture and a medium through which humans and other organisms experience exposure to both natural and synthetic chemicals. Far from its apparent inertness and stability, soil is a dynamic, complex, and highly variable medium. Soils are derived from rocks, and the distinction between soil and rock is somewhat arbitrary.[28] The term *soil* applies broadly to the nonconsolidated component of the earth's crust. Soils are defined by their physical and chemical properties and are classified by their profiles. Toxic chemicals enter soil either directly (dumping or pumping of wastes or as runoff or leachate) or indirectly by airborne deposition (fallout) of particulate matter. Contaminants are removed from soil to air by evaporation, volatilization, or generation of dust. They are removed to surface water and groundwater by runoff and leaching, respectively. They can be taken up by plants or ingested directly by animals, including humans.

The movement of contaminants through soil is called a *plume*. Plumes move both downward and laterally, but it is the lateral movement that can carry contaminants miles from the source. Movement depends on properties of the soil water and on the chemicals and can be very complex and difficult to measure. A hazardous waste site, for example, may contaminate soil with many different chemicals, some of which do not move at all whereas others may move at different speeds, albeit almost always in the same direction. Hydrologists are specialists who study how contaminants move through the soil water.

The ancient Greeks recognized earth as one of the four

essential humors, and today we recognize it as one of the four essential media (air, water, soil, food) through which humans and other organisms are exposed to toxic substances.[18] There is a substantial body of literature on the relation of soil to health; however, much of this literature focuses on the availability of essential trace nutrients rather than on toxicants, for example the valuable monograph by Hopps and Cannon.[13]

Depending on geography and climate, the surface of soil may be barren or covered in vegetation, and it may be substantially altered by human activities ranging from agriculture to pavement or construction. The soil itself may be rich in living plants and animals. Rootlets of plants penetrate the upper layers of soil, and microscopic nematodes and macroscopic earthworms constantly move the soil particles and reconstitute the organic matter. A particularly clear chapter on the ecologic properties of soil is provided by Smith.[27]

Historically, physical and chemical forces, including glaciation, climatic change, erosion, and freezing, have disrupted and pulverized rock into various-sized particles in sizes ranging from nearly 1 cm (coarse gravels) to less than 1 μm (clay particles). The properties of soil depend on this primary structural and chemical composition, the presence and type of organic matter, the vertical profile, the slope, the underlying water and overlying vegetation, and land use.

EXPOSURE TO SOIL CONTAMINANTS

A review of the Exposure Matrix (see Chapter 1) shows that exposure to soil can involve direct dermal contact, ingestion (particularly in children), or inhalation (generation of fine dust producing respirable airborne particulate matter). At first none of these routes seems particularly serious. Most environmental contaminants are only slightly absorbed through the skin; few people other than toddlers ingest appreciable amounts of dirt; and inhalation of dust hardly seems a problem in most urbanized places.

Yet under certain circumstances and for certain chemicals, each of these routes can play an important role in contributing to Total Human Exposure.[3] The ingestion of soil by children proves to be the major route of concern when risk assessments for many soil contaminants are performed.[3,11] When ingestion of household dust (indoor soil) is added, soil can be a very prominent medium and route of exposure.

TYPES OR CLASSES OF SOIL

Soil results from the breakdown of rock, the movement of sand, or the compression of mud. Sedimentary rocks such as sandstones and shales are often freely permeable to water, but igneous (volcanic origin) or metamorphic (slates, marble) rocks are often impermeable and form a bedrock that can at least partly protect underlying aquifers from contamination. Water and leachate move readily through sedimentary formations and along surfaces or fissues through bedrock.

Soils are generally not purely of one particle type. They vary from coarse gravels to sands, loams, and clays, the latter having the smallest particle size. The physical and chemical properties of soil are important. Soils differ in their density and compactness and in their saturation or potential saturation (porosity) by water. Clay's behavior is very different depending on whether it is dry or wet, shrinking and cracking when it is dry and swelling and becoming rubbery when wet. The presence of organic matter is important because organics avidly bind certain chemicals, particularly metals, while increasing the water-holding capacity of soil.

A special type of saturated soil is the sediment on the bottom of bodies of water. Saturated with water and often rich in incompletely decomposed organic matter, these sediments are often a trap for chemical contaminants that in turn have significant impacts on aquatic ecosystems and on humans who exploit their resources.

PHYSICAL AND CHEMICAL PROPERTIES OF SOIL

Depending on the local water table and on its depth, a soil may be saturated or unsaturated. The saturated (vadose) zone's properties are very different from those of the unsaturated zone. The latter has extensive air spaces in which gaseous material may be present. The vadose comprises the zone immediately over the water table or aquifer. Soil water is important in both zones. Chemical interactions between soil particulates and dissolved or volatile material are important aspects of soil chemistry.

Drainage is a property of soil. On the microscopic level drainage is the rate at which the soil pores avoid saturation. On the gross scale it is the amount of water that flows out of the soil and is a function of the moisture content and of air spaces and organic content present. Drainage comprises runoff, internal drainage, and permeability. Runoff depends on the slope, and permeability is a function of soil type and structure. The internal soil drainage determines the downward movement of water through the soil and hence its potential for leaching soluble components.

Drainage characteristics are one basis for soil classification by the U.S. Department of Agriculture. There are seven grades, from excessively drained to well drained to poorly and very poorly drained. There is an entire science of soil classification. The color of a soil often indicates its drainage: reds and yellows reflect good drainage, and grays and green reflect poor drainage with little aeration.

SOIL PROFILES

From the most superficial layer of humus downward, soil is classified by a profile with typically four horizons—O, A, B, and C—each with its subdivisions. The most superficial is the O, or organic, horizon, including the leaf litter and the

Table 45-1. Classifications and descriptions of soils

Classes	Description	Permeability
Coarse grained		
Gravels	Gravel or gravel-sand	Excellent
	Silty or clay gravels	Fair-poor
Sands	Sands	Excellent
	Silty or clay sands	Fair-poor
	Inorganic silts, clay	Fair-poor
Fine grained		
Silts/clay	Clays	Fair-poor
Organic	Peat	Variable

From Brunner DR, Keller DJ: *Sanitary landfill design and operation,* Washington, DC, 1972, US Environmental Protection Agency.

humus. The A horizon, usually within 0.5 m of the surface, is dynamic and is altered by organic matter and water entering from above, which tends to leach out iron and aluminum minerals. The B horizon, usually poorer in organic matter, is likewise influenced by physical processes, and the lower C horizon, or subsoil, is usually paler, generally much thicker in cross-section, and the most stable. In many agricultural and urban areas tillage and construction have greatly altered the natural profile of soils by introducing fill, gravel, or cement or simply by mixing horizons together. Table 45-1 provides a classification and description of soil types.

AQUIFERS

Aquifers are underground reservoirs of water. Their size may be many square kilometers. Sandy soils with abundant interstices or bedrock with openings and fissures may allow accumulation of water. The porosity of rock or soil (percentage of voids or total volume available for water) and its permeability to water (size and connection of pores) are important physical features. Although single openings or fissures may be small, the cumulative volume in a given region can be huge, providing abundant volume for water retention. The shape of soil grains have a major influence on porosity and permeability, and permeability is a nonlinear function of porosity.[28] The water chambers communicate with one another so that contamination at one point in an aquifer may eventually spread, albeit slowly by diffusion, throughout the aquifer.

Coarse sands and gravelly soil or fractured lava provide the most copious aquifers and yield high quantities of water when tapped for municipal supplies or private wells. Silty or clayey soils are very dense, with negligible interstices, and tend to contain little water. Likewise, most metamorphic and igneous rocks have low permeability.

In certain areas an impermeable rock formation traps water below it under pressure, giving rise to an artesian water supply. Alternatively the upper boundary of the saturated zone may contain porous material that holds water by capillarity. This zone does not yield water for wells.

HARDPANS AND LATERITES

Certain soils with very small particle size not only are nearly impermeable to water but are sufficiently compact to interfere with digging and drilling. Roots cannot penetrate these layers, and the resulting hardpan acts in effect as a bedrock. A special case of hardpan occurs when tropical soils undergo laterization. In the absence of alternation of freezing and thawing, hydrologic and chemical processes primarily alter the soil in the tropics. The percolation of rainwater through the soil carries away soluble organic and inorganic matter, leaving behind an excess of insoluble oxides of iron and aluminum that tends to coagulate into a cementlike layer just below the soil surface.

This impermeable layer resists manual agricultural practices and soon impairs the agricultural properties of exposed tropical soils. It is a major limitation to the productivity of tropical soils and contributes to their inability to support the growing population. (See Chapter 61.) This in turn promotes the shifting slash-and-burn life-style because, once cleared, a small tropical farm may have a useful life span of less than a decade, after which it is abandoned for adjacent forest; however, regeneration of forest is slow on the remaining, fertility-deplete hardpan.

SEDIMENTS

A special and important soil is the layer of soil on the bottom of bodies of water, often referred to as the *sediment* because it is actively augmented by the accumulation of organic and inorganic material. The physical properties of sediment can be very variable, but it is saturated with water and can contain very high concentrations of pollutants. Aquatic plants are rooted in this material, and bottom-dwelling (benthic) organisms such as crabs also live there. Sediments are rich in microorganisms, many of which are tolerant of anaerobic conditions and can alter the properties of chemicals. For example, anaerobic bacteria protect themselves from the toxic effects of mercury by methylating it, thereby creating a new pollutant (methylmercury) that bioaccumulates and is generally more toxic to other organisms than was the parent compound.[6] Aquatic organisms such as shrimp readily accumulate contaminants such as PCBs and may be a source of human contamination.[21]

SOURCES OF CONTAMINATION OF SOIL AND GROUNDWATER
Natural contaminants in soil

The earth's crust contains naturally occurring minerals, many of which are toxic. A soil analysis that identifies the presence of a metal, for example, mercury, does not distinguish whether the source is natural weathering of rock, volcanic desposition, or an artificial cause such as automotive emissions or industrial waste. Ramos-Perez et al[24] showed both freshwater and estuarine contamination from metal-rich bedrock in the Virgin Islands. In general, levels of iron, magnesium, and manganese were the highest; however, lead, cadmium, and mercury levels were not reported. Some soils are very rich in arsenic, for example, but others are rich in nickel.

Industrial waste

Industrial waste can contaminate soil both on and off the site. Many industrial facilities dispose of toxic waste on their property. Liquid waste is usually stored in ponds or lagoons, the bottom of which eventually accumulates a sediment with high concentrations of toxic materials. In other cases the waste may have leaked out of drums or may simply have been piled on the ground. Industrial waste has also been transported off site for disposal in what have become de facto hazardous waste sites. Some are indoor facilities such as warehouses in which drums of waste have been stockpiled over a period of years. Others are landfills, and a few are managed as hazardous waste sites. Illegal dumping of hazardous waste has posed a problem, and in some notorious cases tank trucks have simply allowed waste to leak onto road shoulders, contaminating the adjacent soil.

Leachate from landfills

Although municipal landfills are often contaminated with industrial waste or sewage sludge, even "pure" garbage contains metals and other chemicals that can cause soil or water contamination. A study of five municipal landfills showed great variability among sites in metal contamination of leachate. Leachate from all five sites had excessive levels of lead, selenium, iron, and mercury. The concentration of zinc declined with the age of the site. Although the leachate exceeded drinking-water standards, the concentration would generally be diluted when the leachate actually reached a surface water or groundwater supply. Concentrations of metals in leachate moving downward through the unsaturated zone are lowered as metals adsorb to soil particles. This study demonstrated that municipal landfills have the potential to degrade water quality severely.[15]

Landfills and soil and water pollution

Although landfilling is being phased out as the standard means of refuse disposal in the United States, landfills will still be used in specialized circumstances, for example, disposal of incinerator ash. When a former landfill is closed, it is capped with a layer of soil that is then vegetated, in part to stabilize the cap and to reduce the permeation by rainfall or surface water into the landfill material. Water that enters the landfill material can carry toxins laterally off-site or downward into the water table or aquifer. Groundwater is present in the saturated area of soil, and its level varies considerably from place to place and season to season. In general, the upper boundary of the saturated zone is the water table.

Although regulatory responsibility for water pollution does not usually include responsibility for soil contamination, it is apparent that the two are closely connected, soil serving as a source for contamination of water and water as a vehicle for distribution of contamination more widely through soil.

Sludge disposal

Sludge is the semisolid residue that remains after the treatment of sewage and the pumping out of treated water. After 1991 municipalities in the United States were required to find alternatives to ocean dumping of sludge, and application to land became attractive, with or without initial incineration or chemical coagulation. Sludge is rich in organic matter but may also contain various toxic metals, including cadmium, chromium, cobalt, copper, nickel, mercury, and lead. The use of sludge as a fertilizer is questioned because some of these contaminants may be taken up by plants grown or animals grazed on the sludge-amended soil. The hazard depends on the type of sludge and its constituents. Primary, or raw, sludge is the residue of primary waste-water treatment. Secondary treatment, after the settling-out of bacteria-treated, flocculated organic matter, yields activated sludge. Further aerobic, anaerobic, or thermal treatment enhances the decomposition of organic compounds into simpler components, yielding stabilized sludge. High concentrations of metals preclude the use of sludge as a fertilizer for food crops, but the sludge may remain suitable for lawns, shrubs, golf courses, and other uses.

Soil properties also influence the suitability of sludge disposal. Steeply sloping substrates allow rapid extraction of toxins by surface water runoff before the sludge can be stabilized by vegetation. Soils rich in clays tend to have poor aeration and poor drainage and are likely to result in odors as the sludge undergoes further decomposition.[17] (Further details on sludge and on composting of sludge are provided later in Chapter 59.)

LEACHATE TREATMENT

Several technologic approaches are used to treat leachate. It can be purified by ion exchange, biodegradation, filtration, or some combination of adsorption or precipitation; however, prevention of leachate formation and conduction, by adequate coverage of the surface, placement of impermeable barriers, and avoidance of soluble contaminants, is cheaper in the long run and more desirable.

SOILS AND SITING

Health professionals frequently are called on to assist ha community in evaluating proposed siting of potentially hazardous or socially undesirable facilities such as waste-disposal sites, incinerators, and manufacturing facilities. Hydrologic and soil issues often play important roles in determining the utility or safe use of a site. In some cases soil permeability is a desirable feature, but in most cases the presence of bedrock and the isolation of the site from aquifers are the desirable features. Soil characteristics are particularly important in the development of underground storage being considered for disposal of hazardous radioactive wastes. In that case the likelihood that earthquakes may disrupt the integrity of deep-rock storage sites becomes important and is usually the limiting factor.

SOIL PERCOLATION TESTS

In many rural and suburban jurisdictions a permit to build a home on a plot of land is contingent on passing a soil percolation test. The purpose is to ensure that the soil can adequately handle a septic field. A series of six or more uniformly spaced 12-inch-deep test holes is made. Once the hole has been made, the walls of the hole are cleared to ensure a natural interface, and loose material is removed. The surrounding soil is then saturated with water. Subsequently the hole is filled with 6 inches of water, and the disappearance of water is measured over a 30-minute period, providing a semiquantitative estimate of the permeability of soil at the period of greatest water saturation.

ENVIRONMENTAL FATE AND TRANSPORT

Contaminants in soil may be present in the vapor phase in the soil interstices, dissolved in soil water, adherent to soil particulates, bound to micelles, or as solids distributed among the soil grains. The chemical and physical state determines not only the fate and transport of the contaminant but how readily it is taken up by plants or absorbed through the skin and respiratory and intestinal tracts of animals or humans that contact it.

A contaminant entering soil may undergo change or degradation either rapidly or over time. Degradation may proceed spontaneously or may require one or more of the following: moisture, light, ultraviolet light, oxygen, the proper pH, heat, and specific chemical substances. For example, manganese oxides, abundant in the earth's crust, are capable of oxidizing chromium from the trivalent to the more dangerous hexavalent state.

An important feature of soil pollution is the length of time that a toxic chemical remains in the soil. A contaminant may be moved away by physical processes or may be degraded or changed by chemical or biologic processes. It is customary to describe the half-life of a chemical in the soil, although this half-life is actually known for very few chemicals. Half-lives vary with many factors, and the degradation may not follow first-order kinetics, so published half-lives[14] are only approximations. Half-lives may vary greatly, ranging from a few days for volatile organics near the surface and 1000 days for chrysene[17] to about 10 years for dioxins.

The persistence of a chemical in soil is influenced by biologic factors (microorganisms, plants); chemical factors (pH, water, ligands, reactive chemicals); and physical factors (particle size, compactness). Microorganisms, sunlight, chemical reactants, and spontaneous reactions may chemically alter a contaminant, particularly in the upper layers of soil. Plants remove some chemicals and alter others. Volatile compounds may saturate air spaces in soil or leave the soil surface to enter the air. Liquid contaminants may evaporate, and solid or liquid contaminants may become airborne as mists or dusts when the soil surface is disturbed, such as by construction or even hazardous waste clean-up activities.

Contaminants are carried through soil by both downward and lateral movement of water through the soil. Leachate movement is affected by the soil properties and the bedrock. Precipitation impinges on the surface. Some precipitation moves laterally over the surface (runoff), and some enters the surface, where it may be taken up by plants or may continue to move downward and laterally, dissolving some materials, which it carries with it as leachate. Groundwater seeks paths through porous or cracked rocks, moving by gravity or diffusion.

Evapotranspiration is an important environmental variable influenced by the soil, the soil-air interface, and the climate. Soil moisture must be present near the surface. Vegetation may take up the moisture and emit it through the leaves, or water may evaporate directly from the surface. Hot temperatures facilitate evapotranspiration.

SOIL AND SEWAGE

The same properties that allow soil to conduct contaminants allow it to serve as a medium for the dissipation and degradation of sewage. In developed nations most rural homes (and many in small communities) are served by a combination of septic tanks and sewage field. Natural aeration is an important aspect of sewage field soils, and compaction or clogging of the soil pores can interfere with the function of the field. The use of solvents and detergents can greatly reduce the percolation rate through soil.[17]

BIOAVAILABILITY

An animal or person may come in direct contact with contaminated soil, may accidently or deliberately ingest it, or may inhale dust particles when the superficial soil (technically referred to as *surficial*) is disturbed; however, this contact exposure alone is not sufficient to ensure that material reaches the bloodstream and is distributed to target organs. The ability to pass through the skin (dermal uptake), the alveoli, and the intestinal tract depends on the substance and its matrix. The ease with which the contaminant can be extracted from the soil and gain access to the blood is termed *bioavailability*, which depends on the unique properties of each chemical and varies with its chemical and physical state and the properties of the soil, including its organic and water contents.

Many metals salts, such as some chromium compounds, for example, are relatively insoluble in water and have low bioavailability through the skin and intestine. They may be extracted from dust particles deposited in the alveoli, however. Similarly, much of the lead and arsenic occurring as contaminants in soil around mining sites are in a relatively insoluble form with low bioavailability.[9]

Umbreit et al[29] showed that even high levels of dioxin contamination in soil from a Newark, New Jersey, herbicide factory had lower bioavailability than that of similar levels in the more sandy soil of Times Beach, Missouri.[30]

PLANT UPTAKE OF CONTAMINANTS FROM SOIL

Plants extract nutrients from soil through their roots. An extensive agricultural science has investigated the extraction of nutrients such as nitrogen, phosphorus, and potassium from various kinds of soil, and the modifying effect of one substance on the uptake (or bioavailability) of another has been investigated extensively.

Much less is known about the bioavailability and extraction of toxicants from soil. The soil composition and chemistry, including the local concentration of a toxicant in the vicinity of root hairs, determines the uptake of the toxic substance. Matters are seldom simple, however, because the roots are capable of modifying the soil in their immediate vicinity and biochemical processes may selectively concentrate certain chemicals or protect against the uptake of others.

CONTAMINANTS IN SOIL

This section covers a small selection of the many contaminants that can be found in soil. Others are dealt with in Chapter 53.

Naturally occurring metals

Although all but the heaviest elements occur naturally in the earth's crust, some, such as iron, aluminum, silicon, chromium, vanadium, zinc, and copper, are particularly abundant. Iron-rich soils, for example, may contain more than 50,000 ppm. Many of these elements have natural biogeochemical cycles, but most of these cycles have been altered by human activities that speed the release of elements by mining, refining, and smelting them.

Mercury. Mercury is widespread in the earth's crust, although mineable levels occur in only a few countries. The main commercial mercury ore is mercuric sulfide (cinnabar).[22] Natural processes such as erosion and volcanic activity release mercury into the atmosphere; however, approximately 80% of mercury measured in the environment comes from human activities.[23] Inorganic mercurial compounds can be methylated by naturally occurring bacteria, particularly in the relatively anaerobic conditions of sediments in the bottom of bodies of water. The resulting methyl mercury compounds are lipid soluble and tend to bioaccumulate in fish, thereby resulting in significant human exposure.[7] The highest concentrations of mercury generally occur in the upper levels of soil, probably a result of airborne deposition.[4]

Industrial sites that manufacture mercurial products may produce substantial contamination. For example, an abandoned mercurial factory in northern New Jersey caused sediment and soil contamination with concentrations of as high as 18,000 ppm (18% mercury).

Chromium. Chromium may be present in soil in various forms, including both trivalent and hexavalent. There is a strong tendency for trivalent chromium to be oxidized to hexavalent in soil, because of reaction with abundant manganese compounds; however, the chromium may originally have been deposited in the hexavalent form as dichromate salts, which can be completely insoluble, moderately soluble, or highly soluble,[5] depending on the positive ion (for example, sodium, potassium, or calcium).

Hudson County in northeastern New Jersey was home to several major chromate and bichromate producers until the mid-1970s. Chromite ore containing about 50% chromium was processed, and about 2 million tons of the chromate waste (containing as much as 7% chromium) was used as construction fill in more than 180 sites. Many sites have soil concentrations of chromium exceeding 5000 ppm, and at least four sites had levels above 25,000 ppm.[8] Children living in residences built on such soil showed elevated urine chromium levels.[20] Lessons learned from a study of this site include that (1) hexavalent chromium is the most soluble form and poses the health hazard; (2) even if most of the soil chromium consists of trivalent compounds, they may be oxidized to hexavalent under appropriate conditions; (3) high urinary chromium levels may indicate ongoing exposure, but levels return to normal within a few weeks after exposure ceases; and (4) to date there is no documented increased cancer risk attributed to community exposure to chromium in soil.

Lead. Soil contamination by lead poses a significant health hazard, particularly for children. Lead may result from former industrial activities, from battery reclamation, from airborne deposition, and from the degradation of lead-based paints.[1] Factors governing childhood exposure to lead in soil include the amount of soil consumed by a child and the bioavailability of lead. Children are believed to absorb about 50% of ingested lead from their intestines, and this amount increases if the diet is deficient in calcium or iron.[1] The U.S. Environmental Protection Agency[12] has developed a biokinetic model that predicts the distribution of blood lead levels in a population of children exposed to particular amounts of lead in various media, including soil. In general, levels in excess of 500 ppm in soil result in an increase in the number of children whose blood lead level exceeds 10 µg/dL. Below 500 ppm, relatively few children experience significant elevation of blood lead. To provide a margin of safety, a level of 250 ppm in residential soil is usually deemed a level requiring remediation and can be deemed a cleanup level.

Selenium. Selenium is an essential trace element for both animals and plants, and some plants are capable of bioconcentrating selenium. Plants grown on alkaline soils rich in selenium can concentrate as much as 15,000 ppm in their tissues, resulting in a toxic dose to animals or humans that consumes their tissues.[2]

Petroleum hydrocarbons

Petroleum is a complex mixture of organic compounds, and the complexity is enhanced during processing. Petroleum hydrocarbons are defined as the collection of relatively nonbiodegradable oils that can be extracted by chlorofluorocarbons. Petroleum compounds can contaminate soil by leaking from a variety of facilities, including vehicles and underground storage tanks of gasoline or home-heating oil. Petroleum also enters the environment near airports by fuel disposal from circling aircraft. Because the different components of fuels vary in their volatility and their ability to break down, the composition of the hydrocarbons changes as they weather.

Most growing plants do not take up appreciable amounts of these compounds from the soil, so bioaccumulation in the food chain is not an important route of human exposure; however, some are absorbable through the skin, and others can be absorbed through the inadvertent ingestion of soil.

Related compounds are present on the site of former manufactured-gas plants (often referred to as coal gasification facilities). These facilities were major producers of gas for heating and lighting in many parts of the United States and Europe until about the World War I era, when they were largely replaced by other sources. The old facilities were leveled, and the land has undergone other uses, including residential development. The main compounds of concern are benzene, polyaromatic compounds such as benzo[a]pyrene, and heavy metals. Measurements of soil gas and measurements of air levels of benzene in basements can provide evidence regarding the potential for human exposure.

Chlorinated polyaromatics: dioxins and polychlorinated biphenyls

Dioxin, or more specifically 2,3,7,8-tetrachlorodibenzo-*p*-dioxin, along with many other polychlorinated dibenzo dioxins and furans, is a compound with extremely low water solubility and a very long half-life in soil. These compounds strongly absorb to particulate matter.[26] They occur or have occurred as contaminants in herbicides and are produced in combustion or incineration. They are leached only slowly, and by virtue of their lipid solubility, they bioaccumulate to some extent in food chains. Removal from the soil is by biologic breakdown and photolysis, by soil erosion (dust generation), and by emigration or through the food chain.[11] The half-life is estimated to be about 10 years in the subsurface and at least 1 to 3 years on the soil surface.[10]

In general, the concentrations of chlorinated polyaromatics such as dioxins, polychlorinated biphenyls (PCBs), and related compounds are very low, below 1 part per billion. Particulate deposition on the foliage, rather than soil uptake, is probably the main route of plant contamination; however, livestock can bioaccumulate dioxins from plants as well as directly from soil, and milk and meat can therefore be important routes of human exposure.[19] Dioxin levels were higher in cow's milk from the vicinity of municipal waste incinerators than in commercial milk supplies.[25] PCBs and dioxins also accumulate in the sediments of bodies of water. They enter the water either by airborne deposition or by runoff and, once present, adhere to suspended particulates or sink to the bottom. Because of their negligible water solubility and the absence of photochemical degradation, they tend to persist in the sediments or accumulate in the bottom-dwelling (benthic) organisms.

SOIL AS A SOURCE OF HUMAN EXPOSURE
Direct contact with soil

Dermal exposure. The skin is an effective barrier for many chemicals, particularly the heavy metals and polyaromatics. Volatile organic compounds and water-soluble compounds readily penetrate the skin, and even the larger compounds may do so slowly if contact is prolonged.

Ingestion. Small children consume soil both deliberately and inadvertently, and the current estimate for average childhood consumption is about 50 mg/day. Accordingly, the value of 100 mg/day is usually used in risk assessments to estimate what a typical child might consume. Children with pica, however, may consume 1 g/day or more. For certain substances, for example, lead and dioxin, the soil ingestion pathway for children is the most significant route of exposure. Adults generally consume much less soil, although those engaged in gardening or construction may ingest minute amounts of soil that are deposited on their face or hands. Rarely, adults also manifest pica.

Airborne contamination from soil

Dust formation. The finely divided particles on the surface of soil can become airborne when disturbed by construction activities and vehicular or even foot or animal traffic.

Volatilization. Volatile contaminants in soil can enter the air and be inhaled. The importance of volatilization depends primarily on the physicochemical properties of the chemical but also on climatic conditions and physical properties of the soil. Volatilization is generally greater in summer than in winter.

Water contamination from soil

Groundwater. Contaminants in soil may be carried or leached downward into the groundwater and may thereby enter a drinking-water supply for even a remote community. The remediation of contaminated groundwater is often the greatest cost in a proposed hazardous-waste cleanup.

Surface water. Surface runoff readily carries contaminants from the land to nearby bodies of water.

Contamination of food

Plant uptake. The ability of plants to extract contaminants from soil selectively depends on the plant species, the form of metal, and the physical and chemical properties of the soil. Plant uptake is a major route of entrance into the food chain for some soil contaminants[16]; however, airborne deposition on fruits and foliage may be important locally.

Livestock. Animals can directly ingest soil contaminants or can be exposed when drinking water that has accumulated on contaminated soil. Animals also consume plants that may have taken up chemicals and also may breathe dust and accumulate metals.

METHODS FOR EVALUATING SOIL CONTAMINATION
Soil sampling

Questions about exposure hazards from contaminated soil can be addressed in part by sampling and analysis. Sampling begins with a visual inspection and delineation of the site. The actual points at which samples will be taken and the depths to be sampled are developed in a remedial investigation feasibility study.[1] Because of the importance of the soil-air interface, sampling should focus on the upper inch of soil; however, sampling typically is divided into three levels: the upper 6 inches, referred to as *surficial sampling;* 6 to 24 inches; and below 24 inches. Sampling may continue downward as long as significant pollution is encountered. At some sites, sampling may be conducted down to the level at which the water table or bedrock is encountered.

Several kinds of soil-sampling equipment are used. All equipment must be cleansed of any possible contamination prior to use. This cleansing often involves alternated washing with distilled water and acid. Surface samples are usually collected with a trowel. If soils are not densely compacted, the initial sampling of deeper soils may be accomplished by a hand auger. Deeper samples may be obtained by boring using with a hollow-stem auger, a sharp-pointed hollow tube. A split spoon is commonly used for moderately deep samples (4 to 12 feet). Deeper samples are usually obtained by first exposing the site with a backhoe. Information on texture, profile, saturation, and contamination are obtained at the same time. The physical attributes of the soil are described, as is the presence of odor or visible gross contamination. At the same time, specialized measurements, for example, of the soil hydraulic conductivity, may be made.

Once samples have been obtained, care must be taken to avoid contamination of the sample or collecting area. Samples are place into prewashed jars and labeled with the site name, sample number, date, time, and name of sampler.

Chain of custody. This labeling is the beginning of the chain of custody. Each time a sample changes hands, the holder signs over the sample to the new custodian, and each sample is thus accompanied by a list that includes the names of the persons taking the sample, transporting it, receiving it in the laboratory, storing it, digesting and extracting it, and, finally, analyzing it. The chain of custody is a legal document, and failure to maintain a chain of custody often invalidates the sample results, particularly when a legal case is pending.

Quality assurance. Laboratory analyses are only as good as the quality assurance that goes into them. Quality assurance is the full range of activities undertaken to maximize the precision and accuracy of analyses. Laboratory quality control is a major component of a quality assurance/quality control program. Careful recordkeeping ensures that specimens are not mixed up. Appropriately qualified personnel must be selected for each stage from sample collection to sample preparation, analysis, and, finally, supervision and project management.

Analyses are conducted with a variety of specialized samples, including blanks, spiked samples, known standards, and a calibration curve. A field blank is a tube of water that contains no measurable amount of any of the possible analyte (chemicals being analyzed for). It is used to ascertain that no contamination exists in the original sample containers or occurs after a sample has been collected, either during transportation, storage, or handling in the laboratory. Additional blank samples are generated in the laboratory to ascertain that water and reagents are not contaminated. Spiked samples are tubes of soil sample to which a known amount of the substance is added. The analyst then measures the amount of contamination, hoping to recover all of the substance that was added. The percentage of recovery is a measure of how well the laboratory can handle a particular specimen and a particular matrix.

Priority pollutant scan

In certain cases of contamination there is a known source involving one or a few chemicals. In many cases involving hazardous waste sites, however, hundreds of chemicals may be present. Analysis of soil for the many contaminants that could be present in vapor, liquid, or solid form is beyond the capabilities of any analytic laboratory. If a competent laboratory is asked whether a particular substance is detectable, it is possible to receive a reliable answer. It is not possible for the laboratory to characterize the chemicals completely (because there may be thousands) in a soil sample. Therefore the U.S. Environmental Protection Agency has identified a list of 129 so-called *priority pollutants,* which are representative of major classes of inorganic and organic contaminants.

Once collected, a soil is treated in several different ways. Both acid and alkaline extractions are used to identify certain groups of chemicals. Volatile organics and semivolatile and nonvolatile compounds also are identified, as are heavy metals.

Analytic techniques

After the soil has been extracted with different substances, each of the fractions is analyzed with use of a variety of instruments to measure the different types of organic and inorganic contaminants and natural constituents of soil. Some of the new devices, including Fourier transform infrared spectroscopy, thermogravimetric analysis, differential scanning calorimetry, and gas chromatography/mass spectroscopy with differential scanning, as well as more traditional instruments, such as gas chromatographs with various detectors and atomic-absorption spectroscopy, are used.

CONCLUSION

Soil is by no means an inert repository for pollutants. Contaminated soil is often the main source of chemical exposure for humans, and there is an active interchange of chemicals between soil and water, air, and food. Direct contact and ingestion with soil are important exposure pathways in most risk assessments, and inhalation of volatile compounds or dust also may be important. The movement of contaminants through soil is very complex, some moving rapidly and others slowly, and they eventually may reach and contaminate surface or groundwater, on which people rely for drinking and other purposes.

REFERENCES

1. Agency for Toxic Substances and Disease Registry: *The nature and extent of lead poisoning in children in the United States: a report to Congress,* Atlanta, 1988, ASTDR.
2. Agency for Toxic Substances and Disease Registry: *Toxicological profile for selenium,* Atlanta, 1989, ASTDR.
3. Agency for Toxic Substances and Disease Registry: *Health assessment guidance manual, draft,* Atlanta, 1990, ASTDR.
4. Agency for Toxic Substances and Disease Registry: *Draft toxicological profile for mercury,* Atlanta, 1993, ASTDR.
5. Bartlett RJ: Chromium cycling in soils and water: links, gaps, and methods, *Environ Health Perspect* 92:17, 1991.
6. Beijer K, Jernelov A: Methylation of mercury in aquatic environments. In Nriagu J, ed: *The Biogeochemistry of mercury in the environment,* Amsterdam, 1979, Elsevier–North Holland.
7. Burger J, Cooper K, Gochfeld M: Exposure assessment for heavy metal ingestion from a sport fish in Puerto Rico: estimating risk for local fishermen, *J Toxicol Environ Health* 36:355, 1992.
8. Burke T et al: Chromite ore processing residue in Hudson County, New Jersey, *Environ Health Perspect* 92:131, 1991.
9. Davis A, Ruby MV, Bergstrom PD: Bioavailability of arsenic and lead in soils from the Butte, Montana, mining district, *Environ Sci Technol* 26:461, 1992.
10. di Domenico A, Viviano G, Zapponi G: Environmental persistence of 2,3,7,8-TCDD at Seveso. In Hutzinger O et al, eds: *Chlorinated dioxins and related compounds: impact on the environment,* Oxford, 1982, Pergamon Press.
11. Environmental Protection Agency: *A cancer risk-specific dose estimate for 2,3,7,8-TCDD, EPA/600/6-88/007,* Washington, DC, 1988.
12. Environmental Protection Agency: *A biokinetic model for childhood exposure to lead in soil,* release 5, Washington, DC, 1993.
13. Hopps HC, Cannon HL: Geochemical environment in relation to health and disease, Ann NY Acad Sci 199: 1972.
14. Howard PH et al: *Handbook of environmental degradation rates,* Boca Raton, Fla, 1991, Lewis.
15. James SC: Metals in municipal landfill leachate and their health effects, *Am J Public Health* 67:429, 1977.
16. Jensen DJ et al: Residue studies for (2,4,5-trichlorophenoxy) acetic acid and 2,3,7,8-tetrachlorodibenzo-p-dioxin in grass and rice, *J Agric Food Chem* 31:118, 1983.
17. Koren H: *Handbook of environmental health and safety,* Boca Raton, Fla, 1992, Lewis.
18. Lippmann M: *Environmental toxicants: human exposure and their health effects.* New York, 1992, Van Nostrand Reinhold.
19. Nessel CS et al: Evaluation of the relative contribution of exposure routes in a health risk assessment of dioxin emissions from a municipal waste incinerator, *J Exposure Anal Environ Epidemiol* 1:283, 1991.
20. New Jersey Department of Health: *Medical evaluation of children and adults of the Whitney Young Jr. School, Jersey City, New Jersey,* Trenton, 1989.
21. Nimmo DR: Polychlorinated biphenyl absorbed from sediments by fiddlercrabs and pink shrimp, *Nature* 231:50, 1971.
22. National Research Council: *An assessment of mercury in the environment,* Washington, DC, 1978, National Academy Press.
23. Nriagu J, ed: *Biogeochemistry of mercury in the environment,* Amsterdam, 1979, Elsevier-North Holland.
24. Ramos-Perez CR, Gines-Sanchez C, McDowell WH: Influence of bedrock geochemistry on the heavy metal content of stream water, marine water, marine sediments and organisms in St. John, USVI, *Carib J Sci* 25:218, 1989.
25. Rappe C et al: Polychlorinated dibenzofurans and dibenzo-p-dioxins and other chlorinated contaminants in cow milk from various locations in Switzerland, *Environ Sci Technol* 21:964, 1987.
26. Skene SA, Dewhurst IC, Greenberg M: Polychlorinated dibenzo-p-dioxins and polychlorinated dibenzofurans: the risks to human health: a review, *Hum Toxicol* 8:173, 1989.
27. Smith RL: *Ecology and field biology,* ed 2, New York, 1974, Harper & Row.
28. Terzaghi K, Peck RB: *Soil mechanics in engineering practice,* New York, 1967, John Wiley & Sons.
29. Umbreit TH, Hesse EJ, Gallo MA: Bioavailability of dioxin in soil from a 2,4,5-T manufacturing site, *Science* 232:497, 1986.
30. Umbreit TH, Hesse EJ, Gallo MA: Bioavailability and cytochrome P-450 induction from 2,3,7,8-tetrachlorodibenzo-p-dioxin contaminated soils from Times Beach, Missouri and Newark, New Jersey, *Drug Chem Toxicol* 11:405, 1988.

PHYSICAL AGENTS

Chapter 46

IONIZING RADIATION

Joanna Burger

Definitions
Types and sources of ionizing radiation
Human exposure
Dose-response curves
Effects of radiation on humans
    Acute radiation syndrome
    Chronic deterministic effects
    Chronic stochastic effects
Heritable genetic effects
Maximum permissible dose
Health effects other than cancer
    Chromosomal and DNA aberrations
    Immune response
    Growth and development
    Cataracts
    Fertility and sterility
    Life expectancy
Cancer
    Atomic bomb survivors
    Lung cancer
    Leukemia
    Breast cancer
    Cancer in children exposed in utero
Nuclear power and reactor safety
Department of Energy sites
Examples of radiation exposure
    Hiroshima and Nagasaki
    Project Smoky
    Bikini Atoll
    Three Mile Island
    Chernobyl
Prevention of exposure

Ionizing radiation is the form of radiant energy capable of disrupting the atoms and molecules in the tissues through which it passes. Because all living material is composed of atoms joined into molecules, it is vulnerable to ionization by high-energy radiation. These disruptions produce ions and free radicals, which in turn can cause further biochemical damage, including cell death, reproductive effects, and cancer.

Ionizing radiation falls into two broad categories: particulate radiation (principally alpha and beta particles) and electromagnetic radiation (including gamma rays and x-rays, which have extremely high frequency and short wavelengths; Table 46-1). A portion of the ultraviolet spectrum also has ionizing energy but it traditionally comes under the purview of nonionizing radiation. The harmful effects of ionizing radiation have been known since the beginning of the present century. The extensive use of radiation in medicine, science, industry, nuclear energy, and other fields has resulted in the need to study radiation injuries, both immediate and long-term. Moreover, dangerous exposures can occur without human perception or early warning.[16,48] The extensive knowledge about the effects of radiation, coupled with its high hazard potential, provides an important example of environmental exposure for clinicians and public health personnel, in addition to regulators and scientists in governmental agencies.

There are many different sources of ionizing radiation (Fig. 46-1). The objective of this chapter is to describe ionizing radiation; define relevant terms; examine the dose-response curve and exposure measurements; explore the effects of radiation (cancer, reproductive effects, other effects); summarize key epidemiologic studies of radiation exposure; and discuss briefly events such as Hiroshima, Project Smoky, Three Mile Island, and Chernobyl. Finally, the chapter provides guidance on how clinicians can help patients understand exposure and risk associated with radiation.

Several topics are not covered in this chapter. The very real societal problem of safe uses and radioactive waste dis-

Table 46-1. Attributes or different types of radiation

	Alpha	Beta	Neutrons	Gamma	x-ray
Attributes	Helium nucleus Travels short distance	Negatron or positron	Proton +	Electromagnetic radiation electron (photons)	
Mass	1800x electron		1	1800x electron	
Charge	0		−1 or +1	0	
Sources	Natural and artificial heavy elements	Many radionuclides	Artificial Nuclear reactors	Natural Widespread	Artificial x-ray tubes
Shielding	Paper thin	Cardboard	Intermediate	Lead	Lead

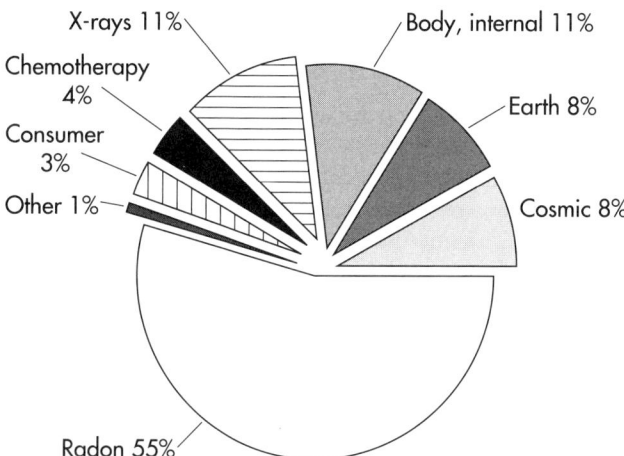

Fig. 46-1. Sources of natural and artificial ionizing radiation (derived from NCRP, 1987). Manmade sources account for 19% of average exposure. Body = internally generated in human body; Earth = natural terrestrial; Consumer = Consumer products; Other = occupational (0.3%), nuclear fallout (0.3%) (Courtesy Environmental and Occupational Health Sciences Institute.)

posal is covered in Chapter 55. Similarly, issues of nuclear power and nuclear safety are not covered.[23] The topics of nuclear war,[14] nuclear winter,[40] and nuclear weapons,[46] although critical environmental health issues, are beyond the scope of this chapter, as are the ecologic consequences of low-level radiation, which can be dramatic, as Woodwell[49] showed in an experimental forest.

DEFINITIONS

The following terminology covers some aspects of the characteristics, measurement, and effects of radiation. The environmental health literature and regulatory framework in the United States persist in using a system of measurements based on centimeters per-gram-per-second (or cgs), but most other countries are using an international system of units (SI units). Thus there are two sets of parallel terminology in common use. Definitions of terms follow:

ALARA The Department of Energy (DOE) policy for regulating radiation releases at its facilities that requires it be as low as is reasonably achievable.[47]

alpha particles Particles with two neutrons and two protons that are emitted spontaneously during the radioactive decay of radionuclides of high molecular weight. They do not penetrate matter easily because of their large size and double-positive charge. Most alpha radiation is stopped by the skin. If inhaled or ingested, however, alpha particles produce a high degree of ionization in immediately adjacent tissues.

background radiation The sum of naturally occurring radioactive materials, including cosmic and terrestrial radiation (such as radon emanating from soil). The DOE includes global fallout and radiation from consumer products in this category.

BAT Best available technology. A DOE approach to controlling radiation emissions.

becquerel (Bq) The International System unit expressing the amount of radioactivity in a given sample of matter. 1 Bq equals the quantity of radioactivity in which there is one atomic disintegration per second. It replaces the old cgs system unit, the curie, everywhere but in the United States. In measurement of radon, 37 Bq/m^3 equals 1 picocurie/liter (pCi/L).

beta Beta particles have the mass of one electron and vary greatly in their ability to penetrate tissues, depending on initial energy and density of matter. As beta particles traverse matter, they lose energy and velocity and the lost energy is emitted as photons or electromagnetic radiation. Only modest thicknesses of commonly available materials are sufficient to stop beta radiation completely. Beta decay can refer to release of either an electron (negatively charged) or a positron.

curie (Ci) The cgs unit of radioactivity. One curie equals the quantity of radioactivity in which there is 3.7×10^{10} atomic disintegrations per second. (Thus 1 Ci = 3.7×10^{10} Bq.) 4 pCi/m^3 = approximately 150 Bq/m^3, and 1 pCi = 0.37 Bq.

derived concentration guide (DCG) Used by the DOE. The concentration of radionuclides in air and water, which would yield a dose of 100 millirem (mrem), or 1 millisievert (mSv), to a human who had continuous exposure.

dosimetry The measurement of a human dose received over a period of time. Radiation badges, for example, measure radiation over a period of a week or a month.

effective dose equivalent (EDE) The sum of exposures received by a tissue obtained by multiplying the dose equivalent by a tissue-specific weighting factor for each radiation type or source. It is measured in rems (cgs) or sieverts (SI). Table 46-2 lists some tissue-specific weighting factors.

gamma rays Electromagnetic radiation emitted as packets of energy (photons) during the nuclear decay of certain radionuclides.

gray (Gy) An SI measure of radiation dose. 1 Gy = 1 J per kilogram of tissue.

Table 46-2. Tissue-specific weighting factors used for estimating effective doses

Organ of tissue	Weighting factor
Gonads	0.25
Breasts	0.15
Red bone marrow	0.12
Lungs	0.12
Thyroid	0.03
Bone surfaces	0.03
Remainder combined*	0.30
Skin	0.01

Modified from US Department of Energy: Radiation protection of the public and the environment, *Federal Register* 58:16268, 1993.
*Based on the five most exposed organs from the following list: liver, kidney, spleen, thymus, adrenal, pancreas, stomach, and intestines.

Table 46-3. Quality factors for different types of radiation used for calculating the dose equivalent from the absorbed dose

Type of radiation	Quality factor
X-rays, gamma rays, beta particles positrons, electrons (for example, tritium)	1
Neutrons <10 keV	3
Neutrons >10 keV	10
Protons	10
Other single-charged particles with rest-mass > one atomic mass unit	10
Alpha particles	20
Other multiple-charged particles of unknown charge and energy	20

Modified from US Department of Energy: Radiation protection of the public and the environment, *Federal Register* 58:16268, 1993.

linear energy transfer (LET) The spatial energy distribution in terms of the average amount of energy deposited in tissue per unit length of particle track. Measured in electron volts (usually kiloelectron volts [keV] or megaelectron volts [MeV] per distance of tissue traversed.

negatron Synonym for an electron or a beta particle with a single negative charge.

rad A cgs measure of the absorbed dose of radiation (corresponds to the SI unit the gray). 1 rad = 100 ergs per gram of tissue = 0.01 Gy.

RBE Relative biologic effectiveness. It allows the doses of different types of radiation to be normalized in terms of risk to humans. The unit is the sievert.

rem The cgs measure of absorbed dose multiplied by a tissue quality factor. Corresponds to the SI unit sievert. 1 rem = 0.001 Sv. Radiation exposure limits are stated in rems. A member of the general population should not be exposed to more than 500 mrem per year. Table 46-3 lists some common quality factors.

roentgen 1 roentgen (R) is the amount of x-radiation that produces one electrostatic unit of change in 1 cm^3 air under standard conditions of temperature and pressure.

sievert (Sv) An SI unit. 1 Sv = the dose in grays multiplied by an appropriate RBE quality factor. Thus 1 Sv of any type of radiation represents the dose that is equivalent in biologic effect to 1 Gy of gamma rays. The corresponding cgs unit is the Rem. 1 rem = 0.001 Sv.

working level (WL) Based on radon exposure of underground miners averaged over 170 hr/mo, an air level of 100 pCi/m^3 of radon gas would result in one working level of exposure. For epidemiologic purposes, residential exposure has been expressed on a cumulative basis in working-level months. (See Chapter 46.)

x-rays Originate in the extranuclear part of the atom. X-rays are produced in an evacuated tube by acceleration of electrons from a heated element to a metal target with voltages in excess of 16 kV.

TYPES AND SOURCES OF IONIZING RADIATION

Ionizing radiation from the decay of radioactive nuclei releases alpha and beta particles and gamma rays (see Table 46-1). The following equations illustrate some of these changes. The emitted particles and rays have characteristic energies.[32] The first illustrates one type of decay of radium 226 to radon 222, releasing an alpha particle with 4.78 MeV energy. The second illustrates the decay of cesium 137 to barium 137, with no change in mass and a gain in atomic number by virtue of loss of a negatron (beta particle) from the nucleus. The negatron carries 0.51 MeV and the gamma rays 0.66 MeV energy.

$$_{88}Ra^{226} \rightarrow {_{86}}Rn^{222} + {_{2}}He^{4} \; (4.78 \; MeV)$$
$$_{55}Cs^{137} \rightarrow {_{56}}Ba^{137} + {_{-1}}B^{0} + gamma \; rays \; (1.17 \; MeV)$$

Ionizing radiation, whether from natural or anthropogenic sources, disrupts the atoms and molecules of biotic material. As radiation impinges on matter and collides with ions, it gives up energy. LET estimates the energy deposited in the tissues. The background level of ionizing radiation includes cosmic rays and natural radium or other radionuclides in the earth's crust.[19] In addition, people generate potassium 40 in their bodies. These sources produce an average population exposure of about 1 millisievert per year.

Most of the background radiation comes from terrestrial radon (about 55%) and cosmic radiation (8%), which vary in intensity as a function of latitude and altitude. Cosmic radiation increases by a factor of three from sea level to 10,000 feet and by a factor of 10% to 20% from 0 to 50 degrees latitude.[26] Other naturally occurring radiation sources are uranium, actinium, and thorium and their decay products.

Man-made radiation sources include nuclear reactors; nuclear weapons; uranium industry (mines, mills, fabricating plants, fuel-reprocessing plants); and high-energy charged particles from accelerators and x-ray devices. X-ray generators accelerate electrons onto a target material in a vacuum. Any device that employs accelerating voltages above approximately 20 kV may generate x-rays of sufficient energy to penetrate the device envelope and present a source of potentially hazardous ionizing radiation leakage.[48] In many devices, some radioactive materials are sealed inside to improve their ionization characteristics. Smoke detectors and alarm systems employ an alpha emitter to ionize the gas between the electrodes.

HUMAN EXPOSURE

Radiation exposure can be short-term (as in an industrial accident or atomic explosion) or long-term (as in household radon or occupational exposure to cosmic radiation among airline employees). Acute exposure can produce immediate effects (the acute radiation syndrome), chronic disease, or diseases such as cancer that become apparent only after a latency period of many years. When radiation exposure is reported in millirems per hour, it is essential to know the duration of exposure to ascertain the total dose.[16]

Estimation of human exposure to ionizing radiation is one of the first steps in determination of risk and ultimately in management or reduction of risk. Estimation of the cumulative dose over some time period is called dosimetry, and for ionizing radiation the absorbed dose (D) is defined as the energy absorbed per unit mass in joules per kilogram (gray) or in ergs per gram (rad). The National Council on Radiation Protection and Measurement[25] has recently calculated the average exposure of the U.S. population to ionizing radiation. For each category the collective effective dose equivalent (EDE) was obtained from the product of the average per-capita EDE received from that source and the estimated number of people so exposed. The average EDE for a member of the U.S. population was calculated by dividing the collective EDE by the U.S. population.

More than 80% of the radiation exposure for the US population comes from natural sources such as radon and cosmic radiation (Table 46-4, Fig. 46-1). The importance of radon as a source of radiation has only recently (in the 1980s) been recognized and is discussed more fully in Chapter 46. Radiation from occupational activities, nuclear power, and nuclear testing contribute negligibly to the average EDE, although they may be very important locally.

Occupational exposure to high levels of radiation has always been of concern, but there has been a concerted effort to evaluate the effects of radiation on entire populations after World War II with the development of the nuclear industry, nuclear weapons, and new medical uses of radiation.[29] Although the average annual EDE is important clinically, there are a number of problems with it. Firstly, there are uncertainties in the data for some consumer products, for exposure of the lung to radon and its decay products, and for the levels of radon and its distribution in the United States.[29] Moreover, these data reflect the average U.S. exposure, not individual exposure. Exposure from medical sources, occupational exposure, consumer products, and radon in the home and workplace all vary markedly among individuals.

DOSE-RESPONSE CURVES

The process of ionization in human tissues may alter the atoms and molecules of the cells to the extent of irreparable damage or death. The clinically relevant aspect of exposure is to determine the relationship between dose and response. Whereas the toxicologic processes by which ionizing radiation causes genetic mutations and cancer is presumed to follow a linear no-threshold dose-response relationship, such is not the case for other kinds of effects. Some interpretations of epidemiologic data suggested that for low-LET radiations, the biologic risk per rad decreases to a greater extent at low dose rates than does the risk with high-LET radiations[48]; however, for leukemia, the atomic bomb survivor studies show that the curve is essentially linear even at very low doses.[16] It is conceptually simple to think of a dose-response curve for a single short-term dose, but the problem is complicated when the dose is a daily, low-level dose.

The National Research Council (NRC)[29] identified five concepts relevant to radiation dose-response (Fig. 46-2):

1. The principal target for radiation-induced cell killing is deoxyribonucleic acid (DNA). It is the most consequential, although not the only, target.
2. With cell lethality as the endpoint, the dose-response relationship for low-LET radiations often approximates a linear-quadratic function of the dose (D). The relative importance of the linear and quadratic contributions varies widely for different cells and tissues. The interpretation of the linear-quadratic formulation is that the characteristic shape of the dose-response curve is proportional to the dose at low doses but is

Table 46-4. Average annual effective dose equivalent of ionizing radiation to a member of the U.S. population

Source	Dose equivalent		Effective dose equivalent	
	mSv	mrem	mSv	%
Radon	24.00	2400	2.00	55
Cosmic	0.27	27.00	0.27	8
Terrestrial	0.28	28.00	0.28	8
Internal	0.39	39.00	0.39	11
NATURAL SUBTOTAL			2.94	82
Medical				
Diagnostic x-ray	0.39	39.00	0.39	11
Radiotherapy	0.14	14.00	0.14	4
Consumer products	0.10	10.00	0.10	3
Occupational	<0.01	0.90	<0.01	<0.03
Nuclear fuel	<0.01	<1.00	<0.01	<0.03
Fallout	<0.01	<1.00	<0.01	<0.03
Miscellaneous	<0.01	<1.00	<0.01	<0.03
ARTIFICIAL SUBTOTAL			0.67	18.39
Total—all sources			3.61	100

Modified from National Council on Radiation Protection and Measurements: *Ionizing radiation exposures of the population of the United States*, Report No 93, Washington, DC, 1987, The Council.

proportional to the square of the dose at higher doses, resulting in the upward bending of the cancer curve.[29]
3. The biologic consequences of a dose vary with the quality of the radiation.
4. Cell sensitivity to radiation varies as a function of stage in the cell cycle (for cell lethality as an endpoint) and the cell division rate.
5. The effect of a given dose may be influenced by the dose rate. The effectiveness of a given dose generally decreases with decreasing dose rate.

Radiation injuries with thresholds include damage to various organs. These are deterministic or nonstochastic effects that show a threshold in the dose-response curve; the nonthreshold, stochastic effects include mutation and cancer resulting from damage to single cells.

In addition to the assumptions involved with dose-response curves in human studies, extrapolations are made from data on laboratory animals. The United Nations Scientific Committee on the Effects of Atomic Radiation has noted three assumptions that are necessary to extrapolate data from other mammals to humans[42]:

1. The amount of genetic damage induced by a type of radiation under a set of conditions is the same in human germ cells as in the test animals.
2. Biologic and physical factors affect the magnitude of damage in similar ways and to similar extents in the test animals.
3. At low doses and low dose rates of LET radiation, there is a linear relationship between dose and the frequency of effects studied.

EFFECTS OF RADIATION ON HUMANS

Effects of ionizing radiation on humans can be divided into somatic effects from short- or long-term exposure and genetic effects, including reproductive effects and cancer.

Acute radiation syndrome

Short-term whole-body exposure to radiation can cause injury or death in humans and other animals, mainly from damage to the gastrointestinal tract and the bone marrow. Severe gastrointestinal symptoms begin on the third day, with death occurring in less than a week. Marrow damage with low white blood cell and platelet counts occurs in the second or third week. At Hiroshima more than half of the blast survivors living in Japanese-style homes within 0.6 miles of the atom bomb epicenter succumbed from radiation illness.[46] Acute exposure in excess of 50 Sv can produce cerebral damage leading to confusion, convulsions, coma, and death. Acute daily exposure in the 10- to 40-R range causes anemia and death, and daily doses of 50 R or greater caused death by infections in beagles.[48] Such cases usually go from the emergency department to intensive care and are not likely to be treated by primary physicians or environmental medicine practitioners.

Chronic deterministic effects

The main effects are thyroid damage, sterility, and cataracts.[26,27,29] Other effects include growth and development effects and life shortening.

Chronic stochastic effects

The major somatic effects include cancer in adults, cancer in children after exposure in utero, and fertility and sterility problems.

HERITABLE GENETIC EFFECTS

Genetic effects of ionizing radiation are mutations in the germ cells that are transmitted from generation to generation. Indeed, as early as the 1920s radiation was used as a means of inducing mutations in experimental organisms to improve breeding. Some radiation-induced changes occur in both germ cells and somatic cells. Chromosomal and chromatid breaks can be readily induced by ionizing radiation, and their number increases linearly with dose.[29] Structural rearrangements in chromosomes can also occur with radiation, proportional to the square of the x-ray dose.

Ionizing radiation can result in changes in the genetic material that can be transmitted from one generation to the next. The two most notable genetic effects are point mutations and aberrations in chromosomes. Although there are mutations and chromosome aberrations that occur spontaneously, the increase caused by man-induced ionizing radi-

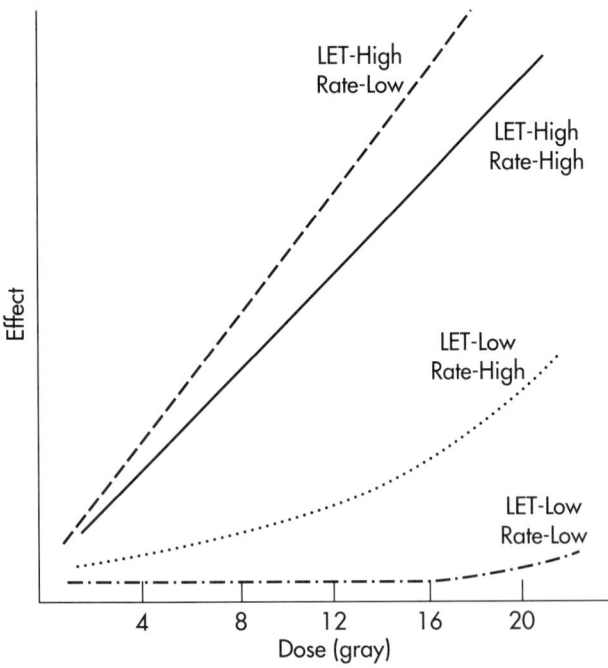

Fig. 46-2. Relationship of dose-rate (dose distribution over time or fragmentation) to effect for high-LET and low-LET radiation. Divided doses enhance the efficacy for high LET radiation and reduce it for low LET. (Redrawn from BEIR IV report, Health risks of radon and other enterally deposited alpha-emitters, Washington, DC, 1988, National Research Council).

ation is of clinical concern. Ionizing radiation has been found to be mutagenic in all organisms studied,[29] and there is no reason to assume that humans are different. Such mutations are expected to be harmful, on average, because most mutations in experimental studies with animals are deleterious. The endpoints used to assess genetic effects of radiation include chromosome abnormalities, altered proteins, congenital malformations, and premature death.

Gene mutations are the most critical targets of ionizing radiation because damage to a single gene may alter or kill the cell, and the heritable effects may be lethal or produce serious abnormalities. A dose of radiation large enough to kill a dividing cell (1 or 2 Sv) suffices to cause dozens of lesions in its DNA.[11] Mutagenic effects on germs cells have been surmised based on studies with somatic cells in which there is approximately one mutation for every 100,000 to 1 million gene loci per sievert.[29] The dose of ionizing radiation that would double the frequency of mutations in the human population is estimated to exceed 1 Sv.[29]

Ionizing radiation can also cause chromosomal aberrations. When chromosomes break and two such breaks occur close together, the broken ends can join incorrectly, causing translocations, inversions, rings, and other rearrangements, which may result in abnormal phenotypic expression. With high-LET radiation the frequency of these events increases steeply as a linear function of dose and independently of dose rate; however, with low-LET radiation the frequency of these events increases less abruptly and is very dependent on dose rate[20] (see Fig. 46-2). In human lymphocytes radiated in culture, the frequency of two-event aberrations approximates 0.1 per cell per Sv in the low-to-intermediate dose range.[20]

MAXIMUM PERMISSIBLE DOSE

The International Commission on Radiation Protection and various federal agencies have estimated the maximal amount to which humans can be exposed without jeopardy to their health. These estimates are expressed as maximum permissible doses (Table 46-5). They reduce but do not completely eliminate the cancer risk.

HEALTH EFFECTS OTHER THAN CANCER

Somatic effects of radiation on humans are changes that affect the individual and can range from cellular to whole organism and can be sublethal or lethal. Somatic chromosome abnormalities can be found in the general population at low levels but are numerous in cancer cells. The most vulnerable tissues are those with the most rapid cell turnover.

Chromosomal and DNA aberrations

The chromosomal aberrations and DNA damage discussed earlier as occurring in germ cells also can occur in somatic cells and in fact have more clearly been demonstrated there.[29] Any cell can be killed by a large enough dose of radiation, but a dose of only 1 to 2 Gy is sufficient to cause human cells to cease to divide.[41] The survival and proliferation of cells decreases exponentially with increasing dose. With high-LET radiation the dose-survival curve is steeper than with low-LET radiation and is relatively independent of dose.[17]

Table 46-5. Maximum permissible doses for different categories of subject and organ

	Occupational (rem/yr)	Community (rem/yr)
Whole body, gonads, bone marrow	5	0.5
Skin, bones, thyroid	15	3.0
Extremities	75	7.5
Other internal organs	15	1.5
Fertile women (over gestation period)	0.5	
Exposure experienced at		
New York City (0 feet above sea level)		0.1
Denver (5280 ft)		0.15-0.2
Kerala (India) mines		1.5-5.0
Population dose limits for genetic or somatic effects (average/year)		0.17

Adapted from National Council on Radiation Protection and Measurements: *Review of the current state of radiation protection philosophy*, Report 43, Washington, DC, 1975, The Council.

Immune response

The cells involved in the immune response exhibit a broad range of radiosensitivities.[3] Some lymphocytes are exceedingly radiosensitive, but plasma cells and macrophages are very resistant. In general, irradiation inhibits the immune response in a dose-dependent fashion,[2] and radiation victims frequently succumb to infection. Recent experiments with animal models, however, have demonstrated that radiation exposure can also be associated with augmentation of the immune system.[2] This phenomenon appears to be due to the loss of a T cell that normally has a suppressive influence. These recent experiments have clinical implications that need further exploration.

Growth and development

Injurious effects of ionizing radiation on the developing brain have been found in the atomic-bomb survivors who were exposed in utero[7,8,34,35] and show a dose-dependent increase in the incidence of severe mental retardation if exposure occurred at gestational age of 16 to 25 weeks. No subjects exposed before 8 weeks or after 26 weeks developed retardation.[31] Analysis of the epidemiologic data shows the maximal sensitivity of the human brain occurs between 8 and 15 weeks of gestation, and new dosimetry techniques suggest that a threshold for the effect may exist in the range of 0.2 to 0.4 Gy.[29,31] Both intelligence-test scores and school performance of children exposed during this critical developmental period were affected.[29]

Cataracts

Cataract formation, or opacification of the lens of the eye, results from the irradiation to the lens in excess of 0.6 to 1.5 Gy, depending on the dose rate and the LET.[18] The threshold for detectable opacities in atomic-bomb survivors was lower (0.6 to 1.5 Gy) than for persons exposed to x-rays to the eye.[18,31] Long-continued occupational exposure to 0.7 to 1.0 Gy of mixed neutron-gamma radiation has been observed to cause cataracts, whereas similar occupational exposure to comparable doses of x-rays or gamma rays alone has not.[18,29] Although detectable damage to the lens can occur from a dose as low as 1 Gy, the threshold for vision-impairing cataracts under conditions of recurrent or protracted exposure is thought to be at least 8 Sv.[18]

Fertility and sterility

The estimated threshold dose equivalent for temporary sterility in the human testis is 0.15 Sv (150 rem); for permanent sterility it is 3.5 Sv (3500 rem) when received as a single dose.[41] The corresponding threshold dose for permanent sterility in the adult human ovary is 2.5 to 6.0 Sv in a single exposure and 6.0 Sv when received in a protracted exposure.[18]

Life expectancy

Evidence from animal studies suggests that for whole-body radiation, life expectancy decreases with increasing dose. Human epidemiologic findings are consistent with the animal studies.[29]

CANCER

The diseases most often studied and of most concern to patients and their doctors are various cancers. Patients with radiation exposure are concerned about future cancer risks, and patients with cancer question whether their disease is related to a possible radiation exposure. The cause of radiation-induced cancer is complex and incompletely understood. The risk of such cancer depends on the type of radiation, the age and sex of the exposed person, the magnitude of the dose to the target organ, the quality of the radiation, the nature and timing of exposure, the presence of other carcinogens or promoters, and individual characteristics of the exposed person.[29] Moreover, determinations of the relative risk from radiation-induced cancers are based on extrapolations from people exposed to large doses. Studies of occupational cohorts include radiologists, radium dial painters, and uranium miners. Epidemiologic studies of patients exposed to radiation for medical purposes, survivors of the atomic bombs at Hiroshima and Nagasaki, uranium miners, and other radiation workers provide evidence of the increased frequency of cancer from radiation. The NRC[29] estimated that if 100,000 persons of all ages received a whole-body dose of 0.1 Gy (10 rad) of gamma radiation in a single brief exposure, there would be 800 extra cancer deaths during their lifetime in addition to the 20,000 cancer deaths that would normally occur in the absence of radiation. Because the most common cancers attributed to radiation also occur in unexposed people, it continues to be a challenge to identify whether a particular cancer was caused by excess radiation or any other environmental factor.

Atomic bomb survivors

There have been extensive epidemiologic studies of the survivors of the Hiroshima and Nagasaki bombings in 1945. These demonstrate that the rate for all cancers and for gastrointestinal-tract, lung, breast, uterus, and ovary cancers are significantly elevated, with relative risks up to 2. The relative risk for multiple myeloma is nearly 3, and that for leukemia is nearly 5. Notably rates of rectal, pancreatic, and prostatic cancer and lymphomas were not elevated.[36]

Lung cancer

As early as 1960 an epidemiologic study of American uranium miners found an excess of lung cancer.[28] The culprit was the alpha-emitting radon gas, a radioactive decay product of uranium. Epidemiologists have used these studies to calibrate the risk from household radon exposure (see Chapter 47). About 20 studies of miners (not just uranium miners) show a consistent excess of lung cancer even in nonsmokers, as well as a synergistic effect of smoking and radon.[33]

Leukemia

Several types of leukemia occur at increased frequency in persons with either acute or chronic radiation exposure. Studies of atomic-bomb survivors and patients who received high-dose radiotherapy for various conditions yield an estimate of about 3 excess cases per 10,000 persons per year per Sv to the bone marrow.[29] The latency for radiation-induced leukemia appears to be relatively short (less than 5 years) in some cases and declines within 15 to 25 years after the exposure.

Although there is no doubt about the increased risk of leukemia associated with high-level exposure to radiation, the association with low-level exposure is controversial. The BEIR V report[29] summarized a variety of studies of populations living near nuclear test sites, nuclear reactors, and nuclear fuel-processing plants. The common thread of these studies is the excess of leukemia cases (Table 46-6), which, although not always statistically significant, seems to be a consistent finding. If there were no relationship, it would be expected that some studies would find slight excesses of different cancers, with no consistent pattern. In view of the consistency, biologic plausibility, and dose-response data, the causal relationship between low-level radiation exposures and leukemia seems inescapable.

Breast cancer

Although breast cancer has traditionally been considered to have few environmental causes (other than diet), short-term and recurrent radiation exposure clearly increases the

Table 46-6. Summary of relative risks of leukemia for populations with low-level radiation exposure

Exposed group	Relative risk
Adults with multiple radiographs	2.4
Utah and Nevada nuclear test sites	2.4
Project Smoky nuclear tests	2.5
British weapons test	3.7
Canadian nuclear cleanup workers	No excess/no statistical power
British reprocessing plants	4.3
Communities near nuclear power plants	Most studies negative

Adapted from National Research Council: *Health effects of exposure to low levels of ionizing radiation (BEIR V),* Washington, DC, 1990, National Academy Press.

risk of breast cancer.[29] This increase has been observed in atomic-bomb survivors, patients receiving chest fluoroscopy or radiotherapy, and radium dial painters. The risk peaks about 5 to 10 years after radiation and persists.

Cancer in children exposed in utero

The Oxford Survey of Childhood Cancers suggested an association between the risk of cancer (mostly leukemia) in childhood with prenatal exposure to x-rays in utero.[37,38] Although initial efforts to confirm this association were mixed, results of a recent reanalysis of cancer cases from these children are supportive.[7]

A New England survey of 1,429,400 children born between 1940 and 1960 in 42 hospitals also showed an excess of cancers among those exposed to diagnostic x-rays in utero.[22] The relative risks for leukemia (1.52) and other cancers (1.27) were not associated with risk factors other than radiation. Because the magnitude of radiation to the fetus is small (5 to 50 mGy), the data imply that susceptibility to radiation-induced carcinogenesis is relatively high during prenatal life.[22,26,27] Furthermore, mortality from cancer appears to be increased in prenatally exposed atomic-bomb survivors even more than four decades after they were exposed.[50] The epidemiologic studies also suggest an association between in utero exposure to diagnostic x-rays and carcinogenic effects in adult life, although the magnitude of the risk is unclear.[29]

NUCLEAR POWER AND REACTOR SAFETY

Although there have been many accidents at private and governmental nuclear reactors, the Three Mile Island and Chernobyl accidents were the major ones capturing public attention and casting a shadow over the safety programs of the nuclear industry. These accidents did more to halt the progress of this industry than all environmental opposition, and indeed the construction of new nuclear facilities is at a virtual standstill in the United States. The DOE, criticized by a National Academy of Sciences panel, shut down some of the Hanford and Savannah River reactors because of uncertainty over safety.[21] The amount of plutonium used by the nuclear industry, projected at 25,000 kg/y, dwarfs the mere 6 kg plutonium in the Nagasaki bomb.[1] Even before these accidents, nuclear scientists predicted that rapid loss of coolant would be the major factor leading to core meltdown,[10] although they considered this event highly unlikely. Ironically, although many new reactors plans have been shelved, old reactors with fewer safety features continue to operate. Although the technology to build safe reactors exists, the industry has yet to provide evidence that they can be maintained and operated safely and that fuel can be recycled to minimize high-level radioactive waste disposal.

DEPARTMENT OF ENERGY SITES

The DOE and its industrial contractors have operated many facilities for the development of nuclear weapons and nuclear energy around the country. From uranium mines to final assembly of bombs, the facilities involve the extraction, purification, handling, and disposal of radioactive substances, particularly those derived from uranium. With increasing public scrutiny of DOE facilities and policies, the magnitude of environmental contamination has become apparent, and there is concern about substantial occupational and community exposure to radioisotopes and hazardous wastes on and adjacent to these sites.[47] Some of the sites, such as Savannah River and Rocky Flats, are huge; others, such as Princeton Plasma Physics, are relatively small.

The DOE proposed several approaches to reducing future releases to "as low as is reasonably achievable," the ALARA policy.[47] This policy requires that the private industrial contractors who operate DOE facilities for the government employ BAT. The DOE policy is aimed at protection of public health and the environment. The DOE also has developed DCGs to facilitate selection of BAT approaches.[47] The DOE guidelines focus particularly on radioactive waste and outline the methods DOE will use for establishing cleanup criteria. The DOE has estimated that a soil concentration of 120 pCi of uranium/g soil would yield an exposure of 100 mrem (0.1 mSv) per year for a person living on the site. The DOE determined that the soil concentration should not exceed 100 pCi/g for any 1-m area or 35 pCi/g averaged over 100 m^2.[47]

The Office of Technology Assessment[30] evaluated the DOE's hazardous waste problems and programs and documented the magnitude of contamination at these sites. It concluded that there were not sufficient resources available to clean up all or even most of the DOE sites and that "the DOE goal . . . to clean up all weapons sites within 30 years— is unfounded because it is not based on meaningful estimates of the . . . level of cleanup to be accomplished." It also found that health threats to adjacent communities had not been adequately examined.[30]

EXAMPLES OF RADIATION EXPOSURE
Hiroshima and Nagasaki

Much of what is known about radiation damage is derived from follow-up studies of the victims of the Hiroshima atomic blast. Many significant reproductive and cancer findings have been reported in the literature. The two atomic-bomb blasts in August 1945 killed more than 100,000 people by several mechanisms, including flash burns caused by thermal radiation.[46] More than 80,000 survivors are enrolled in a life span study,[6] and many epidemiologic studies have documented the nonthreshold linear dose-response relationships between radiation and cancer and other diseases.

Project Smoky

At the Project Smoky bomb test in the 1950s, soldiers were exposed to an atomic test blast at a distance of a few miles. Ten cases of leukemia occurred through 1979 (4.0 expected).[9] Participants have described their role as standing, partly unclad, in full view of the blast and being told at the last minute to hide their eyes.

Bikini Atoll

Marshall Islanders were exposed to iodine 131 from the Bikini bomb test of March 1, 1954. Within 48 hours two thirds of the population on an island 100 miles away suffered nausea, and half developed hair loss. Several children developed hypothyroidism,[13] and a quarter of a century later there was an increased incidence of thyroid cancer.[12]

Three Mile Island

The near meltdown at the Three Mile Island nuclear plant near Harrisburg, Pennsylvania, in March 1979 captured the nation's nuclear accident imagination and dealt a severe blow to the nuclear industry's safety image.[23] A minor failure in the feedwater system, coupled with a faulty pressure-relief valve, allowed the loss of coolant and depressurization of the reactor. Faulty diagnosis and delayed corrective action led to severe core damage.[23] Radioactive gases escaped into the atmosphere, including between 2 million and 13 million Ci xenon and krypton but only about 13 to 15 Ci iodine 131,[5,44] yet the subsequent human exposure was considered to be low[15] although the anxiety and outrage were substantial.

Chernobyl

In 1957 a Soviet nuclear accident in the Ural mountains released about 1 million Ci strontium 90, resulting in the evacuation of people from an area of perhaps 1000 km^2.[39] By contrast the Chernobyl accident was extensively documented. On April 26, 1986, explosions and fires rocked the plant during a test when all safety systems had been inactivated, resulting in extensive local and global contamination through the release of radioactive gases. It required 10 days to seal off the reactor. More than 116,000 people were evacuated, and 32 died (2 immediately, 30 from acute radiation sickness). Heroic measures were taken to prevent marrow depression and cancer. The accident deposited more than 7 million Ci iodine 131, cesium 137, strontium 90, and other radioactive material widely over Europe and even North America, exposing nearly half the world's population.[4] Radionuclides were found in many foods over a period of months in many countries.[43]

PREVENTION OF EXPOSURE

Once exposure has occurred, patients benefit from elimination of future exposure and possibly from screening for adverse effects. Clinicians can certainly help patients make decisions about the costs and risks of medical uses of radiation. The medical and dental professions have an obligation to reduce radiation exposure to their patients and staffs.

There is increasing concern over exposure to radioactive waste. Where people are exposed or potentially exposed to radioactive waste, it becomes necessary to define pathways and estimate the magnitude of exposure, reduce exposure when feasible by interim measures, and require cleanup where necessary.

Patients' concerns about radiation are sometimes exaggerated. Although ionizing radiation is indeed fearsome, particularly as a potent mutagen and carcinogen, it can exert an effect only when there has been actual exposure. The clinician plays a role in evaluating the likelihood and magnitude of exposure and putting the consequent risk into perspective. Because radiation is omnipresent, part of the risk is inescapable. Avoidance of the preventable risks is a reasonable goal.

REFERENCES

1. Albright D, Feiveson H: Why recycle plutonium? *Science* 235:1555, 1987.
2. Anderson RE: Effects of low-dose radiation on the immune response. In Calabrese EJ, ed: *Biological effects of low level exposures to chemicals and radiation,* Boca Raton, Fla, 1992, Lewis.
3. Anderson RE, Warner NL: Ionizing radiation and the immune response, *Adv Immunol* 24:215, 1976.
4. Anspaugh LR, Catlin RJ, Goldman M: The global impact of the Chernobyl reactor accident, *Science* 242:1513, 1988.
5. Auxier JA et al: *Report of the task group on health physics and dosimetry to the President's Commission on the accident at Three Mile Island,* Washington, DC, 1979, U.S. Government Printing Office.
6. Beebe GW, Kato H, Land CE: Studies of the mortality of A-bomb survivors. 6. Mortality and radiation dose, 1950-1974, *Radiat Res* 75:138, 1978.
7. Bithell JF, Stiler CA: A new calculation of the carcinogenic risk of obstetric X-raying, *Stat Med* 7:857, 1988.
8. Blot WJ: Review of thirty years study of Hiroshima and Nagasaki atomic bomb survivors. II. Biological effects. C. Growth and development following prenatal and children exposure to atomic radiation, *J Radiat Res* 16:82, 1975.
9. Caldwell GG et al: Mortality and cancer frequency among military nuclear test (Smoky) participants, 1957 through 1979, *JAMA* 250:620, 1983.
10. Cohen BL: Impacts of the nuclear energy industry on human health and safety, *American Scientist* 64:550, 1976.

11. Cole A et al: Mechanisms of cell injury. In Meyn R, Withers HR, eds: *Radiation biology in cancer research,* New York, 1980, Raven Press.
12. Conard RA: Late radiation effects in Marshall Islanders exposed to fallout 28 years ago. In Boice JD Jr, Fraumeni JF Jr, eds: *Radiation carcinogenesis: epidemiology and biological significance,* New York, 1984, Raven Press.
13. Conard RA et al: *Review of medical findings in a Marshallese population twenty-six years after accidental exposure to radioactive fallout,* Report BNL 5126, Upton, NY, 1980, Brookhaven National Laboratory.
14. Ehrlich PR et al: Long-term biological consequences of nuclear war, *Science* 222:1293, 1983.
15. Fabrikant JI: Health effects of the nuclear accident at Three Mile Island, *Health Phys* 40:151, 1981.
16. Gofman JW: *Radiation and human health,* San Francisco, 1981, Sierra Club Books.
17. Hall EJ: *Radiobiology for the radiologist,* New York, 1978, Harper & Row.
18. International Commission on Radiological Protection: *Non-stochastic effects of ionizing radiation,* ICRP Pub 41, Oxford, 1974, Pergamon Press.
19. Klement AW, ed: *Handbook of environmental radiation,* Boca Raton, Fla, 1982, CRC Press.
20. Lloyd DC, Purrott RJ: Chromosome aberration analysis in radiological protection dosimetry, *Rad Protect Dosim* 198:19, 1981.
21. Marshall E: How safe are Savannah River reactors? *Science* 235:1563, 1987.
22. Monson RR, MacMahon B: Prenatal X-ray exposure and cancer in children. In Boice JD Jr, Fraumeni JF Jr, eds: *Radiation carcinogenesis: epidemiology and biological significance,* New York, 1984, Raven Press.
23. Mynatt FR: Nuclear reactor safety research since Three Mile Island, *Science* 216:131, 1982.
24. National Council on Radiation Protection and Measurements: *Review of the current state of radiation protection philosophy,* Report No 43, Washington, DC, 1975, The Council.
25. National Council on Radiation Protection and Measurements: *Ionizing radiation exposures of the population of the United States,* Report No 93, Washington, DC, 1987, The Council.
26. National Research Council: *The effects on populations of exposure to low levels of ionizing radiation,* Washington, DC, 1972, National Academy Press.
27. National Research Council: *The effects on populations of exposure to low levels of ionizing radiation (BEIR III),* Washington, DC, 1980, National Academy of Sciences.
28. National Research Council: *Health risks of radon and other internally deposited alpha-emitters (BEIR IV),* Washington, DC, 1988, National Academy Press.
29. National Research Council: *Health effects of exposure to low levels of ionizing radiation (BEIR V),* Washington, DC, 1990, National Academy Press.
30. Office of Technology Assessment: *Complex cleanup: the environmental legacy of nuclear weapons production,* Washington, DC, 1991, United States Congress.
31. Otake M, Yoshimaru H, Schull WJ: *Severe mental retardation among the prenatally exposed survivors of the atomic bombing of Hiroshima and Nagasaki: a comparison of the old and new dosimetry systems,* RERF Technical Report 16-87, Hiroshima, 1987, Radiation Effects Research Foundation.
32. Prasad KN: *Handbook of radiobiology,* Boca Raton, Fla, 1984, CRC Press.
33. Samet JM: Radon and lung cancer, *J Natl Cancer Inst* 81:745, 1989.
34. Schull WJ, Otake M: Neurological deficit and in utero exposure to the atomic bombing of Hiroshima and Nagasaki: a reassessment and new directions. In Kriegel H, ed: *Radiation risks to the developing nervous system,* New York, 1986, Gustav Fischer Verlag.
35. Schull WJ, Otake M: *Effects on intelligence of prenatal exposure to ionizing radiation,* RERF Technical Report 7-86, Hiroshima, 1986, Radiation Effects Research Foundation.
36. Shimizu Y, Kato H, Schull WJ: Studies of the mortality of A-bomb survivors. 9. Mortality 1950-1985, Part 2. Cancer mortality based on the recently revised doses, *Radiat Res* 121:120, 1990.
37. Stewart A, Webb J, Hewitt D: A survey of childhood malignancies, *Br Med J* 1:1495, 1958.
38. Stewart A et al: Malignant disease in childhood and diagnostic irradiation in utero, *Lancet* 2:447, 1956.
39. Trabalka JR, Eyman LD, Auerbach SI: Analysis of the 1957-1958 Soviet nuclear accident, *Science* 209:345, 1980.
40. Turco RP et al: Nuclear winter: global consequences of multiple nuclear explosions, *Science* 222:1283, 1983.
41. United Nations Scientific Committee on Atomic Radiation: *Ionizing radiation: sources and biological effects: United Nations Scientific Committee on Effects of Ionizing Radiation,* New York, 1982, United Nations.
42. United Nations Scientific Committee on Atomic Radiation: Genetic effects of radiation. In *Ionizing radiation: sources and biological effects: United Nations Scientific Committee on Effects of Ionizing Radiation,* New York, 1986, United Nations.
43. United Nations Scientific Committee on Atomic Radiation: *Genetic sources, effects, and risks of ionizing radiation: United Nations Scientific Committee on Effects of Ionizing Radiation,* New York, 1988, United Nations.
44. Upton AC: Health impact of the Three Mile Island accident. In Moss TH, Sills DL, eds: *The Three Mile Island nuclear accident: lessons and implications,* New York, 1981, New York Academy of Sciences.
45. Upton AC: Ionizing radiation. In Rom W, ed: *Environmental and occupational medicine,* Boston, 1992, Little, Brown.
46. US Department of Defense: *The effects of nuclear weapons,* Washington, DC, 1964, Atomic Energy Commission.
47. US Department of Energy: Radiation protection of the public and the environment, *Federal Register* 58:16268, 1993.
48. Wilkening GM: Ionizing radiation. In Clayton GE, Clayton FE, eds: *Patty's industrial hygiene and toxicology,* ed 4, vol 1, part B, New York, 1991, Wiley.
49. Woodwell GM: *The ecological effects of radiation,* San Francisco, 1963, WH Freeman.
50. Yoshimoto Y, Kato H, Schull WJ: *Risk of cancer among in utero children exposed to A-bomb radiation: 1950-1984,* RERF Technical Report 4-88, Hiroshima 1988, Radiation Effects Research Foundation.

Chapter 47

RADON

Judith B. Klotz

Description of the agent, its sources, and its distribution
Geologic factors and spatial variation in radon concentrations
    Exposures: extent and variation
Exposure routes
    Biologic dose
Health effects: identification and qualification of lung cancer risk
    Evidence for lung cancer causation and quantitative hazard
    Current basis for protective action
    Histologic types of lung cancer
    Issue of threshold dose
    Extrapolation from mines to residences: differences in populations exposed
    Smoking interaction
    Other cancers
Prevention of exposure
    Radon testing in residents
    Simultaneous actions to address the most highly exposed individuals and the main distribution of the exposure
    Health professionals' role in preventing exposure through motivating citizens to test and fix residences
    Summary and conclusion

Radon poses an environmental risk because of its carcinogenic properties, but the interest in radon extends considerably beyond the issues of exposure to it, its estimated effects, and the means of preventing exposure. Environmental radon is a prime example of a class of environmental hazards, the discovery and control of which differ greatly from those that traditionally come to mind under the category of pollution. First, exposure to radon is predominantly naturally occurring rather than generated by human polluters, even though there are certainly instances in which excess radon exposure results from improper disposal of radioactive waste or, as in underground mines, insufficient industrial hygiene practices. Second, radon exposure is predominantly an indoor problem in private dwellings and in this regard shares many characteristics with other indoor air contamination issues. In particular, high radon concentrations are generally preventable only through the initiative of individual actions by citizens. As such, discovery and mitigation require extensive public education and some private expenditures. Finally, as a recently discovered hazard, the radon problem may be a harbinger of other chemical and physical agents for which the scope of population can only be appreciated as a result of new technology that increases the sensitivity and decreases the difficulty and expense of performing of widespread measurements.

DESCRIPTION OF THE AGENT, ITS SOURCES, AND ITS DISTRIBUTION

Radon is in the decay chain of uranium-238, one of the major natural sources of radioactive isotopes on earth. Given that the half-life of ^{238}U is approximately 9 billion years, this isotope, generated when the planet was formed, is still present on earth in considerable quantities. The entire decay chain of ^{238}U is illustrated in Fig. 47-1. The gaseous and nonreactive characteristics of the noble gas radon result in its easy diffusion through air; it is also soluble in water. When formed in soil and rock from the decay of its parent isotope, radium-226, radon can diffuse from its source. Radon in the ambient air has a stable concentration throughout the world, but the soil gas tends to enter and accumulate in

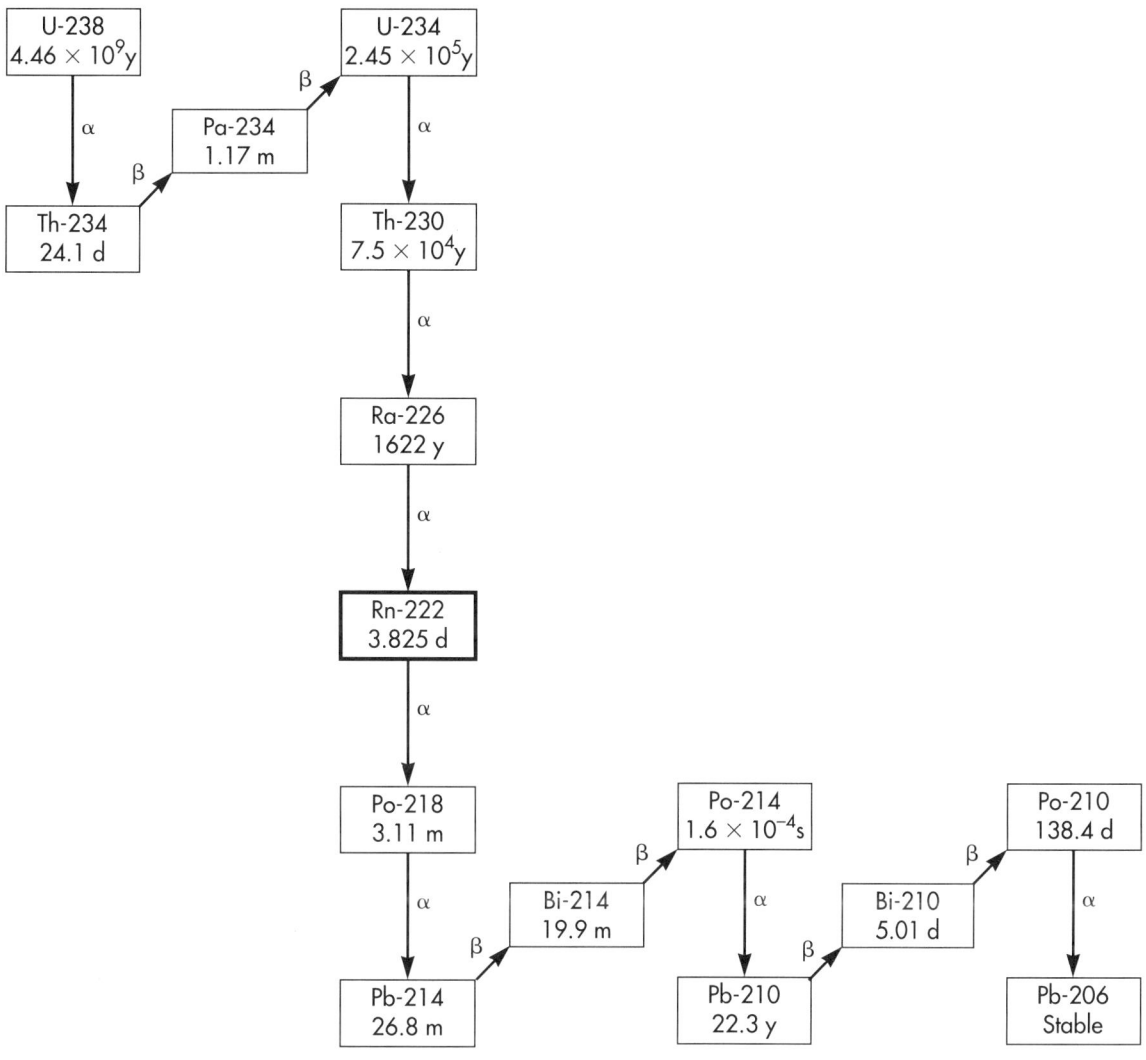

Fig. 47-1. Radioactive decay series showing precursors and decay products of radon-22.

enclosed structures, including mines and buildings, as a result of a combination of diffusion and air-pressure differentials. Because the half-life of radon-222 is about 4 days and because it is not chemically reactive, radon gas itself is very likely to be exhaled after inhalation without having irradiated lung tissue. In contrast, the first few products in the decay chain after radon gas (often called radon daughters or progeny) are short-lived and chemically very reactive isotopes of polonium, lead, and bismuth (Fig. 47-1). These species impart the specifically carcinogenic risk to the population. The polonium decay emits alpha particles, which are highly damaging but penetrate only several cell layers; thus only cells in the immediate vicinity of the radioactive decay are affected. The longer-term decay products at the end of the decay chain, such as polonium-210 and lead-210, present smaller radiation doses to the body than do the short-lived daughters because the overall biologic residence of lead-210 is shorter than the radioactive half-life.

Because radon itself is more inexpensively and reliably measured than its short-lived decay products, it is measured as a surrogate for the more hazardous daughters or progeny. Radon is usually discussed as if it were the hazardous agent, and this chapter reflects that practice.

GEOLOGIC FACTORS AND SPATIAL VARIATION IN RADON CONCENTRATIONS

Factors affecting the likelihood of elevated radon levels in a locality include the type of rock, degree of rock fissuring, and permeability of the soil. In the United States, dwellings built over geologic shear zones, glacial deposits derived from uranium-bearing rocks and sediments, marine black shales, and soils derived from carbonate rocks are particularly prone to excess radon concentrations.[2] Although certain regions of the United States have greater or lesser tendencies for high exposures in residences, there is great variation of radon concentration from house to house on a given street or neighborhood, so the concentrations in one dwelling cannot be reliably predicted from its neighboring buildings.

> **Radon units and equivalents**
>
> Radon concentration:
> 1 pCi/L (picocurie per liter) = 37 Bq/m³ (becquerels per cubic meter)
> 1 pCi = approximately 2 disintegrations per minute
> Concentration of short-lived decay products of Rn-222:
> 1 WL (Working Level) equivalent to 100 pCi/L at equilibrium and to 200 pCi/L at 50% equilibrium (many dwellings)
> Cumulative exposures:
> 1 WLM (Working Level Month) = approximately 5 pCi/L/yr, under typical conditions of equilibrium and 75% of time occupancy of dwellings
> Radiation dose absorbed:
> 1 WLM (5 pCi/L-yr) results in approximately 0.5 rad (500 millirad) of absorbed alpha radiation to the lung.

Table 47-1. Comparative cumulative exposures, in WLM* to radon decay products for occupational, residential, and school settings†

Average concentration (WL*)	Exposure duration (yr)		
	1	4	10
Occupational‡			
5	60	240	600
1 (former standard)	12	48	120
0.3 (current standard)	4	12	40
0.1	1	5	12
0.02	0.2	1	2
Residential§			
0.5	20	80	200
0.1	4	16	40
0.02	1	3	8
School ‖			
0.1	1	3	—
0.02	0.2	0.6	—

*See Box for unit equivalences and conversions.
†Numbers in table are rounded.
Duration assumptions:
‡170 hours per month.
§550 hours per month (75%).
‖ 110 hours per month (15%).

Exposures: extent and variation

Radon concentration in air is presented in picocuries per liter of air (pCi/L) or, in the international system units as becquerels per cubic meter (Bq/m³); 1 pCi/L equals 37 Bq/m³. The typical ambient, that is, outdoor, concentrations, which of course cannot be mitigated, fall between 0.2 and 0.5 pCi/L, severalfold greater than what was traditionally believed before some recent systematic studies were performed by the U.S. Environmental Protection Agency.[4] In residences and other buildings, typical concentrations are 0.5 to 1.5 pCi/L, tending to be higher in parts of the building nearest the soil and in more confined, less ventilated spaces.[13,16] There is also temporal variation in indoor concentrations, influenced by weather, patterns of heating and ventilation, and human use of buildings.

Some special units are traditionally used for characterizing radon exposure. In the United States, concentrations in air of short-lived radon decay products are often expressed in working levels (WL), a unit devised in the 1960s for industrial hygiene use in underground uranium mines of the Colorado Plateau. At radioactive equilibrium of radon-222 and its decay products, 100 pCi of radon gas would generate 1 WL of its daughters. Given that the proportion of decay products is typically less than 50% of such equilibrium because of ventilation and other factors, 1 WL is, in fact, normally associated with more than 200 pCi/L in residences. Typical indoor short-lived decay product concentrations are therefore less than 0.005 WL. (see box)

Risks to individuals and populations are evaluated according to the product of time and intensity of exposure, that is, the cumulative exposure, which is analogous to many other environmental exposures for which long-term rather than short-term concentrations are characteristic. The traditional unit for human cumulative exposure to radon, derived from working populations in underground mines, is the working level month (WLM), which was historically a month of occupational exposure (170 hours) to 1 Working Level. Given that occupancy of dwellings tends to be a much greater proportion of time than that for workplaces (75% to 80% is a reasonable assumption), it is possible to convert residential exposures to the equivalent quantities in WLM. Alternatively, a term such as *pCi/L-yr* or other analogous unit incorporating both intensity and duration of exposure may be used. Typical residential exposures are about 0.2 WLM per year, equivalent to 1 pCi/L-yr. At the current guideline of 4 pCi/L (150 Bq/m³), a person spending 75% of time in his or her residence receives about 0.8 WLM, or 4 pCi/L-yr.

Similarly, exposures in other settings, such as schools and office buildings, depend on the length of occupancy as well as the measured radiation intensities. In large buildings using active ventilation radon concentrations tend to be lower than those in private residences although somewhat higher than outdoor concentrations. Table 47-1 presents some scenarios illustrating relative exposures to individuals in different settings and circumstances. (For public health protection, both the number of people exposed and the amount of exposure to each person in these scenarios should be considered when interventions are designed, as discussed later.)

EXPOSURE ROUTES

The major route of exposure to radon is inhalation of the gas and its decay products derived directly from the soil underneath buildings. A secondary route is inhalation of radon in indoor air derived from household water with groundwater as a source. Volatilization of radon from water occurs easily from household water, especially during showering, dishwashing, and similar activities. (In contrast, ingestion of radon decay products in water and food is not believed to impart a significant dose to the population.[1]) The groundwater source may be the primary one in certain areas of the United States, such as some New England states.

As a rough approximation the ratio of radon in drinking water to air derived from it is 10^{-4}; about 10,000 pCi/L of radon gas in water produces about 1 pCi/L in air. Thus water systems with less than 10,000 pCi/L of radon are unlikely to produce elevated radon in indoor air. In contrast, surface waters have low radon concentrations.[11]

Biologic dose

The amount of radiation from radon decay products that actually reach living human tissue, primarily the lungs, varies greatly among individuals as a result of factors such as physical activity, breathing rate, mouth or nose breathing, and the configuration of the respiratory system (surface-to-volume ratio, for example). Cigarette smoking and other irritants of the respiratory tract can influence the degree of mucous lining and the ciliary action, which can act to expel deposited particles.[12,16]

The lungs receive the overwhelming quantity of radioactivity from radon and its products. About 500 millirad (0.5 rad) is imparted to the lung for each WLM (5 pCi/L-yr) of exposure. Given a quality factor of 20 for alpha radiation, about 10 rem per WLM is absorbed. Much smaller quantities of radioactive dose, some via the long-lived isotopes that appear later in the decay scheme (Fig. 47-1), are distributed systemically.

HEALTH EFFECTS: IDENTIFICATION AND QUANTIFICATION OF LUNG CANCER RISK

The long latency between exposure and clinical onset of lung cancer and the predominance of cigarette smoking as its cause present obstacles to the quantification of the role of radon, particularly its interaction with smoking, in lung cancer etiology. Nevertheless, the occupational data on radon exposure and its effects comprise one of the strongest cause-and-effect stories in environmental epidemiology, based on the exemplary consistency among diverse studies, biologic plausibility, and dose-response exhibited by the radon and lung cancer relationship, so that there is no question that radon is a human lung carcinogen. Some of the controversies that remain involve comparison of the degree of the hazard at the lower radon concentrations found in dwellings with hazards of high radon exposure in the underground mine setting, the interaction with smoking, and the comparative hazard at different ages of exposure.

Evidence for lung cancer causation and quantitative hazard

Evidence from the occupational setting. The evidence on the causal relationship between radon exposure and lung cancer derives principally from working populations, specifically underground miners of uranium, fluorspar, iron, and other minerals.[10] More than 20 well-designed and executed historical cohort studies, that is, epidemiologic investigations in which groups of exposed and unexposed workers were defined on the basis of past records and followed forward in time regarding their health status, have been completed. Not only are results essentially in agreement from studies for many types of underground mines, on different continents, spanning more than three decades, but the dose-response patterns within and among them are remarkably consistent, even though the exposure patterns and study designs varied greatly. Alternative exposures and conditions that could explain the lung cancer excesses among these miners have been effectively ruled out. Both exposures and excess lung cancer rates related to them have declined in underground mines since protective industrial hygiene practices and standards were implemented.

Residential data. Evidence of an association between radon exposure in the home and excess lung cancer has been much more difficult to amass because of the impracticality of defining and following through time a cohort of residents and their pertinent exposures. Instead, the crude method of ecologic analyses of rates of lung cancer in geographic areas has been employed, with varying results.[17] The difficulty in accounting for smoking and other individual determinants of lung cancer greatly limits the interpretation of such analyses of aggregated data; however, studies in which individual cases and controls are defined in the present and exposures are estimated for the past (case-control studies) are viable designs for addressing the question. The relatively smaller exposures to radon normally encountered in dwellings, even most of those in need of remediation, require extremely large numbers of subjects to produce enough statistical power for inferences to be drawn. A few such investigations have already been reported,[8,9,15,19] and many others are under way.[14] Of those already completed, some show an association that is generally consistent with the results of the mining studies (New Jersey and Stockholm, Sweden), but others do not (Shenyang, China, and Winnipeg, Canada).

Current basis for protective action

At the time of writing the strength of the occupational data and the tentativeness of the residential evidence to date, even when consistent with the occupational data, indicate the mining studies to be the appropriate basis for estimating risks of radon exposure. When the factors by which mine and dwelling exposures vary are considered, (such as occupants, time factors, smoking patterns, breathing patterns, and particle and ventilation characteristics), the extrapolation of the radon hazard from underground mines to residences is further validated. The extrapolations are generally performed by using unit risks, that is, the amount of excess risk expressed per unit of cumulative exposure, such as the percentage increase in risk per WLM. A modest decrease in biologic dose estimates per WLM in homes, compared with those in mines, can reasonably be made.[18]

A relative (or proportional) rather than absolute (or additive) risk model appears to fit the data best. A unit risk factor derived from the National Research Council analysis of a combination of mining studies yielded a range of 0.5% to 3% increase of lung cancer risk for *each* WLM (5 pCi/L-yr) of exposure, depending on age and time since exposure. Applying their model to US lung cancer rates and the radon exposure in the population, the National Research Council analysis suggests that for approximately 13,000 lung cancer deaths per year, or about 10% of the total, radon is a contributing factor. Most of these cases probably occur in smokers, on the basis of an assumption of a proportional increase of lung cancer risk in smokers and nonsmokers alike. If one views the effect of radon as an additive risk and also accounts for the differences in dose to the lung between mines and residences, the hazard of lifetime exposure to 4 pCi/L in the living area of one's residence could be estimated as 1.6×10^{-3} additional cases among nonsmokers or about 2.9×10^{-2} additional cases among lifelong smokers.[20]

The dimensions of the excess lung cancer due to radon thus appear to be second only to smoking for the population. Given that the typical lifetime exposure to radon is about 10 to 15 WLM (or 50 to 75 pCi/L-yr) and that radon intensity in dwellings at the current guideline exceed these exposures about fourfold, the excess risk burden on the population and especially on highly exposed individuals is impressive, especially compared with many other environmental contaminants.

Histologic types of lung cancer

Historically, the excess lung cancers observed in underground mines were principally small-cell and squamous (epidermoid) types.[10] Rates of other histologic types have since been observed to be elevated as a result of occupational radon exposure, and consistent patterns have also been seen in some of the residential studies to date, but with much variation among studies.[15,19] The fact that the small-cell and squamous types of lung cancer are also those most frequently induced by tobacco smoking makes the interaction of smoking and radon even more difficult to disentangle.

Issue of threshold dose

Ionizing radiation is the carcinogenic agent for which the absence of a threshold of exposure (level below which there is zero risk) has been classically demonstrated. As such, there is both historical precedent as well as a protective public health rationale for assuming no threshold of exposure for increased risk, in the absence of evidence to the contrary. In practice, such arguments are underscored by the dose-response relationship of radon and lung cancer observed among underground miners and corroborated by many of the residential studies to date. For example, increases of lung cancer risks have been observed in studies of uranium miners[5,10] at cumulative exposures such as 40 WLM, which would occur at a lifetime of residence at the current guideline of 4 pCi/L, or even at ranges of 5 to 20 WLM, typical of all residential exposures. Therefore the threshold controversy is somewhat academic for radon.

Extrapolation from mines to residences: difference in populations exposed

More problematic from practical and policy points of view are the influences of factors such as age and smoking on the hazard to an individual from exposure to radon. Extrapolation from the mining data is necessarily limited to the ages (adulthood before retirement) and sex (male) typified by the population of mine workers. The residential studies are designed in part to address the application of the risks derived from the occupational setting to children and women as well as to the entire population in a nonoccupational setting.

That some studies performed in women have yielded unit risks in the same general range as those for working men suggests that sex may not be a major factor. Because lung cancer has a latency of 5 to 30 years after exposure, the relative vulnerability of children is an important issue in consideration of the population to be protected by testing and mitigating dwellings for radon. Based on sparse data from China, no special vulnerability of child mine workers is evident decades later; however, some agencies have focused on the greater surface-to-volume ratio of children's lungs than that of adults, which theoretically poses a greater likelihood of deposition of radon decay products if they are inhaled.[6] Currently, it appears that attention to childhood exposure is principally warranted because of the general principle of protection of children rather than their special risks of lung cancer at a later date.[20]

Smoking interaction

The mining data suggest a strong positive interaction between tobacco smoke and radon; the consensus at time of writing is for a submultiplicative relationship, that is, the resulting risk of lung cancer in a smoker exposed to excess radon is greater than the addition of hazard from these two exposures separately but less than the risk derived by simply multiplying the effects of the two exposures.[10] Most residential studies to date are consistent with such a conclusion; some appear to suggest that light or moderate smokers bear the greatest relative increased hazard from radon.[19]

Other cancers

There have lately been inquiries into possibilities that other types of cancer in the general population, such as leukemia, might be related to excess radon and other associated natural radiation, although the numerous mining studies did not indicate any such relationship.[3] Pending resolution of this issue, public health measures taken to prevent radon exposures would also protect against other carcinogenic effects.

PREVENTION OF EXPOSURE

The distribution of radon exposure in the population determines the preventive activities that can be effective in avoiding the exposures and the resulting lung cancer risk. It has repeatedly been observed that the distribution of radon in dwellings is log-normal; the distribution therefore has an elongated upper tail of very high exposures, and the arithmetic average exposure is much higher than the median. Although those people in the upper tail of the distribution (including many households that have been featured in media stories on radon) have extremely high exposures and cancer risks, they are relatively infrequent when compared with the segments of the population for which radon exposures are only moderately elevated.

Regardless of the proportion of lung cancer for which radon is a contributing factor, only a portion of such cases of lung cancer, that is, those occurring through scenarios amenable to avoidance or reduction of radon exposure, can be prevented in practice. Assuming a nonthreshold risk pattern as discussed earlier, most of the lung cancer in the population due at least partly to radon occurs in people exposed to relatively low radon concentrations, but each individual supplemental risk is low within this group. In fact, a sizable proportion of the population lung cancer risk is extrapolated to occur in households with background concentrations, that is, about 1 pCi/L or less. The dilemma for the public health professional is that radon concentrations near the background level would be costly to mitigate on a house-to-house basis and the comparative benefit to the *individual* families might be less than that of other health activities competing for their attention and limited money; however, the greatest public health prevention for the *population* as a whole could be accomplished in this group if the distribution were shifted downward by widespread testing and mitigation where appropriate and general use of radon-resistant construction techniques now being developed in localities prone, because of their geology, to high radon concentration indoors.

Since the mid-1980s, trends in technology and costs of radon testing and remediation have made it possible for buildings with excess radon to be discovered and remediated to the current guideline at costs feasible for most households and agencies. Currently, test kits can be obtained by mail or from retailers, exposed to household air for appropriate amount of time, sealed, and sent to laboratories that analyze the detectors and send the results to the consumer.

Radon testing in residences

Worst-case testing, that is, during the heating season, on the lowest livable floor, with windows closed, is appropriate for screening residences to rule out a radon problem; however, such procedures often overestimate the amount of actual, year-round exposure to occupants and should never be used alone as a basis for mitigation; follow-up testing should always be done before any decisions about remediation are made.

Charcoal canisters or their variants can provide reasonable screening tests after a few days of exposure. At time of writing, it is not unusual for the cost of short-term tests to be as low at $20 each. In many dwellings, it may be reasonable and cost-effective to test several parts of a house simultaneously. Longer-term tests of as long as 1 year, such as with the small alpha-track detectors, are more reliable because they integrate radon concentrations over time and can smooth over daily variations due to changes in weather, heating, and ventilation. The US Environmental Protection Agency (EPA) and Centers for Disease Control guidance for testing[21] is to conduct a short-term (usually 2- to 4-day) screening test in the lowest lived-in part of the house (that is, the part of the house frequently used by its occupants that is closest to the soil) and to repeat that test with a long-term or short-term test should the initial screen show levels above the guideline of 4 pCi/L. Some other agencies, including some state governments, recommend that the screening test be conducted in a basement if the house has one. The discrepancy between winter basement and average annual living-area measurements within the same dwelling tends to be greater for houses with higher radon concentrations.[7] Furthermore, in houses with forced-air heating (which tends to distribute the contribution of soil gas throughout the home), there is a greater likelihood that concentrations in all living areas are similar to the lowest-floor readings. The EPA recommends that remediation be conducted if results of a long-term (more than 90-day) follow-up test or an average of two or more short-term tests exceeds 4 pCi/L. Current methods of remediation include sealing openings through which soil gas can enter homes, increasing ventilation of basements, and, particularly, installing subslab or foundation ducts and fans that effectively collect and expel soil gas before it enters the living area of the dwelling. Reduction to radon concentrations to 2 pCi/L or lower is often feasible.[20] *The 4-pCi/L guideline is not based on acceptability of the attendant risk level but on feasibility of testing and remediation:* at the present time, the incremental costs of further radon reduction can be prohibitive. In addition, because of the variability of radon concentrations over time, verification that significant improvement to below this concentration has indeed occurred becomes more difficult and time consuming, involving longer sampling times and more detectors; however, progress in the efficiency and economy of such techniques may enable homes to be reliably brought to even lower concentrations in future years.

In light of the relative importance of air and water as routes of exposure to radon, as discussed previously, exposure reduction can most effectively be conducted by testing indoor air and then addressing elevated water concentrations only if water contributes significantly to the air concentrations. Furthermore, efforts at regulating radon in water, although more administratively straightforward at first glance (involving addition of aeration and other treatment technology at public water-treatment plants), could easily divert resources and attention from the major air route of exposure, unless the overall objective of reduced exposure to people is kept in focus by all agencies concerned.

For all practical purposes, radon reduction and prevention depend on an informed and motivated public. Public health and environmental agencies have struggled since the mid-1980s with issues of how to achieve such motivation while giving appropriate emphasis to other environmental hazards and to other causes of lung cancer. Increased public attention to the issue, as exhibited by consumer use of testing devices and requests for technical assistance, have tended to vary with media stories and with outreach by governmental agencies. Much testing and some decisions to conduct remediation are done as part of real-estate transactions, which typically occur during months other than the heating season in the northern United States.

Simultaneous actions to address the most highly exposed individuals and the main distribution of the exposure

Public health debate regarding radon has often focused on two disparate methods of approaching exposure reduction. The first is identification and mitigation of those at the upper tail of the exposure distribution through aggressive follow-up in the neighborhoods of dwellings with extremely high radon levels or by testing homes in areas where geologic factors suggest that some houses might be affected. At the other end of the scale are the efforts to induce prevention of exposure among the much more numerous new or existing buildings where radon concentrations may be only slightly elevated. Considering the cost per cancer prevented, the former approach of protecting those with the highest individual risk is more efficient, but the latter approach has the potential for protecting a larger segment of the public in the long run. Clearly, both these approaches have value and can be conducted simultaneously, particularly if their respective objectives, strengths, and limitations are recognized.

To accomplish both types of prevention in a coordinated manner, cooperation of the various agencies and health professionals involved in environmental and radiologic health is necessary. In the United States, federal, state, and local governmental agencies have been taking major roles in public advisories, development and distribution of technical materials, training of the public and the radon industry, and, in some states, regulation of the radon industry to protect consumers. Some public agencies are also engaged in predicting where high-radon dwellings are likely to exist or are actively attempting to locate specific residences with extreme problems. State health and environmental radiologic offices and EPA regional offices distribute material to guide consumers in their decisions on testing and fixing their homes, including the revised *Citizens' Guide to Radon*.[21] In fact, the EPA has used radon as a prototype in developing principles and techniques of risk communication.

Health professionals' role in preventing exposure through motivating citizens to test and fix residences

To motivate and guide citizens when market forces such as real-estate transactions are not paramount, health care providers can play a major role in educating individuals, particularly about balancing of health behaviors for preventing lung cancer and regarding concerns about toxins in the environment. Citizens can often be reassured about the extent of the radon hazard to their households and the urgency for remedial action, particularly for a moderately elevated radon level. Unfounded fears of other health effects of radon, such as asthma, can also be put to rest. Even after years of outreach to the public to urge them to test and fix residences, most U.S. households, even in high-radon areas, have not taken the initiative to test.[16] When the radon problem first became general knowledge in the mid 1980s, both panic and apathy by citizens were feared in the public health community. Although some people do overreact to publicity about elevated radon levels in specific homes or neighborhoods or to their own test results, apathy has been far more common, in large part because of many of the characteristics of the problem, with which this chapter began. Radon is naturally occurring, there is no villain, and the problem occurs in the familiar setting of home.[18] Sandman and Weinstein[18] have also investigated psychosocial barriers to testing by citizens. Among their conclusions are that testing is most likely to be encouraged (1) if citizens are reminded personally and locally that their own home may indeed be affected and that testing is necessary to determine whether their home has a radon problem and (2) if assistance is given in identifying and locating appropriate test kits to facilitate actual testing.[18] Although most households that test receive a reassuring result about their radon concentrations, as compared with the current guideline, those that exceed the guideline may need reinforcement of the wisdom of mitigating the problem.

All EPA regional offices and most, if not all, states have materials for citizens to facilitate their finding a test kit, and, if needed, a mitigation firm.

SUMMARY AND CONCLUSION

The indoor radon problem can usefully be considered in the context of other environmental hazards that are not detectable by the senses, require individual citizen action for testing and fixing a condition to prevent exposure, and are not the primary cause of their adverse effect in the population (that is, for lung cancer, it is tobacco smoking). There are several analogies to prevention of the risks resulting from radon exposure through routine application of residence-based inspections and mitigation: termite inspections and smoke detectors are possible models; siting and construction of drinking-water wells and prevention of carbon monoxide poisoning are other models that also involve chemical toxins.

To make wise decisions about the allocation of time and

money for prevention of radon exposures, individuals and their health advocates, including public health agencies, can consider radon exposure in the context of related environmental hazards. The radiation dose from indoor radon greatly exceeds that which most of the population absorbs from other natural sources, medical diagnostic procedures, or emissions from nuclear power plants. With regard to the latter, however, the distinctions must be made between exposures that are under personal control and exposures imposed without one's consent.

Although the cancer risk that can be calculated for typical radon exposures exceeds that which would be extrapolated from most other environmental exposures to chemical carcinogens, for example, through water and outdoor air, it is overly simplistic to show such comparisons without consideration of the following: (1) Contaminants in air and water often have other toxicities in addition to carcinogenicity; (2) aggressive regulation on the state and federal levels of air and water pollution is in large part responsible for reduction of environmental pollution through both enforcement and voluntary compliance, which may never be documented; and (3) as a naturally occurring substance for which baseline exposures cannot be reduced, a significant portion (one third to one half) of radon-related risk cannot be avoided by individual or governmental action. Last, for lung cancer prevention, public health agencies, particularly those with educational components, should incorporate messages on the relative importance of smoking and radon in their communications, including the consensus on positive synergy between radon and smoking.

REFERENCES

1. Crawford-Brown DJ: Age-dependent lung doses from ingested ^{222}Rn in drinking water, *Health Phys* 52:149, 1987.
2. Gunderson LCS: Hidden hazards of radon, *Earth* 1:54, 1992.
3. Henshaw DL, Eatough JP, Richardson RB: Radon as a causative factor in induction of myeloid leukaemia and other cancers, *Lancet* 335:1009, 1990.
4. Hopper R: National ambient radon study, *Proceedings of the 1991 international symposium on radon and radon reduction technology*, Washington, DC, 1991, US Environmental Protection Agency, Office of Radiation Programs.
5. Howe GR et al: Lung cancer mortality in relation to radon daughter exposure in a cohort of workers at the Eldorado Beaver Lodge uranium mine, *J Natl Cancer Inst* 77:357, 1986.
6. International Commission on Radiological Protection: *Cancer risk from indoor exposures to radon daughters,* Oxford, UK, 1987, Pergamon.
7. Klotz JB, Schoenberg JB, Wilcox HB: Relationship among short- and long-term radon measurements within dwellings: influence of radon concentrations, *Health Phys* 65:367, 1993.
8. Letourneau EG et al: Case-control study of residential radon and lung cancer, Winnipeg, Manitoba, *Am J Epidemiol* 10:30, 1994.
9. Lubin J et al: Radon exposure in residences and lung cancer among women: combined analysis of three studies, *Cancer Causes and Control* 5:1, 1994.
10. National Research Council, Committee on the Biological Effects of Ionizing Radiation IV: *Health risks of radon and other internally deposited alpha emitters,* Washington, DC, 1988, National Academy Press.
11. Nazaroff WW et al: Potable water as a source of airborne ^{222}Rn in U.S. dwellings: a review and assessment, *Health Phys* 52:281, 1987.
12. National Council on Radiation Protection and Measurement: Report No 78, *Evaluation of occupational and environmental exposures to radon and radon daughters in the United States,* Bethesda, MD, 1984.
13. Nero AV et al: *Indoor radon and decay products: concentrations, causes, and control strategies,* Washington, DC, US Department of Energy, 1990.
14. Neuberger JS: Residential radon exposure and lung cancer: an overview of ongoing studies, *Health Phys* 63:503, 1992.
15. Pershagen G et al: Residential radon exposure and lung cancer in Swedish women, *Health Phys* 63:179, 1992.
16. Puskin JS: An analysis of the uncertainties in estimates of radon-induced lung cancer, *Risk Anal* 12:277, 1992.
17. Samet JM: Radon and lung cancer, *J Natl Cancer Inst* 81:745, 1989.
18. Sandman PM, Weinstein ND: Predictors of home radon testing and implications for testing promotion programs, *Health Educ Q* 20:471, 1993.
19. Schoenberg JB et al: Case-control study of residential radon and lung cancer among New Jersey women, *Cancer Res* 50:6520, 1990.
20. US Environmental Protection Agency: *Technical support document for the 1992 Citizen's Guide to Radon,* Washington, DC, 1992, Office of Radiation Programs, US Environmental Protection Agency.
21. US Environmental Protection Agency and Centers for Disease Control: *A citizen's guide to radon,* ed 2, Washington, DC, 1992.

Chapter 48

NONIONIZING RADIATION

Joanna Burger
Michael Gochfeld

Radiation and nonionizing radiation
Ionizing radiation
Electromagnetic spectrum
Definitions
Light
    Ultraviolet radiation
    Visible light
    Infrared
    Radiofrequencies and microwaves
    Lasers
    Very low frequency
    Extremely low frequency
Case studies
    Video display terminals
    Cellular phones
    Microwave communication and birth defects
Conclusions

Humans are constantly exposed to both natural and artificial sources of electromagnetic radiation, with both ionizing and nonionizing properties. Radiation is of particular interest to clinicians because of the wide range of radiation types and effects, the potential for increased damage to human health caused by changes in the atmosphere (decreases in the protective ozone layer), and the increase in a wide variety of industrial and electronic devices that are becoming commonplace (for example, microwave ovens, scanning lasers in the stores, high-intensity lamps, video display terminals, cellular phones, and scanning radar for pleasure boats and fisherman). As these uses increase it is imperative to understand their implications for human health, to be able to assess the health effects of their use on people exposed for different periods of time, and to be able to discuss health risks with patients.

In this chapter we describe radiation and nonionizing radiation, define terms used in the field, and examine the biologic and human health risks of nonionizing radiation. (The topics of electromagnetic fields, ionizing radiation, and radon are covered in other chapters. Further details are provided in Michaelson,[19] Plog,[29] and Wilkening.[38])

Major types of nonionizing radiation of clinical interest are light (ultraviolet, visible, and infrared), radiofrequency and microwave, and electromagnetic fields, particularly from electrical power and appliances. One of the concerns with much of the research on nonionizing radiation is that the health physicists who conduct and interpret the research generally think that the public's fears are exaggerated.

RADIATION AND NONIONIZING RADIATION

Electromagnetic radiation consists of vibrating energy waves moving through space at the speed of light and accompanied by a vibrating magnetic field (with wave motion). Electromagnetic waves (or radiation) have three attributes (Fig. 48-1): (1) wavelength, (2) frequency, and (3) amplitude strength. *Wavelength* is the shortest distance between consecutive similar points in the wave pattern. *Frequency* is the number of waves per second. Frequency × wavelength = 186,000 miles per second; hence there is a fixed inverse relationship between wavelength and frequency (Fig. 48-2). Also, in general, the higher the frequency and shorter the wavelength, the higher the quantum energy. *Strength* refers to the intensity or magnitude of the electromagnetic forces. Electromagnetic energy is both wavelike and particulate (photons of energy), and this duality is important for phenomena such as diffraction and photoelectric effects.

IONIZING RADIATION

When there is sufficient quantum energy entering a body, it acts on neutral atoms or molecules with sufficient force to

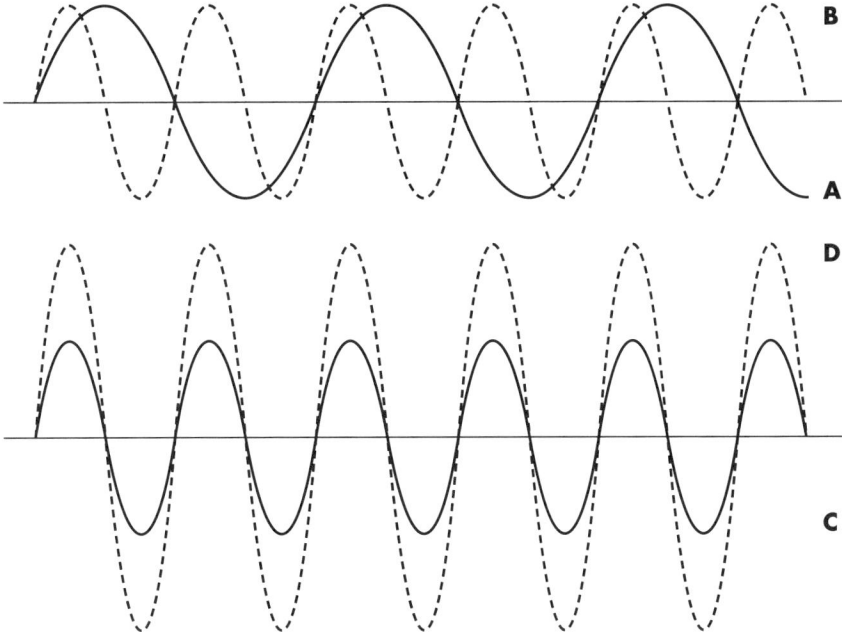

Fig. 48-1. Four electromagnetic waveforms showing variations in wavelength (length between two peaks), frequency (number of waves per second), and amplitude (height difference between negative and positive wave peaks). **A, C,** and **D** have the same frequency and wavelength, and **B** has twice the frequency and half the wavelength of the others. **A, B,** and **C** have the same intensity, and **B** has 1.5 times the intensity. **A** and **C** are 180 degrees out of phase and would cancel each other out if added together. (Courtesy Environmental and Occupational Health Sciences Institute.)

remove electrons, creating an ion. This is the common attribute of *ionizing radiation.* Ionizing radiation has important clinical implications, particularly because of the increase in medical x-ray use and radiotherapy, and is discussed in detail in Chapter 46. Part of the ultraviolet spectrum has sufficient energy to be ionizing, but traditionally it is discussed with the nonionizing radiation. Radiation classed as "nonionizing" (see Fig. 48-2) has lower energy that will not ionize biologic molecules.

Radiation can thus be examined as a continuum from ionizing to nonionizing radiation, from gamma and x-rays through ultraviolet, visible, infrared, and microwave to radiofrequencies and finally very low and extremely low frequencies (including 60-Hz electric fields; see Fig. 48-2). This scale is a continuum, and thus there are only arbitrary divisions between the types of radiation.

These various types of radiation have characteristic wavelengths, frequencies, and energies. It is these differences and the attendant ability to ionize atoms or molecules that lead directly to different biologic and health effects of different parts of the spectrum.

ELECTROMAGNETIC SPECTRUM

Fig. 48-2 illustrates the electromagnetic spectrum. The "packets" of energy are termed *photons,* and the photon energy of electromagnetic radiation is proportional to the frequency of radiation and is thus inversely proportional to wavelength. The shortest wavelengths (gamma rays, x-rays) have the highest energies. Longer wavelengths and lower energies are associated with radio frequency and microwaves. At the extreme are the electromagnetic fields associated with extremely low frequency (ELF) radiation in the electrical frequency range of 50 to 60 Hz. Ultraviolet, visible, and infrared are in the middle of the continuum. Another key characteristic of the electromagnetic spectrum for biologic systems is the depth of penetration of incident radiation through human skin.

UV, visible, and infrared radiation have long been recognized to have important effects, both beneficial and harmful, on human health, and more recently the possible consequences of radiation in the radiofrequency/microwave and in ELF power transmissions have been realized. Our delayed recognition of the potential for health effects of radiation at this extreme of the continuum partly derives from our inability to perceive these wavelengths and from technical difficulties in developing adequate measurement instruments.

Since radiation waveforms oscillate as sine waves or related forms, it is apparent that in most cases the peak intensity does not describe the average intensity estimated by the root mean square, which for a sine wave equals .7 times the peak intensity.

A wide range of health effects have been attributed with varying degrees of confidence to nonionizing radiation. These include thermal, behavioral, CNS, and auditory ef-

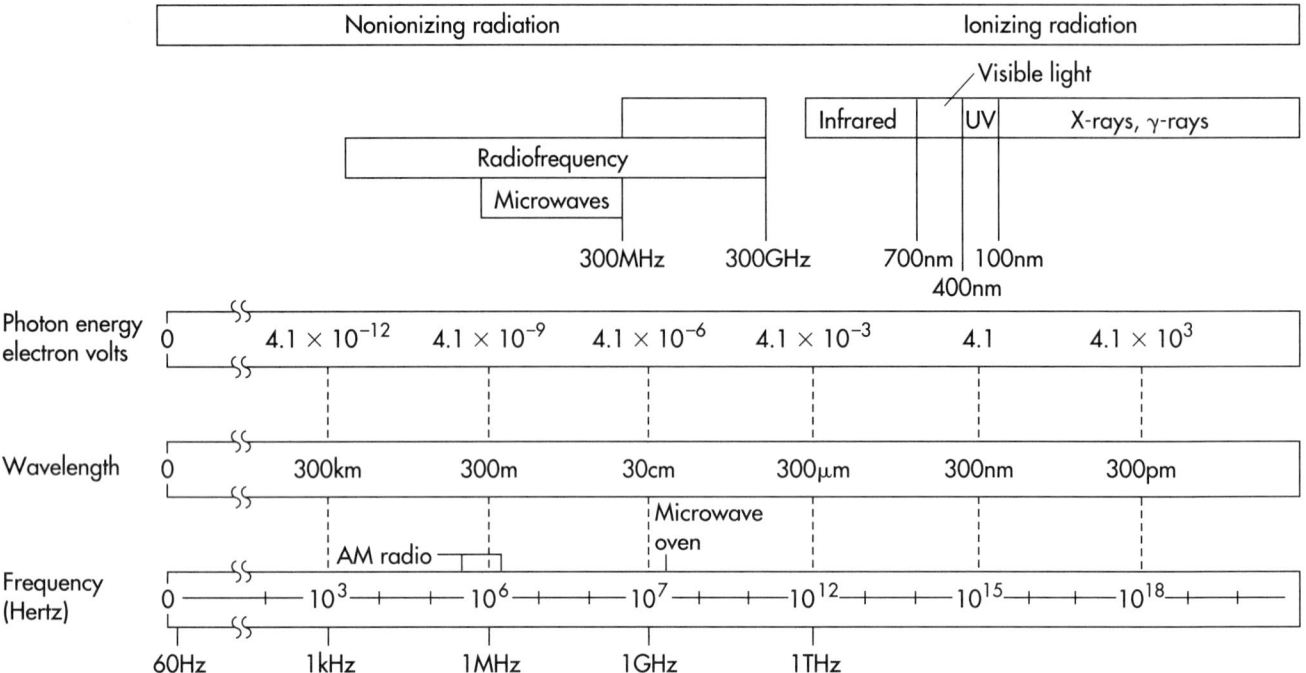

Fig. 48-2. The electromagnetic spectrum, showing subdivisions of the spectrum relative to frequency, wavelength, and energy. (Modified from Wilkening GM: Nonionizing radiation. In Clayton GD, Clayton FE, eds: *Patty's industrial hygiene and toxicology*, ed 4, part B, New York, 1991, Wiley. Courtesy Environmental and Occupational Health Sciences Institute.)

fects; effects on the blood-brain barrier; and immunologic, teratologic, endocrinologic (including effects on biorhythm), developmental, hematologic, and cardiovascular effects. Some of these will be discussed in this chapter. None of the effects attributed to nonionizing radiation are specific or unique to it.

DEFINITIONS

absorbed power mass density Energy absorbed in watts per kg of body weight, also known as the specific absorption rate (SAR).

angstrom Measure of wavelength, and equal to 10^{-4} μm or 10^{-10} meters.

frequency The number of times the electromagnetic wave vibrates or the number of complete cycles per second measured in hertz (formerly called cycles).

gamma e of ionizing radiation with shortest wavelengths and highest energy (see Chapter 48).

gauss (G) A unit of magnetic field strength. 1 G = 10^{-4} tesla.

hertz (Hz) Measure of frequency equal to 1 cycle per second. 1000 hertz (Hz) = 1 kilohertz = 1 kilocycle. 1 megahertz (MHz) = 1 million Hz. 1 gigahertz (GHz) = 1 billion Hz.

infrared (IR) Intermediate-level radiation with wavelength slightly longer than visible light and frequency 3×10^{11} to 4×10^{14} Hz.

intensity For most of the electromagnetic spectrum, the field strength is measured in milliwatts per square centimeter.

ionizing radiation Radiation with sufficient energy to remove electrons (ionize) the atoms or molecules that it strikes. It includes gamma radiation and x-rays with frequency greater than 3×10^{10} and wavelength less than 0.1 μm. It includes part of the UV spectrum (see Fig. 48-2). The photon energy exceeds 10 eV (see Chapter 46).

irradiance Radiant energy falling on a surface such as the skin or eye, measured in watts per cm².

lumen Measure of the flow of visible light. One lumen = the flux of one square foot to a sphere, one foot in radius with a light source of one candle at the center that radiates evenly in all direction.

microwave The component of the radiofrequency portion of the electromagnetic spectrum with wavelength from 1 mm to 10 m and frequency between 3 MHz and 300 GHz.

minimal erythema dose (MED) The least amount of UV light that will produce detectable reddening of the skin. A rough estimate of the intensity of UV.

nonionizing radiation Radiation with insufficient energy to remove an electron from atoms or molecules during collision. As wavelength increases the energy that is imparted decreases.

power density The intensity of radiation measured in mW/cm².

radiant exposure Measured in joules per cm².

Table 48-1. Characteristics of ultraviolet

Ultraviolet radiation	Wavelengths (nm)	Energy range (eV)	Absorbed by
Near or UV-A	320-400	3.1-3.9	
Middle or UV-B	280-320	3.9-4.4	Glass
Far or UV-C	160-280	4.4-7.7	Ozone layer
Vacuum	<160	>7.7	Air

Note: Boundaries are approximate and grade into one another; therefore definitions of the boundary between the different segments vary slightly in different references. For example, Plog (1988) lists Far UV as 200-300 nm and Near UV as 300-400 nm. [Courtesy Environmental and Occupational Health Sciences Institute]
From Wilkening GM: Nonionizing radiation. In Clayton GD, Clayton FE, eds: *Patty's industrial hygiene and toxicology,* New York, 1991, Wiley.

radiofrequency (RF) The portion of the electromagnetic spectrum ranging from about .03 Hz to 300 GHz (wavelength from 1 mm to 10 km).
specific absorption rate (SAR) The whole body average absorbed dosage rate expressed in W/cm².
tesla (T) A measure of magnetic field strength equal to .08 A/m in air. 1 T = 10,000 gauss.
thermal threshold The SAR for RF energy that produces barely the lowest measurable tissue heating.
ultraviolet (UV) Radiation of wavelengths 160 to 400 nm μm and photon energy 3.1 to >7.7 eV. The sun is the major source of UV radiation. The ultraviolet portion of the spectrum is divided into three components: UV-A, UV-B, and UV-C (Table 48-1). Part of the UV spectrum, including all of UV-C, lies in the ionizing radiation domain.
wavelength The shortest distance between similar points in the wave train. Measured in angstroms to kilometers. 1 nm = 1 billionth of a meter.

For convenience, nonionizing radiation will be discussed in terms of light (mainly ultraviolet and infrared), radiofrequency and microwave, and extremely low frequency. Electromagnetic fields associated with electrical power and transmission lines will be discussed in the following chapter (see Chapter 49). A brief description of each type of nonionizing radiation will be followed by a discussion of health effects and epidemiologic data.

LIGHT
Ultraviolet radiation

Ultraviolet is the part of the electromagnetic spectrum bordered by x-rays and visible light, with wavelengths in the 100-nm (photon energy of 124 eV) to 400-nm (3.1 eV range). The higher-energy portion (UV-C) has ionizing properties. Table 48-1 provides a breakdown of the UV portion of the electromagnetic spectrum, showing the different components. The UV range is often divided into vacuum, far (UV-C), middle (UV-B), and near UV-A, in reference to its closeness to the visible range (see Figs. 48-2 and 48-3, and Table 48-1). Vacuum refers to the UV radiation that is completely absorbed by air and can therefore exist only in a vacuum. Vacuum and far UV have energies in the ionizing range. For practical purposes, only UV with wavelengths greater than 160 nm reaches the earth's surface.

Solar radiation, ultraviolet, and the ozone layer. The sun is the major source of UV. The ozone layer, recently of worldwide concern, entirely absorbs solar radiation at wavelengths below 290 nm, which is the higher-energy component of UV. Anthropogenic sources of UV include high- and low-pressure mercury discharge lamps (fluorescent lamps), plasma torches, and welding arcs. Environmental concerns about UV do not so much derive from man-made sources of UV as from man-induced changes in the ozone layer, which in turn increase exposure to UV radiation that reaches the Earth's surface. Even with a normal ozone layer, certain populations have excessive exposure to UV and suffer consequences.

Considerable controversy and discussion surround the issue of the ozone layer and man's culpability reducing the density and effectiveness of this UV filter. In the early 1970s scientists were concerned about the possible impact of supersonic transport aircraft on the ozone layer,[25] but this has paled in comparison to the impact of chlorofluorocarbons (CFCs), which catalyze the degradation of stratospheric ozone. As early as 1980 atmospheric scientists began worrying about the integrity of the earth's ozone layer. Ozone is a reactive oxidant gas produced naturally in trace amounts in the earth's atmosphere,[26] and most is found in the stratosphere (10 to 50 km altitude). Over the past two decades, monitoring of the ozone layer with satellite instrumentation has indicated the catalytic destruction of significant portions of the stratospheric ozone layer, most dramatically seen in the spring Antarctic ozone hole.[39,40]

Determining changes in the ozone layer is difficult, and changes are not uniform over the whole earth.[26] Nonetheless, it has been estimated that ozone concentrations have been reduced by about 2% over the last 20 years.[14]

The ozone layer virtually eliminates all of the UV-C and some of the UV-B that would reach the earth. It has been estimated that a 10% decrease in the stratospheric ozone layer would increase the 305-nm UV-B by 20% but would increase the 290-nm UV-B by 250%.[12] One of the chief culprits in the destruction of the ozone layer are CFCs such as freons, because of their ability to catalyze destruction of ozone.[41] Although CFCs have been banned as spray-can propellants, they are still used in the United States in air conditioning and refrigerators. CFC production continues to grow worldwide at a rate of 5% a year, despite efforts to eliminate their use. Recent international treaties will greatly reduce CFC use, and new chlorine-free refrigerants are being developed. However, even when further use is completely terminated, CFCs will remain in the atmosphere for about a century, because of the slow rate of degradation in the en-

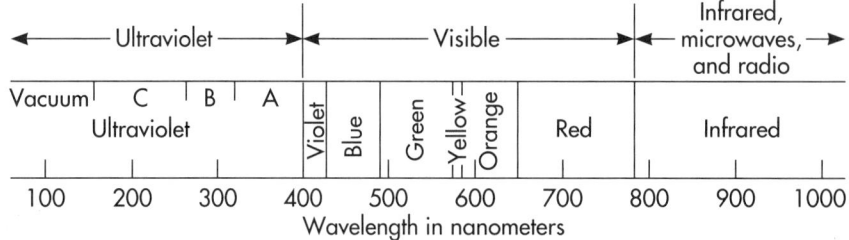

Fig. 48-3. The infrared, visible light, and ultraviolet portions of the electromagnetic spectrum. (Modified from Plog BA: *Fundamentals of Industrial Hygiene,* Washington, DC, 1988, National Safety Council. Courtesy Environmental and Occupational Health Sciences Institute.)

vironment. There are important implications to the resulting increase in UV radiation discussed below and in Chapter 7.

Health effects. Health effects from UV radiation can be classified as those relating to acute exposure and those that appear after a protracted period. Acute effects due to direct UV exposure are usually restricted to the skin and eyes. Immediate changes in the skin occur with exposure to the sun, directly related to intensity and duration of exposure as well as individual susceptibility.

Immediate reactions include darkening of cellular pigment, erythema (sunburn), production and migration of melanin (suntanning), and changes in cell growth in the epidermis. The reactive spectrum of melanin extends to greater than 400 nm.[28]

Sunburn occurs soon after exposure to UV and is a vascular reaction of vasodilation and augmented blood flow. This erythema may occur from 2 to several hours after exposure.[38] Severity depends on skin pigmentation and individual characteristics. In unpigmented skin the minimal dose that provokes sunburn (minimal erythema dose or MED) is about 200 J/ms for wavelengths between 250 and 300 nm, and then increases to $10^5/cm^2$ between 330 and 400 nm.

Suntanning occurs because of increased production of melanin as well as the spread of granules more evenly through the epidermal cells. Continued exposure causes hyperplasia in the epidermis with an increase in shedding of the skin surface cells. This can be followed by skin thickening where there is a thickening of the stratum corneum as a result of UV-induced hyperplasia within the epidermis.[33] Such thickening reduces the amount of UV penetration and plays a significant role in photo-protection.[20]

Acute exposure to UV radiation can also cause ocular damage. Most of the UV radiation is absorbed by the cornea. Small amounts of UV may not produce permanent injury to the eyes, but the only safe procedure is to prevent exposure to UV radiation.[16] Unfortunately, damage can be sustained before the patient is aware of any discomfort during exposure. The potential for strong UV sources (such as lasers) to cause irreversible damage is of concern in the workplace. Effects on the eye can include photokeratitis and conjunctivitis, caused primarily by UV-B and UV-C.

Prolonged exposure to UV, either natural or synthetic, can cause decreased elasticity in the skin, giving the appearance of premature aging, and can cause cataracts.[16] The severity of this finding has only recently become apparent. A study of outdoorsmen on Chesapeake Bay showed a positive association between exposure to UV-B and cataracts.[36] They divided the men into four equal exposure groups and found that the high-exposure quartile had 3.3 times higher relative risk of getting cataracts as the low-exposure group. Energies below 10 mW/cm^2 apparently do not produce cataracts.

Prolonged exposure of the skin to the sun over many years results in elastosis (loss of elasticity), and the skin takes on a wrinkled and leathery appearance.[20] This can lead to premature skin aging, apparent in the faces of farmers, seamen, fishermen, and others who have spent their working lives outdoors exposed to the sun without protection. Likewise, skin on many older people often looks ''younger'' in areas not exposed to the sun, confirming the hazards of exposure to UV radiation (and wind).

Photosensitizing agents may interact with UV to produce more severe results. The combined effect of skin contact with these agents may result in severe irritation and blistering.[38] Moreover, some medicines such as antibiotics are photosensitizing. Clinicians bear a special responsibility to inform patients of these potential hazards. Permissible durations of exposure depend on the wavelength and on the energy reaching the skin (Table 48-2).

Cancer. The relationship between sunlight and skin cancer has been recognized for a century. Chronic and prolonged exposure to UV radiation causes or promotes skin cancer. Increases in skin cancer are a result of both changes in the ozone layer leading to increased exposure for the same duration in the sun and changes in life-style that have increased exposure to the sun. A 1% reduction in stratospheric ozone concentration increases UV-B radiation by 1% or 2%, which will increase nonmelanotic skin cancer rates by 2% to 6%.[37] In Caucasians skin cancer occurs mainly on exposed sites and is related to time spent outdoors. The likelihood of skin cancer is related to pigmentation, and the incidence increases closer to the equator. UV-B light produces skin cancer in animals.

Life-style changes, however, have been far more impor-

Table 48-2. Permissible ultraviolet exposures: allowable exposure is an inverse function of intensity

Allowable exposure	Effective irradiance E^{eff} (uW/cm^2)
8 hr	0.1
4 hr	0.2
2 hr	0.4
1 hr	0.8
30 min	0.7
1 min	50
1 sec	3000

E^{eff} is the irradiance relative to a source of 270 nm, and is a function of the band width of the radiation (the range of wavelengths it comprises), the distribution of energy, and the relative spectral effectiveness of different wavelengths relative to 270 nm. (Courtesy Environmental and Occupational Health Sciences Institute)
From Wilkening GM: Nonionizing radiation. In Clayton GD, Clayton FE, eds: *Patty's industrial hygiene and toxicology,* New York, 1991, Wiley.

tant in the rising skin cancer rates, although this trend may be reversing due to education. The popularity of a "skin tan" as evidence of health, youth, and vigor has contributed to subsequent increases in skin cancer rates. Rates of cutaneous malignant melanoma have risen by a factor of 3.5, and squamous cell carcinoma rates have risen by a factor of 3 over the past 25 years.[8] Mortality rates for malignant melanoma have been rising about 3% per year in the United States.[37] This effect is not just a cohort function of generation as the rates have risen in all age groups.

Considerable controversy surrounds the role of UV radiation and malignant melanomas. Since there is no good animal model for malignant melanoma, data on the relationship between UV radiation and melanomas come from epidemiologic studies. The weight of evidence from several sources indicates that there is a relationship between sunlight exposure (and presumably UV) and melanoma. Several epidemiologic studies have found that the frequency of severe sunburns in childhood is predictive of malignant melanoma risk, whereas neither sunburns nor cumulative exposure during adulthood is predictive.[27]

There is also concern about artificial sources of UV radiation such as occupational exposure to welding equipment, fluorescent lamps, and suntan lamps. UV-A is less carcinogenic, and the newer suntan lamps give off mostly UV-A, whereas the older lamps emitted 65% UV-B. Such studies are difficult to conduct because exposure to natural sunlight must be controlled, and exposure to suntan lamps and to sunlight might be expected to be correlated. Initial concern about the cancerous effects of fluorescent lamps have recently been shown to be unfounded.[11]

Nonmelanotic skin cancer, on the other hand, appears to be more related to cumulative, long-term exposure to sun.[15,34] Rogers and Gilchrest[30] found that people with severe actinic skin damage had 10 times as much risk of basal cell carcinomas as those with no actinic damage.

Prevention of skin cancer is an important clinical objective, and the epidemiologic data indicate that prevention is most effective during childhood. About three-fourths of nonmelanotic skin cancers (and some fraction of melanotic cancers) could be prevented if appropriate sunscreens were used during childhood.[34] Nearly 60% of the total solar UV reaches the earth between 10 AM and 2 PM, depending upon latitude and altitude; therefore, added protection during this time is important. Recently cosmetic manufacturers have started to add appropriate sunscreens to their face creams, but these products are not targeted toward children. Clinicians (as well as television advertisers) bear a special responsibility to emphasize to parents the importance of children using sunscreens all the time, rather than just at the beach.

Another clinical concern is the possibility that outdoor workers who come in contact with chemicals, coal tar derivatives and other chemicals capable of promoting or increasing the rate of skin cancer, are at special risk.

Prevention of UV exposure. Since UV radiation is easily absorbed by a wide variety of materials, prevention of health hazards is straightforward. Prevention of sunburn and suntanning can be accomplished by limiting total time in the sun and the timing of sun exposure (for recreational activities), wearing appropriate clothing, and wearing sunscreen during every exposure. As mentioned, the use of sunscreen and the prevention of erythema in children will be particularly effective in reducing skin cancer risks.

Prevention of ocular problems includes the use of eyeglasses, goggles, and plastic face shields, particularly for industrial and other occupational exposures. Use of UV protective sunglasses is also important in the possible prevention of cataracts. It is necessary to ensure that sunglasses actually protect against all UV wavelengths; otherwise the pupil dilatation that occurs may increase the exposure to UV, leading to damage to the lens and perhaps the cornea.

Benefits of UV radiation. The only benefits of natural UV radiation to man are the synthesis of vitamin D, a substance with an important role in intestinal calcium absorption,[20] and its antimicrobial action. With nonfortified diets, photoproduction of vitamin D in the skin is the chief source of this vitamin. In some countries, such as the United States, there is considerable fortification of vitamin D in the food, and this can lead to overdosing, kidney damage, and elevated serum cholesterol levels.[20]

The elderly, or others confined at home or in hospitals, are at risk for developing vitamin D deficiency. Prevention can include vitamin D supplements or limited exposure to the sun. The level of UV exposure from the sun that is sufficient to provide sufficient vitamin D production, yet avoid damage to the skin or eyes, is not clear and bears further investigation.

Visible light

The visible portion of the electromagnetic spectrum is between 400 and 750 nm (Fig. 48-3). The intensity of visible radiation is measured in units of candles, and the rate of flow of light is measured in lumens.

Health effects. Health effects associated with visible light usually involve ensuring proper lighting to achieve a pleasant and productive environment, and control of visible light radiation to prevent damage to the skin and eyes. Under ordinary circumstances visible light is not injurious to the eyes, although ordinary glare may cause severe visual discomfort or temporary inability to discriminate objects.[38] Exposure of the human eye to high brightness causes physiologic changes such as adaptation, pupillary reflex, partial or full lid closure, and shading of the eyes.[16] Eyes that are in a diseased state are more prone to damage from light in the visible range.[20] Recent attention to seasonal depression syndrome has implicated low light intensity as one etiologic factor.

Prevention. Most temporary damage caused by visible light can be prevented with proper and safe exposure levels. Since the danger of retinal injury is greatest in the blue light range (425 to 450 nm), high-intensity light in this range should be avoided.[16]

Infrared

The infrared region of the electromagnetic region extends from the visible red light region, from 750 nm to 0.3 mm (300,000 nm) (Fig. 48-3), the beginning of microwave. Infrared is normally divided into the near infrared, mid-infrared, and far infrared regions. Infrared exposure can occur from any surface that is at a higher temperature than the receiver. Infrared radiation is emitted from the sun, heated metals, home electrical appliances, incandescent bulbs, furnaces, and occupational sources such as ovens, foundries, welding arcs, IR lasers, welding and soldering devices, and plasma torches.[24] The energy and wavelength characteristics depend on the source temperature.

Infrared radiation can be used for heating applications. Special industrial applications for infrared include (1) drying and baking of paints, (2) dehydrating of textiles and meats, (3) spot heating, and (4) heating of metal parts of shrink fit assembly, thermal aging, brazing, and conditioning surfaces for application of adhesives and welding.

Infrared radiation is measured with spectrophotometers, radiation pyrometers, and stationary or scanning radiometers.[38]

Health effects. Significant IR exposure rarely occurs outside the occupational setting. Infrared radiation is perceptible as a sensation of warmth on the skin. Length of exposure, total amount of energy delivered to the skin, and wavelength of the IR radiation affect the increase in tissue temperature upon exposure.[24] Far-IR radiation is completely absorbed by the skin. Exposure to radiation in the 750 to 1500 nm region can cause acute skin burn and increased persistent skin pigmentation.[16]

Infrared radiation causes health effects mainly to the eye and skin. Thermal damage can occur to the cornea from the energy absorbed in the epithelium rather than in the deep stroma. The main lesions seen are opacities developing just beneath the anterior capsule, whereas the lens was spared.[23] The iris is especially susceptible to damage from radiation below 1300 nm.[24,38] The iris can serve as a heat sink, absorbing IR radiation rather than allowing it to reach the lens.

Thermal injury to the eye is the primary damage caused by IR radiation, but there is some controversy surrounding the relationship between "glassblower's cataract" and IR radiation as its cause.[17,24,38] Cataract formation depends on initial IR-induced heating of the anterior part of the eye (cornea, iris), followed by heat transfer to the lens epithelium. Elevated temperature in the anterior part of the lens is the primary etiologic factor in glassblower's cataract.[38]

Effects of IR radiation on the skin include vasodilation of the capillary beds and increased pigmentation. IR does not normally cause damage to the skin because the skin can dissipate the heat load because of capillary bed dilation, increased blood circulation, sweat, and ambient air movement.

Prevention. Under normal circumstances, precautions taken to prevent UV exposure from the sun will prevent any IR radiation damage. The special case of occupational exposure requires some clinical intervention, especially with respect to ocular exposure. Protective glasses are indicated.[24]

Ultraviolet and infrared radiation combined. Studies from animals have shown that infrared radiation intensifies the effect of ultraviolet radiation of the skin to produce dense matlike fiber deposition in the skin of albino guinea pigs.[13] If these results can be extrapolated to man, the clinical implications of higher levels of exposure to the sun by choice and because of changes in the ozone layer are severe.

Radiofrequencies and microwaves

Radiofrequency radiation ranges from 3 Khz to 300 GHz and includes, in order of decreasing wavelength, short wave > AM > microwave = television > FM > radar. Microwave radiation is included in the range of radiofrequency radiation (see Fig. 47-2), but is considered a special case because of important industrial applications. Microwaves encompass radiation from 10 MHz to 300 GHz. Natural sources of microwaves are the sun and reradiation from the earth. For practical purposes, however, most microwave is anthropogenic. Natural microwave radiation and reradiation create nonionizing electric fields of 100 to 200 V/m^2, whereas the presence of lightning may produce fields as high as 10,000 V/m^2.[38] There has been a 350-fold increase in RF levels over the past 40 years.[20] Measurements made at 486 locations in the United States indicate that the median population exposure to RF in the FM range (88 to 108 MHz) was .005 μW/cm^2, while 0.5% of the population had exposure greater than 1 μW/cm². These are several orders of magnitude below the standard.

Industrial and consumer sources of microwave radiation include microwave ovens, communications and navigational technology (tracking radar, air traffic control radar, weather radar, and UHF TV transmitters), industrial drying equipment, and medical uses (diathermy equipment). Other radiofrequency applications, in addition to microwaves, include radio navigation, LORAN, and amateur radio (Table 48-3). The largest consumer use is in microwave ovens, and there has been considerable concern about potential health hazards. New ovens are designed with adequate shielding and with interlocks that shut off power when the door is opened. Microwave leakage should be negligible in such equipment. Microwave energy has clear advantages over other forms of heating: it is clean and reactive to instant control. It reduces convective heat in the home and workplace.

Microwave or radiofrequency radiation can be transmitted, reflected, or absorbed upon striking biologic tissue, as is true of other forms of electromagnetic radiation. In biologic systems, microwave or radiofrequency radiation induce electric and magnetic fields within the system. Energy is then transferred from the field to the medium and results in attenuation of the field, heating of the medium or tissue, and nonthermal effects. Communication systems are a widespread though weak source of public exposure to microwave.[6]

In 1966 the American National Standards Institute (ANSI) adopted a standard of 100 W/m² of skin as the limit for human exposure, a level that should not raise skin temperature more than 1° C.[6,28] In Eastern Europe and the Soviet Union the standard was 0.1 to 1 W/m², predicated on nonthermal effects reported in research in the 1950s. More recently Eastern European researchers have discounted some of these findings.[35] Absorption of microwave energy varies with frequency and orientation to the source.

Research into mechanisms has covered a variety of molecular and cellular functions.[10] A review of reported biologic effects showed general agreement that effects could be found at doses above 5 W/kg, but there are discrepancies for results reported at much lower doses. In 1982 the occupational standard was revised to limit absorption to 0.4 W/kg (Fig. 48-4), with different energies allowed at different frequencies, and the recommended exposure limit for the general population was 0.08 W/kg.[22]

Recent publicity has revolved around media reports of testicular cancer in police officers using portable radar and brain cancer in people using portable cellular phones. Initial technical reports argue that the energy in these devices cannot cause cancer, but epidemiologic studies are essential.

Health effects. Although there are a number of health effects of radiofrequencies in general, public concern has focused mainly on microwaves. The primary effect of microwaves is thermal; the waves cause heating in tissue through vibration of molecules. "Interpretation of mechanisms . . . is clouded by . . . conflicting reports and opinions."[22] Although radiation energy increases with frequency, in the case of microwave the higher the frequency, the lower the potential health hazard.[16] This is because longer wavelengths penetrate more deeply. Microwave wavelengths less than 3 cm are absorbed mostly in the outer skin; 3- to 10-cm wavelengths penetrate more deeply (1 mm to 1 cm), and wavelengths of 10 to 20 cm can potentially cause damage to internal organs.[38] The human body is transparent to wavelengths greater than about 500 cm.

Health effects from microwaves and radiofrequencies can be classified as reproductive and teratogenic, hematopoietic, immune system, neuroendocrine, behavioral, and psychologic. A prevalent view is that most or all biologic effects of microwave radiation are explainable on the basis of heat disposition in tissues.[38] However, this has been a subject of controversy and is critical because it is easy to measure the dose-response relationship for tissue heating, and if heating is necessary for effect, then one can be confident that there are no health effects at subthermal levels. Much of the controversy over microwave, however, involves intensities that

Table 48-3. Radiofrequencies and microwave designations

Bands	Wavelength	Frequencies	Typical uses
Radio frequency RF			
Low frequency LF	1-10 km	30-300 KHz	Radio navigation
Medium frequency MF	.1-1 km	.3-3 MHz	Loran, AM radio
High frequency HF	10-100 m	3-30 MHz	Amateur radio & CB diathermy
Microwave			
Very high frequency VHF	1-10 m	30-300 MHz	FR, TV, air traffic
Ultra high frequency UHF	.1-1 m	.3-3 GHz	TV, microwave oven telemetry, weather mobile phones
Super high frequency SHF	1-10 cm	3-30 GHz	Satellite communication, ship radars
Extra high frequency EHF	.1-1 cm	30-300 GHz	Radioastronomy

Courtesy Environmental and Occupational Health Sciences Institute
From Wilkening GM: Nonionizing radiation. In Clayton GD, Clayton FE, eds: *Patty's industrial hygiene and toxicology,* New York, 1991, Wiley.

do not cause tissue heating.[22] These are associated with significant effects on the nervous system.

There have been many studies of different frequencies on cells and animals, including work by Adey[2] and Adair and Adams.[1] Both positive and negative studies are reviewed by the NCRP.[22] It seems clear that there are some effects occurring below the thermal threshold in animals, but their significance for humans remains unclear. It is likely that very few people would have significant health effects from exposures well below the thermal threshold, but further research is required with levels around the thermal threshold.

Skeptics argue that there are no known mechanisms for athermal biologic effects, while proponents invoke mechanisms such as resonant responses of biopolymers, particularly at frequencies below 100 GHz,[2,32] or that there is coupling between field oscillations and membranes[3] influencing functions such as calcium transport.

Many different standards have been proposed to protect the public from RF and MW radiation. Since the allowable energy is dependent on frequency, the standards often show different allowable power densities (expressed as W/cm^2) at different wavelengths (see Fig. 48-4).

Lasers

Lasers can be considered separately because of their widespread use for a variety of commercial purposes, including alignment, welding, spectrophotometry, interferometry, flash photolysis, nuclear fission experiments, fiber optics, communications systems, and medical and biologic applications. The term *laser* means *l*ight *a*mplification by *s*timulated *e*missions of *r*adiation. Exposure is almost entirely occupational. The main hazard is to the eye; laser injuries can produce severe burns and permanent blindness.

Very low frequency

VLF comprises radiation with a frequency between 3 and 30 kHz. There has been relatively little study of this portion of the spectrum. However, video display terminals emit some radiation in this portion of the spectrum.

Extremely low frequency

Radiation with a frequency below 300 Hz (including most common electricity with a frequency of 50 to 60 Hz) is labeled ELF. It has extremely long wavelengths, between 3000 and 300,000 km.

Magnetic fields of 50 to 60 Hz. The movement of electric charges, an electric current, creates both an electric field and a magnetic field, which are perpendicular to each other and to the direction in which the waves are traveling (Fig. 48-5). At 50 to 60 Hz there is insufficient energy to heat tissue, and the term *power density* is not applied. Rather, the magnetic field strength is measured in milligauss and is called "flux density." The EMF from electric power and appliances oscillates at 60 Hz, and it is this "flux" that is believed to induce biologic effects.

The earth has a static magnetic field that varies over its surface and averages about 500 mG. Most households have a field strength of 1 to 1.5 mG due to the electrical wiring.

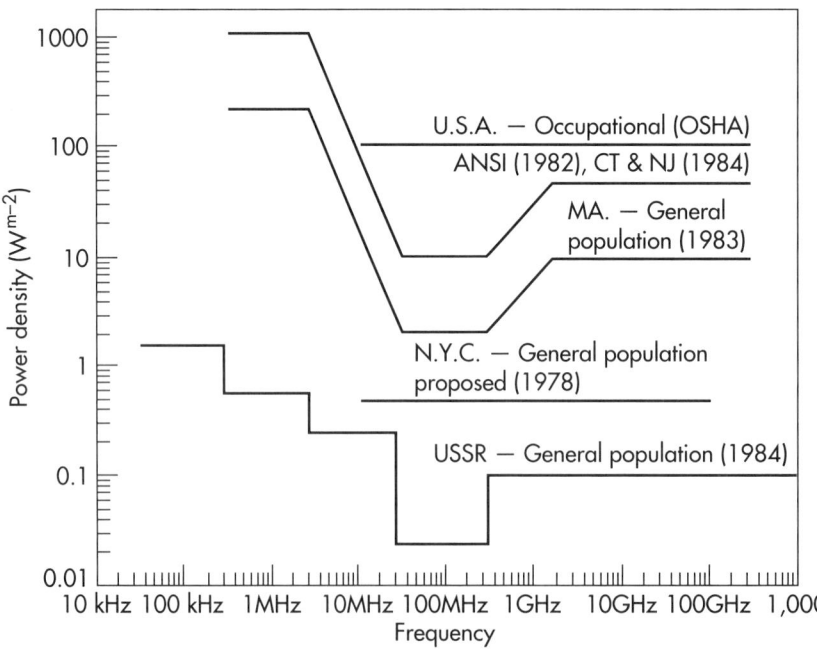

Fig. 48-4. Various standards for protecting people from radiofrequency and microwave radiation showing the allowable power density in watts per square cm at each frequency range. (Modified from Petersen RC: Radiofrequency/microwave protection guides, *Health Physics* 61:59, 1991).

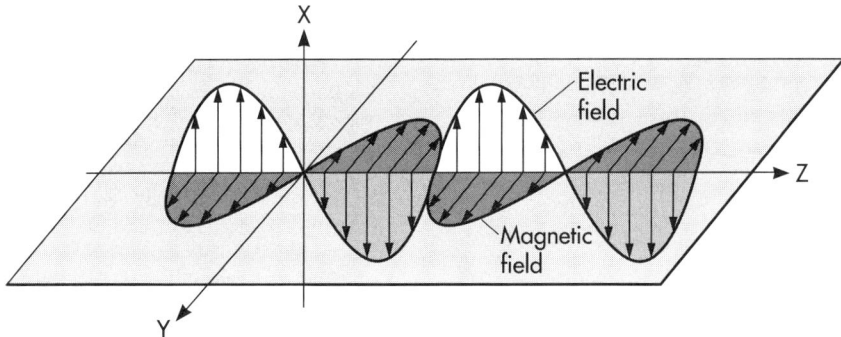

Fig. 48-5. An electric current traveling in one direction generates an electric field and a magnetic field that oscillate in planes perpendicular to the direction of travel and to each other. (Courtesy Environmental and Occupational Health Sciences Institute.)

However, standing close to certain appliances may produce fields of 10 to 50 mG, and lying under an electric blanket yields an exposure to 20 mG. Measurements under high-voltage power lines vary height and configuration, but often exceed 5 mG.

Prevention of exposure requires either source reduction, isolation by distance, or shielding. Electric fields are readily shielded, while magnetic fields penetrate through building materials and the human body. Using a countercurrent system of two wires running parallel but conducting in opposite directions (for example, looping a wire back on itself), the magnetic fields created by each will cancel out.

A variety of cancers (leukemia, brain, male breast) have been reported in groups with occupational exposure to electromagnetic and other nonionizing energy.[18] Occupational exposures to electromagnetic fields tend to be higher than community exposure, although the number of people exposed in the community is much greater. Studies have shown significant increases (about 2 times) in risks of brain cancer with occupational EMF exposure.[18]

Brain cancer deaths occurred in electricians, electronic engineers, and utility company service men with a 50% increased risk in those with known exposure to EMF.[18]

CASE STUDIES
Video display terminals

In the decade since concern was voiced over hazards associated with video display terminals, the sheer numbers of personal computers used in the home, school, and workplace have increased to tens of millions. Several epidemiologic studies have been completed that help put computer/VDT use in perspective. Although concerns were raised regarding both ionizing and nonionizing radiation emanating from the computer screen, most attention has been focused on ergonomic issues regarding how the computer is used (hours per week, type of task) and the physical setting.

VDTs can emit x-ray, UV, and radiofrequency radiation. However, as early as 1980, most models were adequately shielded and did not emit above background. NIOSH published a study[31] evaluating possible association between EMF from VDTs and spontaneous abortion. Telephone operators who used VDTs received higher abdominal exposure to VLF fields (15-KHz range) compared with controls, and there was no difference for ELF fields (45 to 60 Hz). Of 882 pregnancies followed there was no excess risk of spontaneous abortion for women who used VDTs during the first trimester, and no relationship with number of hours of VDT use per week. Most epidemiologic studies include reproduction, and computer use has not shown an increased risk of miscarriage, but at least one study found 1.8 relative risk in women who used VDTs for more than 20 hours per week.[9] The increased risk may have been associated with ergonomic factors, sedentary posture, or socioeconomic correlates of such jobs.

Schnorr et al[31] measured fields in the 1- to 4-mG range. We have measured fields from home computers and found values on the order of 500 mG within 10 cm of the screen, dropping to < 1.5 mG at 42 cm, which is the standard operating distance.

Cellular phones

In early 1993 the media highlighted two cases of brain cancer in people who frequently used portable cellular phones.[5] The proximity of a high-output antenna in close proximity to the head, and the concordance with other studies of brain cancer, prompted concern that there might be a causal relationship. Automobile-mounted mobile phones are considered "safe" because the antenna is remote from the user. Similarly, household portable phones are not implicated because of the low energy transmission between the portable unit and the base. More than 10 million such phones are in use in the United States, but the devices are only a decade old, and most units have been used for less than 5 years; hence there is no way of determining the brain cancer risk at this time. The only consensus at present is that if the association is causal, then increasing distance of the transmitter from the head and decreasing time of use would decrease risk.

Microwave communication and birth defects

The town of Vernon, New Jersey, became a focal point of debate because of a reported excess of birth defects that citizens attributed to the several microwave radioantennas on the hillsides around the town. A committee of epidemiologists was organized to review the data and the EPA made measurements of microwave radiation to which residents might be exposed. As in many such studies of clusters it is difficult to obtain adequate statistical power when only a small community has been exposed; nonetheless the epidemiologists concluded that there was not a significant excess of birth defects, except for Down's syndrome. Fetal deaths were above the New Jersey average, but were the same as the county-wide average.[4] Exposure measurements indicated no exposure in excess of current standards. However, exposure levels were above background for most communities.

CONCLUSIONS

There is substantial public concern regarding exposure to various types of nonionizing radiation. This stems in part from lack of distinction between ionizing and nonionizing, and in part from confusion between different wavelengths of nonionizing radiation. There remains substantial controversy over risks associated with microwave/radiofrequency radiation and with 60-cycle electromagnetic fields. Although the population risks are generally small, there may be subgroups of individuals with unusually high exposure or with unusual susceptibility. Despite the inability of physicists to develop a mechanism, there are a significant number of studies showing excess cancer risk in persons exposed to electromagnetic fields. This will be discussed in Chapter 49.

Although there are no grounds for alarm, neither should society be complacent about the proliferation of new technologies. Judging by the immense number of people who use computers, it is unlikely that any potent health hazard exists, and epidemiologic studies have generally been reassuring. However, long latency conditions (particularly of the visual system) cannot be ruled out yet.

REFERENCES

1. Adair ER, Adams BW: Behavioral thermoregulation in the squirrel monkey: adaptation processes during prolonged microwave exposure, *Behav Neurosci* 97:49, 1983.
2. Adey WR: Frequency and power windowing in tissue interaction with weak electromagnetic fields, *Proc IEEE* 60:119, 1980.
3. Adey WR: Ionic nonequilibrium phenomena in tissue interactions with electromagnetic fields. In Illinger KH, ed: *Biological effects of nonionizing radiation,* Washington, DC, 1981, American Chemical Society Symposium 156.
4. CDC: *Report of Centers for Disease Control consultation on Vernon Township, New Jersey,* Atlanta, 1985, Centers for Disease Control.
5. Elmer-Dewitt P: Dialing "P" for panic, *Time Magazine,* Feb 8, 1993.
6. Foster KR, Guy AW: The microwave problem, *Sci Am* 255:32, 1986.
7. Ghandi OP: Advances in RF dosimetry: their past and projected impact on the safety standards. In Franceschetti G et al, eds: *Electromagnetic biointeraction,* New York, 1989, Plenum Press.
8. Glass AG, Hoover R: The emerging epidemic of melanoma and squamous cell skin cancer, *JAMA* 262:2097, 1989.
9. Goldhaber M, Polem M, Hiatt R: The risk of miscarriage and birth defects among women who use visual display terminals during pregnancy, *Am J Ind Med* 13:695, 1988.
10. Illinger KH: *Biological effects of nonionizing radiation,* Washington, DC, 1981, American Chemical Society Symposium 157.
11. IRPA (International Radiation Protection Association): Fluorescent lighting and malignant melanoma, *Health Phys* 58:232, 1988.
12. Jones RR: Ozone depletion and cancer risk, *Lancet* 443, 1987.
13. Kligman LH: Intensification of ultraviolet-induced dermal damage by infrared radiation, *Arch Dermatol Res* 272:229, 1982.
14. Kripke ML: Impact of ozone depletion on skin cancers, *J Dermatol Surg Oncol* 14:853, 1988.
15. Marks R: Skin cancer—childhood protection affords lifetime protection, *Med J Aust* 147:475, 1987.
16. Langent EJ, Olishifski J, Anderson LE: Nonionizing radiation. In Plog BA, ed: *Fundamentals of industrial hygiene,* Washington, DC, 1988, National Safety Council.
17. Langley RK, Mortimer CB, McCullock C: The experimental production of cataracts by exposure to health and light, *Am Med Assoc Arch Ophthalmol* 63:473, 1960.
18. Lin RS et al: Occupational exposure to electromagnetic fields and the occurrence of brain tumors, *J Occup Med* 27:413, 1985.
19. Michaelson SM, ed: *Fundamental and applied aspects of nonionizing radiation,* New York, 1975, Plenum Press.
20. Moseley H: *Non-ionizing radiation. Medical physics handbooks 18.* Bristol, England, 1988, Hospital Physicists' Association.
21. Nair I, Morgan MG, Florig HK: *Biological effects of power frequency fields and magnetic fields: background paper,* Washington, DC, 1989, Office of Technology Assessment.
22. NCRP: *Biological effects and exposure criteria for radiofrequency electromagnetic fields,* Bethesda, Md, 1986, Natl Council Radiation Protect & Measurements Report #86.
23. NIOSH: *Determination of ocular threshold levels for infrared radiation cataractogenesis.* Cincinnati, Oh, 1980, National Institute for Occupational Safety and Health, Research Report 80-121.
24. NIOSH: *Biological effects of infrared radiation,* Cincinnati, OH, 1982, National Institute for Occupational Safety and Health, Tech Report 82-109.
25. National Research Council: *Biological impacts of increased intensities of solar ultraviolet radiation,* Washington, DC, 1973, National Academy of Sciences-National Academy of Engineering.
26. National Research Council: *Rethinking the ozone problem in urban and regional air pollution,* Washington, DC, 1991, National Academy Press.
27. Osterlind A, Tucker M, Stone B, Jensen O: The Danish case-control study of cutaneous malignant melanoma. II. Importance of UV-light exposure, *Int J Cancer* 43:319, 1988.
28. Petersen RC: Radiofrequency/microwave protection guides, *Health Physics* 61:59, 1991.
29. Plog BA: *Fundamentals of industrial hygiene,* Washington, DC, 1988, National Safety Council.
30. Rogers GS, Gilchrest B: The senile epidermis: environmental influences on skin aging and cutaneous carcinogenesis, *Br J Dermatol* 122:55, 1990.
31. Schnorr TM, Grajewski BA, Hornung RW et al: Video display terminals and the risk of spontaneous abortion, *N Engl J Med* 324:727, 1991.
32. Schwan HP: Classical theory of microwave interactions with biological systems. In Taylor LD, Cheung AY, eds: *The physical basis of electromagnetic interactions with biological systems,* College Park, Md, 1977, University of Maryland Press.
33. Stenback F: Cellular injury and cell proliferation in skin carcinogenesis by UV light, *Oncology* 31:61, 1975.
34. Stern RS, Weinstein M, Baker S: Risk reduction for non-melanoma skin cancer with childhood sunscreen use, *Arch Dermatol* 122:537, 1986.

35. Szmigielski S, Obara T: The rationale for the Eastern European radiofrequency and microwave protection guides. In Franceschetti G, ed: *Electromagnetic biointeraction,* New York, 1988, Plenum Press.
36. Taylor HR, West SK, Rosenthal FS: Effect of ultraviolet radiation on cataract formation, *N Engl J Med* 319:1429, 1989.
37. Urbach R et al: Ultraviolet radiation and skin cancer in man, *Photochem Photobiol* 51:579, 1980.
38. Wilkening GM: Nonionizing radiation. In Clayton GD, Clayton FE, eds: *Patty's industrial hygiene and toxicology,* ed 4, part B, New York, 1991, Wiley.
39. World Meteorological Organization: Ozone trends panel report. In Watson RT, ed: *Global ozone research and monitoring projects,* report no. 18, Geneva, 1988, World Meteorological Organization.
40. World Meteorological Organization: *Scientific assessment of stratospheric ozone: 1989,* vol 1, World Meteorological Organization global ozone research and monitoring project, report no. 20, Geneva, 1990, World Meteorological Organization.
41. World Resources Institute: *World resources 1990-91,* New York, 1990, Oxford University Press.

Chapter 49

ELECTROMAGNETIC FIELDS

Daniel Wartenberg

Studies of adverse health effects associated with electric and magnetic field exposures
Risks, exposure reduction, and the prevalence of the problem

Over the past decade and a half, exposure to electromagnetic fields from electrical distribution systems has emerged as a possible risk factor for certain types of cancers and reproductive disorders. Although the data are still incomplete and in part contradictory, a growing number of studies indicate that exposure to even moderate-strength magnetic fields may be cause for concern. To help clarify the issues involved in this controversy and the possible strategies for reduction of exposures, if warranted, provided here are a brief review of the results of important studies of the association between electromagnetic-field exposure and adverse health effects and the identification of some strategies that can reduce an individual's exposure. Epidemiology and biophysical studies are continuing.

STUDIES OF ADVERSE HEALTH EFFECTS ASSOCIATED WITH ELECTRIC AND MAGNETIC FIELD EXPOSURES

In 1979 Nancy Wertheimer, a child psychologist, and Ed Leeper, an engineer, published a seminal study[7] showing that children in Denver with leukemia tended to live closer to electric transmission lines with a so-called high current configuration (lines that were believed to carry greater electrical current leading to higher electric- and magnetic-field exposures) than did children in Denver without cancer. This surprising result, showing the association between exposure to low-power, nonionizing radiation, which was previously thought to be benign, and childhood cancer, prompted intense scrutiny of the study. Critics questioned whether there was any bias in how the study subjects were selected, whether the rough exposure evaluation (visual inspection of the number, thickness and proximity of electrical wires outside a residence to gauge the so-called current configuration, and proximity to transformers and substations) was valid, whether the exposure assessment had been conducted in an unbiased manner (the case or control status was known by those collecting the exposure data), and whether there was an alternative (confounding) explanation for the observed association. Perhaps traffic volume could be a risk factor; it tended to be higher where there were more electrical lines.

The controversy that ensued prompted a number of scientists to investigate the same phenomenon in more detail.[1,4,5] Scientists developed one series of studies to examine the possible association between residential electric- and magnetic-field exposures and two types of adverse health outcomes: cancer and reproductive effects. Another series of studies was developed to examine occupational exposures and cancer. The advantage of the residential studies is that subjects are less likely to be exposed to substantial levels of other risk factors for the same diseases. Workers who are exposed to electric and magnetic fields (electrical workers, telephone-line workers, radio and television repairers) often are exposed to various organic chemicals that may cause cancer (such as solvents and polychlorinated biphenyls) and to herbicides that are suspected of causing cancer along power line right-of-ways. The advantage of the occupational studies, however, is that the exposures are often substantially higher than those experienced in a typical residential setting, and health outcome data often are easier to obtain.

Since 1979 additional residential studies have been conducted in Rhode Island, Denver, Los Angeles, England, and Sweden. Some of these studies expanded on Wertheimer and Leeper's design by measuring the actual electric and mag-

---

*This chapter was originally commissioned as a brief postscript to Chapter 48 in order to briefly summarize the rapidly evolving epidemiologic literature. It is not intended as a comprehensive account of this very complex field.

netic fields in the residences in addition to using modifications of Wertheimer and Leeper's visual wire-coding scheme. Investigators in these studies found that the wire-coding scheme moderately correlated with measured magnetic fields in the home, but there were substantial variations. Positive associations between the wire-code evaluations and childhood leukemia were reported in most of the studies.[4] Surprisingly, the associations declined when the analyses were conducted with the actual magnetic-field measurements instead of the wire codes and were nonexistent with measured electric fields.[4] One plausible explanation is that the wire codes are indicative of the long-term magnetic-field exposure experienced by residents, but the measurements reflect only a snapshot of exposure on a particular day, failing to capture the seasonal or secular averages. Electric fields are thought not to be a risk factor. One study in Sweden found an association between brain cancer and lymphoma and measured magnetic fields.[6] A few studies have examined cancer rates among residents living close to high-voltage transmission lines, but results are inconsistent.[2] There are fewer studies of cancer in adults and they have yielded weak and inconsistent results, but their study designs were not sufficiently rigorous to rule out an association.

Some of the more recent studies assessed the association between appliance use and cancer. Negative results were obtained in studies of electric-blanket use and leukemia, testicular cancer, and breast cancer; however, one study found an increased risk of childhood cancer associated with the mother's use of an electric blanket during pregnancy. A recent California study found elevated risks of childhood cancer from appliance exposures, including statistically significant risks for use of black-and-white televisions and electric hair dryers.

Concerns have also been raised about the possible association of exposure to electric and magnetic fields and reproductive disorders. Most research has focused on exposures from video display terminals (VDTs). For that exposure, there is limited evidence for a weak association between VDT use and spontaneous abortion and fewer but suggestive findings for an association between VDT use and congenital malformations. Data on reproductive effects from other types of electric- and magnetic-field exposures are too sparse to be reliable.

A substantial number of occupational studies also have been conducted to assess the potential hazard of electric- and magnetic-field exposures. In most of these studies, exposure is characterized imprecisely with use of the job title rather than individual specific measurements or assessments. The job title may suggest a variety of potential exposures in addition to that being studied and may include many workers not exposed to the exposure under study. Nonetheless, independent studies measuring exposure for some of these job titles have confirmed that indeed workers in these jobs typically have higher electric- and magnetic-field exposures than do workers in other jobs. Associations are seen repeatedly between workers believed to be exposed to electric and magnetic fields and both leukemia, and brain cancer.[5] The most recently published study, an investigation of California Edison electrical utility workers from 1960 through 1988, did not show an association between cancer mortality (due to leukemia, lymphoma, and brain cancer) and exposure.[3] Exposure was measured in more detail than in previous studies, and the data were assessed as the mean, median, 99th percentile proportion of time exceeding 1 microtesla (μT), and proportion of time exceeding 5 μT. Still, no associations were found.

In addition, a limited number of studies also suggest an association between electric- and magnetic-field exposure and male breast cancer, an observation that is particularly compelling because a plausible biologic mechanism (suppression of pineal melatonin) had been postulated a priori and is supported by results of animal studies[4]; however, because of the rarity of this disease, many question the strength of the results.

RISKS, EXPOSURE REDUCTION, AND THE PREVALENCE OF THE PROBLEM

In responding to inquiries about the possible effects of magnetic-field exposures, one must assess the type and amount of exposure and the risk that the exposed individual may incur. Unfortunately, to date, there has been little study of the importance of the type of exposure. That is, scientists do not know whether the most relevant aspect of exposure is the overall average magnetic-field strength of the exposure, the variability of the exposure (that is, how often the magnetic-field strength changes), the proportion of time spent above a particular field strength, or some other exposure metric. This lack of information about biologically relevant exposure makes exposure reduction problematic. Most scientists have assumed that the average field strength is the relevant quantity.

On the basis of the assumption that average magnetic-field strength is the most appropriate measure of exposure, current studies indicate that, if there is an association between magnetic-field exposure and cancer, children living in exposed homes, those with two to three times the background magnetic-field strength of 0.05 μT to 2 μT, have approximately twice the risk of developing leukemia as those living in houses with background exposures. It is worth noting that exposure is approximately log-normally distributed, with most homes being at or near background and few houses being far above background. Similarly, workers in occupations with exposure to electric and magnetic fields have approximately twice the risk of developing leukemia or brain cancer as those in occupations without exposure, if there is an association; however, it is important note that both of these risk estimates are approximate, that individual studies vary widely, and that the estimates are predicated on a true association between exposure and disease.

Measures that can be employed to reduce exposure are somewhat limited. Most scientists believe that there are not sufficient, consistent data nor risk to warrant major relocation of electrical distribution systems. Nonetheless, a number of states are implementing regulations regarding the location and design of new or modified high-voltage transmission lines. Some states are conducting surveys of exposures at schools and other locations that children frequent to document the potential problem better.

On an individual basis, exposure to household appliances can be limited if there is a belief that such actions are warranted. For instance, instead of sleeping under an electric blanket the electric blanket may be used to preheat the bed and then unplugged. Electric clocks may be moved from a bedside nightstand to a dresser across the room or maybe replaced with a key wound or battery-driven version. When a microwave oven or other kitchen appliance is used, the user may stand away from it. Television should be watched from at least 4 feet from the screen. A person should not sit within 3 feet of the back of a VDT or computer because the machine backs are not always shielded. In consideration of other exposures, it is useful to note that the magnetic-field strength falls off approximately with the square of the distance from the source. Therefore being 2 feet from a source results in a fourfold greater reduction of the field strength than being 1 foot away from a source. Because it is not easy to shield oneself from magnetic fields, distance from the source is the best protection.

REFERENCES

1. Ahlbom A: A review of the epidemiologic literature on magnetic fields and cancer, *Scand J Work Environ Health* 14:337, 1988.
2. Feychting M, Ahlbom A: *Magnetic fields and cancer in people residing near Swedish high voltage power lines,* IMM-report 6/92, Stockholm, 1992, Karolinska Institute.
3. Sahl JD, Kelsh MA, Greenland S: Cohort and nested case-control studies of hematopoietic cancers and brain cancer among electric utility workers, *Epidemiology* 4:104, 1993.
4. Savitz D: Overview of epidemiologic research on electric and magnetic fields and cancer, *Am Ind Hyg Assoc J* 54:197, 1993.
5. Theriault GP: Health effects of electromagnetic radiation on workers: epidemiologic studies. In *Proceedings of the scientific workshop on the health effects of electric and magnetic fields on workers,* DHHS Pub No 91-111, Washington, DC, 1991, National Institute for Occupational Safety and Health.
6. Tomenius L: 50-Hz electromagnetic environment and the incidence of childhood tumors in Stockholm County, *Bioelectromagnetics* 7:191, 1986.
7. Wertheimer N, Leeper E: Electrical wiring configurations and childhood cancer, *Am J Epidemiol* 109:273, 1979.

Chapter 50

VIBRATION

Donald E. Wasserman

Vibration fundamentals
Hand-arm vibration exposure
Whole-body vibration exposure
Hand-arm and whole-body crossover vibration exposure
Vibration exposure and cumulative trauma disorders
Controlling human exposure to vibration
Medical management
Summary

Since ancient man first took to the sea to fish and to explore, or rode a camel or ox cart for transportation, he has been beset by the effects of motion on his body. Today, as we drive cars; mow lawns; trim hedges; use power tools; ride in an airplane, bus, or train; or engage in a myriad of other activities, we too are beset by a vibration-laden environment.

Although we are in many cases surrounded by vibration in our work and leisure environments, little attention is normally paid to it unless we are disturbed or incapacitated by it, for example, by seasickness while aboard a ship; nausea as an airliner traverses turbulence; or tingling, numbness, and pain in the fingertips after use of a vibrating, hand-held tool on a cold day. What can be gleaned on the human effects of this arcane subject has been derived mostly from focused laboratory, epidemiologic, occupational, military, and aerospace studies.

VIBRATION FUNDAMENTALS[28,31]

Linear vibratory motion of an object begins at some point of reference and moves horizontally, vertically, or laterally. The object can also rotate in the form of pitch, yaw, and roll. For simplicity, only linear motion is considered in human vibration. The quantity known as linear displacement is simply the distance an object has moved away from the reference point. It takes a measurable time for the moving object to go from its starting point to this new position; division of the traveled distance by the traversal time equals the object's velocity, or speed. Velocity is defined as the time rate of change of displacement. A moving object need not maintain a constant speed; it can move slower or faster. The time rate of change of velocity or speed is called *acceleration.* Acceleration is usually the intensity measurement of choice for human vibration, and it is an average type of acceleration, known as root-mean-square acceleration, that is determined.

An object can repeat its motion; this repetition is called *periodic* motion. One full period or cycle of motion is referred to as the frequency of motion; the number of cycles per second is a unit of frequency called a Hertz (Hz). There is no guarantee that an object's motion will be periodic, however; it can have random, or aperiodic, motion. The units of measurement of displacement are distances (inches, feet, meters, centimeters, millimeters). Velocity is distance per second. Acceleration is distance per unit of time divided by time (m/sec/sec or ft/sec/sec); in comparison of gravitational g forces to vibration acceleration, 1 g = 9.81 m/sec/sec.

When objects are subjected to vibration, they often exhibit a strange phenomenon called *resonance,* which can lead to damage to or actual destruction of the vibrating object. This is why, for example, soldiers never march across a bridge. Their marching would cause the bridge's structure to become mechanically excited such that its beams would absorb the vibration energy and internally amplify it uncontrollably. The continuous marching would enhance the vibration, causing the bridge to collapse. Unfortunately, humans and other species exposed to vibration exhibit this same phenomenon at certain resonant frequencies; these frequencies can under certain circumstances represent the Achilles heel of human vulnerability to vibration. Clearly, the human system responds to many vibration frequencies forced on it if the intensity is of sufficiently large magnitude, but at resonance only a tiny magnitude of vibration can cause a large and undesirable response. In the vertical plane the human body responds resonantly in the range of 4 to 8 Hz, nominally at 5 Hz.[4] In both the horizontal and lateral directions, resonance occurs in the 1 to 2-Hz range. In hand-arm vibration (HAV) resonance seems to occur in the 100- to 250-Hz range[23,33] in all directions.

Because humans are sensitive to the frequency of vibration, there is concern about not only the vibration acceleration intensity but also the frequency composition or mixture that a person might receive from driving or being a passenger in cars, trucks, buses, and so on or from operating a power tool, for example. Thus a computed frequency spectrum analysis is needed for each vibration measurement and often provides a unique environmental fingerprint that can then be related directly to various health, safety, and comfort standards and guides.[1,2,13,20]

Vibration is a vector quantity, which means that a measurement has both magnitude and direction. At each measurement point three perpendicular simultaneous acceleration measurements are made, using an internationally agreed-on biodynamic coordinate system of axes.[28] For HAV the measurements are obtained either at the third metacarpal of the hand or hands holding the tool or on the tool handle close to the place at which the tool is grasped. The designated z axis runs parallel to digits along bones of the forearm, the y axis runs across the knuckles, and the x axis runs perpendicular through the palm of the hand. For whole-body vibration (WBV) measurements the designated z axis is from head to toe, the y axis runs across the shoulders, and the x axis runs perpendicular through the sternum. A spectrum analysis is performed for each measurement axis for either HAV or WBV measurements. The results are then compared on an axis-by-axis basis with the appropriate human standard to determine whether the standard has been violated.

HAND-ARM VIBRATION EXPOSURE

In 1862 Maurice Raynaud reported attacks of tingling, numbness, and cold-related idiopathic blanching of the fingers of several housewives seen in his Paris clinic. He reported that these primary Raynaud's disease blanching attacks were emotionally induced.[22] The relationship to vibration was first reported by Loriga in 1911 in a description of Italian miners using pneumatic tools.[16] In 1918 Alice Hamilton reported an 83% prevalence of Raynaud-like symptoms in the hands of limestone cutters and carvers in Bedford, Indiana.[11] Since the historic Hamilton study, many studies have reported an association between use of vibrating pneumatic, electrical, and gasoline-powered tools and Raynaud's phenomenon (later called vibration white finger [VWF]). Typical blanching latencies ranged from 1 to 25 years, and blanching prevalences from 10% to 50% or more after medical exclusions.[21] The first case of diffuse scleroderma and Raynaud's phenomenon due to vibrating-tool use was reported by Leys[15] in 1939, with subsequent confirmation by others.[3] Through the years, not only have other studies shown the association of regular vibrating-tool use with the neuropathy and peripheral vascular condition that characterizes VWF but also HAV became linked to digit osteoarthritis, bone cysts,[8] and repetitive trauma disorders such as carpal tunnel syndrome.[5,35] This complex of conditions is now called hand-arm vibration syndrome (HAVS).

The differential diagnosis of HAVS attempts to exclude the conditions shown in Table 50-1, although it is not always possible to do so.[32] Because there is no single definitive medical test for HAVS the following test battery is usually used to evaluate the patient[21]:

  A. Neurologic-component tests
    1. Light touch
    2. Pain
    3. Temperature
    4. Vibrotactile thresholds
    5. Moberg pick-up test (hand function)
  B. Vascular-component tests
    1. Lewis-Prusik
    2. Allen
    3. Doppler artery delineation

Table 50-1. Exclusion criteria and differential diagnosis for vibration syndrome

Causes of vibration	Differential diagnosis
Primary causes Raynaud's disease	Constitutional white finger

Secondary causes
  Raynaud's phenomenon
  Connective tissue disease
	Scleroderma, systematic lupus erythematosus, dermatomyositis, polyarteritis nodosa, mixed connective-tissue disease

Trauma Direct to the extremities	After injury, fracture, or operation; occupational origin, vibration; frostbite and immersion syndrome
To proximal vessels by compression	Thoracic outlet syndrome (cervical rib, scalenus anterior muscle); costoclavicular and hyperabduction syndromes
Occlusive vascular disease	Thromboangiitis obliterans, arteriosclerosis, embolism, thrombosis
Dysglobulinemia	Cold hemagglutination syndrome: cryoglobulinemia, macroglobulinemia
Intoxication	Acroosteolysis, ergot, nicotine
Neurogenic causes	Poliomyelitis, hemiplegia, syringomyelia
Other	Carpal tunnel syndrome

C. Musculoskeletal component
   1. Grip force
   2. Pinch tests
D. Differential diagnosis
   1. Tinel
   2. Phalen
   3. Nerve conduction (median and ulnar, motor and sensory)
E. Work and medical history

A means of stratifying the extent of HAVS was developed in the early 1970s by Taylor and Pelmear[26] and has been used extensively for several years (Table 50-2). It is heavily based on the patient's vascular assessment, using a latency period defined as the time interval from the beginning of tool use to the appearance of the first white finger tip (stage 1).

In 1986 the Taylor-Pelmear system was revised (Table 50-3) at a Stockholm meeting, because some physicians noted that some of their patients with HAVS remained in the neurologic stages, never advancing to blanching despite continued exposure to vibration. The Stockholm system is currently used and requires separate neurologic and vascular assessment and staging for each hand.[9]

WHOLE-BODY VIBRATION EXPOSURE

The characteristics of WBV exposure are usually quite different from those of HAV exposure. In the latter, tool acceleration levels are often very high (typically several hundred g) over a wide frequency range (typically 5 to 5000 Hz). In WBV, there are low acceleration levels (typically under $1g$) over a much narrower frequency range (typically 1 to 80 Hz). WBV is usually a long-term generalized stressor because it impinges on the entire body simultaneously. Many times, WBV causes diffuse and subtle responses, such as the irritability of people working in a confined space in a building, due perhaps to vibration of one or more roof-mounted unsynchronized air-conditioner compressors; there is no apparent carryover effects when the occupants leave the building. A variety of performance decrements have been reported to occur under WBV, especially in the 4- to 8-Hz resonance band, and thus the concern for safety becomes paramount, especially for vehicle drivers.[10] In the 0.1- to 1-Hz band, kinetosis can develop.[11] Major clinical concerns of WBV exposure are degenerative disk diseases, slipped disks, and chronic back pain, particularly in the lumbar area.[6,12,36] There have been some reports of prostatitis in WBV-exposed workers, especially when tight clothing is

Table 50-2. Stages of vibration white fingers (Taylor-Pelmear Classification System, 1975)

Stage	Condition of fingers	Work and social interference
00	No tingling, numbness, or blanching of fingers	No complaints
0T	Intermittent tingling	No interference with activities
0N	Intermittent numbness	No interference with activities
TN	Intermittent tingling and numbness	No interference with activities
1	Blanching of a fingertip with or without tingling and numbness	No interference with activities
2	Blanching of one or more fingers beyond tips, usually during winter	Possible interference with activities outside work; no interference at work
3	Extensive blanching of fingers; frequent episodes in both summer and winter	Definite interference at work, at home, and with social activities; restriction of hobbies
4	Extensive blanching of most fingers; frequent episodes in both summer and winter	Occupation usually changed because of severity of signs and symptoms

Table 50-3. Stockholm-Revised Vibration Syndrome Classification System

Stage	Signs and symptoms	Interference with activities
0N,0V	No signs or symptoms	None
1N	Intermittent tingling	None
1V	Episodic blanching of one or more fingertips	None
2N	Intermittent numbness; reduced tactile perception	Possible interference with activities involving fine tasks
2V	Episodic blanching of one or more fingers, usually confined to winter	Some interference with social activities
3N	Degraded tactile resolution; intermittent numbness	Interference with activities involving fine tasks at work and at home
3V	Extensive finger blanching, frequent episodes summer and winter	Restriction of hobbies and social activities to avoid vasospasms

worn while they drive.[34] Recent reports of female menstrual disorders, proneness to spontaneous abortion, varicosities, and hyperemesis gravidarum in WBV-exposed women have emerged.[24]

For many years there had been a significant amount of research on WBV by eastern European researchers who claimed that WBV exposures caused a general malaise and debilitating effect in their patients, which they called "whole-body vibration sickness." This condition is characterized by two stages; in the first, symptoms are weight loss, nausea, insomnia, colonic cramps, labyrinth disorders, and a drop in visual acuity. The second stage is characterized by muscular pain and atrophy, trophic skin lesions, and pain in the osteoarticular system.[14]

HAND-ARM AND WHOLE-BODY CROSSOVER VIBRATION EXPOSURE

Rarely do HAV and WBV appear together, except in the form of a crossover exposure that is best described by example. If an operator holds and operates a jackhammer, for example, with outstretched arms, the vibration enters the body through the fingers and moves up the arms (that is, HAV), but some operators rest the jackhammer against their abdomen to damp the vibration, which then becomes WBV. The result could be HAVS and/or serious damage to the omentum and abdomen, because the vibration pathway into the body has been altered.[25,30] Another example is an operator's use of a stand grinder that is bolted to the floor; much of the WBV is coupled and damped into the floor and not necessarily into his entire body; however, it is very possible that this operator will develop HAVS because his fingers and hands must hold and guide the workpiece against the grinding wheel, thus conducting the vibration into his body through the hands.

VIBRATION EXPOSURE AND CUMULATIVE TRAUMA DISORDERS

In recent years cumulative trauma disorders such as carpal tunnel syndrome and low back pain with related disorders, especially when poor ergonomic conditions exist, have been reported not only in the scientific literature but also in the lay press. It is well known that carpal tunnel syndrome can and does appear when no vibration component is present but there is excessive grip force, task repetition, and poor wrist angle (such as ulnar deviation, radial deviation, hyperflexion, hyperextension). Although HAV is a form of repetitive trauma to the hands, in some instances patients are diagnosed with HAVS and not necessarily carpal tunnel syndrome, depending on the situation; it seems that this situation may be due to various factors, such as the tool handle's size and shape, whereby a large handle distributes the vibration across a larger surface area than does a small handle,[28] the type of grip and grip forces used by the operator,[28] and so on. In an attempt to distinguish between the relative contribution of vibration to HAVS and carpal syndrome, one researcher claims that "exposure to vibration does not cause polyneuropathy and at least some of the local neuropathic findings are due to the entrapment of the median or ulnar nerves in the hand and arm. Vibration may cause neurological signs by compression due to tissue swelling and excess collagen formation both intra and extraneurally."[7]

The workplace need not be the only situation in which repetitive trauma exists; for example, in a study of 22 young professional baseball catchers, 13 had abnormal circulation in their left index finger. Of these 13 athletes, 3 had additional findings of impaired circulation in both the radial and ulnar digital vessels and 4 had impaired blood flow in the middle finger, with 1 having additional impairment in the ring finger.[17] It would appear that the repetitive trauma of the ball's striking the gloved hand (impact vibration), as well as the hand/wrist angles and the number of catches, contributed to these findings.

In soccer (and possibly boxing) it appears that even minor head trauma can result in organic brain damage, with neurologic deficits, electroencephalographic disturbance, and neuropsychologic impairment.[27] This damage is associated with the sudden acceleration force. It is also conceivable that head trauma is translated into biochemical and thus central nervous system changes during bus and subway rides and rides on bumper cars at amusement parks, as results of a recent rat study of WBV and neuropeptides might suggest.[18]

CONTROLLING HUMAN EXPOSURE TO VIBRATION[19,21,28,29]

A major objective of vibration control is to protect humans from its effects on health, safety, and comfort. The control is often multifaceted. First and foremost, the vibration must be reduced or minimized as much as possible by source substitution and/or the engineering methods of isolation (modification of the pathway between the vibration source and the exposed person) and/or damping (converting vibration energy into a small amount of heat). In the case of HAV, this reduction means using where and when possible so-called antivibration tools, which are also ergonomically designed to reduce hand, wrist, and forearm trauma. For WBV, this reduction means minimizing vehicle vibration, replacing worn shock absorbers, and maintaining correct tire tread, alignment, and pressure; in fixed structures this means avoiding vibrating surfaces as much as possible by using remote controls or robotics, and isolating and/or damping the sources.

Also important is the use of personal protection. For HAV this means using full-finger protected antivibration gloves, many types of which are available. Antivibration gloves should not be used if the digits are exposed. This is a vain attempt by some glove manufacturers to overcome their problem of poor glove fit by providing maximal tactile feedback without adequate protection of the person. HAVS begins at the fingertip and moves toward the finger root. For

WBV, personal protection means use of air-ride–type seats or mechanically suspended seats, available from many manufacturers.

Adequate work and safety practices should be used. For HAV these practices include keeping the hands and body warm and dry; minimizing the contact time with a vibrating tool; replacing worn tools, chisels, bits, blades, and so on; properly maintaining the tools; letting the tool do the work by minimizing the vibration conducted into the hands by the use of a minimal hand grip force consistent with safe work practices; not smoking; and consulting a physician when the first signs of HAVS appear. For WBV, these practices involve minimizing the actual exposure time, and if the operator has a history of back pain and/or degenerative disk disorders, the potential clinical consequences of continued WBV exposure must be carefully evaluated.[6,12,36] Appropriate health, safety, or comfort standards or guides should be used only after they have been completely read and understood. At this writing there are no mandatory standards for either HAV or WBV; however, the following guidelines are used extensively in the United States:

HAV:
American Conference of Governmental Industrial Hygienists Threshold Limit Values for HAV.[1]
American National Standards Institute, S3.34-1986.[2]
National Institute for Occupational Safety and Health Document 89-106.[20]

WBV:
International Standards Organization, 2631 (same as ANSI S3.18).[13]

MEDICAL MANAGEMENT

At this writing, calcium channel blocker therapy is in use in many situations. Better success has been found with older rather than younger workers. For clinical details and therapeutics, see Pelmear et al.[21]

SUMMARY

In this chapter the salient elements of recognition, evaluation, measurement, and control of human exposure to HAV and WBV found in the workplace and environment are presented. Cumulative trauma disorders of the upper limbs and trunk also are discussed in the context of their interaction with human vibration exposure.

REFERENCES

1. American Conference of Government Industrial Hygienists: *Threshold limit values (TLV) for chemical substances and physical agents: TLV for exposure to hand-arm vibration,* Cincinnati, 1993.
2. American National Standards Institute: *Guide for the measurement and evaluation of human exposure to vibration transmitted to the hand,* S3.34, New York, 1986.
3. Blair HM, Headington JT, Lynch PJ: Occupational trauma, Raynaud's phenomenon, and sclerodactylia, *Arch Environ Health* 28:80, 1974.
4. Coermann R: The mechanical impedance of the human body in sitting and standing positions at low frequencies, *Human Factors* 4:225, 1962.
5. Conner DE, Kolisek FR: Vibration-induced carpal tunnel syndrome, *Orthop Rev* 15:49, 1986.
6. Dupuis H, Zerlett G: *The effects of whole-body vibration,* Berlin, 1986, Springer-Verlag.
7. Färkkilä M: Vibration induced injury, *Br J Ind Med* 43:361, 1986.
8. Gemne G, Saraste H: Bone and joint pathology in workers using hand held vibrating tools, *Scand J Work Environ Health* 13:290, 1987.
9. Gemne G et al: The Stockholm workshop scale for the classification of cold induced Raynaud's phenomenon in the hand-arm vibration syndrome (revision of the Taylor-Pelmear scale), *Scand J Work Environ Health* 13:275, 1987.
10. Griffin MJ: *Handbook of human vibration,* London, 1990, Academic Press.
11. Hamilton A: *A study of spastic anemia in the hands of stonecutters: an effect of the airhammer on the hands of stonecutters,* Industrial Accidents and Hygiene Series No 236/19, Washington, DC, 1918, US Department Labor, Bureau of Labor Statistics.
12. Hulshof C, van Zanten B: Whole-body vibration and low-back pain: a review of epidemiologic studies, *Int Arch Occup Environ Health* 59:205, 1987.
13. International Standards Organization: *Guide for the evaluation of human exposure to whole-body vibration,* 2631, Geneva, 1978.
14. Jakubowski R: General characteristics of vibration at various workplaces in agriculture and forestry, *Med Wicj* 4:47, 1969.
15. Leys D: Diffuse scleroderma and Raynaud's phenomenon from the use of a pneumatic hammer, *Lancet* 2:692, 1939.
16. Loriga G: Pneumatic tools: occupation and health, *Ball Inspet Lorobo* 2:35, 1911.
17. Lowrey C, Chadwick R, Waltman E: Digital vessel trauma from repetitive impact in baseball catchers, *J Hand Surg* 11:236, 1976.
18. Nakamura H: Effects of whole-body vibration stress on substance P- and neurotensin-like immunoreactivity in the rat brain, *Environ Res* 52:155, 1990.
19. National Institute for Occupational Safety and Health: *Current Intelligence Bulletin No 38: vibration syndrome,* DHHS/NIOSH Pub No 83-110, Cincinnati, 1983.
20. National Institute for Occupational Safety and Health: *Criteria for a recommended standard for occupational exposure to hand-arm vibration,* 89-106, Cincinnati, 1989.
21. Pelmear P, Taylor W, Wasserman D, eds: *Hand-arm vibration: a comprehensive guide for occupational health professionals,* New York, 1992, Van Nostrand Reinhold.
22. Raynaud M: *Local asphyxia and symmetrical gangrene of the extremities,* Paris, 1862 (English translation in *Selected Monographs of the New Sydenham Society,* London, 1888).
23. Reynolds D et al: A study of hand vibration in chipping and grinding operations, *J Sound and Vibration* 95:479, 1984.
24. Seidel H, Heide R: Long term effects of whole-body vibration: a critical survey of the literature, *Int Arch Occup Environ Health* 58:1, 1986.
25. Shields P, Chase K: Primary torsion of the omentum in a jackhammer operator: another vibration related injury, *J Occup Med* 31:892, 1988.
26. Taylor W, Pelmear P: *Vibration white finger in industry,* London, 1975, Academic Press.
27. Tysvaer AT: Soccer injuries to the brain: a neuropsychologic study of former soccer players, *Am J Sports Med* 19:56, 1991.
28. Wasserman DE: *Human aspects of occupational vibration,* Amsterdam, 1987, Elsevier.
29. Wasserman D: The control aspects of occupational hand-arm vibration, *Applied Industrial Hygiene* 4:22, 1989.
30. Wasserman D: Jackhammer usage and the omentum, *J Occup Med* 31:563, 1989.
31. Wasserman DE: Vibration: principles, measurements, and health standards, *Semin Perinatol* 14:311, 1990.
32. Wasserman D, Taylor W: Lessons from hand-arm vibration syndrome research, *Am J Ind Med* 19:539, 1991.

33. Wasserman D et al: *Vibration white finger disease in U.S. workers using chipping and grinding hand tools,* vol II, *Engineering,* DHHS/NIOSH Pub No 82-101, Washington, DC, 1982.
34. Wasserman D et al: Vibration exposure in paperboard manufacturing, *J Acoust Soc Am* 76:56, 1984.
35. Wieslander G et al: Carpal tunnel syndrome and exposure to vibration, repetitive wrist movements, and heavy manual work: a case referent study, *Br J Ind Med* 46:43, 1989.
36. Wilder DG, Woodworth BB, Frymoyer JW: Vibration and the human spine, *Spine* 7:243, 1982.

Chapter 51

HEAT STRESS

Francis N. Dukes-Dobos

Safe limits of heat stress
    Heat-stress indices
    Threshold limit values
    Physiologic limits
Populations at risk
Effect of age and gender on heat tolerance
Recognition and first aid of acute heat illnesses and disorders
    Heat stroke
    Heat exhaustion
    Heat cramps
    Dehydration
    Prickly heat (heat rash, miliaria rubra)
    Heat edema
Chronic heat illnesses
Prevention measures
    Acclimation
    Maintenance of body hydration and electrolyte balance
    Education
    Medical oversight
    Heat alert program
Summary

Human beings must keep their body temperature within narrow limits if optimal function is to be maintained. While heat is constantly generated by body metabolism and in the environment the air and radiant temperature, as well as the air movement and humidity vary, the body is equipped with adaptive mechanisms that enable a person to preserve a constant core temperature (t_c).[20] This holds true as long as the environment is cooler than the skin or permits evaporation of sweat from the skin; however, when the climatic conditions exceed the human adaptation capacity, the t_c and the skin temperature rise, creating a stressful condition that is felt as discomfort. When the heat stress exceeds human tolerance limits, heat disorders and illnesses, some of which are fatal, ensue. According to data published by the National Safety Council,[41,42] the 5-year average of fatalities due to excessive heat exposure in the United States was 599 between 1980 and 1984.

With modern technology, heat stress in homes and at work can be prevented by air conditioning and personal protective equipment such as ice vests and water- or air-cooled garments and helmets; however, the cost and energy requirement take air conditioning out of reach for many homes and workplaces. Personal cooling equipment also is costly and can interfere with the performance of skilled work because of its bulkiness. Its weight also is burdensome, and some systems are connected by tubing to compressed air or an ice-water container, which limits mobility. Clothing covered with reflective material gives protection against radiant heat but may cause heat stress by preventing the evaporation of sweat. Consequently, clothing protective against heat stress is worn only in jobs in which heat stress cannot be reduced by other means, and for the time being many people have to live and work exposed to heat stress at times. The questions are, how much heat stress is tolerable, and how can the occurrence of heat illnesses and disorders be prevented?

SAFE LIMITS OF HEAT STRESS

The human body is equipped with physiologic adaptive mechanisms that make it possible to tolerate heat stress within certain limits. Much research has been performed to determine at what level heat stress is considered excessive, that is, gives rise to the risk of heat disorders or causes illnesses.[40] This is a complex problem because of the great individual variability in heat tolerance and because the body's heat exchange with the environment is influenced by numerous factors, the most important being four climatic factors: air temperature, air velocity, air humidity, and infrared (heat) radiation. These four factors can occur in an infinite number of combinations. In addition, to characterize the magnitude of the heat stress imposed on a person, it is necessary to quantify the metabolic heat generated inside the body as well as the heat insulation, radiant heat absorption, reflection and transmission, vapor permeability, moisture absorption, and ventilation properties of clothing.

Measurement of the climatic variables requires a dry-bulb thermometer for air temperature, a wet-bulb thermometer to measure humidity, a globe thermometer to measure heat radiation, and an anemometer to measure air velocity.

Dry-bulb thermometers are like room thermometers and either contain mercury or alcohol in glass or are electric with thermistor or thermocouple sensors.

The wet-bulb thermometer consists of a dry-bulb thermometer that is covered by a wick wetted with distilled water. This thermometer is called a natural wet bulb and is sensitive not only to the vapor content of the air but also to air velocity. Therefore, if the wet-bulb thermometer is to be used for determining the air humidity, the effect of natural air currents has to be eliminated by directing a high-speed air stream, created by an electric fan or by rapid movement of the thermometer, over the wet bulb. Such an instrument is called a psychrometric wet-bulb thermometer.

The globe thermometer[56] consists of a hollow copper globe painted matte black, preferably 6 inches in diameter with a temperature sensor in its center. The globe thermometer also is sensitive to air velocity, which must be taken into consideration in calculation of the mean radiant temperature (MRT)[31]:

$$MRT = GT + 14.4\ V^{0.5}\ (GT - DB)$$

where

GT = heat radiation in degrees Celsius
DB = air temperature in degrees celsius
V = air velocity expressed in meters per second
14.4 = the convective heat transfer coefficient

The anemometer can be either a vane anemometer, which also can identify the direction of air movement, or a hot-wire anemometer, which has averaging capability but is nondirectional.

Measurement of metabolic heat also is not simple. It requires expensive equipment, such as a tight-fitting half gas mask connected, through tubing, with a gas-tight collecting bag and an oxygen and carbon dioxide analyzer and a gasometer.[12] Several innovative instruments are battery driven and portable and include the oxygen analyzer and gasometer. These instruments are quite expensive and not without problems when used in field studies. Therefore, instead of measurement of metabolism, tables containing examples of energy requirements for given activities are used for estimation of metabolism by comparison of the given activity with those listed in the tables. (see Table 51-3.)

The measurement of heat insulation and vapor permeability of the clothing requires a copper mannequin placed in a climatically controlled chamber.[37,55] The mannequin must be able to simulate metabolically generated heat and to exude water to simulate sweating. Both functions must be quantitatively controllable and evenly distributed over the whole surface of the mannequin. Only a few mannequins with these capabilities are available in the United States, Europe, and Japan. Measurements made with those mannequins have been published and are available in tabulated form.[34,44] They can be used for estimation of the insulation and permeability of clothing ensembles.

Clothing ventilation can be measured by any of the gas-dilution techniques described in the pertinent literature.[35,47] Clothing ventilation depends on the porosity of the clothing material, the design and fit of the clothing, the environmental air velocity, and the pumping effect due to body motion.[48]

Heat-stress indices

Several heat-stress indices have been described in the pertinent literature.[8] They combine environmental heat variables—and in some the metabolic heat and clothing properties—into a single number, making it possible to rate and compare the heat stress prevailing at different job sites, even if the proportions of the four components of the climate and the metabolic heat vary at each site. For instance, two heat-stress conditions may have the same index value, even if one consists of heavy work without radiant heat and the other, of light work with high radiant heat. Heat-stress indices also make possible expression of permissible exposure limits as one number.

The various heat-stress indices recommended by different scientists have been evaluated according to their accuracy and practical applicability. None of the indices satisfy all requirements.[8] There are two kinds of indices: rational and empirical.[27]

The rational indices are based on calculation of the heat balance of the body:

$$S = M \pm C \pm R - E$$

where

S = body heat storage (measurable by body temperature)
M = the metabolically generated heat (measurable by oxygen consumption and depending on work intensity)
C = the heat gained or lost by convection (depending on the difference between air temperature and skin temperature and on air velocity)
R = the heat gained or lost by radiation (depending on the difference between skin temperature and the surface temperature of the surrounding solid objects)
E = heat lost by evaporation (measurable by weight loss, and limited by humidity, air velocity, and human sweating capacity)

The first rational heat-stress index, HSI, was developed by Belding and Hatch[6] and is still the most widely used. It can be calculated by the following equation:

$$HSI = \frac{E_{req}}{E_{max}} \times 100$$

where

E_{req} = the amount of sweat evaporation required for elimination of the heat accumulated in the body by exposure to environmental heat and generated by metabolism

E_{max} = the water-vapor uptake capacity of the air; it depends on humidity and air velocity

A nomograph[38] and a computer program[25] are available to calculate HSI. A scale interprets the meaning of the HSI values from 0 to 100. The value of 0 means that there is no thermal strain. From 10 to 30 the heat stress is mild to moderate. From 40 to 60 the heat stress is severe, involving threats to health unless workers are acclimated. Some decrement of physical and mental work can be expected. From 70 to 90 the heat stress is very severe, and only a few people with exceptional levels of fitness can tolerate it. The HSI value of 100 means that this heat stress can be tolerated only by a few young, highly acclimated persons. Beginning with the value of 40, medical selection of workers is recommended. This scale is based on the assumption that sweating 1 L per hour can be tolerated by healthy, acclimated workers for 8 hours a day, over an unlimited period; however, this assumption does not take into consideration that there is a limited ability to replace salt and water lost in the secreted sweat adequately, so the risk of excessive dehydration or electrolyte imbalance must be accounted for. Furthermore, the HSI does not take into consideration the insulation and vapor-permeability properties of the clothing worn by the exposed worker. In addition, the supporting data were derived from experiments on young, healthy subjects, not typical for an average mixed-industrial-worker population. The values of heat-transfer coefficients were based on averages of experimental results and thus are either too high or too low for the majority of a mixed population, leaving the less fit individuals at greater risk.

It must be also realized that any HSI value can be the result of various combinations of E_{req} and E_{max} values. For instance, an HSI of 50 can result from an E_{req} of 300 and an E_{max} of 600, as well as from an E_{req} of 600 and an E_{max} of 1200, yet the two conditions are not equivalent from the point of view of physiologic strain. Furthermore, the HSI is based on the assumption that the mean skin temperature of the exposed person is 35° C (95° F), which is, at best, a good guess and further reduces the predictive accuracy of the HSI. In addition, to obtain an HSI value it is necessary to measure air velocity. Because the speed of air movement fluctuates constantly and also is affected by body movement, an accurate value is almost impossible.

Despite these shortcomings, the HSI is a useful tool for identifying the significance of each factor in bringing about the prevailing heat stress and for calculating the possible benefit resulting from change of any of these factors. It must be emphasized, however, that the actual sweating requirement is always more than the required evaporation because some sweat is always lost to dripping or absorption in clothing rather than evaporation. For all these reasons, HSI is not a practical method for setting safety limits for heat exposure and for monitoring the actual exposure to heat stress. A modified version of the HSI has been adapted by the International Organization for Standardization[23] as a standard method for analyzing the contribution of the different factors of heat stress to the total heat stress. It is based on studies performed in the laboratories of the Center for Bioclimatological Studies under Bernard Metz in Strasbourg, France.[57] This version takes care of the problem of the difference between the required evaporation and the required sweating necessary to achieve the required evaporation for maintenance of heat balance. Therefore this index is called Required Sweating (S_{req}). It also takes into account the clothing effect and the safety of the less acclimated workers; however, calculation of S_{req} uses even more assumed values than the original HSI, and the whole method becomes quite cumbersome even if the equations are calculated by computer.

Empirical indices are based on subjective or objective human responses to heat-stress exposures of different intensity. Subjective responses are verbal ratings of severity of a given heat exposure. Objective responses are changes in physiologic variables, such as heart rate, body temperature, or sweat rate. The most popular empirical indices are the effective temperature (ET),[21] the wet bulb globe temperature index (WBGT),[60] and the predicted four-hour sweat rate (P_4SR).[36] The accuracy of each of these indices is approximately the same; however, the ET and the P_4SR are read from nomographs, whereas the WBGT can be calculated by the use of one of the following two simple equations:

Outdoors in sunshine: WBGT = 0.7 NWB + 0.2 GT + 0.1 DB
Outdoors without
　sunshine and indoors: WBGT = 0.7 NWB + 0.3 GT

This feature makes WBGT more practical, particularly because it made possible development of direct-reading WBGT instruments. An additional disadvantage of the ET and P_4SR nomographs is that their highest air temperature or radiant heat scales do not go beyond 110°C and 130°C, respectively, and extrapolation to higher values is not justifiable without experimental evidence. WBGT also has the advantage that its use does not require measurement of air velocity as a separate climatic variable, because the NWB and GT are sensitive to air speed, as mentioned earlier. For assessment of the value of ET or P_4SR, the air velocity must be measured with a separate instrument. As mentioned previously, this measurement is difficult because of the highly fluctuating nature of this variable.

Threshold limit values

In 1972 the American Conference of Governmental Industrial Hygienists (ACGIH) published a threshold limit value (TLV) for heat stress,[1] based on studies performed at the Cincinnati laboratories of the National Institute of Occupational Safety and Health (NIOSH).[14] This TLV, with slight modifications, was adopted as a standard of the International Organization for Standardization[24] in 1982 and is accepted widely as a guide for safe exposure limits for work in hot environments. The recent modified version of the TLV[2] is shown in Fig. 51-1.

In Fig. 51-1 the hourly time-weighted average (TWA) values of the metabolic heat generated by work are plotted against the hourly TWA-WBGT. There are two limit curves in the diagram shown in Fig. 51-1. The upper curve depicts the exposure limits for acclimated workers; the lower curve, the limits for the unacclimated ones. It is stipulated in the text of the TLV that new workers are considered to be unacclimated during the first week of their employment.

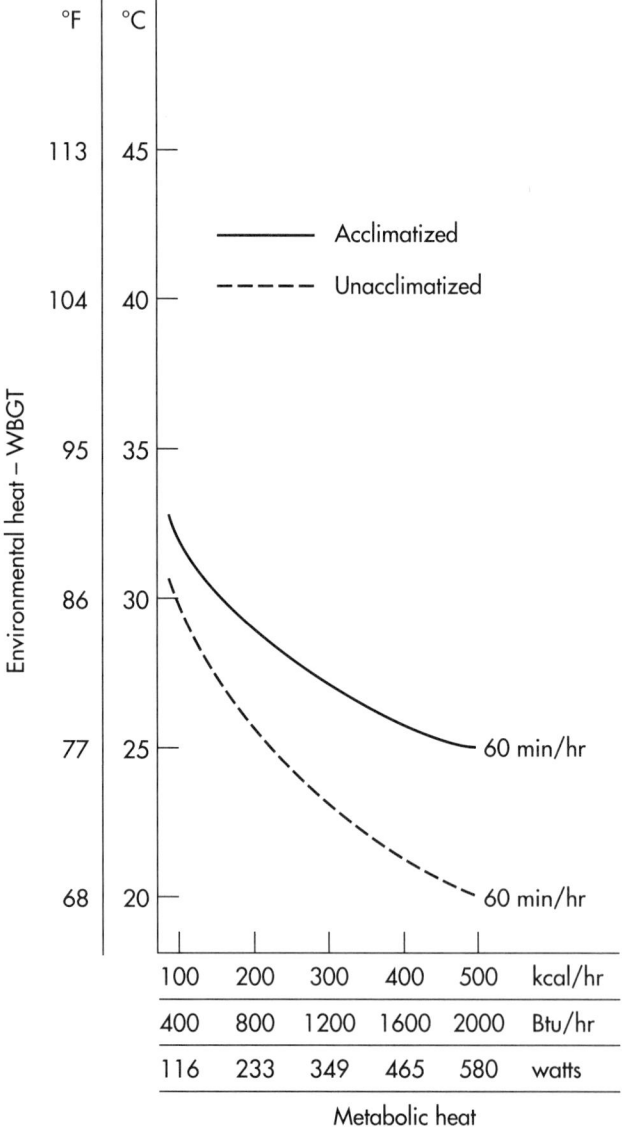

Fig. 51-1. Permissible heat exposure threshold limit values for heat acclimatized and unacclimatized workers. (Adapted from *Threshold limit values for chemical and physical agents and biological exposure indices,* ACGIH, 1992-1993.

The limit values drawn up by the TLV curves shown in Fig. 51-1 are derived from studies performed by Nielsen and Nielsen.[43] They demonstrated that if human beings are exposed to physical exertion in heat, their t_c, measured rectally, slowly increases and reaches a steady state, or equilibrates, after approximately an hour. The equilibrium level, however, is determined solely by the level of physical exertion and is not affected by the level of environmental heat until the heat reaches a critical level. In other words, the equilibrium t_c is not affected by the rise of the environmental heat within certain limits of climatic conditions; however, if the environmental heat is increased beyond this critical level, the equilibrium t_c starts to rise, that is, the equilibrium t_c starts to become affected by the environmental temperature. Lind[32] explored this phenomenon at various work rates and found that the higher the work rate, the higher the equilibrium t_c and the lower the critical temperature. Thus, if environmental heat would continue to increase beyond the critical level, the equilibrium t_c would also increase and eventually may reach or exceed the limit still tolerable without harmful health effects. For instance, at light exercise (180 kcal/hr), the t_c equilibrated at 37.6°C (99.5°F). The critical temperature was 29°C (84°F) in terms of ET index. When the ambient heat was raised by only 5°C (9°F) to 34°C (93°F) ET, the t_c increased to 38.1°C (100.6°F), slightly above the safe limit of 38°C (100.4°F). Lind[32] called the climatic condition below the critical level the "prescriptive zone," suggesting that extended exposures beyond this level should not be permitted because of the health risk involved.

The TLV curves follow the values of the climatic conditions (in terms of WBGT) at the upper limits of the prescriptive zone at each level of work metabolism. The curves have been slightly modified by taking into consideration the difference between the level of acclimation and the clothing worn by Lind's experimental subjects and those of an average worker population.[16] Allowance was also made for shifting the limit values toward the ninety-fifth percentile level instead of the mean. Thus, the TLV values are safe for nearly all workers, that is, the risk that any worker may become affected by a heat illness or disorder when exposed to conditions within the TLV is minimal. As a matter of fact, higher exposures than the TLV are safe for less than an hour if this exposure is compensated within the same hour by exposure to less heat or to rest periods that bring the TWA value down to the TLV limit. (See Table 51-1.)

If a worker is medically screened and it has been established that he or she is more physically fit and heat tolerant than the average worker, exposures slightly above the TLV can be considered safe; however, for complete safety, it is advisable that the worker's oral temperature be monitored to ensure that it does not exceed 37.6°C (99.6°F), corresponding to a t_c of 38°C (100.4°F). This core temperature as a safe limit for prolonged daily exposure has been recommended by an international scientific group convened by the World Health Organization.[58]

Table 51-1. Examples of permissible heat exposure threshold limit values (values are given in °C and [°F] WBGT)*

	Workload		
Work-rest regimen	Light	Moderate	Heavy
Continuous work	30.0(86)	26.7(80)	25.0(77)
75% work—25% rest, each hour	30.6(87)	28.0(82)	25.9(78)
50% work—50% rest, each hour	31.4(89)	29.4(85)	27.9(82)
25% work—75% rest, each hour	32.2(90)	31.1(88)	30.0(86)

Adapted from American Conference of Governmental Industrial Hygienists: *"Threshold limit values for chemical and physical agents and biological exposure indices, 1992–1993,"* Cincinnati, 1992, The Conference.
*As workload increases, the heat stress impact on an unacclimated worker is exacerbated (see Fig. 51-1). For unacclimatized workers performing a moderate level of work, the permissible heat exposure TLV should be reduced by approximately 2.5°C.

Table 51-2. TLV WBGT correction factors in °C for clothing

Clothing type	Clo value*	WBGT correction
Summer work uniform	0.6	0
Cotton overalls	1.0	−2
Winter work uniform	1.4	−4
Water barrier, permeable	1.2	−6

Adapted from American Conference of Governmental Industrial Hygienists: *"Threshold limit values for chemical and physical agents and biological exposure indices, 1992–1993,"* Cincinnati, 1992, The Conference.
Clo, Insulation value of clothing.
*One clo unit = 5.55 kcal/m²/hr of heat exchange by radiation and convection for each °C of temperature difference between the skin and adjusted dry-bulb temperature [$DB_{ad} = (DB + MRT)/2$].

Table 51-2 shows correction factors to be applied to the TLVs when workers wear heavier clothing than the usual lightweight summer uniforms consisting of pants and shirt only. These correction factors are based on the experiments performed recently by Kenney,[26] and Table 51-2 is included in the 1992-1993 edition of the TLV for heat stress.

The TLV also contains guidance for assessment of the metabolic heat generated by muscular work. There are two methods from which to choose. In one method, the work is rated as light, medium, or heavy. Examples are given for each of the three categories to make it possible to rank any job by comparison. The light-work category encompasses work rates to 200 kcal/hr; the moderate work, from 200 to 350 kcal/hr; and the heavy work, from 350 to 500 kcal/hr. The second method (Table 51-3)[30] requires, first, determi-

Table 51-3. Assessment of work load

Average values of metabolic rate during different activities

A. Body position and movement	kcal/min
Sitting	0.3
Standing	0.6
Walking	2.0–3.0
Walking up hill	add 0.8 per meter (yard) rise

B. Type of work		Average kcal/min	Range kcal/min
Hand work	Light	0.4	0.2–1.2
	Heavy	0.9	
Work with one arm	Light	1.0	0.7–2.5
	Heavy	1.7	
Work with both arms	Light	1.5	1.0–3.5
	Heavy	2.5	
Work with body	Light	3.5	2.5–15.0
	Moderate	5.0	
	Heavy	7.0	
	Very heavy	9.0	

Adapted from American Conference of Governmental Industrial Hygienists: *Threshold limit values for chemical and physical agents and biological exposure indices,* 1992–1993, Cincinnati, 1992, The Conference.

nation of the body position or movement and, second, the involvement of the hands, arms, or the whole body in the activity. Metabolic rate values are given for each category in terms of kilocalories per minute, and the two values so derived are added and increased by 1 kcal/min to account for the basal metabolism.

Physiologic limits

Another approach to determination of whether workers are at risk to exceed their tolerance limits to heat exposure is to monitor their physiologic responses. Criteria for such measurements are that they should be socially acceptable and should not interfere with the work to be performed.

Body temperature, as mentioned before, is the critical physiologic response to heat stress. Oral temperature is a good indicator of t_c. It is approximately 0.4°C or 1.0°F lower than rectal temperature but is the measurement of choice to obtain indication of t_c. The subject should not drink or eat anything cold or hot for at least 15 minutes before measurement. The thermometer must be inserted under the tongue, as far as possible, for about 5 minutes, and the mouth must be kept closed as much as possible. This method is preferable to measurement of ear-canal temperature, which tends to be influenced by the ambient temperature unless the ear is covered tightly before the measurement to give the air in the ear canal enough time to take up the temperature of the surrounding skin. In some hospitals, ear-canal thermometers are used routinely, with satisfactory accuracy; however, the room temperature in hospitals is kept constantly at comfort levels, so the conditions are different from those in a hot workshop. Tympanic temperature measurement is not acceptable for routine use because it requires the removal of earwax, and touching the tympanic membrane with the temperature sensor can be painful. The measurement of rectal and esophageal temperature is limited to laboratory use. Measurement of the skin temperature with a sensor that is insulated from the environment can give a good indication of t_c, and such a device is commercially available.[7] As mentioned before, the safe limit of t_c in prolonged daily exposures is 38°C (100.4°F). For shorter periods, an excursion to 38.5°C (101.3°F) can be considered safe, with a warning that the worker needs rest in a cool area to recover.[40]

Heart rate is another measurable physiologic indicator of heat stress to determine whether a heat exposure is within safe limits.[52] A number of commercially available devices can monitor heart rate; however, none is completely accurate. Therefore the recovery heart rate measurement, recommended by Brouha,[9] is still the best approach. This method requires that the worker sit down immediately after completion of a work cycle, and the radial or carotid pulse is measured for 30 seconds after a 30-second waiting period. The pulse is multiplied by two to obtain the first-minute recovery heart rate. In similar fashion, second- and third-minute recovery heart rates are obtained. Brouha's criterion for safe limits is 110 beats per min for the first minute, and the third minute count should be at least 10 beats per minute lower; however, higher first-minute recovery heart rates have been observed in a group of industrial workers by Fuller and Smith,[18] without the workers'[2] oral temperature exceeding 37.6°C (99.6°F). They found that a better indicator is the third-minute recovery heart rate, which should not exceed 90 beats/min.

Brouha[9] also suggested that the 8-hour average heart rate should not exceed 110 beats per minute. The criterion for this recommendation, however, was not the prevention of heat illnesses but to avert accumulation of fatigue, demonstrable by a creeping increase of the heart rate during the day. This increase of heart rate can be interpreted as gradual decrease of fitness, thus making the worker more prone to a heat disorder or illness.

Another physiologic measure of heat stress is sweating. Determination of the amount of sweat secreted within a given period of time requires measurement of the worker's nude body weight at the beginning and at the end of the work period. The weight loss must be corrected by the difference between the weight of the food and fluid intake and the weight of the urine and feces produced during this period; however, if the sweat secreted is in the magnitude of several hundred grams per hour, the error resulting from weighing the workers without removing their clothing becomes insignificant. To reduce the error that accompanies this simplification, the workers are asked to empty their pockets before they are weighed. Furthermore, the work uniform and underwear can be measured before and after work to account for the sweat absorbed by the clothing.

POPULATIONS AT RISK

Every summer, hospital emergency departments and infirmaries of industrial plants treat people suffering from heat illnesses and heat disorders such as heat stroke, which can be fatal, and heat exhaustion, which also may have severe health consequences.[52] Other adverse health effects of excessive heat exposure are heat cramps, dehydration, heat rash, and heat edema, which are categorized as heat disorders rather than illnesses. They are milder, and after recovery they do not leave significant health effects[31]; however, they serve as a warning that there is a risk for more severe health damage.

An increase in the rate of accidents may be another warning of excessive heat exposure. Workers who are under severe climatic stress tend to take shortcuts in maintaining machines, keeping their workplace in order, and following safety rules.[45] Heat stress may also reduce workers' alertness or make them impatient, particularly if they become dehydrated because of excessive sweating and insufficient fluid intake.[40]

The risk of heat stroke in the general population involves mostly the poor and the aged who live in tenements that are not air-conditioned.[10] Some cities have established emergency procedures to make available to old people transportation to air-conditioned shelters during heat waves.

Workers in hot industries, such as steel, iron, and metal smelters; glass-manufacturing plants; brick, earth, and stoneware kilns; paper, textile, and tire factories; canneries; bakeries; and cleaning plants also are at risk for heat stroke as well as for other harmful health effects if preventive measures are not observed.[15] Outdoor occupations such as agriculture, construction, and surface mining expose workers often to extreme ambient conditions, including strong solar radiation. Experienced workers, however, know their tolerance limits and how to protect themselves from becoming overheated. On hot days they slow down, seek shaded rest areas, and wear hats with large brims and light loose shirts. They work in the early-morning hours and cease working before the heat is the greatest in the afternoon. It is the new worker who is at risk of becoming overheated.

Workers who have to wear partially or completely encapsulating protective clothing, as in some operations in chemical plants, at hazardous waste storage sites, in asbestos removal, and at nuclear power plants,[11] are at significant risk of overheating. Usually the material of such protective clothing is impermeable to vapors, thus obstructing sweat evaporation.

People engaged in vigorous outdoor sport activities also are a high-risk population for heat illnesses during the summer.[22] The risk is enhanced by wearing extensive protective gear, such as in football, which interferes with evaporation of sweat. In endurance sports such as bicycling and marathon running, sufficient fluid intake may be difficult; thus dehydration is a major risk factor. Military recruits often suffer heat illnesses or disorders during their drill exercises or when standing in direct sunlight in full uniform.

Pregnant women are at risk for fetal damage during the first trimester if they become overheated. They should be especially careful to avoid exposure to heat stress.[29]

EFFECT OF AGE AND GENDER ON HEAT TOLERANCE

Several studies[4,59] have shown that heat tolerance is in close correlation with aerobic capacity. Because aerobic capacity, in terms of group average, declines slowly but consistently with age[3] beginning at age 20, it could be concluded that the same is true for heat tolerance; however, just as some individuals maintain a relatively high aerobic capacity with aging,[39] so do some people maintain their heat tolerance until a relatively old age.[50] Furthermore, the correlation between age and heat tolerance may vary when a person is resting or is doing physical exercise. During exercise the aerobic capacity plays a major role in heat tolerance, whereas in rest the ability to sweat and to dilate the blood vessels in the skin becomes more important. Curiously, older men's skin blood vessels dilate more than do those of younger men,[19] and women have higher skin temperature in moderate or severe heat stress than do men,[13] suggesting a higher skin blood flow. Older men start sweating later than do the young, and after heat exposure it takes them longer to cool down.[33] On the other hand, women maintain their sweating ability after menopause. Men and women sweat about the same in dry heat,[17] but women tend to sweat more than men do in humid heat. Women, on average, have lower aerobic capacity than have men[3]; however, when men and women with the same aerobic capacity are exposed to the same heat stress, their heat tolerance is about the same.[4]

All these facts lead to the conclusion that, on the average, older people and women have less tolerance to work in heat than do young men. In addition, men over the age of 40 were found to be 10 times more susceptible to heat stroke than were younger men[54]; however, the risk of heat stroke is minimal if the heat stress is kept within the limits of the TLV and preventive measures such as preemployment medical examination and acclimation are observed. In addition, self-selection eliminates people from hot jobs, resulting in a worker population in which even the least heat-tolerant person is able to work without being at risk to be overcome by heat disorders or illnesses.

RECOGNITION AND FIRST AID OF ACUTE HEAT ILLNESSES AND DISORDERS
Heat stroke

When the t_c exceeds about 40°C (104°C), the brain cells cannot continue to function normally. As a result the functions of the body governed by the central nervous system become disorganized. The body's temperature regulation center is in the hypothalamus[20]; when it is damaged, one of the symptoms is cessation of sweating. This creates a vicious circle because when air temperature exceeds skin temperature (approximately 35°C, or 95°F), sweat evaporation is the only route by which heat can be eliminated from the body. Thus the t_c increases even faster than before, and the t_c may rise rapidly to a fatal level.

At the early stage of heat stroke the peripheral vasodilatation, which helps bring the metabolically generated heat to the skin surface, is maximal, which is why the skin of the heat stroke victim is brilliantly red. At a later stage the vasomotor center also is dysfunctional; the victim's skin may become pale and feels cold, and sometimes the patient starts to shiver, which again further increases the body temperature by increasing the internally generated heat.

The longer the body t_c exceeds 40°C (104°F), the more widespread and severe is the cellular damage. Consequently, the victim first becomes disoriented and sometimes mimics the behavior of a drunk person. The victim may wander away from the work site and may lie down in a corner. When detected, the brain damage may have progressed too far, one of the greatest dangers in heat stroke.[14] Workers and supervisors in hot plants should be made aware of this hazard, and workers exposed to high heat stress should never be left alone, which can be ensured by a buddy system.

At a later stage loss of consciousness causes the patient to collapse, and finally convulsions set in. At this stage the cellular damage becomes irreversible, even if the patient survives, which is why it is so important to recognize heat stroke at an early stage and to start to cool the victim immediately. The most advanced technique for cooling is the use of a thermostatically controlled cooling blanket. If it is not available, the victim should be wrapped in a wet sheet after the clothes have been removed, and to accelerate the evaporation, a high-speed fan should be used to blow air toward the sheet. Water must be sprinkled continuously on the sheet to keep it wet. The water should not be colder than 20°C (68°F), or the patient will develop peripheral vasoconstriction, which slows down the transport of heat from the core to the skin. The effectiveness of this method can be enhanced by laying the patient on a hammock instead of a bed, thus also exposing the patient's back to the evaporative cooling.

Immersion in an ice-cooled bath is another alternative for cooling a patient; however, it carries the risk of circulatory shock, and the patient's skin must be constantly massaged to prevent vasoconstriction. It is also difficult to monitor the patient's rectal temperature when he or she is immersed in water, and the patient may become overcooled. Cooling should stop when t_c reaches 38°C (100.4°F), because t_c continues to fall after the cessation of cooling. To obtain t_c values a thermistor thermometer should be inserted 20 cm into the rectum. The patient must be taken to a hospital emergency department as soon as possible so that cooling can be continued under medical supervision. If the victim has cooled successfully by the time he or she arrives to the emergency room, the diagnosis of heat stroke must be based on blood chemistry.[28] If the victim was not involved in vigorous physical activity before the heat stroke, hypokalemia, hypocalcemia, hypophosphatemia, and respiratory alkalosis may be found. If, however, intense physical exertion was the main cause of heat stroke, hyperkalemia, an increased creatine kinase level, and lactic acidosis may be present. If extended forceful exercise was involved, as in military drills or football,[22] heat stroke may be accompanied by rhabdomyolysis, reducing the chance of survival. Myoglobinuria reveals this complication. Disturbance in blood coagulation is typical in heat stroke, consisting of prolonged partial thromboplastin and prothrombin times and a decreased fibrinogen level, with abnormally elevated fibrin split products.[28]

Those with a low level of physical fitness, either temporarily because of recovery from an illness or permanently because of a chronic illness or other causes such as obesity, alcoholism, drug addiction, are at higher risk to become affected by a heat illness or disorder.[28] Another cause of lower tolerance to heat exposure is impaired ability to sweat, either hereditary or acquired as a side effect of skin disorders or use of medications with an anticholinergic effect.

Heat exhaustion

During heat exposure two adaptive mechanisms play the most important roles in the maintenance of the body's t_c within tolerable limits. One is the vasomotor mechanism, which shifts the circulating blood from the deeper tissues to the skin. Blood carries the heat from the internal organs and the muscles to the skin surface, where it can be dissipated to the environment. The other mechanism is sweating, which cools the skin surface by evaporation.

If, during excessive sweating, fluid is not replaced completely, dehydration ensues, leading to diminished blood volume and placing an increased load on the cardiovascular system. To maintain the blood supply to the heart, the muscles, and the brain, the heart beats faster and the vasomotor system contracts the blood vessels in the organs of the digestive and urinary system. This is an undesirable side effect of adaptation to heat, because these organs may become ischemic and suffer cellular damage. Vasoconstriction in the gastrointestinal tract also slows down the absorption of liquids and food from the intestines, causing nausea during attempts to drink water or other beverages in the needed quantity.

If the cardiovascular compensation is not adequate to supply enough blood to the brain, the symptoms and signs of brain ischemia, including feeling of fatigue, headache, dizziness, insecure gait, and finally collapse, occur. At this stage the victim is pale and has clammy skin; a slightly increased body temperature; a fast, shallow pulse; and low blood pressure. These symptoms, however, can be misleading because victims of heat stroke can have the same symptoms if they are in circulatory shock and if body cooling was applied before the diagnosis was made.[16] Furthermore, a person collapsing from circulatory failure without exposure to heat may display the same symptoms. Examination of blood chemistry can help clarify the diagnosis,[28] as described earlier.

The person showing early symptoms of heat exhaustion should go to a cool place, lie supine, and drink cool, lightly salted fluids. If after a rest the person's condition does not improve, he or she should be transported to a hospital emergency department, particularly if he or she has lost consciousness. The person may be injured as a result of collapse and may have other chronic illnesses that may become aggravated by heat exhaustion. Only a thorough medical examination can ascertain that heat exhaustion was the only cause of the person's symptoms. A person who has recovered from heat exhaustion should not be exposed to high heat stress immediately; if the brain was affected because of dehydration or hypernatremia, complete recovery may take several days.[28]

Heat cramps

Muscle cramps are a consequence of the imbalance between the water and salt (sodium chloride) content in the extracellular and intracellular fluids. The potassium balance may also have a role, but it has not been clearly established.[28] The salt concentration of sweat of a person who lives and works in a moderate climate can be as high as 4 g per liter, whereas those adapted to living and working under hot climatic conditions may have as little as 0.4 g salt in 1 L sweat.[31] Salt also is excreted in urine and feces; however, if a person sweats heavily, for example, 1 L per hour, the salt concentration of urine becomes very low and the amount of urine excreted also greatly diminishes. The lowering of the excreted amount of salt in both sweat and urine is a result of adaptive hormonal mechanisms that make it possible for a person to sweat heavily without suffering from salt depletion; however, when the limits of the adaptive mechanisms are exceeded, symptoms of salt depletion become manifest. These symptoms are fatigue, giddiness, loss of appetite, nausea, vomiting, constipation, muscle cramps, and, finally, collapse.

Loss of salt accompanies loss of fluid from the body, with repercussions on the circulation, as mentioned in connection with heat exhaustion.[31] Therefore it is not surprising that many of the symptoms of salt depletion are similar to those of heat exhaustion; however, if a person replaces the water lost by heavy sweating without replacing salt, dilution of body fluids (hyponatremia) may occur. It may be a temporary phenomenon until the excess water is excreted by the kidney. Nevertheless, it has similar effects as salt depletion, most acutely and dramatically manifested in the form of muscle cramps. This temporary phenomenon can occur despite ingestion of enough salt with meals.

Heat cramps occur most often in the extremities used most intensively in the activity performed and also in the abdominal muscles. They are painful and can be temporarily debilitating. If the cramps are mild and not complicated by symptoms of heat exhaustion, recovery can be achieved with rest in a cool place and oral administration of 250 to 500 ml of 0.5% salt solution. The muscle cramps cease, and there are usually no aftereffects, except for minor sensitivity in the affected muscles; however, it is advisable that the patient avoid heat stress for 1 or 2 days or until the electrolyte and fluid balance in the body is fully reestablished, which can be determined by measurement of urine osmolarity and chloride content. In more severe cases, when cramps are extremely painful and spread to a large number of muscles or when symptoms of heat exhaustion also are present, the victim must be taken to a hospital emergency department, where salt can be replaced intravenously, giving immediate relief of the cramps; however, complete recovery may take several days.[31]

Dehydration

Another method to prevent the occurrence of the temporary dilution phenomenon is to restrict water consumption during heavy sweating; however, it carries the risk of dehydration. If dehydration exceeds 1.5% of body weight, symptoms of loss of physical fitness start to occur.[14] Heart rate and body temperature increase faster during exercise, and a feeling of fatigue occurs earlier. When dehydration reaches or exceeds 2.5% of body weight, fatigue becomes excessive and preliminary signs of heat exhaustion may occur.[31] Persons with a lower level of cardiac fitness succumb earlier to heat exhaustion. As mentioned previously, dehydration also makes a person more prone to heat stroke. Thus during heavy sweating for an extended period, fluid replacement becomes a critical issue. Both too little and too much fluid consumption can have deleterious effects, yet thirst is not a good indicator of body hydration; however, if the heat stress remains within certain limits, most workers can learn by trial and error how much to drink without a detrimental effect on their feeling of well-being and fitness.

Table 51-4 shows the levels of rectal and skin temperature increases and the levels of sweat rates considered to be maximal values at rest and work, which are either alerting or dangerous for unacclimated or acclimated persons. At these levels of sweating the risk of excessive dehydration or temporary dilution of body fluids is minimal if drinking water or other nonalcoholic beverages are available in close reach.

Prickly heat (heat rash, miliaria rubra)

Prickly heat is caused by obstruction of the sweat ducts due to the irritating effect of the salty sweat when perspiration occurs continuously during the 8-hour workday in a humid environment. Under these conditions the skin is constantly wet and the salt concentration of the sweat layered over the skin for an extended period increases because of the partial evaporation. Simultaneously, with a prickly feeling on the skin, small papules surrounded by a red halo erupt. If heat exposure continues, the papules develop into vesicles containing clear or milky fluid. They are most often found on the forearms in front of the elbows, on the shoulders and chest, on the waist, and behind the knees. The location of the eruption may be influenced by wet, salty clothing rubbing against the skin. The vesicles can become infected, thus becoming inflamed and itchy.[31]

The most effective and fastest treatment consists of washing off the sweat and salt with antibacterial soap in a cool shower, and, after thorough but gentle drying, prevention of sweating by staying in a cool, comfortable environment. The patient should wear clean underwear, changed daily, and lightweight clothing. A disinfectant and antipruritic lotion can be helpful in eliminating discomfort and ensuring restful sleep.

Heat edema

Swollen ankles and feet are seen most often among people who are suddenly exposed to hot climatic conditions without acclimation. It is a relatively minor disorder but can cause temporary disability because shoes no longer fit. The edema is due to excessive vasodilatation in the skin combined with excessive intake of salt and water. It can become more pronounced if the person has marginal cardiac fitness.[31]

Rest in a cool area may reverse the condition in an otherwise healthy individual overnight, but in a few individuals

Table 51-4. Criteria for thermal limits based on average values

	Heat (nonacclimatized)		Heat (acclimatized)	
	Alert	Danger	Alert	Danger
Rectal temperature increase [°C (°F)]	0.8 (1.4)	1 (1.8)	0.8 (1.4)	1 (1.8)
Skin temperature increase [°C (°F)]	2.4 (4.3)	3 (5.4)	2.4 (4.3)	3 (5.4)
Sweat rate (maximal at rest, g/hr)	260	390	520	780
Sweat rate (maximal at work, g/hr)	520	650	780	1040
Maximal 8-hr sweat production to prevent excessive dehydration	2.60	3.25	3.90	5.20

Adapted from International Organization for Standardization: *Hot environments: analytical determination and interpretation of thermal stress using calculation of required sweat rate,* SO 7933:1989(E), Geneva, 1989, The Organization.

the edema may linger on until acclimation takes place. Reversal of extreme salt intake may hasten the recovery; however, a more thorough examination is necessary if the condition becomes chronic.

CHRONIC HEAT ILLNESSES

If a person works continuously over a long period (months or years) under severe heat stress just below the point that causes an acute heat illness, he or she may suffer from common symptoms such as headache, gastric pain, nausea, dizziness, irritability, sleep disturbance, increased heart rate, decreased libido or impotence, anemia, and hypertension more often than does the average worker. These symptoms may be considered a form of chronic heat exhaustion that, if not relieved by reduction of the worker's heat stress, may lead to an early disability due to damage to the myocardium[14] or to a disease of the gastrointestinal tract.[45] Workers affected by these symptoms should be placed in less strenuous jobs, or jobs should be redesigned to reduce heat load.

Another form of chronic heat illness has been observed among people who move to the tropics from a moderate climate. They suffer more often from skin diseases and sleep disturbances, become more susceptible to minor injuries and illnesses, and may become lethargic because of the extremely hot and humid climate, which leads to avoidance of physical activity and lowered metabolism. Change in the cultural environment and in eating habits may contribute to this syndrome.[31] With the availability of air-conditioned quarters the occurrence of this illness becomes rare; however, residents of desert regions, where the climate is hot and dry, may suffer more often from renal calculi because they become accustomed to drinking little water, which may be a scarce commodity in the desert, thus forcing the kidneys to concentrate the urine to the highest possible degree. They also must sweat constantly, and as a result, their sweat glands may show signs of fatigue or deterioration; thus they become less tolerant to heat. This condition is called anhidrotic heat exhaustion.[31]

Reduced heat tolerance is another form of chronic heat illness that follows an acute heat illness. A person who has suffered from heat stroke, heat exhaustion, or heat cramps is more prone to suffer the same illness again. After a severe case of prickly heat, the sweat glands over a large area of the skin may become dysfunctional, resulting in lower heat tolerance. It appears that some people are genetically more susceptible to a form of heat illness. Anhidrosis is a well-known form of congenital heat intolerance, but it can also develop as the sequela of some skin diseases.

PREVENTIVE MEASURES

NIOSH, in its 1986 revised criteria[40] for heat stress, recommended a number of work and hygiene practices and administrative controls for hot jobs. Most can also be applied to nonoccupational heat stress. The most important ones from the medical point of view follow.

Acclimation

New workers should be gradually introduced to work in a hot job. On the first day, they should work for only 20% of the workday in heat, and the time in heat exposure should be increased by 20% each day. This schedule completes the acclimation procedure within 1 week; however, during the 2 days of the weekend the worker may lose 1 day of acclimation.

After this 1-week period of acclimation the worker's body temperature and heart rate show less of an increase, sweating starts sooner, and a more dilute sweat is secreted in an increased volume.[5] The worker also feels less discomfort and learns how much to drink to prevent dehydration or overhydration. He or she also learns ways in which to dress and to avoid unnecessary physical exertion and heat exposure; however, the level of acclimation is limited to the level of heat stress encountered on the job. If the job's heat load suddenly increases, the worker needs additional time to become fully acclimated.[5] This time, the worker can start to spend 50% of the workday at the hotter job, with a 10% to 20% increment each consecutive day. Thus full acclimation takes only 4 days. Similarly, if a worker returns to the same job after vacation, acclimation can be achieved in 4 days. Acclimation may further increase slowly after the first 4 or 5 days; however, after the first week on the job a worker can be safely exposed to the level of heat stress indicated in the TLV diagram as safe only for acclimated workers.

Maintenance of body hydration and electrolyte balance

There is a difference between the NIOSH recommendation in the Updated Criteria Document[40] and the ACGIH TLV[2] as to how often a worker should drink when exposed to heat stress. NIOSH recommends drinking at least at hourly intervals, but the TLV recommends drinking every 15 to 20 minutes. Both recommendations can be correct, depending on the magnitude of the heat stress to which the worker is exposed. Workers themselves must learn by trial and error what is best for them. If in doubt, workers may check their body weight before and after work to determine how much weight they have lost. Most of their weight loss is due to dehydration, because the food ingested is about the same weight as the waste excreted by bowel movement. If dehydration exceeds 1.5% of body weight, they should try to drink more; however, if they gain weight, they should try to drink less. In principle, drinking small amounts more often is better tolerated than are large amounts at longer intervals.

Both the NIOSH and ACGIH recommend that only the unacclimated worker needs salt supplementation; however, to be on the safe side, it is justifiable to recommend that workers and athletes exposed to high levels of heat stress, who sweat heavily for several consecutive hours drink a 0.1% salt solution (1 g salt per liter). Although, the amount of salt that this solution contains may be somewhat more than that lost by sweating, salt is lost also by urination and bowel movement. Not only does this solution prevent salt-depletion symptoms but it also stimulates drinking. The salt should be completely dissolved in the water, and the water should be kept at about 10°C (50°F). Patients on a salt-restricted diet should consult their physician before drinking salted water or beverages.

Some commercially available salt-containing beverages are sweetened and enriched with other electrolytes, particularly potassium; however, it is difficult to prove or disprove whether potassium supplementation has any beneficial effect, because potassium is stored intracellularly in relatively large quantities when compared with the small amount of potassium excreted in the sweat. Serum potassium levels remain constant during salt loss. The sweeteners added to the commercial beverages, particularly dextrose, provide a quick energy boost to the muscles but also may add unnecessary calories. Because salted fluids are recommended only to those sweating heavily for an extended period, there is a risk that some people who are not sweating excessively and are on a salt-restricted diet also may drink them. This problem could be prevented with a warning label on such drinks.

Use of tablets as a means of salt supplementation is not advisable, because they can cause gastric irritation and nausea.[31] Enteric-coated salt tablets dissolve slowly, if at all, in the intestines; thus they may provide salt not when the sweating takes place but hours later, too late for prevention of heat cramps. It also is difficult to recommend a proper dosage for salt tablets because the rate of sweating may change during the day. In workshops and at outdoor work sites it is necessary to provide drinking stations within easy reach of the workers; if the worker rides in a vehicle, a fluid container in a cooler should be carried along.

Education

Workers, supervisors, and anyone at risk of heat stress should be knowledgeable about the early signs of heat illnesses and disorders and how to prevent their occurrence, as well as how to give first aid when the necessity arises. They should also know how the body adapts to heat exposure and how to increase or maintain heat tolerance and physical fitness. They should be given an opportunity, if possible, to learn what it means when they feel exhausted or overheated in terms of their heart rate and body temperature, which gives them the ability to decide more accurately when to interrupt heat exposure and take a rest until recovery.

Medical oversight

Before placement into a hot job, workers should be thoroughly examined to make sure that they are not heat intolerant, do not have below-average physical fitness, do not suffer from a chronic illness that interferes with adaptation to heat, do not have a history of heat illnesses or disorders, are not incapable of understanding the hazards of working under heat stress and how to cope with them, and are not handicapped to the extent that they cannot escape quickly when a thermal emergency occurs. Pregnant women should not be assigned to jobs with a high risk of heat stress during the first trimester.[40] Subsequently the main problem of heat stress in pregnancy is discomfort.

To ensure that workers maintain their fitness for work under heat stress, they should be periodically reexamined. The optimal time between examinations is 1 year. The physician should be informed about the work demands and the level of heat stress to which the worker may be exposed throughout the year.

Heat alert program

During spring and summer heat waves, the risk of heat disorders and illnesses is greatly increased because workers, as well as the public, are exposed suddenly to higher heat stress than that to which they are acclimated. Installation of a heat alert program[40] in plants that may be affected is therefore recommended. The program should involve representatives of management at different levels, workers, and safety and health personnel. Engineering systems for reduction of heat stress must be double-checked to determine that all are in good working condition and that workers and supervisors are aware of and abide by the preventive practices recommended. Safety and health personnel should be on alert and ready to provide first aid when necessary.

SUMMARY

Almost everyone is occasionally exposed to heat stress. Some people are exposed to hot conditions each summer, and others work in plants in which hot processes place the workers under heat stress all year. Human beings are able to cope with heat stress without adverse health effects to a certain level. There is a great individual variability in heat tolerance, and there are several climatic factors involved in creating heat stress. This variability makes it difficult to determine how much heat a person can tolerate without harmful health effects; however, methods to measure and quantify heat stress and to express the magnitude of heat stress in a single number, called a heat-stress index have been developed.

The most widely accepted and used heat-stress indices, the Belding-Hatch HSI and the WBGT were described previously. It was possible to establish at what combinations of WBGT exposure levels and work intensities the risk of heat disorders or illnesses becomes unacceptable. (See Fig. 51-1) shows these values depicted in two curves, one for acclimated and the other for unacclimated workers. These limit values have been developed and recommended by NIOSH scientists and have been adopted by ACGIH as a TLV and by the International Organization for Standardization as a standard. Heat exposures within the recommended limits are safe for practically all healthy individuals.

REFERENCES

1. American Conference of Governmental Industrial Hygienists: Heat stress. In *Threshold limit values for chemical substances and physical agents, 1972-1973,* Cincinnati, 1972, The Conference.
2. American Conference of Governmental Industrial Hygicnists: Heat stress. In *Threshold limit values for chemical substances and physical agents and biological exposure indices, 1994-1995,* Cincinnati, 1992, The Conference.
3. Astrand I: Aerobic capacity in men and women with special reference to age, *Acta Physiol Scand* 49(suppl):169, 1960.
4. Avellini BA, Kamon E, Krajewski JT: Physiological responses of physically fit men and women to acclimation to humid heat, *J Appl Physiol* 49:254, 1980.
5. Bass DE: Acclimatization to work in the heat. In *Temperature, its measurement and control in science and industry,* New York, 1963, Reinhold.
6. Belding HS, Hatch TF: Index for evaluating heat stress in terms of resulting physiological strain, *Heat Pip Air Condit* 27:129, 1955.
7. Bernard TE, Kenney WL: Rationale for a personal monitor for heat strain, *Am Ind Hyg J* (in press).
8. Beshir MY, Ramsey JD: Heat stress indices: a review paper, *Int J Ind Erg* 3:89, 1988.
9. Brouha L: *Physiology in industry,* New York, 1960, Pergamon.
10. Centers for Disease Control: Fatalities from occupational heat exposure, *MMWR* 33:410, 1983.
11. Cole RD: Heat stroke during training with nuclear, biological and chemical protective clothing: case report, *Milit Med* 148:624, 1983.
12. Consolazio CF, Johnson RE, Pecora LJ: *Physiological measurements of metabolic functions in man,* New York, 1963, McGraw-Hill.
13. Drinkwater BL, Horvath SM: Heat tolerance and aging, *Med Sci Sports* 11:49, 1979.
14. Dukes-Dobos FN: Hazards of heat exposure, *Scand J Work Environ Health* 7:73, 1981.
15. Dukes-Dobos FN, Badger DW: Atmospheric variations: heat. In Key MM et al, eds: *Occupational diseases,* DHEW (NIOSH) Pub No 77-181, Cincinnati, 1977, National Institute for Occupational Safety and Health.
16. Dukes-Dobos FN, Henschel A: Development of permissible heat exposure limits for occupational work, *ASHRAE J* 15(9):57, 1973.
17. Frye AJ, Kamon E: Responses to dry heat of men and women with similar aerobic capacities, *J Appl Physiol* 50:65, 1981.
18. Fuller FH, Smith PE: The effectiveness of preventive work practices in a hot workshop. In Dukes-Dobos FN, Henschel A, eds: *Proceedings of a NIOSH workshop on recommended heat stress standards,* DHHS (NIOSH) Pub No 81-108, Cincinnati, 1980, National Institute for Occupational Safety and Health.
19. Hellon RF, Lind AR: Circulation in the hand and forearm during acclimation, *J Physiol (Lond)* 128:57, 1958.
20. Hensel H: Neural processes in thermoregulation, *Physiol Rev* 53:948, 1973.
21. Houghten FC, Yaglogiou CP: Determining lines of equal comfort, *Trans Am Soc Heat Vent Engrs* 29:454, 1923.
22. Hubbard RW: An introduction: the role of exercise in the etiology of exertional heat stroke, *Med Sci Sports Exerc* 22:2, 1990.
23. International Organization for Standardization: *Hot environments: analytical determination and interpretation of thermal stress using calculation of required sweat rate,* ISO 7933:1989(E), Geneva, 1989, The Organization.
24. International Organization for Standardization: *Hot environments: estimation of heat stress on working man, based on the WBGT-index (wet bulb globe temperature),* ISO 7243:1989(E), Geneva, 1989, The Organization.
25. Kamon E, Rayon C: Effective heat strain index using pocket computer, *Am Ind Hyg Assoc J* 42:611, 1981 (Errata: *Am Ind Hyg Assoc J* 43:A43, 1982).
26. Kenney WL: WBGT adjustment for protective clothing, *Am Ind Hyg Assoc J* 48:A576, 1987.
27. Kerslake DMK: *The stress of hot environments,* Cambridge, UK, 1972, Cambridge University Press.
28. Knochel JP: Heat stroke and related heat stress disorders, *Dis Mon* 35:301, 1989.
29. Lary JM: Hyperthermia and teratogenecity. In Anghileri L, Robert J, eds: *Hyperthermia in cancer treatment,* Boca Raton, Fla, 1984, CRC Press.
30. Lehmann GEA, Muller A, Spitzer M: Der Kalorienbedarf bei gewerblicher Arbeit, *Arbeitsphysiol* 14:166, 1950.
31. Leithead CS, Lind AR: *Heat stress and heat disorders,* Philadelphia, 1964, FA Davis.
32. Lind AR: A physiological criterion for setting thermal environmental limits for everyday work, *J Appl Physiol* 18:51, 1963.
33. Lind AR et al: Influence of age and daily duration of exposure on responses of men to work in heat, *J Appl Physiol* 28:50, 1970.
34. Lotens WA: *Heat transfer from humans wearing clothing,* Soesterberg, the Netherlands, 1993, TNO-Institute for Perception.
35. Lotens WA, Havenith G: Ventilation of rainwear determined by a trace gas method. In Mekjavic IB, Banister EW, Morrison JB, eds: *Environmental ergonomics,* Philadelphia, 1988, Taylor & Francis.
36. McArdle B et al: *The prediction of the physiological effects of warm and hot environments: the P_4SR index,* RNP Rep 47/391, London, 1947, Medical Research Council.
37. McCullough EA et al: Heat transfer characteristics of clothing worn in hot industrial environments, *ASHRAE Trans* 88:1077, 1982.
38. McKarns JS, Brief RS: Nomographs give refined estimate of heat stress index, *Heat Pip Air Condit* 38:113, 1966.
39. Miller JC, Horvath SM: Work physiology. In Helander M, ed: *Human factors/ergonomics for building and construction,* New York, 1981, Wiley.
40. National Institute for Occupational Safety and Health: *Occupational exposure to hot environments: revised criteria 1986,* DHHS (NIOSH) Pub No 86-113, Cincinnati, 1986.
41. National Safety Council: *Accident facts,* Chicago, 1984, The Council.
42. National Safety Council: *Accident facts,* Chicago, 1986, The Council.
43. Nielsen B, Nielsen M: Body temperature during work at different environmental temperatures, *Acta Physiol Scand* 56:120, 1962.
44. Olesen BW, Dukes-Dobos FN: International standards for assessing the effect of clothing on heat tolerance and comfort. In Mansdorf SZ, Sager R, Nielsen AP, eds: *Performance of protective clothing,* STP 989, Philadelphia, 1988, American Society for Testing and Materials.
45. Ramsey JD et al: Effects of workplace thermal conditions on safe work behavior, *J Safety Res* 14(3):105, 1983.
46. Redmond CK et al: Mortality of steelworkers employed in hot jobs, *J Environ Pathol Toxicol* 2:75, 1979.
47. Reischl U et al: Ventilation analysis of industrial protective clothing. In Asfour SS, ed: *Trends in ergonomics/human factors IV,* Amsterdam, 1987, Elsevier.
48. Reischl U et al: Improvement of ventilation by increasing ambient airflow and by opening collar and cuffs of a semipermeable protective garment. In *Designing a better world: proceedings of the 10th International Congress of the International Ergonomics Association,* vol 2, Sydney, 1988, Ergonomics Society of Australia.
49. Richardson IM: Age and work, *Br J Indust Med* 10:269, 1953.
50. Robinson S et al: Acclimatization of older men to work in heat, *J Appl Physiol* 20:583, 1965.
51. Rowell LB: Cardiovascular aspects of human thermoregulation, *Circ Res* 52:367, 1983.
52. Schuman SH: Patterns of urban heat wave death and implications for prevention: data from New York and St. Louis during July 1966, *Environ Res* 5:59, 1972.

53. Shvartz E et al: Prediction of heat tolerance from heart rate and rectal temperature in a temperate environment, *J Appl Physiol* 43:684, 1977.
54. Strydom NB: Age as a causal factor in heat stroke, *Journal of the South African Institute of Mining and Metallurgy* 72:112, 1971.
55. Umbach KH: Physiological tests and evaluation models for the optimization of the performance of protective clothing. In Mekjavic IB, Banister EW, Morrison JB, eds: *Environmental ergonomics,* Philadelphia, 1988, Taylor & Francis.
56. Vernon HM: The measurement of radiant heat in relation to human comfort. *J Ind Hyg Toxicol* 14:9511, 1932.
57. Vogt JJ et al: Required sweat rate as an index of thermal strain in industry. In Cena K, Clark SA, eds: *Bioengineering, thermal physiology and comfort,* Amsterdam, 1981, Elsevier.
58. World Health Organization: *Health factors involved in working under conditions of heat stress, report of a scientific group,* Technical Report Series No 412, Geneva, 1969, The Organization.
59. Wyndham C: The physiology of exercise under heat stress, *Annu Rev Physiol* 35:193, 1973.
60. Yaglou CP, Minard D: Control of heat stress casualties at military training centers, *Arch Ind Health* 16:302, 1957.

Chapter 52

HIGH-ALTITUDE AND AEROSPACE MEDICINE

Lois Bullock

The atmosphere
    Pressure and density
    Temperature
    Composition of the atmosphere
The high-altitude environment
    Physiologic effects of increased altitude
    Acclimatization
    Acute altitude illnesses
    Acute mountain sickness
    High-altitude pulmonary edema
    High-altitude cerebral edema
    Chronic altitude illness—chronic mountain sickness
    Medical disorders affected by high altitude
The aviation environment
    Hypoxia
    Cabin pressurization
    Flight physiology
    Hypoxia at altitude or with slow ascent (slow decompression)
    Hypoxia with rapid decompression
Barotraumas ("trapped gas" illnesses)
    Barotitis media
    Barosinusitis
    Pulmonary overpressure accident
    Decompression sickness ("evolved gas" illnesses)
    Motion sickness
The space environment
    Microgravity
    Atmosphere
    Radiation
    Micrometeroids
Conclusion

The high-altitude environment has only become a concern in the last century as man has tried to reach higher and farther out from his near–sea-level home. As man has ventured "up and out" he has found the environment to be harsh and unforgiving. On the ground the desire to reach the highest peaks presents challenges with decreasing availability (partial pressure) of oxygen, decreasing temperatures, and physical dangers such as avalanches and falls. In the air the decreasing partial pressure of oxygen and low temperatures presented a constant challenge until the development of oxygen equipment and pressurized cabins. Even with these advances aviation still can be unpredictable, with such problems as rapid changes in cabin pressure (failure of pressurization), conflicting spatial orientation inputs, increased radiation exposure, and in high-speed aircraft, rapid acceleration. The "final" frontier of space presents man with even greater challenges, such as microgravity, space sickness, and increased exposure to ionizing radiation.

These high-altitude environments, which are so different from what an average person experiences living near sea level, produce diseases and health concerns unique among any aspect of medicine. It is impossible to present a comprehensive review of these subjects in a single chapter, particularly for the area of aerospace medicine. However, this chapter attempts to present the basics to provide an awareness of the unique conditions and diseases associated with high altitudes.

First, an overview of the atmosphere in which we live will be presented. The second section covers basic principles of high-altitude medicine (traditionally this refers to high altitudes on the Earth's surface rather than aerospace). The third part will touch on several pertinent topics in aviation medicine, dealing with individuals who fly in fixed- or rotary-winged aircraft. The last section will briefly cover space medicine, the newest area of altitude medicine, which deals with those escaping the bounds of Earth's atmosphere.

THE ATMOSPHERE
Pressure and density

A basic knowledge of the earth's atmosphere is necessary to understand the unique diseases associated with venturing into the upper altitudes. The atmosphere extends from the earth's surface to a point we define as "outer space." This point is determined by two factors—thermal (solar) radiation, which tends to expand gases into the vacuum of space, and the earth's gravitation, which tends to pull objects back to the surface.[9,14,43] As one gets further away from the surface of the earth, the gravitation reduces to a level where it no longer is effective in keeping all molecules from escaping into true space. This level, called the "escape level," is about 435 miles (700 km) from the surface of the earth. Above the escape level is a transitional zone where the atmosphere thins out until it becomes true space.

This reduction of gravitation has a strong effect on the nature of the gaseous atmosphere. Both density and pressure decrease in an approximately exponential manner as the distance (altitude) from the earth's surface increases. At sea level atmospheric pressure (or the weight of the air column at sea level) is 14.7 lb/in^2 (1 kg/sq cm) or 760 mm Hg. The reduction of pressure with increasing altitude is shown in Fig. 52-1. At an altitude of 18,000 feet (5486 m) the pressure is half that of sea level (380 mm Hg), and at 33,700 feet (10,272 m) the air pressure is reduced to 190 mm Hg. As pressure is reduced, so is the density of the atmosphere.

This reduction in density by definition means a reduction in the number of molecules in a given volume. This results in a reduced availability of oxygen from the atmosphere (partial pressure), although the composition of air (% by volume) remains about the same. This reduced partial pressure presents a problem of hypoxia as altitude increases. It also means that for gaseous molecules in a closed or semi-closed cavity (such as the middle ear), the volume will increase or decrease in relation to altitude (Boyle's law). Both of these conditions are important in the pathogenesis of diseases at higher altitudes[9,14] and will be discussed further in this chapter.

Temperature

Temperature is also affected by increasing distance from the earth. Temperature cannot be depicted on a simple curve, (see Fig. 52-2), and it shows considerable geographic and seasonal differences. Temperature is affected by different mechanisms at different levels in the atmosphere. For example, the atmosphere just above the earth is warmed both by direct infrared (IR) radiation from the sun as well as convection and reradiation of heat from the earth's surface and reflection of heat from upper layers of the atmosphere. However, as altitude increases, convection and radiation from the earth's surface decline to a point of insignificance. Because of the changing nature of the atmosphere with increasing altitude, it has been broken down into different temperature shells that comprise altitudes of similar temperature phenomenon, also shown in Fig. 52-2. The only shell that will be discussed here is the lowest shell, the troposphere, because the predominance of high-altitude and aviation activity takes place within this shell.

The troposphere is the domain of weather. Clouds are very rarely found above this region. The troposphere has a more or less uniform degree of temperature change with altitude, approximately 2°C/1000 ft (6.5°C/km). However, temperature inversions frequently occur. The upper limit of the troposphere varies with latitude and ranges between

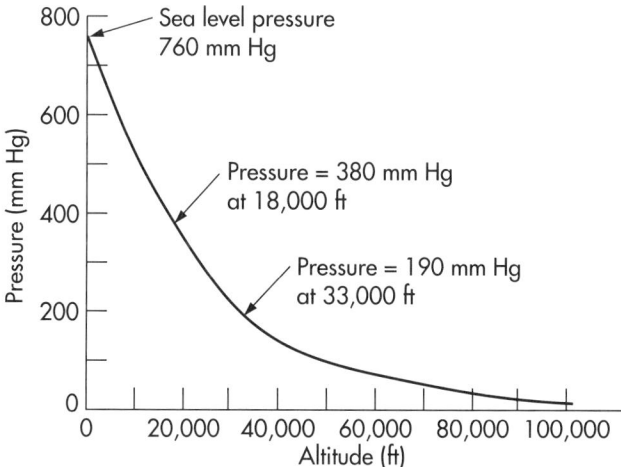

Fig. 52-1. Relationship between atmospheric pressure and altitude.

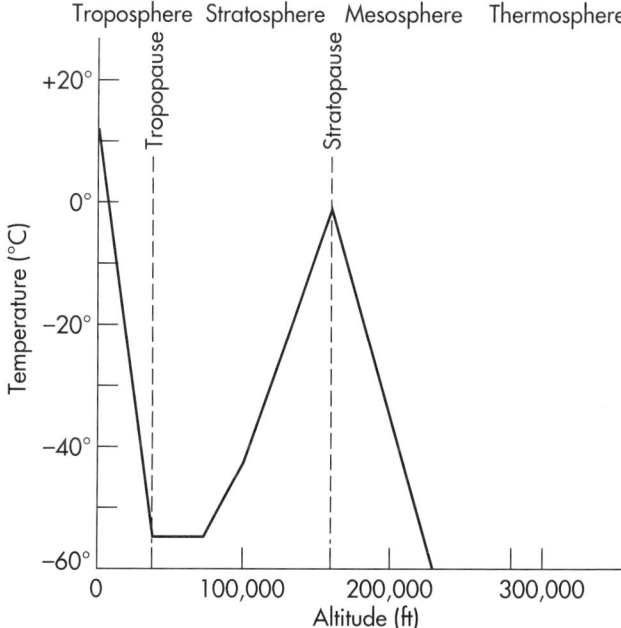

Fig. 52-2. Relationship between ambient temperature and altitude, showing the associated temperature shell.

19,700 and 62,000 feet (6 and 19 km), generally being higher and colder over the equator.

Composition of the atmosphere

The composition of the atmosphere generally remains rather constant until the outer reaches of the atmosphere (above 300,000 feet). It is predominantly a mixture of nitrogen (78.09% by volume in dry air), oxygen (20.95%), argon (0.93%), and carbon dioxide (0.03%), with traces of other gases.[14] The composition does vary somewhat in relation to temperature (increased ability of the air to hold water as the temperature increases) and closeness to the surface of the earth (byproducts of human activity, such as engine exhausts, and natural phenomena, such as volcanoes). However, for practical purposes dry air is generally considered as a mixture consisting of 21% oxygen and 79% nitrogen.

THE HIGH-ALTITUDE ENVIRONMENT

The high-altitude environment includes all mountainous regions, some of which have permanent habitations (such as Denver and many of the ski resort areas in Colorado) and some of which are reached only periodically or rarely by mountain trekkers (such as the peak of Mt. Everest). The atmosphere of this high-altitude environment is mainly affected by decreasing partial pressure of oxygen and decreasing temperature. The effects of these two factors change with increasing altitude. Ranges of high altitude have been defined and categorized in relation to their physiologic effects: moderate altitude, 5000 to 8000 feet (1525 to 2440 m); high altitude, 8000 to 14,000 feet (2440 to 4270 m); very high altitude, 14,000 to 18,000 feet (4270 to 5490 m); and extreme altitude, above 18,000 feet (>5490 m).[26] Since these categories of altitude can be a useful way to remember how to counsel or treat individuals, they will be presented briefly.

The moderate-altitude range (5000 to 8000 feet) includes many well-inhabited and commonly visited areas in the western United States and throughout the world. Most individuals have little or no difficulty ascending to these altitudes, although susceptible individuals may experience mild acute mountain sickness and patients with cardiac or pulmonary disease may experience increased symptoms.

The high-altitude range (8000 to 14,000 feet) includes some well-inhabited and commonly visited areas in the western United States, Europe, and South America, but far fewer than the moderate-altitude range. Notably, there are several ski areas in the Rocky Mountains in the western United States that have lodges located above 8000 feet. However, one reason that there are fewer inhabitants and visitors above the altitude of 8000 feet is that the incidence of high-altitude illness markedly increases. Because of this, 8000 feet is considered the threshold above which altitude-related disease occurs. Above that altitude, the partial pressure of oxygen has decreased enough that there are significant reductions in the arterial Po_2 and oxygen saturation, as shown in Fig. 52-3. This increasing hypoxia is the underlying pathogenesis for most altitude-related disease.

Only a few cities in the world are located in the very-high-altitude range (14,000 to 18,000 feet), and this altitude is barely found in the contiguous United States. However, these altitudes are now commonly reached by mountain trekkers and climbers. Severe medical problems usually occur with rapid ascent to these altitudes (for example, flying from sea level to these altitudes). In Peru one can drive from sea level to almost 16,000 feet in 4 hours. Most of the altitude-related fatalities occur in this altitude range.[26]

The lower limit of the extreme-altitude range (18,000 feet or 5500 m) has physiologic significance in that a prolonged stay above this level results in deterioration rather than the acclimatization seen at the lower levels.[26] As a result, these altitudes are only attained for short periods and only by experienced and previously acclimatized mountain climbers. Even though the physiologic effects are severe in this range, they are probably less of a hazard to the individual than the concomitant severe cold and physical hazards like avalanches and falls.[26]

Physiologic effects of increased altitude

Hypoxia appears to be the underlying etiology for most of the physiologic changes of elevated altitude. Although these changes are attempts to compensate for hypoxia, not all changes are beneficial. These changes include:

1. Reduced resting arterial Po_2 and arterial oxygen saturation, which varies with altitude achieved

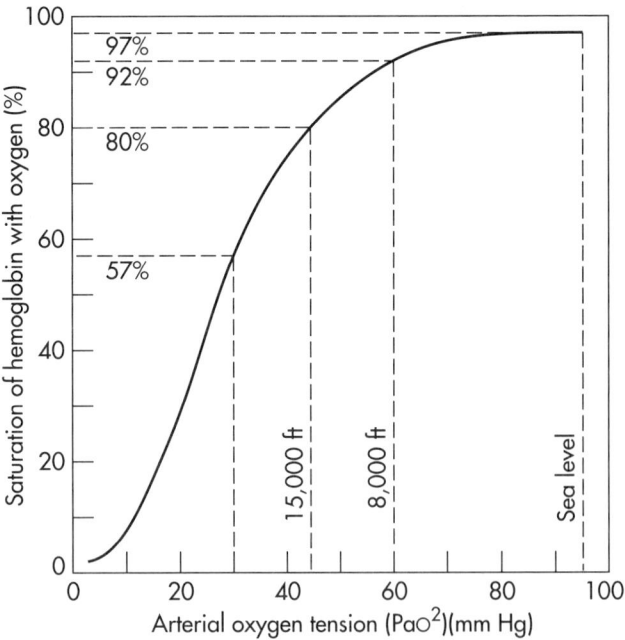

Fig. 52-3. The oxygen-hemoglobin dissociation curve showing the relationship between altitude and saturation of hemoglobin with oxygen.

2. Increased pulmonary ventilation, which seems to persist for the duration of a stay at high altitude[26,30]
3. Respiratory alkalosis, with renal compensation occurring within a few days. This alkalosis tends to shift the oxygen-hemoglobin dissociation curve to the left, which results in increased arterial oxygen saturation for a given arterial oxygen tension.[26]
4. Increased red cell mass occurring after a few days at high altitude
5. Increased sympathetic activity, which gradually decreases with stay at high altitude[21]
6. Reduced exercise capacity.

The underlying etiology of changes in exercise capacity is not completely understood. The primary effect of altitude on exercise capacity is through effects on the cardiovascular system, with decrease in maximum oxygen consumption (VO_2max) and decrease in maximum heart rate. With continued exposure to increased altitude, exercise capacity does seem to improve, but never reaches that attained at sea level.[21]

Acclimatization

Acclimatization involves allowing time for the physiologic adjustments to the hypoxia of increased altitude. The greatest adjustment appears to be increased pulmonary ventilation, which persists throughout the duration of stay at increased altitude. The changes involved in acclimatization occur over time, and the rate and duration of acclimatization vary from individual to individual and with the nature of activities that will occur at the increased altitude (greater physical activity requiring greater time for proper acclimatization).[26] Also, it requires greater stays at intermediate altitude when higher altitudes (particularly over 14,000 feet) will be reached. At altitudes above 18,000 feet, prolonged stays no longer allow acclimatization, but rather result in physiologic deterioration.[26]

There are two methods of acclimatization described in the medical literature—staging and graded ascent. Staging involves a stay of a few days at intermediate altitudes below the final altitude.[15,30,54] The number of intermediate altitude stages required and length of stay at each altitude depend on the ultimate altitude to be attained.[15,54] Graded ascent involves small daily increases in altitude, such as a march to a base camp. With graded ascent, it is important to maintain small increases in altitude, generally less than 1000 feet (300 m) per day at the higher altitudes along with rest days between ascent at altitudes above 14,000 feet (4270 m), to allow for acclimatization to occur.[25,26,30]

Acute altitude illnesses

There are several different entities that are considered acute altitude illnesses. The three most significant medical problems that can be encountered at high altitude are acute mountain sickness, high-altitude pulmonary edema, and high-altitude cerebral edema. These three probably represent a continuum of disease, but their differing symptom complexes, pathogenesis, and slightly differing treatment lend support for an independent presentation of each.

Acute mountain sickness

Acute mountain sickness (AMS) has been known for some time in those living or working in elevated altitudes and has been given many names over the course of time and geographic area. AMS is defined as a symptom complex found in individuals who move to increased altitudes quickly without prior acclimatization. Rate of ascent appears to be the greatest factor in development of AMS, although ultimate altitude and individual susceptibility also play a role.[22] Few serious cases arise below altitudes of 8000 feet, but a majority of individuals will show some symptoms upon rapid ascent to 12,000 feet.[26,39]

Clinical features. The generally accepted criteria for diagnosis of AMS include headache (classically described as throbbing, bilateral, frontal, worse in morning and after exercise), gastrointestinal distress (anorexia, nausea, vomiting), fatigue or weakness, dizziness or lightheadedness, and/or difficulty sleeping that occur in an individual with a recent ascent to high altitude.

The severity of AMS can vary from mild, not interfering with activities, to severe, with disturbed consciousness and often with pulmonary or cerebral edema. Both the symptoms presented and severity experienced vary between individuals but appear to be fairly consistent in any one individual from one altitude experience to the next.[30,50] There also does not seem to be a gender difference for AMS. Symptoms generally develop between 8 and 24 hours after ascent, and typically subside in 2 to 7 days. The fatigue, dyspnea, and disturbed sleep may occasionally persist.[23]

Physical signs of AMS are variable and nondiagnostic, with laboratory studies providing little additional information.

Pathogenesis. The pathogenesis of AMS is generally considered to involve cerebral hypoxia and mild cerebral edema.[5,24,36] Factors that tend to worsen hypoxia tend to increase severity of AMS, and those that tend to reduce hypoxia tend to reduce severity. One example of particular importance is sleep, which increases hypoxia through mechanisms such as hypoventilation and periodic breathing.[30,56] The risk of AMS seems to be associated with the altitude at which an individual sleeps far more than the altitude achieved while awake. Experienced climbers have been well aware of this and have a saying, "Climb high, sleep low."[26] In the Andes, residents label this night sickness "soroche."

A number of investigators have tried to determine specific physiologic differences or risk factors in individuals who develop AMS. These differences found in the responses to high altitude between individuals with AMS and those without AMS appear to be associated with central response to changes in blood gases in AMS,[30] with lower ventilatory response to hypoxia being the major finding.[38,41]

Prevention. The most effective method of preventing of AMS is acclimatization. Unfortunately, it is still often neglected. There are also no sea-level measures that can predict with any consistency those individuals who are more susceptible to AMS.[4] Individuals who have experienced AMS on previous ascent are very likely to have recurrence on their next ascent. In these individuals and in situations where rapid ascent is necessary or likely, prevention can be aided by pharmacologic agents. Both acetazolamide and dexamethasone appear effective in prophylaxis of symptoms in these individuals,[15,23,51] especially in combination with staging.[15]

Treatment. Treatment of individuals who have AMS depends on the nature and severity of symptoms presented. The best and surest treatment is descent, although it is often not convenient and sometimes very difficult (e.g., mountainous regions at night). Mild AMS is often self-treated by the individual, but may also present for treatment. Recommendations for this include acetaminophen, rest, small meals, and avoidance of alcohol.[30] Avoidance of sedatives is important because of the potential to aggravate sleep-induced hypoventilation, resulting in increased hypoxia. Most individuals with mild AMS will recover in a few days whether or not any specific treatment has been given.

More severe symptoms, especially altered consciousness or severe neurologic symptoms (cerebral AMS), should prompt immediate descent.[25] Oxygen should be administered, if available. The use of pharmacologic agents such as acetazolamide[17,19] and dexamethasone[40,51] has been shown to be effective in ameliorating symptoms, but should never replace descent unless symptoms are mild. Dexamethasone tends to have slightly fewer side effects, but has the disadvantage of recurrent symptoms in some individuals upon discontinuing the drug at altitude.[23] Furosemide, although once considered useful in treating AMS, should not be used. The diuresis caused by furosemide may lead to hypotension, dehydration, and hypokalemia, which may complicate the course of the AMS.[19]

High-altitude pulmonary edema

Similar to AMS, high-altitude pulmonary edema (HAPE) occurs most often in unacclimatized individuals who ascend rapidly and engage in strenuous exercise shortly after arrival at altitude; the higher the altitude, the worse the symptoms.[29]

The incidence of HAPE is significantly less than for AMS. Children under 16 years of age, however, appear to have a markedly higher incidence than adults.[29] HAPE can also occur in previously acclimatized individuals who descend to a lower altitude and then reascend after a period of time. Although it is generally considered to take 1 to 2 weeks at the lower altitude before increased susceptibility to HAPE occurs, one study has shown increased incidence with as few as 2 to 3 days at a lower altitude.[53] Similar to AMS, individuals with previous episodes are likely to have recurrences with reascent.

Clinical features. Symptoms will usually begin 24 to 72 hours after ascent. Symptoms classically include dyspnea, tachypnea, dry cough, chest discomfort, weakness, and fatigue. These symptoms may be accompanied or preceded by symptoms of AMS. Typically, the respiratory symptoms worsen at night. The more serious manifestations are disturbances of mental function and consciousness. This is of particular prognostic importance, as those individuals who lose consciousness will die within 6 to 12 hours unless definitive treatment is given.[26,37]

Physical signs include respiratory rate and heart rate, which increase roughly in proportion to severity. Temperature may be elevated, though generally not above 38°C.[26,37] Blood pressure is often low, with symptoms of a shocklike state also present. Marked cyanosis and rales are invariably present. Patients often manifest severe anxiety.

Laboratory abnormalities are not specific but include moderately increased white blood cell count, increase in hemoglobin and hematocrit, markedly decreased PO_2 and PCO_2, and slight increase in pH. Electrocardiographic changes are those of right ventricular strain. Chest x-ray invariably shows infiltrates, typically in the right midlung field, although in more severe cases it can be bilateral. It is typically patchy and does not have the usual findings associated with cardiogenic pulmonary edema. Resolution of infiltrates is rather rapid after descent or oxygen treatment, but may persist if treatment has been delayed.[47]

Death is related to delay in treatment and altitude of occurrence.[26,37,47] Failure to diagnose the condition is a major contributor to delay in treatment. The differential for diagnosis of HAPE includes bronchopneumonia, pulmonary embolism, and high-altitude bronchitis.[37,47]

Diagnostic criteria, as set by the Lake Louise Consensus on the definition and quantification of altitude illness (1992), is the presence of two symptoms (dyspnea at rest, cough, weakness or decreased exercise performance, or chest tightness or congestion) and two signs (rales or wheezing, central cyanosis, tachycardia, or tachypnea).[26]

Pathogenesis. Pathogenesis of HAPE is probably an abnormal degree of hypoxic pulmonary arterial constriction resulting in increased pulmonary arterial pressure.[27,28] Some studies have also found increased concentration of protein in bronchoalveolar lavage fluid, suggesting an increase in permeability of the alveolar membrane, similar to that seen in ARDS (Adult Respiratory Distress Syndrome).[31,52]

Prevention. Acclimatization is again the key to reducing incidence. Education of individuals and physicians is also important for early intervention. In those with previous history of HAPE, nifedipine was shown to reduce the incidence of recurrent attacks.[3,44]

Treatment. The main and most important treatment is descent, particularly while the individual can still walk. If available, high flow (6 to 8 L/min) oxygen with a well-fitting mask should also be given as soon as possible.[26,47] In the field, oxygen flow can be reduced after respiratory rate slows to conserve oxygen. Once descent has occurred, bed rest is also considered essential.[47]

A number of pharmacologic agents have been found beneficial. Morphine sulphate is controversial but may be useful in individuals who are very anxious or agitated. The depression of respiratory function must be kept in mind, with reversal agents such as Narcan available. Nifedipine has been shown to significantly reduce symptoms in individuals, but is recommended only after descent or as a temporizing mechanism in awaiting transport for descent, rather than as a means of continuing ascent.[44] Acetazolamide has also been recommended for use in mild HAPE by the Wilderness Medical Society.[47] Similar to AMS, diuretics such as furosemide should not be used.[19]

An elevated white blood cell count (over 12,000) or a temperature over 100° F suggests coexistent pneumonia, although both can be seen in HAPE alone. In those cases, an appropriate antibiotic should also be administered. In individuals who are comatose, acetazolamide or dexamethasone may be useful in reducing the associated cerebral edema.[26]

Also useful as a temporizing measure, and sometimes as a means of continuing stay at altitude, is a portable hyperbaric chamber, called a Gamow bag. It can be inflated to 2 atm, which corresponds to a reduction in altitude of about 5000 feet for the individual. It has been shown to be very effective in treating symptoms of HAPE with or without supplemental oxygen.[26,47,55] Rebound phenomenon may occur after removal from the device, though this was not found in the protocols used by Taber.[55]

High-altitude cerebral edema

High-altitude cerebral edema (HACE), also called cerebral AMS, is a neurologic syndrome occurring at high altitudes. It is considered by some as end-stage AMS, although other investigators feel that the differing pathologic processes make it a separate entity.

The incidence of HACE is significantly less than for HAPE or AMS, being slightly greater than 1% of individuals studied at high altitude.[23,37] The mean altitude for cerebral AMS is 15,500 feet.[26] Its incidence increases, like other acute altitude illnesses, with rate of ascent and ultimate altitude achieved. Individuals with previous episodes are also probably more likely to have recurrence with reascent.

Clinical features. Symptoms usually begin about 5 days after ascent, although they can appear as soon as 1 day and as late as 13 days.[26] Individuals can also present with symptoms of AMS or HAPE along with HACE, although it has been seen in the absence of any other acute altitude illness.[11,25]

Symptoms of HACE are those of CNS dysfunction. Those most commonly seen include headache, loss of coordination, ataxia, weakness, vomiting, disorientation, irrational behavior, and occasionally hallucinations. Obtundation and coma usually follow these symptoms, but they have been noted to occur as the presenting symptoms, particularly at night.[26]

Signs of HACE can include truncal ataxia, extensor plantar reflexes, hyperreflexia, ankle clonus, and signs of mental dysfunction such as disorientation to time and place. Retinal hemorrhages or papilledema can also be seen frequently.

Laboratory findings include moderately elevated cerebrospinal fluid pressure without abnormalities on fluid analysis, and cerebral edema on CT or MRI.

Pathogenesis. Hypoxia, brain edema, and increased intracranial pressure are the proximate cause of symptoms in most individuals. The edema is probably related to both a vasogenic cause (increased cerebral blood flow) and a cytotoxic cause (cellular swelling secondary to hypoxia).[11,25]

Prevention. Similar to other forms of acute altitude illness, acclimatization and education are the major preventive measures. Individuals with previous episodes of HACE should limit altitude exposure, but those who require or strongly desire reascent should be given prophylaxis with dexamethasone and acetazolamide.[26]

Treatment. Early intervention with immediate descent is key to reducing mortality. High-flow oxygen given with a tight-fitting mask should also be administered as early as possible. Administering dexamethasone, keeping the individual in a sitting position, and encouraging hyperventilation can be beneficial in reducing intracranial pressure. Acetazolamide may be useful as well. More potent diuretics and calcium channel blockers should only be used in the hospital setting, and their effectiveness has not been studied in relation to effectiveness with cerebral AMS.[26] Evaluations that should be included once treatment has begun are computerized tomography, chest x-ray, and complete blood count to rule out coexisting conditions that can mimic cerebral AMS, such as cerebral infarction, pneumonia, or HAPE.[26]

Mortality of HACE appears to be about 13%.[26] In most individuals who recover, the neurologic and retinal effects appear to resolve completely.[11,57]

Chronic altitude illness—chronic mountain sickness

Chronic mountain sickness is an uncommon form of altitude illness that occurs in individuals living at altitude for a length of time and is especially rare in the United States. It was first described in the Andes in the late 1920s by Monge and is often called Monge's disease in the literature. Risk factors for developing chronic mountain sickness are not known with the exception of prolonged exposure to high altitudes over 10,000 feet (3050 m).[26,45,46]

Clinical features. Most cases arise in individuals who have lived at altitude for many years, although a few cases have been seen after only a few years.[46] Cardiopulmonary and cerebral symptoms dominate the clinical picture. Dyspnea, cough, decreased exercise capacity, and fatigability are frequent findings, with cyanosis occurring more variably.

Headache, dizziness, paresthesias, impairment of higher mental functions, and insomnia are common CNS findings.

Physical signs of chronic mountain sickness can include cyanosis of varying degree, clubbing of fingers, evidence of mild congestive heart failure, increased heart rate, increased diastolic blood pressure, and occasionally increased systolic blood pressure. Petechial hemorrhages can also be seen in some.

Hemoglobin and hematocrit studies almost always reveal polycythemia. Chest x-ray usually shows prominence of the pulmonary arteries and accentuation of pulmonary vascular markings. It may also show cardiac enlargement, which is mainly due to right ventricular enlargement.[45,46] Electrocardiographic changes can occur in relation to myocardial changes.

Other conditions must be considered in the differential diagnosis of chronic mountain sickness, especially in the United States. These include sleep apnea syndrome, primary alveolar hypoventilation, hypothyroidism, and chronic obstructive pulmonary disease with CO_2 retention.[20]

Pathogenesis. The exact pathogenesis of chronic mountain sickness is not clear, but the most likely hypothesis is insensitivity to hypoxia and possibly to carbon dioxide.[26,46] The result of this insensitivity is depression of the ventilatory response to hypoxia, worsening the hypoxemia.

Prevention and treatment. Prevention is not really possible since the underlying etiology and risk factors are not known. The only effective treatment is permanent descent to lower, ideally near sea-level, altitudes.[26,45,46] Complete recovery usually occurs in most individuals over a period of months to few years. However, chronic mountain sickness will recur upon return to altitude in most individuals.[46]

Medical disorders affected by high altitude

Individuals with cardiopulmonary and other diseases may be at increased risk for worsening of the medical disorder and possibly increased risk for acute altitude illnesses with ascent to high altitudes. This is particularly true for those disorders associated with decreased arterial oxygen saturation at sea level and/or increased pulmonary arterial pressure, such as primary pulmonary hypertension, cyanotic congenital heart disease, mitral stenosis with pulmonary hypertension, and chronic obstructive pulmonary disease with decreased arterial oxygen saturation. Reduced oxygen saturation at high altitude is harmful to a fetus, so pregnant women should acclimatize carefully.

Individuals with congestive heart failure and coronary artery disease are also likely to be more symptomatic with ascent to altitude. Those with either of these diseases are likely to note reduced exercise capacity.[26,42] Individuals with systemic hypertension may also be affected by increasing altitude. An increase in both systolic and diastolic blood pressure is likely, probably due to the increase in sympathetic activity associated with increased altitude. Limited studies have shown a mean increase of approximately 15 mm Hg for both systolic and diastolic blood pressures, but these have been limited to normotensive or mildly hypertensive individuals.[26]

Sickle crises can also be provoked secondary to the hypoxia of high altitudes in individuals with sickle cell trait as well as sickle cell disease. Usually the crises occur at altitudes greater than 8000 feet. Because of this, individuals with sickle cell disease and those with sickle cell trait who have had crises should not travel to high altitudes.[26]

THE AVIATION ENVIRONMENT

The aviation environment differs significantly from the ground environment because flying has a number of additional physiologic stresses. Individuals today are rarely exposed to elevated altitudes for any extended periods while flying because of pressurized cabins and duration of exposure. The risk of disease from change in pressure and hypoxia is different from that on the ground. These additional stresses vary with the type of aircraft flown, the position of the individual (say, crew member or passenger), the mission of the aircraft, and any emergencies that may occur. Since all aspects of aviation medicine cannot be covered in this chapter, those most pertinent to nonaerospace medicine physicians will be discussed: hypoxia during flying, barotraumas, aviation decompression sickness, and motion sickness.

Hypoxia

Hypoxia still remains a major concern in aviation, although significantly reduced due to aircraft oxygen delivery systems and pressurization of the cabin. Hypoxia can occur during flight due to failure of these systems. The altitudes at which many transport aircraft (commercial and military) fly are much greater than those achievable on the ground, and even subtle effects of hypoxia in the air have the potential to affect aircrew response and thus survivability of crew and passengers, particularly in emergency situations. A brief presentation of cabin pressurization will set the background for this section.

Cabin pressurization

Cabin pressurization is probably one of the greatest and most taken-for-granted advances in aviation. It allows for extended flights at high altitudes while reducing the risk of altitude-related diseases. However, cabin pressurization does have its limitations and problems.

Most jet aircraft pressurization equipment uses bleed air from the jet turbines. The bleed air is very hot and requires extensive cooling before it can be released into the cabin. The basic composition of the air is essentially the same as sea-level air, but because of the high temperature of the air when it enters the pressurization system from the turbines, it is extremely dry. This low humidity is especially important on extended flights because of the drying effect on the exposed mucus membranes and the potential for dehydration.

In addition to the dryness of the air, aircraft are usually not pressurized to sea-level atmosphere; typical pressure ranges from 5000 to 8000 feet above sea level, which is maintained despite the altitude the aircraft attains. The system is called "high differential" because the actual cabin pressure is determined by a predefined pressure differential between the cabin and altitude. Most people who fly have noticed this change in pressure by mild popping or fullness in the ears, and for most this change in altitude is inconsequential. However, there are conditions that can be aggravated even by this change, such as a pulmonary overpressure accident and decompression sickness. Unlike commercial aircraft, many (though not all) military aircraft have low differential pressurization systems, with cabin pressures being more closely related to the altitude of the aircraft. The use of low differential pressurization is related to the risk of loss of pressurization during combat and size of pressurization equipment, especially on the smaller fighter aircraft.[7,14]

Flight physiology

A number of factors affect the severity of hypoxia encountered by the individual, but the greatest and most consistent factors are altitude achieved, duration at altitude, and the rate of ascent. In addition, susceptibility to the effects of hypoxia also depends on a number of individual factors. These include physical activity and fitness (rate of oxygen consumption), cold environment (increased metabolic workload), intercurrent illness (increased metabolic workload), and any medications or alcohol use.

Effect of altitude on maintaining arterial oxygen tension. In the introduction the arterial oxygen saturation–hemoglobin dissociation curve was presented, showing rapid reduction in arterial oxygen saturation with reduction of oxygen tension that accompanies increase in altitude. Table 52-1 shows the percent O_2 requirements to maintain sea-level Po_2. As can be noted, increasing the percentage of O_2 is required with increasing altitude, but there is a point at which even 100% O_2 will not be sufficient to maintain sea-level Po_2. Continuing ascent above about 34,000 feet even with 100% O_2 will result in hypoxia. At these altitudes, positive pressure is required to maintain arterial saturation.

Time of useful consciousness (TUC) and rate of ascent. There are varying definitions for this concept, but the most practical is the period in which the affected individual can act to correct his situation. As with the response to hypoxia described, this varies from individual to individual, but all individuals have a reduced time of useful consciousness (TUC) as altitude increases. At 18,000 feet, TUC averages 20 to 30 minutes for individuals sitting at constant altitude. However, at 36,000 feet, the TUC is only around 1 minute for the same conditions.[9,14] This time can be significantly reduced with factors that increase oxygen consumption (such as physical activity) or with high rates of ascent and rapid decompression, discussed below.

Hypoxia at altitude or with slow ascent (slow decompression)

Slow decompression of cabin pressurization can be very insidious in nature, and significant hypoxia may occur before realization of the situation. Awareness of an individual's hypoxic symptoms is very important in early detection and correction of this problem. This is especially true for some light aircraft and for ballooning, where there are no pressurization systems present but there is the possibility of attaining altitudes that can cause hypoxia.

Clinical features. The specific response to hypoxia varies from individual to individual, but tends to remain the same in one individual on repeat exposures to hypoxia. The primary concern in the aerospace environment is the effects on the central nervous system (CNS). Subclinical effects have been found by investigators at relatively low altitudes. The most notable of these findings are impairment of the ability to learn new tasks, and impairment of memory and cognitive reasoning, at altitudes as low as 8000 to 10,000 feet.[8,10,13,14,16]

Overt clinical effects of hypoxia usually do not present until much higher altitudes. These symptoms include change in personality, lack of insight, poor judgment, euphoria, forgetfulness, mental and muscular incoordination, and eventually unconsciousness and death. Hyperventilation (hypocapnia resulting in cerebral vascular constriction) with hypoxia can produce additional symptoms such as sensory loss, dizziness or lightheadedness, feelings of unreality or apprehension, and paresthesias.

Hypoxia with rapid decompression

One potential failure of cabin pressurization systems is explosive or rapid decompression. Although the likelihood of this type of failure is probably greatest for military aircraft during combat flying, it has been known to occur in commercial aircraft due to stress fatigue of the aging commercial airfleet or acts of terrorism. Rapid decompression is defined as a sudden loss of cabin pressurization resulting in a rapid increase in cabin altitude to that of aircraft altitude. Generally, rapid decompression occurs over a matter of a few seconds to a few minutes. Rapid decompression can also have environmental effects that make awareness of the situation almost unavoidable. These include rushing air current due to equilibration of pressure between the cabin and the alti-

Table 52-1. Percent O_2 required to maintain Po_2 at increasing altitudes

Altitude	Percent O2
Sea level	21
5,000 ft	25
20,000 ft	49
30,000 ft	81
34,000 ft	100
35,000 ft	100% plus positive, pressure breathing

From DeHart RL, editor: *Fundamentals of aerospace medicine*, Philadelphia, 1985, Lea & Febiger.

tude of the aircraft and also due to movement of the aircraft, noise due to aircraft movement and at times from the cause of the rapid decompression (e.g., explosion), and a notable drop in temperature due to both ambient temperature and sudden drop in air density.[7]

Pathophysiology. The main effect of rapid decompression is on reduced arterial oxygen saturation. A rare physical consequence of this is a pulmonary overpressure accident, discussed in the barotrauma section. As noted, the cruising altitude of most transport jets is above 30,000 feet, and at that altitude there is a significant reduction in the available oxygen with decompression. Rapid decompression further complicates the hypoxia normally found when exposed to high altitudes without rapid ascent. The oxygen tension in the lungs will fairly quickly equilibrate with the atmosphere at the aircraft altitude. However, the pulmonary capillary oxygen tension will be much greater from traveling at the cabin altitude. There is a negative gradient from the capillary to the alveoli, so oxygen diffuses down the gradient from the capillaries into the alveoli.[9,13,14] This will further desaturate the blood and cuts the TUC from one-third to one-half that found at altitude.[7,9,14]

Clinical features. In rapid decompression the TUCs are generally so short that often the presenting symptom of hypoxia is unconsciousness in those unable to obtain an immediate source of supplemental oxygen. The severity of hypoxia induced by rapid decompression can be reduced by breathing air enriched with oxygen prior to decompression.[13] However, the greatest determinant for survivability is the rapidity with which supplemental O_2 is started after decompression occurs.[35] However, even if supplemental oxygen is obtained within the recommended 5 seconds, there will still be a lag period where subclinical effects of hypoxia will be present and can affect the individual's functioning.[35] Factors that reduce TUC even further are those that increase oxygen consumption, such as physical activity or extreme anxiety.

BAROTRAUMAS ("TRAPPED GAS" ILLNESSES)

There are a number of organs and cavities in the body that contain air: the respiratory system, including lungs, middle ear and sinuses, and the gastrointestinal tract; each responds to changes in atmospheric pressure. The three major disease entities associated with changes in pressure in these organs will be discussed here: barotitis media, barosinusitis, and pulmonary overpressure accidents.

Barotitis media

Barotitis media is defined as a traumatic inflammation of the middle ear due to differential pressures between the middle ear and the surrounding atmosphere.[1,32] Acute barotitis media is the most commonly encountered aviation-related illness.

Normal anatomy and flight physiology. The middle ear is a semiclosed air-containing cavity. The only opening to atmospheric pressure in the middle ear is by way of the eustachian tube (ET) from the nasopharynx. The proximal two-thirds of the ET has soft walls that are normally collapsed and tends to act like a one-way or "flutter" valve.[1,7,32] On ascent, the expanding gas usually will easily overcome the closure of the ET and can be passively expelled. On descent, the gas in the middle ear contracts due to the increasing pressure. This negative pressure relative to ambient air inside the middle ear, however, cannot be passively overcome due to the "flutter" valve mechanism of the ET.[1] Fortunately, equalization of pressure in the middle ear can usually occur by voluntarily opening the ET through a number of physiologic maneuvers (called "clearing the ears").

Physiologic maneuvers used to clear the ears. There are several physiologic maneuvers used to clear the ears. The most commonly used are simple maneuvers like swallowing, yawning, or jaw movements. These maneuvers use the various soft palate and nasopharyngeal muscles to open the ET. These maneuvers are not effective in some individuals and in some situations. There are two additional maneuvers taught to aviators that raise the pressure in the nasopharynx to facilitate opening of the ET, the Valsalva and Frenzel maneuvers.[14]

The Valsalva maneuver involves increasing the pressure in the nasopharynx to force the ET to open. It is accomplished by exhaling against a closed nose and mouth. The Frenzel maneuver involves closing the glottis, mouth, and nose while contracting the muscles of the floor of the mouth and the superior pharyngeal constrictors.[32] The Frenzel maneuver has the advantages of a lower total opening pressure than the Valsalva and is independent of intrathoracic pressure or respiratory cycle.[32] However, the Valsalva is still probably the most common of these two maneuvers because it is easier to learn and perform.

Pathophysiology

Acute barotitis media. Damage to the middle ear occurs when a pressure differential is not corrected in a timely manner. Armstrong and Heim[1] described the two main causes of acute barotitis media simply as either the failure to open the ET voluntarily when necessary (clearing the ears) or the inability to open the ET.

The first cause, failure to periodically clear the ears, is usually a result of lack of awareness or understanding by the individual. This is much less of a cause in aviators today because of the extensive education received about this problem during most flight training. However, this can be a significant contributor in those who fly occasionally as a passenger on commercial jetliners. Periodically clearing the ears is necessary with descent to maintain pressure equalization between the middle ear and the atmosphere. Even with normal ET function there is a limit to the ability of the previously mentioned maneuvers to open the ET beyond a specific pressure differential between the middle ear and the nasopharynx. This pressure differential, on the order of 80 to 90 mm Hg, is the point above which none of the maneuvers discussed can open the ET and it is considered "locked."[1] Equalization of the pressure differential in these situations requires measures beyond the individual, such as reascent to reduce the pressure differential to the point that the ear can be cleared. The term *ear block* is probably derived from "locking" of the ET, and is the term used by aviators to describe inability to relieve the discomfort in the ears by any of the maneuvers discussed and is usually associated with acute or delayed barotitis media.

The major factor in the second cause of acute barotitis media, inability to clear the ears, is pathology of the upper respiratory tract. The most common pathology is mucosal edema secondary to upper respiratory infections or active allergic rhinitis. This etiology is the predominant cause of acute barotitis media in both aviators and passengers. The mucosal edema reduces the lumen of the tube and increases the pressure required for opening of the ET with descent, making "locking" of the ET more likely.

Both failure and inability to clear the ears can be aggravated by high rates of descent and use of 100% oxygen in flight. High rates of descent cause the pressure differential to increase faster, making it more difficult to keep up with clearing the ears, especially with mucosal edema. The effect of 100% oxygen on the middle ear will be discussed under pathophysiology of delayed barotitis media.

From any of these causes, the resulting relative vacuum of the middle ear produces retraction of the tympanic membrane (TM), engorgement of the vasculature, and resulting transudation of fluid or blood into the middle ear. In severe cases, a large negative pressure differential in the middle ear can cause rupture of the TM or the oval window.[1,32]

Delayed barotitis media. The pressure differentials that cause acute barotitis media generally occur during flight, but cases have been noted where pressure differentials have developed once on the ground. This type of barotitis tends to be less often associated with pathology of the upper respiratory tract. The classic setting for this entity, called "delayed barotitis media," is a long flight where 100% O_2 is used for a portion of the flight, followed by a period of reduced pressure equalization such as during sleep.[6] Using 100% oxygen during the flight enriches the middle ear with oxygen. Since oxygen is more readily absorbed by the middle ear mucosa, a negative pressure differential develops when equalization does not occur. The resulting pathology is similar to that generated during descent, but is usually of a very mild nature and has never been documented to cause rupture of the TM.[32]

Clinical features

Acute barotitis media. Symptoms can vary from mild discomfort and fullness in the ears with mild conductive-type hearing loss to severe pain, significant hearing loss, tinnitus, and vertigo. The symptoms will classically begin prior to landing. Signs include retraction of the TM and engorgement of blood vessels, transudate (which may be serous, serosanguinous, or hemorrhagic), and rupture of the TM in severe cases. The rupture can occur in any portion of the TM and has been described as typically being linear in appearance.[1]

Delayed barotitis media. As noted previously, delayed barotitis media is more often seen in individuals with normal upper respiratory pathology, although it is also increased in those with pathology. The classic onset is after landing, with symptoms presenting after awakening from sleep.[7,32] The symptoms are discomfort or pain and fullness in the ears and mild hearing loss. Physical findings are generally slight, but may include mild retraction of the TM and slight engorgement of the blood vessels.

Prevention. Prevention of acute barotitis media is mainly through education to reduce the numbers of individuals who fly with colds or active allergic rhinitis, especially if rapid changes in altitude are expected during the flight. Also, it is important to educate those individuals who do not routinely fly about the importance of clearing the ears periodically during descent. Passengers frequently use decongestants to prevent these symptoms.

Prevention of delayed barotitis media is through educating individuals about the etiology and clearing ears frequently after landing when 100% O_2 has been in use on a long flight.

Treatment. Symptomatic treatment of the pain and use of topical or systemic decongestants are probably the most commonly used treatments for acute and delayed barotitis media once on the ground. Rebound phenomenon can occur with topical decongestants, which must be considered in their use and in advising individuals. Antibiotics are often used with decongestants in acute barotitis media to reduce the possibility of bacterial overgrowth when there is a transudate present. It is also important to ensure that the individual does not fly until the barotitis media has completely resolved and the TMs move normally on examination.

In those situations other than typical commercial air travel where there is some discretion in the flight plan, there may be the option to reascend until the individual is able to clear the ears. Descent is then reattempted with as slow a change in altitude as possible so the individual is able to continue to clear the ears. For severe cases, even a very slow descent may not prevent recurrence of symptoms prior to landing. Use of a topical decongestant (such as neosynephrine) is also effective in relieving the symptoms so the individual can land, but follow-up evaluation for barotitis must still be accomplished once on the ground. In some cases where there is a flight surgeon (aerospace medicine physician) present with a Politzer bag (a device that allows high amounts of air pressure to be applied to small openings, such as the ET or sinus ostia), politzeration of the affected ETs can provide immediate relief in individuals with severe symptoms.[7] However, it is of little use if treatment is delayed, for the damage to the middle ear will have already occurred.

Barosinusitis

Similar to barotitis media, barosinusitis is a traumatic inflammation of the paranasal sinuses due to pressure differential between the sinus and the atmosphere.

Normal anatomy and flight physiology. The paranasal sinuses are bony cavities in the face and skull which communicate with the nose. The frontal sinus has a fairly long duct that opens into the nose, and the other sinuses have a hole (ostia) in their wall. Unlike the middle ear, the duct or ostia is completely bony. Passive movement of air normally occurs during both ascent and descent.[14]

Pathophysiology. The risk factors are similar to those for barotitis, when there is pathology of the respiratory tract. Again, the most common underlying etiology of barosinusitis is either an upper respiratory infection or active allergic rhinitis, which cause the mucus membranes to swell. Structural pathology like nasal or sinus polyps probably plays a slightly greater role in development of this disease than with acute barotitis media.[7]

Ascent is usually not a problem because the positive pressure within the sinuses often can overcome the pressure of the closed passage (unless severe swelling or blockage is present). Classically, symptoms begin during descent as with barotitis media, through a negative pressure differential created by the increasing atmospheric pressure.[7] The only effective maneuvers to equalize pressure in the sinuses in this case are those that increase the nasopharyngeal pressure, with the Valsalva maneuver providing a far greater increase in this pressure than the Frenzel. Unfortunately, even the Valsalva maneuver is ineffective in many cases.[7,14]

The trauma that results from the negative pressure differential has similarities to that occurring in the middle ear. The negative pressure differential in the sinuses causes vascular engorgement and transudation of fluids or blood into the cavity.

Clinical features. Symptoms, signs, and diagnosis are similar to acute infectious sinusitis. The main symptom is pain, often excruciating in nature, over the affected sinus(es). Signs include percussive tenderness over the affected sinus(es), often with evidence of upper respiratory mucosal inflammation and a possible serosanguinous nasal discharge. The sinuses typically affected are the frontal and maxillary sinuses.[7]

Prevention. Similar to barotitis media, prevention for the majority of cases is through education to reduce flying with colds or active allergic rhinitis.

Treatment. Treatment on the ground is very similar to that of acute barotitis media, with use of analgesics, topical or systemic decongestants, and an appropriate antibiotic.[7] In the air, reascent may be necessary to reduce the severe pain. Slow redescent is necessary, but may not be effective in a number of individuals. As noted above, the Valsalva has limited effectiveness in this condition. In this situation, topical decongestants may be the only means of relief to allow descent. Politzeration, if available, can also provide immediate relief.[7]

Once the symptoms have been controlled, it is again important that the individual does not return to flying until the barosinusitis and underlying etiology is completely resolved. If due to an anatomic abnormality, it may require correction (surgical or otherwise) before the individual can safely return to flying.

Pulmonary overpressure accident

A pulmonary overpressure accident is a rare condition that occurs due to lung damage from expansion of air volume, in aviation usually associated with rapid decompression of the cabin. This condition is seen slightly more frequently (although it is still uncommon) in the deep sea environment.

Normal anatomy and flight physiology. The lungs contain large volumes of air, particularly in the alveoli. The alveoli have relatively narrow passages, the bronchioles, that connect them with the atmosphere via progressively larger airways.[14] In the absence of pathology the air volume changes occurring during normal ascent and descent can be easily compensated for. When problems occur with the lung, it is during ascent (increase in volume of air in the lungs), unlike the previous barotraumas discussed.

Pathophysiology. During a rapid decompression, apparent altitude will change from the cabin pressure altitude, usually about 8000 feet, to the actual altitude at which the aircraft is flying, typically about 33,000 to 40,000 feet (cruising altitude for most commercial airlines). This change generally occurs in a matter of seconds, producing rapid expansion of gas in the lungs. Normally, expansion of lungs and chest wall, and flow of air from the lungs, will compensate for the increase in pressure and volume. If air escape from the lungs is impaired, then damage to the lungs, particularly alveoli, will occur. Air escape can be impaired by conditions that reduce the ability of air to egress (such as asthma, bronchitis, air-containing cysts, or other obstructive airway pathology), by closure of the glottis (as in breath-holding or swallowing), or by the flow restrictions imposed by oxygen equipment that may be in use.[7,14]

The damage to the lung occurs by stretching of the lung tissue beyond its normal limit. Eventually, this stretching will tear the lung parenchyma and result in extra-alveolar gas. Depending on the placement and nature of the tear(s), this extra-alveolar gas can pass into the pleural space, mediastinum, subcutaneous tissue, or torn blood vessels,[7,14] causing subcutaneous or mediastinal emphysema or even air emboli.

Clinical features. Both mediastinal and subcutaneous emphysema are generally benign conditions, unless the latter is accompanied by circulatory compromise. They can be diagnosed by crepitus of the affected areas and x-rays that usually reveal the extrapulmonary gas. Pneumothorax produced by a pulmonary overpressure accident is identical in clinical findings and treatment to pneumothorax from other causes.

The major concern with a pulmonary overpressure accident is arterial gas embolism (AGE), which is often life-threatening. Symptoms will begin almost immediately (within 10 minutes) following a rapid pressure reduction (decompression). Symptoms are predominantly CNS in nature—loss of consciousness, seizures, visual field loss or blindness, weakness, paralysis, or confusion. Symptoms may clear rapidly with descent, so the clinical picture seen by the physician may be significantly milder, suggesting a mild stroke.[7]

The major differential for AGE is neurologic decompression sickness, which is discussed in the next section. The key factor in proper diagnosis is time of onset of symptoms, with AGE occurring rapidly after sudden change in altitude.[7]

Prevention. Prevention is difficult since rapid decompression (the major cause in aviation) is usually a sudden and unexpected event.

Treatment. Descent, if still in the air, is a necessity even before definitive diagnosis has been made. Once on the ground, *ground* transport to the nearest hyperbaric chamber should be arranged as soon as possible. Use of low-flying helicopters should be avoided if ground transportation is at all feasible, since any increase in altitude can potentially worsen the situation. As soon as possible, 100% O_2 using a tightly fitting mask should also be started. Even if the individual becomes completely asymptomatic, arrangement for hyperbaric treatment and use of 100% O_2 should be accomplished. The Trendelenburg position with the individual on his or her left side can be beneficial prior to treatment in the hyperbaric chamber.[7] IV fluids and dexamethasone are also important adjunctive measures and should be started quickly, particularly if there is a delay in obtaining hyperbaric treatment.[7]

Decompression sickness ("evolved gas" illnesses)

Decompression sickness (DCS) is a syndrome arising from evolution of gas bubbles in the body due to reduced atmospheric pressure. The incidence of DCS is much less in aviation than in diving due to protective measures such as cabin pressurization. However, cases still do occur and the key to reducing morbidity and mortality in these individuals is awareness.

There are a number of risk factors in aviation that increase susceptibility to developing DCS. These include altitude (actual exposure, not aircraft altitude in pressurized cabins), duration of exposure, temperature, previous exposure and frequency of exposure to altitude, flying following diving, increasing age, exercise during or after altitude exposure, injury present during altitude exposure, and obesity.[2,34] DCS is extremely rare under 18,000 ft (5486 m), with the notable exception of those who performed diving or other compressed-gas breathing in the previous 24 hours prior to altitude exposure. In these cases, even extremely low altitudes, such as normal cabin pressure of commercial aircraft, can precipitate onset of DCS.

Pathophysiology. This section is a very simple summary of the pathogenesis of DCS, with emphasis on some of the unique features associated with altitude DCS.

Although not completely understood, the basis for DCS is the development of bubbles predominantly of nitrogen. Nitrogen is found in relatively large quantities in the body due to the high percentage of nitrogen in ambient air (79%). With the reduction of partial pressure of nitrogen on ascent, nitrogen is carried from the tissues by the blood and released to the atmosphere from the lungs. However, nitrogen has a limited solubility in blood. As a result, those tissues such as fat with large quantities of nitrogen become supersaturated at increased altitude. Under the right circumstances, which may require bubble nuclei, microbubbles with high concentration of nitrogen can form. These microbubbles grow with continued exposure to reduced atmospheric pressure. This continued growth probably plays a role in those cases of altitude DCS that do not completely resolve with descent.[12] The onset of symptoms appear to occur when they have reached a certain critical size.[7,14] Symptoms are felt to occur secondary to mechanical disruption of tissue or blood flow. The blood-bubble interface also promotes platelet aggregation and vasoconstriction, which further reduces blood flow.

Clinical features. There are several different manifestations of DCS. Golding[18] classified DCS into two main types: type I is mild, involving peripheral limb and joint pain and/or cutaneous involvement without evidence of neurologic involvement, and type II is serious, involving primarily neurologic symptoms as well as other systemic symptoms. The differential diagnosis of the various types of DCS include a number of other diseases. History and understanding of the flight parameters are important in making the proper diagnosis.[58]

Bends (type I). This is the most frequent type of DCS seen in both divers and aviators, comprising about 65% to 70% of all cases of DCS.[7,9,14] It is manifested by pain only, which is usually described as deep and aching but can vary in intensity. The pain tends to be localized around the large joints. It is usually monoarticular, although when it is polyarticular it is usually asymmetrical. Active and passive motion of the joint will aggravate the pain. Local pressure directly over the affected joint will often, though not always, provide some relief. Joints with inflammation due to any cause seem to be more prone to developing bends.

Onset of symptoms usually occurs within 12 hours after exposure to altitude, although the individual may not present for evaluation until 24 or more hours after exposure. The pain can occur on ascent, descent, or after being on the ground.

Neurologic DCS (type II). This form of DCS is far more serious than bends, but is significantly less frequent in occurrence—only about 5% to 7% of the cases of DCS.[7,9,14] There are two forms of neurologic DCS: the central (brain) and the spinal cord.

Spinal cord DCS. This form occurs almost exclusively in divers, being extremely rare following altitude exposure.[7,9,14] The clinical picture is a partial or complete transverse spinal cord lesion. The typical presentation is insidiously progressing sensory loss beginning in the feet and spreading upward. This is usually associated with an ascending weakness or paralysis to the level of the spinal cord lesion. It can also begin with abdominal or thoracic pain.

Brain DCS. This is more commonly seen in aviation and is uncommon after diving exposure.[7,9,14] The clinical picture is of spotty sensory and motor signs and symptoms not attributable to one brain locus. Headache is commonly present, as are visual disturbances. Extreme fatigue or personality changes can occur, and in unusual cases may be the only presenting symptoms.

Chokes. Chokes are rare in both aviation and diving (2%).[7,9,14] This is life-threatening and is due to multiple pulmonary gas emboli. The classic picture is a triad of symptoms including substernal chest pain, dyspnea, and a dry, nonproductive cough, with the pain being worse on inhalation.

Circulatory collapse. This shocklike state is usually subsequent to some other form of DCS, although it has been seen as the only presentation of DCS in some cases. This state is noted by its marked lack of response to fluid replacement.

Minor manifestations—skin bends and pitting edema. Skin bends involves tingling or itching across multiple dermatomes. Normally it is short-lived, passing in 20 to 30 minutes. In itself it is harmless but it may be a harbinger of a more serious form of DCS. If mottling or marbled skin lesions (*cutis marmorata*) follow an episode of skin bends, subsequent neurologic involvement or circulatory collapse can be seen in up to 10% of the cases.[7,48] Swelling and lymphedema may also occur and is rarely associated with serious consequences. It is rarely seen from altitude exposure.

Prevention. In aviation, a major protective factor is the pressurized cabin. In those individuals who will be exposed to high altitudes, as in altitude chamber exposure or flying high-altitude parachute missions, denitrogenation prior to ascent significantly reduces risk of DCS. Denitrogenation involves breathing 100% oxygen for a period of 30 minutes or more, depending on the nature of the mission and expected altitude exposure. Finally, in those individuals who dive, it is recommended that they refrain from flying for at least 24 hours.[48]

Treatment. Initial treatment involves descent, which relieves symptoms in a number of individuals, and administration of 100% oxygen with a tight-fitting mask. The definitive treatment for all cases of DCS is hyperbaric chamber treatment. Transportation to the chamber should be done by ground transport if at all possible, because of the risk of aggravation of symptoms with even slight increase in altitude exposure. In cases of bends pain only, if the symptoms clear while awaiting transport to a hyperbaric chamber, then hyperbaric treatment can be cancelled.[7] However, if there are any doubts, accomplishing hyperbaric treatment is recommended.

Motion sickness

Motion (or air) sickness is a physiologic response to unfamiliar and conflicting sensory inputs. It is often described as "a normal response to an abnormal environment." Incidence of motion sickness varies with the intrinsic susceptibility of the individual (some individuals are very sensitive to motion stimuli, both visual and vestibular, and some individuals rarely develop motion sickness symptoms), the nature of the stimulus (very turbulent flights will result in a significant number of ill individuals, while a smooth flight will result in far less), the nature and intensity of tasks performed, and possibly other environmental factors such as odor or ambient temperature.

Pathophysiology. Earlier theories about the etiology of motion sickness involved primarily the vestibular system (semicircular canals and otoliths), since motion sickness cannot be induced in individuals without vestibular function.[7,14] However, it is not the sole cause, since motion sickness can be induced without vestibular input in some individuals (for example, simulator ride or motion viewed in a large-screen cinema). The exact mechanisms of motion sickness are still not known, but the most widely accepted current hypothesis is the neural mismatch theory. This theory states that motion sickness is induced by conflicting signals from various sensory organs, and that these signals are also in conflict with those that the CNS expects to receive.[14,49] What the CNS expects as signals are based on what has been experienced on the ground over the course of time and are rather accurate with relation to activities occurring on the Earth's surface. The aviation environment, however, often provides completely different sensations.

In the neural mismatch theory the two main types are the visual-vestibular and semicircular canal–otolith mismatch. The mismatch can either be concurrent signals with contradictory information, or signals from one system in the absence of expected signals from the other system. One example, that of visual-vestibular conflict with concurrent contradictory information, is reading a map or text in a moving vehicle (especially an aircraft). In this case the visual cues (the stable book or map) are unrelated to the vestibular motion cues (movement of the vehicle).

Far more detail in describing the visual and vestibular systems is required to truly understand the underlying pathophysiology of motion sickness, and also of a related problem, spatial disorientation. Unfortunately, it is beyond the scope of this chapter. However, excellent presentations can be found in aerospace medicine texts such as *Fundamentals of Aerospace Medicine* edited by DeHart[9] and *Aviation Medicine* edited by Ernsting and King,[14] and these are recommended for further reading on this topic.

Clinical features. The classic features of motion sickness are nausea, vomiting, pallor, and sweating. Other symptoms are more variably present. Usually the onset of motion sickness begins with mild queasiness that can be aborted if the motion is stopped. If not, this progresses to worsening nausea and then vomiting. The severity varies from individual to individual and with the duration and intensity of the stimuli.

Motion sickness often decreases in severity or disappears completely with repeated exposures, as in trained aircrew, although in some people motion sickness is intractable. Individuals vary in how long it takes to adapt, and also how long periods away from flying can be before symptoms of motion sickness recur. Task involvement, such as flying the plane (as in driving a car), also seems to reduce the incidence and severity of motion sickness. Classically, this is shown in pilot training when the queasy student is given control of the aircraft and symptoms often ease or disappear.

A number of studies have looked at various characteristics, mainly behavioral and personality, in an attempt to delineate those likely to be more susceptible to motion sickness. Of the findings, the only aspects pertinent for evaluating and treating those who fly as passengers is the effect of age. Under 2 years of age, motion sickness is very rare; between 3 and 12 years there is increasing incidence with peak at age 12; then slowly decreasing incidence thereafter.[33]

Prevention and treatment. For the passenger a number of measures can be used to reduce the occurrence of motion sickness. Restriction of head movement, for example, leaning the head firmly against the seat, helps reduce potential conflicting sensory cues. Lying down also seems to reduce motion sickness, although on most flights this is not an option. If a clear view of the horizon or other stable visual reference outside the aircraft is available, then focusing on that can be helpful. If there are no outside stable visual references, then closing the eyes will reduce motion sickness. Unfortunately, for most individuals a task like reading worsens motion sickness. Cool air from the vents blown into the face can also help reduce symptoms in some individuals.

Pharmacologic means can be used for both prevention and treatment of motion sickness in passengers. L-scopolamine hydrobromide is probably the most effective medication, but does not have 100% effectiveness in all individuals and situations. It is available in a transdermal patch (Transderm Scop Signal). Side effects include dilated pupils, difficulty focusing, and unpleasant withdrawal. Other medications such as antihistamines (e.g., meclizine or promethazine) can also be used. Oral or transdermal medications are appropriate for prophylaxis, but parenteral delivery of medications is most effective once motion sickness has developed.[7]

THE SPACE ENVIRONMENT

Space presents even more challenges to the human than the high-altitude or aviation environments. Without the use of protective measures, space is truly uninhabitable. Although many advances have taken place since the initiation space exploration programs, there is still much not known about this environment, or the enclosed environment of space vehicles, or of human responses. The information currently available is derived from accomplished space missions, which have generally been short in duration. The individuals participating in these space missions also have been highly selected, meeting stiff physical requirements and undergoing rigorous training prior to departure.

The problems include microgravity, lack of a life-sustaining atmosphere, radiation, and risk of impact with micrometeroids in space. The presentations below are only a brief introduction to each area.

Microgravity

Microgravity, or "zero gravity," is probably the most notable environmental feature of space. Lack of gravity has profound effects on the human body, both physically and physiologically. The major effects include those of the motor system and bone, the vestibular system, and the cardiovascular system, discussed here.

Motor system and bone. Gravity, as known on the surface of the earth, plays a fundamental role in the development of human musculature and bone structure. All movements that occur, even the most simple ones, require compensation for earth's gravitational pull. Most movements, once learned, become second nature and occur without thought. In the weightless environment of space, many movements must be relearned. Weightlessness has benefits, though, allowing for easy manipulation of those objects considered immovable under sea-level gravity.

Unfortunately, prolonged exposure to weightlessness will affect muscle and bone strength. The lack of need for strong antigravity muscles reduces the mass of these muscles, and the significant reduction in the muscle pull on bones leads to loss of bone mineralization and strength. These compensations for weightlessness are probably of little consequence for the individual remaining in space (although there is no experience with individuals with prolonged exposure to the space environment), but become a real problem for the individual returning to earth. Muscular mass and strength appear to return toward normal fairly quickly after returning to gravity, but there is greater concern about bone demineralization.[43]

The vestibular system. Since one of the primary roles of the vestibular system is to provide information about gravity, the lack of gravity has significant effects on its response. The most obvious and operationally significant disturbance of vestibular function is space motion sickness. The pathophysiology of this is probably similar to that induced on the earth, neural mismatch of expected signals. Space sickness is a fairly significant problem for the first few days of entry into space, with about 40% of all individuals developing some symptoms.[9,43] Unfortunately, susceptibility to motion sickness on the ground does not appear to be an adequate predictor of susceptibility to space sickness.[43] The pharmacologic agents used for motion sickness, particularly the L-scopolamine hydrobromide and dextroamphetamine combination, appear to be useful in ameliorating symptoms and are currently the only available measure for treating space sickness.

The cardiovascular system. Similar to other muscles in the body, the heart is affected by weightlessness. There is no longer a static column of pressure that the heart needs to pump against, reducing the force requirements of the beating heart to perfuse the body. The heart becomes deconditioned relative to earth's gravity, and this presents as a problem only after reentry to the earth's atmosphere. Unlike the rest of the muscular system, the heart may take up to 1 month to return to the capacity present before departure into space.[43]

Atmosphere

Provision for a life-sustaining atmosphere is required at all times in space. The main requirements of this environment are pressure and oxygenation, although other factors like control of carbon dioxide and humidity levels play a role. Pressurization and oxygenation have varied on space missions from the currently used sea-level pressure with 22% O_2 in the Space Shuttle cabin to pressures equivalent to altitudes greater than 18,000 feet with 100% O_2 atmospheres found in pressure suits used for EVA (extravehicular activities) and on older space mission flights. At these low pressures, denitrogenation with 100% O_2 prior to exposure and during the flight has allowed successful missions without complications such as decompression sickness.[43]

Radiation

Radiation is probably one of the major environmental hazards after lack of life-supporting atmosphere. In space, the benefit of the protective blanket of earth's atmosphere is absent. Therefore protective measures to reduce exposures are required for missions in space, especially prolonged ones, and may indeed limit the length of time an individual can remain in the space environment. The main classes of radiation found in space are primary cosmic radiations, geomagnetically trapped radiations (Van Allen belts), and radiation from solar flares.

Cosmic radiation. Cosmic radiation consists of particles originating from outside the solar system. These particles are very high in energy and have a low flux density, which means they are virtually unshieldable.[43]

Trapped radiation. Radiation belts around the Earth include electrons and protons of the solar wind. There are two belts, the inner and outer Van Allen belts, that affect mission planning and altitude orbit.[43]

Solar flares. Solar flares are probably considered the most potent of all space radiation hazards. A solar flare is a solar magnetic storm, which produces increased light, solar x-rays, and high-energy protons. These protons are the main concern. With the characteristics of high energy and high flux, these protons can deliver a potentially lethal dose of radiation if exposure occurs.[43]

Micrometeroids

Micrometeroids are also called "interplanetary dust." Although no significant episodes of damage from these particles have been documented in previous space missions, they are still a source of concern for damage to both vehicles and individuals, and protective measures are part of the requirements in design.

CONCLUSION

This chapter has presented a basic overview of the unique conditions and diseases associated with high-altitude and aerospace medicine. The brief review of our atmosphere and descriptions of the symptoms, prevention, and treatment of altitude- and aviation-related illnesses should provide a general background for most physicians. As individuals in greater numbers take to the slopes and the skies, it is likely that physicians of any specialty will encounter individuals who have been or will be exposed to either of these environments. This chapter should provide enough information for general preexposure counseling and/or initial evaluation of individuals with exposure, with an understanding of the need for referral to specialists in these fields if significant pathology should be encountered.

REFERENCES

1. Armstrong HG, Heim JW: The effect of flight on the middle ear, *JAMA* 109:417, 1937.
2. Arthur DC, Margulies RA: The pathophysiology, presentation, and triage of altitude-related decompression sickness associated with hypobaric chamber operation, *Aviat Space Environ Med* 53:489, 1982.
3. Bärtsch P et al: Prevention of high altitude pulmonary edema by nifedipine, *N Engl J Med* 325:1284, 1991.
4. Brown DE: Acute mountain sickness and physiological stress during intermittent exposure to high altitude, *Ann Hum Biol* 16:15, 1989.
5. Carson RP et al: Symptomatology, pathophysiology, and treatment of acute mountain sickness, *Fed Proc* 28:1085, 1969.
6. Comroe JH et al: Oxygen toxicity, *JAMA* 128:710, 1945.
7. Course materials, Aerospace Medicine Primary Course, School of Aerospace Medicine, Brooks Air Force Base, Texas, 1989.
8. Crow TJ, Kelman GR: Psychological effects of mild hypoxia, *J Physiol* 204:248, 1969.
9. DeHart RL: *Fundamentals of aerospace medicine,* Philadelphia, 1985, Lea & Febiger.
10. Denison DM, Ledwith F, Poulton EC: Complex reaction times at simulated cabin altitudes of 5,000 feet and 8,000 feet, *Aerospace Med* 37:1010, 1966.
11. Dickinson JG: High altitude cerebral edema: cerebral acute mountain sickness, *Semin Respir Med* 5:151, 1983.
12. Downey VM et al: Studies on bubbles in human serum under increased and decreased atmospheric pressure, *Aerospace Med* 34:116, 1963.
13. Ernsting J: The 10th annual Harry G. Armstrong lecture: prevention of hypoxia—acceptable compromises, *Aviat Space Environ Med* 49:495, 1978.
14. Ernsting J, King P, ed: *Aviation medicine,* ed 2, London, 1988, Butterworths.
15. Evans WO et al: Amelioration of the symptoms of acute mountain sickness by staging and acetazolamide, *Aviat Space Environ Med* 47:512, 1976.

16. Figarola RR, Billings LL: Effects of meprobamate and hypoxia on psychomotor performance, *Aerospace Med* 37:951, 1966.
17. Forwand SA et al: Effect of acetazolamide on acute mountain sickness, *N Engl J Med* 279:839, 1968.
18. Golding F et al: Decompression sickness during construction of the Dartford Tunnel, *Br J Ind Med* 17:167, 1960.
19. Gray GW et al: Control of acute mountain sickness, *Aerospace Med* 42:81, 1971.
20. Gronbeck C: Chronic mountain sickness at an elevation of 2,000 meters, *Chest* 85:577, 1984.
21. Grover RF, Weil JV, Reeves JT: Cardiovascular adaptation to exercise at high altitude, *Exerc Sport Sci Rev* 14:269, 1986.
22. Hackett PH, Rennie D: The incidence, importance, and prophylaxis of acute mountain sickness, *Lancet* 2:1149, 1976.
23. Hackett PH et al: Dexamethasone for prevention and treatment of acute mountain sickness, *Aviat Space Environ Med* 59:950, 1988.
24. Hansen JE, Evans WO: A hypothesis regarding the pathophysiology of acute mountain sickness, *Arch Environ Health* 21:666, 1970.
25. Houston CS, Dickinson J: Cerebral form of high-altitude illness, *Lancet* 2:758, 1975.
26. Hultgren HN: High-altitude medical problems. In Rubenstein E, Federman DD, eds: *Scientific American medicine,* New York, 1992, Scientific American.
27. Hultgren HN, Grover RF, Hartley LH: Abnormal circulatory responses to high altitude in subjects with a previous history of high-altitude pulmonary edema, *Circulation* 44:759, 1971.
28. Hultgren HN et al: Physiologic studies of pulmonary edema at high altitude, *Circulation* 29:393, 1964.
29. Hultgren HN, Marticorena EA: High altitude pulmonary edema: epidemioloigc observations in Peru, *Chest* 74:372, 1978.
30. Johnson TS, Rock PB: Current concepts: acute mountain sickness, *N Engl J Med* 319:841, 1988.
31. Kawashima A et al: Hemodynamic responses to acute hypoxia, hypobaria, and exercise in subjects susceptible to high-altitude pulmonary edema, *J Appl Physiol* 67:1982, 1989.
32. King PF: The eustachian tube and its significance in flight, *J Laryngol Otol* 93:659, 1979.
33. Lentz JM, Collins WE: Motion sickness susceptibility and related behavioral characteristics in men and women, *Aviat Space Environ Med* 48:316, 1977.
34. Malconian MK et al: Operation Everest II: altitude decompression sickness during repeated altitude exposure, *Aviat Space Environ Med* 48:679, 1987.
35. Marotte H et al: Rapid decompression of a transport aircraft cabin: protection against hypoxia, *Aviat Space Environ Med* 61:21, 1990.
36. Meehan RT, Zaval DC: The pathophysiology of acute high-altitude illness, *Am J Med* 73:395, 1982.
37. Menon ND: High-altitude pulmonary edema: a clinical study, *N Engl J Med* 273:66, 1965.
38. Milledge JS et al: Acute mountain sickness susceptibility, fitness, and hypoxic ventilatory response, *Eur Respir J* 4:1000, 1991.
39. Montgomery AB et al: Effects of dexamethasone on the incidence of acute mountain sickness at two intermediate altitudes, *JAMA* 261:734, 1989.
40. Montgomery AB, Mills J, Luce JM: Incidence of acute mountain sickness at intermediate altitude, *JAMA* 261:732, 1989.
41. Moore LG et al: Low acute hypoxic ventilatory response and hypoxic depression in acute altitude sickness, *J Appl Physiol* 60:1407, 1986.
42. Morgan BJ et al: The patient with coronary heart disease at altitude: observations during acute exposure to 3100 meters, *J Wilderness Med* 1:147, 1990.
43. Nicogossian AE, Huntoon CL, Pool SL, eds: *Space physiology and medicine,* Philadelphia, 1989, Lea & Febiger.
44. Oelz O et al: Nifedipine for high altitude pulmonary oedema, *Lancet* 2:1241, 1989.
45. Pei SX et al: Chronic mountain sickness in Tibet, *Quarterly J Med* 71:555, 1989.
46. Peñaloza D, Sime F: Chronic cor pulmonale due to loss of altitude acclimatization (chronic mountain sickness), *Am J Med* 50:728, 1971.
47. Rabold M: High-altitude pulmonary edema: a collective review, *Am J Emerg Med* 7(4):426, 1989.
48. Rayman RB, McNaughton GB: Decompression sickness: USAF experience 1970-80, *Aviat Space Environ Med* 54:258, 1983.
49. Reason JT: Motion sickness adaptation: a neural mismatch model, *J Royal Soc Med* 71:819, 1978.
50. Robinson SM, King AB, Aoki V: Acute mountain sickness: reproducibility of its severity and duration in an individual, *Aerospace Med* 42:706, 1971.
51. Rock PB et al: Effect of dexamethasone on symptoms of acute mountain sickness at Pikes Peak, Colorado (4,300 m), *Aviat Space Environ Med* 58:668, 1987.
52. Schoene RH et al: High altitude pulmonary edema: characteristics of lung lavage fluids, *JAMA* 25:63, 1986.
53. Scoggins C et al: HAPE in children and young adults of Leadville, CO, *N Engl J Med* 297:1269, 1977.
54. Stamper DA, Sterner RT, Robinson SM: Evaluation of an acute mountain sickness questionnaire: effects of intermediate-altitude staging on subjective symptomatology, *Aviat Space Environ Med* 51:379, 1980.
55. Taber RL: Protocols for the use of a portable hyperbaric chamber for the treatment of high altitude disorders, *J Wilderness Med* 1:181, 1990.
56. Weil JV: Sleep at high altitude, *Clin in Chest Med* 6:615, 1985.
57. Wiedman M: High altitude retinal hemorrhage, *Arch Ophthalmol* 93:401, 1975.
58. Wirjosemito SA, Touhey JE, Workman WT: Type II altitude decompression sickness (DCS): US Air Force experience with 133 cases, *Aviat Space Environ Med* 60:256, 1989.

Chapter 53

CHEMICAL AGENTS

Michael Gochfeld

Classes of stressors
Information resources
　Books
　Computerized data bases
　Hot lines
　Academic and clinical resources
Acute poisonings
Toxicology and risk
Classification or taxonomy of toxic agents
　Classification by source
　Classification by mechanism of action
　Classification by target organ
Chemical structure and toxicology
　Chemical species
　Isomers and congeners
　Toxic effects
Organic chemicals
　Volatile organic compounds
　Pesticides or biocides
　Organometallic compounds
Inorganic chemicals
　Acids and bases
　Gases
　Carbon disulfide
Heavy metals
　Lead
　Mercury
　Cadmium
　Chromium
　Nickel
　Manganese
　Arsenic
　Selenium
　Beryllium
Fibers and crystals

CLASSES OF STRESSORS

The external stressors that harm the body include physical agents (radiation, noise, vibration, temperature); biologic agents (viruses, bacteria, allergens); chemical agents (organic and inorganic); psychosocial factors (stress); and mechanical forces (trauma). Toxicologists focus mainly on naturally occurring and synthetic chemicals. The classes of stressors can interact, any one of them lowering or heightening the body's resistance to a different class. Thus people with chronic, low-level chemical exposure may be more susceptible to infectious diseases.

The chemicals discussed in this chapter are almost all xenobiotics, substances foreign to the human body. Pharmaceutic agents are a familiar class of xenobiotics used for their beneficial effects, but this chapter focuses on substances that mainly cause harm and provides only brief accounts for the more common chemicals of concern to physicians.

There are now many excellent compendia, references, and data bases that provide extensive detail on many toxic substances (see section on Information Resources below), and this chapter provides basic information on the major classes of toxic chemicals and on specific chemicals commonly encountered by patients in their home, community, or workplace.

INFORMATION RESOURCES

For additional information on any of these chemicals or on chemicals that are not covered here, both published sources and referral resources are available (see Appendix C). New books appear several times a year, summarizing the rapidly growing literature on experimental and human toxicology. The clinician will have little trouble obtaining information on the toxic properties of most of the materials encountered by their patients; it is simply a matter of knowing where to look. In the United States, employers who use or produce products and formulations containing hazardous chemicals as active or inert ingredients must provide material safety data sheets (MSDS) for the protection of workers who use these products. The MSDS are usually available to the public also; however, because the chemical compositions of many industrial and consumer products are proprietary, the MSDS may in many cases obscure rather than clarify their effects.[63] Although this information may be difficult to obtain from the manufacturer, in most cases of clinical necessity physicians will be able to obtain information on composition. (In some cases they may be required to sign a statement of secrecy.)

When a product's composition is not available, knowledge of the function of the chemical suggests the effects that it may have; however, even when the available published material shows that a chemical has the effect reported by a patient, the clinician still faces the challenge of assessment of whether the patient has had sufficient exposure to account for his or her disease, symptoms, or concerns.

Books

Lippmann edited *Environmental Toxicants,*[65] a book with detailed chapters on about 25 of the major environmental hazards that physicians are likely to encounter, including air pollution and ozone, asbestos, dioxins, formaldehyde, tobacco smoke, heavy metals, and microwave and electromagnetic fields. *Casarett and Doull's Toxicology*[3] is a widely used resource covering many toxic chemicals and their mechanisms of toxicity. Several books aimed at the environmental and occupational medicine specialist have recently been published as well.[86,87]

A valuable reference is *Clinical Toxicology of Commercial Products,* edited by Gosselin et al.[53] This book not only covers first-aid and emergency treatment of poisonings but lists many consumer products by their trade names, chemical formulations, and ingredients. It also provides names, addresses, and telephone numbers of manufacturers so that they can be contacted about ingredients and hazards. The most recent edition was published in 1984. The *Pocket Guide to Chemical Hazards*[69] (available from The National Institute for Occupational Safety and Health (NIOSH) in Cincinnati) is a valuable quick reference.

Computerized data bases

Many data bases are available on standard or compact disks (for example, from SilverPlatter Information, Inc., 100 River Ridge Drive, Norwood, MA 02062, 800-343-0064; Micromedex Inc., 600 Grant Street, Denver, CO 80203, 800-525-9083; and from the Canadian Centre for Occupational Health and Safety, 250 Main Street East, Hamilton, Ontario L8N 1H6, Canada 800-263-8340). Different data bases cover the hazardous properties of chemicals, technical MSDS, lay-language fact sheets from the New Jersey Department of Health, and information on acute poisonings and chemical hazard response, from the National Library of Medicine (NLM) data bases. The NLM also provides computerized access to its various data bases under MEDLARS (800-638-8480), and increasingly this access is available through public libraries.

The Environmental Protection Agency (EPA) IRIS Chemical Information Data Base[43] is available on compact disk from Micromedex and on standard computer disks from Lewis Publishers, Boca Raton, Florida. It contains both toxicology and EPA risk-estimation data, including cancer potency numbers, unit risk values, and reference doses.

Hot lines

In addition to state and regional poison-control centers, there are nationally available telephone lines. The Chemical Manufacturers Association provides information on a nonemergency basis (800-CMA-8200), and the EPA supports a pesticide information network (800-858-7378).

Academic and clinical resources

About half of U.S. medical schools have at least one clinical faculty member dealing with occupational and environmental medicine and toxicology. About 35 medical schools have clinical services that specialize in this area. In addition, the Association of Occupational and Environmental Clinics (1030 15th Street, NW, Suite 410, Washington, DC 20005, 202-347-4976) has 48 member clinics in 24 states.

Information can also be obtained by contacting various federal agencies, including NIOSH and the EPA. The Agency for Toxic Substances and Disease Registry (ATSDR), part of the Centers for Disease Control (CDC), 1600 Clifton Road NE, E-29, Atlanta, GA 30333) publishes a series of toxicologic profiles on individuals chemicals. More than 150 are currently available. Clinicians anxious to learn more about specific chemicals can obtain the self-study booklets *Case Studies in Environmental Medicine* from ATSDR.

ACUTE POISONINGS

Outside of the workplace, exposure to environmental contaminants in air, water, soil, and food rarely cause acute poisonings, but these poisonings can occur in the event of major industrial, utility, or transportation accidents, includ-

Table 53-1. Toxicity rating for acute chemical exposures

Toxicity rating	Oral lethal dose (g/kg)	Lethal dose for 70-kg adult
6:Super toxic	<0.005	Less than 7 drops
5:Extremely toxic	0.005-0.050	Less than 1 teaspoon
4:Very toxic	0.050-0.500	1 teaspoon to 1 oz
3:Moderately toxic	0.500-5.0	Up to 1 pint or 1 lb
2:Slightly toxic	5-15	1 Pint to 1 quart
1:Practically nontoxic	>15	More than 1 quart

From Gosselin RE, Smith RP, Hodge HC: *Clinical toxicology of commercial products,* ed 5, Baltimore, 1984, Williams & Wilkins.

ing tanker spills, fires, and explosions. These types of poisonings are not covered in this book. The acute lethal potential of a chemical can be determined from its toxicity rating (listed in Gosselin et al[53]; see Table 53-1).

TOXICOLOGY AND RISK

The EPA uses a variety of approaches to determining what levels of contaminants are unsafe. For carcinogens, the Carcinogen Assessment Group (CAG) of the EPA has computed cancer potency values and unit risk values.[43] For noncarcinogens the usual value is a reference dose (RfD).

Cancer potency is an estimate of the number of excess cancers caused per every additional milligram per kilogram per day of the carcinogen. Conversely, the unit risk value for inhalation is the airborne concentration associated with one excess cancer case per million exposed people and is measured as the concentration in micrograms per cubic meter (μ/m^3).

An RfD is calculated by identifying the significant noncancer health effect to be prevented. This is usually the most sensitive, nontrivial endpoint and must be chosen subjectively or by consensus. The literature is then reviewed to find studies in which this endpoint was investigated. The lowest dose at which the endpoint was observed is called the lowest-observed-adverse-effect level (LOAEL), and the highest dose at which the endpoint was not observed is called the no-observed-adverse-effect level (NOAEL). In some studies all doses except the control produce an effect and there is no NOAEL. In that case the LOAEL is used to calculate the reference dose; otherwise, the NOAEL is used. These values are divided by a series of uncertainty factors (see Chapter 3.)

CLASSIFICATION OR TAXONOMY OF TOXIC AGENTS

Although there are 30,000 to 50,000 individual chemicals used in commerce, about 250 account for the vast majority

---

Classification of toxic chemicals by their structure*

Organic chemicals

    Simple aromatics
        Benzene
        Toluene
        Xylene
        Phenols and Cresols
        Chlorobenzene
    Aliphatics
        Methane
        n-Hexane
    Halogenated aliphatics
        Methylene chloride
        Chloroform
        Carbon tetrachloride
        Trichloroethylene
        Trichloroethanes
        Dibromochloropropane
    Alcohols, aldehydes, ketones, and carboxylic acids
        Formaldehyde
        Ketones
        Methyl tertiary-butyl ether
    Nitriles and amides
    Polyaromatic hydrocarbons
        Benzo[a]pyrene
    Chlorinated polyaromatics
        Polychlorinated biphenyls
        Polybrominated biphenyls
        Polychlorinated dibenzodioxins
        Pentachlorophenol
    Pesticides
        Insecticides
            Organochlorines
            Organophosphates

Organic chemicals (continued)

    Insecticides (continued)
        Others
    Rodenticides
    Herbicides
    Fungicides
    Organometallics
        Tetraethyl lead
        Methyl mercury
        Tributyl tin
        Organic manganese

Inorganic compounds

    Acids and bases
        Hydrogen chloride
        Ammonia
    Gases
        Ozone
        Carbon monoxide
        Carbon disulfide
    Heavy metals
        Lead
        Mercury
        Cadmium
        Chromium
        Nickel
        Manganese
    Other elements
        Arsenic
        Selenium
        Beryllium
    Mineral fibers
    Radionuclides

*This is not an exhaustive list but covers the main classes of chemicals discussed in this chapter.

Classification of chemicals by their use

Agricultural chemicals
    Pesticides
    Insecticides
    Herbicides
    Fungicides
    Algicides
    Mitocides, nematocides, acaricides
Automotive products (fuels, coolants, lubricants, de-icers)
Batteries (heavy metals, acids)
Pharmaceutic agents (see pharmacology texts for subclasses)
Cosmetics, deodorants
Detergents, cleansers, bleaches, deodorizers
Disinfectants
Abrasives
Construction materials (asphalts, asbestos, cements, fillers, resins)
Solvents and degreasers (organic, inorganic)
Paints, pigments, dyes, coatings (metal, rubber, silicone)
Adhesives
Art supplies (pigments, glazes, glues, photographic chemicals, engraving chemicals)
Explosives, fireworks

Classification of chemicals by their mechanism of action

Enzyme disruption or inhibition
Enzyme induction
Metabolic poisons
Macromolecular binding (for example, DNA, protein)
Cell membrane disruption
Competitive binding at active sites
Formation of free radicals or active oxygen species
Sensitizers
Irritants

Classification of chemicals by their target organ(s)

Neurotoxins
Hepatotoxins
Metabolic toxins
Reproductive toxins
Genotoxins (including mutagens)
Carcinogens (including initiators and promoters)
Hematotoxins
Cardiotoxins
Endocrine toxins
Teratogens
Nephrotoxins
Pulmonary toxins
Dermatotoxins

of exposures encountered in practice. Gaining a working knowledge of the most common of these is no more difficult than is understanding a like number of pharmaceuticals. These are the substances on which the ATSDR prepares its toxicology profiles. Knowledge of toxic chemicals can be organized by a simple taxonomy. All chemicals in any one of the classes of toxins share certain properties. We can classify chemicals on the basis of their structure, their source, their economic role, their mechanism of action, or their target organ. The lists herein are not intended to be exhaustive.

The box on p. 594 provides a chemical classification based on structure. The box above classifies chemicals by their commercial uses. The box at top right is a classification based on mechanism of action, and the box at right is based on target organs. Because a single chemical can fall in more than one use category, may have multiple mechanisms, and may affect several organ systems, this chapter is organized by chemical structure. Table 53-2 lists the threshold limit values for about 100 common chemicals. These are the levels to which, theoretically, healthy workers can be exposed 8 hr/day and 40 hr/week for a 40-year working lifetime without becoming ill.[4] Many of these are controversial.

Classification by source

In nature, plants and animals synthesize chemicals, some of them highly toxic alkaloids, to keep themselves from being eaten. Many of these naturally toxic substances are harvested by humans for health or other commercial purposes—antibiotics, for example.

Classification by mechanism of action

Much exciting research in modern toxicology focuses on the mechanism by which a bioactive substance interacts with and alters its targets to produce its unwanted effects. Some act at the molecular level; others interfere with biochemical reactions, attack membranes, bind to macromolecules, or are physiologically active.

Classification by target organ

Toxins can act on any organ system in the body. The effects on these target organs are discussed in relevant chapters elsewhere in this book.

CHEMICAL STRUCTURE AND TOXICOLOGY
Chemical species

The same element may appear to exert very different biologic effects, depending on the particular compound in which it is found. One speaks of organic versus inorganic species of mercury, for example. Organic forms of some metals (mercury, lead, tin, manganese) tend to be more toxic than are their inorganic counterparts, but the reverse is true of arsenic. Valence state also is involved; thus trivalent and

Table 53-2. Threshold limit values from the American Conference of Governmental Industrial Hygienists

Chemical	Threshold limit value (mg/m^3/8 hr)	Chemical	Threshold limit value (mg/m^3/8 hr)
Acetone	1780	Lead chromate	0.05
Acrylonitrile	4.3	Malathion	10
Aluminum dust	10	Manganese dust	5
Aluminum salts	2	Mercury	0.01
Antimony	0.5	Methanol	262
Arsenic	0.1	Methyl chloride	103
Arsine	0.16	Methylene chloride	174
Asphalt fumes	5	Methyl isocyanate	0.047
Benzene	32*	Methyl parathion	0.2
Beryllium	0.002	Molybdenum	5
Bromine	0.66	Nickel	1
Bromoform	5.2	Nicotine	0.5
Butane	1900	Nitric acid	5.2
Cadmium dust	0.05	Nitric oxide	31
Calcium carbonate	10	Nitrogen dioxide	5.6
Calcium chromate	0.001	Nitrous oxide	90
Captan	5	Octane	1400
Carbaryl	5	Ozone	0.2
Carbon dioxide	9000	Parathion	0.1
Carbon disulfide	31	Pentachlorophenol	0.5
Carbon tetrachloride	31	Pentane	1770
Chlordane	0.5	Phenol	19
Chlorine	1.5	Phosgene	0.4
Chlorobenzene	46	Phosphine	0.42
Bis chloromethyl ether	.0047	Phthalic anhydride	6.1
Chromium metal	0.5	Platinum metal	1
Chromium III salts	0.5	Platinum salts	0.002
Chromium IV salts	0.05	Pyrethrum	5
Coal dust	0.2	Selenium	0.2
Coal tar pitch	0.2	Silicon	10
Cobalt	0.05	Silver	0.1
Cyanides	5	Sodium hydroxide	2
Dichlorodiphenyltrichloroethane	1	Stoddard solvent	525
Dimethylformamide	30	Strychnine	0.15
Dioxane	90	Styrene monomer	213
Ethanol	1880	Sulfuric acid	1
Ethyl ether	1220	2,4,5-Trichlorophenoxyacetic acid	10
Fiber glass	10	Tetrachloroethane	6.9
Formaldehyde	0.37	Tetraethyl lead	0.1
Heptane	1640	Thallium compounds	0.1
nHexane	176	Tin metal	2
Hydrazine	0.13	Tin, organic	0.1
Hydrogen chloride	7.5	Titanium dioxide	10
Hydrogen cyanide	11	Toluene	188
Hydrogen fluoride	2.6	Toluene diisocyanate	0.036
Hydrogen peroxide	1.4	Trichloroethylene	260
Hydrogen sulfide	14	Vinyl chloride	13
Lead dusts	0.15	Xylene	434
Lead arsenate	0.15	Zinc chloride	1

From American Conference of Government Industrial Hygienists: *1993-1994 Threshold limit values for chemical substances and physical agents and biologic explosive indices,* Cincinnati, 1992, The Conference.
*ACGIH still lists its as 10 ppm despite the OSHA standard of 1 ppm.

hexavalent chromium are different chemical species and have very different toxic properties.[18] Even among the hexavalent chromium compounds the soluble sodium and potassium salts have less toxicity than that of the partially soluble calcium chromates.

Isomers and congeners

The terms *isomers* and *congeners* are important in literature about organic compounds, particularly dioxins and polychlorinated biphenyls (PCBs). Isomers have the same molecular formula but a different arrangement of atoms.

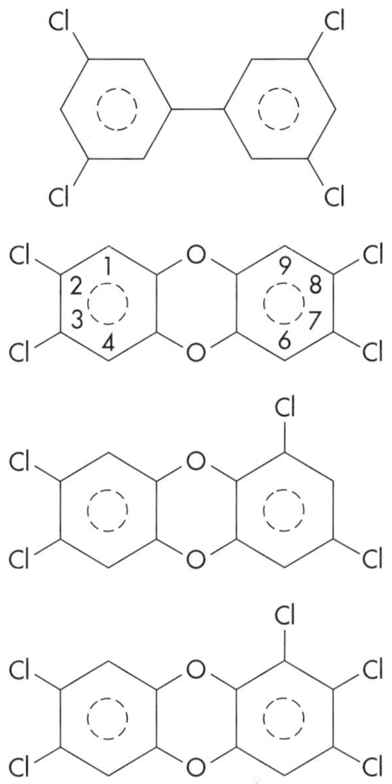

Fig. 53-1. A polychlorinated biphenyl (PCB) and three dioxin compounds. 2,3,7,8-TCDD is 2,3,7,8 tetrachloro dibenzo-*p*-dioxin. 2,3,7,9 TCDD is an isomer; 2,3,7,8,9 PCDD is a congener. (Courtesy Environmental and Occupational Health Sciences Institute.)

Thus butane, a four-carbon compound, can appear as either linear (normal) butane or (branched) isobutane. The behavior in the body and the toxicity may vary greatly among isomers. Congeners are closely related compounds that do not necessarily have the same molecular formula. For instance, dichlorophenol and trichlorophenol are congeners, but 2,4-dichlorophenol and 2,5-dichlorophenol are isomers. Among the dioxins, for example (see Fig. 53-1), 2,3,7,8-tetrachorodibenzo-*p*-dioxin (TCDD) and 2,3,7,9-TCDD differ greatly in their toxicity, although they are isomers. The toxicity of 2,3,7,8,9-PCDD (pentachlorodibenzodioxin) is closer to that of 2,3,7,9-TCDD, although they are congeners. Different dioxin congeners vary more than 1000-fold in their toxicity.[9]

Toxic effects

Although there are many toxic effects, they can be broken down into three main categories: local acute effects, systemic effects, and idiosyncratic effects. Many substances are acutely irritating to the skin, eyes, mucous membranes, and the upper and occasionally the lower airway without exerting systemic effects, but many toxicants are known primarily for their systemic toxicity. A minority of the population (a few percent or less) are hypersusceptible to the effects of chemicals and respond to chemicals that most people find innocuous or respond to toxicants at an unusually low dose. They may exhibit unusual effects that are nonetheless sometimes very serious (for example, anaphylactic reactions to penicillin). Some persons who suffer from multiple chemical sensitivity syndrome fall into this category (see Chapter 30), but other people, by virtue of some genetic or acquired attribute (for example, altered metabolism), may have increased susceptibility to one or more agents.

ORGANIC CHEMICALS
Volatile organic compounds

Low-molecular-weight organics that volatilize readily at room temperature are grouped as volatile organics. Some have boiling points as low as 50°C, and all boil below 260°C. Most common organic chemicals fall in this category. Although there are many hundreds of volatile organic compounds, only a few aromatic, aliphatic, and chlorinated aliphatics are of widespread importance for environmental pathogenesis. At low concentrations, people may detect odors, and as concentrations increase, itching or tingling is sensed and is followed by evidence of irritation, combined with headache and behavioral changes.[67]

Simple aromatics. The most widespread aromatics are benzene, toluene, and xylene, often referred to as BTX. All three compounds are or have been widely used as solvents and degreasers, although most nonessential uses of benzene have been curtailed in industrial countries. Depending on its source, there may be trace amounts of benzene in toluene and to a lesser extent in xylene. The level of this contamination has been reduced greatly with improved manufacturing quality control. There are also trace amounts of toluene in xylene (less than 1%).[11]

They are acutely neurotoxic at high doses. The toxicity declines with the addition of more radicals on the benzene ring. Headaches and lightheadedness are the earliest signs, but high-level exposure, particularly in confined spaces, can progress to confusion, coma, convulsions, and death. All three compounds are readily absorbed from the lungs and intestine and can be absorbed through the skin; however, the skin is also a target organ, suffering from defatting, and a chronic dermatitis is frequently seen in exposed workers. Most home and community exposure levels are insufficient to produce either the acute neurologic or dermatologic conditions, but the possibility should not be ruled out, because high levels of solvent vapors may be inhaled during showering with contaminated water or if a basement has been contaminated from a leaking underground storage tank. Unlike many of the chlorinated aliphatic compounds, hepatotoxicity and nephrotoxicity are not prominent findings. The main concern with BTX exposure hinges on the leukemogenic properties of benzene.

Benzene. Benzene (see Fig. 53-2) is the simplest aromatic and the most carcinogenic. It should not be confused with benzine, which is a mixture of organic solvents containing little benzene. In some countries, benzine is also a synonym for gasoline. Benzene causes leukemia in humans and animals. It is metabolized differently from its relatives

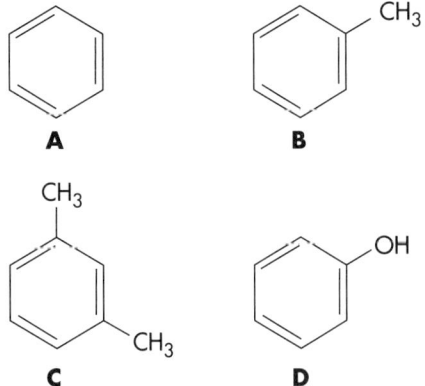

Fig. 53-2. The simple aromatic compounds: (a) benzene, (b) toluene, (c) metaxylene, (d) phenol. (Courtesy Environmental and Occupational Health Sciences Institute.)

toluene and xylene, with which it shares acute neurotoxic properties, acting as a central nervous system (CNS) depressant. (Its toxicity rating is 4.) However, it is the myelotoxic effects of benzene (see Chapter 17) that are of main concern. Of all the known human carcinogens, benzene is the one with the greatest volume of use and the widest distribution.[51] It occurs naturally in petroleum and is therefore a constituent of gasoline at levels greater than 1% (10,000 ppm). It is widely used as a starting material for organic syntheses, particularly in the flavor and fragrance industries; however, its use as a solvent has decreased markedly in the past 20 years. Benzene also is present in a variety of consumer products, such as solvents, and in cigarette smoke. Automobile emissions and leaking underground storage tanks are significant sources of environmental benzene. Water contaminated by benzene can release benzene during showers.

Because it is a carcinogen, it is desirable to eliminate benzene from drinking water, but for practical purposes the maximal permissible level is 5 parts per billion (ppb). Airborne benzene poses a more severe regulatory challenge. The Occupational Safety and Health Administration (OSHA) standard is 1 ppm as an 8-hour time-weighted average. Benzene can be measure in ambient outdoor air, but indoor air concentrations are often much higher and more variable.[94] The EPA conducted a Total Exposure Assessment Methodology (TEAM) study in northern New Jersey in the early 1980s. This included measurements of volatile organics in indoor and outdoor air and in human breath. Benzene was frequently detected in human breath, but there was no relationship with the distance of the person's home to a petroleum refinery. Rather, the higher levels of indoor air benzene swamped any variability induced by ambient benzene levels.[94]

Like many other volatile organic compounds both aromatic and aliphatic, benzene is readily absorbed from air (about 47%) and by ingestion (nearly 100%). Dermal absorption may be as high as 20% to 40% from contact with liquid but is low for contact with vapor.[14] The bone marrow is the main target; depression of bone marrow function leads to fatal aplastic anemia, acute myelogenous leukemia, and certain other cancers[50]; however, once the benzene is taken up by the body, most of it is excreted in expired air, and there is an equilibrium between benzene concentrations in blood and alveoli.[50] It has a half-life in the body of about 2 days, and it does not bioaccumulate. It is metabolized to compounds such as phenol, quinones, and muconic acid and also is eliminated directly via the lungs.

Oral medial lethal doses (LD_{50}s) have ranged from 0.93 g/kg to 5.6 g/kg, and inhalation LC_{50}s have been 10,000 ppm in mice. The EPA-CAG estimates a cancer potency of 2.9×10^{-2} $(mg/kg/day)^{-1}$ for both inhalation and ingestion.[43]

The toxicity of benzene to the bone marrow requires that it be metabolized, and studies of benzene metabolism are critical to understanding its mechanism of action (see Chapter 17). Different animals metabolize benzene differently, which accounts for interspecies variability in susceptibility to leukemia. Unlike many other volatile organics, benzene has low toxicity for the liver, and there is little evidence regarding the effects of long-term low level exposure on the nervous system.

Leukemia. Persons exposed to benzene are concerned about the risks of leukemia. There is some controversy over the risk assessment for benzene.[51] The EPA[43] estimates the risk of leukemia from benzene at 8 in 1 million for a hypothetical person breathing air with a benzene concentration of 1 $\mu g/cm^3$ every day for a 70-year lifetime. The EPA also estimates that a person drinking 2 L water containing 0.66 ppb of benzene[14] for a lifetime increases his or her leukemia risk by 1 in a million (see Chapter 17).

Because benzene itself is short lived in the body, biomonitoring for benzene usually involves measurement of phenol excretion in the urine, preferably of a 24-hour sample; however, phenol itself may be consumed in larger quantities than is benzene, so it is a nonspecific marker. Current studies are exploring alternative biomarkers, for example, muconic acid and related compounds.[96]

Toluene. Toluene (methyl benzene) is a common industrial solvent that is widely used in consumer products. It is one of the most commonly found chemicals at hazardous waste sites. Although volatile, it can persist in moist soils and can move through soil to contaminate water. Absorption of toluene by inhalation can reach 75% and by ingestion approaches 100%.[10] Dermal absorption on contact with liquid toluene is significant, but vapor absorption is probably negligible. Toluene is distributed to fat and the nervous system; it is metabolized and excreted in the urine as hippuric acid. Excretion is essentially 100% within 14 hours after termination of exposure.[10,45]

Toluene is acutely neurotoxic (toxicity rating 4). It is teratogenic, but there is very limited information regarding carcinogenicity. The symptoms of dizziness, weakness, and confusion are nonspecific; however, it also produces a euphoria and is the ingredient responsible for the "high" in glue sniffers.[45] At present it is not listed as "a possible human carcinogen."[10] Long-term or recurrent toluene exposure is associated with neurologic impairment, including both cognitive and motor dysfunction. Whether long-term exposure to toluene causes a dementia or other chronic neurotoxic syndrome is controversial. A chronic solvent syndrome has been reported in several studies following long-term exposure to solvents, including toluene. It includes impairment of memory, cognitive function, and psychomotor function.[70] The ingestion RfD is 300 μg/kg/day, and the long-term inhalation RfD is 1000 μg/kg/day, based on CNS effects and using an uncertainty factor of 100. This dose corresponds to an air level of 3500 μg/m^3.

The myelotoxic properties once ascribed to toluene are now believed to be due to its contamination with benzene, because numerous experimental studies of purified toluene find no evidence for marrow depression and it is not known to cause leukemia.[10]

Xylene. Xylene is almost as widespread in consumer products as is toluene and also is commonly encountered in hazardous waste. There are three isomers of xylene (ortho, meta, and para; see Fig. 53-2). Absorption from the lung is about 64% and from the gastrointestinal GI is as high as 90%. It is also absorbed to a lesser extent through the skin. Xylenes are generally nonmutagenic, but they are teratogenic.[11] There is inadequate evidence regarding carcinogenicity, and it is not classifiable at present. The main effects are acute and chronic neurotoxicity. (See discussion of toluene.) The ingestion RfD is 2000 mg/kg/day, and the inhalation RfD is 400 μg/kg/day.[11] These doses correspond to an air level of 1400 μg/m^3. The acute toxicity (toxicity rating 4) is similar to that of toluene. (See previous discussion.) Xylene is excreted mainly as methylhippuric acid in the urine.[85]

Phenol and cresols. Phenol (carbolic acid) is widely used in commercial and consumer disinfectants and deodorants and is part of some cough medications. Indeed, phenol played a major role in the early development of antisepsis in the nineteenth century. It is also a major metabolite of benzene. Phenol and cresols are not very volatile but are readily absorbed via all routes. Intestinal absorption of phenol is about 100%; pulmonary absorption is as high as 88%, and dermal absorption is about 11%. Phenol is a toxic, irritating, and corrosive material and is acutely toxic to the nervous system, with idiosyncratic responses to relatively low doses also reported. Phenol appears to have cancer-promoting properties, but it is not currently classified with respect to carcinogenicity in humans.[3]

The ingestion RfD is 600 μg/kg/day. There is no separate inhalation RfD. The OSHA permissible exposure limit (PEL) is 19 mg/m^3. An inhalation RfD of 600 μg/kg/day (assuming no ingestion) corresponds to an air level of 2100 μg/m^3, but because the phenol is directly irritating to the respiratory tract, this extrapolation is not protective. Accordingly, dividing the OSHA PEL by 100 yields a more protective air guideline value of 190 μg/m^3.

Chlorobenzene. Chlorobenzene is readily absorbed from the intestinal and respiratory tracts, but data on dermal absorption are inadequate. It is distributed throughout the body, principally to adipose tissue. Results of most carcinogenicity studies of chlorobenzene have generally been negative, but at least one has been positive; hence, chlorobenzene is classified as a possible human carcinogen. It has caused a variety of effects, including reproductive effects. There are no cancer potency data. EPA has derived an ingestion RfD of 30 μg/kg/day and an inhalation RfD of 5 μg/kg/day, which corresponds to an air level of 17.5 μg/m^3.[3]

Other simple aromatics. There are many other aromatic compounds, including ethyl benzene, trimethyl benzene, and nitrobenzene compounds. They are found in varying quantities in a minority of hazardous waste sites.[3]

Aliphatics (alkanes, alkenes, alkynes). Many common compounds fall into the families of the aliphatics, and chlorinated aliphatics are covered in the next section. Gasoline, for example, is a mixture of several alkanes and other organics. The more volatile organics have CNS-depressant properties and are capable of causing headache and dizziness. In liquid form, most are irritating to the skin, extracting lipid and producing irritant dermatitis on repeated exposure. Only two are discussed here.

Methane. Methane, the simplest of the organic compounds, is produced by the incomplete decay of organic material. It occurs naturally in swamps, coal mines, and garbage dumps. It is the explosive fire damp of coal mines, and explosions also occur in garbage dumps if they are not ventilated. Some landfills have facilities for recovery of methane. Its toxicity is mainly due to its replacement of oxygen, hence it is a simple asphyxiant. Although omnipresent, it does not pose a health hazard except in underground mines.

n-Hexane. *n*-Hexane, a widely used solvent, is only occasionally encountered in community exposures. Because hexane is frequently used as a solvent and extractant in analytic laboratories, there is substantial opportunity for occupational exposure. Although it can be present in water supplies, there is no evidence to date of significant environmental exposure. It is unique among the alkanes, causing a dying back axonopathy leading to peripheral neuropathy due to the formation of a unique dihydroxy metabolite. The closely related *n*-pentane, *n*-heptane, and iso-hexanes, although similar in structure, do not form this metabolite and are not known to have the same neurotoxic properties.

Halogenated aliphatics. Chlorinated hydrocarbons are widespread in commerce and are common environmental pollutants. They are found in trace quantities in many municipal and private water supplies. Although most halogenated compounds of concern contain chlorine, there also are some brominated compounds. Many of these compounds are known to be animal carcinogens and possibly or probably human carcinogens. The less toxic compounds, such as 1,1,1-trichloroethane, should be substituted for the more toxic and carcinogenic compounds where possible.

Trihalomethanes. Single-carbon compounds with three halogens (chloroform, dichlorobromomethane, dibromochloromethane, and tribromomethane) make up a subgroup called trihalomethanes, and specific standards limit the combined total of these compounds in drinking water to 100 ppb. The EPA TEAM study in northern New Jersey found that 50% of the population had levels of chloroform in breath exceeding 1 $\mu g/m^3$.[94] Chloroform is neurotoxic, hepatotoxic, and nephrotoxic, the former property accounting for its widespread use as a general anesthetic and the latter two accounting for termination of this use. Ingestion of chloroform has produced cancer in animal studies, but there are no data on animals or humans regarding inhalation of chloroform.[17]

Trichloroethylene. Trichloroethylene (TCE) is one of the most widely used solvents, is carcinogenic in animals, and is commonly detected in well water (see Chapter 42). It affects the skin, nervous system, and myocardium, sensitizing the latter to arrhythmias induced by epinephrine. TCE (under the trade name Trilene) was used as a general anesthetic, particularly for obstetric analgesia, until its relatively high toxicity became known. Irritant dermatitis is characteristic. It is also hepatotoxic and nephrotoxic. Exposure can be estimated by breath analysis. At high doses, TCE sensitizes people to alcohol, much like disulfuran.[25] The main community concern is over long-term, low-level exposure in drinking water. TCE is an animal carcinogen. Occupational epidemiologic studies have suggested a link with cancer, but the results are not clear. Several epidemiologic studies in New Jersey and Woburn, Massachusetts, have shown excess cancers, particularly leukemia, in communities exposed to drinking water contaminated by TCE and other volatile organics, but results of other studies have been negative.[25] Given the current state of knowledge, there are no grounds for complacency but the data do not provide a cause for alarm. Substitution of a water supply with one with lower TCE levels is desirable when possible, but alternative water supplies should be evaluated to ensure that they do not contain other unwanted contaminants. There is some benefit from household filtration systems, provided that they are adequately maintained (see Chapter 42).

Tetrachloroethylene. Tetrachloroethylene, or perchloroethylene, is abbreviated PCE and is also referred to as *Perc*. It is a widely used solvent and is the most common chemical used in dry cleaning. It is commonly encountered at very low levels in drinking water (about 25% of samples). Persons living near dry cleaners have higher exposures than others, and water supplies near hazardous waste sites have higher levels of PCE than those of remote sources. In addition to its neurotoxic and hepatotoxic properties, PCE is an animal carcinogen and teratogen. Epidemiologic studies of dry cleaners have shown an excess of various cancers, but it is not certain that PCE was the offending agent. There is no adequate information, either reassuring or alarming, regarding risks to populations patronizing or living near such facilities,[24] but the excess risk, if any, is very low. PCE is a common trigger for persons with multiple chemical sensitivity, and many of these people report that even dry-cleaned clothes in their closet make them ill.

Methylene chloride (dichloromethane). Methylene chloride, a widely used solvent, can be formed when drinking water is chlorinated, and it is present in incinerator emissions. Background concentrations in the United States are generally in the 30- to 50-parts-per-trillion (ppt) range, with levels as high as 360 ppb measured in New Jersey.[21] Absorption is about 75% from inhalation and 100% from ingestion, with dermal absorption perhaps in the range of 10% from liquid on the skin. Once absorbed, it is distributed throughout the body. It is metabolized to carbon monoxide, carbon dioxide, formaldehyde, and chlorine. Acutely toxic effects primarily involve the nervous system and direct irritation. Methylene chloride is mutagenic, teratogenic, and carcinogenic in animals, but two epidemiologic studies on human populations yielded inconclusive results.[21]

Human volunteers inhaling 40 to 500 ppm (0.1 to 1.7 $\mu g/m^3$) developed carboxyhemoglobin levels of as high as 10%, comparable to those found in smokers.[36] CNS, liver, and kidney effects are found in animals with long-term exposure.

It is a probable human carcinogen, and the EPA-CAG estimated oral cancer potency at 7.5×10^{-3} (mg/kg/day)$^{-1}$.[43] For noncancer effects EPA has computed a long-term RfD of 60 $\mu g/kg/day$, using a safety factor of 100 with an NOAEL of 6 mg/kg/day. There is no separate inhalation RfD. Use of the same value for inhalation yields an allowable air concentration of 210 $\mu g/m^3$.[21]

Vinyl chloride. The monomer vinyl chloride is one of the most widely used raw materials in the plastics industry. It is used to make polyvinyl chlorides. In 1973 an alert physician[35] recognized three cases of angiosarcoma of the liver, hitherto an extremely rare cancer, in workers in one factory. Further research narrowed the search for a culprit to vinyl chloride monomer, which previously had been considered only a mild CNS toxin. Particularly compelling is that vinyl chloride produces the same cancer in animals. The industry was compelled to lower exposure to 1 ppm or less, and within 7 years no additional cases of angiosarcoma were seen. This case provides information on the effectiveness of regulation and on the latency period.[26]

Polyvinyl chloride itself is apparently harmless; however, the vinyl chloride monomer vapor causes lightheadedness and headache and is a mild eye and mucous membrane irritant. Liquid monomer causes a contact dermatitis.

Alcohols, aldehydes, ethers, and carboxylic acids. Many common industrial chemicals fall into the broad categories of alcohols, aldehydes, ethers, and carboxylic acids, and oxidation-reduction reactions convert chemicals from one group to another. Alcohols are often divided into lightweight (methyl, ethyl, isopropyl, and ethylene glycol) and higher alcohols. Methanol is the most toxic and has specific, irreversible neurotoxic effects on the central visual system. Otherwise the toxicity of alkyl alcohols tends to increase with chain length, at least to 5 or 6 carbons.[53]

Formaldehyde. Formaldehyde is one of the most widely used chemicals and is present in many consumer products formulated from resins. It is also used as a disinfectant and germicide. It is very irritating to the eyes, skin, and mucous membranes and can induce asthmatic symptoms. Some people are exquisitely sensitive to formaldehyde, and this sensitivity can be detected with a patch test. It is an animal carcinogen and is suspected to be human carcinogen. It is one substance likely to be responsible for some symptoms of chemical sensitivity.

Ketones. Acetone, methyl ethyl ketone, and methyl-isobutyl ketone are common industrial solvents and reactants that may be present in the air in a community or may occur in hazardous waste. They are readily absorbed by all routes and produce not only local skin conditions but CNS and peripheral nervous system conditions. Pulmonary irritation is a common complaint. Exposure levels can be estimated by measurement of compounds in exhaled breath, but this method is of use only with ongoing exposure. Methyl butylketone causes peripheral neuropathy.

Methyl tertiary-butyl ether. Methyl tertiary-butyl ether has recently come to public attention because it has been added to gasoline (as much as 15% by volume) to increase the oxygen content and therefore the combustion efficiency, thereby lowering carbon monoxide emissions from automobiles. Gasoline-station attendants and some customers around the country have reported a variety of acute symptoms (headache, irritation), perhaps attributed to this additive, and its future use is being reconsidered. The benefits in terms of carbon monoxide reduction may be outweighed by the acutely toxic effects of the additive, and results of an animal carcinogenesis bioassay were positive. Recent rigorous studies comparing reported symptoms with exposure estimates indicate that for most people the methyl tertiary-butyl ether encountered in gas stations is not a cause of symptoms.

Cyanide compounds, nitriles, and amides

Cyanide. Classic poisons such as hydrogen cyanide and potassium cyanide—inorganic compounds—are well known for their effects on the cytochrome system and their blockage of cellular respiration. A number of organic compounds, called cyanogens, can release cyanide either in the environment or in the body. Hydrogen cyanide and potassium cyanide can cause sudden death and, in addition to industrial applications, are used for homicide, suicide, and executions. There are many sources of occupational exposure to cyanide (for example, in electroplating, metallurgy, tanning, photoengraving, and pest control), but the main source of community and household exposure is from hazardous waste, probably through contamination of water. A certain amount of cyanogenic chloride compounds are produced after the chlorination of drinking water. Smoke from fires and, more commonly, tobacco smoke are sources of cyanide.[19] In the body cyanide ions can be converted to thiocyanates or to carbon dioxide, which is rapidly eliminated.

Acrylonitrile. Acrylonitrile, or vinyl cyanide, is used in the manufacture of various polymers. It is a volatile compound readily absorbed through all routes. It has the same acute effects as does cyanide. Warning signs of exposure include headache, irritation of eyes and mucous membranes, and apprehension. It is a possible human carcinogen.

Acrylamide. Acrylamide, a vinyl monomer, is used in production of polymers. It can be absorbed by breathing in dust or through the skin and produces a neurologic syndrome with motor and sensory loss, parasthesias, and weakness. It can progress to tremor and ataxia and can produce permanent neurologic sequelae.[91]

Polyaromatic hydrocarbons. The polyaromatic hydrocarbons are formed during combustion and processing of petrochemical products. They include mainly three- and four-ring compounds, such as the anthracenes, benzanthracenes, and benzpyrenes. Many are known to be animal carcinogens and are probable human carcinogens.

Benzo[a]pyrene. Benzo[a]pyrene (BaP) is the prototype of polyaromatic hydrocarbons. BaP is formed during the incomplete burning of organic matter, including fossil fuel and garbage. It is also found in coal tar pitch, asphalt, creosote, and automobile exhaust. BaP is an important component of cigarette smoke and can be formed during cooking, particularly of meats. Home heating and automobile exhaust are the major sources of BaP.[7]

The main route of entry is through inhalation, although ingestion of contaminated food, water, soil, or dust may be significant in certain cases. Although there are no data for humans, BaP is efficiently absorbed from the intestinal tract (more than 80%) and from the lungs.[7] Because exposure to BaP is widespread and is usually associated with exposure to other toxic materials, there are negligible data on its effects in humans. It is an animal carcinogen and is therefore considered a probable human carcinogen.[7] The American Conference of Government Industrial Hygienists[4] lists it as a suspected human carcinogen.

Animal data on dose-response are scanty. Reproductive or developmental effects have occurred at 10 mg/kg/day by ingestion, and the minimal risk level for noncancer endpoints is considered 10 μg/kg/day.[7] Chronic inhalation exposure at about 10,000 μg/m^3 caused cancer in hamsters. EPA estimates that 2800 μg/L drinking water corresponds to an excess cancer risk of 1 in 1 million.

NIOSH recommends a limit of 100 μg/m^3 (time-weighted average). OSHA established a PEL of 200 μg/m^3. On the basis of this level, the BaP level in homes, schools, or the community should not exceed 2 μg/m^3. The problem in interpretation arises because data exist for total polyaromatic hydrocarbons and not for BaP alone. BaP is the most carcinogenic common ingredient of the polyaromatic hydrocarbon fraction, but it is not the only carcinogen. Gochfeld[48] developed a set of assumptions for polyaromatic hydrocarbons mixtures, based on an estimate that BaP composes only 10% of the total polyaromatic hydrocarbon mixture and that the remainder of the mixture has only 10% of the carcinogenicity potential of BaP. Therefore, the total cancer potency of polyaromatic hydrocarbon mixtures is estimated at 19% ([10% × 90%] + 10%) of pure BaP.

Chlorinated polyaromatics. Some of the most serious environmental contamination problems are due to the chlorinated polyaromatics. The contamination of Hudson River sediments with PCBs from General Electric facilities; dioxin contamination of the Passaic River in Newark, New Jersey, from a Diamond Shamrock plant; and the contamination of Times Beach, Missouri, by waste oil, are widely recognized environmental contamination problems. Nessel and Gallo[74] have provided an excellent review of the dioxins and related compounds such as PCBs, polybrominated biphenyls, and furans. All of the chemicals in this group can cause chloracne.

PCBs. There are 209 different isomers and congeners of PCBs, and their toxicity varies greatly. They were discovered in the nineteenth century and were introduced into U.S. commerce in 1929 for their chemical stability. Commercial mixtures marketed mainly by Monsanto as "aroclors" were widely used in electrical transformers and capacitors because of their high heat tolerance and their low conductivity. PCBs were also used in hydraulic systems as plasticizers, in lubricants and cutting oils as stabilizers, and in carbonless copy paper. They are highly toxic in aquatic ecosystems and to birds and are moderately toxic to humans. They are known to be animal carcinogens. They are highly persistent in the environment, remaining for many years. Originally used as mixtures of the congeners called aroclors, the composition changes because of differential weathering of different compounds; hence the pattern of congeners analyzed may not reflect the actual aroclors that were used decades ago. Therefore the tendency to report analytic results in terms of aroclors has been replaced by isomer-specific PCB analysis; however, it is becoming popular to perform a total PCB analysis first as a screen before an isomer breakdown is sought.[23]

PCBs are commonly found at hazardous waste sites. They pose a problem because temperatures as high as 1000°C are required for complete destruction.

PCBs are stored mainly in fat and can be mobilized from adipose tissues many years after exposure has ceased. The main source of exposure is from consumption of large fish, which often have high concentrations in their tissues; however, occupational exposures and exposures during electrical fires have often caused significant human exposure and illness.

PCBs have been phased out of virtually all uses in the United States, and accordingly PCB levels in the human population have declined dramatically since the 1970s.

Polybrominated biphenyls. Polybrominated biphenyls are not widespread, and evidence of human exposure is infrequent; however, widespread poisoning of animals and humans occurred in Michigan in 1973 when a manufacturer accidentally mixed them in animal food that was widely sold to farmers.

Dioxins and furans. The dioxins, or more strictly the polychlorinated dibenzodioxins and related compounds (such as the *polychlorinated dibenzofurans (PCDFs)*, have become a primary concern in environmental toxicology (see Fig. 53-1),[74] largely because one compound, 2,3,7,8-TCDD, is the most toxic synthetic compound known, at least when tested in guinea pigs. Having gained this reputation, 2,3,7,8-TCDD has become the major contaminant of concern at many hazardous waste sites, in many places where herbicides were manufactured or used, and in the vicinity of active or proposed incinerators.[75] Wherever chlorine comes in contact with heated organic molecules, there is a possibility of formation of these compounds.

Historically, exposure to 2,3,7,8-TCDD has occurred at Nitro, West Virginia, in 1948 at a Monsanto herbicide plant; in Vietnam, in people who handled or were exposed to defoliants; at Times Beach, Missouri, where contaminated oil was used for controlling dust since 1971; in Newark, New Jersey, in the vicinity of a Diamond Shamrock herbicide factory; and at Seveso, Italy, after an explosion at a trichlorophenol plant.[93] In addition, many smaller sources of exposure have resulted in the widespread distribution of 2,3,7,8-TCDD in the environment and its bioaccumulation in the food chain. In the United States the average level of 2,3,7,8-TCDD in the lipid compartment of the serum is on the order of 3 to 5 ppt.[59] In addition, there have been two documented outbreaks of poisoning after ingestion of rice oil contaminated with PCBs and PCDFs because of faulty equipment in the oil-manufacturing facility. The Yusho incident occurred in Japan in 1968, and the Yucheng event occurred in Taiwan in 1979; both words mean *oil disease*. The individuals developed chloracne, hyperpigmentation of the skin, weakness, respiratory disease, immune dysfunction, and neuropathies.

Agent Orange. The defoliant Agent Orange, used extensively in the Vietnam War, contained 50% 2,4,5-trichlorophenoxyacetic acid (2,4,5-T), which was also one of the most common of household herbicides until the mid-1970s, when it was banned. 2,4,5-T was synthesized from trichlorophenol, but in the process two molecules of the trichlorophenol might undergo a condensation reaction forming 2,3,7,8-TCDD. Some batches of Agent Orange contained as much as 50 ppm of TCDD.[74]

Because of the failure of the U.S. Department of Defense to investigate dioxin exposure when it became apparent in 1971, the issues of exposure, cancer among veterans, and birth defects among their children have become the focus of a major public debate, with affected veterans insisting on a definitive study and just compensation. Although results of preliminary studies by the U.S. Air Force of the Project Ranch Hand workers who handled defoliants were negative, more recent follow-up does indicate increased rates of disease. Kahn et al[59] showed that the herbicide handlers still had elevated levels of 2,3,7,8-TCDD in their fat and blood 17 years after exposure terminated. More recent research, still unpublished, indicates that some ground troops in Vietnam had sufficient exposure to TCDD to elevate their risk slightly above average.

Exposure. The dioxins and furans are essentially insoluble in water. They are present in the environment in soil and sediments bound to particular matter and can therefore be suspended in water. They are consumed by organisms and distributed to lipid tissues and thus are readily bioaccumulated. Relatively high levels of TCDD and related compounds have been measured in fish and crabs, and they are significant sources of human exposure. Indeed, contaminated blue crabs in the Passaic River focused attention on the contaminated herbicide manufacturing facility in Newark, New Jersey.

Dioxins and furans are also formed in incineration (see Chapter 41) when organic matter is heated in the presence of chlorine; however, the octachlorodibenzodioxin and other congeners are formed in greater amounts than 2,3,7,8-TCDD.[75]

In addition to industrial accidents involving exposure to trichlorophenol, workers who handled trichlorophenol in the manufacture of herbicides and hexachlorophene were exposed. Some hexachloraphene batches contained significant TCDD as well. Dioxins including TCDD are formed in the process of bleaching paper, which has led to contamination of waste water from paper plants as well as to the presence of minute quantities of dioxins in paper products themselves. The latter has been of particular concern for products used as food containers (see Chapter 43).

Although inhalation of dioxins from incineration emissions may be significant in a few communities,[75] today the major sources of human exposure are ingestion of fish, milk, and meat and accidental ingestion of soil.[93] In general, large, fatty fish are the main culprits, and the larger the fish, the higher the concentrations (not just the total amount). Some people consume high quantities of fish, and for them a reduction in the number of fish, consumption of smaller rather than larger fish, and removal of as much fat and oil as possible reduces intake of TCDD and related compounds.

Toxicity. TCDD exposure causes many physiologic responses in rodents. Among them are death, loss of body weight, increased liver weight, and induction of cytochrome P-450.[74] TCDD is the most potent known inducer of certain enzymes, including cytochrome P-450/1A1, which catalyzes the hydroxylation of BaP and is used as an indicator of TCDD toxicity. TCDD interacts with the estrogen receptor,[46] and it is assumed that most or all of its toxicity is receptor mediated. TCDD is both an animal and human carcinogen. Recent epidemiologic studies of TCDD-exposed workers and Seveso victims have shown elevated risks of several cancers,[29,44] but the results are not consistent. Soft-tissue sarcomas have been reported in most but not all studies, and non-Hodgkin's lymphomas and lung cancer have been reported in several studies. Intestinal cancers have been increased in some subgroups. It is clear that TCDD is not an initiator of cancer, and it appears to act as a promoter. Because of its competition for the estrogen receptor, TCDD has reduced breast cancer rates in some mouse studies and in a recent report of persons exposed at Seveso.[29]

Pentachlorophenol. Pentachlorophenol (PCP) has been widely used as a wood preservative and also in various biocides. In the short term it uncouples oxidative phosphorylation, and it also is a severe respiratory, eye, and skin irritant. It came to widespread attention when babies died from contact with PCP residues in diapers that had been laundered with a fungicidal soap. PCP is also contaminated with small amounts of dioxins, and for that reason its use was banned in the United States in the early 1980s. Some people still have cans of wood preservative with PCP, and treated wood still survives, so there is some movement of PCP in the environment.

Pesticides or biocides

Although the term *pesticide* is often considered a synonym for insecticide, it is actually much broader, including herbicides, fungicides, algicides, acaricides or mitocides, nematocides, rodenticides, and others. The term *biocides* is usually used as a blanket term to avoid confusion. In addition to the toxicity of the active ingredients, many of the vehicles used with pesticides are irritating and sensitizing.

Organochlorine insecticides. Organochlorine (OC) or chlorinated hydrocarbon pesticides are still used worldwide, and although many uses have been phased out in North America, they still have certain applications. The chlorinated ethane compounds include dichlorodiphenyltrichloroethane, better known as DDT. The cyclodienes include some of the most toxic of the organochlorines: dieldrin, aldrin, and chlordane. The hexachlorocyclohexanes include lindane. In the body DDT is broken down into metabolites such as DDE, and it is the latter compound that is measured in most studies.

Exposure. The OC pesticides are persistent in the environment and are lipid soluble; hence they show biologic amplification in the food chain as well as long-term persistence in human adipose tissue. For most people, exposure occurred through the food chain. There are still substantial quantities of OC pesticides in use, but even those phased out 20 years ago are still present in the environment.

Ingestion is the most common route, but exposure during application can result in inhalation of wind-drifted aerosols. These compounds' dermal absorption properties vary. Most of the compounds can be absorbed to some extent from liquid on the skin, but some can actually be absorbed when the powdered form contacts the skin, which has been a major route of occupational exposure; however, a 5% DDT dust has been used in many parts of the world (including on U.S. troops in foreign countries) for delousing purposes, and lindane (in the form of Kwell) has been used to control lice in hair. These compounds have negligible dermal uptake. There is some transplacental exposure of fetuses, and because these lipophilic compounds are excreted in breast milk, it is a potential source of exposure for neonates.

Toxicity. The OC compounds have been developed to kill insects, and they primarily affect the nervous system. Humans with low exposures experience nausea and headache, followed by tremors and paresthesias and then muscle weakness and fibrillation. Although DDT was removed from the market primarily for ecologic reasons, other OC compounds have been removed because of carcinogenicity. DDT, aldrin, and dieldrin are carcinogenic in animals. Not only is chlordane an animal carcinogen but some epidemiologic studies[58] have indicated a link with leukemia and neuroblastoma. Since some OCs are carcinogens, the question of cancer risk has often been raised for populations with any OC exposure. This risk does not appear to be prominent. Probably the main risk for a population with significant OC exposure is adverse reproductive effects, including neonatal exposure through lactation.

Organophosphates. Much of the knowledge of pesticide toxicity is based on studies of parathion. Originally developed as pesticides, their potential as nerve gases for military use led to a proliferation of research and development during World War II.[3] Though the first OP pesticide was marketed in 1944, they came into regular use after the war, with hundreds of congeners now in use. With decisions to phase out many of the environmentally persistent OCs, there was a great increase in OP use, despite their much greater acute human toxicity. These in turn have been replaced for some uses by the less toxic carbamates. The OP chlorpyrifos (marketed under the tradename Dursban) is the most commonly used insecticide against termites and carpenter ants, having replaced chlordane for this function.

Exposure. OPs are used to control insects and other pests on many crops. They tend to have short environmental persistence and are not systemic toxicants. The interval between spraying and time that workers are allowed back into fields is short (generally 2 to 3 days, but it can be much longer for certain applications of parathion). Thus these pesticides do not remain on the surfaces of leafy vegetables and do not accumulate in fruits. Illnesses have been reported to ocur mainly in people who handle, mix, apply, or clean up OP sprays; however, accidental spraying of nearby workers or of residences adjacent to fields has been all too common. Children playing with empty containers or bags that housed OP have been severely poisoned.

Most clinicians encounter pesticide problems from inappropriate application by householders or by commercial applicators in office buildings. Misapplication can include excessive quantities, poor placement, or contamination of ventilation systems.

Absorption occurs through all routes, and skin absorption is relatively high for many OP compounds. Ingestion is sadly common in children because once mixed, pesticides are often stored temporarily in inappropriate containers.

Toxicity. The main effect of the OP compounds is to bind to the active site on the enzyme acetylcholinesterase; thus all pesticides in this group have a common effect. This bond between OP and enzyme is relatively stable, lasting hours to days, compared with microseconds for the physiologic action of the enzyme with acetylcholine. Because acetylcholinesterase is required to break the transient complex between acetylcholine and its receptor on the synaptic membrane or on effector organs or muscles, and in order for recurrent nerve impulses to reach their destination, the anticholinesterase activity essentially blocks the breakup of the transmitter-receptor complex, leading quickly to paralysis.[3]

The body appears capable of adaptation to long-term, low-level OP exposure, perhaps by producing nonspecific cholinesterases, which, unaffected by the OP, can break the transmitter-receptor complex. Thus when long-term exposure depletes cholinesterase levels, they may be much lower than those at which symptoms occur with short-term toxicity. Restoration of normal enzyme levels requires weeks.

The first symptoms are likely to be sweating; nausea; heartburn; intestinal symptoms (cramps, diarrhea); increased salivation and lacrimation. Respiratory difficulty and bradycardia are observed, and in severe cases loss of bowel and bladder control occur in association with pulmonary edema. Although miosis is a classic sign, it is not consistent, and the possibility of poisoning should not be dismissed simply because miosis is not present. Nicotinic effects of OP include muscle twitching and fasciculations and general weakness, which are followed by respiratory paralysis leading to death. The CNS may also be affected with headache, cognitive impairment, anxiety, sleeplessness, and emotional lability. The practitioner should also be aware that in addition to specific OP effects, people with acute exposures may suffer from effects of inert ingredients, which may include irritative effects not characteristic of OP themselves.

With the relatively low levels from environmental exposure likely symptoms are headaches, tiredness, and perhaps salivation and lacrimation.

Evaluation of exposure relies mainly on clinical impression. The OPs are not persistent in the body, and except in cases of recent short-term exposure it is not be possible to detect the parent compound, even with a label. It is relatively simple to measure cholinesterase levels, and a low level is suggestive of excessive exposure or poisoning; however, in the absence of a baseline, it is very difficult to interpret a single cholinesterase reading. A high level may still reflect a decline, whereas a low level may be normal for that individual. For persons who regularly work with OP pesticides, a baseline cholinesterase determination is essential. The cholinesterase in red cells recovers only as new red cells are produced, and most monitoring programs rely on the plasma cholinesterase level, which drops more precipitously and recovers more rapidly.[45]

Other pesticides. Other classes of biocides include the carbamates and pyrethrum and pyrethroid insecticides, organometallic and inorganic metals, and a wide variety of other chemicals used to kill plants and animals. Fumigants such as ethylene dibromide, methyl bromide, and hydrogen cyanide are used to kill insect and rodent pests in stored grain and other foods. These pesticides are acutely toxic to humans, and the bromides are alkylating agents and are suspected to be human carcinogens.

Pyrethrum. Many household insecticides contain pyrethrum, which is derived from certain African flowers of the genus *Chrysanthemum.* They have low potential for systemic toxicity but are potent skin sensitizers. Occasional anaphylactic reactions have been reported.

Rodenticides. Because of the relative similarity of humans and rodents, rodenticides would have the greatest potential for human toxicity. These chemicals are used to fumigate burrows or are distributed as baits. Compounds of several metals, including zinc, thallium, and arsenic, are widely used. The coumarinlike compound warfarin leads to death from hemorrhage. It can also result in human poisoning through accidental ingestion.

Compound 1080 (sodium fluoroacetate) has been used for control of other mammals (such as coyotes); it blocks the tricarboxylic acid cycle, leading to acute symptoms that progress to death.

Herbicides. Herbicides are generally considered to have low potential for systemic toxicity in humans. Many different substances are used to kill vegetation in general and broad-leaved weeds in particular and to sterilize soil.

Chlorophenoxy herbicides. The two best known chlorophenoxy herbicides are 2,4-dichlorophenoxyacetic acid (2,4-D) and 2,4,5-T. They are growth-regulating hormones in plants without apparent hormonal action in animals. They are acutely neurotoxic in high doses and, depending on the formulation, are irritating to the eyes, mucous membranes, and skin; most cause a contact dermatitis. High-level exposure can cause chloracne. These herbicides have been linked with increased risk of soft-tissue sarcoma, particularly in forestry workers. Some studies of farmers have shown increased rates of non-Hodgkin's lymphoma, and there is a possible association with 2,4-D that requires extensive study.

Aminotriazole. Marketed under the name Amitrol, aminotriazole was widely used to control weeds and poison ivy along highway and other right-of-ways. It has relatively low toxicity for humans except that it interferes with thyroid function and has been known to cause goiters in people with long-term exposure.

Fungicides. Among the chemicals used to control molds and other fungi are the organomercurials (particularly methylmercury salts and phenyl mercuric acetate). These compounds were used to treat seeds for long-term storage. The use of pentachlorophenol as a wood preservative relies on its antifungal properties.

Dibromochloropropane. Dibromochloropropane has been used mainly as a nematocide and soil sterilizant. It is a testicular poison, and many workers who manufactured and packaged the product experienced sterility. Sperm counts revealed both oligospermia and azoospermia. In a 10-year follow-up, most of those with oligospermia had recovered to normal levels, but those who were azoospermic remained so.

Organometallic compounds

Some of the most significant environmental toxicants are organic compounds of common metals such as mercury, lead, tin, and manganese. The specific toxic effects of these compounds are discussed herein with their respective metals.

Tetraethyl lead. Tetraethyl lead remains a common gasoline additive in many parts of the world, particularly in the developing nations. It is a major contribution to air pollution and in most people has been the single largest contributor to their body burden of lead.[55] This finding became apparent in the United States after the phase-out of lead from gasoline beginning in the mid-1970s (Fig. 53-3). During the ensuing decade the mean blood lead level in U.S. adults dropped from about 12 μg/dL to 6 μg/dL. An Italian study employing gasoline lead additives with a unique isotopic composition showed that automobile emissions contributed about 5.7 μg/dL to the body burden.[34] Because the lead leaving the tailpipe is converted by combustion to inorganic lead, the toxic effects are actually those of the inorganic compound.

Organomercurials. Organomercurials, particularly the methyl mercury compounds and phenyl mercuric acetate, were widely used for their biocidal properties. As fungicides they were used to treat seed to preserve it over the winter, and major episodes of mercury poisoning resulted from human consumption of treated seed, with epidemics in Iraq and Guatemala and at least one family poisoned in New Mexico. As molluscacides, organomercurials were incorporated in

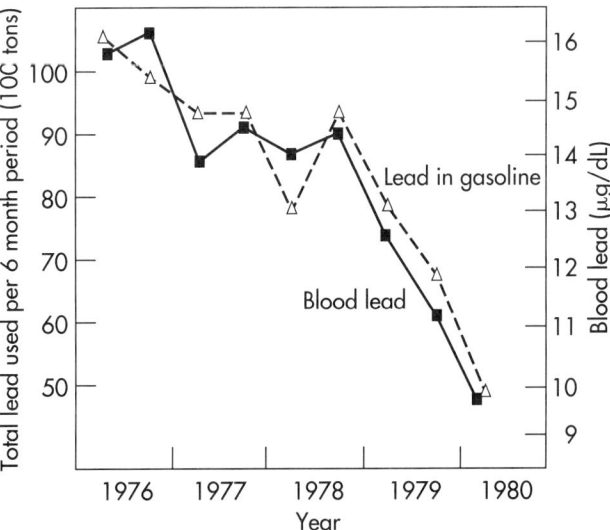

Fig. 53-3. Solid line shows the decline in lead used in gasoline (in 1000 tons/6 months); dotted line shows decline in blood lead (in μg/dL). (From National Health and Nutrition Survey II, Washington, DC, 1986, National Center for Health Statistics.)

marine antifouling paints used on ship hulls to thwart the growth of barnacles. In this role they led to contamination of marine ecosystems. In the United States and some European countries many uses of organomercurials were phased out by 1980.[27]

Other organometallics. Organotin compounds, particularly tributyl tin, have replaced mercury in antifouling paints, but their toxicity to natural aquatic ecosystems is as great as that of mercury, and curtailment of usage is likely to occur.[12,61] Much less is known about their toxicity to humans. Organomanganese compounds, particularly the methylcyclopentadienyl manganese tricarbonyl compound, are being considered for introduction into gasoline as an antiknock agent. Manganese causes a parkinsonian syndrome, but very little is known about the effects of organic manganese on humans, wildlife, or ecosystems, and their use in gasoline is clearly undesirable without extensive testing (see p. 610).

INORGANIC CHEMICALS
Acids and bases

Acids and bases, common reactive compounds including ammonia, hydrochloric, sulfuric, and nitric acids, and lye, are commonly encountered, as are their gaseous precursors, such as hydrogen chloride, oxides of sulfur, and oxides of nitrogen. Some organic acids, such as phenol and formic and acetic acid, also are occasional causes of irritant symptoms, and aqueous solutions of iodine and chlorine also have corrosive properties. The acutely irritant effects of acids and bases on the eyes and skin are well known, and treatment is described in many texts. Not as well known are the results of long-term exposure. Most long-term exposure is confined to the workplace, but some environmental exposure also can occur, particularly through misuse of these materials. Acid salts such as phosphates and sulfates are common in drinking water and generally do not cause illness, although they may have serious ecologic effects.

Acid aerosols, particularly hydrochloric and sulfuric acid, are sometimes components of indoor air pollution. The reported symptoms of eye and mucous membrane irritation are often accompanied by headache and a vague feeling of malaise. Although these are common findings, the mucous membrane irritation is not nonspecific, and the possibility of an airborne irritant such as an acid vapor should be considered.

Hydrogen chloride. Examples of an acid exposure, are industrial or incinerator emissions of hydrogen chloride. Hydrogen chloride is produced endogenously in gastric juice and occurs naturally in most body fluids, which, however, are buffered to prevent harmful effects. Therefore hydrogen chloride is mainly a problem when there has been direct contact with the lungs and mucous membranes. Once in the body, environmental hydrogen chloride is metabolized as is natural hydrogen chloride; however, metabolism does not influence the local toxicity. The odor threshold is unclear, with reports ranging anywhere from 100 to 14,000 $\mu g/m^3$. The effects appear entirely related to local irritation. Reproductive, teratogenic, mutagenic, and carcinogenic outcomes are not at issue for hydrogen chloride. Because local rather than systemic effects are involved, there is no RfD. The state of New York has proposed an ambient guideline concentration of 140 $\mu g/m^3$.[76]

Ammonia. In addition to their use in household cleaners, ammonia and its compounds are widely used in industry, and ammonia gas is used as a fertilizer. Massive acute poisoning episodes have occurred from industrial accidents and tanker derailments. The olfactory threshold is 5 ppm, and most people find levels above 20 ppm distinctly unpleasant. The mixing of household bleaches containing hypochlorite with ammonia is a common source of short-term exposure to the very irritating hypochlorous acid.

Gases

Ozone. The ozone problem is covered in Chapter 40. Ozone is ubiquitous, formed through the photochemical interaction of oxides of nitrogen and sunlight. It tends to peak in the early afternoon on summer days. The major source of oxides of nitrogen has been vehicular emissions, which have been substantially reduced through emission controls.

Ozone is a serious lung irritant, with an OSHA PEL of only 100 ppb (235 $\mu g/m^3$); 100 ppb is also recommended as a ceiling value.[4] Paradoxically the ambient air standard (National Ambient Air Quality Standard) is 120 ppb. This is a rare case of an ambient standard's being less protective than a workplace standard. The possibility that persons with glucose-6-phosphate dehydrogenase deficiency might be more sensitive to the effects of ozone and other oxidizers was explored by Amoruso et al,[5] who showed that rapid reticulocytosis can replace hemolyzed red cells, allowing deficient individuals to adapt to these stresses.

Many studies have shown respiratory impairment on days with high ozone levels, and it is believed to be a significant cause of asthma.[64]

Carbon monoxide. Carbon monoxide is an omnipresent, odorless, and colorless gas released from all forms of combustion, including vehicular combustion, heating, fires, and tobacco smoke. Carbon monoxide is an important toxic in indoor air pollution, particularly from faulty heaters and from tobacco smoke, which contains about 10,000 ppm carbon monoxide. Hemoglobin has a strong affinity for carbon monoxide, and the measurement of carboxyhemoglobin is the standard method of estimation of the magnitude of carbon monoxide exposure. Normal carboxyhemoglobin levels are less than 2%, but smokers may achieve levels of 10%. Occupational standards should maintain carboxyhemoglobin levels below 5%.[68]

The diagnosis and treatment of acute carbon monoxide poisoning are adequately covered in standard medical and emergency medicine texts, yet carbon monoxide remains an important substance in environmental medicine. Many of the issues regarding facility siting, for example, include estimates of carbon monoxide emissions, and concerns regarding health effects are voiced. Outdoor air pollution, even from a fire or incinerator, rarely produces a high-enough level of carbon monoxide to cause acute clinical poisoning.

There is evidence that persons with severe angina may experience symptoms when ambient carbon monoxide levels are elevated to about 4%, which would be exacerbated in a person with a hemolytic anemia. At about 10% concentration of carbon monoxide, persons with lung disease experienced decreased exercise tolerance.[36] Concerns for such health effects have driven regulation. In 1992 the EPA mandated the addition of as much as 15% methyl tertiary-butyl ether to gasoline to improve its combustion properties and diminish carbon monoxide emissions.

Patients with cardiovascular disease have limited compensation when an increased oxygen demand is imposed on the heart, for example, during heavy exercise. During exercise stress testing, carbon monoxide exposure can accelerate the appearance of ST abnormalities indicative of disease and can decrease maximal performance time or time to angina; however, at 100 ppm carbon monoxide (carboxyhemoglobin level below 4%) only minimal changes were observed.[89] At a carboxyhemoglobin level of about 6%, exercise tolerance was significantly impaired.[1]

Carbon monoxide levels above 5% also had acute neurobehavioral effects on vigilance, perception, dexterity, and other tasks. There is also active research on possible relationships between prenatal carbon monoxide exposure (that is, from tobacco smoke) and low birth weight, retarded psychomotor development and sudden infant death syndrome. Not all of the results are in but what is known is sufficient to send a strong message against smoking during pregnancy. A case-control study found no relationship between outdoor carbon monoxide levels and birth weight,[3] but this study does not address the much greater indoor air exposures.

Long-term exposure to carbon monoxide also is of concern. There is conflicting evidence regarding atherogenic properties of carbon monoxide. A comparison of bridge and tunnel workers linked increased carbon monoxide exposure with increased atherosclerosis,[90] while a general study showed an increase in acute disease but not chronic disease. At present it is prudent to consider that carbon monoxide exposure, even at levels associated with moderate smoking, accelerate atherogenesis. There may also be a slight effect of carbon monoxide on pulmonary function, although most studies have been unable to separate carbon monoxide from associated air pollutants that also could affect the lungs.[66]

Carbon disulfide

Carbon disulfide has been widely used in industry, with heavy use in the production of viscose rayon and rubber. It has been used as a fumigant and insecticide. It is well established as a cause of occupational disease; thus, its use has been reduced and it is usually treated with great respect.

There are few circumstances in which humans would be exposed outside of the workplace. It is not used in commercial products. It is present at some hazardous waste sites, and it could be released in a transportation accident. Carbon disulfide is toxic to the heart and irritating to the lungs. Long-term exposure results in a polyneuropathy as well as CNS disease, with some patients exhibiting a parkinsonism-like illness. At lower levels, people exhibit depression, irritability, memory loss, and cognitive impairment.

HEAVY METALS

More than 20 elements are considered heavy metals; they occur naturally in the Earth's crust, but most have relatively restricted commercial use and are not widespread in the human environment. The most important of these metals are lead, mercury, cadmium, nickel, chromium, manganese, and cobalt, and several books on metals,[57] mercury,[78] lead,[83] and chromium[79] summarize knowledge regarding the chemicals in the environment and human exposure. Many heavy metals are essential trace elements but may become toxic at higher concentrations. Copper, iron, and zinc, although potentially toxic, are normally present at relatively high levels in the body. (For information on other metals, see Carson et al[31].) Arsenic and selenium are considered metalloids, capable of forming both anions and cations, and are dealt with in the following section.

The major health problems associated with tin concern tributyl tin and other organic tin compounds. Occasional acute toxicity has been associated with leaching of tin from cans into food, but new technologies have eliminated such leaching in most countries. Copper is an essential element that is regulated by the body. Acute copper toxicity causing intestinal symptoms can occur, particularly from acidic water's leaching copper from pipes or containers. Airborne copper exposures from smelters are a local problem. Otherwise, environmental exposure to copper is infrequently documented to cause health problems. Manganese exposure causes parkinsonismlike disease.

Lead

In the late 1980s lead reemerged as a major environmental toxin causing great concern, particularly for young children.[6,72] Remarkably the level of concern seems to have paralleled that of tuberculosis, reaching a high level in the 1960s and 1970s, then receding as recognition of lead poisoning declined only to reemerge when new research resulted in lower acceptable levels of lead.

Exposure. Lead poisoning has a long history as an occupational disease and was recognized by Ramazzini by 1700.[56] Even today strict OSHA regulations have been necessary to curtail occupational exposures; however, environmental exposure to lead remains a problem. In addition to natural sources of lead, such as that released by volcanoes, lead is introduced into the environment from smelting, soldering, battery reclamation, agricultural chemicals, and industrial waste. The removal of lead paint (deleading) from bridges is a significant source of community exposure[84] as well as occupational exposure.[71] Nearly half of the 1.3 million tons of lead used annually in the 1970s was released into the environment.[83]

Until it was phased out in the United States beginning in the mid-1970s, leaded gasoline was probably the single largest and certainly the most widespread source of lead. As Fig. 53-3 shows, the reduction of lead in gasoline was followed by an immediate and parallel reduction in blood lead levels measured by the National Health and Nutrition Survey. This reduction is widely hailed as the greatest public health success of environmental regulation; however, leaded gasoline is still used in many countries.

Although the use of lead pigments in indoor paint has been banned for many years, many buildings still retain undercoats of leaded paint. These coats are occasionally exposed and may disintegrate. Not only do children eat paint chips but they inhale household dust rich in lead. Moreover the refurbishing of old houses is a common source of nonoccupational adult lead poisoning. Thus both indoor house dust and outdoor soil around houses are significant sources of childhood exposure.

Small amounts of lead are present in drinking water and food; however, where water is slightly acidic (so-called aggressive water) and where pipes still have lead solder or other mobilizable lead, drinking water can contribute significantly to lead intake. A simple rule is to let a tap run for 60 seconds before using it for drinking.

Lead is readily absorbed from the intestinal tract (about 10% in adults but about 50% in children), and absorption is enhanced by dietary deficiencies of iron and calcium. Lead is also taken up from the lung when lead dust is inhaled. There is very little transdermal absorption (less than 0.5% for most lead compounds), although tetraethyl lead is absorbed through the skin. A rapid initial phase of excretion is followed by a slow phase, yielding a half-life in bone longer than 20 years but a soft-tissue half-life of about 19 days.[3,39]

Blood lead levels. Biomonitoring of ongoing lead exposure is usually accomplished by measurement of the blood lead level. This measurement is a relatively simple test, particularly when the level is elevated, but the quality assurance in most commercial laboratories for levels of lead less than 10 μg/dL is poor. Measurements of zinc protoporphyrin or free-erythrocyte protoporphyrin corroborate excessive lead exposure but are not specific. In the absence of ongoing exposure, blood lead levels may be normal despite a high concentration of lead in bone. The bone lead is a dynamic depot from which lead can be mobilized. During the 1960s an average blood level in urban adults was about 15 to 18 μg/dL. By 1980 this average had declined to about 10 μg/dL, and by 1986, to about 5 to 6 μg/dL[49]; however, even into the 1960s blood lead levels of 80 μg/dL in adults and 60 μg/dL in children were considered upper limits of normal, above which symptoms could be expected to occur.[72] As early as 1965, Chisholm argued unsuccessfully that levels greater than 40 μg/dL in children be considered toxic.[33] Through the 1970s and 1980s the understanding of lead in blood in relation to neurotoxicity has been reevaluated.[72] Needleman et al[73] demonstrated that children who had higher lead levels in their deciduous teeth had poorer school performance. Although subsequently criticized, this and Needleman's subsequent studies are generally accepted.[6,20]

Currently a blood lead level above 25 μg/dL in adults is significant and should be investigated, and a level above 40 μg/dL requires intervention. Symptoms consistent with excessive lead exposure can be expected to occur if the blood level is above 25 μg/dL. In children a level above 10 μg/dL is a level of concern that requires a second test and investigation, and a level above 15 μg/dL indicates lead poisoning.[6]

Bone lead stores. Bone is the major depot for lead in the body. A new approach, x-ray fluorescence, can be used to estimate bone lead and hence the body burden.[47] An x-ray beam is aimed at the tibia, and a fluorescence detector tuned to measure emissions from lead is aimed at a right angle.[47] The amount of emission is proportional to the concentration of lead in the bone. The difficulties of this procedure include the high cost and scarcity of the equipment, calibration of the readings to an actual lead concentration, possible variation of bone lead with depth in the bone (meaning that focusing the beam is critical). On the other hand, the correlation with mobilizable lead as measured by lead mobilization tests is reassuring.

The diagnosis and management of lead poisoning have been well covered in a number of books. Diagnostic criteria have changed dramatically (see previous discussion), and diagnostic and treatment capabilities are changing as well. The use of x-ray fluorescence to measure lead stored in bone offers an excellent indication of body burden, which may have a better correlation with long-term exposure and cumulative effects of lead than does a spot blood test.

Lead in children. The major current concern is the relatively large number of children with lead levels above the CDC's criterion for lead poisoning of 15 μg/dL.[6] Chisholm and O'Hara[33] described approaches to management of elevated lead levels, although the recent introduction of oral chelation using 2,3-dimercaptosuccinic acid has significantly altered evaluation and treatment protocols. Needleman[72] has summarized the extensive literature, and the CDC has published an excellent guidebook for prevention of childhood lead poisoning.[32]

Standards and guidelines. There is no reported RfD for lead because of the view that no intake is acceptable. The National Ambient Air Quality Standard is 1.5 μg/m^3, and the water quality standard is 5 mg/L, although a level of 0 is desirable.

Mercury

Sources. Mercury and its compounds are widely distributed in the environment, both through natural processes (erosion, vulcanism) and through industrial contamination and incinerator emissions. Mercury compounds have had many uses, including metallurgy, paint pigments, electronics, batteries, and biocides. The history of mercury use goes back more than 2000 years.[52] Inorganic mercury can be biomethylated in the bottom sediment of lakes by anerobic bacteria, forming the more highly toxic methyl mercury, which is then taken up by fish and bioamplified to the food chain. This process has produced massive outbreaks of severe disease in adults and children as well as a congenital organo-mercury syndrome.[27]

Minamata disease. The dramatic events at Minamata Bay, Japan, were documented by Smith and Smith.[90] Mercury used as a catalyst in the manufacture of acetaldehyde was dumped into the bay, where the process of methylation, bioamplification, human consumption, and environmental disease proceeded over a period of decades. The median mercury level in fish was 11 μg/g.[28] Many hundreds of people became seriously ill, and apparently thousands of more became mildly symptomatic. Cases of fetal death and major congenital malformations were dramatic.[9]

Exposure. The background concentration in air is in the range of 4 ng/m^3 (0.004 μg/m^3). Concentrations in freshwater fish were 0.5 μg/g. Absorption is about 80% by inhalation and 15% by ingestion.[40] The half-life in the body is about 700 days for methyl mercury, about 40 days for inorganic mercury, and 30 to 90 days for elemental mercury. It is eliminated through urine and feces, with urine accounting mainly for inorganic and feces for organic compounds. The EPA has estimated an ingestion RfD of 0.3 μg/kg/day for both organic and inorganic mercury.

Toxicity. Acute toxicity produces severe gastrointestinal symptoms and acrodynia. Organic mercurials cause mainly CNS impairment, including a congenital syndrome resembling cerebral palsy accompanied by blindness and mental retardation. The oral LD_{50} for mercuric chloride is 10 mg/kg in mice and 37 mg/kg in rats. Mercury compounds are mutagenic and teratogenic, but there are limited data on cancer in animals. Data are inadequate to assess it as a human carcinogen, but there are no positive epidemiologic studies.[27] Long-term exposure to inorganic mercury is associated with kidney and nervous system disease. Methyl mercury has profound effects at the subcellular level, binding to the sulfhydryl compound glutathione and interfering with the assembly of microtubules.[54]

Cadmium

Sources. Cadmium is widely used in metal industries, including soldering, alloying, and electroplating, and as a pigment and in batteries. Cadmium is found at many hazardous waste sites, and elevated levels in groundwater or well water are sometimes reported (average U.S. levels are between 0.2 and 0.4 μg/L[31]); however, significant nonoccupational exposure is much less frequent than to lead or mercury.

Exposure. Ambient levels of cadmium in air range from less than 1 ng/m^3 in remote areas to 40 ng/m^3 in urban areas,[16] and a maximum of 7 μg/m^3 has been found. Cadmium absorption is estimated at 50% by inhalation, 6% by ingestion, and less than 0.1% through the skin.[37] It is distributed mainly to the liver and kidney, and it accumulates with age until about 60 years. Its half-life in the body may be as long as 30 years. It induces and binds to metallothionein.[3]

Toxicity. Acute toxicity can occur with industrial exposure or with accidental ingestion. Chemical pneumonitis, pulmonary edema, and metal fume fever may occur at high doses; however, most concern focuses on long-term exposure. Results of tests of mutagenicity are negative, but cadmium is known to be an animal carcinogen, causing sarcomas at the site of injection and lung cancer in rats.[3] Currently cadmium is considered a probable human carcinogen by inhalation but not by ingestion,[37] and some epidemiologic data suggest an association with prostate cancer.[31] At high doses cadmium is teratogenic and a reproductive toxin, but there is inadequate information regarding effects at low doses. Cadmium affects various organ systems, including the lungs and kidney, and effects have occurred at levels below 100 μg/m^3.

Renal effects have occurred with long-term inhalation in the range of 5 to 10 μg/m^3 (equivalent to 1.6 to 3.2 μg/kg/day). Cadmium also causes hypertension.[37] Biomonitoring is currently accomplished by measurement of urinary cadmium excretion and of low-molecular-weight proteins.

For noncancer effects the oral RfD is 1×10^{-3} mg/kg/day (food) and 5×10^{-4} mg/kg/day (water),[43] and there is no inhalation RfD. ATSDR[16] lists an Environmental Media Evaluation Guideline. Inhalation toxicology studies with intermediate to long-term exposure in various species show LOAELs between 10 and 100 μg/m^3. The minimum risk level derived from inhalation is for renal effects and is about 0.2 μg/m^3. The estimated upper bound for a 1 in 10^{-6} cancer risk is 1 ng/m^3.[16]

Chromium

Chromium is widespread in the environment and is frequently encountered as a source of community exposure from industrial waste. Hexavalent chromium is the toxic form, but trivalent chromium is relatively nontoxic (except as a skin sensitizer) and is a required trace element. Trivalent chromium does not cross cell membranes easily and therefore does not enter cells, but hexavalent chromium readily enters cells.[77] In the cell, hexavalent chromium is reduced to trivalent chromium, and there is a question whether the reverse reaction occurs. Hexavalent chromium compounds are mutagenic, teratogenic, and carcinogenic. High exposure to chromium in any form is toxic to the kidney. There is much debate over whether the chromium emitted from incinerator smokestacks is mainly trivalent or hexavalent, because there is active oxidation and reduction at the different stages of the process as well as in the atmosphere and in the soil.[95] Worst-case risk assessments often assume that 100% of the measured chromium is hexavalent and bioavailable, in which case chromium emerges as the single largest contributor to health risk.

Community exposure has occurred in the vicinity of smelters and factories, but most significantly in places such as Hudson County, New Jersey, where waste chromate slag was used for landfill. More than 150 chromium waste sites have been identified in Hudson County, many of them subsequently used for residential, commercial, or recreational purposes.[95]

Absorption varies by compound, but absorption by inhalation is about 2% and by ingestion is about 5%.[18] In occupational epidemiology studies, lung cancer is the main effect. The unit risk value for chromium in air is $1.2 \times 10^{-2}/(\mu g/m^3)^{-1}$. The oral RfD is 5 $\mu g/kg/day$, and there is no separate inhalation RfD. Whether ingestion of hexavalent chromium increases risk of intestinal cancer is controversial, but increased rates have been found in several studies.[18]

Nickel

Nickel has an absorption of about 10% by ingestion. Absorption by inhalation or dermal contact is lower. It is distributed to kidney, lungs, and gonads but not primarily to liver or muscle. It is excreted quickly in the urine. Acute toxicity is infrequent, although workers exposed to nickel carbonyl may have acute respiratory and gastrointestinal symptoms. This compound, common in nickel refining, is not usually identified with incineration. Nickel compounds are known carcinogens, and insoluble compounds tend to be more potent than are soluble ones.[22]

The cancer potency estimated by CAG is 0.84 mg/kg/day for refinery dust.[43] The EPA-CAG developed a unit risk value for nickel in air of 2.4×10^{-4} $(\mu g/m^3)^{-1}$, based on four epidemiologic studies. Nickel compounds are teratogenic and are reproductive compounds. They are also good sensitizers of skin and are toxic to various organs and the immune system.

Air levels of 25 $\mu g/m^3$, corresponding to 8.14 $\mu g/kg/day$ for a 70-kg adult, are considered toxic. The ingestion RfD is 20 $\mu g/kg/day$. There is no inhalation RfD, but if an air level of 25 $\mu g/m^3$ is toxic, an RfD would be approximately 0.25 $\mu g/m^3$ (UF = 10 for LOAEL instead of NOAEL and 10 for protecting the most sensitive individuals).

Manganese

Manganese's absorption efficiency is 70% by inhalation, 3% by ingestion, and less than 0.1% through the skin. Manganese compounds go mainly to the pancreas, liver, kidneys, intestine, and brain.[3] There are many oxidation states for manganese compounds, but the 2+, 4+, and 7+ states are most significant. Its half-life is about 37 days in the body but is longer in the brain. It is excreted mainly by the gastrointestinal tract. Acute toxicity other than metal fume fever is rare. There is inadequate evidence regarding its carcinogenicity, but there are no positive epidemiologic studies. Manganese deficiency is associated with developmental defects, but manganese toxicity has less clear effects. Impaired behavioral performance has occurred in offspring of mice exposed to 50,000 $\mu g/m^3$.[3] Results of most reproductive studies have been negative, but there is some evidence of reduced fertility in males exposed to an average of 940 $\mu g/m^3$.[62]

The main occupational concern has been with chronic manganism, a parkinsonismlike syndrome, but it has occurred only with exposure above 300 $\mu g/m^3$. Iron deficiency increases the absorption of manganese. The EPA has derived chronic RfDs of 200 $\mu g/kg/day$ by ingestion and 0.3 $\mu g/kg/day$ by inhalation.[43]

The organic manganese proposed for addition to gasoline is illustrated in Fig. 53-4. Little toxicologic and no ecologic information has been published on this compound.

Arsenic

Source. Arsenic is widespread in the Earth's crust and is a trace contaminant of many metal ores. It is mostly an unwanted contaminant, but for its commercial uses it is extracted mainly during the smelting of gold, zinc, copper, and lead.[31] Arsenic is incorporated into various biocides and is used in the laboratory and in metallurgy, but it has an important role in the microelectronics industry, where arsine gas mixed with gallium forms gallium arsenide, which is used for doping computer chips.

Arsenic compounds occur in several valence states. Trivalent arsenic is the most toxic and carcinogenic when compared with pentavalent and organic compounds.[13] Indeed, organoarsenicals are widespread in seafood but, unlike or-

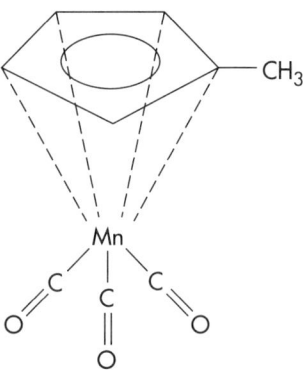

Fig. 53-4. Methylcyclopentadienyl manganese tricarbonyl has been proposed as a gasoline additive to replace tetraethyl lead. Little has been published about its toxicity and nothing about its ecological effects. (Courtesy Environmental and Occupational Health Sciences Institute.)

ganomercurials, are considered to have low human toxicity. Arsenic is an acute metabolic poison, a respiratory asphyxiant that interferes with the electron transport chain and is rapidly fatal at high doses. At lower doses it is a human carcinogen and is toxic to a variety of organ systems, including the skin, liver, and cardiovascular system.[30]

Surprisingly, trace amounts of arsenic appear beneficial to several animal species, promoting healthy growth and development of neonates.[88] Arsenic compounds are added to some livestock feeds. There is no evidence regarding an essential or even a beneficial role in humans.

Exposure. Drinking water usually has low arsenic levels (less than 0.01 ppm), but localized elevations occur where there are natural arsenic deposits or industrial contamination.[13] Soil contaminated by arsenical pesticides has resulted in arsenic contamination of grapes and cereals, leading to cases of arsenic poisoning. The use of arsenicals has been reduced in the past 15 years.[13]

For environmental medicine, there is more frequent concern regarding low-level exposures in food and drinking water and air contamination in the vicinity of smelters. A major episode occurred in Tacoma, Washington, in the mid-1980s, when the community was put in a position of closing a smelter (its major employer) or sustaining an increased risk of lung cancer due to arsenic. The smelter was ultimately closed.

Elevated levels of arsenic are still found in fish and shellfish, particularly from regions such as the Pacific Northwest, where smelting has resulted in water contamination by arsenic. Levels as high as 100 ppm have been documented.[13,81] Also patients who were treated with Fowler's solution (7.6 g/L arsenite) and are at increased risk of skin cancer are still seen. Arsenicals also are still used as anthelmintic drugs.

Depending on the species of arsenic compound, it is readily absorbed from the lungs and intestine. Although air contamination from smelters can be widespread, ingestion is probably the more important route.[13] Trivalent arsenic is transported to the liver and kidneys and can accumulate in the brain, heart, and skin. There is in vivo methylation of trivalent arsenic. Pentavalent arsenic compounds tend to be eliminated more rapidly. Most arsenic is excreted within a few days in the urine as dimethylarsinic acid and methylarsonic acid. Arsenic is also excreted in sweat, nails, hair, and skin. For biomonitoring, a 24-hour urine measurement of arsenic is preferred.

Toxicity. The lower toxicity of organoarsenicals is related in part to their rapid elimination from the body.[13] In cases of severe poisoning there is multiorgan involvement, cardiac failure, coma, and death. Acute treatment with dialysis and chelation with dimercaprol (British antilewisite) are emergency treatments. Such events are likely to involve accidental or intended ingestion of arsenical products rather than environmental exposure.

Arsenic is unusual in that it is a known human carcinogen (based on epidemiologic studies) without an animal model.

Workers with exposure in the chemical industry, smelting, or agriculture had increased rates of respiratory cancer. Hepatic angiosarcoma has been reported to occur in people consuming arsenic-contaminated wine and Fowler's solution. The EPA maximum contaminant level for drinking is 50 μg/L.

Arsenic causes peripheral neuropathy affecting sensory more than motor functions. Gastrointestinal symptoms occur after moderate ingestion. Arsenic dermatitis is seen with occupational exposures, affecting fingernails, toenails, and skin.

Arsine. In addition to its widespread use as a dopant in the microelectronics industry, arsine is generated when acids used to clean metal tanks or vessels extract minute amounts of arsenic to form this highly toxic gas. The main effect is intravascular hemolysis sufficient to produce hemoglobinuria and jaundice. Death can occur from acute renal failure.

Selenium

The biochemistry and toxicity of selenium compounds are very complex and involves organic and inorganic compounds of highly variable toxicity. Its chemistry is similar to that of sulfur. It is also an essential trace element. In addition to its use in dermatology, selenium is used in some insecticides and pigments, in the glass and ceramics industry, and in photoelectric cells. Compounds such as selenium sulfide are not absorbed through the skin, but in general the absorption efficiencies of selenium compounds are not adequately studied. Selenium compounds are distributed to the liver, kidney, spleen, lungs, and pancreas.[8] It is excreted by all routes, mainly in the urine. Acute toxicity includes severe irritation of skin and gastrointestinal tract and cardiovascular effects. The oral LD_{50} for rats was 6700 mg/kg/day for elemental selenium but only 4.8 mg/kg/day for tetravalent selenium.

The oral RfD for selenium is 3 μg/kg/day,[43] and the inhalation RfD is 1 μg/kg/day, which corresponds to an air level for adults of 3.5 μg/m^3, consistent with the observation that 7 to 50 μg/m^3 produced disease.[41] The national drinking water standard is 10 μg/L.

In general, environmental exposure to selenium is seldom high enough to jeopardize human health, and indeed selenium deficiency occurs in some populations; however, aquatic ecosystems have been documented to experience significant excesses of selenium.

Beryllium

Most beryllium compounds (except chloride and nitrate) are insoluble in water. Beryllium is poorly absorbed through the skin (less than 0.01%) and intestinal tract (1%).[15] The main route of concern is inhalation. Once absorbed, it is distributed mainly to the skin, skeleton, lungs, and liver.[3,15] It binds to ferritin instead of metallothionein. It is excreted by the renal tubule[3] and the gastrointestinal tract and has a biphasic excretion, with a half-life of 2 to 4 years.[15] Acute toxicologic effects are rare, even in occupational exposure. Contact dermatitis is the most common skin effect. Beryllium compounds are negative in Ames assay and positive in sister chromatid exchange and other mammalian cell tests.[15] Berylliosis is a chronic inflammatory disease very similar to sarcoidosis. It can be distinguished mainly by a history of significant beryllium exposure and more recently by use of a lymphocyte transformation test.[60] Beryllium has been implicated in lung cancer among exposed workers and assigned a unit risk value of 0.8 $\mu g/m^3$, which places it about halfway on the list of 59 carcinogens evaluated by the EPA.[15]

Disease has occurred with community exposure around a beryllium facility. Air levels of 2.0 $\mu g/m^3$ (resulting in estimated adult intake of 0.65 $\mu g/kg/day$) have been associated with disease. The outdoor air standard is 0.01 $\mu g/m^3$. Ambient air levels of beryllium are generally less than 0.001 $\mu g/m^3$ (less than 10% of standard). Beryllium waste from nuclear weapons industries poses an exposure potential for communities adjacent to Department of Energy facilities.

FIBERS AND CRYSTALS

A variety of fibrous minerals, both natural (such as asbestos) and man-made have a high potential for causing lung disease. Crystalline silica is well known to cause pulmonary fibrosis. These are covered in Chapter 38.

REFERENCES

1. Adams KF et al: Acute elevations of blood carboxyhemoglobin impairs exercise performance and aggravates symptoms in patients with ischemeic heart disease, *J Am Coll Cardiol* 12:900, 1988.
2. Alderman BW, Barron AE, Savitz DA: Maternal exposure to neighborhood carbon monoxide and risk of low infant birth weight, *Public Health Rep* 102: 410-414, 1987.
3. Amdur M, Klaassen CD, Doull J: *Casarett and Doull's toxicology,* New York, 1991, McGraw-Hill.
4. American Conference of Governmental Industrial Hygienists: *1992-1993 Threshold limit values for chemical substances and physical agents and biological exposure indices,* Cincinnati, 1993.
5. Amoruso MA et al: Estimation of risk of glucose 6-phosphate dehydrogenase-deficient red cells to ozone and nitrogen dioxide, *J Occup Med* 28:473, 1986.
6. Agency for Toxic Substances and Disease Registry, Centers for Disease Control: *The nature and extent of lead poisoning in children in the United States: a report to Congress,* Atlanta, 1988, US Public Health Service.
7. Agency for Toxic Substances and Disease Registry, Centers for Disease Control: *Toxicological profile for benzo[a]pyrene.* Atlanta, 1988, US Public Health Service.
8. Agency for Toxic Substances and Disease Registry, Centers for Disease Control: *Toxicological profile for selenium,* Atlanta, 1989, US Public Health Service.
9. Agency for Toxic Substances and Disease Registry, Centers for Disease Control: *Toxicological profile for 2,3,7,8-tetrachloro dibenzo-p-dioxin,* Atlanta, 1989, US Public Health Service.
10. Agency for Toxic Substances and Disease Registry, Centers for Disease Control: *Toxicological profile for toluene,* Atlanta, 1989, US Public Health Service.
11. Agency for Toxic Substances and Disease Registry, Centers for Disease Control: *Toxicological profile for total xylenes,* Atlanta, 1990, US Public Health Service.
12. Agency for Toxic Substances and Disease Registry, Centers for Disease Control: *Toxicological profile for tin,* Atlanta, 1991, US Public Health Service.
13. Agency for Toxic Substances and Disease Registry, Centers for Disease Control: *Toxicological profile for arsenic,* Atlanta, 1992, US Public Health Service.
14. Agency for Toxic Substances and Disease Registry, Centers for Disease Control: *Toxicological profile for benzene,* Atlanta, 1992, US Public Health Service.
15. Agency for Toxic Substances and Disease Registry, Centers for Disease Control: *Toxicological profile for beryllium,* Atlanta, 1992, US Public Health Service.
16. Agency for Toxic Substances and Disease Registry, Centers for Disease Control: *Toxicological profile for cadmium,* Atlanta, 1992, US Public Health Service.
17. Agency for Toxic Substances and Disease Registry, Centers for Disease Control: *Toxicological profile for chloroform,* Atlanta, 1992, US Public Health Service.
18. Agency for Toxic Substances and Disease Registry, Centers for Disease Control: *Toxicological profile for chromium,* Atlanta, 1992, US Public Health Service.
19. Agency for Toxic Substances and Disease Registry, Centers for Disease Control: *Toxicological profile for cyanide,* Atlanta, 1992, US Public Health Services.
20. Agency for Toxic Substances and Disease Registry, Centers for Disease Control: *Toxicological profile for lead,* Atlanta, 1992, US Public Health Service.
21. Agency for Toxic Substances and Disease Registry, Centers for Disease Control: *Toxicological profile for methylene chloride,* Atlanta, 1992, US Public Health Service.
22. Agency for Toxic Substances and Disease Registry, Centers for Disease Control: *Toxicological profile for nickel,* Atlanta, 1992, US Public Health Service.
23. Agency for Toxic Substances and Disease Registry, Centers for Disease Control: *Toxicological profile for selected PCBs (Aroclor-1260, -1254, -1248, -1242, -1231, -1221, and -1016),* Atlanta, 1992, US Public Health Service.
24. Agency for Toxic Substances and Disease Registry, Centers for Disease Control: *Toxicological profile for tetrachloroethylene,* Atlanta, 1992, US Public Health Service.
25. Agency for Toxic Substances and Disease Registry, Centers for Disease Control: *Toxicological profile for trichloroethylene,* Atlanta, 1992, US Public Health Service.
26. Agency for Toxic Substances and Disease Registry, Centers for Disease Control: *Toxicological profile for vinyl chloride,* Atlanta, 1992, US Public Health Service.
27. Agency for Toxic Substances and Disease Registry, Centers for Disease Control: *Toxicological profile for mercury,* Atlanta, 1993, US Public Health Service.
28. Berglund F, et al: Methylmercury in fish, a toxicologic-epidemiologic evaluation of risks: report from an expert group, *Nordisk Hyginisk Tiskrift,* supplement 4, 1971.
29. Bertazzi PA et al: Cancer incidence in a population accidentally exposed to 2,3,7,8-tetrachlorodibenzo-*para* dioxin, *Epidemiology* 4:388, 1993.
30. Bickley LK, Papa CM: Chronic arsenicism with vitiligo, hyperthyroidism, and cancer, *NJ Med* 86:377, 1989.
31. Carson BL, Ellis HV, McCann JL: *Toxicology and biological monitoring of metals in humans,* Chelsea, Mich, 1987, Lewis.
32. Centers for Disease Control: *Preventing lead poisoning in young children,* Atlanta, 1991.
33. Chisholm JJ Jr, O'Hara DM, eds: *Lead absorption in children: management, clinical and environmental aspects.* Baltimore, 1982, Urban & Schwarzenberg.
34. Colombo A, Facchetti S: *The isotopic lead experiment: impact of petrol lead on human blood and air: final report,* Ispra, Italy, 1988, Commission of the European Communities Joint Research Centre.

35. Creech JL Jr, Johnson MN: Angiosarcoma of the liver in the manufacture of polyvinyl chloride, *J Occup Med* 16:150, 1974.
36. Environmental Protection Agency: *Revised evaluation of health effects associated with carbon monoxide exposure,* EPA 600 /9-83-033F, Research Triangle Park, NC, 1983.
37. Environmental Protection Agency: *Health effects assessment for cadmium,* Washington, DC, 1984.
38. Environmental Protection Agency: *Drinking water criteria document for chromium,* Washington, DC, 1985.
39. Environmental Protection Agency: *Lead exposures in the human environment,* EPA/600/D-86/185, Research Triangle Park, NC, 1985.
40. Environmental Protection Agency: *Drinking water criteria document for mercury,* Washington, DC, 1985.
41. Environmental Protection Agency: *Health effects assessment for selenium (and compounds),* Cincinnati, 1986.
42. Environmental Protection Agency: *Estimating exposures to 2,3,7,8-TCDD, Exposure Assessment Group, /600/6-88/005,* Washington, DC, 1988.
43. Environmental Protection Agency: *IRIS Chemical Information Data Base,* Cincinnati, 1989.
44. Fingerhut MA, et al: Cancer mortality in workers exposed to 2,3,7,8-tetrachlorodibenzo-p-dioxin, *N Engl J Med* 324:212, 1991.
45. Finkel AJ: *Hamilton and Hardy's industrial toxicology,* ed 4, Boston, 1983, John Wright-PSG.
46. Gallo MA et al: Interactive effects of estradiol and 2,3,7,8-tetrachlorodibenzo-p-dioxin on hepatic cytochrome P-450 and mouse uterus, *Toxicol Lett* 32:123, 1986.
47. Gerhardsson L et al: In vivo measurements of lead in bone in long-term exposed lead smelter workers, *Arch Environ Health* 48:147, 1993.
48. Gochfeld M: *Residential property action levels and decision trees for preliminary site screening program,* Piscataway, NJ, 1990, Environmental and Occupational Health Sciences Institute.
49. Gochfeld M et al: Temporal changes in blood lead levels of hazardous waste workers in New Jersey, 1984-1987, *Environ Monitor Assess* 25:99, 1993.
50. Goldstein BD: Clinical hematology of benzene. In *Advances in Modern Environmental Toxicology,* vol XVI, *Benzene: occupational and environmental hazards,* Princeton, NJ, 1989, Princeton Scientific Publishers.
51. Goldstein BD, Witz G: Benzene. In Lippmann M, ed: *Environmental toxicants,* New York, 1992, Van Nostrand Reinhold.
52. Goldwater L: *Mercury: a history of quicksilver,* Baltimore, 1972, York Press.
53. Gosselin RE, Smith RP, Hodge HC: *Clinical toxicology of commercial products,* ed 5, Baltimore, 1984, Williams & Wilkins.
54. Graff RD et al: The effect of glutathione depletion on methyl mercury-induced microtubule disassembly in cultured embryonal carcinoma cells, *Toxicol Appl Pharmacol* 120:20, 1993.
55. Grandjean P, ed: *Biological effects of organolead,* Boca Raton, Fla, 1984, CRC Press.
56. Hunter D: *The diseases of occupations,* London, 1974, English Universities Press.
57. Hutchinson TC, Meema KM, eds: *Lead, mercury, cadmium and arsenic in the environment,* SCOPE monograph 31, New York, Wiley.
58. Infante PF, Epstein SS, Newton WA: Blood dyscrasias and childhood tumors and exposure to chlordane and heptachlor, *Scand J Work Environ Health* 4:137, 1978.
59. Kahn PC et al: Dioxins and dibenzofurans in blood and adipose tissue of Agent Orange–exposed Viet Nam veterans and matched controls, *JAMA* 259:1661, 1988.
60. Kreiss K et al: Beryllium disease screening in the ceramics industry: blood lymphocyte test performance and exposure-disease relations, *J Occup Med* 35:267, 1993.
61. Laughlin RB Jr, Linden O: Fate and effects of organotin compounds, *Ambio* 14:88, 1985.
62. Lauwerys R et al: Fertility of male workers exposed to mercury vapor or manganese dust: a questionnaire study, *Am J Ind Med* 7:171, 1985.
63. Lerman S, Kipen HM: Material safety data sheets: caveat emptor, *Arch Intern Med* 150:981, 1990.
64. Lippmann M: Effects of ozone on respiratory function and structure, *Annu Rev Public Health* 10:49, 1989.
65. Lippmann M, ed: *Environmental toxicants,* New York, 1992, Van Nostrand Reinhold.
66. Lutz LJ: Health effects of air pollution measured by outpatient visits, *J Fam Pract* 16:307, 1983.
67. Molhave L: Volatile organic compounds and the sick building syndrome. In Lippmann M, ed: *Environmental toxicants,* New York, 1992, Van Nostrand Reinhold.
68. National Institute for Occupational Safety and Health: *Occupational exposures to carbon monoxide,* Washington, DC, 1972.
69. National Institute for Occupational Safety and Health: *Pocket guide to chemical hazards,* Cincinnati, 1983.
70. National Institute for Occupational Safety and Health: Organic solvents, *Current Intelligence Bulletin,* 1987.
71. National Institute for Occupational Safety and Health: Preventing lead poisoning in construction workers, *National Institute for Occupational Safety and Health Alert,* April 1992.
72. Needleman HL: *Human lead exposure,* Boca Raton, Fla, 1992, CRC Press.
73. Needleman H et al: Deficits in psychologic and classroom performance of children with elevated dentine lead levels, *N Engl J Med* 300:689, 1979.
74. Nessel CS, Gallo MA: Dioxins and related compounds. In Lippmann M, ed: *Environmental toxicants,* New York, 1992, Van Nostrand Reinhold.
75. Nessel CS et al: Evaluation of the relative contribution of exposure routes in a health risk assessment of dioxin emissions from a municipal waste incinerator, *Journal of Exposure Analysis and Environmental Epidemiology,* 1:283, 1991.
76. New York Department of Environmental Conservation: *Ambient concentration guidelines for air pollutants,* Albany, NY, 1989.
77. Nieboer E, Jusys AA: Biologic chemistry of chromium. In Nriagu JO, Nieboer E, eds: *Chromium in the natural and human environments,* New York, 1988, Wiley.
78. Nriagu JO: *The biogeochemistry of mercury in the environment,* New York, 1979, Elsevier.
79. Nriagu JO, Nieboer E, eds: *Chromium in the natural and human environments,* New York, 1988, John Wiley & Sons.
80. Nuclear Regulatory Commission: *Medical and biological effects of environmental pollutants: hydrogen chloride,* Washington, DC, 1976, National Academy of Sciences.
81. Nuclear Regulatory Commission: *Medical and biological effects of environmental pollutants: arsenic,* Washington, DC, 1977, National Academy of Sciences.
82. Nuclear Regulatory Commission: *An assessment of mercury in the environment,* Washington, DC, 1978, National Academy of Sciences.
83. Nuclear Regulatory Commission: *Lead in the human environment,* Washington, DC, 1980, National Academy of Sciences.
84. Prenney B: Community lead exposure, *Am J Ind Med* 23:191, 1993.
85. Riihimaki V et al: Kinetics of m-xylene in man: general features of absorption, distribution, biotransformation and excretion in repetitive inhalation exposure, *Scand J Work Environ Health* 5:217, 1979.
86. Rom W: *Environmental and occupational medicine,* Boston, 1992, Little, Brown.
87. Rosenstock L, Cullen M: *Textbook of clinical occupational and environmental medicine,* Philadelphia, 1994, WB Saunders.
88. Schwartz K: Essentiality versus toxicity of metals. In Brown SS, ed: *Clinical chemistry and clinical toxicology of metals,* Amsterdam, 1977, Elsevier.

89. Sheps DS et al: Lack of effect of low levels of carboxyhemoglobin on cardiovascular function in patients with ischemic heart disease, *Arch Environ Health* 42:108, 1987.
90. Smith WE, Smith AM: *Minamata: words and photographs,* New York, 1975, Holt, Rinehart, and Winston.
91. Spencer PS, Schaumberg HH: Nervous system degeneration producted by acrylamide monomer, *Environ Health Perspect* 11:129, 1975.
92. Stern FB et al: Heart disease mortality among bridge and tunnel officers exposed to carbon omonoxide, *Am J Epidemiol* 128:1276, 1988.
93. Travis CC, Hattemer-Frey HA: Human exposure to 2,3,7,8-TCDD, *Chemosphere* 16:2331, 1987.
94. Wallace L: *The Total Environmental Assessment Methodology (TEAM study) summary and analysis,* Washington, DC, 1987, US Environmental Protection Agency.
95. Witmer C, Gochfeld M, eds: The chromium problem: research needs and risk assessment, *Environ Health Perspect* 92:1, 1991.
96. Witz G et al: The metabolism of benzene to muconic acid, a potential biological marker of benzene exposure, *Biol Reactive Intermed* 4:613, 1990.

Chapter 54

BIOLOGIC AGENTS

Iris G. Udasin

Waterborne infectious diseases
    Giardiasis
    Legionellosis
    Primary amebic meningoencephalitis
Food-borne infectious illness
    Salmonellosis
    Other food-borne diseases
Soil-associated infectious illness
Arthropod vector–borne disease
    Lyme disease
    Rocky Mountain spotted fever
    Plague
Diseases transmitted by animal vectors
    Rabies
Concerns of people exposed to hazardous wastes or sewage
Special considerations for international travel
    Malaria
    Traveler's diarrhea

Historically, infectious diseases constitute one of the oldest environmental health problems. Outbreaks of schistosomiasis, a parasite disease caused by blood flukes, were documented by the ancient Egyptians. This disease continues to affect more than 200 million people worldwide.[32] Human plague, or the Black Death, was mentioned in the writings of Dionysus in the third century, and the first pandemic was well described in the sixth century.[6] This illness is caused by a bacteria, *Yersinia pestis,* and is maintained in nature by a reservoir of infected small rodents and their fleas.

Infectious diseases may be considered to be environmentally transmitted when they are spread by common sources (usually food, water, or soil); by arthropod vectors; by animals; or, occasionally, by fomites. This definition would exclude diseases that are spread by close personal contact or inhaled droplet nuclei.[6] Therefore the bloodborne pathogen, human immunodeficiency virus (HIV), and hepatitis B virus (HBV) are considered only in the context of unintentional needlestick injuries and not in the context of their most common modes of spread via close sexual contact or from shared drug paraphernalia.[10] Similarly, tuberculosis, a major health problem affecting as many as 10 million people worldwide and with 25,700 people each year acquiring drug-resistant strains in the urban areas of the United States, with outbreaks in hospitals, clinics, substance-abuse treatment centers, and prisons, is not discussed here. This disease is spread mainly by droplet nuclei, which are produced and transmitted by talking, coughing, sneezing, and singing.[21,27]

This chapter addresses infectious diseases transmitted by water, food, soil, arthropod vectors, and animal hosts. Special consideration also is given to exposures to waste or sewage material and to issues of concern to travelers or international health. The number of infectious agents (viruses, bacteria, fungi, rickettsiae, parasites, and so on) is too extensive to cover completely, and attention herein focuses on generic features of these diseases and major illnesses. For a more exhaustive discussion the reader is referred to major textbooks of public health and infectious diseases.[31,37] Exposure to infectious agents and allergens via indoor air pollution is treated in Chapter 37.

WATERBORNE INFECTIOUS DISEASES

In 1914 the U.S. Public Health Service adopted drinking water standards with the intention of ensuring aesthetic quality of water and preventing the transmission of waterborne disease. In 1974 the Safe Drinking Water Act was promulgated, establishing maximal contaminant levels of chemicals and also addressing microbial, radioactive, and particulate contamination of water. In 1986 this act was further amended to include criteria that address total fecal coliform contamination and maintenance of a watershed program that minimizes contamination by *Giardia lamblia* and viruses. This act also provides for annual sanitary surveys of water.[42]

In addition to diseases that are spread in drinking water, waterborne illness also is caused by recreational uses of water, including swimming and boating, and through the use of water cooling towers. These pathogens gain access to the body through the oral or inhalation routes. Causes of waterborne diseases include five categories of pathogens: bacteria, viruses, protozoa, parasitic worms, and fungi. The most common pathogens are summarized in Table 54-1.

National statistics have recorded 1702 outbreaks of waterborne disease, causing 542,018 cases of illness and 1089 deaths from 1923 through 1992.[12] Almost all of the deaths occurred before 1940, and most were due to infection with *Salmonella typhi* (typhoid fever). *Salmonella* is no longer a major cause of waterborne illness in the United States but remains a significant cause of food-borne illness. During the years 1981 through 1990, 291 outbreaks of waterborne illness were reported in community (43%), industrial, or institutional (33%) systems; during recreational activity (14%); and from individual (10%) water sources. Most of the community outbreaks occurred in small communities. More than 30,000 rural communities in the United States do not possess safe drinking-water supplies. From 1981 through 1990, contaminated, untreated, or inadequately disinfected groundwater and surface water were responsible for 43% and 24%, respectively, of all water-borne outbreaks.[12]

Traditionally the coliform determination has been used as a general measure of contamination of the water supply. Although several strains of *Escherichia coli* (including a recently isolated strain associated with bloody diarrhea and four deaths during a waterborne outbreak in Missouri) are significant pathogens, not all strains are pathogenic. Coliform count is used as a measure of fecal contamination because *E. coli* is always passed in the normal intestinal tract of humans and other warm-blooded animals. Thus the presence of *E. coli* does not always represent a health hazard; however, the absence usually indicates that the water is free of bacterial contamination.[42,58]

However, most outbreaks of waterborne illness are not caused by *E. coli* and are of undetermined origin. Measures of coliform count do not reflect the level of contamination with viruses. Three agents—hepatitis A virus, Norwalk-type viruses, and rotavirus—have been identified as waterborne causes of gastroenteritis; however, as many as 100 different viruses may be responsible for the outbreaks of undetermined disease. These viruses are often resistant to the usual treatment processes that reduce coliform organisms. Enteric viruses also are spread by person-to-person contact, thus making it difficult to diagnose and prevent the spread of waterborne disease unit it reaches epidemic proportions.[12]

Giardiasis

Giardiasis, which is caused by the flagellated protozoan *Giardia lamblia,* has emerged as a significant cause of waterborne disease that is not detected by the usual coliform counts. *Giardia* cysts have the ability to exist for long periods, as long as 16 days at 8°C and also are somewhat resistant to the chlorination process that destroys coliform organisms. The spectrum of diseases caused by this pathogen ranges from asymptomatic passage of cysts to a chronic diarrheal syndrome with malabsorption and weight loss. *Giardia* infection is more common in young children, particularly those in day-care facilities, than in adults, because of person-

Table 54-1. Important waterborne pathogens in the United States transmitted by ingestion and inhalation

Disease	Pathogen	Source
Bacteria		
Legionnaires' disease, Pontiac fever	*Legionella pneumophila*	Water for cooling systems, hot-water system, shower heads
Campylobacteriosis	*Campylobactor jejuni*	Drinking water, food
Yersiniosis	*Yersinia entercolitica*	Drinking water, milk
Salmonellosis	*Salmonella enteridis*	Drinking water, food sewage
Shigellosis	*Shigella* species	Drinking water, food sewage
Protozoans		
Primary amebic meningoencephalitis	*Naegleria fowleri*	Recreational water use
Giardiasis	*Giardia lamblia*	Untreated water affected by animals
Cryptosporidiosis	*Cryptosporidium* species	Untreated water affected by animals
Viruses		
Gastroenteritis	Rotavirus, Norwalk virus, other viruses	Human feces, sewage, contaminated water, shellfish
Infectious hepatitis	Hepatitis A virus	Human feces, sewage, contaminated water, shellfish

to-person spread and generally poor personal hygiene. The annual incidence of symptomatic illness has been 9.8, 11.6, and 45.7 cases per 100,000 population in Minnesota, Colorado, and Vermont,[4] in contrast to the higher rates seen in developing countries, including 19% in Zimbabwe and 42% in rural Egypt.[57] Brodsky et al[8] performed a now-famous study of travelers to the Soviet Union that indicated that 28% of 1419 tourists were ill with giardiasis related to consumption of water in Leningrad.

Although treatment and filtration of water supplies remove some of the contamination, control of giardiasis is possible only through the identification and proper antibiotic treatment of affected individuals and screening of household members for passage of cysts. Despite these control measures, this disease persists because many animals, including muskrats, cows, goats, and sheep, also are reservoirs of disease. Thus giardiasis remains a common source of morbidity in rural areas, and campers and hikers are at high risk of development of this illness, which has a relatively high morbidity rate but a relatively low case-fatality rate in healthy individuals.[67] Knowledge of local patterns of pathogen or disease occurrence is valuable to increase the likelihood of correct diagnosis of *Giardia* infection in travelers.

Legionellosis

Legionellosis has a unique mode of transmission and is spread by several species of the *Legionella* bacterium. This waterborne illness is transmitted by inhalation of the organisms in droplets of water from aerosol-producing devices. Outbreaks have been reported to be caused by cooling towers, evaporative condensers, and heat-ejection devices. The disease is then transported through ducts and vents in air-conditioning systems. Illness has been reported to spread for miles around contaminated cooling towers.[2,7,14] Because these sources of water are not as strictly monitored as is drinking water, and because this bacterium is difficult to isolate, it is an important environmental pathogen. The first epidemic occurred at an American Legion convention at a Philadelphia hotel in 1976, leading to illnesses and deaths. Subsequently the organism was identified in archived pathology specimens.[20] Approximately 1000 cases of Legionnaires' disease have been reported annually in the United States, and this figure is probably an underestimate. Legionnaires' disease may be caused both sporadically and in epidemics, most commonly during the summer. Control depends on identifying the source of contamination and flushing affected systems with superheated (above 60°C) or hyperchlorinated water.[49]

Primary amebic meningoencephalitis

Primary amebic meningoencephalitis is a rare and often fatal disease that results from infection with the ameboflagellate *Naegleria fowleri*. During 1991, four fatal cases of this disease were reported to occur in healthy children and young adults and have been traced to water-related recreational activities. Central nervous system symptoms occur within 7 days of exposure and are not easily distinguished from bacterial meningitis. The symptoms include headache, fever, anorexia, vomiting, signs of meningeal irritation, and brainstem compression. In most cases diagnosis occurs too late, and death usually occurs within 72 hours after diagnosis.[47]

FOOD-BORNE INFECTIOUS ILLNESS

The food available in the United States is considered to be among the safest in the world. Food safety has been regulated since 1906 with the passage of the federal Food and Drugs Act and the Meat Inspection Act. These laws are administered by the Food and Drug Administration, an agency within the U.S. Public Health Service, the Department of Health and Human Services, and the U.S. Department of Agriculture Food Safety and Inspection Service. The first outbreak of gastrointestinal disease associated with milk was reported in 1923. The surveillance data concerning food-borne outbreaks led to the association between *Salmonella* contamination of milk and infant diarrhea, which resulted in mandatory pasteurization of milk and chlorination of the water supply sooner in the United States than in other countries.[60]

Most reported food-borne outbreaks have occurred as a result of improper holding temperatures, inadequate cooking of food (usually meat or poultry), use of contaminated equipment, infected food handlers, and food obtained from unsafe sources. Many outbreaks have been traced to large institutions, including hospitals, nursing homes, day-care centers, schools, and fast-food outlets. The causative organisms are often undetermined. Among outbreaks in which the cause has been determined, about two thirds of the causes are bacterial. The most common infectious pathogens leading to food-borne disease are summarized in Table 54-2.[29]

Table 54-2. Common infectious causes of food poisoning

Pathogen	High-risk foods
Staphylococcus aureus	Creamy desserts, salads, baked goods, meat
Salmonella typhi	Meat, eggs, milk, cheese
Other *Salmonella* spp.	Meat, diary products
E. coli	Milk, meat, poultry
Campylobacter	Milk, meat, poultry
Bacillus cereus	Rice, vegetables, meat
Clostridium perfringens	Meat, poultry
Clostridium botulinum	Preserved (canned, pickled, cured) meats, smoked or preserved fish and vegetables
Vibrio parahaemolyticus	Shellfish
Shigella	Salad
Viruses (Hepatitis A)	Shellfish
Trichinella spiralis	Uncooked pork, bear
Cestodes	Beef, pork
Clonorchis sinensis	*Crustaceans*

Salmonellosis

Despite improvements in food technology, *Salmonella* species remain the most frequently isolated organisms causing food-borne illness throughout the world. The incidence of disease has continued to increase in the United States and Canada. In 1985 *Salmonella* contamination of an Illinois dairy plant due to improper pasteurization of milk ultimately led to illness in 200,000 people. In New England and the mid-Atlantic states *Salmonella* infection in egg-laying poultry has increased and is sometimes passed on to their eggs.[61] *Salmonella* commonly infects livestock, and it is estimated that 33% of poultry, 15% of pork, and 10% of beef in the United States may be contaminated with *Salmonella*.[60] Marine animals, including whales, dolphins, seals, turtles, crocodiles, fish, shellfish, and fish-eating birds, have been found to harbor *Salmonella*.[38]

Salmonella typhi is a gram-negative, flagellated bacteria that is readily killed by pasteurizing or cooking foods to temperatures above 160°F. It is easily passed to other foods by utensils, surfaces, or food handlers preparing raw meat. The clinical onset of illness is insidious, and the symptoms may vary from a mild febrile illness to a severe illness characterized by long periods of septicemia. Diarrhea is rarely present with this species of *Salmonella*. This disease usually responds to antibiotics such as chloramphenicol, but drug-resistant strains have emerged.[5]

An additional risk factor for the development of clinical illness is the presence of medication-dependent diabetes mellitus. A study in New York City indicated that people with clinical illness caused by *Salmonella* were three times more likely to be diabetic.[59] In view of the increased risk in the diabetic patient, it is crucial for hospitals to maintain careful food-preparation practices.

Other food-borne diseases

Other recent outbreaks of food-borne illness involved food contaminated by *Listeria* species and hamburger meat contaminated with a strain of *E. coli* that caused hemorrhagic cystitis, hemolytic-uremic syndrome, and thrombocytopenic purpura,[45,52-54] which has been linked to fast-food outlets in Canada and the northwestern United States.

Another source of food-borne illness that continues to be important is toxin induced and is found in fish and shellfish poisoning. These food-borne illnesses, which include scombroid, result from microbially generated toxins in food rather than infection of the host, as is summarized in Table 54-3. Because contaminated seafood is difficult to recognize by appearance, odor, or taste, people should be urged to avoid eating fish in places in which proper storage, transport, and preparation of food are impossible.[29]

SOIL-ASSOCIATED INFECTIOUS ILLNESS

Soil-borne parasitic diseases are among the most common infectious diseases worldwide but are usually not prevalent in the United States with the exception of the rural southeast. The most common soil-borne illnesses are summarized in Table 54-4.

Tetanus: Within the United States, tetanus caused by toxins of a bacterium, *C. tetani,* is still present. Although the prevalence is decreasing because of immunization, 110 cases were reported in 1989 and 1990. Most of these cases occurred in adults over the age of 60 or in young children.[46] One case of neonatal tetanus was reported after an nonimmunized woman was delivered of her infant at home and the umbilical cord was cut with unsterile scissors. Puncture wounds account for 52% of reported cases; 23% were from lacerations; and 17% were caused by abrasions. Most were

Table 54-3. Fish and shellfish poisoning

Type of poisoning	High-risk foods
Paralytic shellfish poisoning	Clams, oysters, mussels, scallops
Neurotoxic shellfish poisoning	Bivalves (shellfish)
Mussel poisoning	Mussels
Ciguatera fish poisoning	Reef fish (red snapper, amberjack, barracuda, surgeonfish)
Scombroid fish poisoning	Tuna, albacore, bonito, mackerel, skipjack, mahimahi, and other dark-fleshed fish
Puffer-fish poisoning	Puffer fish, porcupine fish, sunfish

Table 54-4. Soil-associated pathogens

Pathogen	Disease
Parasites	
Ascaris	Pneumonitis; intestinal, pancreatic, and biliary obstruction
	Appendicitis, intussception, volvulus
Hookworm	Intestinal disease, malabsorption, anemia, hypoproteinemia, edema, congestive heart failure
Whipworm	Diarrhea, rectal prolapse
Strongyloides	Intestinal autoinfection, shock, death
Nematodes	Cutaneous and visceral larva migrans
Entamoeba histolytica	Amebic dysentery
Toxocara spp.	CNS disease
Bacteria	
E. coli	Intestinal disease (from fecal contamination)
Clostridium tetani	Tetanus
Bacillus anthracis	Anthrax
Fungi	
Dermatophytes	Ringworm (Tinea corporis, pedis, cruris)

caused by sharp objects, including nails or splinters. Almost half occurred during farming or gardening.

Tetanus infection resulted in 25 deaths during 1989 and 1990. These deaths could have been prevented through routine immunization with booster doses every 10 years and through the prompt initiation of prophylaxis after injury, including immunization in older adults and administration of tetanus immune globulin in adults who are not known to have three prior doses of tetanus toxoid.[1,19]

ARTHROPOD VECTOR–BORNE DISEASE

The term *vector* denotes a nonhuman carrier of infectious organisms that can transmit disease directly to humans. In general, vector-borne disease is of much greater importance in developing countries than in industrialized nations. Malaria, a parasitic disease transmitted by mosquitoes, is one of the most prevalent and serious diseases in the world and is endemic in 102 countries. (It is reviewed in greater detail in the section on travelers' health needs.) Arthropod-borne disease is summarized in Table 54-5.

Lyme disease

The most common vector-borne disease in the United States is Lyme disease, a multisystem disease caused by the spirochete *Borrelia burgdorferi* and spread to humans by bites from infected ticks.[33] The primary vectors are *Ixodes dammini* in the northeastern and midwestern United States and *Ixodes pacificus* on the west coast. The Centers for Disease Control (CDC) have reported that these ticks are established in 17 states (Maine, Massachusetts, Connecticut, Rhode Island, New York, New Jersey, Pennsylvania, Delaware, Maryland, Michigan, Illinois, Wisconsin, Minnesota, Iowa, Washington, Oregon, and California).[35,55] The ticks

Table 54-5. Insect vectors and diseases that they transmit

Vector	Disease	Pathogen
Mosquitoes		
Anopheles	Malaria	*Plasmodium* sp.
Culex	Filariasis	*Wuchereria* sp.
Aedes	Yellow fever, dengue	Arbovirus
Black fly	River blindness	*Onchocerca*
Tsetse fly	Sleeping sickness	*Trypanosoma*
Sand fly	Kala-azar, cutaneous leishmaniasis	*Leishmania*
Gnats	Filariasis	*Mansonella*
Rat flea	Plague	*Yersinia*
	Murine typhus	*Rickettsia typhi*
Body louse	Epidemic typhus	*Rickettsia prowazekii*
	Trench fever	*Rochalimaea quintana*
	Rocky Mountain spotted fever	*Rickettsia rickettsii*
Tick	Lyme disease	*Borrelia burgdorferi*
	Colorado tick fever	Arbovirus
Mite	Rickettsialpox	*Rickettsia akari*

have been found in seven additional states, and their presence is transient and probably related to transport on birds from neighboring states. Spirochete transfer occurs in approximately 10% of people bitten by affected ticks. In New England, the mid-Atlantic states, and the midwest, 1% of larvae, 25% of nymphs, and 50% of adult ticks are infected with *B. burgdorferi*.[55] The prevalence of infection on the west coast is lower.[30] Studies also indicate that there is little risk of infection if the tick is removed in the first 24 hours, 50% risk after 48 hours, and almost universal infection after 72 hours from the time of the tick bite.[9,43]

Disease ranges from mild early disease characterized by development of flulike symptoms and erythema migrans rash, which is usually cured by antibiotics, to multisystem disease affecting 20% to 40% of people, who then develop cardiac, neurologic, and rheumatologic problems.[36] Because of difficult recognition of early disease and the inability to prevent transmission of Lyme disease, many experts are now advocating empirical antibiotic therapy if a tick bite occurs in certain high-risk areas of the country where the probability of Lyme disease is greater than 0.036.[35,62]

Rocky Mountain spotted fever

Although Lyme disease is the most prevalent tick-borne disease in the northeastern and western states, Rocky Mountain spotted fever predominates in the southwest, remains a public health concern in the midwestern and mountain states, and has been reported to occur in the northeast.[34] Its incidence has increased over the past two decades and peaks in the spring and summer.[51]

The major vectors include various ticks, including the dog tick, *Dermacentor variabilis,* and the wood tick, *Dermacentor andersoni.* Ticks transmit the agent of disease, *Rickettsia rickettsii,* among several vertebrate hosts (squirrels, chipmunks, mice, and rabbits), without apparent clinical disease in the host. Dogs and humans develop clinical disease after tick bites.

Clinical disease usually develops abruptly 2 to 12 days after exposure and is associated with high fevers, headache, myalgia, nausea, vomiting, abdominal pain, and conjunctivitis. About 90% of people develop the characteristic petechial rash. Antibiotic treatment should be initiated promptly on the basis of clinical symptoms. No vaccine is available, and prevention is mainly through avoidance and careful removal of ticks.[13]

Plague

Plague, which is of historical importance, is still seen in parts of the United States. In 1992 four cases of human plague were reported in the western states. Flea bites were implicated in most of these cases.[44] The causative organism, the bacterium *Yersinia pestis,* is transmitted by bites from infected fleas. The natural hosts are primarily rodents. Clinical disease in humans is usually in the form of bubonic plague; other complications include septicemia, pneumonia, and meningitis. The pneumonic form of this disease is highly contagious and requires isolation and prompt initiation of antibiotic therapy. Prevention is mainly through education, vector control, and rodent control. Vaccination is advised for people working with the agent in laboratories, in war conditions, or in Peace Corps service in endemic areas.[48]

DISEASES TRANSMITTED BY ANIMAL VECTORS

Throughout history, rats and mice have been highly adaptable creatures, living in both urban and rural areas near structures built by humans. They deliver disease both by being reservoirs of disease and by being mechanical vectors of disease. Their ability to foil most methods of control has led to contamination of water supplies. Leptospirosis, an occupational disease of sewerage workers, among others, is a flulike illness caused by a spirochete transmitted in rat urine. Animal-borne diseases, or zoonoses, are summarized in Table 54-6.

Rabies

The animal-borne disease of greatest concern is rabies, an acute viral infection of the central nervous system that has been reported to occur in animals and human since ancient times.[18] The etiologic agent is a bullet-shaped virus belonging to the family *Rhabdoviridae*. Rabies has a worldwide distribution and has been reported on every continent except Australia. It continues to spread in the United States and Europe.[11,26]

Humans are an accidental host; the major hosts are wild animals and dogs. Each year about 50,000 people worldwide die of rabies. In 1990, 148 cases of rabies in dogs were reported in the United States. With improved immunizations of domestic pets and livestock, dog and cat cases have been markedly reduced, and currently more than half of the reported cases of rabies are in skunks, raccoons, and foxes. Rabid bats have been reported in every state except Alaska and Hawaii and have caused illness in at least 18 humans.

Table 54-6. Animal vectors and diseases that they transmit to humans (Zoonoses)

Disease	Host
Rabies (virus)	Dogs, jackels, wolves, coyotes, foxes, bats, skunks, weasels, mongooses
Psittacosis (Chlamydia)	Birds
Anthrax (bacteria)	Livestock
Brucellosis (bacteria)	Cattle, dogs, goats, pigs, swine
Leptospirosis (spirochete)	Swine, cattle, dogs, rodents
Salmonellosis (bacteria)	Cattle, pigs, poultry
Taeniasis/cysticercosis	Beef, pork
Trichinosis (nematode)	Rats, pigs, bear, horse, walrus
Hydatid disease (cestodes)	Dogs, cats
Lymphocytic choriomeningitis virus (LCMV)	Nude mice

Terrestrial mammals are also important reservoirs of rabies.[50]

Since the mid-1970s, rabies infection has spread northward along the Atlantic coast, reaching upstate New York in 1992.[63] Raccoon rabies has become a serious threat because raccoons readily coexist with humans and live in barns, houses, sheds, old tree trunks, dumpsters and the like. They readily adapt to feeding by humans, and large populations may build up in suburban areas.[25] Many people feed raccoons and encourage their welfare. Similarly, when unwanted raccoons are removed from houses, they may be handled before their release in previously nonendemic areas.[28]

The best control measures include pre-exposure vaccination of pets and people who may work with wild or unquarantined animals. The use of injectable vaccine has virtually eliminated rabies from domestic animals. Wild animals should not be taken in as pets, and people should be urged to avoid handling any animals that are not domestic pets. Efforts to control rabies in wildlife now focus on the distribution of oral virus in baits that are ingested by the target species and lead to immunity.[65] A recent study indicates that this method will be the most cost-effective means of rabies prevention in the future.[63,66]

Muller and Blancou[39] express optimism that pet immunization, oral immunization of foxes, and quarantine measures can eliminate rabies from European countries. With new developments improving the safety of vaccines, the recommendations regarding preexposure and postexposure prophylaxis change fairly frequently. They are published periodically in *Morbidity and Mortality Weekly Report* (MMWR).[64]

CONCERNS OF PEOPLE EXPOSED TO HAZARDOUS WASTES AND SEWAGE

People in all states are concerned about exposure to infectious hazardous wastes during both recreational and occupational activities. The concerns range from needlestick injuries transmitting HIV or HBV to contact with agents known to cause respiratory or gastrointestinal disease. Studies indicate that the likelihood of illness related to bloodborne pathogens is low. The frequency of development of HIV infection after a known needlestick injury in a hospital setting is 1 in 250.[24] The rate is much lower after a needle has been lying on a beach, because HIV usually is infectious for a shorter time outside the body. The frequency of acquiring HBV is about 100 times higher and is a reason to encourage universal vaccination for hepatitis B.[22]

In 1987 the New Jersey Department of Health began a study to determine whether microbial contamination of ocean swimming areas leads to an increase in infectious diseases. It is clear from these studies that the water quality and incidence of infectious illness were low, except during a widely publicized malfunction at a sewage-treatment plant that affected an ocean beach area. Contamination in this setting produced what the Environmental Protection Agency defined as *highly credible gastrointestinal illness* (also known as *stomach virus*).[40]

These studies indicate that the main hazard is fecal contamination, or the development of "night soil." The chief pathogens of concern include *E. coli. Salmonella typhi, Entamoeba histolytica,* poliovirus, and hepatitis A virus. Of particular concern in tropical parts of the world is infection with schistosomes.[32,41,42]

The best method to prevent these diseases is by swimming only in bodies of water known to be free of bacterial contamination, preferably in areas in which the water is chlorinated. People should avoid walking without shoes in questionable areas, and hazardous waste workers and sewage plant workers should use proper protective equipment.

SPECIAL CONSIDERATIONS FOR INTERNATIONAL TRAVEL

Travelers to developing countries are subject to infectious diseases through contaminated food and water as well as through arthropod and other animal vectors. Patients planning to travel often ask physicians for advice about immunizations and prevention of malaria and diarrhea. Currently available and recommended vaccines are listed in *Health Information for International Travel 1994,* a publication of the CDC.[23]

Malaria

Malaria transmission occurs in sub-Saharan Africa, the Indian subcontinent, southeast Asia, Oceania, the Middle East, and Central and South America. The risk varies in different area and depends on the itinerary of the traveler. Malaria is caused by any one of four species of the protozoan parasite *Plasmodium: Plasmodium vivax, Plasmodium ovale, Plasmodium malariae,* and *Plasmodium falciparum,* which causes the most severe illness and is often resistant to prophylaxis and antibiotic therapy. The parasites are transmitted by *Anopheles* mosquitoes. More than 80% of cases in American travelers occur in sub-Saharan Africa. The disease is characterized by fever, anemia, renal failure, pulmonary edema, and death. The best protective measures include use of screens and nets when sleeping, protective clothing, insect repellents, and appropriate preexposure prophylaxis with chloroquine, mefloquine, or doxycycline as per current CDC recommendations outlined in *MMWR* and the *Medical Letter.* These recommendations change as new drugs and new drug resistance emerge. Further information concerning local malaria outbreaks can be obtained by contacting the CDC malaria hotline at (404) 332-4559. Malaria transmission does occur, although rarely, in the United States because vector mosquitos are widespread.[3,15,68]

Traveler's diarrhea

Diarrhea is by far the most common medical problem among people traveling to tropical areas. Traveler's diarrhea is a syndrome characterized by a twofold or greater increase in the frequency of unformed bowel movements. In the healthy traveler, it is usually a self-limited illness but may be associated with nausea, vomiting, abdominal pain, fecal urgency, tenesmus, or the passage of bloody or mucoid stools. The risk of acquisition of this illness is 20% to 50%, depending on the destination and itinerary of the traveler. The highest-risk areas are the developing countries of Latin America, Africa, the Middle East, and Asia. Traveler's diarrhea is mainly acquired through ingestion of fecally contaminated food and water.

The most common causative agent is enterotoxic *E. coli,* which usually produces a watery diarrhea associated with a low-grade fever. Other causative agents include salmonellae (food-borne diarrhea), shigella (bacillary dysentery), *Campylobacter jejuni,* and *Vibrio parahaemolyticus* from raw seafood.

Viral pathogens, including rotavirus and Norwalk-like viruses, have been isolated in as many as 50% of travelers with diarrhea. Parasitic infections, including those caused by *Giardia lamblia, Entamoeba histolytica,* and *Cryptosporidium,* have been recognized.

No data indicate that there are noninfectious causes of diarrhea. Contrary to popular belief, changes in diet, jet lag, fatigue, and the like are not associated with diarrheal illness. The best method of prevention is avoidance of food or water in areas where sanitation is improper by use of bottled beverages, avoidance of uncooked meat, poultry, and seafood, and the use of common sense. Prophylaxis with antibiotics is not recommended, because of the high incidence of side effects, but several antibiotic regimens are effective in treatment of traveler's diarrhea and are periodically updated in the *Medical Letter* and CDC guidelines for international travelers.[16,17,23]

REFERENCES

1. Advisory Committee on Immunization Practices: Diphtheria, tetanus: recommendations for vaccine use and other preventive measures: recommendations of the Advisory Committee on Immunization Practices, *MMWR* 40(RR-10):71, 1991.
2. Addis DG et al: Community acquired Legionnaire's disease associated with a cooling tower: evidence for longer-distance transport of *Legionella pneumophila, Am J Epidemiol* 130:557, 1989.
3. Advice for travellers, *Med Lett Drugs Ther* 34:1–4, 1992.
4. Birkhead G, Vogt RL: Epidemiologic surveillance for endemic *Giardia lamblia* infection in Vermont, *Am J Epidemiol* 129:762, 1989.
5. Blaser MJ, Newman LS: A review of human salmonellosis: infective dose, *Rev Infect Dis* 128:1096, 1982.
6. Blumenthal D: Infectious agents in the environment. In Blumenthal D, ed: *Introduction to environmental health,* New York, 1985, Springer-Verlag.
7. Breiman RF et al: An outbreak of Legionnaire's disease associated with shower use: possible role of amoebae, *JAMA* 263:2924, 1990.
8. Brodsky RE, Spencer AC, Schultz MG: Giardiasis in American travellers to the Soviet Union, *J Infect Dis* 130:319, 1974.
9. Burgdorfer W: Vector/host relationships of the Lyme disease spirochete, *Borrelia burgdorferi, Rheum Dis Clin North Am* 15:775, 1989.
10. Chamberland M: Transmission from health care worker to patient: what is the risk?, *Ann Intern Med* 116:871, 1992.

11. Compendium of animal rabies control, 1992, *MMWR* 41(RR-7):1, 1992.
12. Craun GF: Waterborne disease outbreaks in the United States of America: causes and prevention, World Health Stat Q 45:192, 1992.
13. Doebbeling B: Rickettsial infections. In Last J, ed: *Public health and preventive medicine,* ed 13, Norwalk, Conn, 1992, Appleton & Lange.
14. Dondero TJ et al: An outbreak of Legionnaire's disease associated with a contaminated air-conditioning cooling tower, *N Engl J Med* 302:365, 1980.
15. Drugs for parasitic infections, *Med Lett Drugs Ther* 34(March 17):17, 1992.
16. DuPont HL: Oral aztreonam, a poorly absorbed yet effective therapy for bacterial diarrhea in US travellers to Mexico, *JAMA* 267:1932, 1992.
17. DuPont HL, Ericsson CD: Prevention and treatment of traveler's diarrhea, *N Engl J Med* 328:1821, 1993.
18. Fishbein DB, Robinson LE: Rabies, *N Engl J Med* 329:1632, 1993.
19. Fleming M et al: Tetanus fatality: Ohio, 1991, *MMWR* 42:148, 1993.
20. Fraser DW et al: Legionnaire's disease: description of an epidemic of pneumonia, *N Engl J Med* 297:1189, 1977.
21. Frieden TF: The Emergence of drug-resistant tuberculosis in New York City, *N Engl J Med* 328:521, 1993.
22. Gerbending J: Risks to healthcare workers from occupational exposure to HBV, HIV, and CMV, *Infect Dis Clin North Am* 3:735, 1989.
23. *Health information for international travel 1994,* Washington, DC, 1994, US Department of Health and Human Services, Public Health Service, Centers for Disease Control.
24. Henderson D, Rohey B, Willy M: Risk for occupational transmission of HIV-1 associated with clinical exposures: a prospective evaluation, *Ann Intern Med* 113:740, 1990.
25. Hoffman CO, Gottschang JL: Numbers, distribution, and movement of a raccoon population in a suburban residential community, *J Mammalogy* 58:623, 1988.
26. Human rabies: Texas, Arkansas, and Georgia, 1991, *MMWR* 40:765-76, 1991.
27. Iseman MD: Directly observed treatment of tuberculosis: we can't afford not to try it, *N Engl J Med* 328:576, 1993.
28. Jenkins SR, Perry BD, Winkler WG: Ecology and epidemiology of raccoon rabies, *Rev Infect Dis* 10:S620, 1988.
29. Jong E: Food, fish, and shellfish poisoning. In Jong E, Keston J, McMullen R, eds: *Travel medicine advisor,* Atlanta, 1993, American Health Consultants.
30. Lane RS, Lavoie PE: Lyme borreliosis in California: acarological, clinical, and epidemiological studies, *Ann NY Acad Sci* 539:192, 1988.
31. Last J: *Public health and preventive medicine,* ed 13, Norwalk, Conn, 1992, Appleton & Lange.
32. Li Hsu, SY: Schistosomiasis. In Last J, ed: *Public health and preventive medicine,* ed 13, Norwalk, Conn, 1992, Appleton & Lange.
33. Lyme disease and other spirochetal diseases, *Rev Infect Dis* 11(S6):S1433, 1989.
34. Lyme disease: Connecticut, *MMWR* 37:1, 1988.
35. Magrid D et al: Prevention of Lyme disease after tick bites, a cost-effectiveness analysis, *N Engl J Med* 327:534, 1992.
36. Malawista SE, Steere AC: Lyme disease: infectious in origin, rheumatic in expression, *Adv Intern Med* 31:147, 1986.
37. Mandel GL, Douglas RG, Bennett JE, eds: *Principles and practices of infectious diseases,* ed 3, New York, 1989, Churchill Livingstone.
38. Minette H: Salmonellosis in the marine environment: a review and commentary, *Int J Zoon* 13:71, 1986.
39. Muller WW, Blancou J: Rabies in Europe, *BMJ* 305:725, 1992.
40. New Jersey Department of Health: *Ocean health study: a study of the relationship between illness and ocean water quality in New Jersey,* Trenton, 1992.
41. Okun D: Water quality management, In Last J, ed: *Public health and preventive medicine,* ed 13, Norwalk, Conn, 1992, Appleton & Lange.
42. Olson B: Environmental water pollution. In Rom W, ed: *Environmental and occupational medicine,* ed 2, Boston, Little, Brown.
43. Piesman J et al: Duration of tick attachment and *Borrelia burgdorferi* transmission, *J Clin Microbiol* 25:557, 1987.
44. Plague: US, *MMWR* 41:787, 1992.
45. Preliminary report: foodborne outbreak of *E. coli, MMWR* 42:85, 1993.
46. Prevost R et al: Tetanus surveillance: United States, 1989-1990, *MMWR,* 41(SS-8):1, 1992.
47. Primary amebic meningoencephalitis, North Carolina, *MMWR* 41:457, 1992.
48. Recommendations of the Public Health Service Advisory Committee on Immunization Practices: plague vaccine, *MMWR* 31:301, 1982.
49. Redd SC, Cohen ML: *Legionella* in water: what should be done?, *JAMA* 257:1221, 1987.
50. Reid-Sanden FL, Dobbins JD, Smith JS: ''Rabies surveillance in the United States during 1989, *J Am Vet Med Assoc* 197:1571, 1990.
51. Salgo MP et al: A focus of Rocky Mountain spotted fever within New York City, *N Engl J Med* 318:1345, 1988.
52. Schlech WF III: Expanding the horizons of foodborne listeriosis, *JAMA* 267:2081, 1992.
53. Schuchat A et al: Role of foods in sporadic listeriosis. I. Case control study of dietary risk factors, *JAMA* 267:2041, 1992.
54. Shapiro L, Hager M, McCormick J: Farewell, medium rare, if you're looking for burgers, go for the gray, *Newsweek,* Feb. 22, 1993.
55. Steere AC: Lyme disease, *N Engl J Med* 321:586, 1989.
56. Steere AC, Malawista SE: Cases of Lyme disease in the United States: locations correlated with the distribution of *Ixodes dammini, Ann Intern Med* 91:730, 1979.
57. Sullivan PS et al: Illness and reservoirs associated with *Giardia lamblia* in Egypt: the case against treatment in developing world environments or high endemnicity, *Am J Epidemiol* 127:1272, 1988.
58. Swerdlow D: A waterborne outbreak in Missouri of *Escherichia coli* 0157:H7 associated with bloody diarrhea and death, *Ann Intern Med* 117:812, 1992.
59. Telzak EE: Diabetes mellitus, a newly described risk factor for salmonellosis, *J Infect Dis* 164:538, 1991.
60. Thompson P et al: Foodborne illness: US food legislation, *Lancet* 336:1557, 1990.
61. Todd E: Epidemiology of foodborne illness: North America, *Lancet,* 336:788, 1990.
62. Treatment of Lyme disease, *Medical Lett Drugs Ther* 34:95, 1992.
63. Uhaa IJ et al: Benefits and costs of using an orally absorbed vaccine to control rabies in raccoons, *J Am Vet Med Assoc* 201:1873, 1992.
64. Update on adult immunization: recommendations of the Immunization Practices Advisory Committee, *MMWR* 40:143, 1991.
65. Wandeler AI, Capt S, Kappeler A: Oral immunization of wildlife against rabies: concept and first field experiments, *Rev Infect Dis* 10:S649, 1988.
66. Wiktor TJ, MacFarlan RI, Reagan KJ: Protection from rabies by vaccinia virus recombinant containing the rabies virus glycoprotein, *Proc Natl Acad Sci USA* 81:7194, 1984.
67. Wilson ME: Giardiasis. In Last J, ed: *Public health and preventive medicine,* ed 13, Norwalk, Conn, 1992, Appleton & Lange.
68. Wyler D: Malaria chemoprophylaxis for the traveler, *N Engl J Med* 329:31, 1993.

WASTE

Chapter 55

HEALTH IMPLICATIONS OF SOLID WASTE MANAGEMENT

Michael Gochfeld

Regulatory considerations
    The status of regulations: standards and guidelines
    Standards
Categories of solid waste
    Municipal solid waste
    Residential waste
    Commercial waste
    Institutional waste
    Construction and demolition waste
    Sewage sludge
    Medical waste
    Harbor debris
    Dredge spoilage
    Agricultural waste
    Mining waste
    Hazardous waste
Waste management systems
Source reduction
Reuse and recycling
Pollution from waste management
The technologies
    Incineration
    Composting
Data on facilities operations
Estimating public health risk
Pollution control devices
Emission data
Emissions of public health concern
Toxic hazards from waste management technologies
    Particulates
    Dioxins and furans
    Acid and irritant gases
    Volatile organic compounds
Heavy metals
    Noise
    Odor
    Implications for siting

The estimates of North American garbage production are so staggering that they defy comprehension. Indeed, we become inured to estimates that each American disposes of over 3.5 kilograms of trash each day,[33] up more than 50% from 1970.[26] The United States produces about half the solid waste generated by the developed nations, a sign of economic laxity and also a cause of great financial strain.[21] New York City projected 14 million metric tons of trash per year.[30] The health implications of solid waste include direct effects such as the pollutant burden contributed by various forms of waste management (including incineration, and composting[5]) and the impact of traffic on residential communities, and indirect effects such as the use of money and other resources that society might use more productively.[9]

The politics of waste have become as contentious as the politics of health. The "Green" approach represents the complete solution to the waste management problem in terms of three Rs: source reduction, reuse, and recycling. Alternatives such as incineration are viewed not only as unhealthful, but as thwarting the development of the three R approach.[7] The health implications of waste management are not easily separated from the political and economic aspects.[9,32,35]

There are many ways to collect and process garbage. These can be combined in various systems and on various scales to serve populations of varying size and density.[30,32,35] Landfills, formerly called "garbage dumps" or "rubbish tips," have long been the mainstay of solid waste management. But in many states landfilling is being phased out, and municipalities and counties are required to develop acceptable alternatives, which usually involve multiple approaches.

This chapter reviews some of the approaches, focusing on the health consequences of each. It will cover the different types of garbage or "waste streams," the main environmental hazards associated with waste disposal (chemical contamination of air and water, infectious hazards, noise, and odor), the different waste management technologies, and their consequences.

REGULATORY CONSIDERATIONS

A number of regulatory decisions have changed the options that will be available in the future. These include phasing out of ocean dumping of sewage sludge, closing of most or all hospital incinerators, and phasing out of burning of harbor debris at sea. Individual municipalities and states may have their own waste management regulations, among which recycling ordinances are increasingly common. For example, New York City's Solid Waste Management Act[30] and its implementing regulations require that the city: (1) prevent wastes at the source, (2) reuse, recycle, or compost as much as possible, (3) recover energy, and (4) landfill only material not amenable to other strategies.

The status of regulations: standards and guidelines

Any waste management plan will produce estimates of pollutant emissions into air and waste. Rather than undertake independent risk assessments for each emission and scenario, one can compare the estimated emissions to various regulatory standards or guidelines proposed by federal or state agencies. The ratio of projected emissions or resulting air concentrations to an existing standard or guideline is called a "hazard index." Its reciprocal is called a "protection index." Table 55-1 lists some of the standards and guidelines for different substances. The National Ambient Air Quality Standards (NAAQS) include primary and secondary standards for six criteria pollutants established under the Clean Air Act. Many states have in turn adopted or modified these as state standards or guidelines. Primary standards are health-based; secondary standards deal with visibility, effects on material, and deposition on soil and vegetation. Additional regulations include Prevention of Significant Deterioration (PSD), New Source Performance Standards (NSPS), and National Emission Standards for Hazardous Air Pollutants (NESHAPs 1981, established under Section 112 of the Clean Air Act). The latter covers arsenic, asbestos, benzene, beryllium, mercury, vinyl chloride, and radionuclides.

Standards

Standards governing emissions can be health-based, but in fact are generally based on technological considerations such as the Best Available Control Technology (BACT) and the Lowest Achievable Emission Rate (LAER). As technology changes, as source reduction and source separation of wastes improve, states will regulate more pollutants to achieve even lower levels than at present. This creates a moving target for facility designers.

Table 55-1. Primary and secondary national ambient air quality standards, New York State standards, and related criteria

	Primary NAAQS	Secondary NAAQS	NY State standards 6 NYCRR Pt 237
CO			
8 hr ave	9 ppm	9 ppm	9 ppm
1 hr ave	35 ppm	35 ppm	35 ppm
SO2			
1 yr	80 ug/m^3 (= 0.03 ppm STP)		0.03 ppm
24 hr	365 ug/m^3 (= 0.14 ppm STP)		0.14 ppm
3 hr		1300 ug/m^3	0.50 ppm
NO2			
1 yr	100 ug/cu	100 ug/m^3	0.05 ppm
Ozone			
1 hr	235 ug/m^3	235 ug/m^3	0.08 ppm
PM-10			
1 yr	50 ug/m^3	50 ug/m^3	—
24 hr	150 ug/m^3	150 ug/m^3	—
Pb			
3 mo	1.5 ug/m^3	1.5 ug/m^3	—
TSP			
1 yr			75 ug/m^3
24 hr			250 ug/m^3
Settleable particulates			
30 days			6 mg/cm^2/mo
Hydrocarbons (excluding methane)			
3 hr			0.24 ppm
Beryllium			
1 mo			0.01 ug/m^3
H$_2$S			
1 hr			1 ppm

CATEGORIES OF SOLID WASTE

Solid waste comes from various sources and can be considered in various categories. Table 55-2 shows the estimated breakdown in percentage (by weight) for New York City.[30] Each of these components can be considered as a waste stream, and evaluation requires good data or realistic assumptions regarding the attributes listed in the box on p. 625.

Municipal solid waste

Municipal solid waste varies in composition, by source, from place to place, and even by day of week or month of

Table 55-2. Estimated composition by weight of solid waste generated in New York City[30]

Type	Percentage
Municipal solid waste (residential, institutional, commercial, industrial)	55-60
Construction and demolition waste (including hazardous materials such as asbestos)	15-20
Dredge spoil (for a coastal city with a harbor)	15-20
Sewage sludge	1-2
Medical waste (including potentially infectious material)	1-2
Harbor debris	<1
Agricultural waste	<1
Mining waste (negligible in New York)	
Hazardous waste (not included in solid waste)	

Table 55-3. Composition of a residential waste stream for New York City[30]

Type	Percentage
Food waste	11
Plastic bags	5
Magazines/glossy	4
Textiles	4
Grass and leaves	3
Glass containers	3
Bulk items	10
Newsprint	9
Miscellaneous organic matter	7
Corrugated papers	6
Aluminum cans	0.5
Poisons	0.02
Batteries	0.06
Medical waste	0.02
Pesticides	0.01

Attributes of waste streams requiring evaluation in a waste management plan

Physical attributes
    Density (lbs/yd^3)
    Compactibility
    Heat content (in BTUs)
Combustion attributes
    Temperature
    Residual ash (%)
Chemical composition (%)
    Oxygen
    Nitrogen
    Carbon
    Chlorine
Concentrations of toxic PAHs and metals
Potential for recycling various components
Ease of separation

---

year. There are several sources of data on the composition of various waste streams, including one prepared for New York City[30] (Table 55-3). Airborne emissions can arise at the generation site, during collection, transportation, and tipping, and during various stages of treatment. Regardless of the treatment options chosen, one can identify the emissions that are of public health concern. These fall into several major categories (see below). Public concern over air emissions from waste management focus mostly on incineration,[5] but each treatment option or combination thereof produces emissions of various sorts. Aside from disposal of hazardous materials and metal items, residential and institutional waste is rich in organic materials, which can be either composted or incinerated.

Residential waste

The familiar household waste from private homes and apartments is a mixtures of putrescible waste (mostly food scraps), packaging, newspapers, junk mail and unwanted household items. The composition of a residential waste stream is shown in Table 55-3 based on New York City Department of Sanitation.[30]

Commercial waste

In addition to the above, commercial waste contains office waste such as paper, manufacturing waste, and large amounts of packaging such as corrugated cardboard. Commercial waste can be either source-separated or separated at a transfer station.

Institutional waste

Institutions containing large numbers of people (schools, hospitals, prisons) produce large quantities of waste from a single source. Medical waste (see below) is a special form of institutional waste. There can be an economy of scale in dealing with institutions. A cost incentive/disincentive scheme may encourage institutions to purchase materials and use them in a way that minimizes waste.

Construction and demolition waste

This includes a wide variety of material often saturated with paints or preservatives, and sometimes asbestos. This is bulky material that may have low BTU content and be difficult to incinerate. Contractors are legally required to separate hazardous materials such as asbestos and remove them from the solid waste stream to a separate hazardous waste stream.

Sewage sludge

Municipal sewage is treated in a variety of ways, including chlorination, aeration, and dewatering. After dewatering, the dry treated sludge is usually noninfectious, but residual contaminants include metals and organics. Although this waste was formerly dumped at sea, there is increasing interest in land disposal, including sludge composting for agricultural use and composting for highway construction materials. There is substantial research on the properties of sewage sludge and the conditions under which it can be used on land (see below and Chapter 59).

Medical waste

Medical waste offers a fertile field for source reduction and recycling. Many disposable materials can be replaced with reusable materials. Batteries, needles, polyvinylchloride tubing, and other plastic materials can be reused (if costs are not prohibitive) or recycled. The main public concern and regulatory focus has been over the infectious potential of waste associated with patient contact, yet a large part of the waste from medical facilities does not have infectious potential. Regulations require potentially infectious medical waste to be packaged and destroyed on site or shipped in a secure manner to an approved handler. Some medical waste is shipped to or collected by commercial companies that specialize in medical waste. In addition to potential for infection, medical waste contains large amounts of plastics, which release hydrogen chloride and phosgene when burned.[19,28,35]

Harbor debris

There has been very little study of this waste stream, which contains much scrap metal as well as wood, often waterlogged and saturated with creosote, pentachlorophenol, arsenic, or other preservatives. Presumably much of it can be reused or recycled. This is an important source of waste since most urban areas are situated adjacent to bodies of water; there is high potential for ecosystem contamination.

Dredge spoilage

The U.S. Army Corps of Engineers, charged with maintaining the navigability of coastal and interior waterways, conducts periodic dredging to reestablish deep-water channels for shipping. The sediments of a harbor are often extensively contaminated with heavy metals and polyaromatic hydrocarbons. The U.S. Environmental Protection Agency has designated offshore sites where this material can be dumped. However, the possible resuspension of contaminated sediment in water and the ultimate security of the ocean dump sites is highly controversial, and alternative approaches to managing dredge material are being sought.

Agricultural waste

This includes animal waste from stockyards, vegetation waste after harvesting, as well as container waste (empty bags and cans). Chemical waste such as unused pesticides should be disposed of safely and separately from other farm waste.

Mining waste

Mining waste includes mineral matter such as slag and construction debris. It usually does not enter the municipal waste stream, but is a major source of water pollution.

Hazardous waste

Hazardous waste is dealt with separately in this book. Current regulations governing hazardous waste are intended to keep it separate from the solid waste stream.

WASTE MANAGEMENT SYSTEMS

Although all of the sources described potentially release pollutants, the alternatives for managing the municipal solid waste (MSW) and to a lesser extent sewage sludge have significant health consequences. For the other waste streams the number of technical approaches is more limited. The major components of the MSW are cardboard and paper, textiles, plastic, food and other organic waste, and metals and glass. The major management options are reuse and recycling, incineration, composting, and landfilling, with many variations of these basic themes.

Ultimately one must envision and analyze a three-dimensional matrix of six waste streams handled by various approaches, each combination of waste and technology producing various environmental impacts, both adverse and beneficial, to air, water, soil, food, and human health. Each combination of technologies can be treated as a complete scenario. The hazards associated with each scenario include transportation accidents, occupational injuries, air pollution, water pollution, and aesthetics.

A waste management system embodies waste prevention (including source reduction, reuse, and recycling) and waste treatment (including incineration or waste-to-energy, composting, landfilling, and various modifications of these). The plan should consider the following environmental impacts: (1) air quality, (2) water quality, (3) traffic, (4) noise, (5) odor, (6) socioeconomic effects, and (7) community acceptance.

Therefore, the system must combine a variety of social, transportation, and treatment technologies. Social issues involve the acceptability of particular programs such as mandatory recycling. Transportation alternatives include a variety of vehicles and collection schedules. The treatment technologies include landfilling, incineration, composting, and recycling. For example, for its long-term comprehensive waste management program New York City planned on composting 7% to 14% and recycling 20% to 30% of its waste stream, relying on up to 60% for incineration (or waste-to-energy) facilities. A minimum of 15% of waste (including incinerator ash) required landfilling.[30]

The new combinations of technical approaches require an administrative framework as well. The development of record-keeping and auditing practices as well as new fee structures that provide incentives/disincentives should encourage waste producers, haulers, and managers to choose socially and environmentally preferable approaches.

SOURCE REDUCTION

In both the public and private sector, procurement practices can be controlled to minimize waste. Consumer education programs play a large role in reducing waste, particularly in conjunction with community recycling programs. Incentives for source reduction should encourage replacement of disposables with reusable supplies and equipment[22] and major disincentives for wasteful packaging, which now comprises a major component by volume of the municipal waste stream.

REUSE AND RECYCLING

Many common materials such as metal, glass, plastics, paper, textiles, and bulky items such as appliances are recyclable, and these account for nearly half of municipal solid waste.[32] Although at first many communities relied on voluntary drop-off at recycling centers, new regulations encourage or require communities to develop curbside recycling programs. Recyclables can be source-separated by the consumer-generator and can be collected in compartmentalized trucks to facilitate subsequent separation, or they can be sorted manually or mechanically at the destination site.

A successful reuse/recycling program should be readily accepted by the public, easy to follow, and with goals that are within reach and rewarding to achieve. A public education program must emphasize this approach.[32] In addition to explaining why such a program is necessary, the educational component should clarify how to accomplish source separation, and the message can be spread by radio, television, newspapers, posters, direct mailings, and utility envelope stuffers, in order to reach a wide audience. Equally important is the commitment of the municipality or other jurisdiction to accomplish the collection in a timely fashion. In most cases the collection and recycling is privatized, but it is possible for a public agency to invest in recycling. The success of a program can be evaluated in terms of the percentage of residents who participate and the percentage of their garbage that they can recycle. A common goal for a community is 60% recycling.

Any mandatory program must be coupled with enforcement. There should be incentives for complying (lower cost of disposal) and penalties for noncompliance (refusal of refuse).

Separation is only the beginning of successful recycling. The material must get to the hands of those who can reuse it or change it into a usable product. In some cases the new product may resemble the original (as with paper), or the material may be compounded into an entirely different product from the original, for example, mixing glass fragments into asphalt to produce glassphalt. New reuse/recycling technologies represents a field of rapid technological development. However, even today, there is negligible demand for many recycled items such as plastics and textiles. In some cases this is due to the availability and lower cost of ''virgin'' materials. In some cases the costs of the recycling are still a disincentive. For example, recycled textiles and plastics are currently in low demand.

There is a chicken and egg relationship. Industries will not develop a cost-effective means of recycling a material until there is a sure supply of that material, and communities may not recycle that material until there is a demand. In this case the supply can drive the demand as well as vice versa.

POLLUTION FROM WASTE MANAGEMENT

The data available on pollutants released by working facilities such as solid waste incinerators are scanty. Regulations require facilities to incorporate the Best Available Control Technology (BACT) or to reach the Lowest Achievable Emission Rate (LAER), which is the combination of technologies that produces the least pollution from a particular source. BACT obviously changes from year to year with the introduction of new technology. At any given time, the LAER is the greatest reduction that can be achieved by design, maintenance, and performance strategies.

New York City developed a long-term waste management plan[30] after evaluating 34 different types of waste treatment facilities. The plan estimated air and water pollution with and without incineration. The study included the total environmental ''loading'' or output into all environmental media, as well as predicted airborne concentrations and inputs to water.

Developing and evaluating a comprehensive waste management system requires: (1) confidence that the existing health and environmental guidelines are adequately protective, (2) that there is a procedure for ensuring that all components are maintained and operated according to specifications, and (3) that there is enforcement if the system or any part should prove noncompliant.

One approach to evaluating a municipal or county plan for comprehensive waste management is to evaluate all sources of pollution that contribute to the environmental load of a set of significant pollutants. New York City[30] estimated that of all pollutants examined, only mercury release would pose a significant contribution to the background air pollution. Although the excess mercury was of little concern for human health directly, the airborne deposition or fallout on aquatic systems would lead to bioaccumulation in the food chain, and secondary exposure to people who regularly consume fish and shellfish from the surrounding waters.

Such an analysis necessarily assumes that facilities will be built, maintained, and operated according to specifications in a fashion that will allow them to achieve or better the emission estimates. As in most situations the potential for significant occupational exposure is higher than for community exposure, and clearly attention should be paid to ensuring that workers are adequately protected,[18] even when a particular scenario does not reveal much risk to the community at large.

One approach is to analyze the Hazard Indices for each chemical, the ratio of the projected average emissions to some existing or calculated standard or guideline from a state or federal agency. Where the Hazard Index is less than 0.01, one can be confident that health is not jeopardized. A Hazard Index approaching 1.0 focuses attention on the need to ensure that the facilities operate according to specifications and that efforts to reduce exposure are incorporated. A Hazard

Index greater than 1 indicates an unacceptable condition from the public health perspective. The Protective Index is the reciprocal of the Hazard Index. A PI greater than 100 connotes a large margin of safety. A PI of 1 indicates that the environmental concentrations equal the standard, which usually has a built in margin of safety as well. A PI less than 1 (corresponding to an HI greater than 1) indicates that the standard has been exceeded.

The management of waste can be a noisy and odoriferous operation. The loading and unloading of trucks, the operations of crushers and shredders, all produce noise that may affect operators and nearby residents. Garbage, particularly containing household or other organic waste, becomes odoriferous, and some of the treatments, notably composting, may enhance the odor. The main prevention is to situate noisy and smelly facilities at an adequate distance from residential areas, other workplaces, and recreational areas.

In addition to risks of injury to workers, the transportation of garbage engenders a finite risk of transportation accidents that must be accounted for in a waste management plan.

Estimating exposure for a planned facility usually requires data on the operations of comparable facilities elsewhere. Since technology is always changing, it is often difficult to obtain relevant data, and for most facilities only sporadic data are available for review. Improvements in technology probably mean that relying on data from a plant that is several years old will be conservative since new facilities should perform better.

One limitation on using previously obtained data is that most available reports on pollutants released from waste treatment facilities list only the mean values with little information on the variability or excursion of the data. It would be more appropriate to be able to use the upper 95% confidence limit, for example.

A solid waste plan must be a long-range plan (20 to 30 years), and identify cost-efficient, environmentally sound programs and facilities that will reliably meet projected waste management needs.

THE TECHNOLOGIES
Incineration

The main elements of incineration require a loader, a burner, and a stack. Wastes are emptied into the incinerator usually after some kind of presorting to eliminate bulky and nonburnable items. They then enter a burner where, with or without mixing, they are exposed to high temperatures that oxidize chemicals and ideally break down organic molecules into carbon dioxide or even carbon. The noncombustible material, bottom ash, accumulates in the burner and must be emptied and usually landfilled. The remaining material, including volatile chemicals and very light fly ash, leaves the burner and must be captured by pollution control devices before they escape from the stack. Extensive technological development goes into increasing the efficiency of combustion and reducing the escape of toxic materials. Temperature and residence time in the burner are two of the main factors contributing to successful incineration.

New facilities are often planned as waste-to-energy or energy recovery facilities, harnessing the heat and perhaps gases for some other purposes, such as the generation of electricity.

Composting: (See Chapter 58)

Composting allows organic material to undergo bio- and photodegradation, resulting in simple organic molecules that can actually be beneficial to the environment. Many kinds of organic waste can be composted. The household compost pile of lawn clippings, leaf litter, and kitchen waste is the simplest and most widespread example of composting, with the proviso that after 2 to 3 years the waste can be used for garden mulch. This requires a certain amount of management: liming, and turning, which many householders do not accomplish.

In situ composting is achieved, for example, when grass clippings and leaves are left in place and allowed to decompose naturally. This can be accelerated with various mulching devices that fragment the leaves and grass and reduce damage to lawns. Certain municipalities have terminated the curbside collection of grass and leaves and refuse to accept them at local dumps, thereby requiring in situ treatment.

DATA ON FACILITIES OPERATIONS

Some of the different types of waste management technologies and facility types are described below. Many of these produce no air pollution, and for others there is little actual data on emissions. Where present, the projected emissions data and the air modeling data indicate that most would not contribute significantly to existing background levels of pollutants in residential areas under normal operations according to specifications.[4] However, since most of the estimates are based on mean emission values, the actual exposures may be higher than estimated as much as 50% of the time.

Certain facilities are potentially important sources of particulate and/or sulfur dioxide air pollution, for example, mass burn, refuse derived fuel, waste-to-energy facilities, sludge and medical waste incinerators, ash landfills, and sludge pelletizers. Among incinerators most pollutants showed less than an order of magnitude variation. Lead is an exception, with much higher releases from sludge burning than from most other sources.

The box on p. 629 lists the available waste management approaches. There are several subtypes for most of these.

Truck transfer stations are not expected to contribute significantly to local air pollution, assuming that vehicle exhaust is adequately vented, particularly if the engine is off while the truck is waiting and unloading. However, traffic, noise, odor, dust, and debris may pose a nuisance to the immediately contiguous residents, and vehicle emissions will increase along the route.

> **Waste management components**
>
> Source separation
> Separate collection
> Transfer stations and drop-off facilities
> Material recovery facilities (with or without incineration)
> Special waste processing (medical, harbor debris, sludge)
> Incineration (waste-to-energy, resource recovery)
> Landfilling
> Composting
> Reuse/recycling facilities

Marine transfer station. Air emissions of pollutants are probably insignificant, although windblown debris may be a nuisance and contribute to litter. Local contamination of water by debris and oil may occur. These are noisy operations, but are seldom located in proximity to other human activities.

Rail transfer station. Air emissions of pollutants are probably insignificant. However, these are likely to be noisy facilities.

Materials drop-off (mini-dumps, recycling centers). Air emissions of pollutants are usually insignificant. Traffic congestion and litter are potential problems, and vermin such as rats may be attracted. There is substantial opportunity for material reuse, since a large portion of the residential and commercial waste is completely reusable or repairable.[33]

Household hazardous waste drop-off. Air emissions of pollutants are generally insignificant unless there is spillage or improper treatment or transport. Many communities operate special Household Hazardous Waste Days once or twice a year. However, there is little data available on what is collected or how the community ultimately disposes of it. With rising costs for hazardous waste disposal there must be some way of paying for these programs. In a survey we found that users were more highly educated than the county average but were only slightly above the median income.

Waste oil facility. Air emissions of pollutants are usually minimal since most of the fractions have low volatility. Spillage must be avoided. Much of this material can be recycled.

Mixed waste in-vessel composting. Toxic air emissions of most pollutants is considered insignificant, with the exception of hydrogen sulfide. Dust and particulates can be generated as well as odor. Significant traffic is anticipated.

Leaf and yard waste composting. Toxic air emissions of most pollutants are considered insignificant except for hydrogen sulfide. Dust, mold spores, and other particulates can be generated as well as odor. If vegetation is contaminated with pesticides, toxic leachate may occur.

Sludge composting (see Chapter 58). Specific information on toxic air emissions is limited. Air quality modeling data indicate that toxic air pollutants (for example, hydrogen sulfide, benzene, CO) should not approach the relevant air quality standards, although caution should be taken to ensure that siting avoids elevated receptor populations such as nearby apartment buildings.[30] Odor is a potential problem locally. Various chemicals such as sulfuric acid and hypochlorite may be used to control odors, and then must be disposed of. Chlorine release can exceed the guideline value. Sewage sludge may contain mutagenic substances,[23] and the composting is intended to allow for biological degradation of these materials, rendering them safe for use as compost. This is an area of very active research today.

Sludge pelletizer. Data on this type of facility indicates a potentially significant output of sulfur dioxide and hydrogen chloride with levels exceeding the relevant standards; the data also indicated significant output of chromium, copper, lead, and zinc.[30] Odor is a potential problem locally.

Sludge chemical stabilization. Air emissions of pollutants is considered insignificant, but odor may be a problem. Contributes significantly to copper loading in the environment.

Materials recovery facility. In the absence of combustion, sulfur dioxide emission is not significant.[34] The modeled emissions do not reach levels that would cause a public health threat. Significant truck traffic is anticipated.

Construction and demolition processing. Toxic air emissions are less of a problem than dust and particulates. Asbestos release and wood treated with preservatives are the major concern. Careful storage is important because wet plaster or gypsum can produce significant odors.

Medical on-site chop and bleach. The grinding/disinfection facilities perform a wet operation that should reduce toxic air emissions. Odor complaints among building occupants are a potential problem. Careful transportation and disposal of treated waste is essential. Such facilities are enclosed, and exhaust air is filtered with a High Efficiency Particular filter (HEPA), hence there should be no pollution. However, chlorine release to air can exceed the criterion.

Medical on-site autoclave. An autoclave operates as an enclosed system, but must be properly vented. Common types use steam or ethylene oxide. The bags of treated waste can be handled as nonhazardous solid waste. Significant odor and air contamination occur when the autoclave is opened, particularly if operators must stand close by in an enclosed, inadequately ventilated room. Large regional autoclave facilities are planned for medical waste, and these can be designed specifically to minimize these hazards.

Harbor debris processing. The potential for toxic air emissions depends on how the waste is processed. Wood preservatives are a major concern, and waste burning may release toxic pollutants. The odor potential may be significant.

Dredge spoil dewatering. Lightweight volatile organic compounds may be released. Most contaminants of concern are heavy metals and polyaromatic hydrocarbons with low volatility. However, runoff and leachate of metal-contaminated material and odor are potential problems.

Waste tire processing. This is a grinding operation with the potential for dust and noise but neglible pollutants and odor unless the process overheats. Tires have also been disposed of in lakes and bays to create artificial reefs for fish.

Mass-burn (waste-to-energy) incineration. This category includes the garbage incinerators that have been very controversial. It ranks high among the potential emitters of toxic air pollutants. Nonetheless, the estimated emissions and modeled air concentrations for New York did not exceed relevant standards.[30] For most metals the Protection Index was well above 100. However, for hydrogen chloride, particulates less than 10 μm (PM-10), sulfur dioxide, oxides of nitrogen, dioxin, and arsenic the Protection Indices were <100. For oxides of nitrogen the Protection Index was only 15. This in turn can be expected to contribute to increased ozone levels.

Refuse-derived fuel (waste-to-energy). Another form of incineration, this potentially contributes to significant air pollution. There is little available data to adequately characterize emissions from such facilities, and the technology for energy conversion and pollution control is changing. In one study[30] the Protection Index for most pollutants was greater than 100, but for cadmium, nickel, and oxides of nitrogen it was less than 20.

Sludge incinerator. Based on the scant available data, such facilities could contribute significantly to air pollution. For New York City the modeled air concentrations indicated a Protection Index of only 7 for nickel and 10 for arsenic.[30]

Medical incinerator. Such incinerators potentially contribute significantly to odor and airborne lead. Calcium oxide and carbonate are used for odor control. Large regional incinerators are being planned to reduce the number of point sources. The available data and resultant modeling produced Protection Indices of 4 for hydrogen chloride, 7 for oxides of nitrogen, 9 for dioxin, and 13 for cadmium. Significant technological improvements are required for these facilities, which are necessary to replace obsolete or proscribed hospital incinerators. Protection Indices should at least exceed 10x.

Ash landfill. For any form of incineration, about 25% of the original volume remains as ash, which must be disposed of in some way. Various reuse options are being considered for ash, particularly its use in highway construction materials. However, at present landfilling is the major option. Air emissions of most toxic pollutants is probably insignificant, since most volatile compounds are destroyed in the incinerator, but under certain conditions dust and particulates can be generated as well as odor (depending on the quality of the ash). The main problem is likely to be leaching of toxic heavy metals. This would be one of the main sources of arsenic. Airborne dust carried to nearby residential communities could be significant when trucks disrupt unpaved surfaces.

Municipal solid waste landfill. In most cases toxic air emissions are low except for releases of methane. This assumes that no toxic wastes are dumped. Dust and debris may be generated, and high truck traffic is anticipated. Typical garbage odors represent a mixture of aromatic organic compounds, putrescines, mercaptans, and others. There is a high potential for leaching of hazardous materials into ground water or the runoff of waste into adjacent surface water.

ESTIMATING PUBLIC HEALTH RISK

In addition to the environmental standards, health agencies have estimated the amount or concentrations of material below which no health hazards exist. The plethora of these standards indicates that no single one is satisfactory. For occupational exposures the American Conference of Governmental Industrial Hygienists[1] lists Threshold Limit Values for several hundred industrial chemicals. These are supposed to be values to which most individuals can be exposed for a 40-hour work week over a 40-year working lifetime without adverse health effects. Many of these were adopted by the Occupational Safety and Health Administration (OSHA) as legally enforceable Permissible Exposure Limits (PELs).

Workers are generally the healthiest component of the population and are in the workplace usually for less than 25% of the work week. For the remainder of the time their bodies can readjust to nonexposed situations. People who stay in their homes all the time (168 hours a week), for example, young children, the elderly, or the infirm, would have continuous exposure and might also be more susceptible. There is no generally accepted approach to extrapolating from a PEL or TLV to an acceptable community or residential exposure level. A common rule-of-thumb approach is to divide the PEL by 100 to estimate an appropriate ambient air guideline for residential exposure. However, there are better alternative approaches.

Reference Doses derived by the U.S. Environmental Protection Agency (EPA) estimates the amount of material that can be ingested or inhaled without causing adverse health effects. The method for estimating these is given in Chapter 67. One approach to developing an ambient air guideline is to estimate it from the RfD for inhalation and calculating how much material could be in the air breathed by a person without exceeding the RfD. For example, if the RfD for a substance is 10 mg/kg/day, then a 70-kg adult could take in up to 700 mg/day without exceeding the RfD. Using the standardized estimate for an active adult of breathing 20 m^3 of air per day would result in a maximum allowable concentration of 700/20 or 35 mg/m^3 (assuming that the material were 100% absorbable from the lung).

Recently the Agency for Toxic Substances and Disease Registry[2] has derived its own Environmental Media Evaluation Guidelines (EMEGs) based on Minimum Risk Levels. These do not take into account cancer or special high-exposure subgroups such as children with pica who would

Table 55-4. The media × route matrix for communities potentially exposed to incinerator emissions*

Environmental medium	Routes of exposure		
	Ingestion	Inhalation	Dermal
Air	Particulates TSP	++++ PM-10	Variable Vapors Liquids
Probability	Low	Medium	Very low
Soil	Dirt-on-hands	Re-entrained dust	Muds
Probability	Low	Very low	Low
Water	++++	Showers Aerosols	Liquid
Probability	Low	Low	Low
Food	++++	0	0
Probability	Uncertain	0	0

*From Gochfeld M: A Matrix of Routes and Media of Exposure for Risk Assessment Scenarios, Piscataway, NJ, 1990, Environmental and Occupational Health Sciences Institute.

consume excessive amounts of dirt, paint chips, and other detritus. To date EMEGs have been published for only a few substances.

In evaluating the public health risk from any environmental hazard or facility it is customary to think in terms of sources of contamination, environmental media, routes of exposure, and characteristics of the target population (see Chapter 67). For solid waste management the sources of contamination will be both stationary (the individual operating facilities) and mobile (the collection/transportation component).

The environmental media of concern include air, water (particularly as sources of drinking water), soil, and food.[15,16,24] The routes of exposure are inhalation (of air and dust), ingestion (of food and water), and absorption through the skin (probably negligible for these pollutants). These are summarized in the exposure matrix (Table 55-4). The target populations composed of individual receptors are human (workers on a site, workers near a site, and residents in the community) and nonhuman (wildlife and natural ecosystems). Airborne contamination is considered the major medium of concern, with inhalation as the primary route of exposure.

POLLUTION CONTROL DEVICES

There are a number of issues that must be addressed in the design of pollution control devices (PCDs), and this technology is rapidly changing. The efficiency of devices such as baghouses and electrostatic precipitation (ESP) is directly related to particle size and/or charge and by the airflow rate through the PCD. Baghouse removal efficiency has direct cost consequences, since the greater pressure drop induced by more efficient removal increases operating costs. Scrubbers must be designed to avoid a rapid cooling of the flue gas, which would reduce the exit velocity and plume height and increase nearfield deposition. A new generation of ''dry scrubbers'' is being developed to increase the efficiency of removal of contaminated particulates.

Normally vaporized metals will condense as the flue gas cools and may deposit on particulates and be removed by efficient pollution control devices. Because of its volatility, mercury is a notable exception, and MSW incinerators release significant quantities of mercury. Source separation of batteries is considered a major advantage for removing both mercury and cadmium, as well as nickel, lead, and zinc.

One of the problems with air pollution control devices is that the smallest particles have the largest surface-to-mass ratio. Certain elements that adsorb to these surfaces may be present at very high levels. As the air passes through a PCD the concentration of metals may actually increase, because the smallest particles escape,[36] resulting in a disproportionate amount of the smallest particles with the highest concentrations of toxics. This is referred to as ''enrichment'' and has been reported for dioxins and certain metals.

EMISSION DATA

From an exposure assessment and risk assessment perspective, the main problem in modeling future exposure lies in the paucity of existing data on emissions from comparable facilities. Ideally one would like to have reference facility data that provide information on the statistical distribution of the variable of interest (such as mercury emission) under different operating conditions. A balanced, designed experiment with several replicates of various operating conditions would provide valuable information. Such data are very scarce.[36]

A review of the information available on MSW incinerator operations revealed only a very few reports that provided systematic data on emissions, with even fewer that have attempted to describe operations under various combinations of controlled conditions. Most of these studies turned out to be flawed in one way or another, because one or more of the preset combinations were not achieved.[36]

It is possible to take the mean of a small set of numbers and have it seriously underestimate (or overestimate) the hazard that may occur a significant fraction of the time (say 10% of the time). Assuming that the distribution is log-normal (a common occurrence for comparable environmental data), then the upper 95% confidence limit around the mean value is most likely to be within one order of magnitude of the mean. That is, if the mean is 10, then it is likely that 95% of the values will be below 100.

EMISSIONS OF PUBLIC HEALTH CONCERN

Details on specific pollutants of public health concern are provided in other chapters. Environmental impacts of incineration emissions are associated with heavy metals (from stack and bottom ash), organic products of incomplete combustion (known as PICSs), including particularly the chlorinated polyaromatic compounds such as dioxins, acid gases (SOx, HCl, HF, NOx), and particulates.

For any single incinerator the benefit to risk and cost ratio depends in part on the volume reduction achieved, on the ability to site facilities in appropriate areas, on the effective destruction of organic compounds, on the ability to move metal-contaminated ash to secure sites (either for landfilling or recovery), and on the potential for energy recovery.

Maximizing combustion efficiency requires an appropriate fuel, and a combination of temperature, residence time in the burner, and aeration. This in turn requires attention both to the "hardware" or facility design and to the "software," or maintenance of the facility as well as the feedstock with adequate BTU content. Communities are justifiably concerned over whether a facility, once built, will be maintained and operated according to specifications.

Reduction of emissions, therefore, depends on the initial separation and removal of noncombustibles, possible fuel supplementation, design of the furnace, the boiler, and the stoker/grate, and the installation and maintenance of air pollution control devices such as ESP, baghouses, and acid gas scrubbers.

The availability of recycling options is limited primarily by the available markets and technologies for recycling, and to a lesser extent by behavioral factors, the willingness of generators to source-separate. Nonetheless, heavy emphasis on recycling in schools indicates that the next generation is much more likely to be prepared and even anxious to consider total source separation as a realistic option.[17]

TOXIC HAZARDS FROM WASTE MANAGEMENT TECHNOLOGIES
Particulates

In addition to their direct effect on the respiratory system, particulates serve as nuclei for concentrating heavy metals and organic compounds. Certain organics and metals that vaporize in the incinerator may condense in the pollution control devices or even beyond them in the stack or the atmosphere. The solid particulates can be fractionated by size. Total Suspended Particulates (TSP) includes particles of varying size but sufficiently small to remain airborne for long periods. Particles greater than 10 μm have little likelihood of reaching the lung. Particulate matter less than 10 μm (the PM-10 fraction) is of greater interest because it is inhalable and can reach the trachea and larger bronchi. In recent studies the PM-10 data are often given. However, even more important are particulates less than 5 μm or less than 3.5 μm in diameter, which are likely to evade all of the lung's defense mechanism and reach the alveoli, where adsorbed matter may be absorbed into the bloodstream. These data are seldom given. Up to half of the particles emitted are in the respirable range, and because of their greater surface-to-mass ratio, certain organics, heavy metals, and acid gases adsorb preferentially to this fraction. The National Ambient Air Quality Standard averaged over a 24-hour period is 150 μg/m^3 for PM-10 and TSP. The 1-year average is 50 μg/m^3 for PM-10 and 75 μg/m^3 for TSP.

Dioxins and furans

Probably the most frequent public concern voiced over incineration is the formation and emission of polychlorinated dibenzofurans (PCDFs) and dioxins (PCDDs), particularly 2,3,7,8-tetrachloro dibenzo dioxin (TCDD).[7,31] Although the formation is often assumed to arise entirely from incomplete combustion and chemical reactions in the burner, the scant data available suggest that these chlorinated polyaromatics may be formed beyond the burner in the PCD and stack as the flue gasses cool and phenolic compounds come in contact with chlorine, perhaps in the presence of fine metal particulates. The main source of the phenoloic is likely to be lignin (from paper and wood) reacting with chlorine or HCl released from plastics. Lignin is a polyphenolic compound that is the main source of aromatic hydrocarbons in MSW incineration. Source separation of paper and plastic should greatly reduce the formation of PCDF and PCDD. Nonetheless, some of these compounds are introduced with the feedstock.[11] For example, PCDF in the feedstock accounts for about 4% of the PCDF emitted.

Part of the controversy over emissions of these compounds arises from conflicting data.[3,6] This is partly due to methodology, for if synthesis in the stack is important, there will be a discrepancy depending on whether sampling occurs before the stack or at the stack. Ideally, sampling should be at the top of the stack where the actual emissions are captured, but for convenience stack sampling is usually conducted at or near the base. Haile[20] reported the concentration of PCDD and PCDF in fly ash is about 10 times greater than in the flue gas, but others have found that most of these compounds were emitted in gaseous form. Sampling the ESP plates may not adequately reflect emissions, since ESP are only moderately effective in removing PCDD and PCDF.[11]

Monitoring of PCDD and PCDF levels emitted is complicated by the rather high inter-day variation documented for the Hamilton-Wentworth (Ontario) facility[11] and for the Hampton, VA, facility.[20] Emissions of total PCDD and PCDF per ton of MSW have been reported between 1 and 45 mg/ton.[20,31] The dioxin concentration in flue gas increased fivefold as the temperature dropped from 350°C to 200°C.[8]

Burning paper, wood, vegetable matter, or PVC alone produces a negligible increase in PCDF and PCDD compared with burning a combination of paper or wood with PVC.[31] PVC yields 90% HCl when burned, and this is probably the main chlorine donor. The reactions combining phenolics with HCl are more likely to occur when they are adsorbed to fly ash paricles than when they are in the gaseous state.

Commoner et al (1984),[7] severe critics of incineration,

argue that if the PCDF/PCDD formation occurs after the burner, then regardless of the efficiency of standard pollution control devices, these compounds will be emitted. In that case improved operating conditions must ensure the complete destruction of the phenolic precurors. However, Commoner et al.[7] argue that since phenol is not a limiting factor, even if 0.1% remains this would be 1000 times greater than what was needed to maximize PCDD/PCDF synthesis.

Acid and irritant gases

Sulfur dioxide. Sulfur dioxide is a direct irritant to the eyes, mucus membranes, and lungs. It is also a major contributor to acid precipitation.

Oxides of nitrogen. The family of NOx includes particularly the irritating nitrogen dioxide. These chemicals are associated with respiratory illness and also figure in the photochemical generation of ozone, another irritant.

Hydrogen chloride (HCl). This gas forms hydrochloric acid on contact with moist membranes in the eyes and respiratory tract.

Hydrogen fluoride (HF). This is even more corrosive than HCl, but is emitted in much smaller quantities.

Carbon monoxide (CO). This chemical asphyxiant gas is the classic product of incomplete combustion. It exerts its toxicity by binding with hemoglobin and preventing the transport of oxygen. Humans are normally exposed to relatively high levels of carbon monoxide from automobile combustion and cigarette smoking, and it is unlikely that environmental contamination from incineration or other waste management scenarios would contribute materially to the high background. However, faulty operations could pose a problem to workers at the facility.

Ammonia (NH_3). This is not likely to be emitted by incinerators, but may arise from other waste management activities, particularly composting.

Volatile organic compounds

Many low-molecular-weight aromatic and aliphatic hydrocarbons may escape in the flue gas, through incomplete combustion or chemical reaction, because of inadequate temperature or aeration, excessive airflow, or inadequate mixing or residence time. Some chemical synthesis and condensation reaction may also occur in the hot flue gases. Common volatiles of concern include benzene, toluene, xylene, phenol, vinyl chloride, methylene chloride, trichloroethylene, and chloroform. Two compounds released by burning plastic, acrolein and phosgene, are usually not included in incineration measurements. Both are highly irritating, but both should be destroyed by a properly operating incinerator.

HEAVY METALS

These are of concern because they are not destroyed by incineration. They may be present in bottom or fly ash in elemental form or in inorganic or organic complexes or compounds. They may be vaporized and may be present in stack gases, although most condense and adsorb to particulates. Most data sets provide numbers for at least some of the metals of public health concern (for example, lead, mercury, arsenic, cadmium, chromium, nickel, manganese, beryllium), whereas others such as tin and zinc are often not measured.

Several metals are known or suspected carcinogens, particularly hexavalent chromium (Cr-VI), nickel, arsenic, beryllium[14] and cadmium. For chromium both the trivalent (an essential trace element) and hexavalent (a carcinogen)[13] forms may be present in incinerator emissions, and there is controversy over which prevails.

Other metals measured in some of the incineration studies that pose less of a public health problem from inhalation include cobalt, copper, selenium, and zinc. These are all essential trace elements, and it is unlikely that people would be exposed to toxic amounts from inhalation of waste management emissions. On the other hand, some metals such as tin that may be important are seldom considered.

Noise

A solid waste management system can be noisy. The early-morning clanking of garbage cans being emptied is a familiar sound in many cities. But the transport and unloading of trash and the operation of some facilities may produce noise as well. The system should not result in a residential noise level exceeding 60 dB-A (see Chapter 50). Besides curbside collection noise, the operation of a rail transfer station is likely to be unacceptably noisy.[30] The main protection from noise is "distance," since noise decreases by the inverse square law. Noise barriers commonly used along highways could surround noisy waste facilities. Noise is likely to represent an occupational hazard to workers in the waste management facilities.

Odor

Odors associated with landfilling and composting are often objectionable. However, they may not pose a problem much beyond the site boundary. Odors are mainly a nuisance and a public relations problem, but hydrogen sulfide and ammonia are toxic and odoriferous products of composting. Anaerobic conditions favoring odor formation can be avoided. There is not a generally accepted medical view regarding health hazards of offensive odors per se. Chronic unwanted odors, however, are particularly stressful to communities and have formed the basis of significant community opposition in siting disputes in other areas, even when health is not an issue.

Some small incinerators such as hospital incinerators can produce significant odors that effect other people working in the facility. Again, siting facilities or their exhausts at an adequate distance from receptor populations or fresh air intakes should eliminate the unwanted nuisance effects of odor.

Implications for siting

This chapter has emphasized public health concerns related to the potential toxic emissions to air and water from alternative waste management facilities. In addition, aesthetic, economic, traffic, and other considerations profoundly impact the willingness of a community or governmental jurisdiction to accept any kind of waste management facility.

Regardless of the choice of technology, siting of a facility should take the following into account:

1. Selection of sites that minimize proximity to residential areas and to unrelated areas of employment, and that also minimize exposure to sensitive terrestrial and aquatic ecosystems
2. Adequate size of site to minimize exposure to surrounding communities
3. Adequate distance from high-rise buildings to reduce the impact on elevated receptor populations
4. Adequate stack height; avoiding areas with Federal Aviation Administration regulations on stack heights
5. Involvement of the community in the earliest stages of planning, including a clear presentation of the cost–benefit and risk–benefit considerations
6. Assurance of adequate maintenance and safe operation backed up by posting a bond with the community allowing it to monitor and even shut down a faulty facility

REFERENCES

1. ACGIH: *1993-1994 Threshold Limit Values for chemical substances and physical agents and biological exposure indices,* Cinncinati, 1993, American Conference of Governmental Industrial Hygienists.
2. ATSDR: *Environmental media exposure guidelines,* Atlanta, 1991, Agency for Toxic Substances and Disease Registry.
3. Benfenati E et al: Polychlorinated dibenzo-p-dioxins (PCDDs) and polychlorinated diebenzofurans (PCDF) in emissions from an urban incinerator. 2. correlation between concentration of micropollutants and combustion conditions, *Chemosphere* 12:1151, 1983.
4. Blake DE: Source assessment sampling system: design and development. Report to U.S. Environmental Protection Agency, Washington, DC, EPA-600/7-78-018, 1978.
5. Brunner CR: *Hazardous air emissions from incinerators,* New York, 1985, Chapman & Hall.
6. Choudhry GG, Hutzinger O: *Mechanistic aspects of the thermal formation of halogenated organic compounds including polychlorinated dibenzo-p-dioxins,* New York, 1983, Gordon & Breach.
7. Commoner B et al: *Environmental and economic analysis of alternative municipal solid waste disposal technologies,* Flushing, NY, 1984, Center for Biology of Natural Systems, Queens College.
8. Cooper Engineering: *Air emissions and performance testing of a dry scrubber (Quench Reactor), Dry Venturi and fabric filter system operating on flue gas from combustion of municipal solid waste at Tsushima, Japan.* Report to Contra Costa County CA, 1984.
9. Diaz LF, Savage GM, Golueke G: *Resource recovery from municipal solid wastes,* vol 2, *Final processing,* Boca Raton, Fla, 1982, CRC Press.
10. Dyer FR, Esch VH: Polyvinyl chloride and toxicity of fires, *JAMA* 235:393, 1976.
11. Envirocom: *Report on combustion testing program at the SWARU Plant, Hamilton-Wentworth,* Report to Ontario Ministry of the Environment, ARB-43-84- ETRD, 1984.
12. EPA: *Comprehensive assessment of the specific compounds present in combustion process,* vol 1, *Pilot studies of emissions variability,* Washington, DC, 1983, WPA Office of Toxic Substances.
13. EPA: *Health effects assessment document for hexavalent chromium,* EPA/540/1-86/019, Research Triangle Park, NC, 1984, Environmental Criteria and Assessment Office.
14. EPA: *Health assessment document for beryllium,* EPA/600-8-84/026F, Office of Health & Environmental Assessment, Washington, DC, 1987.
15. EPA: Proposed maximum contaminant levels in drinking water, *Fed Res* 53:31537, 1988.
16. EPA: *Health effects assessment summary tables,* OERR 9200.6-303-(89-2), Cincinnati, 1989, Office of Health and Environmental Assessment.
17. Gochfeld M, Burger J: *The Earth Day 20 school poster contest: how young people view the environment,* New Jersey, 1990, Environmental & Occupational Health Sciences Institute.
18. Gochfeld M, Favata EA: *Hazardous waste workers state-of-the-art reviews in occupational medicine,* vol 5, Philadelphia, 1990, Hanley & Belfus.
19. Gochfeld M, Szenics J: *Emergency guidelines for firefighters* Trenton, NJ, 1993, New Jersey Department of Health.
20. Haile CL et al: *Assessment of emissions of specific compounds from a Resource Recovery Municipal Refuse Incinerator,* Final report to US Environmental Protection Agency, Contract No. 68-01-5915, Cincinnati, 1984.
21. Hershkowitz A: How garbage could meet its maker, *Atlantic Monthly,* June 1993, p 108.
22. Higgins T: *Hazardous waste minimization handbook,* Chelsea, Mich, 1989, Lewis.
23. Hopke PK et al: Multitechnique screening of Chicago municipal sewage sludge for mutagenic activity, *Environ Sci Technol* 16:140, 1982.
24. Lioy P: Assesing total human exposure to contaminants, *Environ Sci Technol* 24:938, 1990.
25. Nessel C et al: Evaluation of the relative contribution of exposure routes in a health risk assessment of dioxin emissions from a municipal waste incinerator, *J Exposure Analysis & Environ Epidem* 1:283, 1991.
26. Nobile P, Deedy J: *The complete ecology fact book* Garden City, NY, 1972, Doubleday.
27. NRC: *Guides for short term exposures of the public to air pollutants. VIII. guide for chlorine,* US EPA Contract No CPA 70-57, Washington, DC, 1973, Committee on Toxicology, National Research Council.
28. NRC: *Chlorine and hydrogen chloride,* Washington, DC, 1976, National Academy of Sciences.
29. NYDEC: *New York State air guide 1. guidelines for the control of toxic ambient air contaminants,* Albany, NY, 1985-1986, Department of Environmental Conservation, Division of Air Resources.
30. NYDS: *Solid waste management plan: environmental impact,* New York, 1991, New York City Department of Sanitation.
31. Olie K et al: Formation and fate of PCDD and PCDF from combustion processes, *Chemosphere* 12:627, 1983.
32. OTA: *Materials and energy from municipal waste: resource recovery and recycling from municipal solid waste and beverage container deposit legislation,* Washington, DC, 1979, OTA-M-93, Office of Technology Assessment.
33. Pringle L: *Throwing things away,* New York, 1986, Thomas Y. Crowell.
34. Sengupta S, Wong KV: *Resource recovery from solid wastes,* New York, 1982, Pergamon Press.
35. Travis CC, Hattemer-Frey HA: *Health effects of municipal waste incineration,* Boca Raton, Fla, 1991, CRC Press.
36. Wartenberg D et al: *How reliable are emission factors: enrichment of metals inversely related to particle size.* Report to New Jersey Hazardous Substances Control Research Center, Newark, 1990.

Chapter 56

COMMUNITY EXPOSURE TO HAZARDOUS WASTE

Michael Gochfeld

Definition of hazardous waste
Federal regulations
Hazardous waste sites
    Chemicals in hazardous waste sites
    Chemical releases
The role of risk assessment
Federal sites: The Department of Defense and Department of Energy
Exposure to hazardous waste
    Concentration
    Exposure
    Internal Dose
    Threshold
Mixtures of chemicals
Health effects from hazardous waste
    Concordance and biologic plausibility
    Exposure
    Temporal relationship
Temporal aspects of exposure
The role of clinicians
    Advising the exposed patient
Evaluation of community exposure to hazardous wastes
    House occupancy scenarios
    Dietary scenario
    Childhood soil scenario
    Vulnerability of the population
Case studies of community exposure to hazardous waste
    Chemical Control, New Jersey
Reducing community exposure
Health surveys and epidemiologic studies
The role of medical surveillance for the community
Special problems
    Leaking underground storage tanks
    Low-level radioactive waste
Prevention of exposure to hazardous waste

Hazardous waste has become one of the major, and potentially most expensive, public health concerns.[64] Wastes produced by the chemical, petrochemical, and pharmaceutical industries over nearly a century have been deposited at many locations both on and off industrial property. In addition, hazardous wastes have been generated in huge quantities at military facilities and at facilities operated by contractors of the U.S. Department of Energy (DOE). Household and municipal waste also contain hazardous materials. The distribution of hazardous waste is not an inevitable consequence of modern society; source reduction and waste minimization are approaches to improvement of the use of resources and manufacturing processes so that less waste is generated.[36] Much of the waste that is generated can be reclaimed and reused or recycled.[45] Waste minimization will inevitably become a critical issue of the 1990s. The Environmental Protection Agency (EPA) has several programs, including a Waste Reduction Innovative Technology Evaluation Program, to evaluate new technologies for waste reduction and a Waste Reduction Assessment Program to encourage the use of waste minimization.[21]

During the 1980s the magnitude of the hazardous waste problem became evident in the United States, and costs in excess of a trillion dollars are estimated if the nation were to undertake complete cleanups at all sites. Although many sites do pose significant or potential hazards to health,[2,3,8,34] there are many sites whose health risks are negligible.[31] On a national basis, people are beginning to question the need and cost-effectiveness of cleaning up every site. Once the most hazardous sites are controlled, greater public health benefits can be achieved by attacking other environmental public health problems with the limited fiscal resources available.

Among the chemical wastes are used solvents, unreacted raw material, low-quality products, sludges and residues from reactor vessels, heavy metals, and other chemicals that a company cannot or chooses not to reuse, reclaim, or recycle. In addition to solid and liquid chemical wastes, there is concern in many communities over radioactive and infectious waste materials.[1,2,4]

The book *Hazardous Waste in America*,[18] by Samuel Epstein and co-authors, stirred controversy over the magnitude of the problem, but many of their observations were subsequently confirmed, and if anything the magnitude of hazardous waste contamination has been underestimated. At the same time, however, the actual health impacts of hazardous waste remain unclear, and the number of people who are or have been exposed to sufficient chemical, radioactive, or biologic waste to actually damage their health is unknown.[56]

The assessment, management, and clean-up of hazardous waste poses a significant hazard to workers,[26,51] but this chapter is concerned with exposure in homes, schools, and communities. Exposure may occur at or near the site where the waste has been generated, along transportation routes, and near sites of ultimate disposal. In communities, hazardous waste has emerged as a major public health concern and political issue. Physicians are increasingly faced with the challenge of evaluating risk in their community and providing expert advice and sound individual counsel on collective and individual risks.[30,32,37]

DEFINITION OF HAZARDOUS WASTE

As defined in the Resource Conservation and Recovery Act of 1976 (RCRA)[59] a solid waste can be called hazardous if its ''quantity, concentration, or physical, chemical or infectious characteristic'' leads to mortality or serious illness or otherwise poses a ''substantial present or potential hazard to human health or the environment, when improperly treated, stored, transported, or disposed of, or otherwise mismanaged.'' This definition is very broad, and more than 50,000 chemicals (raw materials, by-products, solvents, catalysts, and products) that meet this definition are subject to provisions of the Toxic Substances Control Act of 1976.[62] Infectious or medical waste and low-level radioactive waste (LLRW) are components of hazardous waste. Various properties of hazardous wastes that qualify them as ignitable, corrosive, reactive, or toxic are listed in Table 56-1.

The EPA estimates that about 250 million tons of hazardous waste are produced annually in the United States. Although it is usually associated closely with industry, only about 6% of this amount is directly industrial in orgin. Agricultural chemicals and mining waste account for the largest volume production.[15] Table 56-2 provides a breakdown of waste from a sample of the total waste generated for 1979.[31]

Table 56-1. Characteristics of hazardous wastes (used by the U.S. EPA)

Characteristics	Criteria
Ignitability	Liquids with flashpoint below 60°C
	Nonliquids capable of igniting through friction or chemical reaction
	Ignitable compressed gases
	Oxidizing chemicals
Corrosivity	Aqueous wastes with pH less than 3 or above 12
	Liquids that can corrode steel faster than 0.25 inches/yr
Reactivity	Class A and B explosives
	Explosion on direct physical force
	Explosion at normal temperature and pressure
	Chemicals that undergo violent and spontaneous chemical reaction
	Chemicals that react violently with water
	Generation of toxic vapors or fumes when mixed with acids, bases, or water
Toxicity	Waste contains concentrations of arsenic, barium, cadmium, chromium, mercury, selenium, silver, endrin, lindane, methoxychlor, toxaphene, 2,4-dichlorophenoxyacetic acid, 2,4,5-tichlorophenoxyacetic acid, silvex, etc. above some criteria
	A solid waste that fails the extraction procedure (EP toxicity) test

FEDERAL REGULATIONS

Under federal laws the hazardous waste management responsibility has two major divisions. The RCRA governs the production and disposal of hazardous materials. It regulates the management and disposal of hazardous waste by companies producing it. Permits are required for transportation and disposal of hazardous waste, and a manifest system provides for the cradle-to-grave tracking of waste from the site of production to its ultimate disposal, whether on or off site. In theory at least, RCRA could bring to an end the improper handling and disposal of hazardous waste now being generated. By increasing the cost of waste management it might also provide market incentives for waste minimization.

The Comprehensive Environmental Responsibility, Cleanup and Liability Act (CERCLA), the so-called Superfund Act, focuses on remediation of abandoned waste sites. CERCLA has provisions for identifying and characterizing sites, for setting priorities of sites for clean-up, for expending Superfund monies for remediation of sites, and for researching hazardous waste.[44] CERCLA created the Agency for Toxic Substances and Disease Registry (ATSDR) as part of the Centers for Disease Control. It also created the National Priority List (NPL), which has become popularly known as the Superfund List. Under CERCLA, the EPA administers the Superfund, established by a tax on petrochemical and

Table 56-2. Types of hazardous materials

Type	Percentage of total*
Oily wastes	
Sludge	0.7
Waste oil	0.5
Recoverable oil	1.1
Organic wastes	
Solvents	1.0
Organics	0.8
Organic liquids	1.8
Organics and metal salts	0.6
Halogenated solvents	0.6
Biocides, polychlorinated biphenyls	0.1
Contaminated containers	0.8
Waste-water sludges	1.6
Spent caustic acid	0.7
Energy-recoverable waste	0.7
Scrap plastic, rubber	13.7
Inorganic waste	
Inert waste	18.7
Potentially recoverable waste	11.19
Heavy metals	43.5
Water-soluble waste	0.2
Acids and alkalis	1.5
Reactive inorganics	0.1
Miscellaneous	
Dilute aqueous solutions	0.1
Total extrapolated amount	100.0
Major classes of wastes	
Oily wastes	2.3
Organic wastes	22.3
Inorganic wastes	75.2

From Greenberg MR, Anderson RF: *Hazardous waste sites: the credibility gap*, New Brunswick, NJ, 1984, Rutgers University Press.
*Based on a total of 3.5 million tons per year.

chemical industries, which provides the government funds to conduct site investigations and remediation.

The EPA has the responsibility for evaluating the extent of contamination and approving plans for and overseeing remediation, and the ATSDR has responsibility for evaluating hazards to and health of communities. The EPA can also provide grants to communities to facilitate their informed participation in the hazardous waste management and remediation process.[16]

The protection, training, and medical surveillance of hazardous-waste workers is mandated under the Occupational Safety and Health Administration Hazardous Waste and Emergency Response standard (1989 CFR 1910.120).

The Superfund Amendment and Reauthorization Act, particularly its Title III (referred to as SARA Title III), made sweeping changes requiring communities to establish Local Emergency Response Committees (LERC) to review potential chemical release hazards and develop local emergency plans. Any facility experiencing a toxic release had to provide emergency notification to both the state and the LERC. Community right to know was established, and the EPA was required to develop a toxic chemical release inventory.[17]

The EPA is responsible for performing emergency mitigation or removal actions and for planning longer-term remedial actions. If responsible parties can be identified, the EPA can require them to retrieve waste or clean up sites or can conduct the clean-up and then sue the responsible party for damages.[45] Although it is customary to think of a cleanup in which all hazardous material is removed from a site and all contaminated soil or water is either removed or treated, in actuality there are other more common and less complete types of mitigation (see Chapter 57). Often only the most hazardous components are removed and the site is otherwise covered or secured so that waste will not migrate offsite or people will not move on-site to be exposed. On-site containment is increasingly important as the costs for clean-up mount. New technologies (see later) are employed for in situ cleanup of contaminated soil and groundwater.

If the responsible party enters into an administrative consent agreement with either the EPA or a state, it may perform a remedial investigation/feasibility study under the watchful eye of the EPA. If it is approved, the responsible party can then perform the remediation and ultimately have its clean-up or containment certified.

HAZARDOUS WASTE SITES

It is difficult to estimate how many hazardous waste sites exist in the United States. Hart[35] estimated at least 50,000, of which states have listed more than 30,000,[44] yet only about 1200 have been listed on the NPL and are slated for remedial action under Superfund. This list does not include many sites on active industrial properties that are managed under RCRA.

The sites include landfills, drum dumps, abandoned warehouses, and waste-water lagoons.[59] Mounds of mine tailings, weapons bunkers, tanks of nerve gases, rusted 55-gallon drums, and torn bags of unused fertilizer are some of the characteristic findings at such sites. The EPA has established a hazard ranking system (HRS), which includes not only the identification and quantification of contaminants on site but the potential for exposure. The HRS is used to determine whether a site qualifies for the NPL.

Site assessment has become a scientific discipline and is described in more detail in Chapter 57. It embodies the following stages: initial site identification, preliminary site assessment (followed in some cases by emergency interventions), a remedial investigation/feasibility study, and remediation. Many different actions qualify as remediation (see Chapter 57), and it is essential to realize that designation as a Superfund site does not always mean that a site actually poses a significant health hazard or that it will be cleaned up. Indeed, many Superfund sites remain today, unchanged from when they were listed more than a decade ago; some are not even secured and do not adequately warn of the hazards present.[24] In some cases, sites that have been studied

Table 56-3. Top 10 chemicals reported in the First 546 Superfund Sites

Chemicals	Number of sites*
Trichlorethylene	129
Toluene	95
Benzene	94
Lead	93
Chlorotorm	68
Polychlorinated biphenyls	58
Tetrachloroethylene	57
Phenol	55
1,1,1-trichloroethane	54
Chromium	53

Adapted from data in Mitre: Computer printout of National Priorities List: data summaries for the 546 final and proposed sites, report to EPA, McLean, VA, 1983.

have been found to pose less of a hazard than was originally anticipated.[24]

Chemicals in hazardous waste sites

Table 56-3 lists the chemicals found at the largest number of hazardous waste sites. They obviously represent some of the commonest chemicals used in commerce, and the toxic properties of most are well established. Certain sites, however, may have large quantities of chemicals for which there is little toxicologic information.

Of approximately 2000 chemicals on the Department of Transportation's hazardous substance list, the EPA has identified a Hazardous Substance List of about 150 chemicals for analysis in soil and water, including 129 labeled "priority pollutants." These chemicals are the most toxic, the most widely encountered, and/or the most useful surrogates to indicate the presence of extensive contamination.

Chemical releases

A dramatic component of the hazardous-waste picture are the sudden, massive chemical releases resulting from fires, spills, transportation accidents, and industrial explosions. The methylisocyanate release at Bhopal, India, killed more than 2000 people, but there are many releases that kill only a few people or cause illness but do not achieve widespread public attention. There are more than 1000 severe chemical releases, causing about 200 deaths per year.[6]

THE ROLE OF RISK ASSESSMENT

The formal process of risk assessment (see Chapter 58) has been used to set priorities for control of hazardous-waste sites. A well-performed risk assessment can estimate the likelihood that increased rates of diseases (particularly cancer) will occur in a population with actual or potential exposure to hazardous waste. The HRS, discussed earlier, is a very crude form of risk assessment that determines whether a site qualifies for the NPL. Risk assessment is controversial, however, because people question either its ability to provide meaningful estimates of risk or the validity of use of worst-case assumptions in estimation of exposure. In most cases the commonest hazardous materials present can be measured with some precision, but estimation of exposure is rarely simple[42] (see Chapter 57).

FEDERAL SITES: THE DEPARTMENT OF DEFENSE AND DEPARTMENT OF ENERGY

Approximately 10% of the sites on the NPL are federal sites, either military bases (the responsibility of the U.S. Department of Defense) or sites used for manufacturing and testing nuclear weapons and, later, alternate uses of nuclear power (DOE sites, usually operated by a private industrial contractor). Some of the most serious and certainly the most extensive hazardous waste problems occur on these sites.

Nuclear weapons manufacture represents a major industry in its own right. Enormous factories involved in metal fabrication, chemical separation, mineral enrichment, electronics, and so on released large quantities of chemical and radioactive waste. Operated under the aegis of a federal agency, contractors took less care than they would have on privately held sites. As a result most or all DOE weapons sites have significant environmental contamination, and in some cases human receptor populations have been identified.[53] Waste is sometimes exposed on the surface or piled in mounds, or is buried in pits, ponds, and lagoons, where migration into groundwater is a real probability. Some of the most significant sites include the Fernald Field Material Production Center, which produced uranium metal on a 1450-acre site 20 miles northwest of Cincinnati; Rocky Flats, which produced the plutonium triggers adjacent to what is now a densely populated Denver suburb; Hanford, a 360,000-acre site in southeastern Washington, which produced weapons-grade plutonium and has been a major receiver of radioactive waste; Savannah River, which produces tritium and plutonium on a 192,000-acre site and employs more than 20,000 people; and Oak Ridge, a 58,000-acre site 15 miles from Knoxville, Tennessee.[53] The mercury contamination at Oak Ridge is the largest known mercury contamination in the world.

Although DOE has a stated goal of cleaning up all weapons sites within 30 years, the Office of Technology Assessment[53] concluded that it was unrealistic and questioned whether there were sufficient resources to clean up all DOE sites. Moreover, clean-up cannot even begin on many sites until acceptable levels of contamination are defined. Meanwhile, litigation is proceeding at several sites, seeking damages for environmental contamination of property and risk to human health.

EXPOSURE TO HAZARDOUS WASTE

Exposure to hazardous waste can be divided into occupational exposures and community exposures. Workers with potential occupational exposure include those on generator sites, transporters, and those who work on disposal sites, as well as those who investigate and remediate sites. In addition, emergency responders, public safety officials, and government officials are potentially exposed. Protection of hazardous waste workers involves extensive training, determination of their fitness to use respirators, careful selection of appropriate protective equipment, establishment of a standard operating procedures manual that includes appropriate safety planning, and medical surveillance.[51]

Community residents may be exposed because their properties abut hazardous waste sites or contaminated industrial sites, resulting in soil contamination; because they walk or play on or near the site; or because their drinking water or air is contaminated by wastes from the site. Certain groups, such as small children, pregnant women, the elderly, and the infirm, are considered to be at increased risk, either because of their state of health or because they spend many hours per week at home. Sometimes the first sign of a problem arises when household pets become sick after wallowing in puddles of water. Household exposure is usually considered to be long-term, low-level exposure; however, intermittently higher levels may occur under unusually windy and dusty conditions or if fires or explosions occur. If health effects occur they may be acute, short-term events, but most concern focuses on chronic diseases such as cancer. Buffler et al[9] discuss the difficulties in detection of health effects in contaminated communities.

Cancer is one of the main concerns voiced by exposed communities, yet the very long latency of some cancers makes it difficult to ascribe even clusters of cancer cases to hazardous waste or other environmental causes (see Chapter 1). It also makes it difficult to establish responsibility or liability. The legal aspects of hazardous waste liability remain a sticky problem.

The exposure matrix in Table 56-4 shows how contaminants in the environment (air, water, soil, food) can enter the body through the skin, the intestine, or the lung. An exposure pathway comprises a source of environmental contamination, transport of the toxic chemical to a point of potential human contact, uptake by the body, and delivery of a toxic dose to a target organ.[1,42] Exposure may occur directly when people enter the hazardous waste site or indirectly from off-site contamination of soil, water, air, or food. Many sites are attractive nuisances and are used by the nearby community for recreational purposes. Several types of information must be examined to estimate exposure.

Concentration

The environmental media can be analyzed directly to determine the amount of toxic material present in the air (in milligrams per cubic meter), water (in milligrams per liter), soil, or food (in milligrams per gram). Samples are sent to laboratories (in milligrams per liter), to analyze for the 129 different substances that the EPA has designated its Priority Pollutants or for the slightly larger Hazardous Substance List.

Exposure

Estimating how and how much material enter the body is the domain of exposure assessment. The movement of hazardous chemicals in the environment and into and within the body is very complex. Also, what is important at one site (for example, airborne deposition from an incinerator or dust) may not be important at another.

The bioavailability of chemicals (see Chapter 53) influences the likelihood that a material will enter the circulation once contact has been established. For example, soils rich in humus may bind certain chemicals, and even when a child accidently eats the soil, the contaminant may remain in the intestine and be eliminated directly rather than being absorbed.

Internal Dose

The internal dose is a critical value that is difficult to measure directly: how much of a contaminant actually reaches the target site in the body.

Threshold

The dose-response curve for most chemicals and their effects exhibits a threshold, a level below which no harm occurs or is detected. It is difficult to measure directly, and

Table 56-4. Exposure matrix for human exposure to environmental pollutants

	Air	Soil	Water	Food
Skin	Fallout, airborne deposition +	Direct contact ++	Direct contact ++	0
Lungs	Vapors, respirable particles ++++	Airborne dust ++	Aerosols negligible +	0
Gastrointestinal tract	Negligible swallowing of air +	Ingestion ++	Ingestion ++++	Airborne deposition on leaves, soil on roots, food-chain bioamplification* ++++

From Gochfeld M: *An exposure matrix for human exposure to environmental pollutants,* Piscataway, NJ, 1991, Environmental and Occupational Health Sciences Institute.
*Plants can be contaminated by airborne deposition on edible portions or by systemic uptake of material from soil or water.

it is highly controversial whether thresholds for carcinogens exist. Advances in molecular biology have altered the fundamental nature of the threshold arguement, because formerly undetectable changes at the molecular or cellular level can now be measured and can serve as biomarkers of exposure.

MIXTURES OF CHEMICALS

A critical problem with hazardous waste sites is that the chemicals are present in mixtures. A complete analysis of these mixtures is rarely possible, and even if it were, we know little about how mixtures of chemicals influence the toxicity of any components. In some cases, other chemicals may interfere with the metabolism of a contaminant to an active compound or with its degradation and excretion, or there may be competition for active sites.

Additive interactions occur when the combined effects of two or more compounds equal the effect that the same amount of the individual chemicals would cause alone. Synergistic interactions involve two or more chemicals increasing the toxic effects of each other, so the combined effect exceeds the additive effect. The fear of synergism explains why government agencies might strive to be overprotective; however, other interactions can results in subadditive effects, known as antagonistic effects.

HEALTH EFFECTS FROM HAZARDOUS WASTE

It has been very difficult to determine just how much disease has been or will be caused by hazardous-waste exposures. Estimation of exposure has been difficult, and epidemiologic studies are few and far between.[9] Some of these studies, however, have found evidence of human health effects.[39,54] Although there is usually little question regarding the presence of contaminants at hazardous waste sites (but see Gochfeld and Burger[25]), the chemicals must enter the body to cause disease.

Cancer and birth defects are the two concerns most commonly voiced by communities adjacent to hazardous waste sites. Cancer is not a single disease but many different conditions, each with its own biology and natural history. It is difficult to study, because many cancers have long latency periods. The clinician can rarely determine whether a patient has had sufficient exposure to carcinogens to develop cancer; however, research into biomarkers that reflect the cancer process[61]—for example, adducts on the deoxynbonucleic acid (DNA) molecule,[46] DNA-protein crosslinks,[13] and activation of oncogenes[7]—offer promise of an objective estimate of cancer risk.

Some hazardous-waste episodes have been identified by clusters of cancer cases, for example, the twofold excess cases of childhood leukemia attributed to water contamination in Woburn, Massachusetts. The evidence of a causal relation between hazardous wastes and leukemia was deemed sufficient to establish legal liability.

Non-Hodgkin's lymphoma is another group of cancers linked to certain types of occupational chemical exposure.

Bladder cancer and lung cancer are well known to be be caused by certain chemicals in the workplace, but whether exposure at levels usually encountered in the community can cause these cancers is uncertain. The same is true for exposure to hexavalent chromium, which is known to cause lung cancer in industrial settings but remains to be studied in communities with contaminated soil. Until this role has been clarified, it is deemed prudent to reduce exposures by whatever means society can muster.

Although the commonest reproductive effects attributed to hazardous waste exposure are miscarriages and reduced fertility, the most serious concerns involve birth defects and impaired psychomotor development. The latter has come into focus mainly since publications by Needleman[49] have shown that even low-level lead exposure can impair intellectual development in young children.

Many hazardous wastes have significant mutagenic or genotoxic properties.[39] Genetic abnormalities have been reported in some communities, whereas diseases of specific organs such as the liver, kidney, and nervous system could also occur with some of the chemicals listed in Table 56-3.

Chemical sensitivity has emerged as a major national concern.[48] A small proportion of the population reports or develops a variety of symptoms attributed to exposure to chemicals at levels so low that most people find them innocuous. The intolerance includes many foods and food additives, household chemicals, soaps, and perfumes. Some people become incapacitated by this illness, although the relative contributions of physical and psychologic factors are unclear. Often the individual can identify a single triggering cause for his or her disorder, and in a number of cases the triggering cause is exposure to hazardous waste or some acute chemical exposure episode.[20]

Clinicians must be alert to possible adverse effects related to hazardous waste, but establishment of causation in individual cases depends on fitting observations to a series of criteria first formalized by Bradford Hill.[61] Among them are the following factors.

Concordance and biologic plausibility

The reported health effects are those known to be caused by the chemicals to which the community may be exposed, and the damage fits with our understanding of the toxicity of chemicals in animals. Several studies provide consistent results.

Exposure

There is evidence of actual exposure based on measurements of chemicals in air, water, and food, coupled with people being in the right place at the right time.

Temporal relationship

The exposure must precede the outcome, and when there is normally a long latency period, the amount of time elapsed between exposure and outcome must be sufficient.

TEMPORAL ASPECTS OF EXPOSURE

Not only must the cause precede the effect but the duration of exposure must be sufficient for an effect to occur. Generally, biologic responses are proportional to some function of concentration multiplied by duration. Very high doses may produce an effect almost instantaneously, whereas low doses may require a long period of accumulation before a threshold is reached. Very low concentrations may have no effect regardless of the duration of exposure.

The workplace permissible exposure limits promulgated by the Occupational Safety and Health Administration (OSHA) to protect workers are sometimes invoked to evaluate community exposures. One may hear that because the concentration of a contaminant is far below the OSHA standard, it poses no health threat. This is not sufficient, because the OSHA standard is based on healthy adults exposed for a 40-hour week[5,58] and does not apply when exposure significantly exceeds 40 hours. Moreover, these occupational standards do not apply to other segments of the population, such as infants, pregnant women, and the elderly. When such people are homebound, they are exposed for 168 hours per week. Thus a homebound person has four times the duration of exposure of a worker without time free of exposure to eliminate any toxicant.

Several agencies have proposed maximum allowable concentrations or allowable daily intakes for certain pollutants, and they do not entail extrapolation from an OSHA Standard. Where they are not available, a popular rule of thumb is that a standard for protecting people in their homes should be at least 100 times lower than the corresponding occupational standard, and this rule assumes that the occupational standard has a sound biomedical basis.

THE ROLE OF CLINICIANS

Clinicians have the opportunity to document health effects and to document exposure, at least partly, which may be essential to any future epidemiologic investigation of an exposed community and also is important in determining the priority for clean-up. It is also essential for counseling affected individuals. Clinicians should be alert to the possibility of hazardous waste exposure and should carefully document health reports and objective findings, even when it is not yet possible to ascribe them to the presumed exposures. This documentation requires a detailed history, physical examination, and appropriate laboratory tests. If a site is already identified as a hazardous waste site, the EPA, ATSDR, or the corresponding state agency may already have information on contamination.

Advising the exposed patient

In the absence of sound data on exposure and risk, the physician must be careful not to provide unwarranted reassurance or to arouse unnecessary anxiety. Prudence requires reduction of exposures that can be recognized and controlled; however, it is usually not essential to try to avoid every conceivable hazard. The history identifies risky situations and risky behaviors, which can be fit into an exposure matrix (see Table 55-4). Patients can be advised to limit ingestion of contaminated water, to avoid eating fish or produce obtained from or near contaminated sites, to keep children from playing on contaminated soil, and to seek alternative sources of drinking water. The medical examination and testing can provide a basis for reassurance or may identify health effects that require further study. Medical objectivity is essential: the physician should not be overly skeptical or unduly alarmist about the risk of exposure. When there is doubt, environmental medicine specialists at nearby universities or at state agencies; the ATSDR Health Assessments Branch (Atlanta, GA 30333); or the nearest clinic member of the Association of Occupational and Environmental Clinics AOEC (see Chapter 58).

EVALUATION OF COMMUNITY EXPOSURE TO HAZARDOUS WASTES

The first step in evaluation of exposure is the documentation and quantification of hazardous contaminants on a waste site and/or in the air, water, and soil of a community. Sometimes, however, the recognition of a real or apparent excess of mortality, disease, or health effects precedes the study of the hazardous waste site. In some cases the waste site may be in a densely populated urban area, or residences may have been built directly on contaminated soil, for example, on radioactive waste at Grand Junction, Colorado; on chromium waste in Hudson County, New Jersey; and on former coal gas plant sites in many places. The ATSDR was mandated by Congress to perform health assessments (not health studies or screenings) for all sites on the NPL.[1]

The exposure evaluation may be accomplished by a site investigation, exposure assessment and risk assessment, or by some combination of health survey and medical screening. If a risk assessment is to be performed, a series of scenarios regarding potential exposure must be developed. These scenarios are sometimes called realistic scenarios, worst-case scenarios, and ''really worst-case'' scenarios. Problems arise when the realistic scenario produces acceptable risk but the worst case produces unacceptable risks. Also, a risk that is acceptable to the EPA may not be acceptable to the community or individuals.

Some of the assumptions that are made in evaluation of potential risk to a community are indicated herein, with some extreme examples:

House occupancy scenarios

A newborn baby who will live in house for 70 years, sitting on the front porch without ever leaving the house; a 5-year-old who will live in the house 16 hours a day until age 17, then leave and never return; and an adult who will live in the house 16 hours a day for 45 years.

Dietary scenario

A family that obtains 100% of its food from locally caught fish and locally grown milk, meat, and produce; a realistic estimate of the contribution of locally grown produce and fish to overall diet is about 0% in cities and 10% in suburban areas.

Childhood soil scenario

A child with pica who eats 10 g soil per day; an average child in a warm climate who consumes about 50 to 100 mg soil per day playing outdoors for 12 months a year; and an average child in a cool climate who consumes 50 to 100 mg soil per day, playing outdoors 6 months per year.

Similar alternative assumptions must be considered for each cell in the matrix of Table 56-4.[23]

Vulnerability of the population

Not everyone has an equal likelihood of being exposed or harmed. Early risk assessments relied on a hypothetical maximally exposed individual (MEI) who spends all of his or her life at the point of maximal impact of airborne and waterborne contamination, eating contaminated food. Goldstein[29] pointed out why the MEI approach misrepresented community exposure, overestimating in some cases and underestimating in others.

CASE STUDIES OF COMMUNITY EXPOSURE TO HAZARDOUS WASTE

With all the concern over hazardous waste it might be assumed that there were many excellent studies of exposed communities that could be invoked to interpret data. Such studies have proved difficult. In most cases the target community is simply too small to achieve adequate statistical power for an edpidemiologic study. In such cases, negative results of studies are not a basis for complacency. In addition, the number of cases of a disease identified is too small to achieve statistical significance. Communities may justifiably be concerned about only a 50% increase in risk of a serious disease, yet epidemiologic studies may be unable to detect such a subtle difference. There is a high likelihood that such studies will suffer from type II errors, failing to identify a relationship that is real. Once litigation is under way, it becomes even more difficult to study a community objectively. The following are just a few examples of communities exposed to hazardous waste.

Chemical Control, New Jersey

The Chemical Control site fire at Elizabeth, New Jersey, in May 1980 put hazardous waste squarely in the public eye. The 2-day fire damaged more than 40,000 55-gallon drums of chemicals; the combination of leaking chemicals and millions of gallons of water used by firefighters contaminated adjacent rivers; and the plume of smoke from the fire blew over surrounding communities, depositing ash on homes, cars, and playgrounds.[25] For more than a decade prior to the fire the site had been receiving hazardous waste from nearby industries that paid to have the waste destroyed. For more than a year preceeding the fire the State of New Jersey had been supervising a remedial investigation of the site. The clean-up program operated by the State of New Jersey examplifies the problems encountered with hazardous waste clean-up in general. The Chemical Control site was adjacent to an urban receptor community and was at the confluence of two rivers. Although there was an incinerator on site, it was never approved for use, or much of the material could have been destroyed on site.

The contents of each of the 40,000 drums had to be identified so that they could be grouped for shipping. In some cases labels were legible and the company that originally manufactured the material was contacted to retrieve its waste and dispose of it legally. Most drums, however, had to be opened, sampled, analyzed, labeled, and added to a manifest. The clean-up was delayed for months because of difficulties with transportation and location of suitable disposal sites elsewhere. For more than 1 year before the fire, the State and its contractors labored to clean up the site, but by the time of the fire only a small amount of material had actually been moved off site. After the fire, the cleanup proceeded more rapidly, but it still required more than 5 years and cost more than $5 million.

A local community group joined with the State Department of Health to survey people in the exposed community, and two control communities were identified; however, the community-trained interviewers were unable to provide bias free-results and in the end did not even visit the control communities. The study was abandoned, but not before it reported excess rates of respiratory symptoms in the days after the fire, as well as a variety of complaints during the time when the site was operational. At least one death from an acute asthmatic attack was linked temporally to the fire. The National Institute for Occupational Safety and Health documented excessive respiratory disease in firefighters and emergency responders.[14]

Love Canal, New York. For many years Hooker Chemical Company deposited a variety of toxic chemical wastes from its lindane plant in an old canal bed in Niagara Falls, New York. Hooker eventually capped the canal with clay and donated it to the city. Housing and a school were constructed immediately adjacent to the canal. Gross contamination of the surrounding community from a chemical dump site heightened public awareness of community exposure to hazardous waste.[41] Several observational studies identified significant associations between exposure to mothers and low birth weight[28,63] and an excess of chromosomal abnormalities,[57] but these results were considered controversial because of inadequate controls.

The State of New York evacuated the homes closest to the canal and purchased them. In 1988 the State approved the area for reoccupation, although it does not yet certify its safety.

Woburn, Massachusetts. An excess of childhood leukemias was linked to contaminated well water. This situation attracted great public attention (second only to Love Canal), and ultimately the community was awarded a substantial settlement. Lagakos et al[40] found a positive association between contaminated well water and childhood leukemia, other illnesses, and adverse reproductive outcomes.

Lowell, Massachusetts. Ozonoff and associates[55] found a higher rate of respiratory and irritant symptoms in residents near a paint waste site than in a comparable control neighborhood. They concluded that either the general population appears to react to levels much lower than those considered effective in the occupational setting or such effects last longer than generally thought.

Santa Clara, California. Trichloroethylene and other volatile compounds contaminated drinking water in this South Bay county because of runoff from an electronics-manufacturing firm. Residents suspected an excess of adverse reproductive outcomes, and indeed the State Department of Health found a 2.6-fold excess of major cardiac anomalies among infants born in 1981; however, with the spatial distribution of these births comparison of the contamination of the water did not support a causal relationship. The spontaneous abortion rate was increased twofold and the overall congenital anomaly rate threefold over those in the comparison area. The investigators concluded that the excess was not due to recall bias or confounding factors. They concluded, however, that there was insufficient exposure data to assess the relationship between exposure and outcome.[11]

Polychlorinated biphenyl in North Carolina. Polychlorinated biphenyl contamination of a roadside community by illegal leakage of waste from tank trucks was not reflected in elevated breast milk levels.[60]

Times Beach, Missouri. Waste oil contaminated by chemical waste from herbicide manufacturing was used for dust control in and around horse rinks in several Missouri communities. The herbicide waste contained relatively high levels of 2,3,7,8-tetrachlorodibenzo-*p*-dioxin (TCDD), and soil levels of TCDD exceeded 1 part per billion. Although health effects were not documented, the EPA recommended evacuation of the entire town, and the U.S. government purchased the homes.

Smith Hall, New Jersey

In the late 1970s four cases of lymphomas (four distinct histologic types) occurred in occupants of a university laboratory-and-classroom building. The public ascribed the cases to wastes from an animal laboratory, but none of the cases occurred in persons working with the animals. Numerous other illnesses were subsequently attributed to the exposure, but a physician's review of the medical records indicated that some of the putative cases were misreported (for example, several so-called ovarian cysts proved to be Bartholin's gland cysts). A survey by the State Department of Health raised the suspicion of exposure to laboratory waste as a cause and prompted improvement in building structure and maintenance to reduce further contamination; however, causality was not demonstrated with a high degree of probability.

REDUCING COMMUNITY EXPOSURE

Clinicians should realize that when a risk assessment identifies an elevated risk for a community or when there is obvious contamination, intervention is called for, even before site remediation occurs. A household or community may be warned or ordered to discontinue use of water for drinking, cooking, and even for bathing or showering. Communities with well water may have emergency hook-up to municipal water (assuming that the municipal water is not contaminated). If the water is contaminated with volatile substances, residents should not use it for showering because such use may entail high exposure, but otherwise, well water can be used for showering and bottled water for drinking and cooking.

Fencing and sign-posting of a site to keep people out should be undertaken immediately. Although they are required for Superfund sites, they are often not achieved.

Physicians should reenforce public health advisories against consuming fish or other foods from contaminated waters and produce grown on contaminated soil. The responsible public health agency should issue such advisories in a timely fashion.

If dust is blowing from a contaminated site, emergency capping of the site is required. Physicians can help their patients provide evidence of such exposure.

Soil contamination poses a difficult problem because there are many communities with soil contamination but no obvious exposure pathway. In such cases, risks are likely to be overestimated.[31] Different agencies have different guidelines for identification of contaminated soil. When soil is contaminated above a certain level, it must be treated (by either physical, biologic, or chemical treatment or removal) to lower the level to a certain set standard (which is not always the same level that is considered hazardous). A number of companies that have contaminated adjacent residential properties have had to remove the top layer of soil and replace it with clean soil.

HEALTH SURVEYS AND EPIDEMIOLOGIC STUDIES

When a community learns about a significant exposure to hazardous wastes, it is likely to call for a health survey, but public health agencies are likely to voice reluctance about such surveys and are often not able to conduct an adequate epidemiologic study. The ATSDR has the responsibility for performing at least an initial health assessment, evaluating data on environmental contaminants that might pose a current or future public health threat.[1]

Health surveys are more detailed, hands-on investigations of health. Such studies could include surveys and questionnaires but might also include studies of birth or death certificates, data from birth-defects or cancer registries, or comparisons of disease incidence or mortality in the affected community with that for a comparable community or the state. Unfortunately, in the absence of more detailed exposure data the exposure status of the individuals who become ill can rarely be determined and such studies are very likely to be inconclusive.[24,27]

For a survey to be successful the community should be involved at all stages in its planning, implementation, and interpretation. Otherwise they may respond with skepticism when the results of the study, particularly when results are negative, are released.[31]

A health study could include medical screening of the community ranging from questionnaires and laboratory tests to complete medical examinations. The latter are sometimes undertaken to establish the prevalence of certain exposures or conditions and may serve either to reassure or to alarm the target community.

Careful attention must be given to design of such studies, particularly to the manner in which either negative or positive outcomes will be explained to the community, to government, and to responsible parties. Inadequately planned surveys may fail to uncover significant exposure, may provide spurious results that later undermine the community's efforts, and may discourage both the community and public health officials; however, because in many cases further exposure is terminated, a health survey, if it is to be conducted, should be conducted in a timely manner before evidence of exposure fades.[24]

To design an effective health study it is essential to determine how the results will be interpreted. Often this interpretation requires use of existing health data or study of an appropriate control community, and often the survey is complicated by pending or future litigation. A survey that finds no evidence of damage might be welcomed as reassuring by one community and received as unwelcome and harmful to pending litigation by another.

THE ROLE OF MEDICAL SURVEILLANCE OF THE COMMUNITY

Whereas a single cross-sectional medical screening examination may determine the extent to which a community population has been exposed or harmed, ongoing medical surveillance involves periodic, often lifelong examination of affected or exposed individuals to detect evidence of disease and provide intervention or treatment.

Many legal cases seeking damages from hazardous waste generators or waste sites include ongoing medical surveillance as part of the damages sought. To be scientifically valid, medical surveillance must have adequate sensitivity, specificity, and predictive value. The World Health Organization outlined criteria for medical screening, which can be adapted for determination of whether medical surveillance of an exposed community is warranted.

The predictive value of any test procedure or program hinges not only on the sensitivity and specificity of the test but on the prevalence of the underlying condition being sought. In this case, the relevant prevalence is significant exposure to one or more toxins. If such exposure has occurred, medical surveillance can detect pathophysiologic changes.[19,26] If significant exposure has not occurred, the community should be reassured rather than put into a potentially stressful program that cannot afford them real benefit.

Although medical surveillance is warranted only in special cases, it is certainly prudent to develop a registry of all residents in a community, including information such as dates and location of residence, data on soil and water contamination, age, time spent in home, and current health status. Maintenance of the registry would allow the identification of the potentially exposed residents at a future date when more is known about the hazard or when some people begin to show signs of illness.

On the other hand, in the case of significant exposure to a toxic agent, at least baseline medical testing may be valuable. If the agent can produce disease at a later date (such as carcinogens and reproductive toxins), follow-up examination may be warranted; however, when these conditions have a very low prevalence (that is, when the risk is low), the predictive value of even a positive test result is likely to be low. Probably a more fruitful endeavor would be to establish a long-term trust fund to provide medical services and compensation for exposed residents. An alternative suggestion, advanced by Louria et al,[43] is to focus community attention on health promotion to reduce other risk factors.[24]

SPECIAL PROBLEMS
Leaking underground storage tanks

Leaking underground storage tanks at abandoned gasoline stations and leaks from old oil storage tanks are an all-too-frequent problem. Homeowners complain of oily odors in their basements, and often they can see gross signs of contamination. An entire house may become unlivable or the quality of living may suffer. Sometimes, real health hazards, such as elevated levels of benzene in the shower, can be identified. In other cases the main consequence is economic.

Even when the offending tank has been removed, a substantial amount of soil clean-up may be required or groundwater contamination may require remediation. Many thousands of gallons may be lost into the soil before the problem is recognized. Often the site is abandoned and no responsible party can be identified.

Various procedures are available to minimize the risk of future leaks. Gasoline stations are required to undergo periodic pressure testing of their tanks to ensure that there are no leaks. Metal tanks can be protected from corrosion by connecting them to an electric current (cathodic protection). Double-walled tanks and tanks made of synthetic resins resist corrosion and leakage.[12]

Low-level radioactive waste

The disposal of radioactive waste is a major national concern. High-level waste, such as uranium wastes, spent nuclear power rods, and other material containing more than

100 nCi of alpha-emitting isotopes with half-life greater than 20 years must be disposed of at a very few sites, such as DOE's Hanford facility. Low-level radioactive waste (LLRW) is defined as any waste that is not classified as high level; and most radioactive waste is LLRW, including, for example, gloves and syringes used in biomedical research or clinical services and animal or human tissue containing radionuclides. About half the LLRW is generated from commercial nuclear reactors. The other half is from industrial and medical by-products. Most radionuclides in LLRW require only marginal shielding and decay rapidly, and they are believed to represent trivial risks to public health.[10] In 1980 Congress shifted responsibility for the disposal of LLRW to the states.[10,50]

Although the radiation risks from high-level waste are real and clear, there is a tendency to assume that LLRW carries similar risks. The public has an aversion to any radioactive waste, which has been supported by scientists' declarations of a linear no-threshold cancer risk from radiation, that is, any amount of radiation causes some effect. This has made it virtually impossible for states to site LLRW disposal facilities.

In 1991 there were three active sites licensed and willing to receive LLRW,[24] but as of 1993 only only the Barnwell, South Carolina, site, scheduled to close in 1994, was receiving such waste, and the cost escalated to more than $2000 per drum of radionuclide-contaminated material. It now costs more to dispose of a radioisotope than to purchase the pure reagent. This has already provided a strong incentive to reduce the use of radioisotopes, and alternatives to radioisotopes in biomedical research are rapidly emerging, providing an example of an economic incentive leading to source reduction in a hazardous waste.

PREVENTION OF EXPOSURE TO HAZARDOUS WASTE

Garrett Hardin[33] argued that our climate of regulation promoted rather than penalized waste generators by allowing them to spread the cost over society. By the late 1970s the EPA and several states, led by New Jersey, had active programs to discover and control hazardous waste sites. In the early 1980s Love Canal, the Chemical Control fire, and the book by Epstein et al[18] raised public awareness of the magnitude of the hazardous waste problem, and specific medical evaluation approaches for populations exposed to hazardous waste were described.[22]

The increased cost and regulation of hazardous waste disposal have made waste minimization more attractive and ultimately an economic necessity.[36] In 1984 the Hazardous and Solid Waste Amendments to RCRA stated "that it is to be a national policy of the United States that, where feasible, the generation of hazardous waste is to be reduced or eliminated." The Office of Technology Assessment[52] concluded that industry has been slow in achieving waste minimzation yet that waste minimization may actually reduce costs.

REFERENCES

1. Agency for Toxic Substances and Disease Registry: *Health assessment guidance manual,* Atlanta, 1990.
2. Andelman JB, Underhill DW: *Health effects effects from hazardous waste sites,* Chelsea, Mich, 1987, Lewis.
3. Baker D, Greenland S: *Stringfellow health effects study: an epidemiological health survey of residents of Gel Avon and Rubidoux, California.* Los Angeles, 1986, California Department of Health Services.
4. Bartlett KG, ed: *Hazardous waste management,* vol 1, *law of toxics and toxic substances.* Boca Raton, Fla, 1984, Lewis.
5. Bingham E: Standards, regulation and public health, *Med Clin North Am* 74:527, 1990.
6. Blinder S: Deaths, injuries, and evacuations from acute hazardous materials releases, *Am J Public Health* 79:1042, 1989.
7. Brandt-Rauf P: Oncogene proteins as molecular epidemiologic markers of cancer risk in hazardous waste workers, *State-of-the-Art Reviews in Occupational Medicine* 5:59, 1990.
8. Budnick LD et al: Cancer and birth defects near the Drake Superfund site, Pennsylvania, *Arch Environ Health* 39:409, 1984.
9. Buffler PA, Crane M, Key M: Possibilities of detecting health effects by studies of populations exposed to chemicals from waste disposal sites, *Environ Health Perspect* 62:423, 1985.
10. Burns ME: *Low level radioactive waste regulation,* Chelsea, Mich, 1988, Lewis.
11. California Department of Health Services: *Pregnancy outcomes in Santa Clara County, 1980-1982: reports of two epidemiological studies,* Epidemiological Studies Section, 7540-958-1301-5, Berkeley, 1985.
12. Cheremisinoff PN, Casana JG, Ouellette RP: *Underground storage tanks guidebook,* Northbrook, Ill, 1987, Pudvan.
13. Costa M et al: Preliminary report on a simple new assay for DNA-protein cross-links as a biomarker of exposure experienced by welders, *J Toxicol Environ Health* 40:217, 1993.
14. Costello RJ, Melius J: *Technical assistance determination report: Chemical Control, Elizabeth, New Jersey,* TA 80-77, Cincinnati, 1981, National Institute for Occupational Safety and Health.
15. Environmental Protection Agency: The birth of a program, *EPA Journal* 1:14, 1987.
16. Environmental Protection Agency: Technical assistance grants to groups at National Priorities List Sites, U.S. Environmental Protection Agency Interim Final Rule, *Federal Register* 53:9736-9755, 1988.
17. Environmental Protection Agency: *Toxic Release Inventory results, Region III,* Washington, DC, 1993.
18. Epstein SS, Brown LO, Pope C: *Hazardous waste in America,* San Francisco, 1982, Sierra Club Books.
19. Favata E, Gochfeld M: Medical surveillance of hazardous waste workers: ability of laboratory tests to discriminate exposure, *Am J Ind Med* 15:255, 1988.
20. Fiedler N, Maccia C, Kipen H: Evaluation of chemically sensitive patients, *J Occup Med* 34:529, 1992.
21. Freeman HM: The US EPA waste minimization research program. Proceedings of the 6th Hazardous Materials Management Conference International, Atlantic City, NJ, 1988.
22. Gochfeld M: Assessment of clinical toxicity in populations exposed to hazardous wastes. Proceedings of the International Congress on Industrial Hazardous Waste, New Jersey Institute of Technology, Newark, 1982.
23. Gochfeld M: *An exposure matrix for human exposure to environmental pollutants,* Piscataway, NJ, 1991, Environmental and Occupational Health Sciences Institute.
24. Gochfeld M, Hazardous waste. In Rosenstock L, Cullen M, eds: *Textbook of clinical occupational and environmental medicine,* Philadelphia, 1994, WB Saunders.
25. Gochfeld M, Burger J: Investigations and activities at Superfund sites, *State-of-the-Art Reviews in Occupational Medicine* 5:127, 1990.

26. Gochfeld M, Burger J: Criteria and alternatives for the medical surveillance of communities exposed to hazardous waste. In Mehlman M et al, eds: Proceedings, Princeton, NJ, 1995, Princeton Scientific Publications.
27. Gochfeld M, Favata EA, eds: Hazardous waste workers. *State-of-the-Art Reviews in Occupational Medicine* 5:1, 1990.
28. Goldman LR et al: Low birthweight, prematurity and birth defects in children living near the hazardous waste site, Love Canal, *Hazardous Waste* 2:209, 1985.
29. Goldstein BD: The maximally exposed individual, *Environ Forum* (Nov/Dec) 13, 1989.
30. Goldstein BD, Gochfeld M: Role of the physician in environmental medicine. In Upton A, ed: *Medical clinics of North America,* vol 74(2), *Environmental Medicine,* Philadelphia, 1990, WB Saunders.
31. Greenberg MR, Anderson RF: *Hazardous waste sites: the credibility gap,* New Brunswick, NJ, 1984, Rutgers University Press.
32. Hance BJ, Chess C, Sandman PM: *Industry risk communication manual: improving dialogue with communities,* Boca Raton, Fla, 1990, Lewis.
33. Hardin G: Tragedy of the Commons, *Science* 162:1243, 1968.
34. Harris R, Highland J: Adverse health effects at a Tennessee hazardous waste disposal site, *Hazardous Waste* 1:183, 1984.
35. Hart FC: *Preliminary assessment of cleanup costs of national hazardous waste problems,* report to the US EPA, Feb. 23, 1979.
36. Higgins T: *Hazardous waste minimization handbook,* Chelsea, Mich, 1989.
37. Hogan MD et al: Disease-causing effects of environmental chemicals, *Med Clin North Am* 74:461, 1990.
38. Houk VS: The genotoxicity of industrial wastes and effluents: a review, *Mutation Res* 277:91, 1992.
39. Johanson WG: An analysis of a health effects survey conducted by residents living near a toxic waste site, master of public health thesis, Houston, 1991, University of Texas School of Public Health.
40. Lagakos SW, Wessen BJ, Zelen M: An analysis of contaminated well water and health effect in Woburn, Massachusetts, *J Am Statistical Assoc* 81:583, 1986.
41. Levine AG: *Love Canal: science, politics, and people,* Lexington, Mass, 1982, Lexington Books.
42. Lioy PJ: Assessing total human exposure to contaminants, *Environ Sci Technol* 24:938-945, 1990.
43. Louria D, Bogden J, Gochfeld M: *Health promotion versus medical surveillance for reducing health risks of communities near hazardous waste sites.* Newark, 1993, University of Medicine and Dentistry of New Jersey.
44. Lucero G et al: *Superfund Handbook,* ed 3, Chicago, 1989, Idleyard Austin.
45. Majumdar SK, Miller EW, Schmalz RF: *Management of hazardous materials and wastes,* Lafayette, Pa, 1989, Pennsylvania Academy of Science.
46. McDiarmid MA, Strickland PT: DNA adducts as markers of exposure in hazardous waste workers, *State-of-the-Art Review in Occupational Medicine* 5:49, 1991.
47. Mitre: Computer printout of National Priorities List: data summaries for 546 final and proposed sites, Report to EPA, McLean, Va, 1983.
48. National Research Council: *Multiple chemical sensitivities,* Washington, DC, 1992, National Academy Press.
49. Needleman H: *Human exposure to lead,* Boca Raton, Fla, 1992, CRC Press.
50. Nuclear Regulatory Commission: *Managing low-level radioactive waste: a proposed approach,* Washington, DC, 1980.
51. Occupational Safety and Health Administration: Standard on hazardous waste operations and emergency responses, final rule. *Federal Register* 54:CFR 1910. 120, March 6, 1989.
52. Office of Technology Assessment: *Serious reduction of hazardous waste,* OTA-ITE-317 Washington, DC, 1986, US Office of Technology Assessment.
53. Office of Technology Assessment: *Complex cleanup: the environmental legacy of nuclear weapons production,* OTA-O-484 Washington, DC, 1991, US Congress.
54. Ozonoff D: Medical aspects of the hazardous waste problem, *Am J Forensic Med Pathol* 3:343, 1982.
55. Ozonoff D et al: Health problems reported by residents of a neighborhood contaminated by a hazardous waste facility, *Am J Ind Med* 11:581, 1987.
56. Phillips AM, Silbergeld EK: Health effects studies of exposure from hazardous waste sites: where are we today? *Am J Ind Med* 8:1, 1985.
57. Picciano D: Pilot cytogenetic study of the residents living near the Love Canal, *Mammalian Chromosome News* 21:86, 1980.
58. Plog BA: *Fundamentals of industrial hygiene,* ed 3, Chicago, 1988, National Safety Council.
59. Resource Conservation and Recovery Act, PL 94-580, 90 Stat 2795, 1976.
60. Rogan WJ et al: Chromatographic evidence of polychlorinated biphenyl exposure from a spill, *JAMA* 249:1057, 1983.
61. Schulte PA: A conceptual framework for the validation and use of biomarkers, *Environ Res* 48:129, 1989.
62. Toxic Substances Control Act, PL 94-469, 90 Stat 2003, 1976.
63. Vianna NJ, Polan AK: Incidence of low birth weight among Love Canal residents, *Science* 226:1217, 1984.
64. Wilkes A, Kiefer I, Levine B: *Everybody's problem: hazardous waste,* SW-826, Washington, DC, 1980, US EPA Office of Solid Waste.

Chapter 57

ASSESSMENT AND REMEDIATION OF HAZARDOUS WASTE SITES

Michael Gochfeld
Joanna Burger

Site assessment
Setting priorities
   Environmental equity
   Ecological risk assessment
Cleanup criteria
Approaches to site remediation
Types of treatment
   Soil and water treatment
   Liquid hazardous waste
   Thermal technologies
   Chemical treatments
   Stabilization
   Dilution approaches
   Biological treatment
   Landfilling of hazardous waste
Social considerations

Example of technologies used to remediate petroleum contaminated soils

Biological treatment
   Bioremediation in situ or ex situ
   Composting
   Land farming
Physical treatment
   Soil flushing or washing
   Vacuum extraction
   Solvent extraction
   Air/steam stripping
Chemical treatment
   Hydrogen peroxide catalysis
   Chemical treatment in situ
High temperature treatment
   Incinerator
   Infrared thermal treatment
   Vitrification in situ
   Plasma-fired reactor
   Electric reactor
Low temperature treatment
   Low volatilization
   Radio frequency in situ
Stabilization/solidification
   Asphalt incorporation
Excavation/containment
   Capping
   Slurry Wall
   Reuse without treatment

Although the assessment and remediation of hazardous waste lies in the domain of the regulator, the engineer, and the environmental scientist, clinicians benefit from knowledge about how sites are evaluated and from understanding the benefits and drawbacks of available remediation methods. Clinicians may evaluate and educate hazardous waste workers or patients who live near a site slated for remediation, and they may participate in the public decision making process when there is a choice of technologies. This chapter introduces a few major alternative treatments for hazardous waste (see box).

Modified from a report to the New Jersey Department of Transportation from the New Jersey Institute of Technology, "Alternate Technologies for the Remediation and Disposal of Soils Contaminated with Petroleum Hydrocarbons and Chlorinated Hydrocarbons" (1991).[11]

The first step in managing hazardous waste is to curtail the production of future waste. All other activities become insignificant if the rate of new hazardous waste production is not drastically slowed. There are four waste reduction strategies: process elimination, process alteration, reuse of waste as is, and recycling into new material.[9,13] Some states (e.g. New Jersey) have model pollution prevention laws.

SITE ASSESSMENT

There are several phases involved in the management of hazardous waste sites, including site identification, preliminary assessment, remedial investigation, and remediation.

Identification. Sites are identified by the public, by investigators, by the media, and by responsible parties. In some cases extensive detective work is required to determine who owned a site when waste was deposited, and often it is impossible to determine whose waste is present on a site. All identified sites are listed on the CERCLIS—a list of more than 30,000 sites that have been investigated or require investigation under the Comprehensive Environmental Responsibility Liability and Cleanup Act (CERCLA)[12] (see Chapter 55).

Preliminary site assessment (PSA). The EPA or corresponding state agency determines if there is a potential hazard to health or the environment. This may result in an emergency remediation, or the hazard ranking system (see below) may be implemented at this stage to determine whether the site should be listed on the National Priority List (NPL) (see Chapter 56).

A remedial investigation/feasibility study (RI/FS) is then conducted, usually by private contractors. This phase documents the type and extent of contamination and outlines the types of remediation required. Recommendations may range from simple enclosure and warning signs to complete removal of waste, treatment of soil and ground water, and capping.

During the RI/FS (or occasionally the preliminary site assessment), the hazard ranking system is applied and yields three scores involving estimates of: (1) the capability of hazardous chemicals to migrate offsite (i.e., become airborne or waterborne); (2) the likelihood that humans (technically known as "receptors") will contact contaminated air, water, soil, or food; and (3) a composite measure of the fire and/or explosion hazard. Finally, a report is generated in the public domain.

Either the responsible party (RP) or a governmental decision tree for treating hazardous waste sites are shown in Fig. 57-1. They include management on site versus offsite, and various cleanup options include landfilling, treatment (removal and/or destruction), and reuse.

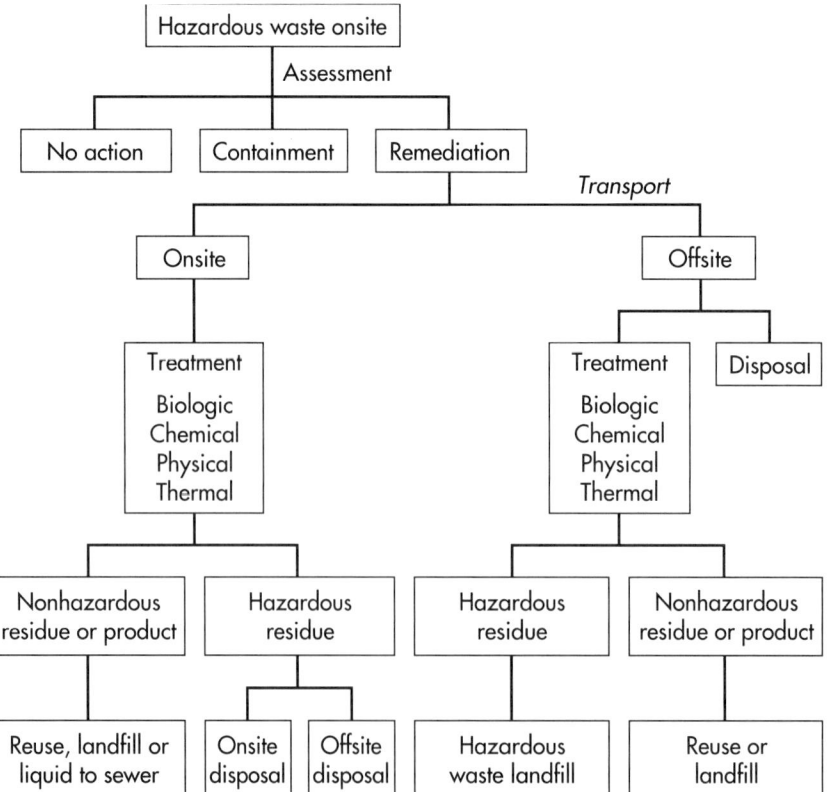

Fig. 57-1. Flow chart outlining main management decisions for hazardous waste. (Courtesy Environmental and Occupational Health Sciences Institute.)

SETTING PRIORITIES

Whether a site requires remediation (either emergency or routine) depends on the magnitude of the hazard, the potential for exposure, and the number of susceptible people potentially exposed, as well as possible impacts on sensitive ecosystems. The site assessment and the hazard ranking system provide some of the data necessary to make these determinations. Risk assessments are often used to rate overall risk to a population, and if risk assessments are done in a standardized fashion for many sites they can help set priorities for remediation.

Environmental equity

The distribution of both hazardous waste sites and susceptible populations varies between communities and geographic regions. The U.S. government's recent report on environmental equity[10] recognizes that poor and minority communities are more likely to have significant hazardous chemical exposure,[2] and at the same time have greater susceptibility to disease and less access to medical care. The residents in these communities have more limited recreational and travel opportunities and are therefore more likely to approach being the theoretical "maximally exposed individual." It is now recognized that remediation priorities need to address equitable risk allocation within society.

Ecological risk assessment

Although decisions regarding hazardous waste management have most commonly been made in response to direct threats to human health, there is an increasing realization that threats to natural ecosystems are critical as well and also represent indirect threats to human health and well-being. In some cases animals can be used to monitor contaminated sites and to estimate exposures[18] and for general environmental quality biomonitoring[21] predicated on the recognition that the overall biochemistry and physiology of animals and humans is very similar.[6] Ecologic risk assessment is emerging as a discipline and modifying the more traditional health risk paradigm.[19] The health of an ecosystem involves many species rather than just one, and the endpoints used in risk assessment are more complex to evaluate.[17,21] Moreover, whereas human risk assessments are usually based on a single temporal scale, the "average" 70-year life span, a variety of temporal scales must be considered for ecologic risk assessment.[3]

CLEANUP CRITERIA

The PSA and RI/FS provide data that must be incorporated into major decisions that will affect many people and cost millions of dollars. Soil may have to be excavated and removed; water may have to be pumped and treated. Criteria must be developed to (1) determine whether current contamination levels warrant remediation (setting of action levels) and (2) set the "target goals" for cleanup; that is, the levels to which contamination must be reduced before the site is certified as acceptable.

Regulators, responsible parties, and the public need to know "how clean is clean?" When is a site safe? When is it safe to shower, to drink the water, to play in the yard, to garden? There is no simple answer to these questions.[14]

An early approach to determining the hazard potential of soil was to subject it to a standardized *extraction procedure* (EP Toxicity Test) and measure the amount of contaminants that could be removed from the soil. If levels of contaminants were excessive, the soil was deemed hazardous. EPA expanded this approach with a *toxic characteristics leaching procedure* (TCLP), which added 38 organic chemicals to the smaller list of chemicals measured in the EP test.[14]

Another more straightforward determination of hazard involves the direct analysis of soil to measure the concentration of specific substances, for example, lead or dioxin. The TCLP is more applicable to hazardous waste sites where there are large numbers of substances present, while direct measurement is more often applied when a site contains one or a few known contaminants. As early as 1977 Cleland and Kingsbury[5] provided the EPA with estimated permissible concentrations of contaminants in air, water, and soil that were not deemed toxic to humans or ecosystems. However, these have not been widely used in site assessment.[14]

New Jersey[16] promulgated soil cleanup levels after considering a number of approaches. One was to require that a responsible party clean up "to background." Thus for metals that occur naturally in soil, there is some average background level, below which cleanup would not be feasible. However, there are separate backgrounds for urban versus rural areas, and it is not often feasible to expect urban soils to reach rural levels. For petroleum hydrocarbons the NJDEP assumed a background of 100 ppm, consistent with the widespread distribution of hydrocarbons in today's environment, even though these do not occur naturally. Although the public is uncomfortable when any toxic material is detected in soil, the NJDEP[16] reasoned that improved analytic methodology assured that a growing number of substances would be detected at lower and lower levels. Ideally, cleanup would be set at levels that do not pose a health hazard to anyone and are not an ecologic threat.

Risk assessment methodology has also been used to evaluate hazardous waste sites (see Chapter 55). This is limited, however, by the alternative "exposure scenarios" that one can choose, and it is important to develop site-specific scenarios if the risk assessment is to assist in determining cleanup levels.[16] Moreover, the projected use of the site is relevant; it is not necessary to clean up an industrial site to the same level as a residential site.[14] If certain sites are subsequently used for housing or recreation, however, additional extensive cleanup might be required.

APPROACHES TO SITE REMEDIATION

In the United States compliance with environmental regulation has spawned a sophisticated industry for site evaluation, remediation, and cleanup. New technologies are developing rapidly. Throughout the 1980s federal and state regulatory agencies placed a premium on cleaning up contaminated sites with the aim of eliminating all future exposure and restoring any site to background conditions, thereby allowing any future land use. The immense cost and constraints on transportation and ultimate disposition of waste, have led to increasing emphasis on alternative forms of treatment in situ, at the original site. This means that in some cases future uses of the land will be limited by deed restrictions, a bitter pill for some land owners and environmental regulators.

The options for remediating a contaminated site range from no action to complete cleanup. The hazardous waste may be treated, and treatment can occur at the original site or at some other site. Many new technologic approaches are being explored to facilitate remediation, particularly in situ. Some technologies are developed primarily for emergency responses (e.g., transportation spills, fires), whereas others are more appropriate for long-range management of a site. New technologies must be considered for the combined chemical and radioactive waste plaguing Department of Energy sites.[20]

Hazardous waste management is conducted on active industrial sites under the Resource Conservation and Recovery Act (RCRA) and on abandoned sites under CERCLA. The basic technologies available are the same, but they differ in scale and in preference. Some are well-designed to operate on a daily basis as part of an industrial waste water treatment system, for example. Facilities decontamination has become a growth industry, independent of the emergency response and cleanup. In a growing number of states industrial property must be certified as free from significant contamination before it can be sold.

TYPES OF TREATMENT

Hazardous waste treatment can be divided into *physical* treatments (absorption, flotation, evaporation, filtration, sedimentation, stabilization), *chemical* treatments (acid-base neutralization, precipitation, oxidation, *photochemical* reactions), *biologic* treatment (microbial degradation), and *thermal* treatment (incineration, volatilization). Stabilization or solidification includes formation of cement, use in lime or thermoplastic material, vitrification, plasma arc solidification, and encapsulation.[13] Nuclear wastes can also be treated in a variety of ways, including storage for four or more half-lives and physical dilution.

Ground water treatment

A variety of technologies must be evaluated depending on the extent, depth, and type of contamination.[7] Automatic skimmers are used to recover floating hydrocarbons such as oil products from surface waters. For contaminated ground water, siphons and pneumatic pumps are used to recover substances that are heavier and lighter than water, respectively. Air stripping towers remove volatile organics from waste water or ground water. A strong vacuum applied to the soil surface or through a well creates an underground vacuum that enhances volatilization of chemicals into the soil gas compartment (see Chapter 45), and draws the gas to an extraction point and ultimately to the surface. Appropriate for the lighter fractions of petroleum hydrocarbons, this technology cannot remove the heavier components efficiently.

Traditionally, companies have been called in to "pump and treat" the ground water, ultimately recharging the "clean" water back into the aquifer. This system does not seem to be effective in the long term, because of recontamination from adjacent soil. It has been used with short-term success in removing chlorinated hydrocarbons and petrochemical products from ground water, but its success depends on the hydrogeology of the site, the physicochemical characteristics of the soil, and the extent and distribution of contamination. EPA[8] concluded that the program at Savannah River would not meet its goal of 99% extraction over a 30-year pumping period. Pump and treat facilities can incorporate ultraviolet light, ozonation, and chemical treatments to break down contaminants, and are usually monitored by a series of ground water monitoring wells.[20]

Leaking underground storage tanks. Many underground storage tanks used for gasoline and petroleum products at distributors and residential sites have developed leaks, resulting in contamination of water, soil, and basements. The investigation and remediation of these tanks have become a specialty area. Tanks can be pressure tested to determine whether they are leaking. Leaky tanks can be pumped out and then dug up, but the surrounding soil then requires some form of decontamination.[4] Such soils can be removed in bulk to disposal sites and replaced with clean soil. In situ thermal volatilization offers an economic alternative to removal.

The oil, often referred to as "product," can seep through to bedrock and can contaminate ground water. Recovery of product requires drilling a well through the water table to bedrock, pumping the soluble fraction out of the ground water, and then recovering the "product" from soil immediately above the water table.

New approaches involve vapor extraction of the gaseous and liquid product from the soil to the point where the equilibrium may actually favor the movement of "product" out of the water into soil. The underground vacuum actually encourages the volatilization of lighter organics, facilitating their extraction. This technique offers great promise in permanently removing contaminants in the more mobile fractions, and appears to have few drawbacks other than price.

Other technologies in various stages of development and implementation include solvent application and extraction (solvents forced into soil under pressure and then retrieved, pulling certain contaminants out of the soil), high-pressure surfactant cleaning, and hydroblasting.

Liquid hazardous waste

Many industrial facilities have stored liquid wastes on site in lagoons or impoundments. Under RCRA stringent requirements have been imposed on this form of disposal. Liquid wastes can be treated in several ways. Dewatering eliminates the aqueous phase, leaving behind a dense slurry with high concentrations of contaminants. This can be disposed of more economically than the original large volume. Pressure filtration can force more water out of this slurry, leaving behind a solid cake on the filter, and allowing the liquid effluent to be discharged to a sanitary sewer or municipal water treatment facility.

Thermal technologies

This class of technologies involves the application of heat to chemically alter toxic materials, rendering them environmentally safe. Incineration is the best known of these and is highly controversial because of concerns regarding the release of toxic air pollutants and the production of hazardous ash with bioavailable components, leading to a possible moratorium on the development of new incinerators.[22]

Mobile incinerators. Incineration involves the complete combustion of organic materials to carbon and water vapor. This in turn requires that the material be burnable (have adequate BTU value), that it be adequately mixed with air, that it be heated to a sufficient temperature, and that it remain in the burner for a sufficient time (''residence time'' is on the order of seconds). In reality combustion of organics is seldom complete, so that a variety of organic and inorganic molecules may be released to the atmosphere as vapor or adsorbed to fly ash. Of particular concern is the failure to destroy toxic metals and the persistence or formation of polychlorinated dioxins and furans (PCDDs and PCDFs). These chlorinated polyaromatics (including the PCBs) require very high temperatures to achieve complete destruction.

Thermal oxidizers. This technology can be used as a small-scale incinerator built into an industrial system, or as an inline pollution control device. Specialized burners capture oxygen from the emissions to enhance combustion efficiency even at low temperature. These devices are aimed at reducing emissions (odor, smoke, NO_x, SO_2), without relying on scrubbers or catalysts. The economy lies in capturing the BTU value of the hydrocarbons and any oxygen remaining in the emission stream as well as the opportunity for heat recovery. They can be used for liquid and gaseous waste streams.

Commercial hazardous waste incinerators. A few large corporations have constructed hazardous waste incinerators to meet the needs of their own corporation and have marketed this service to other industrial clients. These incinerators must manage liquids and sludges as well as solids and must accept drums as well as loose material. Special approval is required for an incinerator to handle PCBs, dioxins, radioactive materials, or medical wastes. To certify a hazardous waste incinerator one must meet an elaborate protocol. The waste type and quantity must be known in advance, and it must be sampled and analyzed before being accepted for destruction. The incinerator manager must follow up with a certificate of receipt and destruction, so that the generator can conclude their cradle-to-grave manifesting responsibility.

Chemical treatments

Many approaches are available to chemically alter hazardous materials. Neutralization of acids and bases, precipitation out of liquid phase, oxidation reactions, and photochemical degradation are the main approaches. Chemical treatments can render materials suitable for recycling as well. Under natural conditions many hazardous materials undergo chemical alteration.

Stabilization

Stabilization involves ''locking'' the hazardous chemicals into a matrix that keeps them away from air, water, the food chain, and people. Vitrification requires high temperature to form a glassy substance primarily from inorganic materials. The glass is durable, and is resistant to physical and chemical forces. It can be disposed of as solid waste or used in construction. Chips of glass can be incorporated into asphalt or cement and used for highway construction, enhancing the durability of these materials. Hazardous wastes, particularly in solid form, can be incorporated directly into construction materials.

Plasma arc technology employs a 7000°C torch to turn the solid material into a plasma that will cool into a rock-hard substance. The procedure generates little gaseous contamination, but requires much energy input. It is being used to process hazardous ash from incinerators.[1]

Dilution approaches

Dilution reduces the concentration of contaminants in soil or water by adding uncontaminated material rather than by removing contaminants. It increases the volume of material that must be disposed of, but allows disposal as a nonhazardous waste.

Soil. One approach that makes great sense from a policy viewpoint but that seems to enrage the public is to take contaminated soil and mix it with larger amounts of ''clean'' or less contaminated soil, thereby diluting the pollutants, and ultimately reducing their concentration below some action level. Thereafter, the soil can be treated as any other soil. Once the concentration has been lowered to a point where no one would have been concerned in the first place, it seems rational to use the soil, recognizing that few soil samples in the United States, whether in urban or agricultural areas, are free of detectable man-made contaminants.

Solid waste. Companies that generate solid hazardous wastes can mix these with other solid wastes that are nonhazardous until the contaminant level has been reduced to a concentration below regulatory concern.

Liquid dilution. As an alternative to dewatering liquid waste, when pollutants are water soluble, dilution with fresh water can reduce the concentration of hazardous material below a level of regulatory concern, at which point it can simply be pumped into a sewage facility. This approach results in an extravagant waste of fresh water and does eventually result in the same level of input of the toxic material to the environment.

Biological treatment

A variety of organisms are being sought or engineered for their ability to degrade hazardous materials. Certain bacteria specialize in removing chlorine from organic compounds, a detoxifying process, yet others can add methyl groups to mercury, which enhances its toxicity. Researchers seek natural microorganisms that proliferate in the soil of hazardous waste sites on the assumption that they either need or tolerate high concentrations of chemicals. Genetic engineering of *Pseudomonas* is being developed for potential detoxification of wastes.[15]

Landfilling of hazardous waste

Prior to the 1970s communities tended to mix hazardous wastes indiscriminately, particularly household hazardous waste and solid waste. With the phasing out of landfills as the preferred approach to solid waste management, the landfill retains a specialized role as a repository of certain hazardous wastes, including bottom ash from incinerators and and sludge. It is likely that future hazardous waste management will include landfilling for certain purposes. The construction of secure landfills has been challenging, since the site must provide barriers to keep wastes from migrating or leaching offsite or into the ground water. Operating a landfill requires some recycling capability.

A secure chemical landfill requires a site that is not in close proximity to residential areas and preferably does not overlie an aquifer used for drinking water. In many places landfilling is a suitable approach for at least part of the hazardous waste solution.

SOCIAL CONSIDERATIONS

Remediation of hazardous waste is important and beneficial in reducing the potential for human exposure and environmental degradation. Ideally, regulatory influences on hazardous waste management ought to be congruent with public health benefits, but this is not always the case.

The remediation should:
1. Eliminate the potential for significant human exposure to toxic chemicals
2. Satisfy the aesthetic and economic needs of the community
3. Allow a site to be returned to other beneficial uses
4. Provide a definitive solution rather than simply move the problem elsewhere
5. Be socially and fiscally responsible
6. Not increase air, water, or soil contamination

The overall benefits should outweigh the overall risks.

One problem, however, is that there is an asymmetry in who gets the benefits and who suffers the risks. The issue of environmental equity (see p 649) is predicated on one community not benefiting at the expense of another.

Before undertaking remediation, it should be clear that there are significant hazards or other socio-economic factors that warrant intervention. Often there is a transient increase in pollution during a removal or remediation procedure; hence it is sometimes better to let sleeping pollution lie.

Many remediation technologies are satisfactory for reducing the level of air, soil, and water contamination (and thereby of food chain contamination as well). They differ in cost and permanence, and in their removal efficiency. Digging up and transporting soil may be more efficient at removing the last vestiges of contamination than in situ treatment, but it may not be necessary.

One of the lessons of the 1980s is that management of any site must involve community participation at an early stage (see Chapter 66). The public's expectations and desires are as important to successful cleanup as are regulatory levels of contaminants.[20]

The remediation of hazardous waste sites has become a major industry that is spawning a wealth of new technologies. As in many aspects of society, the appearance of technologic solutions may drive policy, without adequate attention to social, economic, and health issues. Society needs to make a major investment in risk management policy, to determine whether projected costs of remediation are matched by benefits experienced by different stakeholders (communities, governments, workers, businesses) in different currencies (health, freedom from anxiety, money). Any remediation process must be evaluated periodically to ensure that it does more good than harm.

REFERENCES

1. ATSDR: "Artificial lightning" could revolutionize waste disposal, *Hazardous Substances/Public Health* 3(2):1, 1993.
2. Bullard RD: *Dumping in Dixie: race, class and environmental quality,* Boulder Colo, 1990, Westview Press.
3. Burger J, Gochfeld M: Temporal scales in ecological risk assessment, *Arch Environ Contam Toxicol* 23:484, 1992.
4. Cheremisinoff PN, Casana JG, Ouellette RP: *Underground storage tanks guidebook,* Northbrook Ill, 1987, Pudvan Publishing.
5. Cleland JG, Kingsbury GL: Multimedia environmental goals for environmental assessment, National Technology Information Service PB276920, Washington, DC, 1977.
6. Colborn, T, Clement C: *Chemically-induced alterations in sexual and functional development: the wildlife/human connection,* Princeton, NJ, 1992, Princeton Scientific Publishing.

7. EPA: Guidance on remedial actions for contaminated ground water at Superfund Sites, Environmental Protection Agency, Cincinnati, OH EPA/540/G-88/003, 1988
8. EPA: Case study for the Savannah River Plant A/M Area site, in evaluation of ground water extraction remedies, Environmental Protection Agency, Cincinnati, OH, EPA/540/2-89/054B, 1989.
9. Higgins, T: *Hazardous Waste Minimization Handbook,* Chelsea, Mich, 1989, Lewis Publishing.
10. Johnson BL, Williams RC, Harris CM, eds: *National minority health conference: focus on environmental contamination,* Agency for Toxic Substances and Disease Registry, Princeton, NJ 1992, Princeton Publishing.
11. Librizzi W, ed: Alternate technologies for the remediation and disposal of soils contaminated with petroleum hydrocarbons and chlorinated hydrocarbons, Report to NJ Dept Transportation from New Jersey Institute of Technology, Newark, NJ 1991.
12. Lucero G. et al: *Superfund handbook,* ed 3, Chicago, 1989, Sidley and Austin.
13. Majumdar SK, Miller EW, Schmalz RF: *Management of hazardous materials and wastes,* Lafayette Pa, 1989, Pennsylvania Academy of Science.
14. Menzie CA, Burmaster DE: Overview of soil clean-up levels and risk-based decision making, Proceedings of the sixth Annual Hazardous Materials Management Conference International, Atlantic City, NJ, 1988.
15. Molhot B: Innovative biotechnologies for detection and disposal of hazardous materials and wastes. In Majumdar SK et al, eds: *Management of hazardous materials and wastes,* Lafayette Pa, 1989, Pennsylvania Academy of Science.
16. NJDEP: Summary of Approaches to Soil Cleanup Levels, New Jersey Department of Environmental Protection, Trenton, NJ, 1987.
17. NRC: Testing for effects of chemicals on ecosystems, National Research Council, National Academy Press, Washington, DC, 1981.
18. NRC: Animals as sentinels of environmental health hazards, National Research Council, National Academy Press, Washington, DC, 1991.
19. NRC: Issues in Risk Assessment, National Research Council, National Academy Press, Washington, DC, 1993.
20. OTA: Complex Cleanup: The environmental legacy of nuclear weapons, Office of Technology Assessment, Washington, DC, 1991.
21. Peakalll D: *Animal biomarkers as pollution indicators,* London, 1992, Chapman & Hall Ecotoxicology Series 1.
22. Schneider K: Administration to freeze growth of hazardous waste incinerators, *New York Times,* May 18, 1993, p 1.

Chapter 58

ENVIRONMENTAL AND HUMAN HEALTH PERSPECTIVES ON MUNICIPAL COMPOSTING

Jim Cook
Jan Beyea

Composting could be an excellent alternative to landfilling or incineration for dealing with the biodegradable fraction of residential, restaurant, and commercial wastes.[1] Humus from composted organic materials can be used on farms and commercial forests, helping to restore our depleted, eroded soils. Today society robs from the soil and sends to landfills or incinerators nutrients and organic materials that should be returned to the soil, closing the loop. If done right, composting fits naturally with recycling—and can become the next big step after recycling.

Issues of public acceptance and the need to minimize risks to human health and the environment will be crucial in the development of municipal composting as a viable solid waste strategy. Risks associated with production and use of composts include human pathogens and a variety of inorganic and organic compounds.[4,6] Potential risks of ecologic damage from nonhuman pathogens present in composts have not been addressed in the literature. Indeed, it appears that the organisms present are generally beneficial to the soil ecology.[8]

Many primary human pathogens—viruses, bacteria, protozoans, and helminth parasites—may be present in compost feedstocks. Most of them are effectively destroyed at the elevated temperatures characteristic of active composting (45 to 60°C), although contamination by incompletely composted material may occur. Although compost workers have not been reported to suffer from an elevated incidence of exposure-related infectious disease,[4,6] regular immunization of employees may be appropriate, similar to policies for sewage treatment workers.[12]

As is the case whenever vegetative materials decay, a variety of human pathogens thrive during composting and may be present in finished composts.[6] Although generally not infectious to healthy people, airborne bacteria and fungal spores can cause inflammation, chronic mucous membrane irritation and bronchitis, and the development of allergic reactions. Various components of these organisms are responsible: endotoxins (from gram-negative bacteria), proteases (from *Bacillus* spp.), fungal β-1,3-glucans, and mycotoxins (such as aflatoxin from *Aspergillus flavus*).[6,11]

Exposure to high concentrations of spores of the thermophilic fungus *Aspergillus fumigatus* and related species can lead to the infection "brown lung," which is well known among farmers.[6,11] Although spore concentrations downwind of *unenclosed,* windrow composting facilities may be significantly above background, they are probably not high enough to put healthy people at significant risk. However, immunocompromised individuals, those with primary (especially lung) infections and those treated with immunosuppressive drugs such as corticosteroids or antibiotics,[6,12] are more susceptible to *Aspergillus* spp., and they may be at significant risk for infection downwind of these facilities.

Enclosed composting facilities do not appear to pose a risk even to immunocompromised individuals, because downwind spore concentrations are not significantly above background levels.

A variety of volatile inorganic and organic compounds are formed during the composting process, and many of them are malodorous, especially those containing nitrogen, sulfur, or selenium. Under aerobic composting conditions these compounds are rapidly degraded. However, they can accumulate if facilities are not operated properly and conditions become anaerobic. Many of these compounds are very unpleasant for workers, and some are toxic at high enough concentrations.[6] Furthermore, inattention to odor control and consequent odor complaints by residents have been the major issue in most cases where composting facilities have been forced to close. Effective methods of odor control are air management with biofilters or chemical scrubbers.

Certain components of compost feedstocks may contain low levels of toxic and carcinogenic inorganic and organic substances, and sorting "mistakes" may contribute additional contaminants. Generally, contaminant levels are lower when residents separate organic feedstocks for composting than when post-collection separation techniques are used on mixed wastes.* Although volatile organic compounds (mostly solvents) are largely lost and/or degraded during composting, they can potentially impact the health of workers, and good ventilation (and air filtration) is important to minimize risks.[3,6] However, a variety of toxic metals and organic compounds may persist in municipal composts, and they could conceivably impact the human food chain and the general environment.

It is important to consider the net, long-term change in the soil concentrations of these persistent species that would result from ongoing compost usage on a large scale. Short-term application of composts with elevated contaminant levels will have a minor impact on soil contaminant levels. Long-term application, however, could lead to accumulation above current soil levels in rural areas, requiring consideration of ecologic and human-health impacts.

Current soils are far from perfect, however, and it is appropriate to compare contaminant levels in composts to ambient levels in the soils that will receive those composts. Compost used on some agricultural lands may represent an improvement, even if contaminant levels are higher than those in pristine soils. Similarly, suburban and urban soils can be so contaminated that even the use of low-grade composts would improve them.

The concentrations of some potentially toxic metals—particularly cadmium, lead, and mercury—in composts derived from mixed-waste feedstocks are substantially higher than current concentrations of those metals in most agricultural soils. However, the concentrations of cadmium and lead in composts made from source-separated feedstocks are generally lower than those in mixed-waste composts.[4,13,14] For this reason, environmentalists tend to favor source-separated composting. Metal levels in source-separated composts are much lower than EPA's limits for sewage sludge; lead levels are a third of EPA's limit (300 ppm), and the levels of the other metals are a tenth or less of the corresponding limits.

Relatively few data are available on the occurrence of toxic organic compounds in compost feedstocks, finished composts, and soils[3]. Potential contaminants include polychlorinated dibenzodioxins and dibenzofurans (dioxins and furans), polychlorinated biphenyls (PCBs), polycyclic aromatic hydrocarbons (PAHs), and a variety of other compounds. Other potential organic contaminants, motor oil, pesticides, herbicides, and fungicides, could be introduced accidentally at concentrations high enough to increase soil levels (recalling that farmers and the general public intentionally and accidentally introduce such contaminants to agricultural and other soils on regular basis).

Since dioxins and furans have been considered to include the most toxic and carcinogenic compounds known, considerable information is available about them. The main sources are combustion and a variety of industrial processes, and atmospheric deposition appears to be the major input of most dioxins and furans to U.S. soils.[5] Overall, 30 million tons per year of compost may eventually be produced and returned to our nation's soils. Given current levels of dioxins and furans in composts, we expect that this would be a minor component of the annual input of these compounds to agricultural and silvicultural soils. Locally, however, compost application rates may be higher than the national average. Even so, we estimate that the amounts of most dioxins and furans added to the soil would be less than current atmospheric deposition at compost application rates up to 10 tons per acre per year.[5,7,9,10]

In any case, focusing on making cleaner compost will help ensure increasing public acceptance, markets, and ecologic benefits. Three options for improvement are available: separation by residents before collection, improved separation at composting facilities, and attention to the design of products and paper packaging that may end up in compost. Success will mean that organic resources that were once buried or burned will be returned to the land.

REFERENCES

1. Beyea J et al: Composting plus recycling equals 70 percent diversion, *BioCycle:* May:72, 1992.
2. Beyea J, Conditt M: *Wet bag composting demonstration project,* National Audubon Society, Procter & Gamble, International Process Systems, Waste Management, McDonalds, Greenwich Audubon Society, and the Town of Fairfield, Conn, 1993.
3. Epstein E: Neighborhood and worker protection for composting facilities: issues and actions. In Hoitink HAJ, Keener HM, editors: *Science and engineering of composting: design, environmental, microbiological and utilization aspects,* Worthington, Ohio, 1993, Renaissance Publications.

---
*References 2, 3, 4, 13, 14.

4. Epstein E et al: Trace elements in municipal solid waste compost, *Biomass and Bioenergy* 3:227, 1992.
5. Fiedler H, Hutzinger O: Dioxins: sources of environmental load and human exposure, *Toxicological and Environmental Chemistry* 29:157, 1990.
6. Gillett JW: Issues in risk assessment of compost from municipal solid waste: occupational health and safety, public health, and environmental concerns, *Biomass and Bioenergy* 3:145, 1992.
7. Harrad SJ et al: Levels and sources of PCDDs, PCDFs, chlorophenols (CPs) and chlorobenzenes (CBzs) in composts from a municipal yard waste composting facility, *Chemosphere* 23:181, 1991.
8. Hoitink HAJ, Boehm MJ, Hadar Y: Mechanisms of suppression of soilborne plant pathogens in compost-amended substrates. In Hoitink HAJ, Keener HM, editors: *Science and engineering of composting: design, environmental, microbiological and utilization Aspects,* Worthington, Ohio, 1993, Renaissance Publications.
9. Kjeller L-O et al: Increases in the polychlorinated dibenzo-*p*-dioxin and -furan content of soils and vegetation since the 1840s, *Environmental Science and Technology* 25:1619, 1991.
10. Koester CJ, Hites RA: Wet and dry deposition of chlorinated dioxins and furans, *Environmental Science and Technology* 26:1375, 1992.
11. Millner J et al: Bioaerosols associated with composting facilities. Report from a January 25-27, 1993 workshop convened in Beltsville, MD by the Composting Council, the U.S. Environmental Protection Agency and the U.S. Department of Agriculture (in preparation).
12. Ontario Ministry of the Environment: *Interim guidelines for the production and use of aerobic compost in Ontario,* PIBS 1749, Toronto, Ontario, Canada, 1991, Ontario Ministry of the Environment.
13. Prince J: Separation strategies: effect on the quality of recyclables and compost, *Resource Recovery* July:70, 1992.
14. Richard TL, Woodbury PB: The impact of separation on heavy metal contaminants in municipal solid waste composts, *Biomass and Bioenergy* 3:195, 1992.

Chapter 59

REUSE OF SLUDGE

Mark G. Robson

What is sludge?
The disposal problem
Beneficial reuse of sludge
Contaminants in sludge
Health risk assessments
Some examples of metal contamination
    Cadmium
    Lead
    Pathogens
    Bacteria
    Protozoa
    Helminth worms
Conclusion

WHAT IS SLUDGE?

There are a number of byproducts and wastes that come under the broad name of "sludge." For this discussion we will be referring to the sludge byproducts that are from sewage treatment. The issue of sludge reuse has become more important as thousands of communities across the country consider doing something beneficial with their sewage sludge and as opportunities for disposal of sludge diminish. As we improve the levels of waste water treatment, the quantities and volumes of sludge are increasing. The process of decomposition required to release the nutrients in sludge are complex.[5]

Sludge is the semi-solid residue derived from the treatment of waste water. Sludge can be described as liquid sludge with 5% solids, dewatered sludge with 12% to 30% solids, and dried sludge with 60% to 80% solids. In many cases the sludge products contain a significant concentration of valuable plant nutrients, such as nitrogen (up to 10%), potassium, and phosphorous. Unfortunately, sludge, especially that which has little pretreatment, can contain a number of undesirable contaminants such as heavy metals, pesticides, chemicals, and pathogens.

THE DISPOSAL PROBLEM

The disposal of sludge has been a major problem for local governments and industries for a number of years. The problem became more severe when state and federal governments banned the use of ocean dumping for the disposal of sludge. The practice of ocean dumping began as early as 1924. The EPA began a formal permit process in 1972. While Congress banned ocean dumping in 1981, challenges in the court have allowed the process to continue until fairly recently. However, it is expected to cease completely by the mid-1990s.

BENEFICIAL REUSE OF SLUDGE

As the opportunity to dump sludge becomes limited, various ways of destroying or reusing sludge have been considered. Incineration and landfilling are two alternatives, but reuse is gaining popularity, and sludge products for use as fertilizers and soil conditioners are entering the market at a steady pace. Sludge has been incorporated into pellets, composted, and packaged in several ways.

Reuse of the sludge, even into beneficial products, still has a number of concerns, which range from practical considerations of cost and processing to health concerns regarding the presence of toxins and pathogenic agents in the sludge products.

Sludge products are sold as fertilizer products and soil conditioners in most states; they are often sold and used based on their nutrient content. In many states the nutrient guarantee is usually very low or nonexistent; hence regulation based on the nutrient value is nonexistent. While there are still serious concerns regarding sludge as a fertilizer on foods, it can be safely used on lawns and nonfood crops, as long as enrichment by cadmium is not a problem.

CONTAMINANTS IN SLUDGE

A number of compounds and metals are of concern in sludge products, including metals, PCBs, pesticides, and pathogens.

Because of the potential health problems, many crops, both commercial and home garden, are not suitable for growth on land treated with sludge, particularly vegetables such as tomatoes, squash, and sweet corn, leafy vegetables, and root crops such as carrots or beets grown for direct human consumption.

In addition to health considerations, odor is also an issue. There are few practical options available to control odor problems associated with sludge, except isolation by distance.

HEALTH RISK ASSESSMENTS

In developing risk assessments for the use of sludge-derived products, several interesting complications arise. In most cases a risk assessment is based on exposure to a particular hazard via a specific medium, such as air and drinking water. In the case of sludge there are many more pathways. Below is a list of pathways, modified from a list developed by EPA[8,9]:

1. Sludge → Soil → Plant → Human toxicity
2. Sludge → (Soil) → Human toxicity (direct ingestion)
3. Sludge → Soil → Plant → Animal → Human toxicity
4. Sludge → Animal (direct ingestion) → Human toxicity
5. Sludge → Soil → Plant → Animal toxicity
6. Sludge → Animal toxicity (direct ingestion)
7. Sludge → Soil → Plant toxicity (phytotoxicity)
8. Sludge → Soil → Soil biota toxicity
9. Sludge → Soil → Soil biota toxicity → Predator toxicity
10. Sludge → Dust → Human inhalation
11. Sludge → Particulate resuspension (inhalation)
12. Sludge → Vaporization (inhalation)
13. Sludge → Surface runoff → Surface water → Human toxicity
14. Sludge → Surface runoff → Aquatic food chain → Human toxicity
15. Sludge → Ground water (ingestion) → Human toxicity

Uncertainties associated with the extrapolation of sludge research include issues of uptake of metals by particular plants; bioavailability of metals in sludge and soil by direct ingestion; the changes in bioavailability of metals over time with changes in soil chemistry; the biomagnification of cadmium through the food chain and the bioavailability of cadmium due to interactions with other metals; background levels of lead in soil; contamination due to chemical fertilization; adverse ecologic effects of pathogens; the occurrence of protozoa in treated sludge; and the aquatic toxicity from runoff. Sludge-grown vegetables fed to rats did not cause evident toxic damage, but did increase mutagens in urine and cadmium levels in kidneys.[1]

SOME EXAMPLES OF METAL CONTAMINATION

Cadmium

Cadmium is a compound of concern when reusing sludge. Cadmium has historically been associated with electroplating, galvanizing, color pigmentation, battery manufacture, and in the mining and smelting process for lead and zinc. Discharge of industrial waste water into sewage systems results in cadmium contamination of the resulting sewage.

Cadmium is found in air, water, soil, plants, and animals. It is not an essential metal to any organism. It can accumulate in the liver and in the kidney. While acute effects of cadmium, such as nausea and abdominal pain, are unlikely to be seen as a result of sludge use, cadmium could accumulate in the body where there is a long half-life. The synthesis of cadmium-binding metalloprotein in the liver and the kidneys enhances the accumulation and retention of cadmium.

Lead

Lead also poses a problem for sludge use. Approximately 70% of the lead exposure for the general population is via diet. Food products that are grown in sludge-amended soil with a high lead concentration can pose a health risk, if the lead is taken up by the plant.

Pathogens

Pathogen exposure can cause disease and illness. Pathogens and associated diseases have been summarized by EPA[8,9] and are listed below:

Bacteria	Diseases
Salmonella spp.	Salmonellosis (food poisoning), typhoid fever
Shigella spp.	Bacillary dysentery
Yersinia spp.	Acute gastroenteritis (including diarrhea, abdominal pain)
Vibrio cholerae	Cholera
Campylobacter jejuni	Gastroenteritis
Escherichia coli	Gastroenteritis

Viruses	Diseases
Poliovirus	Poliomyelitis
Coxsackie virus	Meningitis, pneumonia, hepatitis, fever, common colds, etc.
Echovirus	Meningitis, paralysis, encephalitis, fever, common colds, diarrhea
Hepatitis A virus	Infectious hepatitis
Rotavirus	Acute gastroenteritis with severe diarrhea
Norwalk agents	Epidemic gastroenteritis with severe diarrhea
Reovirus	Respiratory infections, gastroenteritis

Protozoa	Diseases
Cryptosporidium	Gastroenteritis
Entamoeba histolytica	Acute enteritis
Giardia lamblia	Giardiasis (including diarrhea, abdominal cramps, weight loss)
Balantidium coli	Diarrhea and dysentery
Toxoplasma gondii	Toxoplasmosis

Helminth worms	Diseases
Ascaris lumbricoides	Digestive/nutritional disturbances, abdominal pain, vomiting, restlessness
Ascaris suum	May produce symptoms such as coughing, chest pain, and fever
Trichuris trichiura	Abdominal pain, diarrhea, anemia, weight loss
Toxocara canis	Fever, abdominal discomfort, muscle aches, neurologic symptoms
Taenia solium	Nervousness, insomnia, anorexia, abdominal pain, digestive disturbances
Necator americanus	Hookworm disease
Hymenolepis nana	Taeniasis

Yates[10] identified the major considerations for land disposal of sewage sludge.

Clinicians should be aware that

1. Pathogens (especially parasites and, to a lesser extent, viruses) can survive in the environment for months to years.
2. The number of pathogens is reduced during each stage of sewage (sludge) treatment, but sewage treatment does not completely inactivate all pathogens, and even composted sludge cannot be guaranteed to be free of all pathogens.
3. The absence of indicator bacteria in sludge does not guarantee the absence of pathogenic microorganisms.
4. Viruses have been detected in ground water beneath sites where sewage sludge is being applied.
5. Shallow ground waters are more vulnerable to contamination than deep ground waters.
6. Coarse-textured or fractured soils allow pathogens to be transported more readily than fine-textured soils.
7. Areas with high rainfall and/or that irrigate have a higher potential for ground or surface water contamination because pathogens can be carried with the water.

Certain parasites (such as tapeworms) that may be present in animal waste can also pose a threat to human health.

There are several environmental factors that influence the potential for human exposure to pathogen exposure in sludge.

On the positive side:
1. Viruses are inactivated (killed) more rapidly at high temperatures than low temperatures.
2. Exposure to ultraviolet (sunlight) can reduce the number of viruses and bacteria.

Obviously, all of the above are generalities, and the interactions between these factors must be considered for a given site. A very general description of a site that would have a relatively high potential for human exposure to pathogens might be as follows: application of liquid sludge to a sandy soil with a shallow (less than 50 feet) water table in a cool environment. Domestic wells in close proximity to the sludge-applied land, especially if down-gradient, may be vulnerable to contamination.

Careful site selection and management of sludge application combined with monitoring of the sludge quality can lead to a beneficial use of material that would otherwise be wasted. Properly treated sludge material can be used as a beneficial soil conditioner; this use will serve as a reasonable alternative to disposal as well as take advantage of the beneficial nutrients contained in the sludge. However, you must keep in mind that there is no such thing as a zero-risk situation.

CONCLUSION

Sewage sludge treatment is an evolving technology and future uses of sludge for fertilizer is certain to occur. Caution is important and at present, it is not recommended for use on food cropland.

REFERENCES

1. Boyd JN et al: Safety evaluation of vegetables cultured on municipal sewage sludge-amended soil, *Arch Env Contam Tox* 11:399, 1982.
2. Chaney RL: Twenty years of land application research—part 1, *BioCycle* 9:54, 1990.
3. Chaney RL: Public health and sludge utilization—part 2, *BioCycle* 10:69, 1990.
4. Chaney RL: Scientific analysis of proposed sludge rule, *BioCycle* 7:80, 1989.
5. Hartenstein R: Sludge decomposition and stabilization, *Science* 212:743, 1981.
6. Motto HL et al: *Sludge composting and utilization,* NJAES Project Report 03543, Rutgers University, 1984.
7. NJDEP: *White paper on beneficial use of sewage sludge,* Trenton, NJ, 1990, New Jersey Department of Environmental Protection and Energy.
8. USEPA: *Pursuing beneficial uses of sludge,* conference proceedings, EPA 503/9-91/002, Washington, DC, 1989, EPA.
9. USEPA: *Development of risk assessment methodology for land application and distribution and marketing of municipal sludge,* EPA/600/689/801, Washington, DC, 1989, EPA.
10. Yates M: Land disposal of sewage sludge, *Environmental toxicology newsletter,* vol 12-2, 1992, University of California.

Chapter 60

INCINERATOR WASTE EXPOSURES

Eddy Bresnitz

Incinerator operation
    Municipal solid waste
    Hazardous waste
    Biomedical waste
    Exposure pathways
    Potential health effects
Epidemiologic data
Statutory background for incinerator operations
Research needs and summary

The disposal of both municipal solid waste and hazardous waste has become a prominent public health issue over the past decade. Incineration, as one step in the waste management system, is perceived by the public as being particularly risky to health; however, the few epidemiologic studies of exposure to incinerator by-products suggest minimal if any health hazards to either workers or neighboring residents. Nevertheless, proposals to build new refuse-derived fuel plants or hazardous waste incinerators usually stimulate strong protests from community residents, their rallying cry: "NIMBY (Not in my back yard!").

The relationships between exposures to incinerator waste by-products and potential health effects are complex and depend on the specific waste stream, the existing incineration technology, the likely exposure pathways, and the methods of waste by-product disposal. Health risk assessment must account for variations within each of these areas and is often based on incomplete and/or theoretic exposure assessment.[25] For example, exposure data may be derived from air monitoring of stack emissions in trial burns conducted during ideal conditions of incinerator operation.[28,29] Health risk projections, both carcinogenic and noncarcinogenic, based on these data fail to account for day-to-day variations in the waste stream composition, malfunctions in the incineration process, poor combustion conditions, and exposures through indirect pathways, such as the food chain or contaminated drinking water. Also, failure to assess additional exposure sources outside the waste stream may contribute to underestimates of disease risk. Depending on its assumptions, risk assessment also can overestimate risk.

This section describes and considers the process of incineration as a stage in solid-waste management. It reviews incinerator technology, the types of waste streams and incinerator hazardous by-products, exposure routes, potential health effects and relevant epidemiologic data, the statutory and regulatory background for incinerator operation, and, finally, the key elements in prevention of human and environmental exposures (see also Chapter 4).

INCINERATOR OPERATION

Incineration is a process that burns (oxidizes) organic matter and reduces its volume. The waste stream is arbitrarily classified as municipal solid waste, industrial or hazardous waste, and biomedical waste.[23] This categorization may be artificial because the by-products of incineration of these waste streams differ qualitatively for some substances but only quantitatively for others. A small percentage (0.2% to 0.4%) of the MSW stream consists of hazardous waste, mostly derived from household and office waste and small commercial generators (less than 220 lb/month). Hazardous waste accounts for the bulk of residual postincineration waste (landfill) disposal in the United States, with 392 million tons buried in 1987, compared with 148 million of municipal solid waste.[34]

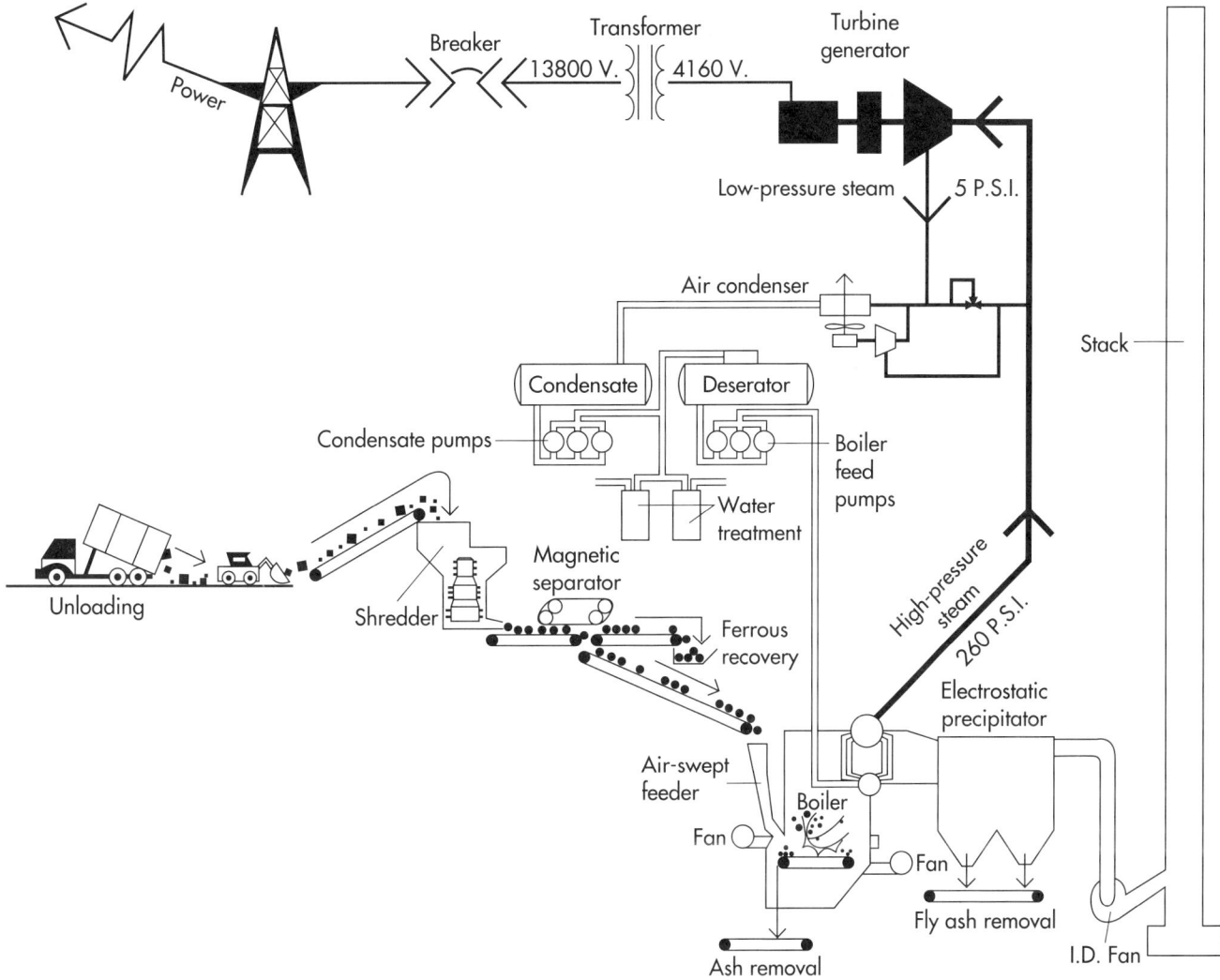

Fig. 60-1. Schematic of refuse-derived fuel-burning plant. (From Mozzon D, Brown DA, Smith JW: Occupational exposure to airborne dust, respirable quartz and metals arising from refuse handling, burning and landfilling. *Am Ind Hyg Assoc J* 48:111(2), 1987.)

The stoker type of incinerator is the major type of mass-burn incinerator in operation in the United States. Waste is fed either in batch fashion or, more commonly, continuously into a hopper that feeds the combustion chamber (Fig. 60-1). A continuous-feed mass-burn incinerator can handle about 200 to 300 tons of MSW daily.[34] A facility may have more than one functioning incinerator. In 1989, there were 210 MSW incinerator sites in the United States, with 450 operating units burning a total of 105,000 tons daily.[23] The Environmental Protection Agency (EPA) arbitrarily defines an incinerator facility as small, large, or regional if it burns less than 200, 200 to 2000, or more than 2000 tons daily, respectively.

Fig. 60-2 schematically outlines the four major operations of a waste incineration system: waste preparation, combustion, air pollution control, and residue and ash handling.[22] Process component options also are outlined. It is beyond the scope of this section to discuss the selection criteria for choosing among these options.

Municipal solid waste

MSW (household waste, nonhazardous waste from commercial operations, public street waste) is increasingly being disposed of through mass-burn incineration (5% to 10%) instead of in landfills (85%).[23] Table 60-1 lists the average physical composition of MSW in the United States in 1987, although there is a considerable amount of waste-stream heterogeneity.[34] With the increasing use of source separation (recycling programs) in communities throughout the United States, the proportion of glass, plastics and metal products in MSW should decrease. Municipal waste incineration reduces the volume of waste by 70% to 90%, often cogenerating energy, usually in the form of electricity via steam production. It should be emphasized that incineration does

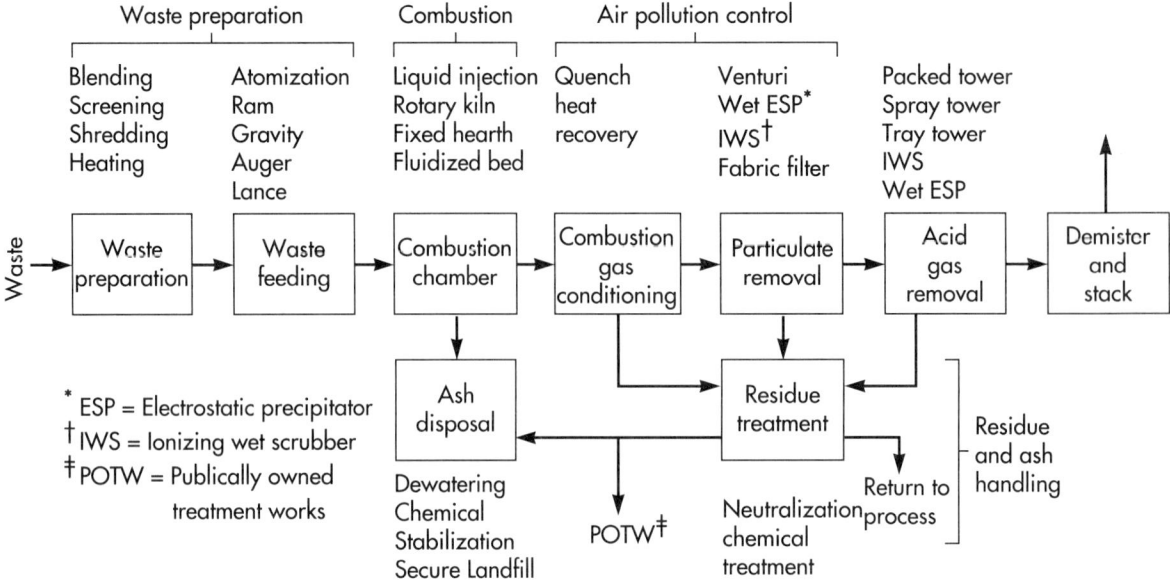

Fig. 60-2. Incineration subsystems and typical process component options. (From Oppelt ET: Air emissions from the incineration of hazardous wastes. *Tox Ind Hlth* 6:23(5), 1991.)

Table 60-1. Physical composition of municipal solid waste, United States, 1987

Substance	Percentage
Paper	37.1
Garbage	8.1
Woods and weeds	17.9
Fiber	2.1
Leather and rubber	2.5
Plastic	7.2
Glass	9.7
Metal	9.6
Incombustible	1.8
Other	0.1
Water content	23.0

Modified from Last L, Wallace R, eds: *Maxcy-Rosenau-Last public health and preventive medicine,* ed 13, East Norwalk, Conn, 1992, Appleton & Lange.

not eliminate waste, it only reduces its volume and changes its form. In the process, potentially hazardous substances are destroyed, created, or concentrated into more readily disposable waste residues, such as fly ash, bottom ash, and adsorbed gases and vapors.[6,16,30]

Fly ash is the fine particulate, incombustible material that emerges from the combustion chamber and either is collected at various points in the incineration process by electrostatic precipitators, fabric filters, and scrubbers or that escapes from the stack. Bottom ash refers to the particulate solid residue that falls to the bottom of the boiler grate. Combustion gases, consisting mainly of hydrogen chloride, carbon monoxide and nitrogen oxides, are collected by scrubbing or by neutrifying with lime[8] or a caustic soda solution such as sodium hydroxide.

Ash by-products contain concentrated collections of solid particulates and dust with adsorbed heavy metals such as mercury, lead, cadmium, chromate, arsenic, and zinc.[6,19] These metals, if vaporized in the incineration process, are also collected during the scrubbing phase of waste stream processing. The concentrations of heavy metals vary among these different waste by-products. As would be expected, incinerator workers who are required to clean boilers, precipitators, and scrubbing units are at particularly high risk for airborne exposures,[12,18] as are workers who have to move the ash mechanically, such as tractor-trailer operators.[5]

Hazardous waste

The Resource Conservation and Recovery Act (RCRA) of 1976, significantly amended by the Hazardous and Solid Waste Amendments of 1987 defines waste as hazardous when it poses a threat to human health or the environment, based on the criteria of ingnitability, corrosivity, reactivity, and toxicity.* In addition, a waste is deemed hazardous if it is a chemical listed under RCRA or under the Clean Water Act; a mixture of hazardous and nonhazardous waste; or waste derived from certain specified processes. Sewage sludge is not defined as hazardous waste.

Hazardous waste incinerators have performance standards distinct from those related to MSW incinerators.[23] Hazardous wastes are burned principally as fuels in industrial boilers and furnaces and less commonly in waste incinerators.[2] The principal by-products of the combustion pro-

---

*40 CFR § 261.

Table 60-2. Most frequent hazardous waste incinerator stack emissions

Volatile compounds	Semivolatile compounds
Benzene	Naphthalene
Toluene	Phenol
Carbon tetrachloride	Bis(2-ethylhexy)phthalate
Chloroform	Diethylphthalate
Methylene chloride	Butylbenzylphthalate
Trichloroethylene	Dibutylphthalate
1,1,1-Trichloroethane	
Chlorobenzene	

Modified from Oppelt ET, Air emissions from the incineration of hazardous waste, *Toxicol Ind Health* 6:23, 1990.

cess are water vapor, carbon dioxide, inert ash (containing metals) partially burned components, and reaction organic compounds such as hydrogen chloride and nitrogen oxides. Certified incinerators must destroy and remove 99.99% of each principal organic hazardous constituent (POHC) in the waste stream.[22,37] In addition, they must remove at least 99% of hydrogen chloride from the exhaust gas and have particulate matter emissions no greater than 180 mg/m^3.

Heavy metals in airborne emissions and in ash residuals are as much of concern in by-products of hazardous waste incineration as in MSW incineration. This is particularly true for lead in industrial processes using hazardous waste as a fuel.[22]

Organic products of incomplete combustion (PICs) from hazardous waste incinerators have potential toxic effects that raise the concerns of environmentalists, community residents, and regulators. PICs are defined as "organic compounds which are present in the emissions from the incineration process, which were not present or detectable in the fuel [wastestream] fed to the incinerator."[22] The PICs may derive from incomplete destruction of POHCs, newly created compounds, or from contaminated scrubber water. Table 60-2 lists the compounds most frequently found in stack emissions from incinerators or boilers burning hazardous wastes. This list represents only a small fraction of the total PICs and was determined from EPA field tests.[22]

Biomedical waste

BMW is defined as "any solid waste . . . generated in the diagnosis, treatment, . . . or immunization of human beings or animals, in research pertaining thereto, or in the production or testing of biologics."* About 10% of nonhazardous waste consists of BMW.[11]

BMW is not considered hazardous waste in the United States and as such is regulated as solid waste. The only exception is if the BMW is treated in an incinerator that burns more than 100 kg/mo of RCRA-defined hazardous waste.[23] Nevertheless, or as a result of a lack of strict hazardous waste regulation, studies indicate that BMW incinerators emit significant amounts of toxins, including heavy metals, hydrogen chloride, and dioxins.[11]

The potential emission of airborne bacteria from BMW incinerators has been of special concern. Several studies have examined this issue and have noted that BMW incinerators contain viable bacteria in the exhaust flue gases but not in the waste ash.[1,3,4,27] The air in the room housing the incinerator has been the source of bacteria, for the most part.[3] Investigators have noted the elimination of bacteria when temperatures in the primary combustion chamber exceed a certain level.[3,4,27] No epidemiologic data suggest that BMW incinerators are a source of infectious hazards to surrounding communities.

Exposure pathways

Modern incinerators increase the concentrations of toxins in the ash by reducing concentrations of airborne pollutants through quantitatively more efficient air pollution control technologies. Thus, incineration should be viewed not as a waste-disposal method but as a waste-modification method. Changes in the quality of ash shifts the toxic burden from the atmosphere to landfills, where potential leaching of hazardous substances into the groundwater increases the likelihood of food-chain contamination.[6,33] Ingestion of contaminated water leached from ash landfills[17] and food tainted through either airborne emissions or uptake from contaminated nutrients and water from the soil[32] may increase the body burden of incinerator-derived toxic wastes. In fact, the increasing efficacy of current technologic methods to reduce airborne emissions from incinerators suggests that the bulk of potentially toxic exposures to the public will derive from contamination of the food chain. This is true for heavy metals in addition to organic compounds such as dioxins.[9]

Dioxins are a group of polychlorinated chemicals consisting of different forms of polychlorinated dibenzo-*p*-dioxins (PCDDs) and polychlorinated dibenzofurans (PCDFs).[36] The National Toxicology Program considers 2,3,7,8-tetrachlorodibenzo-*p*-dioxin (TCDD) a potent chemical carcinogen.[21] Mixtures of PCDDs and PCDFs are often expressed as TCDD toxic equivalents, or TEQs, and are found in soil samples worldwide. Studies of TCDD levels in samples taken from soil of communities near incinerators have revealed concentrations similar to background levels in soil from rural and urban areas.[35] Air concentrations of TEQs near incinerators are also similar to background urban air levels, indicating that incinerators are not a prime source of dioxin pollution.

For the most part, the food chain is the major pathway of human exposure to dioxins, as it is for other organics such as pesticides and polychorinated biphenyls.[9,20,36] Travis and Hattemer-Frey[36] list five known TCDD sources that account "for a *maximum* of (only) 11 percent of total annual TCDD input into the US environment."[36] These sources include MSW incinerators, motor vehicles, hospital waste incinera-

---

*40 CFR § 259.30(a).

tors, residential wood burning, and pulp-and-paper-mill effluent. Surprisingly, hazardous waste incinerators emit only minimal amounts of these toxic pollutants. Additional potential sources include forest fires, metal-processing and treatment plants, pentachlorophenol production, and others.

Potential health effects

The adverse health effects of exposure to heavy metals are described elsewhere in this book (Chapter 23). Analyses of various incinerator waste by-products have demonstrated the presence of potential carcinogens, such as the dioxins and polynuclear aromatic hydrocarbons, in incinerator waste.[16] The bulk of these analyses have used the Ames testing method to assess mutagenicity. Studies of samples of airborne incinerator dusts,[24] ambient dust in the vicinity of an incinerator,[38] MSW incinerator ash[14,31] and urine of MSW incinerator workers[26] have demonstrated increased mutagenicity in comparison with control samples. In most cases, simultaneous testing with mutagen promotors (promutagens) demonstrated enhancement of the mutagenic ability of the sample tested.

Pani et al[24] studied both suspended and settled 24-hour dust samples from a MSW incinerator in Trieste, Italy. They were able to demonstrate a dose-response curve of mutagenicity in total and respirable (less than 3.5 μmol particles) suspended dust as well as in settled dust collected in the incinerator. The high mutagenic activity of dust extract was virtually eliminated when a sample of settled dust was reheated to a high temperature (above 350°C), indicating that the sample probably contained mutagenic compounds found in incompletely burnt material leaking from the ovens.

A study by Watts[38] demonstrated significant dose-response mutagenicity activity in extracts of samples of ambient air collected near a MSW incinerator; however, the authors could not attribute the source of mutagens to emissions from the incinerators.

MSW incineration ash also has been shown to have mutagenic potential. Silkowski et al[31] show varying levels of mutagenic activity in MSW ash, depending on the type of substance (organic solvent, water, or acidified water) used to extract the mutagens from the ash. The influence of the type of extractant has important implications for the level of mutagenicity of landfill leachate.

In one of the few human studies of biologic indices of exposure to genotoxic agents, Scarlett et al[26] compared the proportion of MSW incinerator workers with significant urinary mutagens with a control group of water-treatment plant workers. The incinerator workers, particularly at one facility, were almost 10 times more likely to have urinary mutagens in a sample collected at the end of the day than were the water workers. Age minimally increased the proportion of workers with urinary mutagens. Smoking, use of wood stoves, alcohol consumption, and consumption of fried meats had no effect on the proportion of workers with urinary mutagens in either group. Repair workers in the incinerator plant appeared to have the greatest likelihood of having positive assay results. Additional studies are desirable to confirm this observation.

Overall, the studies employing the Ames bacteriologic assay support the conclusion that different incinerator waste components have the potential to induce cancers in humans; however, only a handful of epidemiologic studies have assessed this issue.

EPIDEMIOLOGIC DATA

The studies that have been done have focused on MSW incinerator workers. In the only mortality study of municipal waste workers, Gustavsson[13] noted an excess of deaths due to ischemic heart disease and lung cancer in workers in Sweden. There was no attempt to correlate potential exposures (incinerator or lifestyle) with incidence of disease.

The National Institute for Occupational Safety and Health (NIOSH) has conducted five Health Hazard Evaluations of waste incinerators in the 1980s. The most complete was done in Philadelphia in 1988.[5] After an Agency for Toxic Substances and Disease Registry site survey of a Philadelphia trash-burning incinerator, 89 of 105 active employees were assessed for potential health effects. Comparison of the 86 males in the cohort, divided into potentially high- and low-exposure groups, revealed no clinically significant differences in mean blood or serum measurements of many substances. Eight individuals had an elevated biologic index indicating exposure to a heavy metal; however, these evaluations were unrelated to the individuals' exposure classification. Differences in pulmonary function related to smoking status only. Thirty-four percent of the workers had evidence of hypertension, which was associated with significant proteinuria in both exposure groups. Of the many airborne samples taken by NIOSH, results of four personal breathing zone tests—one for lead in a welder, one for phosphorus, and two for total airborne particulates—were elevated above Occupational Safety and Health Administration or American Conference of Governmental and Industrial Hygienists standards. The environmental monitoring results indicate generally low levels of exposure among all the workers, although working conditions during the sampling period most likely did not reflect the usual operations at the plant. Although these data are limited, they do not support significant clinical effects secondary to airborne exposures in active municipal incinerator waste workers.

In another study, Elliott et al[7] studied the incidence of laryngeal and lung cancer between 1974 and 1987 in geographic areas adjacent to solvent and oil waste incinerators in Great Britain. Expected values were based on national rates, and the data were adjusted for socioeconomic status and lag time between incinerator start-up and cancer incidence. There was no evidence of a relationship between disease risk and distance from the 10 incinerators included in the study.

Although much has been written about the potential health effects on community residents exposed to incinerator waste by-products, no other epidemiologic studies address this issue. Communities that decry MSW incineration perceive their risks as principally stemming from exposure to airborne pollutants. As described previously, the air concentrations of the most feared pollutants in the vicinity of incinerators, namely dioxins, are not increased above background levels.[35] Other airborne pollutants, mainly the criteria pollutants (lead, carbon monoxide, nitrogen oxides, and total suspended particulates), generally fall well below National Ambient Air Quality Standard levels as a result of efficient air-quality control technology in the combustion and waste-gas conditioning processes.[16]

More significant health hazards stem potentially from leaching of toxic substances from terrestrial ash landfills. There have been no epidemiologic studies to assess the health risks of these hazards. It is unlikely that any epidemiologic study could adequately address this issue given the nearly impossible task of estimating the degree of exposure attributable to landfill leachate. As a result, a discussion of potential adverse health effects must be limited to effects on other biologic systems (see earlier) and theoretic risk assessment modeling, which may underestimate the true risk of disease.[6,37]

STATUTORY BACKGROUND FOR INCINERATOR OPERATIONS

The regulation of incinerator toxic emissions is grounded in several laws passed in the 1970s and 1980s.[10] These laws empowered the EPA, which was established in 1970, to regulate the type and quantity of air and water pollutants. The authority to license and monitor incinerators is delegated to state environmental agencies that are bound to follow EPA guidelines. The major relevant legislation includes the Toxic Substances Control Act of 1976 to regulate disposal of chemicals*; the Clean Water Act to control chemical leaching from waste effluent†; the Clean Air Act of 1971 significantly amended in 1990, to regulate air pollution and incinerators‡; and the RCRA§ of 1976 to manage ash waste.

The major elements of RCRA are subtitles C and D. Subtitle C¶ outlines hazardous waste regulations. The majority of regulations for MSW management are set by state agencies, not by the EPA. In contrast, most of the rules pertaining to hazardous waste control are promulgated by the EPA. Subtitle D sets out guidelines for disposal of nonhazardous solid waste that includes "any garbage, refuse, sludge from a waste treatment plant, water supply treatment plant, or air-pollution control facility and other discarded material."§ The 1984 amendment to RCRA specifically excluded MSW incinerators from the stringent control required of hazardous waste if a municipality set up inspection procedures that ensured exclusion of hazardous waste from the MSW stream.[23]

The Clean Air Act initially regulated only particulate-matter emissions.* The Act considers incinerators as hazardous pollution point sources and was amended in 1990 to require the EPA to establish performance standards to regulate emission levels of toxic air pollutants from new and existing "municipal waste combusters."† MSW incinerators must comply with a performance standard that requires the lowest emission that can be achieved by the best system of emission reduction (section 129). Incinerators must have reliable, continuous emission-monitoring systems in place and must maintain good combustion practices. These operating practices form the foundation for compliance with the Clean Air Act and include control of the feedstock composition and flow (through source reduction and recycling), incinerator operator certification and training, adequate burn-temperature maintenance and incinerator air supply, and flue gas measurements and limits on carbon monoxide emissions.

The Clean Air Act also regulates the levels of lead and heavy metal emissions; the release of particulates, dioxins, and acid gases (such as oxides of nitrogen, SO_2, and HCl) into the atmosphere; and ash disposal. Although residual fly and bottom ash contain higher concentrations of toxic elements than does unburned waste, the EPA has no policy on whether MSW ash should be considered hazardous waste. Currently, MSW bottom and fly ash are mixed with non-burned waste and buried in nonhazardous landfills. There are no regulations to stabilize the ash to prevent leaching of toxic heavy metals and other hazardous chemicals into the groundwater.

RESEARCH NEEDS AND SUMMARY

The most relevant health research needs in the field of incinerator waste by-products are cohort epidemiologic morbidity-and-mortality studies of both MSW and hazardous waste workers and improved exposure assessment, taking temporal and spatial variability into account. Given the small size of most incinerators, registries of potentially exposed individuals, such as those organized by the Agency for Toxic Substances and Disease Registry, would be most appropriate. Collection of personal and environmental monitoring data, as well as lifestyle risk-factor data, would be important for correlation of disease with exposure. In contrast, health studies of communities adjacent to incinerators or landfills are unlikely to yield useful or meaningful data, given the problems with estimating valid exposure or exposures.

Increasingly, incinerators are becoming a key element in the management of municipal and hazardous wastes; however, their use must be viewed as only one part of the waste-

---

*15 USC § et seq.
†USC § 1301 et seq.
‡42 USC § 7601 et seq.
§42 USC § 6903.
¶42 USC § 6921-6931.

*42 USC § 7411(b).
†42 USC § 7429.

management system. If incineration is viewed as a method of waste control instead of waste disposal, public health authorities and society are not likely to view incinerators as the solution to the increasing scarcity of landfills, which should lead to new and improved methods of combustion, air pollution controls, monitoring of emissions, and ash management. As Denison and Silbergeld[6] advocate, society must consider all steps in the product cycle, including production and use, not just waste management. "Only comprehensive source-based strategies are likely to prove successful in achieving significant reductions in the metal content of MSW and incineration by-products." Society needs to take a more primary preventive approach to waste management by reducing the availability of toxins in our consumer products. A primarily preventive attitude must replace the trash-and-burn attitude that is prevalent at all levels.

REFERENCES

1. Allen RJ et al: Emission of airborne bacteria from a hospital incinerator, *JAPCA* 39:164, 1989.
2. Behmanesh N, Allen DT, Warren JL: Flow rates and compositions of incinerated waste streams in the United States, *J Air Waste Mgmt Assoc* 42:437, 1992.
3. Blenkharn JI, Oakland D: Emission of viable bacteria in the exhaust flue gases from a hospital incinerator, *J Hosp Infect* 14:73, 1989.
4. Blenkharn JI, Oakland D: Safety and efficacy of clinical waste incineration, *J Hosp Infect* 17:311, 1991 (letter).
5. Bresnitz EA et al: Morbidity among municipal waste incinerator workers, *Am J Ind Med* 22:363, 1992.
6. Denison RA, Silbergeld EK: Risks of municipal solid waste incineration: an environmental perspective, *Risk Anal* 8:343, 1988.
7. Elliott P et al: Incidence of cancers of the larynx and lung near incinerators of waste solvents and oils in Great Britain, *Lancet* 339:854, 1992.
8. Frame GB: A comparison of air pollution control systems for municipal solid waste incinerators, *Air Poll Contr Assoc* 38:1081, 1988.
9. Fries GF, Paustenbach DJ: Evaluation of potential transmission of 2, 3, 7, 8-tetrachlorodibenzo-*p*-dioxin-contaminated incinerator emissions to humans via foods, *J Toxicol Environ Health* 29:1, 1990.
10. Gaba JM, Stever DW: *Law of solid waste, pollution prevention and recycling,* Deerfield, Ill, 1992, Clark Boardman Callaghan.
11. Glasser H, Chang DP, Hickman DC: An analysis of biomedical waste incineration, *J Air Waste Mgmt Assoc* 41:1180, 1991.
12. Gostin J: Northwest incinerator and NIOSH activities, Unpublished Report of Occupational Health Services, Inc, 1988.
13. Gustavsson P: Mortality among workers at a municipal waste incinerator, *Am J Ind Med* 15:245, 1989.
14. Kamiya A, Ose Y, Sakagami Y: The mutagenicity of refuse leachate from a municipal incinerator, *Sci Total Envir* 78:131, 1989.
15. Landrigan, PJ: Incompletely studied hazards of waste incineration, *Am J Ind Med* 15:243, 1989 (editorial).
16. Lisk DJ: Environmental implications of incineration of municipal solid waste and ash disposal, *Sci Total Envir* 74:39, 1988.
17. Lisk DJ et al: Element composition of municipal refuse ashes and their aqueous extracts from 18 incinerators, *Bull Environ Contam Toxicol* 42:534, 1989.
18. Mozzon D, Brown DA, Smith JW: Occupational exposure to airborne dust, respirable quartz and metals arising from refuse handling, burning and landfilling, *Am Ind Hyg Assoc J* 48:111, 1987.
19. Mumma RO et al: National survey of elements and radioactivity in municipal incinerator ashes, *Arch Environ Contam Toxicol* 19:399, 1990.
20. Nessel CS et al: Evaluation of the relative contribution of exposure routes in a health risk assessment of dioxin emissions from a municipal waste incinerator, *J Exp Anal Environ Epidemiol* 1:283, 1991.
21. National Toxicology Program: *Sixth Annual Report on Carcinogens: summary 1991,* NIEHS Publication, Research Triangle Park, NC, 1991.
22. Oppelt ET: Air emissions from the incineration of hazardous waste, *Toxicol Ind Health* 6:23, 1990.
23. O'Reilly JT: *State and local government solid waste management,* Deerfield, Ill, 1991, Clark Boardman Callaghan.
24. Pani B et al: Mutagenicity test of extracts of airborne dust from the municipal incinerator of Trieste, *Environ Mutagen* 5:23, 1983.
25. Roffman A, Roffman HK: Air emissions from municipal waste combustion and their environmental effects, *Sci Total Environ* 104:87, 1991.
26. Scarlett JM et al: Urinary mutagens in municipal refuse incinerator workers and water treatment workers, *J Toxicol Environ Health* 31:11, 1990.
27. Scott GM, Jones GH: Emission of viable bacteria in the exhaust flue from a waste incinerator, *J Hosp Infect* 16:183, 1990 (letter, comment).
28. Sedman RM, Esparza JR: Evaluation of the public health risks associated with semivolatile metal and dioxin emissions from hazardous waste incinerators, *Environ Health Perspect* 94:181, 1991.
29. Sedman RM, Esparza JR: Evaluation of volatile organic emissions from hazardous waste incinerators, *Environ Health Perspect* 94:169, 1991.
30. Shane BS et al: Organic toxicants and mutagens in ashes from eighteen municipal refuse incinerators, *Arch Environ Contam Toxicol* 19:665, 1990.
31. Silkowski MA, Smith SR, Plewa MJ: Analysis of the genotoxicity of municipal solid waste incinerator ash, *Sci Total Environ* 111:109, 1992.
32. Stern AH, Munshi AA, Goodman AK: Potential exposure levels and health effects of neighborhood exposure to a municipal incinerator bottom ash landfill, *Arch Environ Health* 44:40, 1989.
33. Takeshita R, Akimoto Y: Leaching of polychlorinated dibenzo-*p*-dioxins and dibenzofurans in fly ash from municipal solid waste incinerators to a water system, *Arch Environ Contam Toxicol* 21:245, 1991.
34. Tanaka M, Takatsuki H, Itokawa Y: Solid and radioactive waste disposal. In Last L, Wallace R, eds: *Maxcy-Rosenau-Last public health and preventive medicine,* ed 13, East Norwalk, Conn, 1992, Appleton & Lange.
35. Travis CC, Hattemer-Frey HA: A perspective on dioxin emissions from municipal solid waste incinerators, *Risk Anal* 9:91, 1989.
36. Travis CC, Hattemer-Frey HA: Human exposure to dioxin, *Sci Total Environ* 104:97, 1991.
37. Travis CC et al: Potential health risk of hazardous waste incineration, *J Hazardous Materials* 14:309, 1987.
38. Watts R: Use of bioassay methods to evaluate mutagenicity of ambient air collected near a municipal waste combustor, *Air Poll Contr Assoc* 39:1436, 1989.

Part VI

PREVENTIVE APPROACHES IN ENVIRONMENTAL MEDICINE

Chapter 61

GLOBAL ASPECTS OF ENVIRONMENTAL HEALTH

Joanna Burger
Michael Gochfeld

The global environment
    Climate change
    Stratospheric ozone
    Acid precipitation
    Land-use changes
Global issues in environmental health
Demographic factors
    Migrations and refugees
    Population levels
    Overpopulation and poverty
    Overpopulation and war
    Overpopulation, poverty, and violence
Food and potable water
    Sustainable agriculture
    Pesticides
    Climate and agriculture
    Sustainable energy
    Coastal resources
    Biodiversity
    Global economic issues
Toward a global synthesis
Conclusion
Acknowledgments

Clinicians recognize the relationship between economic issues, public understanding, and delivery of health care. This chapter explores the complex interrelatedness among many factors, social, economic, agricultural, ecologic, industrial, and climatic, that influence /environmental health on an international and global scale over a very long time frame, affecting people in both the developing and developed nations.[104] This chapter expands both the spatial and temporal scale of environmental medicine.

The growing interest in environmental health on an international scale has paralleled other concerns regarding the world ecosystem. On the one hand, dramatic changes in Eastern Europe have led to recognition of major environmental disasters,[53] with the extent of air pollution just being recognized.[52] On the other hand, the North American Free Trade Agreement has led to concerns regarding the impact on environmental quality in developing nations[19] as well as on jobs in the United States.

Practitioners of environmental health have expanded their horizons to other countries and regions, but only recently have they gone beyond a focus on specific geographic areas to encompass global issues. Rather than examining environmental health issues only from the perspective of a city, state, or nation, we will examine global factors influencing health and disease, seeking commonalities that to a large extent transcend national concerns. Issues in environmental health that might not be important for any one region take on added significance when considered globally.

Such an environmental synthesis has been seriously impaired by the real disparities between the priority environmental health issues in different parts of the world.[99] In industrialized countries environmental health focuses on exposure to toxic chemicals, radiation, chemical causes of cancer, reproductive disorders, and chemical sensitivity. Parts per million of metals and pesticides, and parts per trillion of dioxin in soil, food, and drinking water become critical issues. However, in developing countries environmental health priorities include sanitation, potable water, and vector control. Individuals are more concerned with the basic availability of food, soil, and water rather than whether they are chemically contaminated. Even these issues have not been examined globally in light of our changing environment. Overpopulation is a problem worldwide, although it poses more severe immediate problems in developing nations. A valuable catalog of environmental changes is provided annually by the World Resources Institute in collaboration with the United Nations Environmental Program (UNEP).[36]

In this chapter we discuss the relationship of humans in a world ecosystem, confronted by global demographic and climatic changes and the interrelationship of these global changes: the effects of population, land use, and climate on food, energy, sustainable agriculture, and other human endeavors.[56,99]

An ecosystem is a geographic entity comprising both abiotic (soil, water, atmosphere) and biotic (microorganisms, plants and animals, including humans) components. Energy flows through the trophic levels of ecosystems, from the primary producers (usually green plants that fix solar energy), through primary and secondary consumers, which, after death, are broken down by decomposers. In this pathway, with its thousands of variations, solar energy is eventually dissipated, but matter (carbon, sulfur, phosphorus, nitrogen, and many other elements) is recycled. Decomposers restore the elements to soil, making them available for future generations of organisms.

By global we mean the sum total of the ecosystems of the Earth, including all the abiotic and biotic components. Indeed, global considerations extend from the ocean depths and soils through the Earth's atmosphere to the sun. When the whole world is the ecosystem of interest, then inputs and outputs in the form of energy, and movement of materials through different parts of the ecosystem, become of paramount importance. It becomes necessary to consider a broad spatial scale[28] and a long-term temporal scale.[8]

Ecologists have led the way in scaling up from individuals (humans or other organisms) to whole populations, communities, and ecosystems. Only recently have environmental health practitioners been drawn into these issues. As recently as 1983 Moriarty[60] lamented the lack of involvement of toxicologists with basic ecologic principles. Environmental health practitioners and indeed many ecologists have concentrated on the health of the individual, and then extrapolated to populations and communities. The jump from communities to ecosystems, regions, and the world has been a substantial extrapolation.

Two major developments link the concerns of environmental medicine and ecology: the rapid evolution of environmental risk assessment (health risk assessment) throughout the 1980s,[65,70,97] and the emergence of serious attention to ecologic risk assessment in the past decade.*

One model of environmental health examines humans exposed to environmental toxins.[60] More recently environmental scientists have put the environment in the model (Fig. 61-1), and other organisms are increasingly recognized as part of the system and as having pivotal roles in predicting future environmental problems. Furthermore, there are feedback loops between all parts of the system, making the consideration of the health of other organisms in the system an important goal in itself. This approach has led to important understandings of the causes of human illnesses, and to subsequent interventions and regulations to prevent environmental disease.

However, we argue in this chapter that we also need to examine the problem of environmental change and environmental health from the top down, from the global environment to the community. Both approaches are necessary, but the global approach has been sadly neglected by environmental health.

THE GLOBAL ENVIRONMENT

The recent emergence of the study of how the Earth's ecosystem operates and responds to global change has involved large-scale cross-disciplinary and multidisciplinary research in addition to progress in traditional single-discipline approaches.[58] Marked changes in the Earth's environ-

---

*References 9, 67, 71, 73, 92.

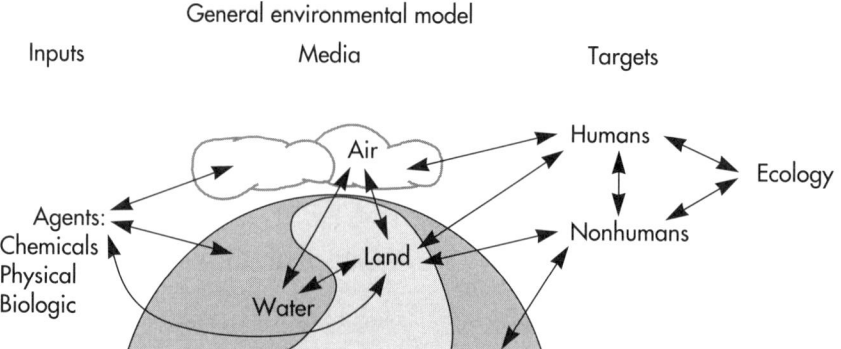

Fig. 61-1. A general model of environmental interactions showing the input of chemical, physical, and biological agents, their distribution through environmental media, and their ultimate impact on human and nonhuman biota and on ecological relationships. (©J. Burger, by permission of the Environmental and Occupational Health Sciences Institute.)

ment have been observed, and these will accelerate as human population increases.[86] Direct and indirect feedbacks link humans and the terrestrial ecosystems they live in with global changes, including fluxes of water, energy, nutrients, and greenhouse gases.[80]

There are two major types of global change related to demographic change: climate change and land-use change. They both lead to shifts in the Earth's ecosystems that in turn influence sea level, temperatures, rainfall, agriculture, land mosaics, and biodiversity[75] (Fig. 61-2). These have an impact on human health issues, influencing the availability of food, energy, potable water, and exposure to toxic agents (metals, pesticides, oil, and other chemicals).

Climate change

The Earth's climate is directly related to physical features of the Earth and its atmosphere, and the energy from the sun. Two changes, depletion of the ozone layer and accumulation of greenhouse gases, are global concerns, while a third, acid precipitation, is primarily regional.[66,68] In 1989 the National Institute for Environmental Health Sciences held a conference on *Global Atmospheric Change and Human Health* that highlighted the complex interrelationships between the physical world and human activity patterns such as energy consumption and industrialization, which in turn influence health. Goldstein[31] noted that while climatologists focus on how these activities increase carbon dioxide and affect climate, environmental health specialists are concerned as well with the direct release of irritant gases such as oxides of sulfur and nitrogen, air pollutants that have direct, negative impacts on health. Moreover, depletion of the ozone layer directly affects human health issues such as increases in skin cancer due to increased penetration of high-energy ultraviolet radiation.

The normal pattern of climate is a function of the solar energy entering the Earth's atmosphere and being absorbed, radiated, or reflected (Fig. 61-3).[85] Incoming solar radiation is reflected by the atmosphere (25%), absorbed by the atmosphere (25%), absorbed by the Earth's surface (45%), or reflected by the Earth's surface (5%).[85] This process leaves room for man-induced changes caused by increases in greenhouse gases (carbon dioxide, methane, chlorofluorocarbons) and land-use changes (mainly deforestation). The main contribution to global warming is increased atmospheric carbon dioxide from the burning of fossil fuels.

The greenhouse effect operates because some gases and particles in the atmosphere allow more sunlight to filter through to the surface of the planet, but reflect back to Earth much of the radiant infrared energy that would otherwise escape through the atmosphere back into space.[40,41,85]

This creates a one-way mirror effect. The higher the concentration of ''greenhouse'' material in the atmosphere, the less infrared energy can escape, and the more heat is trapped in the lower part of the atmosphere, thereby increasing the Earth's temperature and leading to a warmer climate.

This phenomena is well understood and accepted by atmospheric scientists.[40,41,85] What is at question is how much the Earth's average temperature will change with a given increase in the concentration of the greenhouse gases, hence the debate over the time scale of change. There is a need to link the predictive climatologic models with data from ecologic studies in order to determine the most significant impact on natural and human-altered ecosystems.[81]

Absorptive properties of the atmosphere have varied spatially and temporally through the course of the Earth's history. A natural greenhouse effect has operated over eons to gradually alter climate (Fig. 61-4). Thus many thousands of years ago tropical environments extended far north of their current limits. Dramatic cooling occurred over a period of millennia, resulting in ice ages that pushed the tropical frontier many thousands of miles toward the equator. More than 10,000 years ago that frontier began to move poleward again. Thus major shifts in climate are not new to our planet.

Other agents can influence climate. For example, volcanic eruptions release particles that have the reverse effect of absorbing sunlight and producing a cooling effect. When Mount Pinatubo in the Philippines erupted in 1991 there was a significant, but short-lived, cooling of the Earth and acceleration of ozone depletion.[34] These disruptions of the normal balance in the atmosphere are normally short-lived, and climate soon returns to pre-eruption conditions.[51] An extra-global event that can also cause these shifts is the breakup of an asteroid, now postulated to have occurred at the end of the Jurassic Period (60 million years ago). The resultant

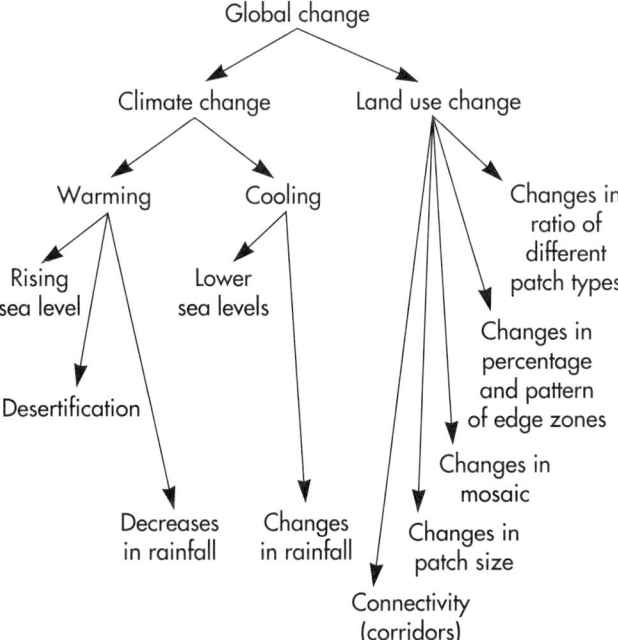

Fig. 61-2. Model of global changes and related processes, showing the consequences of climatic and land use changes. (©J. Burger, courtesy the Environmental and Occupational Health Sciences Institute.)

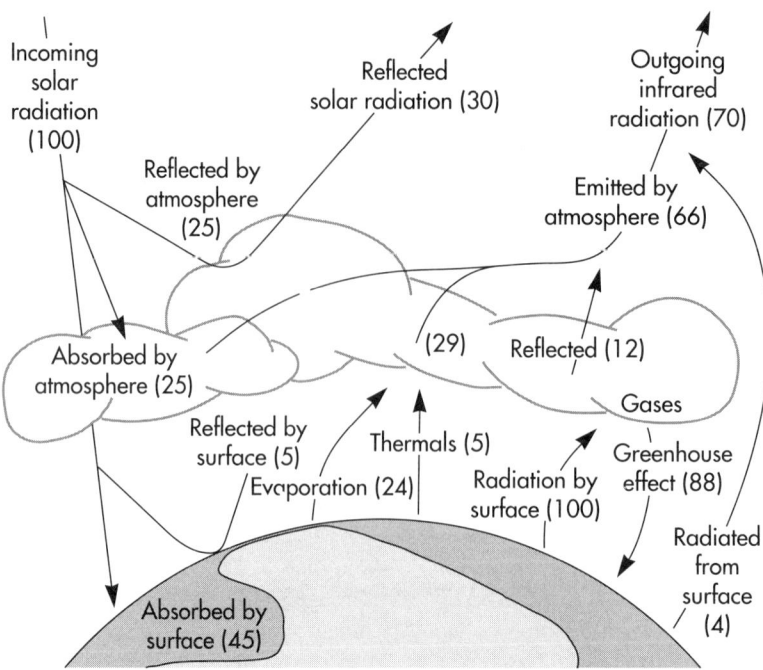

Fig. 61-3. Schematic representation of the global greenhouse effect showing the percentage (in parentheses) of solar energy and Earth's radiant energy, following various pathways of absorption and reflection. (Modified from Schneider SH: The greenhouse effect: science and policy, *Science* 243:771, 1989; courtesy the Environmental and Occupational Health Sciences Institute.)

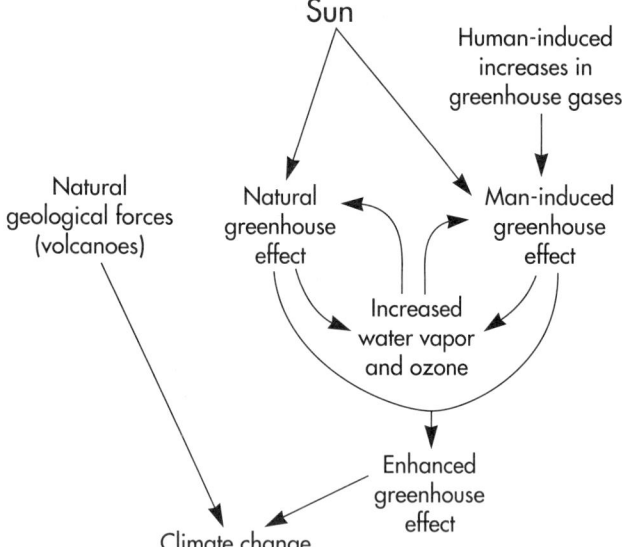

Fig. 61-4. Model for factors affecting the greenhouse effect. (Modified from Hammond AL: *World resources 1990-1991*, New York, 1990, Oxford University Press; © J Burger, courtesy the Environmental and Occupational Health Sciences Institute.)

cloud of particles over the Earth's surface is believed to have cooled the Earth significantly, reduced photosynthesis and plant productivity, and eliminated the large herbivores and carnivores of the day, hence the extinction of the dinosaurs.

What is of concern is the speed of change and the likely unidirectionality of the man-induced greenhouse effect caused by rapid increases in the greenhouse gases occurring over a period of decades, which in turn also increase water vapor, leading to an enhanced greenhouse effect. The speed of change is important, not only because it affects our ability to shift large, coastal population centers to higher ground and alters the venue for agriculture, but also because it affects the ability of native vegetation and other biomes to adapt and flourish.

Man-induced increases in greenhouse gases are clear. There has been between 3.5% to 102% increase in the four major greenhouse gases (carbon dioxide, methane, chloroflurocarbons or CFCs, and nitrogen dioxide) since 1850 (Table 61-1).[80] Human contributions stem from energy use (mainly carbon dioxide), industrial production (CFCs), deforestation (mainly carbon dioxide), and agriculture (mainly methane, Table 61-2). Gasoline-burning vehicles, industrial emissions, and incineration contribute to nitrogen dioxide.

The CFCs have a long residence time in the atmosphere, during which they absorb the infrared energy reradiated from the Earth's surface, thereby trapping heat. However, they provide double jeopardy, for when they finally do break down, they yield free radicals that in turn break down stratospheric ozone, leading to increased penetration of short-wavelength ultraviolet light. CFCs have increased more dramatically than the other substances (Fig. 61-5), leading to worldwide attempts to quickly phase out their use.[68] The 1987 "Montreal Accords" called for a 50% cut in CFC use by 1998 and provided technical assistance to developing

Table 61-1. Trace gas concentrations and trends*

Gas	Concentrations		Trends from 1975-1985 (%)	Predictions for mid-21st century
	Pre 1850	1985		
CO_2	275 ppmv	345 ppmv	+4.6	400-600 ppm
Methane	0.7 ppmv	1.7 ppmv	+11.0	2.1-4 ppmv
Nitrogen dioxide	0.285 ppmv	0.304 ppmv	+3.5	0.35-0.45 ppmv
Chlorofluorocarbons	0	0.60 ppbv	+102	2.9-7.8 ppbv

ppmv, parts per million by volume

*From Ramanathon V: The greenhouse theory of climate change: a test by an inadvertent global experiment, *Science* 240:293, 1988. Courtesy Environmental and Occupational Health Sciences Institute.

Table 61-2. Contributions to global warming by greenhouse gases and human activity; overall percent warming by activity in parenthesis*

Sector	CO_2	Methane	Ozone	Nitrous oxide	Chlorofluorocarbons
Energy (49)	35	4	6	4	—
Deforestation (14)	10	4	—	—	—
Agriculture (13)	3	8	—	2	—
Industry (24)	2	—	2	—	20
Overall (100%)	50	16	8	6	20

*From Hammond AL: *World resources 1990-91,* New York, 1990, Oxford University Press.

nations that require substitutes. By 1990, however, the urgency of the problem prompted the United Nations to obtain agreement from 93 countries for a complete phaseout of all CFCs by 2000.[4] Goldstein[31] cautions that it is essential to study the properties and potential hazards of substitutes for CFCs. For instance, one proposed substitute is hydrochlorofluorocarbons, which degrade rapidly, but the impact of their degradation products on both atmospheric quality and human health requires study.

The increase of these greenhouse gases has driven the climate system out of equilibrium by warming the surface-trophosphere system and cooling the stratosphere. The predicted changes during the next few decades alone could far exceed climate variations throughout recorded history.[80]

Several different computerized atmospherc general circulation models (GCMs) have used past increases in greenhouse gas concentration and surface temperature to predict the extent of climate change.[40,41,72] There is much disagreement about these models,[5] and the predictions that each makes differ dramatically. Nonetheless, there clearly has been a change in greenhouse gases and mean temperature, and this is already reflected in sea-level changes.

The models predict that there will be a mean global change of 4°C (best estimate) by the year 2100[41] (Fig. 61-5), based on an average 0.3° increase in temperature per decade, greater than has occurred over the last 10,000 years.[41] These increases could be reduced with decreases in greenhouse gas emissions. However, atmospheric concentrations of the long-lived greenhouse gases adjust very slowly to changes in emissions. For example, a 60% decrease in emissions from human activities is required immediately to stabilize their concentrations at today's levels.[41]

The contribution of human activities to global warming includes energy use, deforestation, agriculture, and industry (see Table 61-2). Clearly, increases in CO_2 are most severe, and these are coming largely from energy uses. Energy use and industry contributed to over 70% of the global warming so far experienced.

Unfortunately for the modeling, an increase in mean global temperatures does not result in the same changes worldwide: high northern latitudes warm more than the global mean in winter; land surfaces warm more rapidly than the oceans; and continental interior regions warm diffcrently from coastal regions. By the year 2030 estimates for climate change include the following[57,76]:

1. Central North America will experience warming from 2 to 4°C in the winter and 2 to 3°C in the summer accompanied by a 5% to 10% decrease in summer precipitation.
2. Warming will vary from 1 to 2° in southern Asia, with increases in precipitation of 5% to 10% in the summer.
3. Southern Europe will experience warming of 2°C in the winter and 2 to 3°C in the summer, with an increase of 5% to 15% precipitation in the summer.
4. Australia will experience an increase in summer of 1 to 2° with a 2°C warming in winter.

Attempts to predict climate changes over entire continents are difficult, and vary markedly (Table 61-3). None-

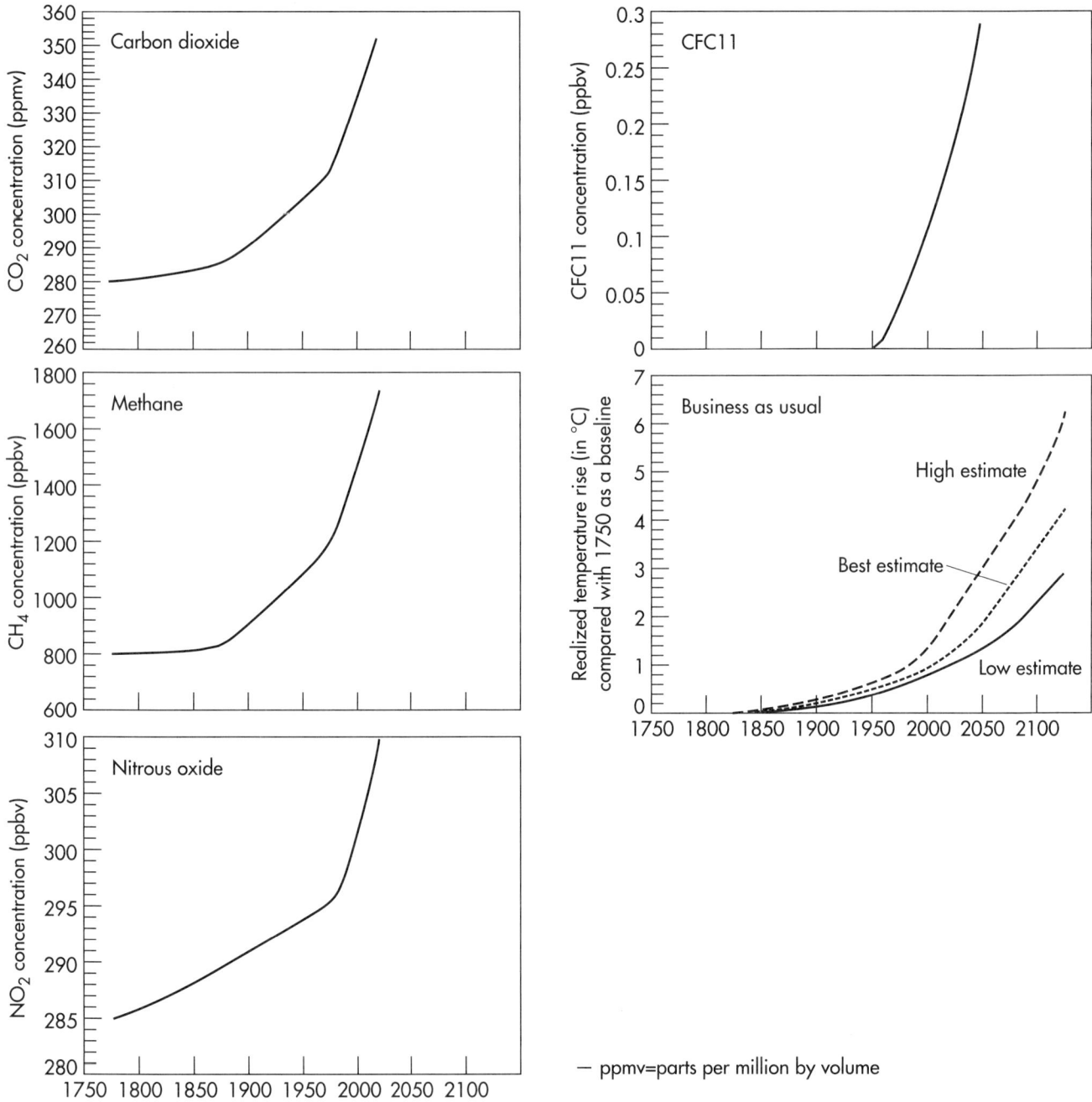

Fig. 61-5. Changes in greenhouse gases and temperature since the year 1750, with estimates or measurements of concentration. Three scenarios are used for plotting temperature rise. Ppmv = parts per million by volume. (A composite of curves from Houghton JT, Jenkins GJ, Ephraums JJ: *Climatic change,* New York, 1990, Cambridge University Press. Courtesy Environmental and Occupational Health Sciences Institute.)

theless, the changes in most places are dramatic. Furthermore, marked differences in soil moisture are projected that will change agricultural practices on a worldwide scale[85] (Fig. 61-6).

The effects of these warming climates on the Earth's ecosystems and on the human condition are enormous. First, there is a predicted change in sea level that will dramatically change our coastal landscapes (Fig. 61-7). The best estimate predicts at least an 80-cm rise in sea level by the year 2100.

Other predictions are more alarming. Although sea-level rise will cause difficulties worldwide, they will be greatest in temperate regions, where many of our most populous cities are situated on low-lying coasts. This in turn will affect coastal fishing and other coastal activities.

The combined changes in temperature, rainfall, and soil moisture will have marked effects on agriculture, which in turn will affect food supply and may ultimately lead to mass migrations. In the United States alone there will be a new

Table 61-3. Projected change in land area with and without climatic change* under different scenarios

	Areas of irrigation (million hectares)		With climatic change	
	1980	Projected in 2000 without climate change	Projected % of landmass with 4°C temperature increase in summer	Projected % of landmass with decreased soil moisture
Europe	17	19	100 (50)	100 (80)
Asia	140	165	80 (40)	70 (60)
Africa	11	15	15 (30)	80 (30)
North America	29	35	100 (15)	90 (50)
South America	8.5	11	5 (60)	40 (35)
Australia/Oceania	2.0	25	0 (70)	30 (55)
USSR	20	23.5	100 (30)	100 (80)

*Modified from Hammond AL: *World resources 1990-91,* New York, 1990, Oxford University Press. (Courtesy Environmental and Occupational Health Sciences Institute.)

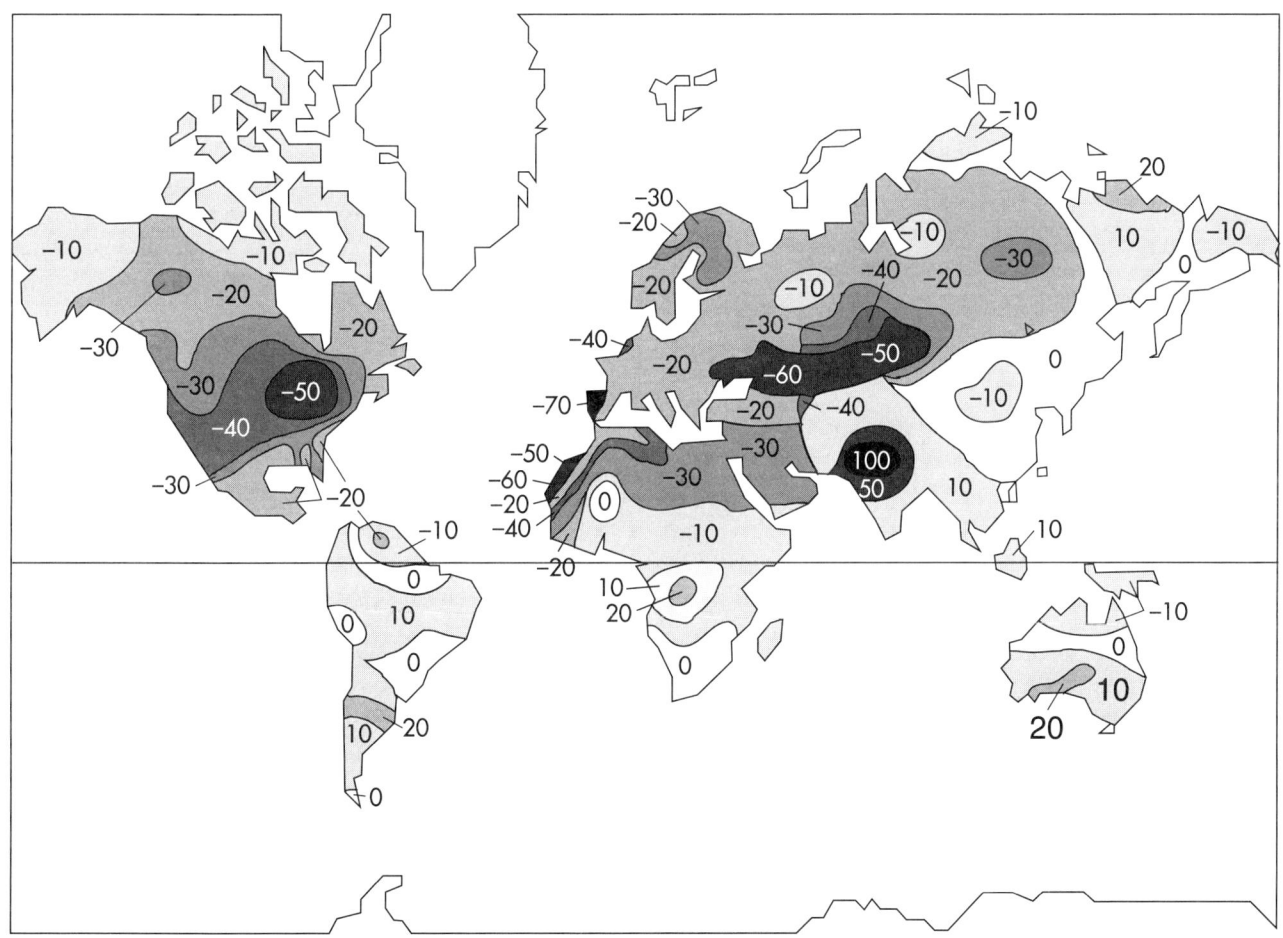

Fig. 61-6. Percent shifts in soil moisture worldwide as predicted by current general circulation models. (Redrawn from Schneider SH: The greenhouse effect: science and policy, *Science* 243:771, 1989; courtesy Environmental and Occupational Health Sciences Institute.)

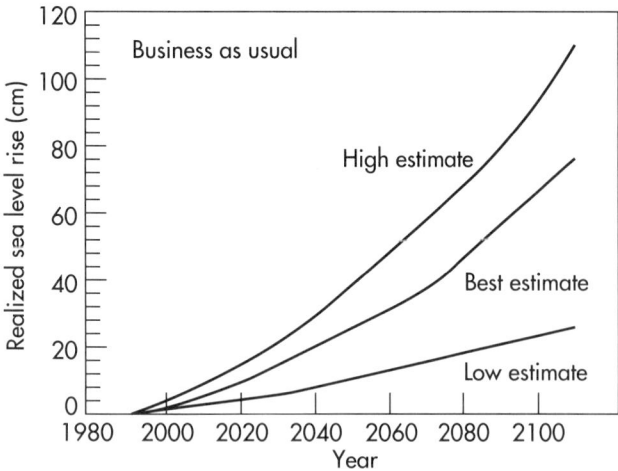

Fig. 61-7. Predicted changes in sea level with current emission levels. (Modified from Houghton JT, Jenkins GJ, Ephraums JJ: *Climatic change*, New York, 1990, Cambridge University Press. Courtesy the Environmental and Occupational Health Sciences Institute.)

Table 61-4. Effect of climate change on irrigated and rain-fed acreage in the United States; based on Global Climate Models of Goddard Institute of Space Studies,[1] with an average annual temperature increase of 3.5 to 53° C, with a doubled CO_2 forecast

	Base acreage (millions)		Change from base* (millions of acres)	
	Irrigated	Rain-fed	Irrigated	Rain-fed
Corn belt	—	95.5	—	+1.53
Lake states	—	33.8	—	+0.14
Southeast	1.72	10.8	−0.06	−3.78
Delta	3.11	16.8	+1.08	−11.68
Northern plain	10.28	91.4	+3.94	−1.12
Southern plain	5.31	49.4	+1.50	−12.40
Mountain	16.14	5.5	−2.69	+1.46
Pacific	7.73	1.9	−0.21	+1.03
Northeast and Appalachia	—	19.5	—	−5.68
TOTAL	44.29	324.63	+3.56	−40.50

*Princeton Geophysical Fluid Dynamics models predict an increase of irrigated acreage to 9.46, and a decrease in rain-fed of 27.26 million acres. Courtesy Environmental and Occupational Health Sciences Institute.

increase in lands requiring irrigation, with a large decrease in the acreage of agricultural land that is rain-fed, requiring increased energy-dependent irrigation (Table 61-4).[1] This results from the decreases in rainfall and soil moisture. This parallels increased needs for water for sanitation and drinking that tracks increases in human populations in naturally arid areas (for example, the southwestern United States). The effects of global warming on agriculture and our food supply will be discussed below.

In addition to agricultural changes, climate change will affect other components of terrestrial ecosystems. The distribution of forests will change, and the ranges of disease vectors may shift dramatically, some increasing, others decreasing. Changes in the structure and function of ecosystems, population dynamics, and biodiversity are likely consequences.

Oceanic warming may exceed that currently seen with the El Nino–Southern Oscillation phenomenon, whereby warm tropical surface waters penetrate deeply into temperate waters. The sudden appearance of warm, nutrient-poor surface water leads to the massive die-off or emigration of fish, which in turn can lead to the total collapse of a fishery. Fish-eating seabirds suddenly deprived of food undergo massive mortality, leading to a decline in guano production (for fertilizer), an important export product of a number of nations.

Stratospheric ozone

Ozone depletion is another problem that has engendered confusion and controversy. The public reads on the one hand that increased levels of ozone cause disease, and on the other that reduction in ozone threatens the environment. The physician may need to explain that breathing in ozone is harmful to health and is associated with increased asthma and other respiratory diseases, while ozone in the stratosphere (12 km and more above the Earth) plays an essential role in modulating solar radiation. Ozone absorbs ultraviolet light, which in turn damages DNA and is a major cause of skin cancer. As early as the 1970s the destructive effect of chlorofluorocarbons on atmospheric ozone was recognized and phase-out of these chemicals was recommended.[63]

Acid precipitation

Acid precipitation has tended to be a regional concern for areas immediately downwind of major industrial and urban areas. Despite political rhetoric there is evidence of substantial impacts on forests and forestry, on inland lakes and fisheries, with less documented impacts on agricultural practices or direct human health.[23,66] Acid aerosols speed the formation of atmospheric ozone, and together these produce respiratory irritation and contribute to asthma and other respiratory morbidity. Moreover, acidity increases biomethylation and bioavailability of heavy metals to aquatic ecosystems.

Much remains to be learned about climate and health, requiring research in climatology, air pollution, epidemiology, phototoxicology, and computer modelling.[31]

Land-use changes

Land-use changes are an equally important part of global change, but have received much less attention in public debate. Recent human history reveals escalating impacts and transformations of the Earth.[94] The driving force for these changes relate largely to the need for food by the exponentially increasing world population (Fig. 61-8), particularly in the developing nations, and to the hunger for an increased standard of living leading to resource exploitation in the industrialized nations (Fig. 61-8). Other factors also affect land-use changes, such as energy use, settlement patterns,

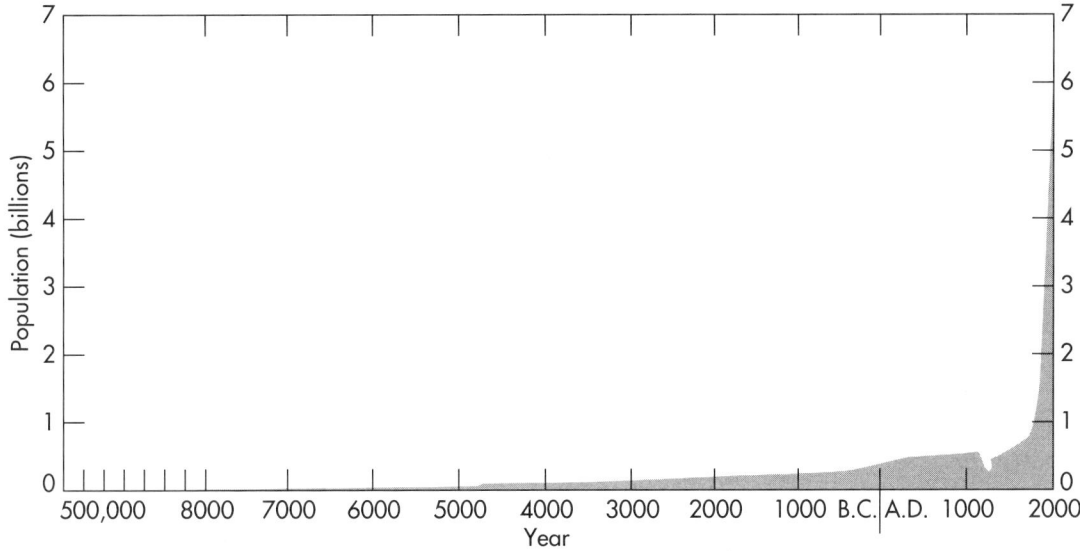

Fig. 61-8. Human population trends over time. Note dip due to plague in the 1300s. (With permission of the Environmental and Occupational Health Sciences Institute.)

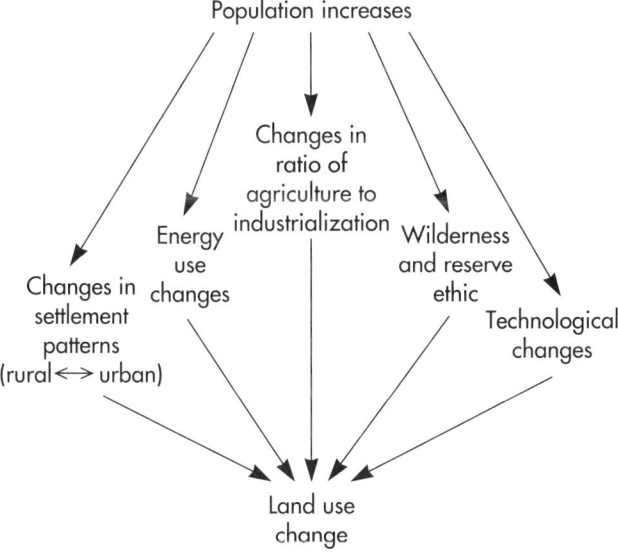

Fig. 61-9. Impact of population increases on various socioeconomic and technological changes ultimately affecting land use changes.

wilderness ethics, technological changes, and a change in the ratio of agriculture to industry (Fig. 61-9).

Humans have changed the landscape markedly, mainly since the agricultural revolution, when land was cleared for farming or grazing. But even then the changes were small and did not begin to be important until there were large population increases, industrialization, and massive migrations around the globe. Thus large-scale land-use changes are fairly recent. The process has further escalated with large-scale deforestation in the past 40 years.

A cautionary note, however, should be interjected. Conventional wisdom held that the "New World" was relatively pristine until the explorers arrived from the Old World to break the tranquility of the inhabitants. Recently, however, Turner and colleagues[93] have proposed that Native Americans had already significantly altered their landscape. Before Columbus arrived North and South America contained a wide range of land types from less disturbed to totally transformed landscapes. Most of the more heavily populated and altered landscapes were in the tropics.[93] In these tropical regions the Amerindians employed a wide range of agricultural techniques such as irrigated terraces, sculptured fields, gardens, orchards, and managed wetlands. The main Amerindian population concentrations in 1492 were in Mexico (17 million) and in the Andes (16 million), with an estimated total of 54 million.[17] Given that the estimates for the world population in 1650 was only 500 million,[21] the Amerindian population probably accounted for about 10% of the world total in 1492. Between 1492 and 1650 an estimated 75% of these people from Mexico to Argentina were eliminated, largely through the introduction of diseases that were previously unknown in the New World.[17]

Landscape patterns. Recent interest in biodiversity, endangered species, and endangered habitats has prompted ecologists to examine the structure and functional aspects of landscape patterns.[43] Landscape structure is measured by the distribution of energy, nutrients, species, and the kinds and configurations of component patches.[27] A *patch* is a community or species assemblage surrounded by a dissimilar community. Thus, from an environmental health perspective, a patch could be a town, village, farm field, pasture, toxic waste dump, forest, or lake. From an endangered or other species point of view, patches are like islands.[87] As such, organisms can be "marooned" on a patch that gradually decreases in size, leading to ever-decreasing access to food, water, mates, and genetic diversity.

Important elements of landscapes are patch types, patch size, pattern or mosaic of patches, and connectivity (how patches are connected).[20] *Mosaic* refers to how the different patch types are distributed in space. Are forests surrounded by farms, cities, lakes, or other habitats? Are lakes surrounded by cities, toxic waste dumps, landfills, airports, or forests? Connectivity describes the connections between patch types. Are there thin belts of forest between large forests? Are there streams or rivers connecting lakes? Can organisms get off their "island" and enter more propitious surroundings?

Initially ecologists were convinced that corridors were a conservation bargain because animals could move between habitat patches that were small. Thus they would not be isolated from potential mates, food, or other needs. Recently, however, the concept of corridors has come into question.[88] Corridors, by their very definition, are narrow belts of habitat between other larger, dissimilar patches. The surrounding patches may be hostile in terms of environmental factors, people, or predators. Plants or animals that require large patches for survival may be lured into these corridors and fail to reach another large patch or face disturbances they are unable to cope with.

The questions of patch type, patch size, and connecting corridors are also of interest to humans in a variety of aspects. Considerable planning is required to link various types of human patches (residential areas, shopping centers, farms, landfills) with appropriate patches, creating corridors (often roads, railroads, canals). Similarly, the types of corridors we create between human patches can result in human environ-

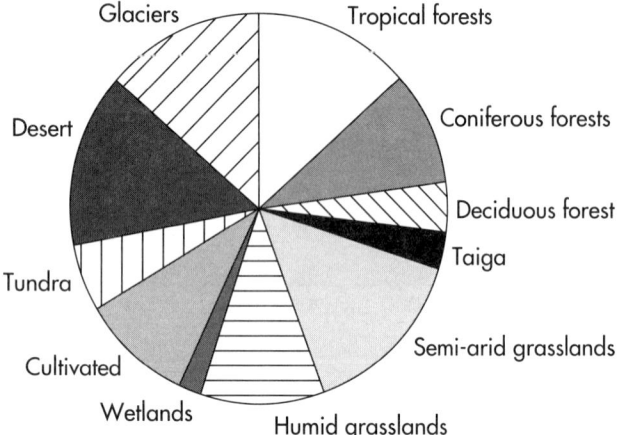

Fig. 61-10. Total acreage of the world by major biome or habitat type (Modified from Ehrlich PR, Ehrlich AH, Holdren JP: *Ecoscience: population, resources, environment,* San Francisco, 1977, WH Freeman. Courtesy Environmental and Occupational Health Sciences Institute.)

Table 61-5. Population, urbanization, and land-use changes since 1960*

	World	Africa	North and Central America	South America	Asia	Europe	USSR	Oceania
Land area (hectares)	13,076,536	2,963,627	2,137,796	1,753,473	2,678,653	472,960	2,227,200	788,660
Population density 1989 (per 1000 hectares)	398	212	197	166	1,139	1,050	128	33
Urban population as percent of total								
1960	34.2	18.3	63.2	51.7	21.5	60.9	48.8	66.3
1975	38.5	25.3	67.1	64.5	25.3	68.8	60.0	71.8
1990	42.7	34.5	71.0	76.1	29.9	73.1	67.3	70.9
Annual population change from 1960-1990 (%)								
Urban	2.6	5.0	1.9	3.7	3.2	1.1	2.1	2.1
Rural	1.4	2.1	0.7	0	1.7	−0.7	−0.5	1.2
Percentage of labor force in:								
Agriculture 1960	60	78	18	44	75	28	42	27
1980	51	69	12	29	66	14	20	20
Industry 1960	18	8	32	22	10	39	29	32
1980	21	12	29	26	15	39	39	28
Services 1960	22	14	50	33	15	33	29	41
1980	28	19	58	45	19	47	41	52
Land-use change since 1975								
Cropland	+27	+4.6	+2.1	+14.1	+0.8	−1.0	0	+14.0
Pasture	− 0.2	−0.5	+2.5	+ 4.0	−1.2	−3.4	+0.2	− 3.8
Forest	− 2.1	−4.0	−2.2	− 4.5	−1.5	+1.3	+1.9	− 6.7
Other	+ 1.3	+1.9	+0.5	+ 3.1	+1.3	+2.5	+2.6	−14.3
Wilderness as percent of total	39	31	42	24	14	4	34	30

*From Hammond AL: *World resources 1990-91,* New York, 1990, Oxford University Press. Courtesy the Environmental and Occupational Health Sciences Institute.

mental health problems if they are not wide enough and protected from surrounding land uses.

All of these landscape elements are important to human environments. From a global perspective, for both humans and other organisms, the total acreage as well as the relative change in different habitat types is important (Fig. 61-10). The relatively rapid change in land-use patterns is a critical factor (Table 61-5). Since 1975 there has been a net increase in cropland in the world, with a corresponding decrease in forests and pastures.[36]

There has also been a rapid change in the percentage of people living in urban rather than rural areas (Table 61-5). In 1960 34% of the world's population lived in urban areas; by 1990 this had risen to 43%,[36] with a projection of 50% by 2000.[104] This change has been particularly marked in Africa. Rapid shifts from rural to urban areas usually are ccompanied by increased problems with housing, food, potable water, and sanitation.[36] Urbanization is associated with increasing employment in marginal and hazardous industries with negligible access to health care. This has been exacerbated by the exportation of the most hazardous industrial operations from the industrialized to the developing nations, fostered by the rise in multinational corporations.

GLOBAL ISSUES IN ENVIRONMENTAL HEALTH

The global changes in climate and land-use patterns have profound implications for human health as well as for environmental quality. Gordon[33] argued that public health has tended to lose sight of imperative issues in environmental health, traditionally one of the mainstays of public health.[80] Studying environmental quality is essential not only because other species can serve as indicators or early warnings of impending human health problems and as models for understanding human responses to a myriad of chemicals, but because we depend on the Earth's ecosystem for our existence.

The major impacts of global change from an environmental health perspective concern human population levels and its distribution worldwide patterns, food supply and potable water, energy and biodiversity. These are necessarily interrelated, and there are feedback loops, both negative and positive, among all these components. Yet we can initially examine each separately.

DEMOGRAPHIC FACTORS
Migrations and refugees

Elementary schoolers learn that immigrants to the United States came largely to escape stresses such as war, religious or political persecution, famine, and/or to seek economic opportunity. Civil strife almost invariably creates refugees, and the health of refugees becomes a significant public health problem. The World Health Organization estimates no fewer than 15 million persistent refugees in various parts of the World,[98] with at least an additional 50 million people displaced, but not living in refugee camps. Many of these are "ecological refugees."[4] Refugees frequently bring with them disease and then find themselves facing poverty and malnutrition. Refugee camps generally are on marginal lands unsuited to agriculture.

Migration has played a prominent role in human evolution, yet for most of the past 2000 years, most populations were sedentary. Migrating groups tended to be small, limited by the size of social groups and modes of transportation, and by lack of knowledge about the relative conditions in distant lands. Significant migrations allowed the colonization of Europe from Africa, and the movement of humans out of Asia, across the Bering land bridge into the New World.

Certain agricultural processes resulted in annual migrations of herders among different pasture lands, mimicking the natural migration of herds of ungulates in tropical Africa and the Arctic. Since the mid-1850s, however, the rate of migration worldwide has remained relatively high (Fig. 61-11).[21] Increases in population levels, and concentrations of people in urban, industrialized areas have created some of our major environmental health problems: lack of potable water, exposure to industrial chemicals, exposures due to energy use, and air pollution.

Even within the United States regional intermigration has been prominent. For example, the population of Florida jumped 20% from 1980 to 1986, making it the fifth-largest state. Arizona, Texas, and Nevada were among the top five gainers[2] as well, all states in which there is a significant shortage of water.

At the time of this writing (1994), United States media are highlighting the magnitude of "illegal immigration," which contributes more to population growth than intrinsic reproduction. Legal immigrants to the United States are screened for infectious diseases, while illegal or undocumented immigrants are not. Unable to risk confrontations with the law, undocumented immigrants are willing to accept hazardous employment, thereby impeding efforts to improve workpace health and safety. Even the shipment of

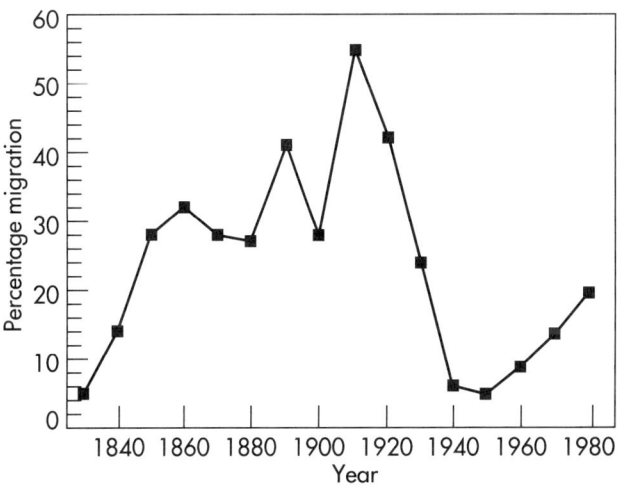

Fig. 61-11. Total immigration rates worldwide since 1830, showing peak during World War I. (Modified from Ehrlich PR, Ehrlich, AH, Holdren JP: *Ecoscience: population, resources, environment,* San Francisco, 1977.)

large quantities of food from growing areas to consuming cities has entailed exposure to new chemicals (for example, fumigants such as ethylene dibromide) designed to preserve crops during storage. All of these problems have increased disproportionately to increases in population. The problems are due not only to an increase in production of harmful environmental agents, but to the massive problems created by the necessity to safely dispose of these agents in crowded environments.

Furthermore, we have failed to develop locations and the means to safely dispose of our wastes while concentrating people in urban areas. Thus the input of hazardous materials and conditions exceeds the output and contributes to the urban crisis, a complex of socioeconomic, health, and environmental concerns.

In the present century one of the most severe environmental health problems concerns the presence of hazardous waste sites. In developed nations this is largely a result of industrial contamination on public as well as private land,[37] but it is increasingly important in developing nations with little or no environmental or hazardous waste infrastructure. The main approach to hazardous waste today is new technologies for remediation and cleanup, while the emphasis on pollution prevention is still in its infancy.

Hazardous waste is now being recognized as a valuable commodity, and companies and countries bid for the opportunity to sell services and land for waste disposal. This became apparent with the opening of Eastern Europe and the discovery of major hazardous waste sites, particularly in East Germany. Latin American nations are receiving waste ostensibly for recycling, but statistics on the amount of material and its fate are unavailable. Hazardous waste disposal that costs $2000/ton in the United States costs only $2.50/ton in Africa.[62] In 1988, however, many African nations signed a treaty restricting trade in hazardous waste. The impact of massive, long-distance transport of waste, and deposition of waste in new locations, including vulnerable coral atolls in the Pacific, pose challenges for environmental policy, and raise environmental health questions for the recipient populations as well as the people and ecosystems along the route of transport.

Although starvation, persecution, war, and repression are proximate factors leading to refugees, excessive population density is usually the ultimate factor, increasing the demand on and competition for limited space and resources.

Population levels

Underlying all of the environmental ills is the unbridled growth of human population worldwide,[38] a topic that has been downplayed in the past decade, perhaps because of the seductive impact of technologic and agricultural developments.[4] Tyler and Herold[95] provide an excellent primer on how population grows and on the relative contribution of mortality reduction (prolongation of life) and fecundity enhancement. The World Health Organization lists the ''slowing down and eventual halt of population growth'' as a number-one priority.[99]

For most of human history population levels were relatively small, stable, and limited to tropical and subtropical regions of the world (see Fig. 62-8). In the past century or two the human population has increased exponentially—the population explosion. About 5% of the people who have ever lived during the 5 million years of human evolution are alive today.[21] The World Commission on Environment and Development[104] concluded that ''in many parts of the world the population is growing at rates that . . . are outstripping any reasonable expectations of improvements in housing, health care, food security or energy supplies.'' It is instructive to examine the time required for human population to double, and it has changed dramatically (see box).[21,103]

The number of people per decade added to the world population amounted to 750 million (1970s), 840 million (1980s), and a projected 960 million (1990s). The present growth rate is 1.8%, up from 1.7% in 1980, due to increases in birth rates in China and decreases in death rates in India. The fact that the doubling time appears to have stabilized is hardly grounds for complacency.

In 1960 Deevey[16] recognized that human population growth had not been constant, but had shown three surges that correspond to cultural (living in groups), agricultural (about 8000 BC), and industrial-medical (after 1800 AD) revolutions. Whereas the cultural and agricultural revolutions were followed by long periods of relatively stable populations, this has not been the case for the industrial revolution (Fig. 61-12).

Initially, at the dawn of human evolution, human populations were confined to Africa, and numbers were low. For most of human history culture was transmitted orally and may have consisted of information about hunting, food gathering, food preparation, rules of social conduct, and identification of enemies. Consequences of this cultural revolution appear to have been small in terms of population size. However, this was not the case for the agricultural revolution,[21] which was accompanied by a dramatic change in birth rate.

Doubling the human population

Date	Population	Doubling time
8000 BC	.05 billion	
1 AD	.2 billion	1500 yr
1650 BC	.50 billion	200 yr
1850 AD	1 billion	80 yr
1900 AD	1.6 billion	
1930 AD	2 billion	45 yr
1975 AD	4 billion	36 yr
1980 AD	4.5 billion	
1992 AD	5.45 billion	36 yr

Evidence from surviving populations of hunter-gatherers, from the demography of extinct human populations inferred from fossils, and from the behavior of nonhuman primates supports the view that our ancestors probably "spaced" their births because there was no reliable source of soft diet for children under the age of 3 and they were nursed by their mothers. Widespread agriculture and new sources of food eliminated this constraint.[16]

With the industrial-sanitation-medical revolution came a decrease in death rate at all ages and an immigration of rural people to towns and urban centers. On a worldwide basis the lack of knowledge on how to control family size, coupled with reductions in infant mortality and improved medical care prolonging life (and particularly reducing death from puerperal sepsis), facilitated rapid population increases.

At any point in time the rate of population growth is a function of intrinsic birth rate, mortality, and immigration patterns. Actual population growth in a year is measured by

$$b - d + i - e$$

where b = births, d = deaths, i = immigrants, and e = emigrants. Although the total population at any point in time is of concern, particularly with regard to the health care needs of an aging population, it is the proportion of the population in the reproductive age group that is most critical. Extension of life increases the elderly, but has a minimal impact on the reproductive age group. Population biologists and human demographers can use the age structure of a given population to predict future population growth (Fig. 61-13). An age structure with a high proportion of people in

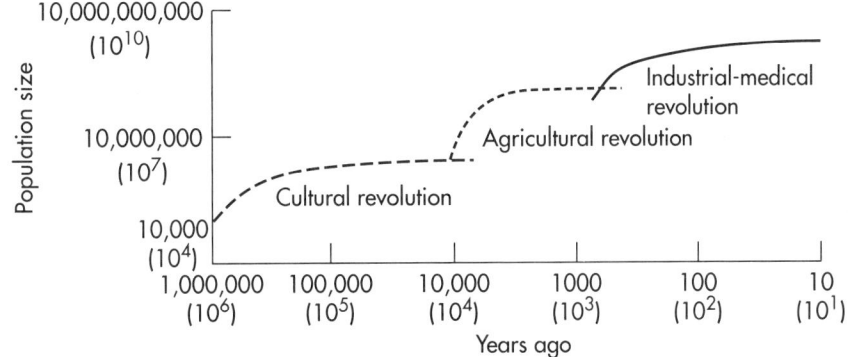

Fig. 61-12. Surges in human population growth reflecting three major sociocultural revolutions. (Modified from Ehrlich PR, Ehrlich AH, Holdren JP: *Ecoscience: population, resources, environment,* San Francisco, 1977, WH Freeman. Courtesy Environmental and Occupational Health Sciences Institute.)

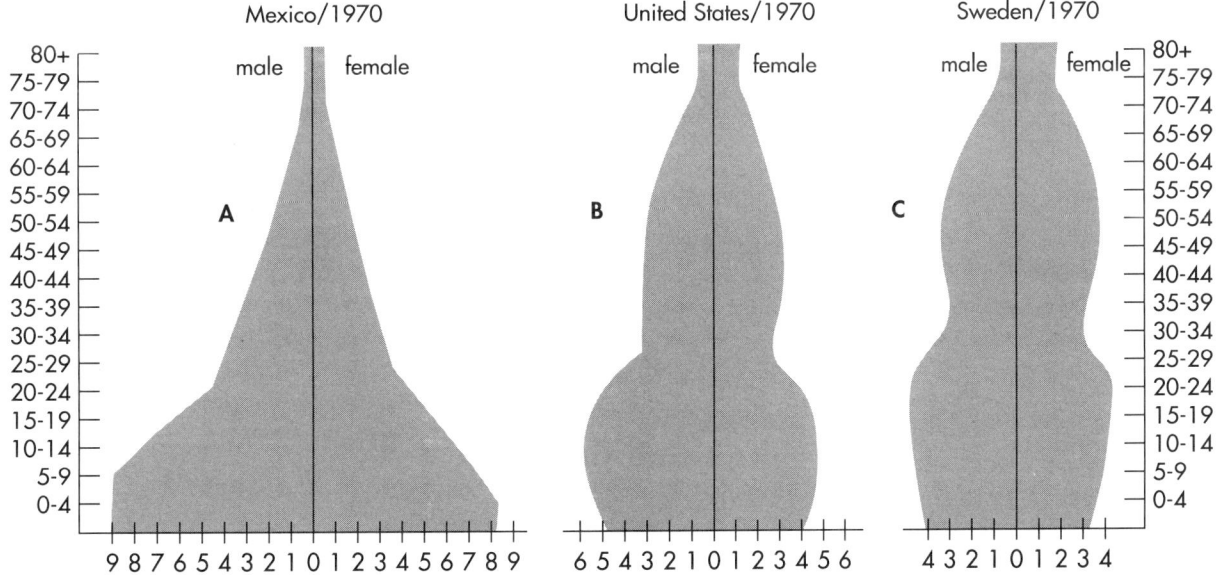

Fig. 61-13. Typical age structure of different human populations, showing rapidly expanding population of Mexico, stable population of U.S., and declining population of Sweden. (Modified from Hammond AL: *World resources 1990-1991,* New York, 1990, Oxford University Press.) (Courtesy Environmental and Occupational Health Sciences Institute.)

the prereproductive stage is increasing and will soon have a high proportion of women in the reproductive phase. Age structures that are more narrow (*B* on Fig. 61-13) can be stable. Those with constrictions (*C* on Fig. 61-13) may suggest a period of high mortality for one age group (as occurs during a war), low birth rate (as may occur during a famine), or high infant mortality.

The number of women in the reproductive age is a good indication of future population growth, given similar birth rates. Projections of the number of women in this age group vary (Fig. 61-13). The growth in this age group is higher in less developed than in developed countries. In addition, the age at first reproduction is a critical parameter, for the earlier one reproduces, the more offspring one can have in a lifetime. The ultimate example is the rodent (*Microtus*), in which females can become pregnant before they are weaned. In human populations, however, adolescent fertility is a major contributor to population growth.[21]

The number of women using contraception is a significant predictor of population growth. It ranges from 60% to 80% in developed nations, while developing nations have percentages as low as 1% (certain African countries) and as high as 50% (Mexico, Indonesia, Malaysia) up to 60+% (Costa Rica, Colombia, Thailand). Despite the removal of much United States support of family planning programs during the 1980s, many developing countries greatly increased birth control practices during this period.[45] This indicates widespread acceptance of the importance of population control and provides a basis for optimism. However, it is necessary to expand practices because even a 70% contraceptive use prevalence does not halt population growth.

Increases in human population put additional demands on agriculture (considered below) and add stress on undeveloped wild lands. Land previously considered marginal may be forced into use, with increased possibilities of disastrous crop failures.

Overpopulation and poverty

There are complex relationships between overpopulation and poverty. Throughout the world the two are closely associated. Only with the extreme deprivation of prolonged famine leading to serious malnutrition is there a physiologic inhibition of reproduction. Indeed, our reproductive capabilities have probably evolved to function even in times of food stress. Some argue that poverty leads to overpopulation and that improved standards of living will suppress reproduction. Improved economic and social standards lead to improved hygiene, which, coupled with better medical services, reduces infant and childhood mortality. Thus a couple would not need to have as many children in anticipation of a high loss rate. This reasoning is attractive in that reducing poverty will also allow people to purchase more goods and services and contribute to economic growth. It is probably flawed in most cases, however, since if the high mortality were operational, it would not lead to exponential population growth. It does not explain why couples in most countries produce an excess of children over any realized death rate. It also does not fit with observations in the United States that for a greater part of the twentieth century people with higher incomes had larger families, and that economic hardships and uncertainties associated with depression and war led to delayed initiation of families and smaller family size.

Many demographers and population ecologists[21] hold the reverse view that excess population growth is an outcome of poverty mainly because of lack of access to birth control, and contributes to poverty by increasing the number of mouths to feed on limited resources. Many countries have responded to this view and have active fertility regulation programs and in some cases incentives. Although only China has developed a firm "regulatory" approach, many other nations are examining incentive/disincentive systems. During the 1980s the United States interfered seriously in population control programs around the world, undoubtedly contributing in part to an actual increase in population growth rate during that decade. At the same time some states

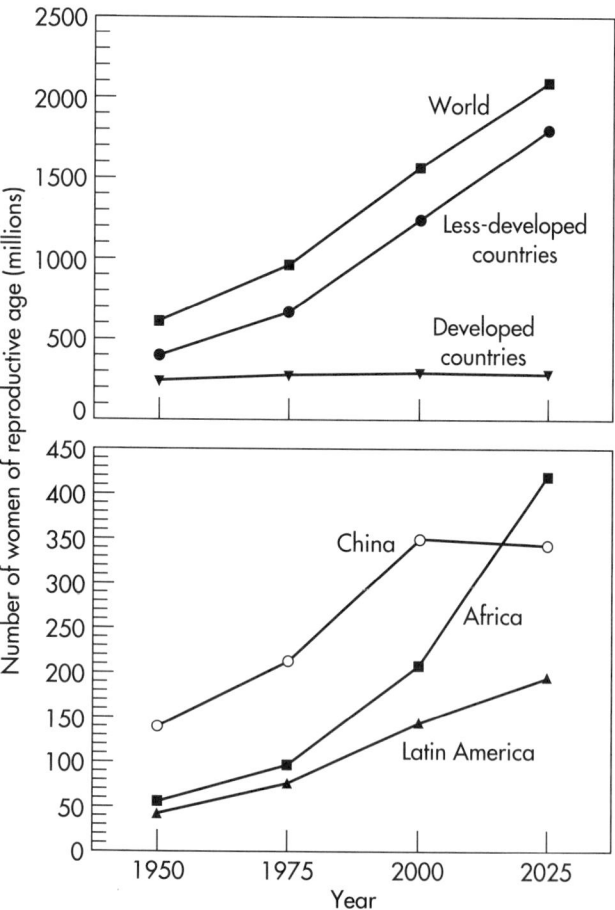

Fig. 61-14. Number of women of reproductive age comparing developed and less-developed countries (*upper*) and three developing areas (*lower*). (Modified from Hammond AL: *World resources 1990-1991,* New York, 1990, Oxford University Press.) (Courtesy Environmental and Occupational Health Sciences Institute.)

have explored welfare disincentives and no longer reward people for having children that they cannot support financially.

Overpopulation and war

The cyclical interactions of population, environment, and health become conspicuous in times of war or civil strife. Historically ecologic conflicts (competition for hunting grounds, agricultural land, and access to water and other resources) have led to battles among tribes, clans, ethnic groups, and nations. War produces refugees and most recently has increased the potential for intentional or inadvertent exposure to toxic chemicals. The recent Gulf War (1991) resulted in substantial air pollution from oil well fires in Kuwait that caused black rain over Turkey, covering a large area, contaminating water supplies, and creating panic.[25] More recently high rates of illness among American troops stationed in the Middle East are being reported in the media, the true extent of which remains to be determined. War also disrupts water and sanitation systems and inadvertently or intentionally affects agriculture and food supplies, as in the use of defoliants to destroy crops in Vietnam to deprive the enemy of food.

Overpopulation, poverty, and violence

The above section treated war as an ecologic consequence of overpopulation and increasingly scarce resources. Overpopulation, increased population density, and poverty also affect violence per se. Although not the first to discuss a biologic basis for crime, E. O. Wilson[101] provided a sociobiologic framework for understanding war and violent behavior. This engendered long-lasting and often acrimonious controversy over biologic determinism and the inevitability of violent behavior.[54]

Both parties are right. Human behavior has a strong evolutionary and biologic basis, yet humans have been successful at modifying their environment (for better or worse) and can modulate their biologic heritage.

Violent crime has become a major concern for preventive medicine worldwide, and a variety of biologic, psychologic, and socioeconomic theories have been adduced to explain the mounting tide of criminal behavior. All of these factors interact to increase rates of violence. When poverty leads to lack of opportunity to reach personal goals through legitimate, socially acceptable behavior, crime becomes an attractive alternative.[78]

However, there is increasing evidence that crowding and density per se may contribute to violent behavior independent of poverty. Beginning nearly a half-century ago, behavioral ecologist David E. Davis and his students published the famous "Baltimore rat study" and experimental studies with mice.[15] Among their observations were that increased crowding contributed to violent and agressive behavior and to biologic stress involving the pituitary-adrenal axis, which in turn produced illness. Parental neglect, social withdrawal, and "psychotic" behavior were observed as was a decline in birth rate.[9,10] Demographers were quick to develop this into an apochryphal vision of what overpopulation would do to humans, in a framework of what is called "density-dependent selection" or a "negative feedback loop." Galle et al[30] conducted an ecologic study of the density of Chicago communities (persons per room, rooms per building, admissions to mental hospitals) and found, as in the rat studies, a direct relationship between human density and social pathology. However, unlike rats, human birth rates increased with density, disturbing evidence of a positive feedback loop. Where, for example, crowding delayed sexual maturity in rodents, it had no such effect in humans. As noted, age at first reproduction is a critical parameter in population growth.

FOOD AND POTABLE WATER

One of the world's chief environmental health concerns is access to adequate amounts of healthful, uncontaminated food and water. In many less developed countries the concern may be for food and water that is free of infectious disease agents and/or vectors, whereas in developed countries concerns revolve around contamination from a variety of toxins. However, even developing nations have had their share of food-borne toxic disasters, such as methyl mercury poisoning from contaminated seed grain in Iraq and Guatemala (see Chapter 43).

In many parts of the world people do not have access to safe drinking water, a problem particularly acute in rural areas of developing nations (Table 61-6). Although in many countries urban areas have access to relatively safe drinking water, in most rural areas of Africa, Central America, and South America there is little access to safe drinking water (Table 60-6).[36]

The distinction between the environments of industrial and less developed countries with respect to types of environmental problems was easier to make in past decades, but atmospheric transport patterns make it more likely that pol-

Table 61-6. Access to safe drinking water in 1985 on a worldwide basis; given are median percent (range in parenthesis) for countries*

	Urban	Rural
Africa	73 (13-100)	35 (12-98)
North and Central America	95 (51-100)	47 (13-100)
South America	87 (49-100)	30 (8-94)
Asia	95 (25-100)	68 (17-100)
Europe	100 (94-100)	100 (65-100)
USSR	100 (-)	100 (-)
Oceania	94 (91-95)	45 (15-60)

*From Hammond AL: *World resources 1990-91,* New York, 1990, Oxford University Press. Courtesy Environmental and Occupational Health Sciences Institute.

lutants that enter the air over industrialized nations will fall on land even hundreds of miles away. The most profound example of this was the Chernobyl disaster, which yielded airborne radionuclides (particularly ^{137}Cesium and ^{131}iodine) that spread westward over Europe, contaminating both air and food chains.[96]

Access to sufficient quantities of safe, uncontaminated food has occupied the energies of mankind for millennia. Other than the few cultures that continue to maintain a hunter-gatherer lifestyle, most human populations depend on agriculture in terrestrial environments, or on resources harvested from the oceans. Most of the world's human food energy comes from cereals such as rice (21%) and wheat (20%), with only a small percentage coming from fish and livestock (Table 61-7).[21]

The world's dependence on cereals, which do not contain nutritionally complete proteins, requires that certain essential amino acids must be supplied by other foods, such as animal protein (even in small quantities) or legumes. In the developed nations people are bombarded with health messages calling for reductions in red meat in the diet. Although developing nations have no surfeit of animal protein there is an ecologic imperative for relying on vegetable rather than animal protein. Every trophic transition, from sunlight to green plant, from green plant to animal proteins in livestock, and from dietary protein to the human diet, entails substantial inefficiency. At each transfer only 10% of available energy is utilized. Thus where land and fertilizers are scarce, families profit by consuming vegetable protein directly rather than by feeding it to animals. The nutritional and ecologic tradeoffs must be considered in developing planning and education programs, particularly for impoverished subsistence agricultural areas.

Sustainable agriculture

Although for many decades the emphasis was on transforming all economies to large-scale agriculture or industry, with massive inputs of capital, nutrients (fertilizers), and irrigation, there is increasing recognition that less highly developed, less "modern" forms of agriculture are more sustainable in the long run. With the recent recognition of global changes in land-use patterns and continued exploitation of nonrenewable resources, there is a developing ethic concerning sustainable development,[56,89] and about sustainability of the biosphere in general.[77]

Although there is much discussion about the definition of *sustainable*[100] and the degree to which a system can be called *sustainable* while receiving some inputs from the outside, there is general agreement that sustainability is a goal we must strive for. The nature and the seriousness of the global environment-development crisis is being acknowledged in both national and international circles.[89] Indeed, even the World Bank has declared that forest conservation and sustainable forest management are to be conditions for extending loans to developing countries.[47] One could only hope that this goal is applied to developed countries as well. Certain forestry and fishery practices treat those resources as nonrenewable to be extracted and traded as quickly as possible, with no attention to sustainability.

The interest in sustainability has been fueled by national farm crises, industrial and agricultural pollution, the failure of economic growth to keep up with population growth, and the increasing frequency of national disasters and the recognition of a worldwide biodiversity crisis. The emphasis of agricultural production is shifting from maximization to regeneration and optimization while maintaining sustainability and minimizing environmental damage.[22] With the recognition that farmers control some 30% of the Earth's surface, more than any other group,[13] comes the realization that we must understand the cultural as well as scientific basis of farming methods. Although sustainable agriculture practices can vary greatly, there are several common features:

1. Minimum till farming, with little disruption of root systems and thus little erosion
2. Integrated pest management with little reliance on chemicals
3. Mixed cropping, both spatially and temporally, to minimize disease, enhance soil fertility, and contribute to diet diversity
4. Animal waste used as fertilizer, obviating the need for external inputs (purchased fertilizer) while at the same time reducing the negative effects of overfertilization
5. Minimal use of agrochemicals

In contrast, "modern" agriculture uses primarily large-scale monoculture (increasing susceptibility to disease vectors), massive tilling, massive irrigation and water extraction, reliance on machinery that requires nonrenewable fossil fuels, reliance on pesticides, and livestock requiring grain, and fails to maintain genetic diversity. The use of fossil fuels contributes to a range of other problems (pollution, transport of oil) in the immediate future, while a reduction in genetic diversity poses potential hazards for the distant future. This was the misplaced promise of the so-called Green Revolution.

Overreliance on only a few agricultural species leaves us vulnerable to massive crop failures if this species becomes

Table 61-7. Source of human food energy*

Food	Percent of energy supplied
Cereals	56
Roots and tubers	7
Fruits, nuts, vegetables	10
Sugar	7
Fats and oils	9
Livestock and fish	11

*From Hammond AL: *World resources 1990-91,* New York, 1990, Oxford University Press. Courtesy Environmental and Occupational Health Sciences Institute.

susceptible to some disease. Similarly, the use of monocultures increases the need for agrochemicals to control pests that are free to spread over large croplands uninterrupted.

Pesticides

From an environmental health perspective with respect to "modern" agriculture, the use of pesticides and other chemicals can cause direct problems in terms of toxicity to applicators, immediate reactions in consumers, and long-range problems due to chronic exposure.

Agricultural workers are exposed mainly through the skin or through inhalation, whereas consumers are exposed through ingestion. Problems can arise immediately from ingestion, or from bioaccumulation over time. Recently scientists have begun to emphasize the levels of toxins such as metals in the agricultural food chain,[91] and pesticides are being studied from an ecologic risk perspective[35,49,50] rather than only from a single-species approach. Moreover, household use of pesticides is a potential danger not only to applicators but to occupants, particularly small children.

Pesticides are not just features of agriculture in developed countries (Table 61-8); they are heavily marketed and utilized in many countries in Africa, Asia, and Central and South America. In many of these countries the regulations governing their use are less stringent than in more-developed countries as they strive to equal production rates of developed countries, and this creates additional environmental health problems for humans as well as wildlife.

The pesticide hazard to health in developing nations is greater than in the industrial nations, but pesticide regulation in the United States has not been universally effective. The deregistration of pesticides by the Environmental Protection Agency has proceeded slowly. Regulatory loopholes exist, such as the right to use up stocks of a banned pesticide that are already on hand. Thus pineapple growers in Hawaii are still using the dangerous organochlorine pesticide heptachlor, which they claim are from stocks on hand when the pesticide was banned in 1982. The feeding of heptachlor-contaminated pineapple tops to dairy cattle resulted in significant human exposure, which led to the ban.[24] Additionally, children are at greater risk from pesticide ingestion, not only because of different susceptibilities, but because their eating habits differ and are less diverse than adults.[69] Young children often restrict food intake to a few food types for many weeks at a time.

Many of the more hazardous substances that are now banned in the United States continue to be produced for sale in countries where they are not regulated. In the past few decades developing countries have received thousands of tons of pesticides as donations from developed countries. These excess pesticides, aging, obsolete, dangerous after years of faulty storage, and deemed dangerous to the environment, are posing a serious human health hazard, especially in Africa.[44] These pesticides provide not only an immediate problem when they are used, often because of improper labeling or lack of training of users, but create a disposal problem if this becomes necessary. Problems with these pesticides include fires caused by improper storage in Mozambique, and acute poisoning of workers in Yemen.[44]

In the late 1960s pesticides such as DDT came under scrutiny because of their environmental impacts on wildlife and their persistence in the food chain. Once in the environment they were not broken down, and their effects continued to be felt long after they were no longer used.

The newer classes of agrochemicals, carbamate and organophosphorus insecticides, are far less persistent,[49] but many of the latter are more acutely toxic to humans. Despite the extensive tests such chemicals receive, most tests still rely on a few species and are conducted in laboratories without follow-up in the field. This contrasts with drug development, where laboratory testing must be followed by clinical trials.

The wholesale use of pesticides has potential effects on wildlife and entire ecosystems.[49] In most cases these effects have been examined in ecotoxicology tests on single species.[60] Yet determining the effects of agrochemicals on a variety of organisms and ecosystems is necessary before the

Table 61-8. Agricultural inputs in 1987*

	Total cropland (ha)	Irrigated land as proportion of cropland	Average annual fertilizer use (kg per ha)	Range of average annual pesticide use (metric tons, active ingredients)
World	1,473,699	15	91	
Africa	185,424	6	19	23-21,400
North and Central America	273,853	9	83	859-373,333
South America	141,972	6	39	658-46,698
Asia	450,920	31	93	234-159,267
Europe	140,100	12	228	1,508-98,733
USSR	232,570	9	114	535,400
Oceania	48,860	4	34	1,793-65,200

*From Hammond AL: *World resources 1990-91,* New York, 1990, Oxford University Press. (Courtesy Environmental and Occupational Health Sciences Institute.)

full effects can be fairly ascertained. Pesticides have already had the effect of fostering successful resistance species, much as inappropriate antibiotic use has led to the emergence of resistance strains of microorganisms.

Climate and agriculture

In addition to the environmental health problems created by agriculture and associated agrochemicals and fuel usage, consider what global climate change will do to agriculture. Land may be arable or suitable for agriculture or it may be unsuitable, or suitable only with major manipulation (such as irrigation). Land also may or may not be available. Increasing human population increases the density of people per hectare. Certain inheritance patterns result in dividing land among children, such that each generation has a smaller base of support than the previous one.

By the middle of the next century there will be an increased worldwide need for irrigatation imposed by a rise in global temperatures and a decrease in rainfall. At the same time there will also be a very large decrease in rain-fed agricultural lands (see Table 61-4). Irrigation requires a source of surface or well water, and often energy to pump the water into the field (even if the energy is provided by human muscle).

This change in the usable agricultural land will have profound consequences: not only frank starvation, but environmental health problems associated with food deprivation, including increased disease susceptibility of underfed people. Human ecologists speak of a "food gap," the difference between the amount of food needed and the amount available. The current food gap of 10 million tons of maize equivalents will widen over the next 30 years to 245 unless something is done (Fig. 61-15). This can be mitigated temporarily by an increase in food production but in the long run there must be a decrease in human fertility or the food gap will continue to widen.[4] There are limits to our ability to increase food production, including physical and chemical constraints that decrease land suitability, as well as simple reduction in the availability of arable land (Table 61-9). This balance may be further disrupted by massive land-use changes. On most continents of the world only 4% to 21% of the total land area has no inherent soil or physical constraints to agriculture. Physical constraints include steep slopes, shallow soil, poor drainage, and tillage problems. Much of this land is vulnerable to erosion and is only marginally useful for agriculture. Observations of South American farmers struggling up fields cleared to the top of 60-degree mountain slopes highlights the unsuitability of existing farmland and the unavailability of additional space.

Current global warming scenarios present us with a picture of even further decreases in tillable land, shifting usable land (to higher latitudes), and desertification (encroachment of nonarable desert) on some heretofore usable land. This means that we will not only have to cope with the food shortages that already exist in many nations, but face accel-

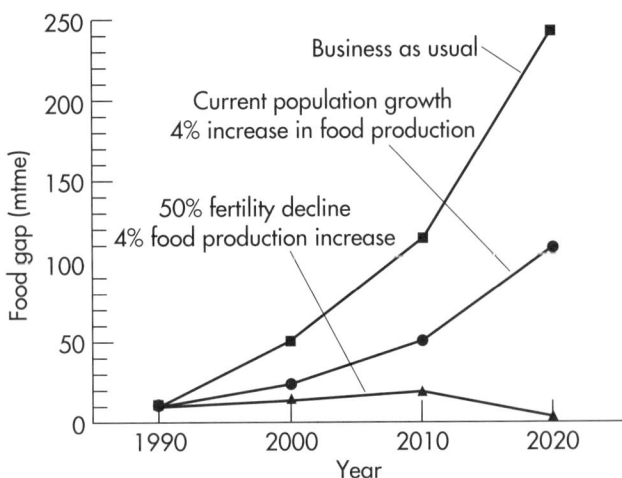

Fig. 61-15. Predicted food gap in millions of tons of maize equivalent under a business-as-usual scenario, and with an increase in food production and decline in fertility. (Based on data in Hammond AL: *World resources 1990-1991,* New York, 1990, Oxford University Press.) (Courtesy Environmental and Occupational Health Sciences Institute.)

erated food shortages and the spectre of large population shifts in quest of new agricultural lands, or more likely urban jobs.

Biotechnology. Just as the Green Revolution was cited prematurely as a solution to world food shortages, new foods generated by biotechnology are being hailed as a solution to the problem. Far from signaling an end to starvation, however, biotechnology carries its own potential problems. Engineered foods may not fit the cultural demands of populations. Herbicide-resistant plants may escape and outcompete other foodstuffs. Bovine somatotropin offers the promise of increasing milk production, but the economic consequences of increasing the production of cheap milk will cause the failure of many small dairy farms during the introductory period.[48]

Deforestation. Tropical forests occupy 13% of land and embody 40% of the Earth's plant carbon. Intact forests absorb up to 3% of atmospheric carbon dioxide, while the burning of forests as in slash-and-burn agriculture, or even the slower decays of downed timber, release carbon dioxide to the atmosphere. During the 1980s the deforestation rate increased nearly 100% worldwide and over 180% in South America. Deforestation is thus a major influence on global climate and also deprives indigenous humans and wildlife of food and shelter. Forest destruction decreases evapotranspiration and rainfall, increases susceptibility to erosion, and can result in the formation of a nontillable hardpan through laterization. Moreover, rainforest soils tend to be fragile, infertile soils, incapable of sustaining high-yield agriculture without substantial energy input.

Sustainable energy. Overall the world must be in energy balance. It cannot consume more than it harnesses or produces. North America, Europe, and Australia are already

Table 61-9. Physical and chemical soil constraints*

	Total land area	No inherent soil constraints	Physical constraints				Chemical constraints
			Steep slopes	Shallow soil	Poor drainage	Tillage problems	
Africa	3,011,330	442,733	260,864	397,812	198,239	111,779	1,784,393
Central America	273,999	58,592	68,810	44,139	15,417	18,671	70,308
South America	1,898,326	207,647	328,981	192,612	212,775	26,976	2,524,788
Southeast Asia	897,615	33,111	261,439	90,678	108,628	75,797	744,454
Southwest Asia	678,017	45,557	161,378	173,856	6,070	6,421	96,360

*From Hammond AL: *World resources 1990-91,* New York, 1990, Oxford University Press. Courtesy Environmental and Occupational Health Sciences Institute.

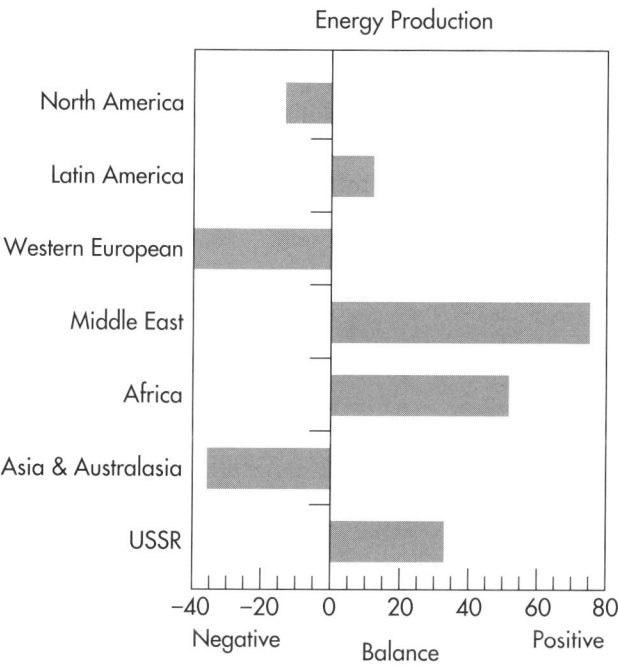

Fig. 61-16. Contrast of positive energy balance (mainly in the Middle East and Central Africa) areas and negative balance (Western Europe, Australia, and Asia). (Computed from data in Hammond AL: *World resources 1990-1991,* New York, 1990, Oxford University Press.) (Courtesy Environmental and Occupational Health Sciences Institute.)

in negative energy balance,[36] consuming up to 40% more energy than they produce (see Fig. 61-16). The world's reliance on fossil fuels continues to increase. These nonrenewable resources are costly to explore, exploit, and transport, and their use in coal-burning power plants and motor vehicles are among the major sources of air pollution and acid precipitation.[32] Moreover, although many of us remember the political debate over the exploitation of oil in Alaska, few realize that predictions show these fields will be depleted in a mere 25 years. Indeed, the World Watch Institute raised the question of whether misuse of energy represented a threat to national security.[4] The air pollution resulting from burning fossil fuel is linked to increasing respiratory disease. In many parts of the world where people cannot afford to purchase these products they cut trees for firewood or charcoal, thereby placing yet another demand on forests. In many poorly ventilated households, the burning of wood or charcoal creates intense indoor air pollution, including carcinogens. The morbidity attributable to this cause is little understood, particularly because smoking is also common in these populations.

With few local exceptions sustainable sources of energy such as wind, geothermal, solar, and biomass have not been developed as alternatives to fossil fuels, despite the fact that the cost per kW-hour is now similar to electricity generated from coal.[4] Alternative sources of energy coupled with energy conservation are necessary for any nation, even those few with large oil reserves.

Coastal resources

Present global change models predict a significant rise in sea levels over the next century (see Fig. 61-7). This will have a number of significant environmental health effects: mass dislocation of people currently living in low-lying coastal areas, changes in fish stocks and their spawning grounds, changes in migratory patterns of fish caused by changes in sea temperatures (the latter two will change their food potential), and increased contamination of fish stocks because of the resuspension of toxins currently on land. This latter effect is one not usually considered. The future of fish populations and fisheries involves interactions between environmental quality and fishery practices driven in turn by cultural markets for specific foods. Some of these changes may lead to decreases in fish stocks, providing a food gap for some peoples. Just as ecologists must determine viable population sizes for terrestrial animals, marine resources require the same considerations.[90] Many fishery cultures throughout the world fished for centuries without depleting their stocks. However, the increased range of new vessels coupled with improved technology have allowed countries to harvest fish stocks beyond the point of recovery. Thus fisheries are being treated as a nonrenewable resource. The blue-fin tuna, for example, much prized as a delicacy in Japan, is being hunted to extinction, managed only by a commission made up of those with commercial interests in overexploiting this species.[83]

If there should be a continued rise in sea level for decades and centuries, water will cover some of our coastal population centers, including large industrial complexes, landfills, and other low-lying contaminated areas. Should these be covered with water there will be immediate increases in toxins in estuarine and coastal waters, with subsequent transfer of certain chemicals to fish tissue. Even today there are serious concerns about toxic chemicals in our fish,[7,18,26] and these will intensify with global warming, sea-level rises, and increased industrial and agricultural pollution.

Biodiversity

The recognition of the massive land-use changes around the globe in the face of expanding human populations coupled with the knowledge of the recent loss of species worldwide has prompted interest in maintaining biodiversity.[102] Although initially this interest was sparked by concern for tropical forest ecosystems, we are now recognizing that other habitats (and their species) are in even more danger. Janzen[46] recently proposed that dry tropical forests may be the most endangered tropical ecosystem. Coastal and estuarine systems, on which many of the world's nations are dependent for food, are also threatened with loss of diversity. Even understanding the extent of biodiversity requires the systematic cataloging of species and ecosystems.[5]

There are many arguments for maintaining biodiversity[102]:

1. Maintaining ecosystem integrity
2. Maintaining community structure as long as we do not know or understand the role of particular organisms within the system. This carries an implicit assumption that some species may play pivotal or "keystone" roles such that should they become extinct the system will be seriously impaired.
3. Maintaining genetic diversity. Although this argument can be made on the basis of preserving the ecosystems themselves, it is often made on the basis of preserving genetic diversity so that we may someday discover new food plants, industrial products, and pharmaceuticals.

This last argument is the one most often used in the defense of protecting biodiversity. From an environmental health prospective it is an imperative, since we may obtain valuable chemicals from yet undiscovered plants. Many large pharmaceutical companies are now instituting natural products divisions. The recent discovery, exploitation, and eventually synthesis of taxol, a potent anticancer drug isolated from yew trees, argues persuasively for exploring and protecting biodiversity.

The ultimate hope is that not only will we be able to develop new agricultural, industrial, and medical products from among the vast array of species, but once these chemicals are discovered, we will be able to manufacture them rather than exploit them to extinction. This latter point is critical, for otherwise we are protecting biodiversity today only to destroy it tomorrow if the chemicals become useful.

Global economic issues

Clinicians are no strangers to economic issues, and it is instructive to consider important ways that economic institutions provide incentives that increase many of the problems discussed. The International Monetary Fund and the World Bank provide loans for many projects that have multiple negative impacts, although the latter agency has begun to give stronger weight to environmental issues. Impoverished nations find it attractive to sell massive amounts of raw materials, particularly timber to forest-starved developed nations, for needed foreign currency. Thus forestry is practiced on a nonsustainable basis. There is clearly an economic incentive to exploit resources rapidly for short-term monetary gain and invest it elsewhere, rather than to husband a resource as a longer-term investment. Only when the economic incentive changes will countries have a vested interest in husbanding resources for long-term harvest and return.

In a classic paper Hardin[36] pointed out that our social structure encourages individuals or companies to misuse public lands (as for grazing and waste disposal) at a fraction of their true value. Costanza[14] pointed out that economic incentives were social traps promoting misuses of resources, and that an equitable distribution of costs, taxing those who misuse resources rather than encouraging them, is essential for halting environmental degradation.[11]

TOWARD A GLOBAL SYNTHESIS

It is becoming increasingly clear that the world behaves as one ecosystem, a concept originally identified by Lovelock[55] with his Gaia Hypothesis. The health of the environment is intimately tied up with our own health. In no branch of medicine is this more clear than in environmental health. On a global scale human populations have been growing and developing such that we possess the ability to alter our environments markedly. In the end all of these become economic issues involving how much and how long society is willing to pay for environmental quality, as well as questions of who will pay and who will benefit.

Although land use changes have been occurring gradually for centuries, they have accelerated in the last century to the point where we affect our climate, food supply, and water, and this requires intervention from health and environmental professionals. In addition, we have begun to change the world's climate through the addition of greenhouse gases and the depletion of atmospheric ozone, in such large quantities that our global climate balance has been altered.

Some of the human effects on global change can be altered through decreases in emissions, decreases in production of toxins, development of sustainability in agriculture, fisheries, forestry, energy use, and protection of endangered species[84] and habitats. Although many of the changes are impossible to reverse, their progression can be slowed or halted. However, this ultimately requires dramatic, worldwide changes in fertility patterns, and population stability as well as international accord. We will never return to pre-industrial revolution population levels, but further growth can be slowed or halted. If this is not accomplished voluntarily, it will be imposed by food shortages and war. Some of the land-use pattern problems can be addressed through the new and emerging fields of ecologic engineering[59] and restoration ecology.[12] Many of these interrelationships and suggestions for solutions have been summarized by Myers.[61] Nonetheless, the environmental health practitioner must work with and interpret the environment as it now exists.

Land use and climate changes are not in themselves independent since the elimination of forests changes the reflectivity and absorption of the Earth's surface, which in turn changes the climate still further. Both of these factors affect where people live and their community patterns, as well as their agricultural possibilities.

Global patterns of air and water movement over the face of the Earth affect the movement and distribution of pollutants. When outputs in one part of the world are large, these materials are transported to other parts of the world. Air pollution (including acid rain) no longer affects the health of those nations responsible, but falls on other nations, transferring the health care problems elsewhere.

Toxic chemicals that enter the food chain in one part of the world make their way to other parts, either directly through our exportation and importation of food, or indirectly through intermediaries. For example, fish that pick up toxins on their wintering grounds transport them to their spawning grounds; migratory birds exposed to heavy metals or pesticides on wintering grounds in Latin America carry them thousands of miles northward, where they are hunted and eaten by indigenous peoples in the Arctic. Whales and other large marine organisms wander the world picking up and transporting pollutants; cows grazing in Poland pick up cesium emitted from Chernobyl and transfer it to their milk. People in many parts of the world eat these organisms and are themselves exposed.[7,79]

Environmental health practitioners must now consider the global environment when examining and treating patients and planning preventive health programs. Furthermore, global changes in temperature, sea levels, greenhouse gases, and land use all affect environmental health and will continue to do so as the changes escalate.

CONCLUSION

It has been said in many ways, by many voices, for a long time, that humankind and all other life are facing a serious ecologic crisis.[34] Compared with the situation on Earth Day 1970, global environmental quality had sadly deteriorated by 1990: "Measured on virtually any scale, the World is in worse shape than it was 20 years ago."[39] The clinician is faced not only with the health consequences of environmental degradation, but with playing an important educational role for their patients and colleagues. Physicians are often called on to serve on government committees, and many medical societies have environmental committees. These provide a forum for a medical voice to be heard.

Population regulation must be fostered, and many nations have given this high priority.[29] The World Commission on Environment and Development[104] and World Watch Institute[4] have explained the linkages between population, environmental quality, resource availability, and health. Sustainable development is being sought on many levels, and the 1992 United Nations Conference on Environment and Development in Rio de Janeiro represented a major step in this direction, one in which the United States played a small but obstructive role.[74]

Additional research will improve the predictive value of the climatic and population models used for planning and will play a role in the interactions among nations. It is important to realize that thus far published predictions of population growth have underestimated world population at any point in time. For example, Frejka[29] reported several estimates placing the world population of humans at 5 to 6 billion by 2000. It already exceeds 5.5 billion in 1993 and will probably exceed 6.3 billion by 2000. Overpopulation is the key environmental health issue because it affects the existence and health of our ecosystems and leads to increased demand for chemicals and other resources of all kinds.

International organizations of physicians and other health professionals concerned with public health and preventive medicine offer an opportunity for the voice of physicians to be heard and to influence government policy worldwide. A model exists in the efforts of International Physicians for Prevention of Nuclear War. Introduction of environmental health curricula into medical training throughout the world is an important step, for primary practitioners are the ones who see the immediate consequences of environmental health problems (IOM 1988).

ACKNOWLEDGMENTS

Over the years we have profited from discussions about global change, sustainability, environmental pollution, and environmental health with: Caron Chess, Keith Cooper, Michael Gallo, Bernard Goldstein, Michael Greenberg, Stephen Handel, Herb Lowndes, Jane Lubchenko, Bertram Murray, Joel O'Connor, David Polichansky, George Rhoads, Don Stone, Dan Wartenberg, Nicholas Wright, and many others.

REFERENCES

1. Adams RM et al: Global climate change and US agriculture, *Nature* 345:219, 1990.
2. Associated Press: Florida 5th in population, *Sun-Sentinel,* Dec. 31, 1986, p 1.
3. Broecker WS: The biggest chill, *Natural History* 10:74, 1987.
4. Brown LR: *State of the world,* New York, 1991, WW Norton, World Watch Institute.

5. Brun DA, Wiersma GB, Rykiel EJ Jr: Ecosystem biomonitoring at global baseline sites, *Environ Monit Assess,* 17:3, 1991.
6. Bryson RA: Will there be a global "greenhouse" warming?, *Environ Conserv* 16:97, 1989.
7. Burger J, Gochfeld M: Fishing a superfund site: dissonance and risk perception of environmental hazards by fisherman in Puerto Rico, *Risk Anal* 11:269, 1991.
8. Burger J, Gochfeld M: Temporal scales in ecological risk assessment, *Arch Environ Contam Toxicol* 23:484, 1992.
9. Christian JJ. The adreno-pituitary system and population cycles in mammals, *J Mammal* 31:247, 1950.
10. Christian JJ: Phenomena associated with population density, *Proc Natl Acad Sci USA* 47:428, 1961.
11. Clites AH, Fontaine TD, Wells JR: Distributed costs of environmental contamination, *Ecological Econ* 3:215, 1991.
12. Cohen T: Ecological restorations, *Tech Review* Feb/Mar:20, 1992.
13. Coleman DC, Hendrix PF: Agroecosystem processes, *Advances in Ecol Res* 13:1, 1981.
14. Costanza R: Social traps and environmental policy, *BioScience* 37:407, 1987.
15. Davis DE: The characteristics of rat populations, *Quart Rev Biol* 28:373, 1953.
16. Deevey ES: The Human Population, *Scientific American,* Offprint #608, San Francisco, 1987, WH Freeman.
17. Denevan WM: *The native populations of the Americas in 1492,* Madison, Wis, 1992, University of Wisconsin Press.
18. DeVault DS: Contaminants in fish from Great Lakes harbors and tributary mouths, *Arch Environ Cont Toxicol* 14:587, 1985.
19. Dorman P: NAFTA: a great leap backwards, *New Solutions* 3:81, 1993.
20. Dunning JB, Danielson BJ, Pulliam HR: Ecological processes that affect populations in complex landscapes, *Oikos* 65:169, 1992.
21. Ehrlich PR, Ehrlich AH, Holdren JP: *Ecoscience: population, resources, environment,* San Francisco, 1977, WH Freeman.
22. Elliott ET, Cole CV: A perspective on agroecosystem science, *Ecology* 70:1597, 1989.
23. Elsworth S: *Acid rain in the U.K. and Europe,* London, 1984, Pluto Press.
24. Environment Hawaii: Heptachlor use: has it stopped yet. *Environ Hawaii Newsletter* June 1993, p. 3.
25. Evliya H: Black rain in turkey, *Environ Science and Tech* 26:873, 1992.
26. Fogarty MJ, Rosenbert AA, Sissenwine MP: Fisheries risk assessment sources of untertainty, *Environ Sci Tech* 26:440, 1992.
27. Forman RTT, Godron M: Patches and structural components for a landscape ecology, *BioScience* 31:733, 1981.
28. Fox J: The problem of scale in community resource management, *Environ Manage* 16:289, 1992.
29. Frejka T: *The future of population growth: alternative paths to equilibrium,* New York, 1973, J Wiley.
30. Galle OR, Gove WR, McPherson JM: Population density and pathology: what are the relations for man? *Science* 176:23, 1972.
31. Goldstein BD: Global atmospheric change and research needs in environmental health science, *Env Health Persp* 96:193, 1991.
32. Goldstein BD, Greenberg M: Environmental applications and interventions in publich health. In, Holland, Detels, Knox, editors: *Oxford textbook of public health,* ed 2, New York, 1991, Oxford University Press.
33. Gordon LJ: Does public health still include environmental health and protection?, *J Public Health Policy* winter:407, 1992.
34. Gore A: *Earth in the balance,* New York, 1992, Houghton Mifflin.
35. Greig-Smith PW: A European perspective on ecological risk assessment, illustrated by pesticide registration procedures in the United Kingdom, *Environ Toxicol Chem* 11:1673, 1992.
36. Hammond AL: *World resources 1990-1991,* New York, 1990, Oxford University Press.
37. Hardin G: The tragedy of the commons, *Science* 162:1243, 1968.
38. Hardin G: Nobody ever dies of overpopulation, *Science* 171:527, 1971.
39. Hayes D: Earth Day 1990: society's challenge, *Environ Sci Tech* 24:403, 1990.
40. Houghton JT, Callander BA, Varney SK: *Climate change 1992,* New York, 1992, Cambridge University Press.
41. Houghton JT, Jenkins GJ, Ephraums JJ: *Climate change,* New York, 1990, Cambridge University Press.
42. Houghton RA: The global effects of deforestation, *Environ Sci Tech* 24:414, 1990.
43. Hudson WE: *Landscape linkages and biodiversity,* Washington DC, 1991, Island Press.
44. Jain V: Disposing of pesticides in the third world, *Env Sci Tech* 26:226, 1992.
45. Jamison E: *World Population Profile: 1989,* Washington, DC, 1989, U.S. Dept. Commerce.
46. Janzen DH: Tropical dry forests: the most endangered major tropical ecosystem. In *Biodiversity,* Washington DC, 1988, NAS Press.
47. Josephson J: Sustainable forest management in cold and warm lands, *Environ Sci Tech* 26:1892, 1992.
48. Kalter RJ: The new biotech agriculture: unforeseen economic consequences, *Issues in Science & Technol* 2:125, 1985.
49. Kendall RJ, Akerman J: Terrestrial wildlife exposed to agrochemicals: an ecological risk assessment perspective, *Environ Toxicol Chem* 11:1727, 1992.
50. Kendall RJ, Lancher TE Jr: Ecological modelling, population ecology, and wildlife toxicology: a team approach to environmental toxicology, *Environ Toxicol Chem* 10:297, 1991.
51. Kerr RA: Pinatubo global cooling on target, *Science* 259:594, 1993.
52. Levy BS, ed: *Air pollution in Central and Eastern Europe: health and public policy,* Boston, 1991, Management Sciences for Health.
53. Levy BS, Levenstein C: *Environment and health in Eastern Europe,* Boston, 1991, Management Sciences for Health.
54. Lewontin RC, Rose S, Kamin LJ: *Biology, ideology, and human nature,* New York, 1984, Pantheon Press.
55. Lovelock JE: *GAIA, a new look at life on earth,* Oxford, 1979, Oxford University Press.
56. Lubchenco J et al: The sustainable biosphere initiative: an ecological research agenda, *Ecology* 72:371, 1991.
57. Mohnen VA, Wang W: An overview of global warming, *Environ Tox Chem* 11:1051, 1992.
58. Mooney HA: Emergence of the study of global ecology: is terrestrial ecology an impediment of progress?, *Ecol Applic* 1:2, 1991.
59. Mitsch WJ: Ecological engineering: the roots and rationale of a new ecological paradigm. In Etnier C, Guterstam B, editors: *Ecological engineering for wastewater treatment,* Stockholm, Sweden, 1991, Bok Skogen.
60. Moriarty F: *Ecotoxicology: the study of pollutants in ecosystems,* New York, 1983, Academic Press.
61. Myers N: *GAIA: an atlas of planet management,* New York, 1984, Doubleday.
62. Nash NC: Latin nations getting others' waste, *New York Times* Dec 16, 1991, p. A10.
63. National Research Council: *Stratospheric ozone depletion by halocarbons: chemistry and transport,* Washington, DC, 1979, National Academy of Sciences.
64. National Research Council *Testing for effects of chemicals on ecosystems,* Washington, DC, 1981, National Academy Press.
65. National Research Council: *Risk assessment in the federal government: managing the process,* Washington, DC, 1983, National Academy Press.

66. National Research Council: *Acid deposition: atmospheric processes in Eastern North America,* Washington DC, 1983, National Academy Press.
67. National Research Council: *Ecological knowledge and environmental problem-solving: concepts and case studies,* Washington, DC, 1986, National Academy Press.
68. National Research Council: *Rethinking the ozone problem in urban and regional air pollution,* Washington DC, 1991, National Academy Press.
69. National Research Council: *Pesticides in the diets of infants and children,* Washington DC, 1993, National Academy Press.
70. National Research Council: *Issues in risk assessment,* Washington, DC, 1993, National Academy Press.
71. Norton SB et al: A framework for ecological risk assessment at the EPA, *Environ Toxicol Chem* 11:1663, 1992.
72. Ojima DS et al: Critical issues for understanding global effects on terrestrial ecosystems, *Ecol Applic* 1:316, 1991.
73. O'Neill RV et al: Ecosystem risk analysis: a new methodology, *Environ Toxicol Chem* 1:167, 1982.
74. Parsons EA, Haas PM, Levy MA: A summary of the major documents signed at the earth summit and the global forum, *Environ* 34:12, 1992.
75. Peters RE, Lovejoy TE: *Global warming and biodiversity,* New Haven, 1993, Yale University Press.
76. Poiana KA, Johnson WC: Global warming and prairie wetlands, *BioScience* 41:611, 1991.
77. Risser PG, Lubchenco, Levin SA: Biological research priorities—a sustainable biosphere, *BioScience* 41:625, 1991.
78. Rosenberg ML, Mercy JA: Violence: assaultive violence. In Last JL, Wallace RB, eds: *Public health and preventive medicine,* New York, 1992, Appleton-Lange.
79. Rosenberry M, Burmaster DE: A note: estimating exposure concentrations of lipophilic organic chemicals to humans via raw finfish fillets, *J Expos Analy Environ Epidemiol* 1:513, 1991.
80. Ramanathan V: The greenhouse theory of climate change: a test by an inadvertent global experiment, *Science* 240:293, 1988.
81. Root TL, Schneider SH: Can large-scale climatic models be linked with multiscale ecological studies, *Conservation Biology* 7:256, 1993.
82. Rosenau MJ: *Preventive medicine and hygiene,* ed 3, New York, 1918, D. Appleton.
83. Safina C: Bluefin tuna in the western Atlantic: negligent management and the making of an endangered species, *Conservation Biology* 7:229, 1993.
84. Schaffer ML: Minimum population sizes for species conservation, *BioScience* 31:131, 1981.
85. Schneider SH: The greenhouse effect: science and policy, *Science* 243:771, 1989.
86. Shaw RP: Rapid population growth and environmental degradation: ultimate versus proximate factors, *Environ Conserv* 16:199, 1989.
87. Simberloff DS: Experimental zoogeography of islands: effects of island size, *Ecology* 57:629, 1976.
88. Simberloff D, Farr JA, Cox J et al: Movement corridors: conservation bargains or poor investments, *Cons Biol* 6:493, 1992.
89. Simon D: Sustainable development: theoretical construct or attainable goal?, *Environ Conserv* 16:41, 1989.
90. Soule ME: *Viable populations for conservation,* Cambridge, 1987, Cambridge University Press.
91. Stevens JB: Disposition of toxic metals in the agricultural food chain. 2. steady-state bovine tissue biotransfer factors, *Environ Sci Technol* 10:1915, 1992.
92. Suter GW, Loar JM: Weighing the ecological risk of hazardous waste sites, *Environ Sci Technol* 26:432, 1992.
93. Turner BL II, Butzer KW: The Columbian encounter and land-use change, *Environ* 34:16, 1992.
94. Turner BL et al: Two types of global environmental change, *Global change* 1:14, 1990.
95. Tyler CW Jr, Herold JM: Public health and population. In Last JM, Wallace RB, eds, *Public health and preventive medicine,* ed 13, New York, 1992, Appleton & Lange.
96. United Nations: *Sources, effects, and risks of ionizing radiation,* New York, 1988, United Nations Scientific Committee on the Effects of Ionizing Radiation, United Nations.
97. Wartenberg D, Chess C: Risky business, *The Sciences* March/April 1991:17, 1992.
98. World Health Organization: *Global estimates for health situation assessment and projections—1990,* WHO/HST/90.2, Geneva, 1990, Division of Epidemiologic Surveillance.
99. World Health Organization: *Report of the WHO commission on health and environment—summary,* Geneva, 1992, WHO.
100. Wilcox BA: Defining sustainable development, *Environ Sci Technol* 26:1902, 1992.
101. Wilson EO: *Sociobiology: the new synthesis,* Cambridge, 1975, Harvard University Press.
102. Wilson EO: *Biodiversity,* Washington, DC, 1988, National Academy Press.
103. World Almanac: *The world almanac and book of facts—1993,* New York, 1993, World Almanac.
104. World Commission on Environmental Development: *Our common future,* Oxford, 1988, Oxford University Press.

Chapter 62

ENVIRONMENTAL HEALTH SURVEILLANCE

Lora E. Fleming
Jessica Herzstein
Stuart L. Shalat

Definitions
Goals of health surveillance
Preventive strategies in surveillance: sentinel health events
Issues in environmental surveillance
Environmental surveillance and clusters
Elements of surveillance
Implementation of a surveillance program
    Definition of disease
    Defining the surveillance population
    Establishing a disease sentinel
    Data management and confidentiality
    Exposure
    Analysis
Conclusions

Modern society affords multiple and increasingly numerous opportunities for environmental exposure with the potential for adverse health effects. Disease may result when people in the community are exposed to contaminated drinking water, toxic materials in hazardous waste sites or toxic landfill, toxic materials emanating from an incinerator or an industrial process, or toxic substance spills or releases. Increasingly, public concern is focused on the relationship between exposures or potential exposures and disease.

Environmental disease surveillance extends beyond risk assessment to address the question: Is the environmental exposure (for example, a hazardous waste site) associated with an increased incidence of disease among residents in the vicinity of the exposure? Surveillance thus involves analysis of exposures and exposure routes, of disease types and disease rates, and collection of environmental monitoring data. Clinicians play important roles in collecting health data, including providing accurate diagnoses and complete vital statistics data; alerting public health authorities about potential health hazards and clustering of disease; and educating patients and community leaders about health surveillance and environmental hazards (see Chapter 10). This chapter addresses the goals of health surveillance in environmental medicine, preventive strategies and sentinel health events (SHEs), clinical issues in surveillance, investigation of disease clusters, and the design of surveillance systems.

DEFINITIONS

Surveillance, as defined in the *Dictionary of Epidemiology,* is "the ongoing scrutiny [of the occurrence of disease and injury], generally using methods distinguished by their practicality, uniformity, and frequently their rapidity, rather than by complete accuracy. Its main purpose is to detect changes in trends or distributions in order to initiate investigative or control measures." The Center for Disease Control and Prevention has defined surveillance as "the ongoing, systematic collection, analysis and interpretation of health data. This information is used for planning, implementing, and evaluating public health interventions and programs."[28]

In the strictest sense medical surveillance results in the identification of individual disease cases (index cases) and the prevention of further cases (through isolation of contacts in infectious disease or control of hazards in occupational and environmental disease).[50] The goal is to reduce the disease incidence. In contrast, the objective of monitoring is primary prevention, in which a disease is anticipated before it occurs and irreversible damage is avoided. Screening involves both detection of risk for disease (such as through genetic testing) and identification of disease (or a higher probability of disease, which requires confirmatory testing) before the person would normally seek medical care and at a time when intervention is beneficial. Screening programs aim to reduce the prevalence of disease. Whereas surveillance indicates the periodic ongoing evaluation of individuals, screening refers to a cross-sectional evaluation of a population.[22]

Criteria for the validation and screening procedures have received wide acceptance.[30,41] It is important, for example, that acceptable therapy for the condition be available, that therapy improve survival and/or function, and that screening lead to an improvement in outcome among those in whom early diagnosis is achieved; however, many tests and procedures still commonly used in evaluating asymptomatic persons have not met these criteria.[41] Clinical guidelines on the examination of asymptomatic persons have been developed by the Canadian Task Force on the Periodic Health Examination (1979), the American Cancer Society (1992), the American College of Physicians (1989), and other sources.[42] The U.S. Preventive Services Task Force has developed rigorous clinical guidelines for the secondary prevention of a wide array of conditions, based on a systematic review of evidence of clinical effectiveness.[42] The guidelines are practical strategies of proven efficacy for screening, counseling, and immunizations and serve as comprehensive recommendations for clinicians providing preventive services for any age group.

GOALS OF HEALTH SURVEILLANCE

An ideal surveillance system identifies populations with an elevated risk for disease or exposure and institutes primary prevention practices (such as prevention of disease by eliminating exposure prior to the occurrence of disease). Surveillance protocols may detect, for instance, an occasional excessive exposure as evidenced by subclinical health effects or changes in biomarkers. The testing that is part of surveillance examinations may reveal early reversible changes (such as abnormal liver function tests) at a time when intervention can prevent irreversible end organ disease due to the toxin.

Surveillance most commonly involves secondary and tertiary prevention, that is, detection of disease once the disease process is underway and early signs and/or symptoms are present. For example, data bases on hazardous waste workers attempt to collect information on health status and exposures to discover adverse health effects related to chemical exposures and protect future workers. Surveillance is usually instituted during exposure or even after hazards are controlled. For example, after the atomic bomb blasts of Hiroshima and Nagasaki, extensive surveillance was instituted to observe both acute and subsequent causes of morbidity and mortality due to the effects of radiation on the human population. These forms of surveillance can identify early disease processes for which successful interventions are available. Cures or significant reductions in morbidity and mortality can be affected.

Finally, surveillance of exposed populations often leads to knowledge about the prevention of disease that can be applied to other populations. This is especially true when a disease is linked to a new exposure. For example, methyl mercury was not known to cause significant human disease until 1954, when extensive human environmental exposure through the consumption of contaminated fish in Minamata, Japan, resulted in severe irreversible methyl mercury poisoning in adults and children.

In addition, education about healthy life-styles and behaviors may result in the lowering of risk for other exposed persons. (See the SHEs below.) Thus surveillance aims to ensure that diseases do not claim new victims.[50] Once an increased incidence of disease has been found in a population with certain exposures, surveillance of similarly exposed persons (for example, with exposure markers and biomarkers) may lead to early detection of risks associated with development of disease and an intervention may reduce this risk.

An important complement to health surveillance is hazard surveillance, which involves the collection and analysis of information about the type, dose, and duration of exposures. A thorough assessment of hazards and potential hazards is the first step in the design of a health surveillance program. Hazard surveillance promotes disease prevention, because the data can be analyzed and controls put in place prior to the occurrence of symptoms or signs of disease. This form of surveillance attempts to identify hazards that may merit an intervention, for example, the precise nature of airborne toxins in a community exposed to emissions from an industrial plant.

PREVENTIVE STRATEGIES IN SURVEILLANCE: SENTINEL HEALTH EVENTS

Many worksites developed company-based occupational health surveillance programs in the 1970s and 1980s after the initiation of medical surveillance for 27 physical or chemical hazards mandated by the Occupational Safety and Health Administration. The surveillance also provided data to analyze the health effects related to occupational exposures. Federal statutes on toxic substances that cover, for example, chemical use, manufacture, and assessment and hazardous waste site clean-up (including Superfund), as well as state legislation, have also encouraged surveillance for the early recognition of adverse health effects. Index cases identified through medical screening are useful in the development of strategies to prevent future illness (such as with tuberculosis).[31,50]

In 1983 Rutstein et al[38] presented the concept of the SHE in occupational disease:

A disease, disability, or untimely death which is occupationally related and whose occurrence may: (1) provide the impetus for epidemiologic or industrial hygiene studies; or (2) serve as a warning signal that materials substitution, engineering control, personal protection, or medical care may be required.

The National Institute for Occupational Safety and Health has implemented a medical surveillance system based on the sentinel event: Sentinel Events Notification System for Occupational Risks (SHEs).[7] This system uses occupational physicians in the community as event reporters. The initial list of work-related conditions has been updated and expanded.[34] Sentinel event strategies have now been extended to environmental health practice.[2] The Agency for Toxic Substances and Disease Registry is developing national exposure and disease registries.[3] Disease surveillance systems incorporating SHEs offer some important advantages over strategies aiming to study disease occurrence in relation to environmental hazards.[2]

ISSUES IN ENVIRONMENTAL SURVEILLANCE

Increased public awareness of environmental health problems and highly publicized litigation around such well-known environmental disasters as Love Canal, New York, and Bhopal, India, have led to increased interest in environmental surveillance by the general public.[12,23,25,29] This interest can in turn place huge pressures on clinicians and public health officials to investigate any perceived environmental exposure–disease connection.[36,37] Therefore, it is crucial that all parties realize some of the inherent limitations of environmental surveillance.[20]

In general, environmental toxin exposures are significantly lower, even in the worst scenarios, than occupational toxin exposures. Occupational exposures are regulated and experienced at levels of parts per million, and environmental exposures are regulated and usually experienced at levels of parts per billion; environmental exposures are usually at least a thousandfold lower than occupational exposures, even in the worst cases. Therefore, the amount of disease expected is significantly less with environmental toxic exposures because most toxins follow a dose-response pattern. This means that, as opposed to occupational toxin exposures, environmental exposures are so low that a much larger group of people needs to be studied to find detectable increases of a specific toxin-induced disease.

In addition, environmental toxin exposures often occur via oral routes (such as contaminated water and food) and to a lesser extent via inhalation and dermal routes; occupational exposures are predominantly inhalational and dermal exposures. These different routes of exposure can lead to different toxin interactions. In addition, these exposures can occur over considerable lengths of time; it is often difficult or impossible to define the time of onset, duration, or dose of exposure from toxins in environmental exposure situations.

Furthermore, because many populations are extremely mobile in modern society, defining the exposed population can be very difficult, especially when chronic diseases and diseases with long latency periods (such as cancer) are examined. Finally, as opposed to occupational toxins that potentially expose a well-defined group of workers, environmental toxins potentially expose entire populations of people, including the elderly, children, those with preexisting diseases, and pregnant women (see Chapter 28).

ENVIRONMENTAL SURVEILLANCE AND CLUSTERS

Individual clinicians who observe their own clinical practice and public health personnel working with established environmental surveillance systems will inevitably become involved in the investigation of disease clusters.[1,19,20] A disease cluster is an excess of disease (death) in time and/or space; an aggregation is a group of individuals with a shared exposure.[1,9,36,40] Disease clusters are noted by clinicians, community residents, and public health officials when they present as an excess of a rare disease (for example, angiosarcoma of the liver due to vinyl chloride); a striking excess of common disease (such as the classic church-picnic gastroenteritis epidemic); or a relative excess in an uncommon population (for example, lung cancer in a young population).

Investigations of disease clusters seek to prove the existence of the cluster and uncover a shared past exposure (for example, aggregation) among the individuals suffering from the same disease. There are, however, several inherent difficulties associated with the investigation of disease clusters.

The major limitation of cluster investigation is that the majority of disease clusters ultimately are due to random chance, not a shared exposure.[36,39] In other words, many groups of people who share a similar disease in time and place ultimately have not shared a similar environmental exposure. The number of disease clusters due to chance statistically increases when surveillance systems are in operation. This finding is true with both systematic surveillance systems and those established due to heightened public awareness. Even when a plausible shared exposure is identified for a given disease cluster, ultimately the results of a particular cluster investigation can be considered only hypothesis generating, because chance cannot be excluded as cause.[1,19,36] Furthermore, the concept of chance as the cause can be very difficult to communicate to patients and to communities in which the disease cluster has occurred, especially in the present atmosphere of heightened environmental awareness and litigation.[19,23]

Further practical difficulties include the low number of cases usually associated with environmental disease clusters, which makes statistical analysis difficult and often uninterpretable.[45] Especially with environmental exposures, as mentioned earlier, the exposures are often relatively small over long, undefined periods, and the affected populations are mixed, mobile, and not easily defined. Investigation of chronic disease clusters are especially difficult because of the extended periods from uncharacterized exposures with highly mobile populations.[20]

Furthermore, because of public interest and extensive tort litigation, these investigations readily become difficult political situations for the investigators. All of these factors make the investigation of environmental disease clusters unappealing to many epidemiologists and public health officials.[35-37] Nevertheless, because of public concern and historical discovery of disease-toxin connections through disease cluster investigations (such as the methyl mercury health effects in Minamata and radiation effects in Hiroshima), these investigations will continue.[1,20]

Recently there has been considerable interest in disease cluster investigations, especially the establishment of investigational protocols by the Centers for Disease Control and others.* These protocols allow systematic investigation as well as educated expectations for all involved. It is hoped that in the future these protocols will aid clinicians, public health officials, and the general public in understanding the process and limitations of disease cluster investigations.

ELEMENTS OF SURVEILLANCE

The question of how to deal with situations in which environmental factors are suspected of causing human disease is as old as the practice of medicine. Hippocrates stated: "One should consider most attentively the waters which inhabitants use, whether they be marshy and soft, or hard and running from elevated and rocky situations."[27] In attempts to determine the role of environmental factors in disease causation today, this advice is still sound.

All too often scientists are urged to rush to conclusions about outbreaks of disease suspected to be environmentally associated. Before expensive laboratory tests are ordered or significant effort and expense of any description are undertaken, three questions should be asked. Is there a true elevation of the disease rate in the population? Does a significant potential source of exposure to the population exist? Is there biologic plausibility to the hypothesized exposure-disease relationship?

Two situations can give rise to the call for surveillance. The first is a suspected elevation in the rate of disease. The second is the discovery of a suspected source of exposure. Whichever issue initiated the recognition of the situation, that question (exposure or disease rate) should be answered first. Only if the answers are in the affirmative should any further action be anticipated.

Biologic plausibility also is an important consideration in the relation of environmental exposures to human disease. Can the environmental exposures identified, operating via the hypothesized routes of exposure, conceivably cause the disease under consideration? Clearly, if there is an established causative relationship in animals or humans, the credibility and rationale for establishing surveillance are enhanced; however, the absence of an association does not preclude the desirability of creation of a surveillance system. It does, however, entail the burden of developing a hypothesis about the potential mechanism for the exposure/disease relationship.

There is a significant difference between observing a so-called cluster of disease and/or a common-source environmental exposure (an aggregation) and proving that the two are causally linked. The path from cluster investigation to causation often leads to the establishment of some form of surveillance. (See previous discussion.) Although clinicians are essential to surveillance activities and may often feel impelled by the situation to undertake such endeavors, an appreciation of the magnitude of the time and resources required is essential.

Several issues must be examined to determine the need for a surveillance program. The nonuniform distribution of disease in the general population raises an alarm. As previously discussed, clusters are fairly frequent events.[20] It is crucial to verify the existence of the condition described, because it is not uncommon for a variety of illnesses to be reported in a cluster. The diagnosis must be as clear, unambiguous, and objectively documented as possible.

IMPLEMENTATION OF A SURVEILLANCE PROGRAM

Six steps are involved in establishing a surveillance program: (1) identifying the disease in question, (2) identifying the population base[32] to be monitored, (3) selecting a sentinel system that can be used to identify disease outcome or outcomes, (4) establishing a data management system, (5) monitoring the environment and/or the population for exposure, and (6) selecting the methods for data analysis.

Definition of disease

It is critical to decide a priori which diseases will be included in the surveillance. As previously discussed, this decision must be made in as objective a manner as possible. Any information on biologic plausibility should be used to guide this decision. New diseases and complex, amorphously defined syndromes should be avoided.

Previously it was thought that identification of a single disease entity gave more credibility to such investigations. It is now apparent, however, that multiple outcomes can be of legitimate interest in certain circumstances. For example, non-Hodgkin's lymphoma, soft-tissue sarcoma, and breast cancer all have been linked with exposure to pesticides.[46-48] In such circumstances it should be realized that the inclusion of multiple outcomes does not appreciably affect the cost of the surveillance.

Defining the surveillance population

An essential part of surveillance is the decision at the onset about whom to include. The concept of population

---
*References 4, 10, 13, 14, 18, 19, 21, 33.

base includes by inference a location- and time-specific population.[32] To the extent that any subgroup is excluded or not represented, the results of the surveillance can be biased and invalid.

The types of records that are most useful in defining the population are census data, voter registration lists, and school enrollment records. Information on age distribution, gender, and race or ethnicity is essential to develop appropriate denominators for the calculation of rates of the illness under investigation. The primary exception to this approach occurs in the study of adverse reproductive outcomes, which would include spontaneous abortions, stillbirths, congenital malformations, and pregnancy complications. The population of interest is limited to pregnant women. The surveillance of this information is specialized and is only obtainable through a primary source (such as hospital or physician records) or a secondary source (for example, birth-defects registries).

Establishing a disease sentinel

Once the population base is defined, it is necessary to establish a method that provides a census of disease in the selected population. The goal is to establish a sentinel system that would positively identify each individual in the population base who develops the disease of interest. Both primary (hospital and physician records) and secondary sources (registries) can be used for this purpose. Although local medical facilities capture most of the cases, it is not unusual, particularly in rural or even suburban areas, for people to travel significant distances for treatment of serious illness. If this possibility is a concern, the extent of such loss of case identification must be calculated or the cases must be tracked.

The most objective form of the diagnostic information must be used in surveillance. In the absence of pathologic specimens, which permit independent evaluation, original laboratory reports are useful. Summaries such as medical records are often not reliable sources of information. They may contain layers of supposition, particularly if the situation has been covered in the media. Maximization of the accuracy of the diagnostic information appreciably enhances the usefulness of the surveillance data.

Data management and confidentiality

It is essential that the data collected be treated with the same confidentiality afforded to other patient medical information. Access to information must be limited to authorized personnel. In some states access is limited to governmental agencies, although this arrangement is not ideal from the reseacher's perspective. Legitimate researchers whose protocols are approved by a human-subjects review board are usually allowed access. Some states take the additional step of requiring physician approval to use a patient's health data. This process can be cumbersome and an additional burden on physicians. In addition, it can be argued that it takes the decision away from the individual whose records are at issue. It must be kept in mind that surveillance is a first step in establishing knowledge about disease and is not an end in itself.

Exposure

It is not an uncommon scenario for a community to suddenly discover that it is located near a source of pollution. The source may be a waste site, such as the Love Canal toxic waste site in Niagara Falls, New York; the location of illegal dumping of hazardous waste, such as Times Beach, Missouri; an industrial accident such as that in Seveso, Italy; or an industrial site such as the Department of Energy facility in Fernald, Ohio. The result of such realizations is often the call for studies of possible adverse health effects in the exposed population.

The surveillance system can provide a method for quantification of health outcomes and the general level of risk; however, unless this information can be linked to data on exposure, the researchers may not have data to address a putative causal association with health problems. Assessment of exposure and human health effects including federal government activities in these areas and relevant case studies have been reviewed in the arena of hazardous waste management.[3] In reality, there need to be significant data supporting the existence of important health problems before such exposure investigations can be fiscally justified.

Assessment of exposure can be performed by measuring levels of contaminants in the environment and by assessing internal exposure through the use of biomarkers of exposure in individuals. Biomonitoring involves the measurement of either the concentration of the toxin or its metabolites or the biochemical effects (such as methemoglobin formation or cholinesterase inhibition) that have been correlated with exposure concentration (see Chapter 63).

Analysis

Analysis of the data generated during the surveillance investigation is best performed by an experienced biostatistician.

CONCLUSIONS

Environmental surveillance systems provide information critical to planning, implementing, and evaluating public health programs and interventions. Surveillance systems can generate early information on the presence of health problems resulting from environmental pollution and provide important insight into previously unrecognized exposure-disease relationships. Surveillance extends beyond the collection and analysis of data to the direction of active prevention programs that aim to reduce or eliminate the occurrence of exposure-related conditions and diseases. Individual clinicians can play important roles in disease and exposure surveillance, keeping in mind that successful surveillance involves immense time and resources and potentially complex political pressures.

REFERENCES

1. Acheson ED: Clinical practice and epidemiology: two worlds or one? *Brit Med J* 1:723, 1979.
2. Aldrich TE, Leaverton PE: Sentinel event strategies in environmental disease: *Annu Rev Public Health* 14:205, 1993.
3. Agency for Toxic Substances and Disease Registry: *Policy and procedure for establishing a national registry of persons exposed to hazardous substances: National Exposure Registry,* Atlanta, 1988, US Public Health Service.
4. Agency for Toxic Substances and Disease Registry: CLUSTER Software, 1991.
5. Andelman JB, Underhill DW: *Health effects from hazardous waste sites,* Chelsea, Mich, 1987, Lewis.
6. Anderson HA et al: surveillance of environmental disease: the Wisconsin initiative, *Wis Med J* 89:120, 1990.
7. Baker EL: Sentinel event notification system for occupational risks (SENSOR): the concept, *Am J Public Health* 79(suppl):18, 1989.
8. Baker EL: Surveillance of disorders caused by occupational hazards: principles and practice: a review, *J R Soc Med* 419:418, 1991.
9. Caldwell GG: Time-space cancer clusters, *Health Environ Digest* 3:1, 1989.
10. Centers for Disease Control: Guidelines for investigating clusters of health events, *MMWR* 39 (RR-11):1, 1990.
11. Citizens Fund: *Poisons in our neighborhoods: toxic pollution in the United States,* Washington, DC, 1990, The Fund.
12. Cohen G, O'Connor J, eds: *Fighting toxics,* Washington, DC, 1990, Island Press.
13. Elliott P, ed: *Methodology of enquiries into disease clustering,* London, 1989, Small Area Health Statistics Unit, London School of Hygiene and Tropical Medicine.
14. Enterline PE: Evaluating cancer clusters, *Am Ind Hyg Assoc J* 46:B10, 1985.
15. Environmental Protection Agency: *The Toxic Release Inventory: a national perspective.* Washington, DC, 1989, Government Printing Office.
16. Environmental Protection Agency: *Toxics in the community: national and local perspectives,* Washington, DC, 1990, Government Printing Office.
17. Favata EA et al: Clinical experiences: development of a medical surveillance protocol for hazardous waste workers, *Occupational Medicine: State of the Art Reviews* 5:117, 1990.
18. Fiore BJ, Hanrahan LP, Anderson HA: State health department response to disease cluster reports: a protocol for investigation, *Am J Epidemiol* 132:S14, 1990.
19. Fleming LE, Ducatman AM, Shalat SL: Disease clusters in occupational medicine: a protocol for their investigation in the workplace, *Am J Ind Med* 22:33, 1991.
20. Fleming LE, Ducatman AM, Shalat SL: Disease clusters: a central and ongoing role in occupational health, *J Occup Med* 33:818, 1991.
21. Frumkin H, Kantrowitz W: Cancer clusters in the workplace: an approach to investigation, *J Occup Med* 29:949, 1987.
22. Gochfeld M: Medical surveillance and screening in the workplace: complementary preventive strategies, *Environ Res* 59:67, 1992.
23. Goldman BA: *The truth about where you live: an atlas for action on toxins and mortality,* New York, 1991, Times Books.
24. Goldsmith JR, ed: *Environmental epidemiology: epidemiological investigation of community environmental health problems,* Boca Raton, Fla, 1986, CRC Press.
25. Hadden SG: *A citizen's right to know: risk communication and public policy,* Boulder, Colo, 1989, Westview.
26. Halperin WE et al: Medical screening in the workplace: proposed principles, *J Occup Med* 28:547, 1986.
27. Hippocrates: *On airs, waters, and places,* translated and republished in *Medical Classics* 3:19, 1938.
28. Klaucke DN et al: Guidelines for evaluating surveillance systems, *MMWR* 37(S-5):1, 1988.
29. Legator MS, Harper BL, Scott MJ, eds: *The health detective's handbook: a guide to the investigation of environmental hazards by nonprofessionals,* Baltimore, 1985, Johns Hopkins University Press.
30. Marfin AA, Schenker M: Screening for lung cancer: effective tests awaiting effective treatment, *Occupational Medicine: State of the Art Reviews* 6:111, 1991.
31. Matte TD et al: Guidelines for medical screening in the workplace, *Occupational Medicine: State of the Art Reviews* 5:439, 1990.
32. Miettinen OS: *Theoretical epidemiology,* New York, 1985, Wiley.
33. Monson RR: *Occupational epidemiology,* ed 2, Boca Raton, Fla, 1990, CRC Press.
34. Mullan RJ, Murthy LI: Occupational sentinel health events: an updated list for physician recognition and public health surveillance, *Am J Ind Med* 19:775, 1991.
35. Neutra RR: Counterpoint from a cluster buster, *Am J Epidemiol* 132:1, 1990.
36. Rothman KJ: Clustering of disease, *Am J Public Health* 77:13, 1987.
37. Rothman KJ: A sobering start for the cluster busters' conference, *Am J Epidemiol* 132:S6, 1990.
38. Rutstein DD et al: Sentinel health events (occupational): a basis for physician recognition and public health surveillance, *Am J Public Health* 73:1054, 1983.
39. Schulte PA, Ehrenberg RL, Singal M: Investigations of occupational cancer clusters: theory and practice, *Am J Public Health* 77:52, 1987.
40. Smith PG, Schottenfeld D, Fraumeni J, eds: *Cancer epidemiology and prevention,* New York, 1982, WB Saunders.
41. Spitzer WO, Brown BP: Unanswered questions about periodic health examination, *Ann Ind Med* 83:257, 1975.
42. US Preventive Services Task Force: *Guide to clinical preventive services,* Baltimore, 1989, Williams & Wilkins.
43. US Public Health Service: *Healthy people 2000: national health promotion and disease prevention objectives,* Pub No (PHS) 91-50213, Washington, DC, 1991.
44. Walsh JME: Cancer screening in older adults, *West J Med* 156:495, 1992.
45. Wartenberg D, Greenberg M: Detecting disease clusters: the importance of statistical power, *Am J Epidemiol* 132:S156, 1990.
46. Wigle DT, et al: Mortality study of Canadian male farm operators: non-Hodgkin's lymphoma mortality and agricultural practices in Saskatchewan, *J Nat Cancer Inst* 82:575, 1990.
47. Wolff MS, et al: Blood levels of organ organochlorine residues and risk of breast cancer, *J Nat Cancer Inst* 85:648, 1993.
48. Woods JS et al: Soft tissue sarcoma and non-Hodgkin's lymphoma in relation to phenoxyherbicide and chlorinated phenol exposure in western Washington, *J Nat Cancer Inst* 78:899, 1987.
49. World Health Organization: *Congenital malformations worldwide.* Amsterdam, 1991, Elsevier.
50. Yodaiken RE: Surveillance, monitoring, and regulatory concerns, *J Occup Med* 28:56, 1986.

Chapter 63

BIOMARKERS

Paul A. Schulte

Potential uses of biomarkers in environmental medicine
    Definition of biomarkers
    Exposure assessment
    Mechanisms of toxicity
    Delineation of preclinical effects
    Risk assessment
    Identification of susceptible subpopulations
Operational use of biomarkers
Validation of biomarkers
    Reliability
    Validation of markers of exposure
    Validation of the relationship between biologic changes and disease
    Validation of markers of susceptibility
A framework for considering biomarker use
Ethical and legal issues in the use of biologic markers

Biologic markers can provide clinical information relating to exposure, toxicity, pathophysiologic mechanisms, preclinical effects, susceptibility, and risk assessment.* Biomarkers are used in environmental epidemiology studies, in disease diagnosis and surveillance, and in intervention trials of exposure or disease control. There are ethical, legal, and social issues that must be confronted by the medical practitioner who uses biomarkers. In this chapter the following topics are addressed under three general headings: potential uses for biomarkers in environmental medicine, validation of biomarkers, and ethical and legal issues in the use of biomarkers.

---

*References 9, 13, 17, 20, 22, 33, 36, 51.

POTENTIAL USES OF BIOMARKERS IN ENVIRONMENTAL MEDICINE
Definition of biomarkers

The term *biologic marker* or *biomarker* refers to any indicator of events in biologic systems or samples. These events may range from death and clinical disease to changes in genetic material and molecular constituents. It is the latter genetic, biochemical, and cytologic markers that have received the most attention in recent years, as technology has driven the focus toward the identification of disruptions in cellular and subcellular processes.

Biomarkers have been defined as follows by the National Research Council[29]:

It is useful to classify biologic markers into three types—markers of exposure, of effect and of susceptibility—and to describe the events peculiar to each type. A *biologic marker of exposure* is an exogenous substance or its metabolite(s) or the product of an interaction between a xenobiotic agent and some target molecule or cell that is measured in a compartment within an organism. A *biologic marker of effect* is a measurable biochemical, physiologic, or other alteration within an organism that, depending on magnitude, can be recognized as an established or potential health impairment or disease. A *biologic marker of susceptibility* is an indicator of an inherent or acquired limitation of an organism's ability to respond to the challenge of exposure to a specific xenobiotic substance.

These three types of biomarkers (exposure, effect, and susceptibility) present a continuum of events between exposure and disease.

Examples of biomarkers of exposure include the measurement of the actual substance (for example, lead or PCBs) or a metabolite (phenol or muconic acid from benzene) or a subtle biochemical effect that is relatively specific to the exposure. Indeed, many biologic markers of exposure are actually the results of subtle or "early" effects. For example, the use of zinc or erythrocyte protoporphyrin or delta aminolevulinic acid as markers of lead exposure reflect the effects of lead on blocking various steps in the heme synthesis pathway, resulting in the buildup of these precursors that are then measured in blood or urine. Similarly, the use of red cell or serum cholinesterase to estimate exposure to organophosphate pesticides reflects the basic toxic effect of these substances that bind relatively irreversibly to cholinesterase.

An important attribute of biomarkers of exposure is their "specificity." Thus lead has many biologic effects, some of which (such as peripheral neuropathy) are not specific to lead, whereas others (such as zinc protoporphyrin) are nearly unique to lead. In the final analysis only the measure of lead itself provides an absolutely unique biomarker for lead exposure (and even that requires consideration that some of the lead we measure in blood today may have been recently mobilized from bone, thus reflecting exposures that occurred many years prior to the exposure of current interest, perhaps even in utero).

An exciting area of research is the development of molecular markers of exposure, for example, specific adducts on DNA. The recent demonstration of increased DNA-protein crosslinking in welders[8] suggests that this molecular lesion may be relatively specific to certain carcinogens.

The designation "biologic markers of effect" can be confusing because it is very broad. Thus every physiologic or biochemic endpoint that we measure (for example, blood creatinine, forced vital capacity, urine specific gravity) can be considered a biomarker of one or more effects from one or more chemicals. Several recent studies provide exhaustive lists of markers that can be used to evaluate pulmonary toxins,[31] immunotoxins,[30] and reproductive toxins.[32]

Exposure assessment

The clinician faces an ongoing challenge in attempting to link specific health effects with an environmental exposure(s). Major factors in this decision making process include an inadequate knowledge base about environmental exposures and related health effects and a lack of objective data to link a health effect with a particular environmental exposure. The current generation of biologic markers has the potential to indicate minute interactions of xenobiotics and critical macromolecules. It is now possible to identify the concentration of a foreign compound or xenobiotic at the zeptomole (1 in 10^{21}) level.[4] Clearly, the ability to analyze far exceeds the current understanding of the health significance of the findings.

Nevertheless, the new analyses make it possible, for example, to determine more accurately who among residents around a point source of pollution have had recent exposures to specific xenobiotics. To be clinically useful, biomarkers of exposure should have certain characteristics.[6] First, there should be a clear relationship between the systemic dose of the xenobiotic being studied and the measured levels of the biomarkers. Second, variations in the levels of biomarkers or biomarker levels should be as specific to the chemical of interest as possible. The EPA has categorized biomarkers as those that are compound-specific (for example, benzene, trichloroethylene, acrylamide, styrene, nicotine, and lead) and those that are indicators of relevant classes of compounds (for example, dioxins, PCBs).[11] Third, the most promising markers of exposure are those that are identifiable in close temporal proximity to the exposure. For the purposes of etiological research and historic risk assessment, estimates of past human exposures are important. This can be achieved with the use of biomarkers in conjunction with other tools for exposure assessment such as historic ambient monitoring, plant record review, job exposure matrices, and activity diaries.

Biomarkers for exposure have been used as an indicator of biologic dosimetry. The concept of biologic dosimetry has evolved from one oriented toward the accurate and systematic determination of dose toward one that describes dose in terms of a defined biological response.[27]

Mechanisms of toxicity

Historically, epidemiology has used inferential statistics to determine the link between an environmental exposure and a resultant disease. This approach has led to many of the advances in the last 100 years of public health. Many of these successes have occurred without knowledge of the mechanism underlying the exposure-induced toxic effect. Such mechanisms were often hypothesized but not well understood. It is now beginning to be possible to define a detailed continuum of events for various environmental diseases.

For example, exposure to carcinogenic aromatic amines in cigarettes and in the workplace are well documented causes of bladder cancer. However, a more detailed picture has evolved by understanding various mechanisms of action. For example, 4-aminobiphenyl in cigarette smoke has been found to bind to hemoglobin (and to DNA). The risk of bladder cancer has also been found to be increased in individuals exposed to aromatic amines and who have the slow acetylator phenotype. Vineis and Ronco[58] have shown that the formation of 4-aminobiphenyl hemoglobin adducts is greater in slow than in fast acetylators. The use of quantitative fluorescence image analysis and multiple bladder cell surface markers has allowed for the determination of which atypias in exfoliated cells are likely to be precursors of malignant diseases. The p53 tumor suppressor gene has been found to associate with high-grade tumors, indicating those patients with the worst prognosis. Hence it is possible to distinguish the following heuristic continuum for aromatic amine-induced bladder cancer (see Table 63-1).

Table 63-1. A detailed continuum of events for aromatic amine-induced bladder cancer

	Cancer marker	Reference
Exposure ↓		
Internal dose ↓	Urinary benzidine	Lowry, 1980
Biologically effective dose ↓	Hemoglobin adducts; DNA adducts	Vineis and Ronco, 1992; Talaska et al, 1991
Altered structure/function ↓	p300, DNA hyperploidy	Rao, 1993
Clinical disease/prognosis	p53 mutation	Sarkis et al, 1993

Delineation of preclinical effects

The depiction of a heuristic continuum between a xenobiotic exposure and resultant effects provides for the potential to identify intermediate, prodromal, or preclinical changes indicative of disease, or a warning of imbalance in homeostatic mechanisms. Identification of these earlier changes may offer the opportunity to intervene while the process is reversible.[9] Biologic markers of early disease processes will help ensure that the efficacy of environmental controls is evaluated promptly; there would be no need to wait for clinical disease to manifest. A decrease in preclinical disease rates could be considered evidence of disease prevention. Hence biologic markers could constitute an early warning system to identify hazards or risks.[36]

With valid markers of preclinical disease, it should no longer be necessary to wait for disease to occur before evaluating an association between an exposure and a disease. If a preclinical change predictive of disease is identified and validated, then the same clinical and epidemiologic methods used in traditional epidemiology can be used to determine an association between an exposure and the preclinical stage of disease. This is illustrated in the work of Hemstreet et al,[16] in which DNA hyperploidy was shown to increase the bladder cancer risk in workers exposed to 2-naphthylamine. Eventually, it should be possible to use early effect markers as dependent variables that appear very early in the exposure-disease continuum, that is, closer to the time of exposure.

As with validated exposure markers, exposure characterization is no longer limited to an ecologic assessment, in which subgroups of subjects are lumped into one or a few categories of presumed exposure.[20] It is increasingly possible to evaluate the dose of a xenobiotic in target tissues: these are the true "exposures" that result when subjects with different work practices, physiologic and metabolic characteristics, other important exposures, or perhaps "life-style characteristics" are studied.

The classic epidemiologic paradigm of a dichotomous exposure and disease classification (exposed or not, diseased or not) worked well in the past when exposures were large and effects detectable by astute clinicians and epidemiologists. Those days are gone in many countries. Today exposures are generally less intense and effects subtler in many workplaces and environments. Large exposures still occur in developing countries and in small businesses in developed countries. However, in most occupational settings today courts and regulatory agencies are increasingly inclined to rely on evidence that accounts for the magnitude of occupational risks in light of other intervening factors. Current clinical and epidemiologic research can best provide this evidence when techniques are used that measure valid biologic markers of exposure, effect, and susceptibility.[51]

Risk assessment

Risk assessment[14,34] (see Chapter 3) is the characterization of the potential adverse health effects of human exposure to hazardous substances. Risk assessments are conducted when there are inadequate data about risks at certain levels of exposure. Extrapolations from high doses to low doses and across species are a component of risk assessments. Biologic markers can be useful in the risk assessment process by fostering insights into mechanism, by aiding in appraising comparability between species, and by providing intermediate indicators of toxicity in lieu of traditional health endpoints.[36,51,54]

The ability to provide mechanistic and toxicologic detail also makes the use of biologic markers in risk assessments the source of problems. Hattis and Silver[14] have described this paradox and relate it to the difference in goals between analysis in basic science and epidemiology versus risk assessment. Biomedical research aims to collect information on health outcomes and causal connections. In contrast, risk assessments identify the shape of the exposure–disease relationship and the time scale involved. To overcome these differences in goals, biomarker research in human populations needs to pay more attention to modeling biologic processes rather than conforming to a limited number of statistical models.[14]

Identification of susceptible subpopulations

The tools of molecular biology and analytical chemistry allow researchers to identify a degree of interindividual variability not previously imagined.[21] This variability is such that within the category of homo sapiens, it is unlikely that, except for genetic twins, any two people have the same genetic makeup. The biochemical individuality that people are born with is compounded by the differences in their environmental exposures and accrued life experiences, serving to further heighten this variability.[13]

During this century biologists have accepted the notion of biochemical individuality and rejected the notion of "essentialism" (the belief that everything is a product of a limited number of fixed unchanging forms). The term *popula-*

tion thinking represents this acceptance. As Mayr[26] describes:

Population thinkers stress the uniqueness of everything in the organic world. What is important for them is the individual, not the type. They emphasize that every individual in sexually reproducing species is uniquely different from all others, with much individuality even existing in uniparentally reproducing ones. There is no typical individual, and mean values are abstractions. Much of what in the past have been designated in biology as classes are populations consisting of unique individuals.

It is now necessary to seek new means to accommodate the accumulating knowledge of biologic phenomena at the molecular level. Until recently analysis of variation at the DNA level was limited because the exact molecular structure of a lesion was not always apparent in the small amounts of genetic material available for study.[1] However, Mullis et al[28] described a new technology, the enzymatic amplification of DNA by a process called "DNA polymerase chain reaction" that is capable of increasing the amount of a selected target DNA sequence in any sample by enzymatically synthesizing many copies of the target DNA segment. This technology has provided the capability to identify smaller changes in DNA structure. Widespread use of this technique will allow the detection of more variation than we knew existed. We need to be able to describe this genetic variation, determine which gene components are associated with disease (and with exposure), and then address what we have learned at the policy level.[19]

OPERATIONAL USE OF BIOMARKERS

A whole set of practices for using biomarkers has evolved under the heading of "molecular epidemiology." Key to this effort is consideration of biomarkers as supplements to the conventional tools of epidemiology.[48]

Validity and practicality are critical to all potential applications of biomarkers. Validity pertains to both the laboratory characteristics of the marker assay and its predictive value in populations.[49] Practicality refers to the ease and acceptability with which a marker can be obtained from patients or research subjects and the cost of gathering specimens and conducting assays.[15]

VALIDATION OF BIOMARKERS

The key to the validation of markers is the determination of the validity of the marker assay.

Reliability

Marker validity also depends on the reliability of the assay; that is, the degree to which a marker will be a valid representation or predictor of an event is influenced by the reliability with which it can be measured. Reliability encompasses the unsystematic, random variation observed after repeated measurements.[23,39] In the measurement of continuous variables, such as with most biologic markers, errors of various kinds are inevitable, and the absolutely correct measurement can never be determined.[24] If a measure of a biologic marker yields results that differ markedly from one occasion to another, it is of little value in environmental research.

It is possible to use quantitative indices of the extent of random variation of a biologic marker. These indices can be used to determine whether the reliability of a given measure is sufficient for the purpose being considered. The two most common indices are the standard error of the measurement and the reliability coefficient.[25] To assess random errors, multiple measurements are needed to compensate for the fact that the random error in the arithmetic mean of several measurements is likely to be much less than the random error in an individual measurement.[25] The reliability coefficient is technically known as the intraclass coefficient of variability[10] and ranges from 0 to 1. If each measurement is identical, then the intraclass coefficient is 1.0. Fleiss[10] recommends that unreliability be controlled by conducting pilot studies and replicating measurement procedures on each study subject. In some cases the measurement of the amount of a marker is not an end in itself but a step to calculate some other value, thereby propagating measurement errors.[25]

Validation of markers of exposure

$$\text{Exposure} \rightarrow \text{Internal dose} \rightarrow \text{Biologically effective dose}$$

Markers of exposure may be validated by assessing the relationship of an exogenous exposure and internal dose or biologically effective dose.[22,44,48] Critical in such research is the need to have an effective exposure assessment. This may require a combination of personal and environmental monitoring and questionnaires, record review, and modeling to reconstruct exposure history. The approach also requires understanding of the pharmacokinetics involved for the particular xenobiotics being studied. Related to this is the need to understand the natural history of the marker and utilize it in the validation study. For example, in the study of hydroxyethyl hemoglobin adducts in workers exposed to ethylene oxide, we used the life span of the erythrocyte (approximately 4 months) as the time span in which to reconstruct exposure.[49] There is also a need to account for factors that might influence the appearance of a marker. In the aforementioned study, an exposure response relationship was found, at levels below the permissible exposure level, when mean values were adjusted for important covariates such as age, cigarette smoking, and education.

Validation of the relationship between biologic changes and disease

$$\text{Early biologic effects} \rightarrow \text{Altered structure function} \rightarrow \text{Disease}$$

The lack of validation information in this category often bears much of the criticism about using biologic markers.[47]

The often repeated question is, "What do they mean concerning health and disease?" These types of validation studies are difficult to accomplish because of the temporal factor. To identify an early change, that is, a change in pathogenesis or a change predictive of disease, generally requires a prospective study design. This is difficult as evidenced, for example, by the fact that there still is little consensus on their predictive value despite the large number of studies on cytogenetic markers. Since most of the studies have been cross-sectional, they suffer from temporal ambiguity levels of the marker and the presence of disease are determined simultaneously. To perform the appropriate prospective studies of sister chromatid exchanges or any proposed marker of early effect would take a large population and a relatively long time. The best and possibly only example of such a study is the Nordic prospective study on the relationship between peripheral lymphocyte chromosome damage and cancer morbidity in occupational groups.[38] Ten laboratories in four Nordic countries participated in a study of a combined cohort of persons (mostly from occupational groups) who had been cytogenetically tested. The cohort will be followed prospectively for cancer morbidity. The cohort is comprised of 3190 subjects of whom 1986 subjects (62%) have been scored for chromosome aberrations and 2024 subjects (63%) scored for sister chromatid exchanges.

Validation of markers of susceptibility

Exposure → Susceptibility → Disease

Biologic markers of susceptibility may result from inherited or acquired processes.[48] Susceptibility may influence any of the other markers in the continuum between exposure and disease. Thus they may influence the extent to which a xenobiotic enters an individual, is transported, reacts with critical macromolecules, causes reversible and irreversible biologic changes, causes disease, and influences disease prognosis.

Susceptibility markers may be used to determine why, of two similarly exposed individuals, only one develops the disease in question. This is referred to as "effect modification" in epidemiology. *Effect modification* is a term encompassing both statistical and biologic aspects. Statistically, the examination of joint effects of two or more factors is often discussed in the context of effect modification. Conclusions depend on the statistical method (multiplicative or additive) used to model interaction. From the biologic perspective, effect modification answers the question of why two similarly exposed individuals both do not develop a disease. The answer in part is individual variability in metabolic and detoxification capabilities or other biologic mechanisms mediating susceptibility.

For example, the issue of the acetylation phenotype and bladder cancer in aromatic amines illustrates the influence of susceptibility.[57] Despite a plethora of studies, the scientific literature is still inconclusive as to the extent to which being a slow acetylator modifies one's risk of bladder cancer. Generally, most studies have been too small, had weak exposure characterization, and were too poorly designed to determine whether exposure or susceptibility was the key factor or how much importance should be attributed to each factor.

In what may be viewed as a classic study, Vineis and Ronco[58] showed an example of how partial validation of a susceptibility marker may occur without using disease as the outcome. Vineis and Ronco[58] compared the formation of hemoglobin adducts (which are documented surrogates for DNA adducts and hence believed to be involved in carcinogenesis) between individuals exposed to 4-aminobiphenyl and who were slow or fast acetylators. They found that the slow acetylator had an average of 1.5-fold greater frequency of adducts than the fast acetylators. Despite these encouraging efforts at validation, few markers of susceptibility have been validated and none are ready for use in population screening.[34,50] Nonetheless, one of the greatest contributions of molecular epidemiologic research should be a heightened ability to disentangle genetic and environmental factors.

A FRAMEWORK FOR CONSIDERING BIOMARKER USE

Too often in recent years discussion of biomarkers has been unfocused. This has not led to clear thinking of issues or heightened efforts for their use in research, intervention, or clinical practice. The effective use of biomarkers is a collaborative venture between different disciplines. To foster collaboration it is useful to have a framework in which to consider and discuss with some specificity the type of marker and the use for which it is intended.

It is possible to consider biomarkers in terms of a continuum of events between exogenous exposure and resultant disease. This continuum can be considered one axis of a matrix and the type of study involving the marker as another axis.[52] Four study types may be considered: laboratory studies, where markers are developed; transitional studies, where markers are characterized for their use in population studies; etiologic studies, which are case-control, cohort, and prevention trials; and applied studies such as screening programs. The resultant matrix of biomarkers and study types can provide researchers, program managers, clinicians, and decision makers with a frame of reference for discussing projects and describing collaborations.

Biomarkers can be used in a cross-sectional monitoring program, for example, to determine whether a community has had excessive exposure. A common example would be blood lead monitoring to determine whether a particular group of children has had excessive exposure. A different application is the use of biomarkers to track ongoing exposure or diminution of exposure in a workplace or community-based population. Validated biomarkers of effect can also be used to screen asymptomatic individuals for early disease or disease risk.[12,46]

ETHICAL AND LEGAL ISSUES IN THE USE OF BIOLOGIC MARKERS

Although biologic markers provide tremendous opportunities for disease prevention, their use also raises a number of additional ethical and legal issues and creates new responsibilities.[3,35,40,45] These issues can be discussed in the context of marker development and marker use. When developing and validating markers, research involving animals may be required. Such research is of great benefit to human health and should be continued. However, care should be taken that marker research is performed, in a peer-reviewed fashion, on animal models appropriate for the development of a marker and for the extrapolation of results to humans.

Some of the critical questions in research on biomarkers are: How is the current state of knowledge about the markers most accurately reported to subjects when securing their consent to participate? In developing study protocols, what actions will be taken for people with extreme results? In general, subjects should be notified if subsequent research identifies a predictive risk associated with markers that are used in validation studies. At the end of the studies subjects should be informed of the results. Thought needs to be given to how to inform subjects of study results involving markers that can be construed as early disease and that can inadvertently trigger statutes of limitation considerations related to compensation issues. Finally, the collection and handling of biomarker data should adhere to good practices for privacy and confidentiality.

The potential for the unethical use of biologic markers is great. This issue has been raised most pointedly with markers of susceptibility that might be used in genetic screening in the workplace.[35,50] If these markers correlate with particular racial or cultural characteristics, the potential exists that individuals and groups already burdened by discrimination may face further burdens. In addition, because of individual variability, there may be a false assurance that workers who "pass" such a screening tests will constitute a hardier group, and thus the temptation to place them in the most hazardous jobs or to relax environmental engineering controls might increase. Insurers, litigants, and researchers may have interests in data on susceptibility marker determinations for use in rate setting, litigation, or environmental epidemiology.

Examples of genetic testing for biomarkers of susceptibility include the screening for glucose-6-phosphate dehydrogenase deficiency (for susceptibility to oxidants) and alpha-1-antitrypsin deficiency (for susceptibility to pulmonary irritants). Indeed, the exclusion of women from jobs believed to pose a fetal hazard is based on a presumed genetic susceptibility. For various reasons none of these tests have proven to have scientific merit. The Supreme Court in the case of Johnson Controls struck down the restriction of women from jobs solely on the basis of "fetal protection."

The intentional or inadvertent disclosure of the findings of research or practice involving markers of exposure, disease, and susceptibility could have a chilling effect on a worker's ability to get or keep a job, or to obtain health insurance. A major issue is what to do with employees who manifest altered markers in the absence of diagnosed disease. Findings of workers with excess frequencies of various markers may put an ethical obligation on employers to provide follow-up monitoring. In terms of workers' responsibilities the question arises about whether they have a responsibility to disclose the results of marker evaluations performed on them to insurers or potential employers. The use of biologic markers in occupational health also must be considered in terms of worker monitoring. Two legal issues have emerged: the rights of those monitored and the use of monitoring as a primary control strategy.

Ashford et al[3] and Rothstein[35] have comprehensively identified many issues surrounding the rights of monitored workers. Ashford et al[3] concluded that "discriminatory practices and consequential tort suits, deterioration of labor-management relations, and agency sanctions may follow poorly conceived and poorly executed human monitoring." They believe that when the costs of worker removal are fully internalized in cost of production, monitoring for biologic markers as a primary control strategy will not be as economically attractive as proponents have argued. That debate still continues.

In conclusion, it is important for clinicians and scientists in environmental medicine to be aware of the social power of biologic marker data. To the practitioner, these data may appear as neutral pieces in a larger puzzle, but to many segments of society other interpretations and uses are possible. The social and ethical issues mandate consideration prior to using markers in health surveillance, screening programs, or clinical research. By anticipating the implications of a biomonitoring program, the practitioner can begin to realize the potential role of biomarkers in addressing environmental health issues.

REFERENCES

1. Arnheim N: New technologies for studying human genetic variation. In Woodhead AD, Bender MA, Leonard RC, eds: *Phentotye variation in populations,* New York, 1988, Plenum Press.
2. Ashby J: Monitoring human exposure to genotoxic chemicals. In Foa V et al, eds: *Occupational and environmental chemical hazards: cellular and biochemical indices for monitoring toxicity,* Chichester, England, 1987, Ellis Horwood.
3. Ashford NA et al: *Monitoring the worker for exposure and disease: scientific legal and ethical considerations in the use of biomarkers,* Baltimore, 1990, Johns Hopkins University Press.
4. Abel-Baky S, Giese RW: Gas chromatography electron capture negative-ion mass spectrometry at the zeptomole level, *Anal Chem* 63:2986, 1991.
5. Bi WF et al: Field molecular epidemiology: feasibility of monitoring for the malignant bladder cell phenotype in a benzidine-exposed occupational cohort, *J Occup Med* 35:20, 1993.
6. Bull RJ: *Decision model for the development of biomarkers of exposure,* EPA 600/x-89/163, Las Vegas, Nev, 1989, US Environmental Protection Agency.
7. Cartwright RA et al: The role of N-acetyltransferase in bladder carcinogenesis: a pharmacogenetic epidemiological approach to bladder cancer, *Lancet* 2:842, 1982.
8. Costa M, Zhitkovich A, Toniolo P: DNA-protein cross-links in welders: molecular applications, *Cancer Res* 53:460, 1993.

9. Cullen MR: The role of clinical investigations in biological markers research, *Environ Res* 50:1, 1989.
10. Fleiss J: Statistical factors in early detection of health effects. In Underhill DM, Radford ED, eds: *New and sensitive indicators of health impacts of environmental agents,* Pittsburgh, 1986, University of Pittsburgh.
11. Fowle JR, III, Sexton K: EPA priorities for biologic markers research in environmental health, *Environ Health Perspectives* 98:235, 1992.
12. Gochfeld M: Medical surveillance and screening in the workplace: complementary preventive strategies, *Environ Res* 59:67, 1992.
13. Hattis D: The use of biological markers in risk assessment, *Stat Sci* 3:358, 1988.
14. Hattis D, Silver K: Use of biomarkers in risk assessment. In Schulte PA, Perera FP, eds: *Molecular epidemiology: principles and practices,* San Diego, 1993, Academic Press.
15. Hayes RB: Biomarkers in occupational cancer epidemiology: considerations in study design, *Environ Health Persp* 98:149, 1992.
16. Hemstreet GP et al: DNA hyperploidy as a biological marker for biological response to bladder carcinogen exposure, *Int J Cancer* 42:817, 1988.
17. Henderson RF et al: The use of biological markers in toxicology, *Crit Rev Toxicol* 20:65, 1989.
18. Hernberg S: Report of Session 1. In Foa V, Emmertt EA, Maroni M et al, editors: *Occupational and environmental chemical hazards: cellular and biochemical indices for monitoring toxicity,* Chichester, England, 1987, Ellis Horwood.
19. Hornig DF: Conclusion. In Brain JD et al, eds: *Variations in susceptibility to inhaled pollutants,* Baltimore, 1988, Johns Hopkins University Press.
20. Hulka BS, Wilcosky T: Biological markers in epidemiologic research, *Arch Environ Health* 43:83, 1988.
21. Janetos AC: Biological variability. In Brain JD et al, eds: *Variation in susceptibility to inhaled pollutants,* Baltimore, 1988, The Johns Hopkins University Press.
22. Landrigan PJ: Relation of body burden to ambient measures. In Gordis L, editor: *Epidemiology and health risk assessment,* New York, 1988, Oxford University Press.
23. Last JM, ed: *A dictionary of epidemiology,* New York, 1983, Oxford University Press.
24. Lowry LK et al: Chemical monitoring of urine from workers potentially exposed to benzidine-drived azo dyes, *Toxicol Letters* 7:29, 1980.
25. Massey BS: *Measures in science and engineering,* Chichester, England, 1986, Ellis Horwood.
26. Mayr E: *The growth of biological thought,* Cambridge, 1982, Harvard University Press.
27. Mendelsohn ML: An introduction to biological dosimetry. In Gledhill BL, Mauro F, eds: *New horizons in biological dosimetry,* New York, 1991, Wiley-Liss.
28. Mullis K et al: Specific enzymatic amplification of DNA in vitro: the polymerase chain reaction, *CSH Symp Quant Biol* 51:263, 1986.
29. National Research Council: Biological markers in environmental health research, *Environ Health Persp* 74:1, 1987.
30. National Research Council: *Biologic markers in immunotoxicology,* New York, 1992, National Academy Press.
31. National Research Council: *Biologic markers in pulmonary toxicology,* New York, 1989a, National Academy Press.
32. National Research Council: *Biologic markers in reproductive toxicology,* New York, 1989b, National Academy Press.
33. National Research Council: *Environmental epidemiology,* vol 1, *Public health and hazardous wastes,* Washington, DC, 1991, National Academy Press.
34. Office of Technology Assessment: *Medical monitoring and screening in the workplace,* OTA-BA-455, Washington, DC, 1990, US Government Printing Office.
35. Omenn GS: Predictive identification of hypersusceptible individuals, *J Occup Med* 24:369, 1982.
36. Perera FP: The potential usefulness of biological markers in risk assessment, *Environ Health Persp* 76:141, 1987.
37. Rao JY et al: Alterations in phenotypic biochemical markers in bladder epithelium during tumorigenesis, *Proc Nat Acad Sci* 90:8287, 1993.
38. Hagmar L et al: Cancer risk in humans predicted by increased levels of chromosomal aberrations in lymphocytes: Nordic study group on the health risk of chromosome damage, *Cancer Res* 54:2919, 1994.
39. Rothman KJ: *Modern epidemiology,* Boston, 1986, Little, Brown.
40. Rothstein MA: *Medical screening of workers,* Washington, DC, 1984, Bureau of National Affairs.
41. Saiki RK, Arnheim N, Erlich HA: A novel method for detection of polymorphic restriction sites by clearance of oligonucleotide probes: application to sickle cell anemia, *Bio Technology* 3:1008, 1985.
42. Sarkis AS et al: Nuclear over expression of p53 protein in transitional cell bladder carcinoma: a marker for disease progression, *J Natl Cancer Inst* 85:53, 1993.
43. Schulte PA: Methodologic issues in the use of biologic markers in epidemiologic research, *Am J Epidemiol* 126:1006, 1987.
44. Schulte PA: A conceptual framework for the validation and use of biologic markers, *Environ Res* 48:129, 1989.
45. Schulte PA: Contribution of biological markers in risk assessment, *Environ Health Persp* 76:141, 1987.
46. Schulte PA: A conceptual and historical framework for molecular epidemiology. In Schulte PA, Perera FP, eds: *Molecular epidemiology: principles and practices,* San Diego, 1993, Academic Press.
47. Schulte PA: Biomarkers in epidemiology: scientific issues and ethical implications, *Environ Health Persp* 98:143, 1992.
48. Schulte PA: Use of biological markers in occupational health research and practice, *J Toxicol Environ Health* 40:359, 1993.
49. Schulte PA et al: Biological markers in hospital workers exposed to low levels of ethylene oxide, *Mutation Research* 278:237, 1992.
50. Schulte PA, Halperin WE: Genetic screening and monitoring of workers. In Harrington M, ed: *Recent advances in occupational health,* vol 3, Edinburgh, 1987, Churchill Livingstone.
51. Schulte PA, Mazzuckelli LF: Validation of biological markers for quantitative risk assessment, *Environ Health Persp* 90:239, 1991.
52. Schulte PA, Rothman N: Design and conduct of molecular epidemiologic studies. Presentation at the Conference "Molecular and biochemical methods in cancer epidemiology and prevention—path between the laboratory and the population," Naples, Fla, Sept. 23, 1992.
53. Schulte PA, Singal M: Interpretation and communication of results of medical field investigations, *J Occup Med* 31:589, 1989.
54. Shields PG, Harris CC: Molecular epidemiology and the genetics of environmental cancer, *JAMA* 246:681, 1991.
55. Talaska G, Al-Juburi AZSS, Kadlubar FF: Smoking-related carcinogen-DNA adducts in biopsy samples of human urinary bladder: identification of N-(deoxyguanosin-8-yl)-4-aminobiphenyl as a major adduct, *Proc Natl Acad Sci USA* 88:5350, 1991.
56. Talaska G, Dooley KL, Kadlubar FF: Detection and characterization of carcinogen-DNA adducts in exfoliated urothelial cells from 4-aminobiphenyl-treated dogs by 32P-postlabeling and subsequent thin-layer and high-pressure liquid chromatography, *Carcinogenesis* 11:639, 1990.
57. Talaska G et al: Detection of carcinogen-DNA adducts in exfoliated bladder cells of cigarette smokers: association with smoking, hemoglobin adducts, and urinary mutagenicity, *Cancer Epidemiol Biomarkers Prev* 1:61, 1991.
58. Vineis P, Ronco G: Interindividual variation in carcinogen metabolism and bladder cancer risk, *Environ Health Persp* 98:95, 1992.

Chapter 64

HAZARDOUS MATERIALS EMERGENCY MEDICAL RESPONSE

Patricia H. Hiatt
Kent R. Olson

Approaching the scene
    Goals
    Recognition and identification
Scene organization
    Hot zone (exclusion zone)
    Warm zone (decontamination zone)
    Cold zone (support zone)
    The incident command system
Response
    Hazard assessment
    The concept of secondary contamination
    Resources
    Response personnel
    Protective equipment
    Victim management
Summary

Emergencies involving hazardous materials are commonplace today. Views of the scenes of these emergencies, available almost nightly on television news, focus primarily on workers in "moon suits" at the site of a leaking tank or railroad car. Although their activities receive considerably less coverage on the news, health care professionals play a crucial role in the mitigation of these incidents.

Many different individuals and organizations must work together as a team to ensure appropriate and efficient management of a hazardous materials incident. Some of the important roles include not only stopping the chemical release but also protecting the responders at the site and treating any victims of the original release and any responders who become injured in the line of duty. The details of risk management in the emergency response setting are provided in (Chapter 65.)

This chapter serves as an introduction for medical professionals to the hazardous materials response process, and it emphasizes the roles of health care providers, from the emergency medical service (EMS) through the hospital emergency department (ED). As is true for all others involved in the process, health care providers responsible for treating persons exposed to hazardous materials need special training, preparation, and resources.

The U.S. Environmental Protection Agency (EPA), Department of Transportation (DOT), and other state, federal, and local agencies have developed numerous definitions and lists of hazardous materials. In fact, the lists have become so numerous that the State of California publishes a List of Lists so that users can determine which agencies consider which materials hazardous. For the purposes of this chapter, we assume that a hazardous material is one capable of causing harm to people, property, or the environment. People can be harmed because of either the physical hazards (flammability and reactivity) or health hazards (corrosivity or toxicity) of a chemical compound or mixture.

The most succinct definition of a hazardous material comes from the U.S. Occupational Safety and Health Administration (OSHA): "A hazardous chemical means any chemical which is a physical hazard or a health hazard."[7]

OSHA further defines both *physical hazard* and *health hazard*, but for the purposes of this review, it is sufficient to understand that any flammable, reactive, corrosive, or toxic chemical (that is, a substance or material) is likely to be considered a hazardous material.

A hazardous material incident involves release of a hazardous material, with the subsequent potential for that material to affect human health or damage the environment. An incident can occur during transportation, production, storage, or use of a hazardous material. Spills, leaks, fires, and other release mechanisms have the potential to produce damage to people, property, and the environment. The types of hazardous material incidents vary considerably, depending on the nature and quantity of chemical or chemicals released, types of hazards created, nature of the environment affected, and the response efforts required to mitigate the release and its effects. The resolution of a hazardous material incident may be as simple as immediate control of the chemical release or as complicated as long-term rehabilitation of injured people or a damaged environment. Although all hazardous aspects are considered during the mitigation of an incident, protection of human health is a priority (with the primary concern being the health of the responders) and the area of practice of medical professionals. This chapter reviews hazardous materials response activities, with an emergency medicine focus.

APPROACHING THE SCENE
Goals

The DOT is instrumental in regulating the vast quantities of hazardous materials transported throughout the country and preparing for hazardous material incidents. The DOT *Emergency Response Guidebook,*[28] an orange, pocket-sized paperback, is standard issue for police, sheriff, fire, and EMS agencies. DOT recommendations for approaching the scene have become adopted as practice by most agencies that respond to incidents. Their guidelines include the following:

- Approach cautiously. Resist the urge to rush in; you cannot help others until you know what you are facing.
- Identify the hazards. Placards, container labels, shipping papers, and/or knowledgeable persons on the scene are valuable information sources. Evaluate all of them and then consult the recommended guide page before you place yourself or others at risk.
- Secure the scene. Without entering the immediate hazard area, do what you can to isolate the area and ensure the safety of people and the environment. Move and keep people away from the scene and the perimeter. Allow room enough to move, and remove your own equipment.
- Obtain help. Advise your headquarters to notify responsible agencies and call for assistance for trained experts.
- Decide on site entry. Any efforts you make to rescue persons or protect property or the environment must be weighed against the possibility that you could become part of the problem.
- Above all, do not walk into or touch spilled material. Avoid inhalation of fumes, smoke, and vapors, even if no hazardous materials are known to be involved. Do not assume that gases or vapors are harmless because of lack of smell; odorless gases or vapors may be harmful.

Recognition and identification

Although there are several ways to determine that hazardous materials are present at an incident (for example, the presence of 55-gallon drums, vapor clouds, odor, irritation, or injured or dead people or animals), identification of the chemical or chemicals present is key to mitigation. Placards or labels on vehicles, containers, or buildings are the most obvious signs that hazardous materials are involved and can provide clues to the hazards involved and even the identity of the material. In addition to placards and labels, shipping papers and material safety data sheets (MSDSs) are used to identify hazardous materials.

DOT requires placards and labels on vehicles and containers used in transporting hazardous materials. DOT placards and labels contain an identification number and coded information on hazards. The United Nations (UN) or North American (NA) identification number is a four-digit number that corresponds to a specific chemical or class of chemicals. (The number is sometimes preceded by the designation UN or NA, but the numbers in both systems are identical; the UN system is replacing the NA.) Hazard information is presented in three ways: color coding (for example, red placards denote flammable materials), symbols (skull-and-crossbones denotes a poison), and numerical hazard class (class 7 denotes a radioactive material). Placards incorporate numerous mechanisms for identifying the chemical and its hazards: color coding, symbols, hazard classification, and exact numerical identification. Fig. 64-1 presents an example of a DOT placard. In addition to placards, DOT also requires that hazardous materials shipments be accompanied by a manifest called shipping papers. Shipping papers, which are carried in the cab of trucks transporting hazardous materials, provide more specific identification information, including a telephone contact. In fact, recent legislation requires that these papers include a 24-hour telephone contact for an in-

Fig. 64-1. Example of a U.S. Department of Transportation (DOT) hazardous material transportation placard.

Identification of Health Hazard Color Code: BLUE		Identification of Flammability Color Code: RED		Identification of Reactivity (Stability) Color Code: YELLOW	
Signal	Type of Possible Injury	Signal	Susceptibility of Materials to Burning	Signal	Susceptibility to Release of Energy
4	Materials which on very short exposure could cause death or major residual injury even though prompt medical treatment were given.	4	Materials which will rapidly or completely vaporize at atmospheric pressure and normal ambient temperature, or which are readily dispersed in air and which will burn readily.	4	Materials which in themselves are readily capable of detonation or of exposive decomposition or reaction at normal temperatures and pressures.
3	Materials which on short exposure could cause serious temporary or residual injury even though prompt medical treatment were given.	3	Liquids and solids that can be ignited under almost all ambient temperature conditions.	3	Materials which in themselves are capable of detonation or explosive reaction but require a strong initiating source or which must be heated under confinement before initiation or which react explosively with water.
2	Materials which on intense or continued exposure could cause temporary incapacitation or possible residual injury unless prompt medical treatment is given.	2	Materials that must be moderately heated or exposed to relatively high ambient temperatures before ignition can occur.	2	Materials which in themselves are normally unstable and readily undergo violent chemical change but do not detonate. Also materials which may react violently with water or which may form potentially explosive mixtures with water.
1	Materials which on exposure would cause irritation but only minor residual injury even if no treatment is given.	1	Materials that must be preheated before ignition can occur.	1	Materials which in themselves are normally stable, but which can become unstable at elevated temperatures and pressures or which may react with water with some release of energy but not violently.
0	Materials which on exposure under fire conditions would offer no hazard beyond that of ordinary combustible material.	0	Materials that will not burn.	0	Materials which in themselves are normally stable, even under fire exposure conditions, and which are not reactive with water.

NATIONAL FIRE PROTECTION ASSOCIATION
IDENTIFICATION OF THE FIRE HAZARDS OF MATERIALS

NFPA 704
HAZARD SIGNAL SYSTEM

Flammability (Red)

4–Highly flammable and volatile
3–Highly flammable
2–Flammable
1–Low flammability
0–Does not burn

Health Hazard (Blue)

4–Extremely hazardous
3–Moderately hazardous
2–Hazardous
1–Slightly hazardous
0–No health hazard

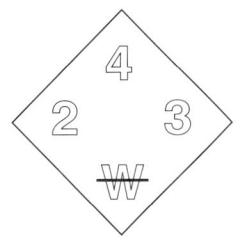

Reactivity (Yellow)

4–Highly explosive, detonates readily
3–Explosive, less readily detonated
2–Violently reactive but does not detonate
1–Not violently reactive
0–Normally stable

Other Hazards

☢ – Radioactive
OX – Oxidizer
W̶ – Water reactive

Fig. 64-2. National Fire Protection Association (NFPA) System 704.

dividual knowledgeable about the material and its hazards. When they are available, shipping papers also provide information useful to incident mitigation.

MSDSs are multipage chemical-specific information documents required by OSHA. Although the format and quality of information in MSDSs are highly variable, the main categories of information that must be included are: material and manufacturer identification, ingredients, physical data (such as boiling point and water solubility), appearance and odor, health hazard data, reactivity data, spill or leak procedures, special protection information, and special precautions. MSDSs must be available on site when hazardous chemicals are used or stored. They are also often carried with hazardous materials shipments.

The National Fire Protection Association (NFPA), a nongovernmental professional association of firefighters and hazardous materials responders has created a system to identify and rank the hazards of materials at fixed facilities. Although the NFPA is not a regulatory agency, NFPA standard 704 has been adopted by many local government agencies. Standard 704 ranks the hazards in three categories: health, flammability, and reactivity. Presented in a diamond divided into four sections (Fig. 64-2), the three categories are color coded (blue for health, red for flammability, and yellow for reactivity) and contain a numerical ranking (0 to 4) to between no hazard (0) to extreme hazard (4). With respect to health, the numeric ranks discern chemicals that "offer no hazard" (0) to those that "on very short exposure could cause death or major residual injury even though prompt medical treatment were given" (4). The bottom of the diamond is available to identify special hazards, such as radioactivity. Symbols similar to those used on DOT placards are used to denote these hazards.

Although these identification systems are primarily used on scene at an incident, medical personnel should not hesitate to use them also. For example, shipping papers may contain information on the manufacturer and/or another knowledgeable contact. In many instances, major chemical producers have medical personnel on staff (and on call) to assist with patient management. Likewise, the MSDS itself contains a section on treatment. Although it may only contain first aid information, it may also contain more specific antidote or treatment information that is not common medical knowledge.

SCENE ORGANIZATION

The scene of a hazardous material incident is organized by establishing areas for incident mitigation, decontamination, and support activities. These three areas—the hot zone, the warm zone, and the cold zone, respectively—also indicate boundaries of exposure risk, from high exposure (or likelihood of exposure) in the hot zone, to significant risk of exposure in the warm zone, to unlikely risk of exposure (assumed safety) in the cold zone. Fig. 64-3 depicts the basic scene organization of a hazardous materials incident.

Hot zone (exclusion zone)

The hot zone is the area immediately surrounding the hazardous material incident and that area in which human health is thought to be at risk of exposure to hazardous chemicals. The hot zone may be cordoned off with barriers or tape, but even then, its boundaries are not set and can be reestablished (larger or smaller) on the basis of incident mitigation. Only persons with specialized hazardous material training can enter the hot zone. Although some of these persons may be trained as paramedics, only limited medical care can be provided in the hot zone while protective clothing and equipment are worn.

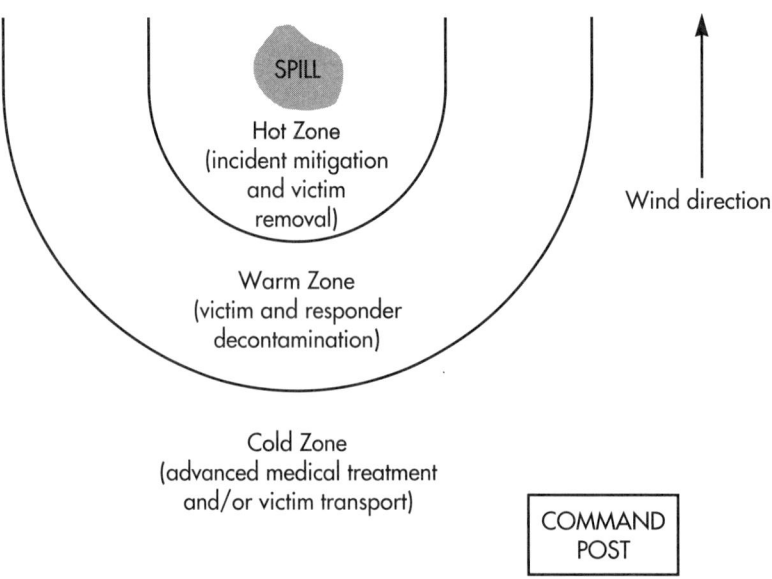

Fig. 64-3. Hazardous materials incident scene organization.

Warm zone (decontamination zone)

The warm zone is established beyond the point at which responders are likely to face direct exposure to the hazardous material involved. Although exposure is still possible, and even likely because of decontamination activities, the warm zone provides a buffer between the hot zone and the cold zone in which activities can be performed without immediate or overwhelming risk to the responder. Although EMS responders may be in the warm zone, there are still significant limits as to the medical care that can be provided, because respirators and gloves interfere with even the most basic care, such as taking a pulse.

Cold zone (support zone)

The cold zone is the area of a hazardous material incident assumed to be and should be maintained free from hazardous material contamination. In the broadest sense, the cold zone is unlimited; there is no outer boundary to the safe area. But because all support activities and equipment are maintained in the cold zone, it is advantageous to cordon off the cold zone to minimize interference from bystanders. Within the cold zone, an operations headquarters or command post should be established. A staging area where ambulances, equipment, and additional personnel are assembled and prepared also is set up. Because the cold zone is set up away from the dangers of chemical exposure, protective clothing is not required. More sophisticated medical management can be performed by rescuers operating in the cold zone, because movement is unencumbered and more medical equipment is available.

The incident command system

The Incident Command System (ICS) is an organization scheme used to ensure efficient, effective management of hazardous material incident mitigation operations. The ICS is similar to the command-post method used by fire departments to organize firefighting operations, and as noted in Fig. 64-3, a Command Post is established in the cold zone. The Command Post functions as an operations headquarters. Under the ICS, one individual, the incident commander (IC), is in charge of the scene and makes all decisions and authorizes all actions related to response. The IC designates responsibility for certain specific details to subordinates, who in turn establish teams of their own to assist in a specific capacity. For example, a health officer is in charge of assembling medical personnel and reporting back to the IC. Regardless of the size of an incident, use of the ICS assures that all responders use common terminology, know his or her responsibilities on the basis of title in the structure, and need to report to only one supervisor. The ICS is actually a theory of united response. Regardless of the number of units and original departments involved, in the ICS structure, the most senior individual is the IC and all directions and responsibilities flow up to that one person, regardless of day-to-day or organizational-chart reporting schemes.

Although titles and activities of each ICS change, the underlying key elements include the use of common terminology; modular organization, with each person reporting to only one supervisor and each supervisor responsible for a manageable number of persons (optimum: five); and integrated communications.

Although ICS should be used in hazardous material incident responses of all sizes, the system is especially useful in large-incident response for organizing personnel from several different agencies or departments into one team.

RESPONSE
Hazard assessment

The health hazard posed by a chemical is a function of exposure (the amount of that chemical that a person may come into contact with) and its toxicity (the inherent ability of the chemical to do harm). The toxicity of a chemical can vary, depending on the route of exposure (see Chapter 53).

$$\text{Hazard} \approx \text{toxicity} \times \text{exposure}$$

In contrast to traditional medical terminology, evaluation of hazardous materials incidents focuses on exposure as a function of the amount of chemical in a person's immediate environment, rather than on dose, the amount of chemical entering the body. Thus hazard potential is related to the concentration of the chemical at the site of an incident or other affected areas (typically expressed in units of milligrams per cubic meter of air or milligrams per liter of water rather than human doses (such as milligrams per kilogram of body weight or milligrams per deciliter). The level of exposure is estimated from the concentration of the chemical and the length of exposure.

Once the chemical is identified with use of the labeling systems previously described (such as the DOT placard or shipping papers), a number of references can be consulted to identify potential hazards associated with exposure to the agent (see Appendix C). The potential for human health effects can be evaluated by comparison of the concentration of the hazardous material, usually determined by on-scene monitoring or by modeling of the release and movement of the chemical through the environment, with information from various exposure guidelines.

The most common exposure guidelines include threshold limit values (TLVs), the permissible exposure limits (PELs), immediately-dangerous-to-life-or-health (IDLH) values, and emergency response planning guidelines (ERPGs).

TLVs are worker-protection guidelines expressed as air concentrations of hazardous chemicals. TLVs are established by the American Conference of Governmental Industrial Hygienists (ACGIH). Although the ACGIH is not a government agency and TLVs are not legally enforceable standards, TLVs have been adopted as worker-protection standards by several government agencies, including some individual states. ACGIH has established three categories of exposure guidelines: the TLV time-weighted average (TLV-

> **ACGIH occupational exposure guidelines**
>
> Threshold limit value (TLV): the time-weighted average concentration for a normal 8-hour workday and a 40-hour workweek, to which nearly all workers may be repeatedly exposed, day after day, without adverse effect.
>
> Short-term exposure limit (STEL): the concentration to which workers can be exposed for a short period of time without suffering from irritation, chronic or irreversible tissue damage, or narcosis of sufficient degree to increase the likelihood of accidental injury, impair self-rescue, or materially reduce work efficiency, and provided that the daily TLV is not exceeded. A STEL is defined as a 15-minute time-weighted average exposure that should not be exceeded at any time during a workday. Exposures at the STEL should not be longer than 15 minutes and should not be repeated more than four times per day. There should be at least 60 minutes between successive exposures at the STEL.
>
> Ceiling: the concentration that should not be exceeded during any part of the working exposure.

> **AIHA emergency response exposure guidelines**
>
> ERPG-1 is the maximal airborne concentration below which it is believed that nearly all persons could be exposed for as long as 1 hour without experiencing symptoms other than mild transient adverse health effects or perceiving a clearly defined objectionable odor.
>
> ERPG-2 is the maximal airborne concentration below with it is believed that nearly all persons could be exposed for as long as 1 hour without experiencing or developing irreversible or other serious health effects or symptoms that could impair their abilities to take protective action.
>
> ERPG-3 is the maximal airborne concentration below with it is believed that nearly all individuals could be exposed for as long as 1 hour without experiencing or developing life-threatening health effects.

TWA, commonly called TLV), the short-term exposure limit (STEL), and the ceiling (see box above). It is important to observe that if any one of these three TLVs is exceeded, a potential hazard from that substance is presumed to exist.

PELs are occupational exposure standards set and enforced by OSHA. The PEL is very similar to the TLV in that it is set for 8-hour-per-day, 40-hour-per-week exposures, but although TLVs are recommended by the ACGIH, PELs are air concentrations that by law must not be exceeded.

Although there are criticisms of both ACGIH's TLVs and OSHA's PELs,[8,26,35] the ACGIH TLVs appear to be updated more frequently than are the OSHA PELs and therefore may be preferable guidelines with respect to prediction of adverse health outcomes.

IDLHs are air concentrations of hazardous chemicals that are thought to pose an immediate danger to life or health. IDHLs are established by the National Institute of Occupational Safety and Health Administration (NIOSH). The IDLH concentrations ''represent the maximum concentration from which, in the even of respiratory failure, one could escape within 30 minutes without a respirator and without experiencing any escape-impairing (such as, severe eye irritation) or irreversible health effects.'' NIOSH is an independent research organization that provides guidance to OSHA but is without regulatory authority.

ERPGs are the only exposure guidelines developed expressly for use in cases of hazardous materials incidents. ERPGs are established by the American Industrial Hygiene Association (AIHA). Although AIHA has established ERPGs for fewer than 50 chemicals (when compared with approximately 300 each for TLVs and PELs), they are the most appropriate exposure standard to use in the management of exposures due to a hazardous materials incident. AIHA has established three different levels of standards, differentiated by the health effects expected by exposure at three different concentrations of the chemical (see box above). Exposure at ERPG-1 is expected to produce minimal (if any) effects, and exposure at ERPG-3 could produce more significant adverse health effects, approaching those that would be life threatening.

Although the existence of exposure guidelines makes it convenient to say that exposures below such levels are safe, this assumption cannot be made. Each type of exposure guideline—and in fact, the guidelines for each individual chemical—are based on unique toxicologic effects and specific conditions. For example, TLVs and PELs are established for healthy working adults and may not provide adequate protection for children, the elderly, or individuals with preexisting health problems, especially from prolonged exposure to a hazardous material. Within each system, exposure guidelines can be based on eye irritation, systemic effects, or simply good housekeeping practices.

An additional confounding factor in the use of occupational exposure standards for evaluation of hazardous material incident exposures is that hazardous material incidents usually involve short-term, one-time exposures. Health effects associated with long-term exposure (such as cancer and neuropathy) are probably not relevant to hazardous material victims but may be the basis for the occupational exposure limit.

The concept of secondary contamination

Primary contamination refers to direct contact of the victim with the hazardous material. Secondary contamination refers to the transfer of material from the victim to personnel or equipment. The potential for secondary contamination has implications for decontamination and triage of victims and for the protection of rescue and health care personnel. When

> **Chemicals with serious potential for secondary contamination**
>
> Highly toxic liquids and solids or finely divided solids (for example, organophosphate pesticides concentrated acids and alkalis, cyanide salts, hydrofluoric acid, phenol, and aniline)
> Radioactive liquids and dusts
> Certain biologic agents (for example, harmful viruses and bacteria)

> **Chemicals with no or little potential for secondary contamination**
>
> Gases (for example, carbon monoxide and arsine)
> Vapors (unless they condense to a liquid state on clothing or skin)
> Substances without serious toxicity or skin absorption (for example, propylene glycol and motor oil)

> **Hazardous material resources for the health care provider**
>
> *Books*
>   *ATSDR Medical Management Guidelines* (Agency for Toxic Substances and Disease Registry, Atlanta, Ga)
>   *DOT Emergency Response Guidebook* (U.S. Department of Transportation)
>   *NIOSH Pocket Guide* (National Institute of Occupational Safety and Health)
>   Olson KR, editor: *Poisoning and Drug Overdose* (Appleton & Lange, Norwalk, Conn)
>
> *Computer data bases*
>   NLM: Toxline, HSDB (National Library of Medicine)
>   Poisindex (Micromedex, Denver, Colo)
>
> *Telephone hotlines*
>   Poison Control Centers (American Association of Poison Control Centers, Washington, DC) (See Appendix III)
>   CHEMTREC (Chemical Manufacturers Association, Washington, DC): (800) 424-9300
>   Agency for Toxic Substances and Disease Registry, Atlanta, Ga: (404) 639-0615

chemicals that pose a risk of secondary contamination are involved in an incident, special attention must be paid to determining the extent of victim contamination and therefore the need for decontamination. When the incident involves a chemical with little risk of secondary contamination, victims may need only minimal or no decontamination. In these cases, attention should be paid to ensuring prompt medical attention to those in need in lieu of performing unnecessary or excessively lengthy decontamination. Immediate victim decontamination is recommended for materials that pose risks of secondary contamination, eliminating both the potential for rescuer contamination and further exposure to the victim.

A substance poses a risk of secondary contamination if it is both toxic and likely to be carried on the clothing, skin, or hair of victims in sufficient quantities to threaten other personnel. Every effort must be made to decontaminate contaminated victims before they are transported to a medical care facility.

Substances that present the most serious risks of secondary contamination are presented in the box. In the next box are examples of substances with little or no risk of secondary contamination. Note that although several of the substances listed are highly toxic (for example, arsine and carbon monoxide), they do not pose risks of secondary contamination because these chemicals do not contaminate the victim; therefore, they cannot secondarily contaminate rescuers.

Not all hazardous material victims pose a risk of secondary contamination. Regardless of a material's potential for secondary contamination, only victims who are actually contaminated pose a risk. Exposed victims who do not carry solid, liquid, or condensed vapors on their clothing, skin, or hair do not pose a risk.

Secondary contamination also poses a risk in cases of ingestion. Ingested materials can react with stomach acid to produce noxious gases, which can endanger both the victim and rescuers. Vomitus may off-gas the hazardous material or a reaction product. Toxic vomitus should be quickly isolated in closed containers.

Previously published documents on hazardous materials have recommended zipping patients into body bags to minimize the transfer of chemical from patient to rescuer. This technique is not completely effective for prevention of rescuer exposure, and it may pose a significant risk of increased dermal absorption to victims. Body bags are not recommended as an alternative to thorough decontamination.

Resources

The box above lists references of particular interest for hazardous material incident response. These resources should be reviewed and used prior to actual use in an emergency to ensure that they contain the information desired; some are designed for emergency use and others are more applicable for chronic exposure consultations.

Role of poison control centers. Poison control centers (PCCs) play a unique role in hazardous materials incident response. They are able to assist a wide range of the professionals involved in the incident and are commonly contacted by hazardous materials technicians, ambulance personnel, exposed victims, and the media.

The regional PCC (see Appendix III) can provide information about the health effects of the chemicals and specific treatment advice, including recommendations for decontamination, use of antidotes, and multicasualty triage (see box).

Forty-two U. S. PCCs are certified by the American Association of Poison Control Centers. Certified centers meet strict operating criteria, including experienced and specially trained staff, 24-hour operation, and access to qualified medical toxicologists. Each PCC staff member handles an average of 5000 calls per year, involving a variety of toxic drugs and poisons. Specialists in poison information are experienced in assessing immediate health risk and knowledgeable about the indications and doses of antidotes. In 1990, PCCs handled more than 25,000 human environmental exposures, including hazardous materials incident calls.[20] PCCs have access to numerous books, journals, and computerized information retrieval resources such as Poisindex. The PCC may be able to assist in confirming the identity of a chemical substance and in most circumstances can contact the manufacturer for more information on ingredients. Once the identity of the substance is known, the PCC can locate information about its acute health effects and appropriate treatment. The PCC can also make an estimation of its potential for secondary contamination and provide guidelines for decontamination. In addition, on the basis of the chemical's physical state, its acute toxic effects, and the potential for secondary contamination, the PCC may be able to advise on-scene personnel about the necessity for protective gear.[5]

After any large incident, the PCC is likely to be contacted by citizens, local hospitals, news media, and public health officials.[27] The PCC is often viewed by these entities as an impartial and trusted information resource.[14] Moreover, the traditional role of PCCs in providing advice for immediate treatment of acute poisoning exposures has recently been challenged by the recognition that the public as well as physicians increasingly look to the PCC as a source of information about long-term, low-level exposures to such materials as asbestos, radon, and other environmental hazards. In a 1988 report the Institute of Medicine (IOM) identified a critical need for a credible and accessible source of information in occupational and environmental medicine.

PCCs can attest to this need because they have found that after years of assisting in emergency response activities, they are increasingly consulted about long-term chemical exposure. The San Francisco Bay Area Regional Poison Control Center, through its state-funded Toxic Information Center (TIC), responded to 6000 calls about such topics in 1990. Tables 64-1, 64-2, and 64-3 present information on the nature of TIC consultations, topics of concern, and the background of TIC callers. Until it was closed in 1991 because of state budget cutbacks, the TIC saw a continual increase in demand for its service from its inception in 1984. In a 1990 follow-up to its 1988 report, the IOM described the TIC model as one of two possible mechanisms for providing physicians with this needed information. Debate at the national level has begun to focus on how the federal government can assist physicians and the public in using PCCs or specialized toxic-information centers to obtain information about environmental hazards.

Table 64-1. Nature of concern, TIC consultations, 1990

Concern	Percentage of consultations
Health effects (toxicology)	31
Hazardous waste	17
Hazardous material regulations	14
Occupational health	14
Hazardous material spill	8
Soil, water, or air pollution	4

Table 64-2. Subject of TIC consultations, 1990

Subject	Percentage of consultations
Pesticides	36
Solvents	15
Gases	10
Corrosives	8
Asbestos	7

Table 64-3. Background of caller, TIC consultations, 1990

Background	Percentage of consultations
General public	46
Government employee	16
Employee or employer	11
Fire department	5
Physician	4
Media	2

Advice available from regional poison control centers

Assistance with identification
Contacts with manufacturer
Health effects
Potential for secondary contamination
Decontamination advice
Necessity for protective gear

Response personnel

Police, firefighters, and hazardous materials technicians. As first responders, response personnel from law enforcement, the fire department, and hazardous material teams all have the same initial priorities when they arrive on the scene of a hazardous materials incident.

First Responder Responsibilities
  Approach cautiously
  Identify the hazards
  Secure the scene
  Obtain help
  Decide on site entry

Hazardous materials response training for the these responders is mandated by OSHA. Regulations outlined in 29 CFR 1910.120 designate numerous levels of training based on expected responsibilities on scene. In addition, NFPA, a nongovernmental association of fire service and hazardous materials professionals, has developed Standards of Professional Competence for hazardous materials responders.[22] These competencies exceed the regulatory requirements and provide detail for the regulations in 29 CFR. The titles and levels of training, which range from first responder, awareness level to IC, include

---
First responder
  Awareness
  Operational
  Technician
  Specialist
  Instant commander

The first-responder level of training is further divided into two programs: the awareness level and the operations (or operational) level. The awareness level is the most basic level of training, which simply introduces the student to terminology and overall hazardous material scene organization. The responder at the awareness level must demonstrate competency in understanding what hazardous substances are and the risk associated with them in an incident, understanding the potential outcomes associated with an emergency when hazardous substances are present, recognizing the presence of hazardous substances at an emergency, identifying the hazardous substance present, and realizing the need for additional resources and making additional communications to obtain such assistance.

The next step, the operations level, is for responders who will be used to provide assistance to the responders. At the operations level, students are taught how to select and use personal protective equipment; basic decontamination techniques; how to control, contain, or confine the hazardous material; standard operating procedures; and hazardous materials terminology. At the operations level, responders act to implement directions provided by others but are not directly responsible for mitigation. Operations-level responders are taught defensive measures to rectify effects of an incident without trying to stop the release.

At the technician level, hazardous material responders are capable of taking direct action to mitigate a hazardous material incident. The hazardous material technician has competency in implementing an emergency response plan; identifying the hazardous material, using field instruments and equipment; functioning independently in an ICS system; selecting and using personal protective equipment; understanding hazard and risk assessment techniques; performing complex control, containment, or confinement operations; understanding and implementing decontamination procedures; understanding basic chemical and toxicologic terminology; and understanding termination procedures.

At the specialist level, hazardous materials responders are trained to perform the same actions as the technician but in addition have specialized chemical knowledge and can act to supervise on-scene activities and interact with other responders.

Hazardous materials response technicians are commonly firefighters with more than 200 hours of special education and training. Although these "first responders" are not always first on the scene, firefighters, police and sheriff's officers, and other public safety personnel are trained to await the arrival of the hazardous material response technicians before attempting any type of mitigation. Technicians are organized into teams of at least four members who perform normal firefighting duties but are on call for hazardous material incidents.

EMS personnel. Emergency medical technicians (EMTs) who respond to hazardous materials incidents must also have special training. Their specific training is based on the role that EMTs are expected to play at an incident and depends highly on local practice. Some EMTs are trained to assist with incident mitigation and victim decontamination, and others are reserved for medical treatment only. This training is commonly obtained through classes with other responders (fire and police) according to the OSHA regulations discussed earlier. Although the aforementioned goals for approaching the scene apply to all responders, specific responsibilities for EMTs are focused on victim management (see box).

EMT hazardous materials incident responder responsibilities

Protect oneself
Obtain toxicity and medical treatment information
Determine the potential for secondary contamination
Perform or ensure decontamination (depending on level of training)
Provide basic and advanced life support
Transport victims to the hospital

> **Emergency department personnel responsibilities**
>
> Determine the potential for secondary contamination
> Ensure that victims have received decontamination (if appropriate)
> Obtain toxicity information
> Provide supportive and antidotal emergency care
> Perform laboratory testing
> Determine the need for observation, admission, and follow-up care

The EMT at a hazardous material incident will likely function only in the cold (support) or warm (decontamination) zones. Basic medical care may be rendered in the hot zone by hazardous material technicians with limited EMT training. OSHA does not require separate hazardous materials training for EMTs, but the NFPA has established competencies for EMTs who respond to hazardous material incidents.[23] The two levels of competence (level I and level II) for EMS hazardous material responders can be achieved by EMTs with either basic life support or advanced life support training. The EMS/HM level I responder operates in the cold zone. In addition to EMS training, the EMS/HM level I responder will have special training in toxicology, chemical and physical properties, response planning, pesticide labels, and responder medical monitoring. At the EMS/HM level II responder level, responders are able to provide patient care in the warm zone. The level II responder has the training and knowledge of a level I responder, plus knowledge of risk assessment, decontamination, personal protective equipment, ICS, technical information, research, and medical monitoring. Because only limited medical care can be administered while chemical protective clothing and respiratory equipment are worn, most EMTs operate in the support zone, where no special protective clothing is necessary. Even these EMTs would benefit from minimal hazardous materials training.

ED staff. ED personnel (physicians, nurses, and technicians) involved in providing medical treatment to victims of hazardous materials incidents also need to have specific goals to guide their activities. These goals or responsibilities are listed in the box above. Although no federal regulations require hazardous material training for ED staff, it is prudent to consider training if staff are expected to respond to a hazardous materials incident. Federal regulations for firefighters and EMS personnel state that "training shall be based on the duties and function to be performed by each responder of an emergency response organization,"[7] and ED staff likewise would be well served to learn how to plan for a response and how to treat hazardous material victims.

Protective equipment

Once hazardous materials have been identified as being involved in an emergency, all rescue operations must await the arrival of properly trained and equipped responders. Until field testing indicates otherwise, all environments involving hazardous materials must be assumed to pose a risk to the health of responders. To provide assistance or to mitigate damage without becoming part of the problem, responders must use protective equipment—respirators and chemical-protective clothing—to guard against exposure and adverse effects.

Respiratory protection. Air-supplied respirators may be air-line or self-contained. Although commonly used during hazardous waste site clean-up, the air-line respirator is not used at the site of a hazardous material emergency. The air-line respirator consists of a mask or facepiece that seals around the face and supplies air through an air hose connected to an air compressor at a distant site. Because the air hose may be degraded by chemicals or heat and the hose may become tangled, the air-line respirator is not practical for emergency operations during a hazardous material incident.

The self-contained air-supplying respirator, or self-contained breathing apparatus (SCBA), is commonly used by firefighters when performing firefighting functions. It also provides protection against the inhalation of hazardous chemicals at a hazardous material incident. An SCBA consists of a facepiece that seals, a tank of compressed air carried on a backpack, and an air-supply hose that runs from the supply tank to the facepiece (Fig. 64-4, B). Because the system is self-contained, portable, and frequently used by firefighters, SCBA is most often used in hazardous material incident responses. The specific type of SCBA recommended today is pressure demand. Although air is always flowing into the facepiece, providing (positive) pressure, the flow increases in response to inhalation (demand). This type of SCBA not only provides fresh air but also protects against the infiltration of hazardous chemicals into the breathing space around the facepiece.

Air-purifying respirators do not provide an independent air supply to the user; they simply filter the ambient air. They can be very simple, such as a dust mask that filters out large sawdust particles from air that a carpenter breathes, or very complicated, such as a full-facepiece respirator with numerous cartridges to filter hydrocarbon vapors, asbestos fibers, and acid mists from the air that a hazardous waste worker breathes (Fig. 64-4, C). The conditions for safe use of an air-purifying respirator are often difficult to guarantee at the scene of a hazardous material incident. Safe use of an air-purifying respirator requires an adequate concentration of oxygen (19%), identification of the chemical contaminant and its concentration in the air, contaminant concentration below the NIOSH IDLH, and low relative humidity.

Protective clothing. Protective clothing is constructed in two basic forms: encapsulating and nonencapsulating. An encapsulating suit is one in which gloves, feet, and a face shield are built so that the entire suit is airtight. Encapsulating suits are impermeable to hazardous chemicals in the

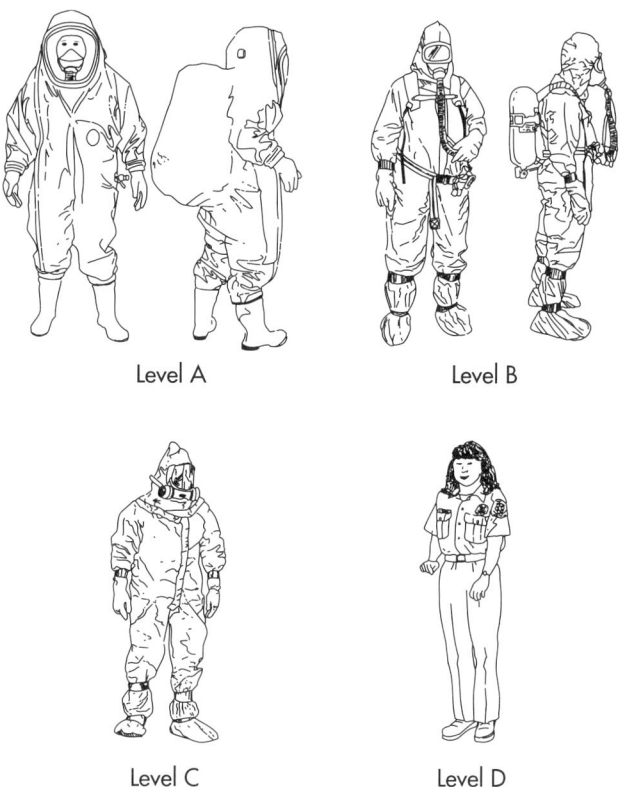

Fig. 64-4. Examples of U.S. Environmental Protection Agency (EPA) levels of protective clothing.

solid, liquid, and gaseous phases. Because the entire body is covered by an encapsulating suit, an air supply must be contained inside. As the user exhales supplied air, the suit will balloon. Although encapsulating suits have one-way, pressure-activated exhaust valves, these valves are not operational until the suit has a pronounced amount of inflation.

The EPA has established a classification system to address the amount of protection afforded by specific combinations of protective clothing and respirators. The EPA defines four levels of protection, from A, affording the most protection, to D, providing the least. Fig. 63-4 presents examples of the protective clothing for each EPA level of protection. Level A consists of a positive-pressure demand SCBA and a fully encapsulating chemical-resistant suit. Level B consists of SCBA and a nonencapsulating chemical-resistant suit. Level C consists of an air-purifying respirator and nonencapsulating chemical-resistant suit. Level D consists of work clothes such as steel-toed boots or aprons that do not provide any specific respiratory or skin protection against hazardous chemicals.

NFPA has established performance standards for protective clothing. These standards complement the EPA levels A through C equipment designations by specifying performance criteria for the suits used in emergency response operations. NFPA 1991 establishes standards for vapor-protective suits, the equivalent of an EPA level A suit. NFPA 1992 establishes standards for liquid splash-protective suits, the equivalent of EPA level B protection. Both standards require documentation of performance in several areas, including chemical-permeation resistance, pressurization, water penetration, tear strength, abrasion resistance, flammability resistance, cold temperature performance, and flexural fatigue.

Structural firefighters' protective clothing (turnouts or bunker gear) is heat- and flame-resistant clothing that firefighters wear for firefighting. This clothing does not afford protection from chemical exposure; however, if the chemical is not corrosive to or absorbed by the skin but creates only an inhalation hazard (for example, carbon monoxide and arsine), the turnout/SCBA ensemble can provide minimal protection when urgent victim rescue is needed.

Limitations. Although chemical-protective clothing provides clear advantages to hazardous materials responders, use of such equipment also places a significant physical burden on the wearer. In addition to the training required for hazardous material responders to use personal protective equipment such as respirators and chemical-resistant suits, physical examinations are critical. Similar to a pre-placement physical examination, a pre–hazardous material response physical examination ensures that no preexisting disease or condition would inhibit response activities or place the responder at risk for medical complications. Prior to use of respiratory protection, pulmonary function tests must confirm pulmonary status. Likewise, a physical examination including an electrocardiogram and a treadmill test should be considered to ensure that the tremendous physical burden of the equipment is acceptable. A complete blood count, chemistry panel (liver and kidney function), urinalysis, chest radiograph, and specific laboratory tests based on chemicals likely to be encountered should also be performed prior to response activities. Responders should undergo this testing both before response activity and periodically during the response career.

Additional monitoring may be performed during a response and after any suspected chemical exposure. Many response teams have developed exposure logs to record all hazardous material response activities regardless of medical evaluation. These logs can provide insight into determining cause of disease or preventing adverse effects in years to come (see Chapter 53).

Heat stress. Heat stress is a serious risk for any personnel using bulky or encapsulating clothing.[3,13,32,33] Normally during warm weather or with strenuous exercise, sweating is followed by evaporation, which is a highly efficient cooling mechanism to maintain the body core temperature. Because chemical protective clothing does not allow outward movement of moisture, it blocks evaporative cooling. Although the user may sweat heavily (which contributes to dehydration), there is no reduction in core temperature. On a hot day and during heavy physical exertion, personnel in protective gear may become overheated within 15 to 30 minutes. Consequences of heat stress include confusion, dizziness, syncope, and heat stroke. Heat stroke is a life-threatening syndrome characterized by extreme hyperthermia (temperature above 40°C), which may result in multiple-organ-system failure, including brain damage, cardiac arrest, renal failure, and coagulopathy.[25]

Treatment of heat stress includes rest, fluid replacement, and applied evaporative cooling by spraying the victim with water and fanning him or her. Severe heat stress may be prevented by a strict protocol for personnel using protective gear that includes frequent breaks with removal of the gear, mandatory drinking, use of replacement teams, and physical monitoring (mental status, vital signs). Heat stroke is a medical emergency and requires rapid cooling and hospital evaluation.

Victim management

At the scene. EMS personnel arriving at the scene of a hazardous materials incident have several important goals for victim management. To manage victims efficiently and protect rescuers, it is crucial to determine the chemical or chemicals involved and the potential risk of secondary contamination.[30] Victims exposed to only gas or vapors are not likely to carry significant amounts of chemical outside of the hot zone and do not pose a serious threat of contaminating others; however, victims whose skin or clothing is soaked with solid or liquid material (including condensed vapor) may contaminate response personnel by direct contact or off-gassing vapors. The risk for secondary contamination determines the need for and extent of decontamination procedures. In some cases, advanced medical care and hospital transport may have to be delayed until the victim can be decontaminated.

Rescuers may not enter the hot zone until it has been determined that there is no toxic hazard or they are adequately protected.[5] In most circumstances, prehospital medical providers do not have the necessary training to enter the hot zone in chemical-protective clothing or with use of respirators. Therefore, they must await specially trained and outfitted hazardous materials personnel. Although some hazardous material personnel may be trained as paramedics, most are at the EMT-1 (basic life support) level.

Because of the constraints of bulky protective gear, only very limited medical care can be provided in the hot zone. If the victim is unconscious, rescuers should quickly ensure a patent airway, taking care to stabilize the cervical spine if trauma is suspected. Gross contamination may be removed by brushing it off or cutting away contaminated clothing. Bleeding may be reduced by direct pressure. The victim may then be carried or dragged out of the hot zone. If awake, the victim may be able to assist with removal of his or her own contaminated clothing and, if ambulatory, can be led to the decontamination area.

Victims with exposure to only gas or vapors and without evidence of skin or eye contamination or irritation do not need decontamination and may be transferred immediately to the support zone (see later). All others should undergo basic decontamination.

The decontamination area may be set up in any convenient location that is safely out of the hot zone. If possible, the decontamination area should be established outdoors, where natural ventilation enhances the dispersion of any off-gassing vapors. Personnel in the decontamination zone are also required to wear protective gear. Generally it is recommended that the level of gear be no more than one level below that worn in the hot zone (which usually means EPA level B); however, if the risk of inhaling off-gassing vapors is low (the chemical is not highly volatile or the decontamination area is set up outside, with good natural ventilation), it may be acceptable to use a lower level of protection (such as an air-purifying respirator).

Advanced medical care is still difficult in this area, although it may be possible, depending on the circumstances, to insert an artificial airway, administer supplemental oxygen or nebulized bronchodilators, and assist ventilation. Direct pressure can be applied to control heavy bleeding. Rescuers wearing respirators and heavy gloves will find it very difficult to insert an intravenous line or perform endotracheal intubation. Expensive electronic equipment such as cardiac monitors should generally not be brought into this area, because it may be difficult to decontaminate later.

Even victims with serious trauma or medical complications (such as seizures) may have to wait for advanced medical care until decontamination is completed, depending on the concentration of the chemical and its potential for secondary contamination.

Decontamination is the removal of hazardous materials from personnel to the extent necessary to prevent potential adverse health effects.[28] Patients who are able and cooperative may remove their own clothing and assist with basic decontamination. Contaminated clothing should be removed and double bagged. Jewelry and valuables should be placed in a separate bag for easy retrieval later.

Exposed areas should be flushed with plain water for 3 to 5 minutes. The length of time for flushing may vary with the chemical and the circumstances of exposure. Concentrated or strongly alkaline materials may require 10 to 15 minutes or longer, whereas vapor exposure with only mild skin or eye irritation may be treated with a shorter flush. For removal of oily or otherwise adherent chemicals from the skin or hair, mild soap or shampoo is used.[19] Any liquid hand or dishwashing soap is satisfactory; there is no evidence that tincture of green soap or abrasive soaps are better. Only soft-bristled brushes should be used; abrasive brushes or decontamination devices may enhance skin penetration and injury. Bleach or vinegar should not be used on the hair, eyes, or skin; these so-called decontamination solutions are meant for equipment, not patients. In only a few circumstances, specialized solutions may be used to neutralize or remove a chemical from the skin (such as calcium or magnesium solutions for hydrofluoric acid, polyethylene glycol or isopropyl alcohol for phenol).

Emergency response personnel should not be misled by cautions regarding water-reactive materials. Many chemicals can react violently with water, creating an explosion or toxic gases; however, this caution applies mainly to addition of water to a large spill (that is, in fighting a fire). It does not apply to the victim in the decontamination zone whose contaminated clothing has been removed and who has very little of the material left on or around his or her body; such a person needs the water flush to dilute and remove residual material. There is no significant risk of creating a reaction hazard by adding water to this small residual chemical. It should be kept in mind that there is a small amount of water (moisture) on the skin naturally, which is already reacting with the residual chemical.

Exposed or irritated eyes should be flushed with plain water or saline for at least 5 minutes. An attempt should be made to remove contact lenses if present. Any residual chemical material in the conjunctival sacs should be sought and removed. If corrosive exposure is suspected or there is persistent pain, the eye irrigation should be continued while the patient is transported to the hospital.

In cases of ingestions, vomiting should not be induced. Vomiting is relatively ineffective in emptying the stomach, and it can be dangerous (for example, if the material is a corrosive).[24] If the victim is awake and can swallow, activated charcoal (50 to 60 g in a water slurry) should be administered. Activated charcoal absorbs many poisons and is relatively easy to administer. If the ingested substance is a corrosive, charcoal may obscure the view if endoscopy is performed later at the hospital to determine the extent of injury.

When decontamination is complete, or if decontamination is not required, the victim should be transferred to the support zone. Because the support zone is established well away from the danger of direct chemical exposure, primary contamination is unlikely. Victims who have already undergone decontamination and those with exposure to only gas or vapors pose no serious risk of secondary contamination. Therefore, personnel in the support zone do not need specialized protective clothing. There are occasional exceptions, such as heavy victim exposure to a potent organophosphate pesticide or other oily or adherent material. In such cases, even if basic decontamination has already been performed, it may be prudent for the support-zone team to wear disposable aprons or gowns and gloves.[5]

It is in the support zone that advanced medical treatment can be provided, including endotracheal intubation, intravenous access, cardiac monitoring, and administration of specific drugs if appropriate. Aerosolized bronchodilators such as metaproterenol (Alupent) or albuterol (Proventil) can be administered by metered-dose inhaler or preferably by hand-held nebulizer. These medications may provoke cardiac arrhythmias in victims intoxicated by halogenated, aromatic, and other hydrocarbon solvents.[1,2]

The comatose patient should be evaluated for possible opioid overdose or hypoglycemia, and naloxone (Narcan) and dextrose should be administered according to usual protocols. The possibility that coma or seizures may be a result of a head injury rather than chemical poisoning should be considered. Specific antidotes should be administered (Table 64-4) if indicated and within the prehospital scope of practice.

Emergency response personnel should determine whether continued decontamination is needed, possibly because of corrosive exposure to the eyes or skin or heavy contamination with an oily or adherent material.

Victim transport. The base station and the receiving hospital should be informed of the number and condition of the patients, the chemicals involved, and the extent of prior decontamination. Generally, no special preparation of the ambulance is needed if decontamination has already been performed[5]; however, if the victim ingested a chemical, the ambulance should be equipped for possible vomiting of toxic material. Toxic vomitus can directly contaminate personnel and equipment. In addition, it can off-gas volatile vapors, a dangerous situation in the small, poorly ventilated patient-care area of the ambulance. A number of chemicals can be converted to poisonous gases by the action of stomach acids, for example, cyanide salts create hydrogen cyanide gas,[34] and sodium azide can produce hydrozoic acid gas.[10] The floor of the ambulance should be covered with plastic or other protective material, and several absorbent

Table 64-4. Some examples of antidotes for hazardous materials intoxications

Chemical	Antidote
Carbon monoxide	Oxygen
Cyanide	Sodium thiosulfate, sodium and amyl nitrite
Hydrogen fluoride	Calcium
Methemoglobin inducing agents	Methylene blue
Organophosphate or carbamate pesticides	Atropine, pralidoxime

---

Suggested equipment for an outdoor decontamination area

Gurney with plastic tub or run-off collector
Hose attached to a lukewarm water source, with a shower or spray nozzle
Mild soap or shampoo
Soft-bristled brushes
Disposable chemical-resistant jumpsuits (for example, of Tyvek or Saranex)
Chemical-resistant gloves (for example, of butyl rubber) in various sizes
Splash-protective face shields or eye protectors
Plastic garbage bags to store removed clothing and valuables
Disposable towels
Oxygen tanks and delivery supplies

---

towels and opened plastic bags should be readied to soak up and isolate vomitus quickly.

Exposures to hazardous materials may involve several or perhaps even hundreds of possible victims. The goal of triage is to identify those victims with the most serious injuries who can benefit most from rapid treatment and transport. Whenever possible, on-scene personnel should consult with the base-station physician regarding triage criteria. The regional PCC (see Appendix B) may be able to provide triage guidelines based on the chemical's routes of exposure, potential for secondary contamination, acute health effects, warning properties, and potential for delayed onset of toxicity. In general, asymptomatic patients who have had no direct chemical exposure or only brief exposure to gases or vapors can be observed without immediate treatment.

ED. Hospital preparation for the hazardous material victim should include protocols for obtaining information from on-scene personnel and the regional PCC, facilities for decontaminating the unexpected contaminated victim, and management of specific chemical exposures, including stocking of appropriate antidotes.

Although basic decontamination should be carried out prior to victim transport, there are circumstances in which it may not have been done. For example, a contaminated victim might be brought directly to the ED by a co-worker. Thus, it is necessary to plan for the unexpected arrival of a potentially contaminated victim.[12]

Indoor decontamination facilities create a potentially serious risk of inhalation exposure for hospital personnel, especially if the material is highly volatile. Many existing hazardous materials protocols call for shutting off the ventilation system to protect the remainder of the hospital from cross-contamination; however, it compounds the inhalation risk for ED personnel.[12,21] Very few hospitals have the financial resources to construct a properly ventilated separate decontamination room or to train and fit-test their staff to use self-contained breathing apparatus or air-purifying respirators.

It is safer and more practical to perform basic decontamination outside in a naturally ventilated area adjacent to the ambulance entrance.[5] Suggested equipment for an outdoor decontamination area is listed in the box.

Basic decontamination should be performed as previously described. Patients with exposure to only gas or vapors and with no evidence of skin or eye irritation or contamination do not need decontamination. They may be transferred immediately to the critical care area.

After, decontamination, local hazardous materials experts (such as the hazardous material team or health department) should be consulted for assistance with the decontamination or disposal of contaminated clothing or medical equipment. Although many items can be decontaminated with a simple soap-and-water wash, others can not be effectively decontaminated. Materials that cannot be decontaminated—for example, some leather items—may need to be disposed of or incinerated.

Medical care may be started while rapid decontamination is performed; however, in some circumstances, decontamination may take priority over treatment. For example, a victim heavily contaminated with a highly toxic organophosphate insecticide poses a great risk for secondary contamination of health care personnel; touching the patient must be delayed until staff are appropriately gloved and gowned and the patient decontaminated. Similarly, a person soaked with a flammable material cannot be treated with direct-current countershock until decontamination has been carried out.

As long as appropriate decontamination efforts have been completed before entry to the critical care area, there should be no need for special equipment or precautions such as covering floors and walls with plastic or shutting off the ventilation system; however, if the patient has ingested a chemical, there should be preparation to isolate any toxic vomitus quickly. (See discussion of ingestion exposure later.) ED staff in the critical care area should not have to wear specialized protective gear, but water-resistant gowns, latex gloves, and eye-splash protection are prudent.

The airway, breathing, and circulation should be evaluated and supported. The trachea should be intubated if indicated by severe respiratory distress or apnea. Supplemental oxygen should be administered. Ventilation should be assisted with a bag-valve mask device or a mechanical ventilator if necessary. Intravenous access should be established, cardiac rhythm should be monitored continuously, and frequent monitoring of the airway and vital signs should be performed. Many chemicals can cause progressive airway injury or systemic illness several minutes to hours after the original exposure. The possibility of multiple exposures or multiple-system injuries should be kept in mind. For example, smoke inhalation can cause immediate dramatic airway injury due to thermal and irritant chemical injury and coma from systemic asphyxiants such as carbon monoxide and cyanide.

Comatose patients should be evaluated for possible opioid overdose or hypoglycemia, and naloxone (Narcan) and dextrose should be administered according to usual protocols. Seizures should be treated with the usual anticonvulsants (diazepam, phenytoin, or phenobarbital). The possibility that coma or seizures may be a result of a head injury rather than chemical poisoning should be considered, as should the possibility of alcohol or other drug intoxication.

Hypotension should be treated with intravenous boluses of saline (250 to 500 ml up to a total of 1 to 2 L in adults) as well as dopamine or other inotropic drugs if needed. Persistent hypotension may be caused by hypothermia or hyperthermia, both of which can be a complication of the exposure. Hypothermia should be considered if the victim was stripped and decontaminated with cold water or in a cold setting. Hyperthermia can be caused by some poisons (such as dinitrophenol) and is also a complication of wearing level A or B encapsulating chemical suits, especially on a hot day.

Ventricular arrhythmias that occur after exposure to hydrocarbons (most commonly, chlorinated, fluorinated, or aromatic solvents) may be caused by excessive myocardial sensitivity to catecholamines and may respond more favorably to β-blockers (such as esmolol, propranolol) than to lidocaine and other traditional antiarrhythmics. Arrhythmias following hydrogen fluoride (hydrofluoric acid) exposure may be caused by hypocalcemia and should be treated with intravenous calcium.[6]

There are very few established antidotes for poisoning.[11] (See Table 64-4.) The regional PCC should be contacted if the specific chemical agent is known.

For symptomatic patients with inhalation exposures, supplemental oxygen should be administered and a chest radiograph should be made. Oxygen saturation should be monitored by pulse oximetry or measurement of arterial blood gases. These monitoring techniques may be unreliable in patients with carbon monoxide poisoning or methemoglobinemia; in such cases a direct measurement of oxyhemoglobin saturation should be obtained with a cooximeter.[31]

Wheezing should be treated with aerosolized bronchodilators (such as metaproterenol and albuterol). Bronchodilators are β-adrenergic stimulants and may provoke ventricular arrhythmias in patients with cardiac sensitization after halogenated, aromatic, or other hydrocarbon exposure.[1,2]

Patients with potentially serious exposure should be observed for at least 4 to 6 hours and admitted for treatment or further observation if there are progressive symptoms or if the chemical agent is suspected of causing delayed pulmonary edema. Agents commonly associated with delayed-onset pulmonary edema include phosgene and nitrogen oxides (nitric oxide, nitrogen dioxide).[29] These agents are poorly soluble in water, and unlike more soluble gases, such as ammonia or hydrogen chloride, they do not produce rapid onset of upper airway irritation or respiratory distress. Thus, patients may be inadvertently sent home only to develop pulmonary edema as late as 24 hours after exposure.

Chemically induced noncardiogenic pulmonary edema (chemical pneumonitis) is not effectively treated by administration of digoxin, afterload reduction, or diuretics. Although corticosteroids and antibiotics have been commonly recommended for treatment of chemical pneumonia, there is little credible evidence of benefit.[29]

Chemical burns may behave differently from thermal burns. Often, the extent and depth of injury are not immediately apparent. In addition, absorption of the corrosive chemical may cause acute or delayed systemic toxicity.[9]

Patients with exposure to a highly corrosive, penetrating, oily, or persistent chemical may require additional decontamination to prevent further injury or systemic absorption (see box on next page). Common sites of residual contamination include the axillae, groin, hair, ears, nostrils, fingernails, and toenails. These patients are not likely to pose a risk of secondary contamination at this point, but if the material is highly contaminating (for example, parathion, radioactive dust) it may be prudent for caregivers to wear gowns and gloves as mentioned earlier.

Special decontamination solutions may be used for a few specific chemicals (for example, calcium for hydrogen fluoride[6] and polyethylene glycol or isopropyl alcohol for phenol[15]).

Eye injuries can be catastrophic. Alkaline materials may continue to produce corrosive injury for several hours.[4] Adequate eye irrigation must be ensured. Contact lenses should be removed, exposed eyes should be irrigated with water or saline dribbled from intravenous tubing or a soft plastic irrigating lens (such as a Morgan Lens). An ophthalmic anesthetic, such as 0.5% tetracaine, may be necessary to alleviate blepharospasm, and lid retractors may be required to allow adequate irrigation under the eyelids. Any residual chemical material in the conjunctival sacs should be sought and removed. If the chemical is an acid or alkaline product, the pH of the conjunctival sac should be checked frequently, and irrigation should continue until the pH nears 7 to 7.5.

After irrigation, the visual acuity should be tested and the eyes should be examined with a magnifying device or a slit lamp with fluorescein staining to evaluate corneal injury. Small corneal defects may be treated with topical ophthalmic antibiotic ointment or drops and an oral analgesic medica-

> **Examples of chemicals that cause systemic toxicity after dermal exposure**
>
> Lindane and other chlorinated hydrocarbon insecticides
> Organophosphate and carbamate pesticides
> Phenol
> Hydrofluoric acid
> Formaldehyde
> Methylene chloride
> Dinitrophenol

tion. The patient should return within 24 hours for reevaluation. An ophthalmologist should be consulted immediately if the patient has severe corneal injury.

Patients who have ingested toxic materials are at risk for corrosive injury as well as systemic absorption. Emesis should not be induced, because of the risk of aggravation of corrosive injury and because it is relatively ineffective. Gastric lavage should be performed with a small flexible tube to remove and dilute the material in the stomach, then activated charcoal, 50 to 100 g, should be administered through a gastric tube. If the amount ingested was small (such as a swallow), activated charcoal should be administered orally without prior gastric emptying.

Ingested chemicals and their reaction products from contact with stomach acid may be hazardous to ED personnel through direct contact or by inhalation. For example, ingested cyanide is converted to highly toxic hydrogen cyanide gas in the stomach.[34] Staff must take measures to isolate toxic vomitus or gastric washings,[21] which can be done by attaching the lavage tube to isolated wall suction or other closed container.

The use of gastric lavage for ingested corrosive materials is controversial. Opponents argue that the lavage tube may further injure the chemical-damaged esophagus or stomach. On the other hand, blind gastric tube placement and stomach emptying are routinely performed prior to endoscopy anyway, and it is better to remove the liquid corrosive from the stomach as early as possible. Dilution with a glass of water is an alternative but is not as effective as lavage. If a corrosive product was ingested, endoscopy should be considered to evaluate the extent of gastrointestinal tract injury.

Activated charcoal is capable of absorbing most poisons and should be given as early as possible. Even poisons listed as having a relatively poor adsorption to charcoal (such as cyanide and alcohols) are still bound to some extent, and charcoal may be life saving in these patients.[18] It should be noted that charcoal may obscure the endoscopist's view and may have to be washed out prior to endoscopy.

Depending on the chemical exposure and the patient's symptoms and signs of toxicity, useful routine tests include a complete blood count; measurement of glucose, electrolytes, and liver enzyme levels; renal function tests; urinalysis; and an electrocardiogram. Chest radiographs and measurement of arterial blood gases are recommended for severe inhalation exposure. Occasionally, a specific blood or urine toxicologic test may be indicated.

Laboratory results may be normal immediately after the exposure. Abnormal findings are often delayed for several hours or even days, depending on the specific chemical exposure. For example, chest radiographs may not show signs of pulmonary edema until 12 to 24 hours after a phosgene exposure.[29] Signs of liver injury may not appear until 2 to 3 days after exposure to a hepatotoxic agent. The regional PCC can assist with the selection and interpretation of routine and specialized toxicology tests.

SUMMARY

Effective and efficient hazardous material incident response requires extensive planning, training, and the cooperation of large numbers of individuals with different backgrounds. Regardless of the specific duties assigned to an individual responder, the primary goal is to protect oneself. Hazardous materials victims can be assisted only when rescuers' safety is ensured. A downed responder, whether a firefighter or medical professional, is of no assistance and in fact only escalates the problem.

Emergency medical responders, including health professionals, must have special training, preparation, and access to resources. The response to a hazardous material incident requires substantial advance education and coordination of responsibilities and capabilities among personnel (police, firefighters, hazardous material technicians, EMS personnel, and ED staff) as well as toxicologists, risk-assessment experts, and scientists. A cohesive team response and communication with off-scene support are essential components of successful hazardous materials emergency response.

SUGGESTED READINGS

Binder S: Deaths, injuries and evacuations from acute hazardous materials releases, *Am J Public Health* 79:1042, 1989.

Bronstein AC, Currance PL: *Emergency care for hazardous materials exposure,* St Louis, Mosby, 1988.

Agency for Toxic Substances and Disease Control: *Managing hazardous materials incidents,* Vol I, emergency medical services: a planning guide for the management of contaminated patients, Atlanta, 1992.

Agency for Toxic Sustances and Disease Control: *Managing hazardous materials incidents,* vol II, hospital emergency departments: a planning guide for the management of contaminated patients, Atlanta, 1992.

Agency for Toxic Substances and Disease Control: *Managing hazardous materials incidents,* vol III, medical management guidelines for acute chemical exposures, Atlanta (in preparation).

Chemical Manufacturers Association: *Medical response to chemical emergencies,* 6 modules, Washington, DC, 1992, The Association.

National Fire Protection Association: *NFPA 1991, vapor-protective suits for hazardous chemical emergencies, 1990 edition,* Quincy, Mass, 1990, The Association.

National Fire Protection Association: *NFPA 1992, liquid splash-protective suits for hazardous chemical emergencies, 1990 edition,* Quincy, Mass, 1990, The Association.

National Fire Protection Association: *NFPA 471, Recommended practice for responding to hazardous materials incidents,* Quincy, Mass, 1992, The Association.

National Fire Protection Association: *NFPA 472, standard for professional competence of responders to hazardous materials incidents,* Quincy, Mass, 1992, The Association.

National Fire Protection Association: *NFPA 473, standard for professional competencies for EMS personnel responding to hazardous materials incidents,* Quincy, Mass, 1992, The Association.

Plante DM, Walker JS: EMS response at a hazardous material incident: some basic guidelines, *J Emerg Med* 7:55, 1989.

Stutz DR, Janusz SJ: *Hazardous materials injuries: a handbook for prehospital care, ed 3,* Beltsville, Md, 1992, Bradford Communications.

Sullivan JB Jr, Krieger GR, ed: *Hazardous materials toxicology: clinical principles of environmental health,* Baltimore, 1992, Williams & Wilkins.

REFERENCES

1. Antti-Poika M, Heikkila J, Saarinen L: Cardiac arrhythmias during occupation exposure to fluorinated hydrocarbons, *Br J Ind Med* 47:207, 1990.
2. Bass M: Sudden sniffing death, *JAMA* 212:2075, 1970.
3. Beckett WS et al: Heat stress associated with the use of vapor-barrier garments, *J Occup Med* 28:411, 1986.
4. Borak J, Callan M, Abbot M: *Hazardous materials exposure,* New York, 1991, Brady.
5. California Emergency Medical Services Authority: *Hazardous materials medical management protocols, ed 2,* Sacramento, Calif, 1989, Health and Welfare Agency.
6. Caravati EM: Acute Hydrofluoric acid exposure, *Am J Emerg Med* 6:143, 1988.
7. Code of Federal Regulations, Labor, 29 1910, Washington, DC, 1990, Office of the Federal Register National Archives and Records Administration
8. DeSilva P: TLVs to protect "nearly all workers", *Appl Ind Hyg* 1:49, 1986.
9. Edelman PA: Chemical and electrical burns. In Archauer BM, ed: *Management of the burned patient,* Norwalk, Conn, 1987, Appleton & Lange.
10. Emmett EA, Ricking JA: Fatal self-administration of sodium azide, *Ann Intern Med* 83:224, 1975.
11. Gosselin RE, ed: *Clinical toxicology of commercial products,* ed 6, Baltimore, 1988, Williams and Wilkins.
12. Gough AR, Markus K: Hazardous materials protections in ED practice: laws and logistics, *J Emerg Nursing* 15:477, 1989.
13. Hensley E: Personal cooling: preventing heat stress in chemical protective clothing. In Conference Proceedings, Haztech International, Denver, Colo, 1986, Colorado Ground Water Association.
14. Hiatt PH, Blanc PD, Olson KR: The toxic information center of the San Francisco Bay Area Regional Poison Control Center: an occupational and environmental health resource center model, *Am J Ind Med* (in press).
15. Hunter DM et al: Effects of isopropyl alcohol, ethanol, and polyethylene glycol/industrial methylated spirits in the treatment of acute phenol burns, *Ann Emerg Med* 21:1303, 1992.
16. Institute of Medicine: *Report of a study: meeting physicians' needs for medical information on occupations and environments,* Washington, DC, 1990, National Academy Press.
17. Institute of Medicine: *Role of the primary care physician in occupational and environmental medicine,* Washington, DC, 1990, National Academy Press.
18. Lambert RJ, Kindler BL, Schaeffer DJ: The efficacy of superactivated charcoal in treating rats exposed to a lethal oral dose of potassium cyanide, *Ann Emerg Med* 17:595, 1988.
19. Lavoie FW et al: Emergency department decontamination for hazardous chemical exposure, *Vet Hum Toxicol* 34:61, 1992.
20. Litovitz TL et al: 1991 Annual Report of the American Association of Poison Control Centers National Data Collection System, *Am J Emerg Med* 10:452, 1991.
21. Merritt NL, Anderson MJ: Malathion overdose: when one patient creates a departmental hazard, *J Emerg Nursing* 15:463, 1989.
22. National Fire Protection Association: *NFPA 472, standard for professional competence of responders to hazardous materials incidents,* Quincy, Mass, 1992, The Association.
23. National Fire Protection Association: *NFPA 473, standard for professional competencies for EMS personnel responding to hazardous materials incidents,* Quincy, Mass, 1992, The Association.
24. Olson KR, ed: *Poisoning and drug overdose,* San Mateo, Calif, 1990, Appleton & Lange.
25. Olson KR, Benowitz NL: Environmental and drug-induced hyperthermia: pathophysiology, recognition, and management, *Emerg Med Clin North Am* 2:459, 1984.
26. Roach SA, Rappaport SM: But they are not thresholds: a critical analysis of the documentation of threshold limit values, *Am J Ind Med* 17:727, 1990.
27. Tong TG: Role of the regional poison center in hazardous materials accidents. In Sullivan JB Jr, Krieger Gr, ed: *Hazardous materials toxicology: clinical principles of environmental health.* Baltimore, 1992, Williams & Wilkins.
28. U.S. Department of Transportation: 1990 emergency response guidebook, DOT P 5800.5. Washington, DC, 1990.
29. Wald PW: Respiratory effects of acute toxic inhalations: smoke, gases, and fumes, *J Intensive Care Med* 2:260, 1987.
30. Walter FG et al: Hazardous materials incidents: a one-year retrospective review in central California, *Prehosp and Disaster Med* 7:151, 1992.
31. Watcha MF, Connor MT, Hing AV: Pulse oximetry in methemoglobinemia, *Am J Dis Child* 143:845, 1989.
32. White MK, Hodous TK: Physiological responses to the wearing of fire fighter's turnout gear with neoprene and Gore-Tex barrier liners, *Am Ind Hyg Assoc J* 49:523, 1988.
33. White MK, Ronk R: Chemical protective clothing and heat stress, *Prof Safety* 29:34, 1984.
34. Windholz M, ed: *The Merck Index* ed 10, Rahway, NJ. 1983, Merck & Co, Inc.
35. Ziem GE, Castleman BI: Threshold limit values: historical perspectives and current practice, *J Occup Med* 31:910, 1989.

Chapter 65

CHEMICAL DISASTER PREPAREDNESS

Thomas R. Parker

Background
    What is a chemical disaster?
Health risk assessment of the Cantara incident
    Toxicologic assessment of MITC in air
Hazard identification and reduction
    Risk management and prevention plans
    Emergency planning levels
Emergency response and risk management
    Emergency response preparation
    Contingency planning: the RAPID plan
    Contingency planning: the internal plan
    Regional planning: the issue of air monitoring
    Levels of concern
    Information resources
Summary

On a July evening in 1991 a Southern Pacific freight train lost an engine and several rail cars over the sharply curving Cantara Loop bridge near the foot of Mount Shasta, California. One of the tank cars, which ruptured as it plunged into the Upper Sacramento River, was filled with 20,000 gallons of the pesticide methyldithiocarbamate, commonly called "metam."[20]

As the tank car bled its contents into the currents of the Sacramento River, the metam reacted with river water and formed methylisothiocyanate (MITC). MITC is a chemical cousin of methylisocyanate, which was released in Bhopal, India. Once in river water, some MITC evaporated into the air, potentially exposing nearby residents as well as riparian plants and animals to the hazardous effects of the pesticide.

What developed has been called California's worst inland environmental disaster involving chemicals.[23] During the 6 days following the spill, over 400 residents along the river received medical treatment or first aid in an evacuation shelter, and more than 80 patients were treated in emergency rooms at one of three hospitals.[20] Thousands of fish and many other aquatic organisms and land animals were killed along 45 miles of river habitat.

There was a delay in warning the people in the downstream town of Dunsmuir. The placards on the ruptured tank car did not precisely identify the chemical inside as metam. Once identified, it was learned that the chemical metam was not found on the EPA's list of extremely hazardous substances, and that no "level of concern" had been established. Protective "action levels" had to be calculated directly from the available toxicity data, with precious little time. The hazard inherent in the transportation of toxic chemicals had now become an imminent—and uncalculated—risk of human chemical exposure and disease. Compounding the risk to the public and the environment from exposure to MITC was the delay caused by initial confusion among those responding to the emergency.

This chapter illustrates how toxicologists and physicians in the Office of Environmental Health Hazard Assessment (OEHHA) assisted in the response to the MITC spill at Cantara and how they are addressing potential future chemical exposure incidents through planning and preparedness.

BACKGROUND

Accidental releases of hazardous chemicals are not unusual.[2] In 1991 more than 25,800 hazardous material incidents were reported to the National Response Center in Washington, D.C. Among these reports, 893 involved injury, 352 involved evacuation, and 97 involved death.[5]

Along with the Cantara incident, some other examples of chemical emergencies and disasters are as follows.

- In June 1992 a tank car derailed from a trestle, spilling about 26,000 gallons of benzene into the Wisconsin River, causing a 10-hour evacuation of more than 50,000 people. About 25 people were hospitalized, with dizziness, headache, and eye irritation among the chief health complaints. A liquid petroleum gas tank car came very close to rupturing and exploding in the same accident.[25,26]
- In November 1984 bromine from an industrial plant in Geneva, Switzerland, was accidentally vented to the atmosphere in a densely populated portion of the city. Approximately 25,000 persons were exposed to bromine concentrations that exceeded the short-term exposure limit of 0.3 ppm. The factory was evacuated, and people were asked to take shelter indoors and to close all windows. Numerous telephone calls to the police, fire, and hospital services paralyzed the telephone network, severing communication between the hospital, the first-aid teams, and the Swiss Toxicological Centre in Zurich. Ninety-one exposed persons visited the hospital; and, for the 59 patients whose symptoms were recorded, eye and upper airway irritation and cough were the most prevalent complaints.[17]
- In December 1984 over 2000 persons lost their lives in Bhopal, India, as about 40 tons of methylisocyanate were accidentally released into the atmosphere from a pesticide plant at night.[4] In terms of chemical injury and loss of life, the Bhopal disaster stands as the most tragic in history.

What is a chemical disaster?

The term *disaster* has no shortage of definitions. For this chapter, use the definition offered by Leonard and Teitelman[15]: "... A disaster means any community or regional event that disrupts community function and activities and causes concern for the lives, health, and property of the citizens of a community." The authors further define a *mass casualty incident* as an incident producing many casualties but not necessarily covering a wide geographical area. The terms are sometimes used interchangeably. As a practicality, this chapter makes little distinction between chemical disasters and mass casualty incidents of chemical cause, since comprehensive prevention planning reduces the risk of occurrence of both, and well-orchestrated emergency management and preparedness measures mitigate the potential for tragedy for both.

HEALTH RISK ASSESSMENT OF THE CANTARA INCIDENT*

In response to the Cantara incident the central goal of OEHHA toxicologists and physicians was to determine the nature and extent of health risks posed to the community from exposures to released chemicals, primarily MITC. A risk assessment for environmental exposures is typically conducted in four steps: hazard identification, exposure assessment, toxicological and dose-response assessment, and risk characterization. Hazard identification involved decisions about which among the released chemicals and degradation products presented the greatest toxicity and relative exposure. Metam and MITC were the most important and received most attention.

Ideally, exposure assessment would be performed by air and water monitoring, but monitoring was not initially available, and environmental concentrations of metam and MITC could only be estimated by theoretical modeling. Since previously established safe exposure levels and protective action concentration levels did not exist for either metam or MITC, responders had to estimate these levels from the available scientific data.

Toxicologic assessment of MITC in air

Immediately after the spill, we collected and evaluated the medical and toxicologic information reported in the published literature as well as the data submitted for registration of the pesticide metam. Such serious, irreversible health effects as birth defects and tissue injury were emphasized. Effects that might strain available medical services from large-scale self-presentations, such as respiratory irritation, nausea, and vomiting, were also considered.

In order to evaluate the potential for noncancer health effects, an assumption was made that exposures must be above certain minimum thresholds to have an effect. Our objective was to determine the concentration level at which adverse health effects would not be anticipated in essentially any members of the public. Such *reference exposure levels,* or RELs, are estimated from the literature as the no observed adverse effects levels, or NOAELS, divided by appropriate safety factors to compensate for uncertainties in relating animal toxicology studies to human exposure outcomes.

Based on comparisons among lethality studies in animals, MITC is significantly more toxic than metam when tested at high concentration levels for short-term exposures. The literature investigation revealed that acute, high doses of MITC in animals elicited responses such as skin and eye irritation, dyspnea, vomiting, diarrhea, ataxia, convulsions, and death.

The MITC 1-hour animal exposure studies were examined, and no observed adverse effect levels, or NOAELS, of

---

*Adapted from DiBartolomies M, Alexeeff G, Fan A, Jackson R, *Evaluation of the Health Risks Associated with the Metam Spill in the Upper Sacramento River,* 1992, Office of Environmental Health Hazard Assessment, draft.

Table 65-1. One-hour NOAEL-based reference exposure levels for methylisothiocyanate (ppb)

Species	Endpoint	NOAEL concentration	Reference exposure level (REL)
Rat	Lethality	207000	2070
Rabbit	Birth defects	72,000	720
Cat	Lacrimation, salivation	70	0.7
Cat	No effects	35	0.4

the most sensitive species at selected endpoints were found. Then reference exposure levels were calculated by dividing the NOAELS by appropriate safety factors (Table 65-1). Reference exposure levels were calculated that were then employed as protective action levels, to assist local responders to the Cantara MITC incident.

HAZARD IDENTIFICATION AND REDUCTION

In planning for and managing chemical disasters, the cooperation of clinicians and toxicologists is essential. They play important roles in: (1) assisting with the identification and reduction of hazard, and (2) preparing for emergency response and participating in risk management (see Chapter 64).

Hazard reduction is the optimal risk control strategy. Proactive programs in disaster planning operations, which are designed to prevent or minimize chemical releases, are the most effective means for protecting community health and safety and the environment.[1a,20,21,24]

Risk management and prevention plans

As an example of proactive planning in California, local emergency planning authorities are empowered by state law to request risk management and prevention plans from fixed-site facilities that use sufficiently large quantities of hazardous chemicals.[24] The elements of a risk management and prevention plan for a specific facility can include such information as the following:
- A structured assessment of chemical hazards
- A personnel training program for the prevention of, and response to, chemical emergencies
- Schedules for regular testing of the program
- Procedures for reducing the probability of chemical accidents
- An analysis of potential off-site health consequences

Emergency planning levels

Emergency planners can estimate human and environmental exposures from potential chemical accidents, but the impact of exposure at projected concentration levels is often unclear. Unfortunately, not much guidance is currently available to local emergency planners who wish to understand and anticipate potential human health effects from the accidental release of toxic chemicals. Much of the data available to local emergency planners were generated in the occupational setting, where we would not ordinarily encounter highly sensitive individuals. In fact, available health data and regulatory standards do not as a rule apply to sensitive individuals, including those with preexisting conditions and certain age-defined populations (see Chapters 28 and 29).

In California the Chemical Emergency Planning and Response Commission recognized this problem and identified a need for a process to calculate scientifically sound concentration levels for acute chemical exposure of the public. The commission identified the 48 chemicals of greatest concern and apportioned them into three groups on the basis of suspected hazard (see box). The Office of Environmental Health Hazard Assessment developed methods for establishing emergency planning values, and the latter are currently being tested.

---

48 Chemicals recommended for investigation by the Chemical Emergency Planning and Response Commission

Immediate action (25)	*As soon as possible (17)*	*Future investigations (6)*
Acrolein	Bromine chloride	Acetaldehyde
Ammonia	Butadiene	Aldicarb
Arsine	Chlorine dioxide	Benzene
Boron trifluoride	Chloropicrin (gas)	Bromine
Carbon disulfide	Chloropyrophos	Butane
Chlorine	Ethylene	Chloroform
Ethyleneimine	Fluorine	
Ethylene oxide	Formaldehyde	
Hydrazines	Methane	
Hydrochloric acid	Methylene chloride	
Hydrofluoric acid	Mevinphos	
Hydrocyanic acid	Paraquat	
Hydrogen sulfide	Pentachlorophenol	
Methyl bromide	Phenol	
Methyl isocyanate	Styrene	
Nitric acid	Tetraethyl lead	
Nitrogen dioxide	Vinyl chloride	
Nitrogen trioxide		
Parathion (methyl)		
Phosgene		
Phosphine		
Propane		
Sulfur dioxide		
Sulfuric acid		
Toluene diisocyanate		

Source: California Planning and Response Commission: 48 chemicals recommended for further investigation, Governor's Office of Emergency Services, 1990.

The final form of these methods will enable local planners to understand the theoretical risk to the public posed by chemical release, and thereby to maximize prevention and hazard reduction planning by evaluating health consequences of potential releases.

EMERGENCY RESPONSE AND RISK MANAGEMENT

As important as hazard identification and reduction are, they cannot, of course, prevent all chemical accidents. From Cantara it is learned that which chemical, or even in which medium an emergency chemical release will occur, cannot be anticipated.

Emergency response preparation

Readiness is more than just availability. Response plans must be in place and well rehearsed. Much confusion exists during the early stages of a the disaster.[15] The precious first minutes of a chemical disaster are likely to be chaotic, with poor information from the incident scene and inadequate communications. Those assisting emergency responders must be able to rely on training as well as practical response, or "contingency," planning. They must also be prepared to work with industry experts and all levels of government officials. In the words of Makris,[16] "Chemical emergency planning is most effective where industry, government, the medical community, public interest groups, and others . . . coordinate their responsibilities cooperatively." The integration responsibilities of emergency response team members are detailed in Chapter 64.

Contingency planning: the RAPID plan

Following the Cantara incident, the Rail Accident and Immediate Deployment or RAPID plan was developed in California in order to bring those state governmental agencies that have an emergency response role into the emergency response system in an orchestrated manner and to integrate this system with local emergency response.[20,23] The RAPID plan, which is published in the form of a "working" draft, coordinates 17 state governmental agencies under a single director within the state's incident command system. The impact assessment function is organized into four groups. These groups are human health effects, environmental fate and transport, laboratory support, and cleanup technology.[7]

The responsabilities of the human health effects assessment group are as follows.

1. *Assist responders in determining type of information needed to evaluate public health threat.* In order to assess risk, we must know which chemicals are involved, and what chemical exposure concentrations to the public might be predicted, and for what time durations. Therefore, we must first be prepared to assist certain responders by suggesting the kinds of information we need. What is the concentration of the chemical, and what has the chemical mixed with? What is the concentration of chemicals in the plume? What is the plume movement? How many persons may be exposed to the plume? These are types of information that on-scene responders may be in the best position to obtain quickly.

2. *Predict the effects on human health from the chemicals of concern.* "The successful management of a major toxic release will . . . depend on a rapid and complete assessment of the health hazard, a process which must begin as soon as possible and be updated as the emergency unfolds."[6] This is the *risk characterization* portion of the risk assessment, and it focuses first on acute data (human if available), then longer-term consequences from short-term exposures; and last, chemicals with potential carcinogenicity. We have a wide variety of toxicologic and medical databases at our disposal, including computer information databases and 24-hour emergency information hotlines such as CHEMTREC. Good information exists for many, but not all, toxic chemicals used in commerce.

3. *Determine action levels.* Early in a chemical emergency, a possible question to be posed by incident command is "Should we evacuate or shelter-in-place?" or simply, "What is the evacuation level?" As urgent as these questions are, we cannot answer them directly. We can, however, suggest approximate concentrations at or above which protective action of some kind should be considered. Along with chemical gas concentration, incident commanders must consider other factors in the decision on whether to evacuate people, shelter-in-place, or simply isolate the hazard and deny entry. Some of these factors are[9]:
   - Concentration and expected duration of toxicant exposure
   - Number of people exposed
   - Availability of suitable escape routes
   - Special institutions such as schools, hospitals, and prisons
   - Weather conditions

Additionally, real-time monitoring of toxicants released in the atmosphere is not usually available. Large uncertainties in assumptions used to make predictions of exposure concentrations may lead to lower confidence in these estimated levels. Potential health effects, at specified concentration levels, are thus only one of many considerations folded into decisions about protective action. The health professional should make any recommendations advisedly.

Actually, much prescriptive-action-level information is readily available to the local responding agency. The U.S. Department of Transportation publishes "Initial isolation and protective distance" information for each of the chemicals it considers to be an "inhalation hazard."[9] The publication stresses, however, that the table is useful for only the first 30 minutes of a spill incident. Perhaps the best known action levels are *levels of concern*. The U.S. Environmental Protection Agency defines levels of concern as "... the concentration of an extremely hazardous substance ... in air above which there may be serious irreversible health effects or death as the result of a single exposure for a relatively short time."[11] These levels of concern can be based on such existing values as Emergency Exposure Guidance Levels or EEGLs,[19] Emergency Response Planning Guidelines or ERPGs,[1] or calculated as one tenth of the Immediately Dangerous to Life and Health values.[11,18] Levels of concern are examined more thoroughly later in this chapter. The levels of concern are not meant to be equated with action levels, especially if time permits a close examination of the supporting data.

For chemical emergencies for which published guidance levels are either nonexistent or are based on faulty supporting data, it may be appropriate to estimate *reference exposure levels*. The reference exposure level can be calculated as the NOAEL concentration at the desired endpoint (see Table 65-1) divided by the appropriate safety factors.[20] Special attention should be paid to the quality, quantity, and suitability of the research data used to estimate reference exposure levels.

4. *Risk communication.* The communication of risk to the general public is a vital component of our responsibilities under the RAPID plan. Through the public information liaison, toxicologists and physicians can inform the public of the best estimate of actual risks to those exposed as well as the most prudent precautions to prevent or minimize effects from a chemical toxicant (see Chapters 3 and 64).

5. *Technical assistance to local agencies and hospitals.* The RAPID plan includes preparations to offer advice to local health departments as well as local physicians and hospitals on such diverse topics as symptoms, possible treatments, and risk communication suggestions, working closely with poison control centers.

6. *Assist in the selection of sampling plans and control techniques.* An overall sampling plan addresses public health as completely as possible, including sensitive community receptors. When control techniques are under consideration possible breakdown products and risks associated with the mitigation process are identified.

7. *Predict long-term health effects.* Risk characterization also involves determining whether any segments of the exposed population might suffer long-term consequences from brief exposures. This analysis may be performed retrospectively, as an epidemiologic study.

Contingency planning: the internal plan

The goal is to reach a state of internal preparedness to provide information on hazardous material risk, medical treatment, and environmental fate to assist command, local physicians, and other agencies in responding to emergency releases of hazardous substances in the environment.

The emergency contingency plan involves the following elements: establishing an internal training program and a duty officer system using scientific professionals trained to respond to chemical emergencies; providing assistance in risk characterization through verification of action levels, recommendation of protective action levels and safe community levels, and assessment of environmental fate; and coordination and consultation in the treatment of chemical injuries, the collection of information resources, the training of health professionals, and epidemiologic investigations.

Regional planning: the issue of air monitoring

In order to estimate exposure to toxicants during a hazardous material incident, responders first make estimates about the rate and mass of escaping toxic gas, local wind conditions, and local topography. A computer program such as ALOHA is used to plot concentration versus population. Since this method has several elements of uncertainty, actual air monitoring would be preferred. Baxter[6] stated that actual air sampling would be invaluable, but "... the duration of most releases, with the possible exception of uncontrollable fires ... may be far too short to enable the mobilization of scientists with appropriate equipment." The problem of trying to mobilize equipment and human resources in time to be of value in a fairly short-duration chemical release is a challenge to emergency planners. Even when appropriate equipment and personnel are available, they may be too far from the incident to be used in time, or worse, the incident commander may not even know that the resources exist.

One answer to the problem is to identify the specific emergency air monitoring capabilities, including specialized equipment and personnel, from federal, state, and local governmental agencies, as well as from industry, all within a confined geographical area, such as, the San Francisco Bay Area. This kind of regional planning has the additional benefit of acquainting experts, responders, and decision-makers from a spectrum of diverse governmental agencies and industries.

Levels of concern

As mentioned earlier, many responders will consider the levels of concern (the concentrations above which members of the exposed population may experience irreversible injury or even death) as a protective action level. The kinds of protective action options available to incident command include evacuation, sheltering-in-place, and isolation of the hazard area. The EPA equates the level of concern principally as one tenth of the Immediately Dangerous to Life and Health, or IDLH, concentration.[11] We suggest caution with this algorithm, however, as IDLH values vary considerably among chemicals in severity of toxic effects.[3] The EPA also states that other exposure guidelines can be used to estimate the LOC, including Threshold Limit Values (American Con-

Table 65-2. Information resources

Type	Resource	Description
Telephone assistance	CHEMTREC 1-800-424-9300	Chemical and response advice from Chem. Manufacturer's Assn. specialist[9]
	National Response Center 1-800-424-8802	Chemical and response advice from U.S. Coast Guard specialist[9]
	Poison Control Center (consult local listing)	Provides advice for managing victims of hazardous materials exposure[10]
Computer databases	Integrated Risk Information System	EPA database of specific risk information on over 400 chemicals. Gives reference doses for noncarcinogens[8]
	Chemical Hazard Response Information System	U.S. Coast Guard database on emergency response and chemical hazards for over 1,000 chemical[3]
	Registry of Toxic Effects of Chemical Substances	NIOSH database providing toxicity data on over 100,000 potentially toxic chemicals[8]
Computer programs	Computer Aided Management of Emergency Operations (CAMEO)	Provides information on chemicals, industrial facilities, transportation data, contact persons, response resources, and other subjects[12]
	Areal Locations of Hazardous Atmospheres (ALOHA)	Estimates airborne pollutant concentration downwind from a spill using gaseous dispersion model[13]
Handbook	Guidebook for First Response to Hazardous Material Incidents	Provides numerical index of hazardous materials and includes suggested initial action to be taken for accidental releases[9]

ference of Governmental Hygienists), Emergency Exposure Guidance Levels (National Academy of Sciences), and the Emergency Response Planning Guidelines published by the American Industrial Hygiene Association.

Information resources

Numerous information resources are available to the medical responder to chemical emergencies (Table 65-2). For information in an emergency, 24-hour information hotlines are available such as the Chemical Transportation Emergency Center, usually called CHEMTREC, or the National Response Center.[9] CHEMTREC, which is a service of the Chemical Manufacturer's Association, provides immediate chemical information on an urgent basis for incident command, and includes information from over 400,000 Material Safety Data Sheets. The Chemical Manufacturer's Association has introduced a new service in concert with CHEMTREC called MEDTREC.[14] Physicians and toxicologists would normally contact CHEMTREC (Table 65-2), and if more detailed medical advice were required, CHEMTREC specialists would contact MEDTREC through the San Francisco Poison Control Center. MEDTREC offers a training package for physicians entitled Response to Chemical Emergencies.[14]

Along with emergency information hotlines, several medical and toxicologic computer databases exist* which can provide toxicologic, medical, environmental, and regulatory information about thousands of chemicals (see Table 65-2).

Among those to consider for consultation are databases from NIOSH (Registry of Toxic Effects of Chemical Substances), from the EPA (Integrated Risk Information System as well as Oil and Hazardous Material Technical Assistance), and the U.S. Coast Guard (Chemical Hazard Response Information System).[8] Many of these databases can be acquired individually from the original sources, or several can be acquired simultaneously from commercial vendors of CD-ROM databases (see Appendix C).

SUMMARY

Accidental releases of chemicals are not unusual events. Toxicologists and clinicians can help reduce overall chemical hazard and risks through planning and preparedness. Preparation to assist responders involves characterizing risk through contingency planning, training, and information management. Response plans should be well rehearsed. Large-scale multidisciplinary plans should include general instructions for all participating agencies. Agency-specific incident contingency plans contain specific elements that support the general responsibilities outlined in multidisciplinary preparedness plans. Personnel and equipment resources can be identified and shared within a geographic region by industry and all levels of government. A variety of information resources are available to the health professional assisting in a response to a chemical emergency.

---

*These computer databases are described as examples only. In the interest of brevity, not every database is included in this discussion. Mention of commercial information resources does not constitute endorsement by the Office of Environmental Health Hazard Assessment.

REFERENCES

1. AIHA (American Industrial Hygiene Association): *Emergency response planning guidelines,* Cleveland, 1991, AIHA.
1a. Alexeef G et al: Dose response assessment of airborne methyl isothiocyanate (MITC) following a metam sodium spill, *Risk Anal* 14:2, 1994.

2. Alexeeff G, Lewis D, Lipsett M: Use of toxicity information in risk assessment for accidental releases of toxic gasses, *J Haz Mat* 29 387, 1992.
3. Alexeeff G, Lipsett M, Kizer K: Problems associated with the use of immediately dangerous to life and health (IDLH) values for estimating the hazard of accidental chemical releases, *Am Ind Hyg J* 500:598, 1989.
4. Amdur M: Air pollutants. In Amdur M, Doull J, Klaassen C, eds: *Toxicology: the basic science of poisons,* ed 4, New York, 1991, Pergamon Press.
5. ATSDR (Agency for Toxic Substances and Disease Registry): Preparing for the unthinkable, *Hazardous Substances and Public Health* 2:1, 1992.
6. Baxter P: Responding to major toxic releases, *Ann Occup Hyg* 34:615, 1990.
7. Cal/EPA (California Environmental Protection Agency): *Railroad accident prevention and immediate deployment (RAPID) plan* Sacramento, Calif, 1993, Department of Toxic Substance Control.
8. Deck K, Bonzo S: *Some publicly available sources of computerized information on environmental health and toxicology,* Atlanta, 1990, Centers for Disease Control.
9. DOT: *Emergency response guidebook,* DOT P 5800.5, 1990, U.S. Department of Transportation, Office of Hazardous Materials Transportation, Washington, DC 20590-0001.
10. EMSA (California Emergency Services Authority): Hazardous materials emergency management protocols. Koehler G, California Emergency Services Authority, Sacramento, CA (1991)
11. EPA, FEMA, DOT (U.S. Environmental Protection Agency, Federal Emergency Management Agency, U.S. Department of Transportation): *Technical guidance for hazards analysis: emergency planning for extremely hazardous substances,* 1987
12. EPA, NOAA 1990a: *Computer aided management of emergency operations,* user manual, v1.0 1990
13. EPA, NOAA 1990b: *Areal locations of hazardous atmospheres,* user manual, v5.0 1990
14. Hartman S: Chemical Manufacturer's Association, personal communication, 1993.
15. Leonard R, Teitelman U: Manmade disasters, *Crit Care Clinics* 7:293, 1991.
16. Makris J: Chemical emergency planning and the medical community, *Health and Environment Digest* 55:1, 1992.
17. Morabia A et al: Accidental bromine exposure in an urban population: an acute epidemiological assessment, *Int J Epidemiol* 17:148, 1988.
18. NIOSH (National Institute for Occupational Safety and Health): *Pocket guide to chemical hazards,* NIOSH #90-117, 1990
19. NRC (National Research Council) committee on toxicology: *Criteria and methods for preparing emergency exposure guidance level (EEGL), short-term public emergency guidance level (SPEGL), and continuous exposure guidance level (EEGL) documents,* Washington, D.C., 1986, National Academy Press.
20. OEHHA (Office of Environmental Health Hazard Assessment): *Evaluation of the health risks associated with the metam spill in the upper Sacramento River,* External review draft. DiBartolomies M, Alexeeff G, Fan A, Jackson R. Office of Environmental Health Hazard Assessment, California/EPA, Berkeley, CA (1992a)
21. OEHHA (Office of Environmental Health Hazard Assessment): *Guidelines for determining emergency planning levels for acute chemical exposures,* final draft. Parker T, Alexeeff G, Lipsett M, Jackson R. Berkeley, Calif, 1992b, Office of Environmental Health Hazard Assessment, California/EPA.
22. Reference deleted in proofs.
23. OEHHA (Office of Environmental Health Hazard Assessment): *Improving transportation safety and response: results of the Cantara and Seacliff hazardous materials incidents,* draft. Russel H. Berkeley, Calif, 1993, Office of Environmental Health Hazard Assessment, California/EPA.
24. OES (Office of Emergency Services): *Guidance for the preparation of a risk management and prevention program:* Lercari F, Sacramento, Calif, 1989, Governor's Office of Emergency Services.
25. Reisch M: Rail benzene spill forces major evacuation, *Chemical and Engineering News* 70:5, 1992a.
26. Reisch M: Wisconsin train accident costly, but not deadly, *Chemical and Engineering News* 70:18, 1992b.

Chapter 66

HELPING PATIENTS ADOPT HEALTHFUL LIFE-STYLE CHOICES

Dennis D. Tolsma
Jessica Herzstein

The case for behavioral risk reduction
Gaps in progress
Strategies and settings
    Community-based health promotion
    Health promotion in schools
    Work-site wellness
    Health promotion in health care settings
Conclusion

Health promotion and education have become central elements of the nation's health strategy. In 1990 the Secretary of the Department of Health and Human Services released *Healthy People 2000,* a set of national health goals and objectives for the year 2000; this major policy document strongly confirms the high priority on health promotion set a decade earlier by the U.S. Surgeon General in Healthy People objectives for 1990. The foreword acknowledges the importance of health behavior choices in its opening sentences:

Americans today are taking a more active interest in their health than ever before. They are coming to realize the influence that they, themselves, can have on their own health destinies and the overall health status of the Nation.[39]

This emphasis was carried forward in the Clinton administration's health reform proposals. Both clinical preventive services and health education were included in the planned "guaranteed National benefit package." In addition, the section on health research initiatives anticipated expanded research on health and wellness promotion, and the section on public health initiatives detailed enhanced efforts to inform and educate consumers and health care providers about their roles in preventing and controlling disease and the appropriate use of medical services.

Clinicians and other health care workers can offer invaluable support to patients, families, and communities in undertaking health promotion strategies. Many already do so, and many others are asking how best to undertake such interventions. This chapter outlines the status of health promotion and education in the United States, with special emphasis on efforts in health care settings.

THE CASE FOR BEHAVIORAL RISK REDUCTION

A multitude of factors influence health: personal factors, such as genetic, physiologic, psychologic, and demographic variables; environmental factors, such as hazards encountered in work, community, home, and recreation; and societal factors, such as cultural and socioeconomic variables. Individual choices of health behaviors are typically not independent of societal factors, and risk reduction thus must take this interdependence into account. Nevertheless the practice of medicine and public health must recognize that health behaviors have become steadily more important as underlying causes of preventable morbidity, premature death, and reduced quality of life.

In 1984 former President Carter convened a health policy consultation, entitled Closing the Gap, at the Carter Center of Emory University. The report of that consultation marked the first comprehensive attempt to quantify all of the generic (underlying) risk factors that contribute most to 14 leading causes of morbidity and mortality. On the basis of these reports, a panel of experts identified alcohol, tobacco, injury, and unintended pregnancy as the highest-priority precursors. (Three other precursors that ranked nearly as high were overnutrition, including obesity and high serum cholesterol levels; handguns; and dental problems.) To the final list were added two generic health problems: gaps in primary care and mental health issues (violence, depression, and substance abuse).[12] Virtually all of these priority precursors are either directly behavior choices (for example, smoking) or risk factors in which behavioral choice plays a major role (such as unintended pregnancy).

A few illustrations from the Carter Center analyses show the range of behavioral risks that influence health. For example, the diabetes analysis found that "prevention of obesity may reduce the incidence of type II diabetes by one half and gestational diabetes by as much as one third."[15] It also estimated that if all the 1 million diabetics who continue to smoke were to stop, the incidence of peripheral vascular disease could be reduced by 30%. Another analysis reviewed the health impacts of smoking, diet, and alcohol on major cancers. Overall, 24% of cancer deaths, 21% of life-years lost before age 65, 21% of hospital days, and 16% of direct medical care costs were attributable to these behavior-related precursors.[32]

Cardiovascular disease remains the leading cause of death in the United States. The Closing the Gap analysis of cardiovascular disease calculated that smoking is the cause of 30% of premature deaths due to cardiovascular disease (defined as potential years of life lost before age 65). Similarly, 18% of life-years lost because of cardiovascular disease was attributed to high blood pressure, and 9% to elevated cholesterol. These three variables accounted for more than half of each measured health burden of cardiovascular disease.[46] Metaanalyses of studies of exercise and heart disease also conclude that moderate-to-vigorous physical activity reduces the risk of coronary heart disease, that the relative risk of this factor is of the same order of magnitude as those of moderate smoking and an elevated cholesterol level, and that an estimated 20,000 fewer persons would die each year if half those persons without leisure-time physical activity began to participate in a moderate exercise program.[6] These types of data argue that nonpharmacologic measures, that is, counseling for nonsmoking and protective behavioral choices in exercise, diet, and weight loss, are important clinical strategies and can reduce the health impact of cardiovascular disease substantially.

A summary analysis combining the findings of the 14 individual Closing the Gap analyses suggests that "approximately two thirds of deaths in the United States are attributable to a preventable precursor.[2] Six precursors—tobacco, alcohol, injury risks, high blood pressure, overnutrition, and gaps in primary prevention—accounted for three fourths of the preventable health impact. Tobacco was the strongest precursor for deaths, life-years lost, and hospital days. Four precursors that are strongly related to personal health behavior—tobacco, high blood pressure, overnutrition, and alcohol—accounted for approximately 1 million preventable deaths, nearly 4 million potential years lost, and 45.5 million days of hospital care.[2]

There is no doubt that changing behavior is a formidable goal; in fact, many people, including a large number of health care providers, do not believe that behavior change can be accomplished. Yet the reality is somewhat different. Accumulating evidence indicates that health behavior choices are modifiable and sometimes change at a pace that equates to rapid social change. Examples in daily life are numerous: jogging and fitness, at least among the middle class; reduced social acceptability of drinking and driving, paralleled by declines in the proportion of intoxicated drivers in fatal crashes; a rising prevalence of seat-belt use, after years of public education culminating in the passage of state laws requiring seat-belt use; and rising use of infant safety seats in cars, now a regular practice in most families.

Perhaps the most striking example of population behavior change in public health is the 25-year decline in cigarette smoking. From 1965 to 1987, the overall prevalence of smoking dropped from 40% to 29%; for men the drop was almost 20 percentage points, from 50.2% to 31.7%.[28] Clearly, despite the addictive potency of tobacco, millions of individuals quit smoking, millions more were deterred from starting, and the population prevalence of a major hazardous behavior changed in a significant way.

GAPS IN PROGRESS

If health promotion is a good thing, it follows that society would wish its benefits to reach everyone. Unfortunately, not all parts of society adopt or maintain healthful behaviors at the same rate, and some of the most vulnerable social groups typically lag behind. Again, smoking provides an object lesson. Although overall rates of smoking have declined among both men and women, the rate of decline has been lower for women, particularly for young women, with obvious consequences for the health of both these women and their infants.[22] There is a higher prevalence of smoking in people of racial and ethnic minorities, and these smokers often quit less often than do those in nonminority groups.[22]

Socioeconomic variables are important factors influencing both the adoption of health practices and the success of intervention strategies. The association of poverty with mortality and illness has been clear for a long time. Survival rates have been shown to vary in direct relation to family income: the lower the income, the lower the survival rate.[4] At least 23 health problems are more frequent at lower socioeconomic levels in the United States.[18]

Formal educational attainment appears to have a particularly strong association with personal behavior choices.

Again with smoking as an example, the less education people have, the greater the likelihood that they are current smokers. This inverse pattern has been observed consistently in both the United States and Canada for cigarette smoking, lack of physical activity, lack of seat-belt use, and safety practices (such as having a smoke detector in the home).[37] The opposite pattern has been noted for alcohol use and for driving after excessive alcohol use.

STRATEGIES AND SETTINGS

As already noted, personal, environmental, and societal factors have impact on individual health behavior choices. Therefore, successful health promotion efforts need to include interventions that address all of these spheres of influence; however, the relationships can be complex. One model arrays the determinants of behavior into five groups:

1. Intrapersonal factors: characteristics of the individual such as knowledge, attitudes, behavior, self-concept, and skills (includes the developmental history of the individual)
2. Interpersonal processes and primary groups: formal and informal social network and social support systems, including the family, work group, and friendship networks
3. Institutional factors: social institutions with organizational characteristics and formal (and informal) rules and regulations for operation
4. Community factors: relationships among organizations, institutions, and informal networks within defined boundaries
5. Public policy: local, state, and national laws and policies[23]

Although not all of these factors may be accessible to the readers of this book who wish to promote healthy lifestyles, it is important to recognize them as matters that can reinforce or can negatively affect practitioner efforts.

The primary focus of this chapter is on health education and promotion in health care delivery setting; however, there is a variety of other settings in which interventions can appropriately, economically, and effectively be mounted.[3] There is general agreement that, in addition to health care delivery settings, communities, schools, and work sites are most appropriate for health promotion activities.

Community-based health promotion

In community health in general, and even more so in health promotion, many community institutions and resources are essential partners. These institutions include public health departments, voluntary and civic organizations, academic centers, medical societies, and hospitals.

An example of such a partnership in community health promotion programs is Planned Approach to Community Health (PATCH), a collaboration between state and local health departments and the Centers for Disease Control and Prevention. Some 17 states and more than 50 communities are involved. One of its basic tenets is local ownership.[20] The health department partners work with community residents and institutions to define local priorities, set measurable objectives, collect community data, and undertake health promotion programs. The use of data collected from the local community, including a behavioral risk factor survey, vital statistics, and opinion leader interviews, has helped to gain support for PATCH objectives and strategies within the community. This planned approach has also been successful in gaining intersectoral cooperation, for example, in school health education, highway safety, and work-site smoking policies.

According to a Department of Health and Human Services study, racial and ethnic minorities experience more than 58,000 excess deaths from chronic diseases when compared with the more favorable mortality rates of nonminority populations, and many are attributable to behavioral risk factors.[29] Addressing the health promotion concerns of minorities in a culturally sensitive, responsive fashion is essential. In one program that explicitly sought community involvement, African-American residents of an Atlanta neighborhood designed and implemented the Community Health Assessment and Promotion Project in cooperation with the staff of a nearby teaching hospital. Community concern about high blood pressure led to support for a weight loss and exercise program. Results of the interventions included a significant loss of weight when compared with a control population. Perhaps because of a concerted effort to develop culturally appropriate strategies, these community-guided interventions were able to avoid one of the shortcomings of many minority health promotion programs: falloff in participation rates.[9]

Broad participation is a vital ingredient of successful community health promotion programs.[21] All recent intervention trials in cardiovascular disease have drawn on both behavioral theory and community organization research to incorporate community health promotion strategies in their approaches. Community organization skills and principles reinforce the efforts of health promotion practitioners in disseminating health information, motivating decisions to adopt healthful behaviors, providing opportunities to change behavior, and maintaining such changes.[44]

The health promotion model cited in the previous section suggests that behavior is determined by multiple influences; the community is a particularly appropriate setting to organize interventions at several levels. Medical personnel should be aware of the valuable assistance that they can lend to those responsible for community health promotion, for example, by providing leadership in support of community and organizational change strategies.

Health promotion in schools

Equipping youth to make healthful behavior choices is an important responsibility of adolescent health care, one that school health education and services can substantially support. Some early behavior choices, such as sexuality, drug use, and drinking and driving, can have a direct and immediate impact on the current health status of young people. Lifelong maintenance of other protective health behaviors (such as nonsmoking and regular aerobic exercise) contributes to life expectancy and the quality of life that they will have as adults.

Regrettably, surveys of adolescent behavioral risks and their perceptions of their risks offer evidence that an alarming fraction of students are engaging in behaviors that increase health risks. For example, in one survey of 8th- and 10th-grade students, 56% of the students reported that they had not worn a seat belt during their most recent trip in an automobile. About 25% of boys and 42% of girls indicated that they had seriously considered suicide at some point in their lives. Among eighth-graders, 51% said they had tried smoking tobacco, 77% said they had used alcohol, and 15% said they had tried marijuana. Significant majorities of respondents had correct perceptions of sexual risk factors for human immunodeficiency virus infection, and smaller majorities understood sexually transmitted disease signs; however, a large fraction of the respondents were unsure or had incorrect perceptions. Widely varying percentages reported having received instruction in school, depending on the health topic surveyed. The area for which health education was reported most frequently was the effects of tobacco, alcohol, and drugs.[30]

Traditionally, school health has three basic areas: school health education, school health services, and school health environment; however, experts today broaden the framework to include physical education, school food services, counseling, on-site health promotion for faculty and staff, and integrated school and community health promotion efforts.[1]

To ascertain the effectiveness of school health education, the Centers for Disease Control and Prevention has supported several controlled trials of comprehensive health curricula. The results convincingly document that well-planned school health education can accomplish improved health knowledge, attitudes, and behaviors. For example, in a major study of fifth- and sixth-grade children in four curricula, educationally significant improvements were observed at 3-year follow-up. As expected, it was relatively easy to produce knowledge gains with a few hours of instruction, but these curricula also accomplished positive changes in health behavior and health attitudes, with maximal impact reached at about 50 hours, the optimal "dose" of this "intervention."[7] A longitudinal study of a high school–level curriculum yielded similar findings; the program improved attitudes (especially by preventing deterioration in health attitudes that occurred in control groups) and improved several priority behaviors (notably self-reported use of illegal drugs).[13]

Teenage pregnancy is a serious problem in the United States; most pregnancies among women under 20 years of age are unintended. In this area as well research indicates that school-based health promotion can be employed to good effect. A program named School and Community Program for Sexual Risk Reduction among Teens was developed and tested in a South Carolina county. Compared with three control counties, which experienced net increases in the estimated pregnancy rate among females aged 14 to 17, the study population reduced its pregnancy rate by 54%.[42] An essential lesson from this study was the need to combine both specific educational messages and skills training with strong efforts to secure broad community involvement, including parents, teachers, representatives of churches, and community leaders.

Forty-eight million children and youth attend school daily, providing a ready opportunity to address their health needs. Although many states have general policies encouraging school health education, only 27 have specific health education requirements for high school graduation. The nation's health objectives for the year 2000 include measurable targets both for high-school graduation rate (90%) and for the proportion of schools (75%) providing quality school health education.[39] Health care practitioners can make an important contribution to ensure that their communities offer good school health programs. They can do so both by volunteering to help in health classes and, equally importantly, by lending their individual and collective professional voices to reinforce school boards, administrators, and teachers who aim to promote better school health.

Work-site wellness

Health promotion and health education programs conducted in the work setting—often also called life-style programs or work-site wellness programs—compose one of the most active areas of health promotion. One survey of the nation's largest corporations, the *Fortune* 500 list, found that two thirds of these corporations have health promotion programs. Many of these programs are slated for expansion, and one third of corporations without programs indicated that they plan to initiate them.[16]

More than half of American workers are employed at work sites with 50 or more employees. The 1992 National Survey of Worksite Health Promotion Activities documents the nature and extent of health promotion activities in work sites of this size. The survey indicates that 81% offer at least one health promotion activity, up from 66% in 1985. The six most commonly offered activities are job hazards and injury prevention (64%), exercise and fitness (41%), smoking control (40%), stress management (37%), counseling about alcohol and other drugs (36%), and back care (32%).[38] In both the *Fortune* 500 survey and the broader work-site survey, organizational size is an important factor in initiating programs: the larger the employer, the more likely it is to offer health promotion activities. Small businesses have found it more difficult to staff and finance these activities, but some have found ways to draw on offerings of health departments and voluntary associations or to form consortia to share the cost of organizing activities.

Business leaders cite a wide variety of perceived benefits as reasons to support health promotion at the work site: job satisfaction, morale, employee health improvements, improvements in productivity and in factors that influence productivity (such as absenteeism and turnover), and reductions in medical care costs.[35] Most respondents in the work-site survey were satisfied that benefits outweighed costs; in fact, ''improved employee health'' was cited more frequently than ''to control health care costs'' as the reason for initiating activities.[38]

One criticism of health promotion at the work site is that it can divert attention to changing the behavior of workers exposed to hazards rather than addressing the issue of hazard control directly. In addition, risk assessment and risk reduction should not be allowed to translate into personal coercion, compromise of health care benefits, or discrimination in hiring. One guard against inappropriate practices is the leadership provided by the emergence of national and regional organizations of professionals in workplace health promotion, whose membership establish and adhere to standards for sound programs. Worker participation in planning programs and ensured confidentiality also are critical elements in the institution of ethical and successful work-site health promotion program.

Despite a growing number of studies indicating that cost savings result from work-site health promotion programs, health economists have suggested caution regarding the economic benefits of work-site programs. Given the practical limits to research in the work setting, the lack of sound evidence of cost savings does not mean that there are none but rather reflects the need for careful reading and additional evaluation. Data that fall short of absolute proof of cost savings may still give corporate decision makers enough confidence in the positive benefits of the program to warrant the investment.[11]

Among the better-known programs nationally are the Live for Life program of Johnson & Johnson, the AT&T Total Life Concept program, The Employee Health Improvement Program of the Du Pont Company, the Employee Health Promotion program of the Group Health Cooperative of Puget Sound, and the Blue Cross–Blue Shield of Indiana program.[27]

Several trends that affect work-site health promotion and that may be significant in relation to the national health care reform debate have emerged in recent years. First, employee-assistance programs (EAPs) have traditionally focused on providing assessment, short-term counseling, and referral of employees with substance-abuse and mental health problems; health promotion programs have focused on educational interventions aimed at employee populations.[45] Today some EAPs are moving from a case-finding approach toward broad-scale education and prevention. Second, health promotion programs are focusing increased attention on the organizational environment, for example, corporate culture, health-related policies, and health benefits design in support of health promotion.[31] Third, there is a trend toward linking health promotion with preventive screening activities provided as part of employee health services or by outside providers; typically, cancer and heart disease are the focus of these types of programs.[10] Finally, there is a growing integration of worker protection activities and health promotion, EAPs, and employee health activities.[17]

A model for implementation of workplace health promotion would combine behavioral- and environmental-change strategies—for example, offering both smoking-cessation programs and protective ventilation of hazardous operations—developed with input from both labor and management.[14]

Health promotion in health care settings

A modest fraction of health care expenditures is devoted to prevention. A recent study estimates that about 3% of the nation's health care expenditures support prevention; even if prevention expenditures from private and insurance sources are not as well documented, the total is unlikely to exceed 5%.[5] Clearly a much smaller fraction supports health promotion in health care settings, despite its enormous potential and visible national endorsements.

A principal finding of the 1989 *Guide to Clinical Preventive Services* is that ''conventional clinical activities (e.g., diagnostic testing) may be of less value to patients than activities once considered outside the traditional role of the clinician (e.g., counseling and patient education). This suggests a new paradigm in defining the responsibilities of the primary care provider.[40] The report also recognizes that clinicians may not currently possess all the skills needed to assist patients in changing behaviors and that patients also need to develop new skills for a changing and more participatory role in patient-physician encounters. Fig. 66-1 portrays a number of behaviors and behavior-related processes that can be productively assessed and modified in a health care setting.

A body of literature regarding successful strategies for medical personnel to use in counseling patients and helping accomplish behavior change has emerged in recent years. Some reports describe methods aimed at specific risk factors, such as smoking[19] and exercise.[36] Others detail counseling models, such as direct patient-physician counseling and reinforcement by office staff.[43] Many health professionals, in addition to medical and dental practitioners, are able to provide health promotion services. Among them are nurses, occupational therapists, certified nurse-midwives, certified physician assistants, registered dental hygienists, registered dietitians, and other allied health professionals. The principles and rationale for patient education and behavioral counseling, including the role of the clinician, have been reviewed in depth by Russell.[33]

Although work-site health promotion aims to improve health through primary prevention and early detection strat-

> **Primary prevention**
>
> Use of seat belts and child safety restraints
> Nutrition: diet and weight control
> Tobacco use
> Substance use
> Stress reactions
> Physical activity
> Immunization status
> Home safety
>
> **Secondary prevention**
>
> Behavior patterns linked to high blood pressure
> Behavior patterns linked to elevated serum cholesterol
> Substance abuse (early stages)
> Care-seeking behaviors
>
> **Tertiary prevention**
>
> Cardiac rehabilitation
> Substance abuse (symptomatic)
> Allergen exposure (avoidance)
> Diabetic diet and compliance

Fig. 66-1. Examples of behaviors and behavior-related processes that may be effectively addressed by health promotion in health care settings.

egies oriented to a worker population, the clinician, especially in primary care settings, can provide much-needed education, behavioral counseling, and support on a one-to-one level. The clinician must first master skills in interviewing, problem identification, and behavioral counseling.[33] Some patients should receive treatment of psychologic problems as a first priority and prescription of a health behavior program may be wisely deferred in such cases. Clinical scenarios that often require psychologic counseling include alcohol and drug dependence, clinical depression, nutritional syndromes such as anorexia and bulimia, and current life crises.

The *Guide to Clinical Preventive Services*[40] recommends extensive preventive services, performed at regular intervals and aimed at primary and secondary disease prevention and health promotion. These guidelines are typically presented for specified age groups, with additional services as indicated by gender. The *Guide* also offers specific additional actions for patients assessed as ''high risk.'' Among the recommendations for a periodic visit for patients aged 40 to 64 are screening (for example, history: tobacco, alcohol, and drug use; laboratory and diagnostic procedures: mammogram every 1 to 2 years for women older than 50 who are not at increased risk); Counseling (for example, diet and exercise: fat—especially saturated fat, cholesterol, complex carbohydrates, fiber, sodium, and calcium); and immunizations (for example, tetanus-diphtheria booster every 10 years).

In cases in which individuals have increased susceptibility to environmental exposures because of host factors, the clinician's recognition of this disease risk and initiation both of steps to reduce exposure and of education and behavioral counseling are critical. Environmental exposures compound preexisting risk. Examples of susceptibility include exposure to ultraviolet light or carcinogenic chemicals in persons with xeroderma pigmentosa; exposure to carbon tetrachloride in patients who consume alcohol; and exposure to asbestos or coal dust among patients who smoke tobacco.

Clinicians have successfully guided life-style intervention strategies in a variety of areas, such as dietary fat reduction, cardiovascular fitness, smoking cessation, and management of stress. Most commonly, clinicians target these life-style activities to those who have conditions related to these risks. For example, weight loss and physical activity would be prescribed for someone with hypertension, stress management and dietary counseling are important treatments for someone with irritable bowel syndrome, and smoking cessation and stress management are often pursued among patients with asthma. Clinicians should not lose sight, however, of the important influences on future health status of pursuing patient counseling with otherwise-healthy patients whose history includes unhealthful life-style choices.

On both an empirical and a theoretical basis, patient education is strongly supported by evidence of effectiveness. A metaanalysis of 102 studies of education and counseling for prevention offers two generalizations about effectiveness. First, no single channel of education is inherently superior to another. Additional exposure to any intervention may be more important than the educational approach adopted. Second, application of five educational principles was predictive of intervention effectiveness: reinforcement, feedback, individualization, facilitation, and relevance.[26]

Reinforcement is activity intended to reward desired behaviors. *Feedback* is activity to demonstrate to patients the degree to which they are achieving progress in making the behavior change they desire. *Individualization* involves tailoring the intervention so that it allows each patient to set the pace of learning and makes it possible to get answers to questions throughout the process. *Facilitation* denotes the degree to which an intervention provides the means for patients to take action or reduces barriers to action. *Relevance* refers to actions to make the learning process appealing to the learner through content and methods derived from assessment to patients' needs, capabilities, and interests.[26]

Empirically the patient-education literature of the past decade has provided numerous examples of careful patient-education studies that measured a range of specific health outcomes. These measurable outcomes range from care utilization, in Zapka and Averill's study[47] on self-care of colds; costs, in Vickery and colleagues' study[41] of health maintenance organization self-care education; adherence to prescribed regimens, in Morisky and colleagues' work[25] on antituberculosis drugs; behavioral risk reduction, in Sanders and colleagues' randomized controlled trial[34] of antismoking advice by nurses and Coates and associates' review[8] of changes in high-risk behavior in men at risk of acquired immunodeficiency syndrome; and health status and mortality reductions in Morisky and colleagues' controlled trial[24] documenting a 50% reduction in mortality among inner-city hypertensive women receiving a patient-education program.

In addition, patient counseling can play a positive role in health care reform strategies. A number of personal health behaviors affect the health care system; examples include ability and motivation to seek and use appropriate health care and preventive services, deterring both overuse and underuse of the health system; choices to adopt or maintain protective health practices that reduce demand on health services; skills that support adherence to preventive and therapeutic regimens, which can reduce unnecessary services; and skills and motivation to keep appointments, which promotes efficiency in service delivery.

The barrier is not a lack of availability of preventive technologies. Rather, issues such as education and attitudes of providers; motivation and expectation of patients; and aspects of health care organization, including access and reimbursement, impede successful incorporation of health promotion in health care settings. The health system is a long way from accomplishing its potential in health promotion.

CONCLUSION

The primary care provider can play a major role in achieving the nation's health goals by ensuring that the majority of patient encounters include an assessment of behavioral factors that affect risk (see Fig. 66-1) and education about behavioral modification when indicated. Successful behavioral counseling involves steps such as identification of the problem and of treatment goals, behavioral diagnosis, intervention plan, progress review, maintenance program, and process review. These components have been mastered by many clinicians involved in preventive health care delivery.[33] Health promotion can be targeted at a number of levels to suit the needs of apparently well individuals and those with preexisting conditions or known risk factors. Depending on the current state of health, health promotion activities can be aimed at primary prevention (reduction of risks before the onset of disease), secondary prevention (improvement in outcome related to early diagnosis), and tertiary prevention (improvement in outcome after the disease process is well underway).

Clinicians have significant opportunities to make a positive contribution to their patients' health by directing health promotion efforts toward healthful behavior choices. A number of useful references and resources are now available to assist in the development of health promotion in communities, schools, workplaces, and health care settings. The steady growth of health promotion policy and practice affords new opportunities and challenges for health practitioners.

> A 1994 publication of the U.S. Public Health Service, *Clinician's Handbook of Preventive Services,* is an excellent reference that can be ordered from the U.S. Government Printing Office, Mail Stop SSOP, Washington, D.C. 20402-9328.

REFERENCES

1. Allensworth DD, Kolbe LJ: The comprehensive school health program: exploring an expanded concept, *J Sch Health* 57:409, 1987.
2. Amler RW, Eddins DL: Cross-sectional analysis: precursors of premature death in the United States, *Am J Prev Med* 3(5 suppl):181-187, 1987.
3. APHA Technical Report: Criteria for the development of health promotion and education programs, *Am J Public Health* 77:89, 1987.
4. Berkman LF, Breslow L: *Health and ways of living: the Alameda County study,* New York, 1983, Oxford University Press.
5. Brown RE et al: *National expenditures for health promotion and disease prevention in the United States: final report of a contract,* Washington DC, 1991, Batelle.
6. Centers for Disease Control and Prevention: Public health focus: Physical activity and the prevention of heart disease, *MMWR* 42:669, 1993.
7. Christenson GM et al: Preface to results of the school health education evaluation, *J Sch Health* 55:295, 1985.
8. Coates T, Stall R, Hoff C: *Changes in high risk behavior among gay and bisexual men since the beginning of the AIDS epidemic: Office of Technology Assessment report,* Washington DC, 1988, US Congress.
9. Curry R: *Mobilizing a minority community to reduce risk factors for cardiovascular disease: an exercise-nutrition handbook,* Atlanta, 1989, Emory University School of Medicine and the Centers for Disease Control.
10. Eriksen MP: Cancer prevention in workplace health promotion, *Am Assoc Occup Health Nurs J* 36:266, 1988.
11. Fielding JE: The proof of the health promotion pudding is . . . , *J Occup Med* 30:113, 1988 (Editorial).
12. Foege WH, Amler RW: Introduction and methods, *Am J Prev Med* 3(5 suppl):3-6, 1987.
13. Gold RS et al: Summary and conclusions of the THTM evaluation: the expert work group perspective, *J Sch Health* 61:39, 1991.
14. Green LW, Kreuter MW: *Health promotion planning: an educational and environmental approach,* ed. 2, Mountain View, Calif, 1991, Mayfield.
15. Hermann WH, Teutsch SM, Geiss LS: Diabetes mellitus, *Am J Prev Med* 3(5 suppl):72, 1987.
16. Hollander RB, Lengermann JJ: Corporate characteristics and worksite health promotion programs: survey findings from fortune 500 companies, *Soc Sci Med* 26:491, 1988.
17. Jordan-Marsh M, Vojtecky MA, Marsh DD: Workplace health promotion/protection: correlates of integrative activities, *J Occup Med* 29:353, 1987.
18. Kaplan GA et al: Socioeconomic status and health, *Am J Prev Med* 3(5 suppl):125, 1987.
19. Kottke TE et al : Attributes of successful smoking cessation interventions in clinical practice: a meta-analysis of 42 controlled trials, *JAMA* 259:2882, 1988.
20. Kreuter MW: PATCH: Its origin, basic concepts, and links to contemporary public health policy, *J Health Educ* 23:135, 1992.
21. Labonte R: Community health promotion strategies, *Health Promotion* 26:5, 1987.
22. Mason JO et al: Health promotion for women: reduction of smoking in primary care settings, *Clin Obstet Gynecol* 31(4):989, 1988.

23. McLeroy KR et al: An ecological perspective on health promotion programs, *Health Educ Q* 15:351, 1988.
24. Morisky DE et al: Five-year blood pressure control and mortality following health education for hypertensive patients, *Am J Public Health* 73:153, 1983.
25. Morisky DE et al: A patient education program to improve adherence rates with antituberculosis drug regimens, *Health Educ Q* 17:253, 1990.
26. Mullen PD, Green LW: Educating and counseling for prevention: from theory and research to principles. In Goldbloom RB, Lawrence RS, eds: *Preventing disease: beyond the rhetoric,* New York, 1990, Springer-Verlag.
27. Opatz JP: *Health promotion evaluation: measuring the organizational impact,* Stevens Point, Wisc, 1987, National Wellness Institute.
28. *Reducing the health consequences of smoking: 25 years of progress: a report of the Surgeon General,* US Dept of Health and Human Services Pub No. (CDC)89-8411. Atlanta, 1989, Centers for Disease Control.
29. *Report of the Secretary's Task Force on Black and Minority Health,* vol 1, US Dept of Health and Human Services, Washington DC, 1985, Government Printing Office.
30. Results from the national adolescent student health survey, *MMWR* 38:147, 1988.
31. Roman PM, Blum TC: Formal intervention in employee health: comparisons of the nature and structure of employee assistance programs and health promotion programs, *Soc Sci Med* 26:503, 1988.
32. Rothenberg R et al: Cancer, *Am J Prev Med* 3(5 suppl):30, 1987.
33. Russell ML: *Behavioral counseling in medicine,* New York, 1986, Oxford University Press.
34. Sanders D et al: Randomised controlled trial of anti-smoking advice by nurses in general practice, *J R Coll Gen Pract* 39:273, 1989.
35. Sciacca JP: The worksite is the best place for health promotion, *Personnel Journal* 66:42, 1987.
36. Simons-Morton BG, Pate RP, Simons-Morton DG: Prescribing physical activity to prevent disease, *Postgrad Med* 83:165, 1988.
37. Stephens T, Schoenborn CA: *Health habits in the US and Canada,* DHHS Pub No (PHS)88-1429, Hyattsville, Md, 1988, National Center for Health Statistics.
38. US Department of Health and Human Services: *The 1992 national survey of worksite health promotion activities,* Washington, DC, 1993, Government Printing Office.
39. US Department of Health and Human Services, Public Health Service: *Healthy people 2000:* national health promotion and disease prevention objectives: full report with commentary, DHHS Pub No (PHS) 91-50212, Washington, DC, 1990, Government Printing Office.
40. US Preventive Services Task Force: *Guide to clinical preventive services,* Baltimore, 1989, Williams & Wilkins.
41. Vickery DM et al: Effect of a self care education program on medical visits, *JAMA* 250:2952, 1983.
42. Vincent ML, Clearie AF, Schluchter MD: Reducing adolescent pregnancy through school and community-based education, *JAMA* 257:3382, 1987.
43. Vogt HB, Kapp C: Patient education in primary care practice, *Postgrad Med* 81:273, 1987.
44. Wakefield MA, Wilson DH: Community organization for health promotion, *Community Health Stud* 10:444, 1986.
45. Ware BG: Workplace health promotion: issues for the future, *HealthLink* 3:3, 1987.
46. White CC et al: Cardiovascular disease, *Am J Prev Med* 3(5 suppl):43, 1987.
47. Zapka J, Averill BW: Self-care for colds: a cost-effective alternative to upper respiratory infection management, *Am J Public Health* 69:814, 1979.

Chapter 67

HEALTH RISK COMMUNICATION

Virginia H. Sublet
Max R. Lum

What is risk communication?
Why should physicians learn about risk communication?
    Useful information resources
    How are people exposed?
    How are hazardous waste sites assessed?
    Who is the public?
    How do people perceive risk?
    Tips to earn trust and credibility
    Basic risk communication issues
Principles of risk communication

The objective of this chapter is to provide health professionals with an understanding of health risk communication principles and how these can be helpful in addressing concerns about health risks related to environmental exposures. Health risk communication principles can be applied to many areas in medicine.

WHAT IS RISK COMMUNICATION?

Risk is defined as the possibility of suffering a loss or an effect because of some event. Communication is defined as the exchange of information. Risk communication can be described as the exchange of information about a possible effect caused by some event. Applied to the field of public health, risk communication is the exchange of information about some health risk from exposure to a hazardous substance.

Risk communication is a two-way process.[8] It does not involve merely presenting information to the public or the patient. It does however involve an interactive process between the individual or source with a message and a receiver or patient with viewpoints to express. The interaction of the two is necessary to resolve differences and come to consensus about a particular risk of concern. Risk communication is a component of risk management, which is the selection of risk control options. The clinician can utilize the basic concepts of risk communication in helping individuals to understand health risks related to exposure, to control those risks, and to adopt healthful behaviors (see Chapter 66).

WHY SHOULD PHYSICIANS LEARN ABOUT RISK COMMUNICATION?

Research has shown that physicians are the most trusted resources available to the public.[10] Physicians and other health practitioners are increasingly receiving questions from their patients and the community about health risks related to hazardous substances due to escalating concerns about these exposures.

Why is the medical community so revered? Health practitioners fulfill a number of roles for their patients, including the gatekeeper of health, the educator, and the trusted confidant. Furthermore, clinicians are a source of special knowledge respected by patients. The clinician is also an investigator and is capable of identifying sentinel cases of disease. For centuries practitioners have advised patients about medications, diseases, symptoms, and treatments. This role is now expanding as patients ask their practitioners about health risks associated with environmental or occupational exposures. In this regard physicians face a dilemma because most have not received training in environmental health, toxicology, or risk communication.

Useful information resources

There are a number of different factors that can influence how effectively the health care professional addresses health risk communication issues. Familiarity with several types of information can increase the competence of the answers and the confidence of the health professional's delivery when he or she speaks with the worried patient. These information resources include laws and agencies that deal with hazardous substances, the toxicology of hazardous substances found in the community, the manner by which people become exposed in the community, the process of hazard assessment in the community, the constitution of various public agendas that may motivate people, the community's perception of risk, and the basic principles of health risk communication.

Familiarity with the local, county, state, and federal laws (such as SARA Title III, CERCLA, OSHA Hazard Communication Std.) that regulate hazardous substances in the environment can be helpful (see Appendix A). This knowledge can save the physician time in an emergency situation because the laws that regulate hazardous substances in the environment require companies to provide information about chemical exposure to the public (which they previously did only on a voluntary basis).

Federal agencies that deal with hazardous substances in the environment or the occupational setting include the Occupational Safety and Health Administration (OSHA), to which occupational exposures and exposure conditions are reported, the U.S. Environmental Protection Agency (EPA), regional EPA offices that provide information about remediation activities in the community, the National Institute for Occupational Safety and Health (NIOSH), and the Agency for Toxic Substances and Disease Registry (ATSDR), which addresses public health issues related to exposures. State, county, and local health departments can be helpful during emergency incidents and provide other environmental services such as industrial hygiene assessments of certain chemicals in homes or at local sites for hazardous waste. The regional poison control centers across the United States operate 24 hours a day, provide information about household products and other hazardous substances, have professionally trained staff, and provide services without cost to the caller (see Appendix B). The Local Emergency Planning Committee has information about all local companies including an inventory of where and what hazardous substances are stored or utilized. Familiarity with these agencies and resources can be helpful during a crisis, as well as in the diagnosis and surveillance of environment related disease.

How are people exposed?

A number of factors influence how people are exposed. These include the environmental or occupational pathway of exposure (air, water, soil, and biota), the biological routes of exposure, and the toxicity and chemical properties of the substances in question (see Chapter 4).

Knowledge of these parameters equips the clinician with powerful tools for diagnosing environmentally related disease and provides the background for communicating with patients about the risk of exposure associated with a toxic agent.

How are hazardous waste sites assessed?

There are approximately 40,000 hazardous waste sites in the United States. A hazardous waste site may be a landfill, an incinerator, or hazardous waste found at an abandoned facility. Of these sites approximately 1250 are on the Environmental Protection Agency's National Priority List (NPL). Those sites on the NPL require cleanup action. A number of assessments are done on hazardous waste sites that are being remediated. These include preliminary assessments, geologic surveys, a remediation investigation and feasibility study, a risk assessment, and public health assessments. The results of the risk assessment, which characterize the exposure risk through mathematical and statistical modeling, are used by the EPA in determining the type of remediation that will be done at a site. In addition, public health assessments are conducted at these sites by the ATSDR. The public health assessments evaluate available environmental data, health outcome data, and community health concerns to make a judgment about the health status of the community located in proximity to a hazardous waste site. ATSDR also responds to petitions from any citizen in the United States with concerns about public health effects at hazardous waste sites. If a clinician has patients who have been exposed at a site, the health assessment also provides a good history of the site and information on what has been done to clean up the contamination.

Who is the public?

When communicating with the community, it is imperative to know who the "publics" or stakeholders are in the community. Included in the "publics" are the residents, civic organizations, elected officials, regulatory agencies, federal facilities, the media, and activist groups. The roles of the "publics" need to be identified. For example, who are the citizen action groups? Are they local or part of a national organization? Do they work with communities to help resolve environmental issues or do they have their own agenda? Who are the leaders in the community? Are regulatory agencies or federal installations from the Department of Energy or Department of Defense located in the community? The media is an additional "public" group that may influence other groups by the reporting of community events. The roles of the different publics must be considered in the risk communication process because these stakeholders determine the acceptability of the solution(s) under consideration at a hazardous waste site.

Members of any community are a composite of different backgrounds, perceptions, and varied personal agendas. These factors influence their perspectives in any situation. The greatest concerns of communities include health effects, safety, environment, economics, aesthetics, and process issues. These concerns are viewed subjectively. For example, communities want to know if their health will be affected by the site. Is it safe to live in the area? Has the environment been contaminated to the point where the fish and garden produce should not be eaten? Will the town become deserted as people move away? What about property values? These complex factors all come into play as the community reacts to an environmental hazard.

Working with the stakeholders successfully is very difficult for federal agencies. One way ATSDR has found to learn about the community and the priorities of the different stakeholders within the community is to develop a dialogue with the members at the beginning of any site work. ATSDR uses public meetings, public availability sessions, and community assistance panels to help establish a relationship with the community and build credibility. Public meetings allow citizens to ask questions in an open forum. Another mechanism used by ATSDR to communicate with communities is public availability sessions, which offer one-on-one consultations for anyone in the community. The objective is to provide a more private opportunity for residents to discuss public health concerns with the Agency. The public availability session is similar to visiting one's health practitioner, but the trust and credibility already established in the practitioner–patient relationship does not exist. Community assistance panels (CAPs) consisting of community residents have also been used successfully by ATSDR. The CAPs are particularly helpful for federal agencies, which characteristically have low credibility with communities, and seek to work with the residents to show their empathy and caring. Members of the CAP are chosen from the community, participate with ATSDR during each step of its study, and are given quarterly updates of ATSDR progress at the site of concern.

How do people perceive risk?

Scientific experts and the public perceive risk differently. In 1990 the EPA's Scientific Advisory Board conducted a study to decide which environmental problems pose the greatest risk to human health.[13] At the same time the public's concerns about the environment were assessed in a 1990 Roper poll.[14] The Scientific Advisory Board's priority list of environmental problems included toxic air pollutants, radon indoor air pollution, drinking water contamination, occupational exposure to hazardous chemicals, application of pesticides, global warming, habitat depletion, and stratospheric ozone depletion. The public viewed hazardous waste, occupational exposure to toxic chemicals, oil spills, and nuclear power plants as being much more important than most of the categories chosen by the experts. Occupational exposure to toxic chemicals was the only category that was near the top of both lists.

Other data further substantiate the dichotomy between the experts and the public. For instance, it is well known that exposure to radon kills more people every year than all of our hazardous waste sites combined, yet millions of people have chosen not to evaluate their homes for exposure to this hazardous substance. Smoking-related morbidity and mortality far outweighs any known environmental risk from a hazardous waste site. Therefore, the risk that is most dangerous to life or health is not necessarily the risk that angers or frightens the public the most.[17]

Scientists think of risk as a hazard (based on mortality and morbidity statistics).[7] They see the exposure risk objectively as it affects a large population. The public sees exposure risk subjectively. Communities are not concerned with large populations. Communities want to know, how will this hazard affect me, my family, and my neighborhood?

The public perception of risk also includes concern or outrage factors that are directly derived from psychological processing or intuitive reasoning.[16] The concern people have about the exposure risk depends on their judgment of the risk. The person decides based on his background, education, personal experience, personal values, and common sense whether the risk is something to be considered or dismissed. Once an intellectual choice has been made, the person decides how concerned he is about the risk based on several concern or outrage factors in conjunction with inferential reasoning skills.[9,21,22] Unfortunately, scientists have often ignored the concern factors and the public has not understood the hazard factors in most instances.

The main outrage factors that influence how people perceive risk are summarized below.[2,15,20]

1. Voluntary risks are accepted more readily than those that are imposed and involuntary.
2. Risks under control of the individual are more readily accepted than risks under the control of others.
3. Risks that seem fair are more acceptable than those that are unfair. Workers in an industry may be willing to live in an environmentally polluted area because they receive a monetary benefit. The rest of the community, however, will find this contamination unfair. Equity issues also come into play here. For example, where will the incinerator be located, in the rich or poor community? Is this decision arrived at fairly?
4. Risks that are ethically objectionable will seem more risky than those not viewed as ethically objectionable. Many people feel that pollution is morally wrong. As a result, much of the public feels that pollution is an unacceptable risk and want it stopped no matter what the cost in comparison to the benefit.
5. Unfamiliar risks are more objectionable than familiar everyday risks. The high-tech chemical company down the street is seen as a greater risk than household exposure to radon.
6. Natural risks are more acceptable than artificial or man-made risks. Radon in homes is not considered to be nearly as risky as radon from uranium mines.

7. Dreaded risks pose a greater threat than familiar risks. Cancer or AIDS are dreaded diseases in comparison to emphysema, which in reality may be as serious.
8. Information from a trustworthy source is more readily believed than information from other sources. Advice from one's doctor is accepted more easily than advice from an acquaintance.

Trust and credibility are the key issues in risk communication. The ability to establish constructive communication is determined in large part by whether the clinician or expert is perceived as trustworthy. Research indicates that people's assessment of how much someone can be trusted and believed is based on empathy/caring, competence/expertise, honesty/openness, and dedication/commitment.[3] Of these factors, empathy/caring is the most important and is assessed within 30 seconds. Trust and credibility are difficult to achieve, and if once lost they are even more difficult to regain. Below are a number of ways to improve credibility and trust. These were originally developed by the Environmental Communications Research Program at Rutgers University[6] and have been modified slightly for this document.

Tips to earn trust and credibility[6]

1. Demonstrate competency—investigate the data and information regarding the risk concern.
2. Be caring. Your attitude pervades your words. Though the concern may seem unreasonable, it is still the concern of the patient.
3. Encourage public involvement. From the beginning, making the community part of the investigation is imperative to the resolution of the problem.
4. Be honest. When you do not know the answer, be sure to say so.
5. Pay attention to process. Explaining how you arrived at your decision is extremely important.
6. Explain your procedures. How did you obtain the information about the exposure risk? What kinds of medical procedures are necessary to assess the problem? What legal issues must be considered?
7. Be forthcoming and encourage public involvement from the beginning.
   - If people are at risk, tell them about it.
   - Is it a known risk? If so, consider informing the public; they can understand.
   - If it may be released by the media, do it first.
   - If no data or poor data are available, explain what you are doing to deal with the problem.
   - If you do not trust the data, tell the public what you are doing but do not release the data.
   - Release information before final risk management decisions are made.
   - If you cannot give information about the problem right away, talk about what you are doing but do not remain silent.
8. Emphasize building trust as much as the evaluation of scientific data.
9. Do not promise what you cannot deliver, people will not forget.
10. If you do not know the answer, say so, but find out and follow up.
11. Provide information that meets the needs of the concerned individuals. Do not decide what you think they need to know, listen to what they want to know.
12. Get the facts straight. Check and recheck data before they are presented.
13. Coordinate with others that may be involved at a site.
14. Do not give mixed messages. If it is a minimal risk, why wear protective clothing to take samples?
15. Listen to what stakeholders are telling you.
16. Acknowledge uncertainty of the data.
17. Do not minimize the risk.
18. If trust is low,
    - Acknowledge it.
    - Tell how you will avoid the problem in the future.
    - Ask how you can regain trust.
    - Respond personally, not just in a group setting.
    - Be patient.

Basic risk communication issues

Effective risk communication is difficult for a number of reasons. It depends on the source, channel, message, and receiver. The following are risk communication issues as identified by Lusch and Lusch.[12] The source or expert may be viewed as untrustworthy. Scientific experts often disagree about the data and what they mean, causing confusion for the receiver. The expert may have limited means to address the risk in terms of authority or resources. The person delivering the message may fail to disclose the limitations for addressing risk problems. The expert may have limited understanding of the interests, concerns, fears, values, priorities, and preferences of individuals and groups. Legal and technical language may reduce the effectiveness of the message. Explaining the risk itself is often the most difficult factor because studies conducted to assess the risk are often complex and difficult to understand. Failure to disclose limitations of risk assessments/public health assessments and resulting uncertainties also contribute to problems for the source because the public may reach faulty conclusions without knowledge or understanding of this concept.

The channel or mechanism used to disseminate the message may pose additional challenges to effective risk communication. The media may have biased viewpoints and the reporting of the event may reflect drama, disagreements, and conflicts. The media may disclose information prematurely, which may cause the public to accuse the source of the message of dishonesty and coverup. Oversimplifications, distortions, and inaccuracies in interpreting the technical risk information may support inaccurate conclusions on the part of the public.

The message itself may be a concern. The public will not understand the main message if it is not simply constructed. The lay public cannot comprehend the technical language or jargon of experts. Deficiencies in scientific understanding, data, models, and methods result in large uncertainties in risk assessment and public health assessments, which are difficult to explain simply to a layperson.

The receiver of the message may also influence the success of the risk communication process. People may have inaccurate perceptions of risk as shown by the opinions of experts versus the public. People may have set agendas, values, or viewpoints that are difficult or impossible to change. The need for the public or the patient to be part of the investigation from the beginning, even though they may not understand the integral procedures being conducted, will determine how readily the community accepts the solution. Feelings of injustice and immorality will influence the layperson's reaction to the message. The public's emotions are sometimes difficult to address and, if feelings are ignored because the risk is thought to be negligible, emotions will escalate. The important questions are, Will the exposure cause me to get cancer? Will my unborn child be malformed? Will my child get sick? Exaggerated expectations about the effectiveness of regulatory action are also a problem. People want to simplify the situation involving risk of adverse effects following exposure and be told it is safe or hazardous, but the complexities involved in determining the impact of the contaminant of concern on the health of a community of individuals makes it difficult or impossible to categorize health risks on this basis.

Risk acceptability depends on the level of the risk, as well as the benefits, practical alternatives, the voluntary/involuntary nature of the risk, and community values.[19] The person chosen to present the information needs to be trusted by the community if the effort is to be successful. What tools does the risk communicator use to explain environmental risk? An exposure risk of 1 in 1,000,000 is difficult for people to understand in their everyday experience. Risk communication experts originally encouraged the description of an exposure risk situation through use of the common comparisons of risk to illustrate how the exposure risk in question related to a common risk.

However, experience has shown that risk comparisons should be used with caution, particularly in a low-trust and high-hostility situation. This is especially true when the comparison seems to minimize the risk by equating it to a seemingly trivial event. This angers the stakeholders because they see the comparison as an effort to persuade people that the risk is smaller than they thought. People usually seek enough knowledge to establish their own sense of the seriousness of the risk. Concentration, probability, and quantity are risk-related numbers that have been used to help conceptualize risk. The use of voluntary risks (e.g., smoking) compared with involuntary risks (e.g., pollution) may cause citizens to reject the comparison as invalid. Some experts have developed a graded system of risk comparisons that may be used. These are ranked from the most to least useful below[4]:

1. Comparisons of the same risk at two different times or with a standard. The risk of exposure to hazardous substances such as dioxin is 40% what it was before the scrubbers were installed. Exposure of the patient is within the acceptable limits imposed by the Occupational Safety and Health Administration.
2. Comparisons of the risk of doing something versus not doing it. If the most advanced emission control equipment is purchased, the risk will be reduced. If we do not buy the equipment, the risk will be lowered.
3. Comparisons of average risk at a particular time or location. The risk posed by the emissions of ammonia to the nearest home is 90% less than at the plant gate.
4. Comparisons of risk with cost, risk–benefit, and etiologic factors in illness. To reduce the risk posed by chlorine by 50% will cost $100. X-rays produce far less lung cancer than exposure to natural background levels of geologic radon.
5. Comparisons of unrelated risks. For example, compare the risk for tobacco-related health effects as compared to disease caused by pollutants from the company next door. These comparisons are not recommended.

The use of risk comparisons is not prohibited, but the expert must realize the potential negative impact of the use of comparisons to explain exposure risk. Risk acceptance depends on the level of the risk and the public values. The most important factor is the presence of a trusted community representative to relay this information to the community.

PRINCIPLES OF RISK COMMUNICATION

1. Background: The message should be grounded in an understanding of the patient or the community's needs and concerns.
2. Outline: It is important to think about the available data and the bottom-line message to be presented, as well as what people expect and need to know.
3. Message: In developing the message, make a strong introduction. Remember that trust and credibility are quickly assessed, and include a statement of personal concern in the opening. If you are representing a group or organization, state your intent or purpose. Also describe the format of the meeting. You should expect people to assimilate no more than 3 take-home points from a presentation at a meeting or discussion with a patient. The message must be simply constructed. This main statement followed by explanation to support the primary message is important. Examples help illustrate the main message and further substantiate its validity. The message should end with a conclusion and information about future action. Be sure to provide information about the

background or assessment of the exposure of concern. Where does the data come from? Why are uncertainty factors used? What is the toxicity of the contaminants of concern? What is the alternative to the hazard? What is being done to control the problem? What kind of medical evaluation and treatment is reasonable and available for those exposed? Will testing help to determine whether and to what extent the community was exposed?

4. Avoiding mistakes:
   - Remember the differential knowledge of the source and the receiver.
   - The message must be based on a common language that people can understand without difficulty. This should probably be aimed at the sixth-grade level.
   - The use of jargon or technical language used by experts must not be employed.
   - Avoid charged language, which will increase the concerns of the receiver (i.e., toxic, hazard, poisonous).
   - Simple graphics are worth a thousand words.
   - Determine if English is the first language of the receiver. If not, you may need translation.
   - The outrage factors must be considered in the overall message about the risk.
   - Risk comparisons should be used with caution.
   - Abstract concepts should not be included in the message.
   - Complex numbers are difficult to explain because people want a bottom-line answer. Is it safe or a hazard?
   - Zero risk should be realized as an impossible goal.
5. Practice: Test the message on someone who is not technically trained. Prepare for questions. Practice again with someone else, then rework the message based on comments. Talk to others who have dealt with this exposure risk to determine any lessons that may have been learned from the experience. Do cultural issues influence how the message is perceived?
6. Presentation: Be aware of body language. Does the source feel comfortable in addressing the patient or other receiver? Does the source feel more comfortable behind a desk? Does the presenter listen well to the receiver's concerns and maintain eye contact? Humor should be avoided except in special situations. Think about the unexpected things that might happen. What are the potential sources of conflict? Be caring and honest. Listen carefully to what the receiver asks about the exposure risk.
7. Answering the tough questions. Lack of preparation for questions in clinical practice or at a public meeting can destroy the opportunity to reduce concern and conflicts.

The media plays an important role in educating the lay public about exposures to environmental hazards. The media focuses public attention on specific environmental issues and away from others. Several publications address the importance of understanding the media's view of environmental issues[18] and the steps involved in developing an interview strategy.[1,5]

Experience at ATSDR in addressing public concerns has generated the following general guidelines for developing a good risk communication program:

1. Become knowledgeable of other credible sources involved at the site.
2. Define the issue accurately and honestly.
3. Understand the health risk communication process.
4. Carefully plan messages, materials, and strategies.
5. Help resolve conflicts between stakeholders.
6. Demonstrate personal involvement-accessability.
7. Do not promise what you cannot deliver.
8. Simplicity is key.
9. Take the initiative. Act first not later.
10. Use evaluation to obtain feedback to improve the program.

REFERENCES

1. McLouglin B: *Communicating with power,* New York, 1990, Barry McLoughlin Associates.
2. Covello V: The perception of technological risks, *Technology, Forecasting, and Social Change: An International Journal* 23:285, 1983.
3. Covello V: Risk communication, trust and credibility, *J Occup Med* 35:18, 1993.
4. Covello V, Sandman P, Slovic P: *Risk communication, risk statistics, and risk comparisons: a manual for plant managers,* Washington, DC, 1988, Chemical Manufacturers Association.
5. Donovan E, Covello V, *Risk communication student manual,* Washington, DC, 1989, Chemical Manufacturers Association.
6. Hance BJ, Chess C, Sandman P: *Improving dialogue with communities: a risk communication manual for government,* Trenton, NJ, 1988, New Jersey Department of Environmental Protection.
7. Reference deleted in proofs.
8. Improving Risk Communication, National Research Council, p. 21, 1989.
9. Kahneman D, Tversky A: Prospect theory: an analysis of decisions under risk, *Econometrica* 47:263, 1979.
10. McCallum D et al: *Public knowledge and perceptions of chemical risks in six communities: analysis of a baseline survey,* Washington, DC, 1990, EPA.
11. McCallum DB, Covello VT: What the public thinks about environmental data, *EPA Journal,* May/June: 22, 1989.
12. Lusch R, Lusch VN: *Principles of Marketing,* Boston, 1987, Kent Publishing.
13. Roberts L: Counting on science at EPA, *Science* 249:616, 1990.
14. Roper Poll, March 1990.
15. Sandman P: *Explaining environmental risk,* Washington, DC, 1986, EPA.
16. Sandman P: Facing public outrage, *NAPEC Quarterly* vol 1, issue 1, 1990 from *EPA Journal,* 1987.
17. Sandman P: Facing public outrage, NAPEC Quarterly, vol 1, issue 1, 1990 from *EPA Journal,* 1987.
18. Sandman PM: *Explaining environmental risk,* EPA, pp 1-13, 1986.
19. Slovic P: Perception of risk, *Science* 236:280, 1987.
20. Slovic P, Fischhoff B, Lichtenstein S: Facts and fears: understanding perceived risk. In Schwing RC, Albers WA Jr: *Societal risk assessment: how safe is safe enough?,* New York, 1980, Plenum Press.
21. Tversky A, Kahneman D: Availability: a heuristic for judging frequency and probability, *Cognitive Psychology* 4:207, 1973.
22. Tversky A, Kahneman D: Judgement under uncertainty: heuristics and biases, *Science* 185:1124, 1974.

Appendix A

ENVIRONMENTAL LEGISLATION

Gary Walker
Joyce Martin

National Environmental Policy Act
Environmental compliance statutes
Environmental enforcement provisions
Major federal programs
    Federal Water Pollution Control Act (Clean Water Act)
    Clean Air Act
    Comprehensive Environmental Response, Compensation, and Liability Act (CERCLA or Superfund)
    Resource Conversation and Recovery Act
    Occupational Safety and Health Act
Other important federal programs
    Toxic Substances Control Act
    Federal Insecticide, Fungicide, and Rodenticide Act
    Safe Drinking Water Act
    Emergency Planning and Community Right-to-Know Act of 1986

Environmental law is a system of federal, state, and local statutes, regulations, and judicial decisions intended to protect the environment and related public health and safety. Congress and state legislatures have enacted environmental statutes and laws, and federal and state agencies, along with city and county governments, have adopted regulations and rules protecting the environment. In addition, state and federal courts have decided cases involving environmental laws and regulations, thereby adding to our understanding of how environmental law is applied.

During the 1970s and 1980s the federal government and many state governments enacted dozens of new environmental laws and adopted related administrative regulations implementing the federal statutes. Because of the complexity of these laws and regulations, this chapter presents only an overview of the major environmental laws and applicable regulations. Throughout the chapter, the term *person* includes any individual, corporation, partnership, association, state or federal agency, or any agents or employees of such entities.

NATIONAL ENVIRONMENTAL POLICY ACT

The first contemporary federal law specifically addressing protection of the environment was the National Environmental Policy Act of 1969 (NEPA), which establishes broad goals intended to protect and preserve the country's environmental and natural resources. NEPA requires that all federal agencies analyze alternatives to proposed federal action based on the environmental effects of such action prior to making a decision on the action. The act requires agencies to include an environmental impact statement (EIS) in every recommendation regarding proposals for federal legislation and other major federal actions significantly affecting the quality of the human environment. The EIS must be distributed internally within the agency, to other agencies, and to the public.

NEPA is essentially a procedural statute in that it requires agencies to follow a process in examining the potential environmental impact of governmental action, but the substantive standards by which the proposed action will be evaluated are left to other environmental laws. However, NEPA has forced the review of thousands of federal agency actions, including even agencies that are not directly involved in environmental regulation.

Other major environmental laws may provide certain procedures for complying with the statute, but they also provide substantive environmental protection standards with which governmental agencies and private persons and entities must comply.

ENVIRONMENTAL COMPLIANCE STATUTES

Most major environmental statutes require the U.S. Environmental Protection Agency (EPA) to identify harmful substances and to regulate the handling, emission, discharge, or disposal of those substances. Other significant environmental statutes identify activities harmful to the environment and either regulate or prohibit such activities through other environmental agencies.

Virtually all environmental laws in this country rely on a set of eight general regulatory approaches, which include the following compliance requirements:

1. Notifying, monitoring, and self-reporting current and proposed activities that may have significant environmental effects
2. Imposing controls at the point at which the substance is disposed of, discharged, or released into the environment
3. Placing regulations on the industrial process to reduce the quantity of pollutants and to prevent their release into the environment
4. Imposing product and packaging regulations to minimize waste generation and disposal problems
5. Prohibiting or restricting activities that in themselves have a negative environmental impact
6. Regulating the transportation of regulated substances
7. Requiring clean-up of past pollution
8. Requiring responsible parties to pay directly for clean-up or to compensate other parties that have undertaken clean-up[1]

In addition to requiring compliance with environmental regulations, most major environmental statutes also provide mechanisms for enforcing compliance.

ENVIRONMENTAL ENFORCEMENT PROVISIONS

Although national standards are established by EPA under federal statutes such as the Clean Air Act, the Clean Water Act, and the Resource Conservation Recovery Act (RCRA), those standards are implemented through state permit programs. These federal laws allow the states to set standards that must be as strict as, and may be more strict than, federal standards. EPA approves state programs and in some cases can replace a deficient state program with a federal one.

Environmental enforcement, more so than other regulatory laws, relies primarily on the use of permits. A permit is an individualized enforcement tool that allows EPA and other agencies to define a statute's requirements specifically for one industry or one regulated substance. The permit, in conjunction with the applicable statute and agency regulations, constitutes the law for that industry or substance, and violations of the permit are enforced as strictly as violations of the statute or regulations.

When a person violates an environmental statute, regulation, or permit, the EPA and other environmental agencies have a full range of sanctions available, including administrative orders and fines; civil court injunctions, fines, and damages; and criminal penalties for knowing or negligent violations.

MAJOR FEDERAL PROGRAMS
Federal Water Pollution Control Act (Clean Water Act)

Water pollution laws are among the oldest in the country, dating to the Refuse Act of 1899, which focused on protection on navigation in U.S. waters; however, the existing water regulation system contained in the Clean Water Act was not enacted until 1972. The goals of the act are improving water quality to provide for protection of fish, shellfish, and wildlife and for human recreation, and eliminating discharges of pollutants into U.S. waters.

The primary regulatory mechanisms of the Clean Water Act include the following.

National pollutant discharge elimination system (NPDES) permitting. It is illegal for any person to discharge any pollutant from a point source into waters of the United States without a permit, which sets limits on the types and levels of pollutants that may be discharged. The permit also requires the discharger to report to the permitting agency the volume and type of discharge, as well as any failure to meet pollution discharge limits. A *point source* refers to any discrete conveyance (such as a pipe) from which pollutants are or may be discharged into U.S. waters, which includes navigable waters, ditches, marshes, and almost any wet area.

Under the act most states have assumed primary responsibility for enforcing the NPDES program, but the EPA retains independent enforcement authority over the permitting program in states that have not assumed responsibility for enforcing the program.

In acting on an application for a permit the EPA must give public notice of the permit application and must provide 30 days for public comment prior to action on the permit application. After the agency's decision either to issue or to deny a permit, a discharger may may appeal the decision.

National discharge limitations. The Clean Water Act uses two primary approaches to establish discharge limits into U.S. waters. First, the act requires the EPA to establish nationally applicable, *technology-based effluent limitations* for direct industrial discharges on an industry-by-industry basis, for discharges by publicly owned treatment works (POTWs), and for industrial discharges into POTWs to protect POTW operations and prevent discharges of pollutants that cannot be treated adequately by POTWs. These limitations establish the minimal level of treatment for all discharges, requiring discharges to be treated by methods that are technologically and economically achievable.

The second approach of the act focuses on water quality, rather than simply on discharge treatment technology. Water quality standards limit discharges based on their effect on a specified level of quality in the receiving water. Water quality standards are determined on the basis of the permissible effluent concentration limits necessary to support the designated use of the receiving body of water, such as for water supply, recreation, agriculture, or propagation of fish or wildlife.

States are required to establish water quality standards subject to EPA approval, and if they fail to do so, the EPA will implement its own program. Moreover, states are required to enforce a statewide antidegradation policy designed to maintain and protect existing in-stream uses and existing high-quality waters. Water quality standards may require much higher treatment than technology-based effluent limitations.

The 1977 amendments to the act require such higher treatment for certain priority toxic pollutants and require new, higher performance standards for 21 major industries. With respect to toxic pollutants, states are required to identify all bodies of water that do not meet applicable water quality standards, even with the application of technology-based effluent limits. States must identify individual point-source dischargers blocking the attainment of standards and develop individual control strategies for each such discharger.

Regulation of municipal and industrial stormwater discharges. Although stormwater discharge may contain harmful and even toxic pollutants, only certain municipal and industrial stormwater discharges are regulated by the Clean Water Act. The 1987 amendments to the act regulate

1. Discharges associated with industrial activity
2. Discharges that had NPDES permits as of February 1987
3. Discharges from municipal separate storm-sewer systems serving a population of more than 100,000
4. Other discharges that EPA or an NPDES administrator determines to contribute to water quality violations or that are significant contributors of pollutants

Dredged or fill disposal permitting and wetlands protection. The Clean Water Act requires a special permit from the U.S. Army Corps of Engineers with stringent requirements for dredging or disposing of dredged or fill material into navigable waters, including wetlands adjacent to such waters. Dredged material is material excavated or dredged from a water body, and fill material is any material used to replace water with dry land or to change bottom elevation. Dredging and filling in navigable waters are regulated by the Corps and the EPA, and states may regulate such activity in nonnavigable waters.

Oil and hazardous substance spills. The Clean Water Act prohibits discharges of oil or hazardous substances into waters in quantities that may be harmful to the public health or welfare. The discharger must immediately notify the appropriate agency of any spill of a reportable quantity of hazardous substances or when there is a visible sheen of oil on water.

Strict liability for clean-up costs is imposed on the owner or operator of the vessel or facility from which oil or hazardous substances are discharged. An owner or operator is liable to the United States and/or the state for the cost of clean-up, damages from injury, or loss of natural resources, as well as for penalties.

Clean Air Act

Congress first attempted to control air pollution in 1955, but that legislation proved ineffective, resulting in enactment of the Clean Air Act of 1970, which was amended in 1977 and greatly expanded by the Clean Air Act Amendments of 1990. The goal of the Clean Air Act, as amended, is to respond to the impact of air pollution on public health, welfare, and the environment.

National ambient air quality standards. The Clean Air Act creates national standards for emission of hazardous air pollutants and for new stationary air pollution sources. Notwithstanding the creation of these national standards, the act gives the states the primary responsibility for enforcing air quality laws, and requires the states to meet National Ambient Air Quality Standards (NAAQSs) by a certain time.

The act requires the EPA to establish the NAAQSs for six pollutants that are dangerous to human health or welfare: ozone, carbon monoxide, small particulate matter, sulfur dioxide, nitrogen dioxide, and lead. The two types of NAAQS are primary standards, which are set at a level to protect persons with medical conditions that may be aggravated by pollution and individuals with normal health, and secondary standards, which are established to protect the public welfare (crops, livestock, structures, and so on) from any known or anticipated adverse effects of such pollutants. Primary standards are set with use of health protection as the only test. Cost and the technical feasibility of meeting those standards may not be considered. The Clean Air Act requires review of the NAAQS for adequacy every 5 years.

Under the 1970 amendments each state is required to implement the NAAQS through adoption of a state implementation plan intended to allow local tailoring of air standards to the types of sources and existing levels of pollution within a state. Once EPA has approved the state implementation plan, it becomes the primary mechanism by which the act is enforced under both state and federal law.

To protect areas of the country in which the air is cleaner than that required by national standards, the 1977 and 1990 amendments to the Clean Air Act require the EPA to place each region that complies with NAAQSs into one of three classes. Class I includes national parks and wilderness areas, in which little air quality deterioration is allowed, class II includes areas in which moderate increases in ambient concentrations are allowed, and class III includes areas in which larger increases are permissible to allow industrial development, provided that it does not cause a violation of an NAAQS.

New source performance standards. The Clean Air Act requires the EPA to adopt new source performance standards (NSPSs) for new or modified stationary air pollution sources, such as boilers, utilities, and industrial plants. Those standards must reflect the best available control technology, taking into consideration the cost of compliance. NSPSs for three pollutants resulting from combustion of fossil fuels—particulates, sulfur dioxide, and nitrogen dioxide—must be reduced by a certain percentage below the level that would have resulted without technologic control methods.

National emission standards for hazardous air pollutants. The EPA also is required to set national emission standards for hazardous air pollutants for which no NAAQS had been established and that could be anticipated to cause an increase in mortality or serious illness. The 1990 amendments to the Clean Air Act specify 189 substances as toxic air pollutants that EPA must regulate through technology-based and, when necessary, more stringent health-based standards.

1990 Clean Air Act amendments. In addition to the aforementioned provisions of the 1990 amendments to the Act, those amendments also set new attainment deadlines, create a uniform permitting program that expands the types of stationary sources subject to emission controls under the nonattainment program, and establish timetables and standards to measure progress toward the goals of the Act. In addition, the 1990 amendments address prevention and remediation of acid rain, stratospheric ozone protection, strengthened mobile source emission control, and increased enforcement authority.

The permitting program. The permitting program created by the 1990 amendments is similar to the NPDES permit program under the Clean Water Act in that states are intended to be the air permitting authorities. Also, as in the NPDES permit program, new air permits must contain all the requirements of the Clean Air Act, such that the permits themselves become legally enforceable. Nearly all sources that emit air pollutants are required to obtain permits.

All permit applications, as well as proposed and final permits, submitted to permitting agencies must be reviewed by the EPA and by affected states, that is, those states that are contiguous to the issuing state or within 50 miles of the applicant. The EPA may veto the issuance of a permit by any state and may revoke permits already issued.

The 1990 amendments also add special air-quality and technology-based requirements for new or modified pollution sources in nonattainment areas, that is, where air quality is lower than required by the Clean Air Act. Requirements of the 1990 amendments focus on the specific pollutant involved relative to the extent to which that pollutant exceeds the NAAQS. The 1990 requirements apply to each of the six aforementioned pollutants for which EPA was required to adopt NAAQSs, and those requirements are more rigorous in areas of greater nonattainment.

Acid rain. Acid rain is thought to be caused by sulfur oxide emissions, largely from increased coal combustion. This acid precipitation, which falls frequently in the eastern United States and Canada, renders lakes so acidic that they cannot support fish life. Recent research also suggests direct adverse effects on plant life and indirect adverse effects on soil, crop yields, and buildings. In addition, at least 100 million people in the United States alone are exposed to significant levels of acid rain particles, the health effects of which are not fully known.

The 1990 amendments set total national limits on emissions of particles that cause acid rain and are intended to reduce emissions of sulfur dioxide by 10 million tons annually and emissions of oxides of nitrogen by 2 million tons each year. The acid rain provisions do not replace prior controls but add a new layer of regulations that must be met.

Pursuant to the 1990 amendments, the EPA issues sulfur dioxide emission allowances to pollution sources, which essentially authorize such sources to emit specified levels of sulfur dioxide. The amendments create an allowance trading system designed to permit utilities and other power producers to transfer sulfur dioxide emission authorization. To the extent a source can operate with fewer allowances, it can sell them or bank them for the future. The EPA is required to establish an allowance auction system.

Stratospheric ozone protection. Depletion of the ozone layer increases the level of detrimental ultraviolet radiation, which is linked to skin cancer and reduced crop production. The 1990 amendments provide for the elimination of known and suspected ozone-depleting substances, which the amendments place into two classes. Class I includes chlorofluorocarbons, halons, and carbon tetrachloride, all of which must be phased out in stages by January 1, 2000, and methyl chlorofluorocarbons, which must be phased out by January 1, 2002.

Class II substances are hydrochlorofluorocarbons and other substances that the EPA finds to harm the ozone layer significantly. Production of class II substances will be capped January 1, 2015, and terminated January 1, 2030.

Mobile source emission control. Among the primary pollutants from mobile source emissions are carbon monoxide, hydrocarbons, oxides of nitrogen, and particulate matter. The 1990 amendments enhance EPA regulation of mobile source emissions of these pollutants by strengthening requirements applicable to urban buses, fleet vehicles, and trucks and by expanding EPA regulation of vehicle fuel. The EPA must adopt rules requiring new, light-duty vehicles to have on-board refueling emission-control systems, and such light-duty vehicles are subject to a phased-in reduction of emissions of these pollutants, beginning in 1994. In addition, diagnostic systems to identify emission-related failure or dysfunction are required in vehicles in model year 1994 and later.

The EPA also must adopt regulations for emissions from intercity buses, locomotives, and new engines used in locomotives and for certain ozone nonattainment areas that will require use of reformulated gasoline in those areas. The EPA is also required to establish a demonstration program in California for alternative-fuel vehicles.

Comprehensive Environmental Response, Compensation, and Liability Act (CERCLA or Superfund)

The Comprehensive Environmental Response, Compensation, and Liability Act of 1980 (CERCLA) was created to allow the federal government to clean up leaking hazardous waste sites. Although CERCLA was substantially expanded by the Superfund Amendments and Reauthorization Act of 1986 (SARA), it continues to focus primarily on old waste sites. CERCLA is also known as the "superfund" law because of the more-than-$5 billion Hazardous Substances Trust Fund (created by section 111 of the act), which is used to pay for removal and remedial actions to clean up releases of hazardous substances to the air, water, or land.

Because CERCLA deals with all three environmental media, it is much broader than the Clean Air Act or the Clean Water Act. Moreover, CERCLA is broader than those acts in that it governs virtually any type of facility and defines hazardous substances more broadly than does any other act. Pursuant to section 101(14) of the act, hazardous substances include all substances designated as hazardous or toxic by EPA under the Clean Air Act, Clean Water Act, RCRA, and Toxic Substances Control Act (except that petroleum and natural gas are expressly excluded). In addition, the EPA's list of hazardous substances includes a number of other substances that could present a substantial danger to health or the environment.

The primary regulatory mechanisms of CERCLA include the following.

Information gathering and establishing priority sites. The EPA is given broad authority to conduct inspections at sites at which hazardous wastes are or were generated, stored, treated, disposed of, or transported to or from. Section 103 of CERCLA requires owners and operators of hazardous waste storage, treatment, or disposal sites to notify the EPA of the types, amounts, and possible releases of such substances from those facilities. The EPA also may request and obtain all records regarding operations at those facilities. From this and other related information, the EPA develops the National Priorities List of hazardous sites that may be eligible for clean-up using funds from the $5 billion trust fund.

Releases and types of clean-up. EPA action and private liability for clean-up under CERCLA are triggered by the release or threat of release of a hazardous substance into the environment. Section 101(22) of CERCLA broadly defines *release* of a hazardous substance to include virtually any way in which a substance can enter the environment. The EPA has authority to deal with an emergency by seeking a judicial order or issuing an administrative order requiring persons involved in the release to take certain actions. The EPA can enter a facility to determine the need for response as well as to inspect the premises and collect samples.

Section 104 of the Act establishes the federal authority to take emergency action to remove hazardous substances and to remedy leaking sites. A removal is a short-term, immediate response such as taking leaking containers of hazardous waste away from a site, and a remedy is a long-term, more expensive action such as extensive excavation of an abandoned hazardous waste site.

Section 121 of CERCLA imposes stringent clean-up standards, in which the preferred remedies are those that permanently and significantly reduce the released hazardous substance. On-site remedial technologies are preferred to off-site transport and treatment. If the remedial action leaves material on site, the government is required to review the remedial action at least once every 5 years and will take further action if necessary. Thus, potentially responsible persons are subject to potential future liability even after a remedial action is completed.

Responsible parties and liability under CERCLA. CERCLA makes persons who are responsible for releases of hazardous substances liable for the costs of clean-up and restitution. Section 107 of the Act provides that owners and operators of hazardous storage, treatment, and disposal sites, as well as generators and transporters of hazardous substances, are liable for costs of removal or remedial action, other necessary cost incurred by other persons in clean-up, and damages to natural resources resulting from hazardous releases.

Courts have held CERCLA liability to extend to the following persons:
1. Current owner or operator
2. Past owner or operator at the time of disposal
3. Generator or transporter
4. Lessor and lessee
5. Successor and assignee
6. Shareholder, director, or officer
7. Lender or creditor (based on active participation by the lender in the management of the vessel or facility).

However, the 1986 amendments create an exception for "innocent landowners," who acquire property and, after all appropriate inquiry into the previous uses of the property, have no reason to know that hazardous substances have been disposed on the property. Innocent landowners also may include a government entity that acquired the property involuntarily or through eminent domain and an owner who acquired the property by inheritance or bequest.

CERCLA liability is not based on fault or negligence but on strict liability, such that a person may be liable even though he or she may have exercised the highest degree of care in handling the hazardous substance that ultimately was released. Moreover, CERCLA liability is generally joint and several, that is, each person is liable for the full amount of the clean-up costs. Joint-and-several liability allows the government to recoup clean-up costs without having to sue each potentially responsible person and without having to establish the degree of responsibility of each person. Persons who pay for such clean-up may sue other persons responsible for the release.

Private rights of action. In addition to government action for clean-up costs, private parties may bring suit to recover from the responsible parties the costs of responding to a release of hazardous substances. Prior government approval is not required before a private action is brought to recover response costs; however, only the federal government may bring an action for injunctive relief under CERCLA. The statute does not create a private cause of action for injunctive relief.

In addition to private actions to collect clean-up costs, the 1986 amendments authorize citizen suits to challenge the sufficiency of remedial action before clean-up is completed. In a citizen suit, if a court finds that the remedies being applied are inadequate in protecting health or the environment, the clean-up can be modified prior to completion.

Settlements. Section 122 of CERCLA directs the EPA to pursue settlement agreements whenever practicable and in the public interest to expedite effective clean-up and minimize litigation. The EPA must notify each potentially responsible party (PRP) of the names and addresses of all other PRPs, the volume and nature of substances contributed to the facility by each PRP, and a ranking by volume of the substances at the facility, to the extent such information is available.

When a PRP receives notice that the EPA wants to begin settlement negotiations, he or she has 60 days to make an offer to undertake or finance the response action. If the PRP agrees to settle with the EPA, section 122(c) of the act authorizes EPA to include a promise not to seek additional clean-up costs from the party involved in the settlement. Moreover, section 113(f) protects the PRP who settles from actions by other PRPs for contribution.

Resource Conservation and Recovery Act

The RCRA was enacted in 1976. The Act, which has been amended several times since its adoption, addresses problems involved in the disposal of hazardous waste, which includes medical waste. Hazardous waste includes any solid waste that, because of its concentration, quantity, or its chemical, physical, or infectious characteristics, may cause or contribute to increased mortality or serious illness or may pose a significant hazard to human health or the environment. With many sites, the most serious risk is toxic substances infiltrating groundwater and contaminating public drinking water.

Historically, much hazardous waste has been transported from the generation site by independent transporters to off-site disposal locations, which have a typical active life of 20 years. Disposal sites often routinely received hazardous waste from a variety of transporters, often without knowledge of identity of the generator or the nature of the waste. With no requirement of maintaining adequate records, there was little means of determining the environmental risk of the waste. Moreover, once a site becomes inoperative, subsequent owners of the site may not learn of its use as a hazardous waste site.

The RCRA addresses these problems by establishing comprehensive cradle-to-grave control of current hazardous waste by regulating generators and transporters of hazardous waste, and owners and operators of treatment-storage-and-disposal (TSD) facilities. The primary regulatory mechanisms of RCRA include the following.

Identification of hazardous waste. Section 3001 of RCRA requires the EPA to establish criteria to identify hazardous waste. Before a material can be classified as hazardous waste, it must first fall within the RCRA definition of *solid waste,* which includes

any garbage, refuse, sludge from a waste treatment plant, water supply treatment plant or air pollution control facility and other discarded material, including solid, liquid, semisolid, or contained gaseous materials resulting from industrial, commercial, mining and agricultural activities and from community activities but does not include solid or dissolved material in domestic sewage, or solid or dissolved materials in irrigation return flows or industrial discharges, which are point sources subject to permits under section 402 of the Federal Water Pollution Control Act, as amended, or source, special nuclear, or byproduct material as defined by the Atomic Energy Act of 1954, as amended.

This broad definition applies to almost all waste, no matter what its physical form, including liquid and contained gases; however, EPA rules exclude many materials from regulation as hazardous waste to exclude minor hazardous substances and focus instead on substances that have a major adverse impact on human health and the environment.

Under the RCRA the EPA regulates two types of hazardous waste. Listed wastes are those that appear on any of the four lists published in the hazardous waste regulations at 40 C.F.R. part 261, subpart D. Characteristic wastes are those wastes not specifically listed but covered because they are ignitable, corrosive, reactive, or toxic.

Hazardous waste management program

Generators and transporters. Generators are entities that create hazardous waste, usually within their business operations. Section 3002 of the RCRA imposes requirements on generators of hazardous waste, including reporting, labeling, record-keeping, and use of appropriate containers for hazardous waste. The Act uses a hazardous waste manifest, which stays with the waste at all times to track the hazardous waste to its proper disposal. Generators may not transport, treat, store, or dispose of hazardous waste without an EPA identification number. Generators also must follow the manifest requirements to track the journey of the hazardous waste from its creation through transportation and storage to its final disposal site. Those requirements include (1) using an acceptable manifest (a paper form to record pertinent information); (2) designating an EPA-approved facility as the waste's destination; (3) providing copies of the manifest for the generator, each transporter, the designated facility, and return to the generator; and (4) signing the manifest and obtaining the signature of the transporter.

Before transferring the hazardous waste to a transporter, the generator must package and label the waste according to EPA standards. The generator may store hazardous waste on-site for as long as 90 days without qualifying as a TSD facility and without being required to obtain a TSD permit or interim status. Interim status allows a facility to store waste prior to receiving a permit. The generator storing hazardous waste for 90 days or less is required to label, store, and manage the waste properly pending shipment of the waste to a permitted facility within 90 days. Pursuant to the 1984 amendments to the RCRA, the EPA applies slightly less stringent requirements to small-quantity generators (those that produce less than 1000 kg of hazardous waste per month).

The RCRA defines a transporter as any person engaged in the off-site transportation of hazardous waste by air, rail, highway, or water and includes both interstate and intrastate transport. Section 3003 of the Act requires transporters of hazardous waste to use the same manifest system as generators and requires similar labeling, handling, and record-keeping by transporters.

Transporters must have an EPA identification number and can accept hazardous waste for transport only if a manifest has been signed by the generator of the waste. Transporters must deliver the entire shipment of hazardous waste either to the next transporter or to the designated facilities, and if the shipment cannot be delivered, transporters must contact the generator for further instructions. Transporters are subject to both EPA and Department of Transportation regulations.

TSD Facilities. The last stage of the cradle-to-grave regulation of hazardous waste is contained in section 3004 of the RCRA, which governs TSD facilities.

Treatment is defined broadly to include facilities in which hazardous waste is subjected to any method or process designed to alter the waste physically, biologically, or chemically, to make it nonhazardous or less hazardous, or to recover energy or resources from the waste. *Storage* involves holding the hazardous waste for a temporary period of time before transferring the waste to another entity or site. *Disposal* involves intentionally placing the hazardous waste into or on land or water, where the waste will remain after closure of the site.

EPA regulations require TSD facilities to comply with the waste manifest system and to maintain certain other records. TSD facilities also must obtain a permit from the EPA or an EPA-authorized state. 1984 amendments to section 3004 of the RCRA require new or expanded TSD facilities to have double liners, leachate collection systems, and groundwater monitoring systems unless the EPA deter-fjmines that a facility has an equally effective alternative design. The amendments also require the owner or operator of a TSD to provide proof of financial ability to comply with applicable RCRA standards and prohibit continued dumping of liquids and certain other types of waste after certain dates.

All TSDs are subject to closure requirements when they no longer accept hazardous waste. Closure activities include completing treatment and disposal practices and preparing a detailed plan for closure. In addition, TSDs must provide for groundwater monitoring and for maintaining other monitoring and waste-containment devices for 30 years after closure of the facility.

Regulation of nonhazardous solid waste. Subtitle D of the RCRA makes states responsible for nonhazardous solid waste. The EPA's role in this regulation is limited to its adoption of standards for nonhazardous waste disposal sites. Facilities that do not meet the standards are automatically classified as open dumps, which must either be closed or placed on an enforcement schedule to meet standards; however, unlike other RCRA standards, the EPA has no authority to enforce these standards, which are left to the states to enforce.

Medical waste. Of special interest to physicians and other health care providers is the Medical Waste Tracking Act of 1988, which added medical waste to the list of hazardous waste regulated by the EPA under the RCRA. Under this act, the EPA established 2-year demonstration projects in New York, New Jersey, Connecticut, and states bordering the Great Lakes. In 1991, the Act was extended by 2 years so that Congress could amend the RCRA to create a permanent medical waste program for the entire country.

The Act requires the EPA to regulate infectious waste, human blood and blood products, pathologic waste, patient-care and laboratory sharps, and contaminated animal remains. As with other hazardous waste covered by the RCRA, this Act requires special containers, labeling, transportation, and waste manifests for all medical waste.

Occupational Safety and Health Act

The Occupational Safety and Health Act (OSH Act), enacted in 1970, is largely a labor-related statute but also has significant environmental aspects. The OSH Act and other environmental statutes such as the RCRA, the Clean Air Act, and the Clean Water Act each deal with many of the same health hazards and issues, such as asbestos, carcinogens, vinyl chloride, hazard labeling, and the like. The primary difference between the OSH Act and the other statutes is that the OSH Act focuses on these issues in the workplace. Although the EPA enforces the other environmental statutes, the OSH Act is enforced by the Occupational Safety and Health Administration (OSHA) within the U.S. Department of Labor.

Purpose, scope, and duties. Section 2(b) of the OSH Act states the purpose of the act, to ensure as far as possible that workplaces in this country are safe and healthful. The act has been broadly construed to apply to all private-sector employers whose business affects interstate commerce. The OSH Act excludes governmental employees, although federal employees are covered pursuant to presidential order in 1980, and 23 states have OSHA-approved employee health and safety plans.

The OSH Act imposes two obligations on employers. The general duty clause in section 5(a)(1) of the act requires employers to provide employment and a place of employment "free from recognized hazards that are causing or likely to cause death or serious physical harm." In addition, section 5(a)(2) requires employers to comply with specific, detailed health and safety standards adopted by OSHA pursuant to section 6(b) of the OSH Act.

OSHA standards. OSHA standards that apply to virtually all employers are known as general-industry standards, but certain industries such as shipbuilding, construction, and paper mills have their own health and safety standards, referred to as specific-industry standards. Specific standards have priority over general ones in these industries, but general-industry standards apply in these industries when there is no specific-industry standard applicable to a particular safety issue.

OSHA standards govern matters such as environmental hazards involving ventilation, air contaminants, and exposure to hazardous and toxic substances; fire safety and other physical and structural hazards; health and medical issues; and personal protective equipment. OSHA health standards often can be characterized as air-containment standards or general environmental and health standards. Both involve, among other elements, medical surveillance, record-keeping, monitoring, and physical review.

Of increasing importance in OSHA is the hazard communication standard (29 C.F.R. part 1910), which requires employers to inform workers of hazardous chemicals in the workplace. Employers comply with the standard by maintaining material safety data sheets, ensuring proper container labeling, and providing training on each hazardous chemical.

OSHA inspections. The OSH Act provides for OSHA inspection of workplaces to ensure compliance with the act. When a violation is found, the OSHA inspector is authorized to issue a written citation and provide the employer with a proposed penalty and a correction date. The employer can contest the existence of the violation, the amount of the penalty, and the time for correction. Under certain circumstances, the employer can obtain variances from a standard. In all violation cases, section 9(b) requires the employer to keep the employees informed of the status of the violation, case, or variance.

OTHER IMPORTANT FEDERAL PROGRAMS
Toxic Substances Control Act, 15 U.S.C. §§ 2601-2629

The Toxic Substances Control Act of 1976 controls toxic substances by requiring manufacturers to test potentially hazardous chemical substances and by regulating their production, use, distribution, and disposal.

Section 4 of the act authorizes the EPA to require manufacturers to conduct tests on new substances to determine their effects on human health and the environment. Section 5 requires manufacturers to give notice to the EPA prior to manufacturing a new chemical substance and to provide the EPA with premanufacture notification of results from any tests required under section 4. Limited exemptions to premanufacture notification are available, such as in situations in which the EPA determines that a new substance will not pose an unreasonable risk to health or the environment, for certain research and development uses of small quantities of a chemical, and for certain test marketing if it does not pose unreasonable risks.

Section 6 empowers the EPA to remove substances from the market or to restrict the production, use, or distribution of a substance that poses unreasonable risk of injury to human health or the environment. Using this authority, the EPA has banned production of use of such substances as polychlorinated biphenyls, chlorofluorocarbons, and asbestos.

Federal Insecticide, Fungicide, and Rodenticide Act

The Federal Insecticide, Fungicide, and Rodenticide Act (FIFRA) in section 136 requires that all new pesticides be registered with the EPA prior to use. The manufacturer must provide the formula of the product, a label that complies with the Act, and the results of all tests of the pesticide. The registration is approved unless the EPA determines that the pesticide presents an unreasonable risk of harm to humans or the environment.

Section 136 requires the EPA to classify pesticides as general or restricted. Restricted products may be used and applied only by certified applicators. Other restrictions relate to issues such as application methods and amounts, geographic area of use, and limitation of use to specified pests.

FIFRA also provides the EPA with a wide range of cancellation and suspension authority to stop the distribution, sale, and use of pesticide products that pose a substantial question of human or environmental safety. The process normally gives the pesticide registrant the right to notice of the intended action and an opportunity to present evidence opposing the proposed action, but in emergency suspensions these rights may be circumscribed. The EPA has used this authority to cancel the registration of pesticides such as DDT, kepone, and chlordane.

In addition to regulation under FIFRA, pesticides also may be regulated under other environmental statutes, such as the Clean Air Act, the Clean Water Act, and the OSH Act, as well as by the Food, Drug and Cosmetic Act when the pesticide appears in food products.

Safe Drinking Water Act

The Safe Drinking Water Act (SDWA) was enacted in 1974 to ensure safe drinking-water supplies, protect the purity of aquifers, and prevent contamination of drinking water by regulating the underground injection of waste. The Act requires the EPA to identify substances that contaminate drinking water and to set maximum contaminant levels (MCLs) for each of those substances.

MCLs apply to public water systems that supply water at least 60 days per year to at least 15 connections or to 25 or more persons. States are allowed to implement the SDWA if their water standards are no less stringent than the federal standards.

The primary focus of underground injection-control regulations is on hazardous waste disposal and mining and gas-production processes. In addition to injection-control programs, the EPA is authorized under the SDWA to designate an aquifer as the sole source of an area's drinking-water supply to provide special protection for that aquifer beyond that in other parts of the SDWA.

Emergency Planning and Community Right-to-Know Act of 1986

The Emergency Planning and Community Right-to-Know Act (EPCRA) was passed as part of the 1986 Superfund Amendments. EPCRA requires state and local governments to prepare hazardous chemical emergency plans to respond to releases of such chemicals. Sections 301 to 303 of the act require the creation a state emergency response commission in each state and designation of emergency planning districts with local planning committees.

Pursuant to the EPCRA, the EPA has adopted a list of extremely hazardous substances, and section 302 of the act requires that all facilities with such substances above a specified quantity notify the state commission, the local planning committee, and the local fire department of the presence of those substances. Such facilities also must notify the commission and committee of releases of such substances. In addition, the EPCRA requires certain manufacturing facilities to report annually on total annual releases of certain chemicals.

The EPCRA provides the public and certain individuals, such as firefighters and health care professionals, with new rights of access to information on hazardous chemicals. The law also provides relatively severe civil and criminal penalties for violations of the statute or its regulations.

REFERENCE

Environmental Law Handbook, ed 11, Rockville, Md, 1991, Government Institutes, Inc.

Appendix B

POISON CONTROL CENTERS

Paytricia Hiatt
Kent Olson
Virginia H. Sublet

Poison control centers first came into existence around 1953 to help physicians deal with poisoning of adults and children in the United States. In 1957 the National Clearinghouse for Poison Control Centers (Division of Poison Control, Food and Drug Administration Bureau of Drugs) was created to aid centers by providing information about the toxicity of household products and treatment and to help analyze poisoning reports from these centers. Because of federal funding limitations the National Clearinghouse curtailed many of its services by the early 1980s. In 1983 the American Association of Poison Control Centers (AAPCC) was established as the professional organization for poison control centers. The AAPCC has developed a National Data Collection System to tabulate various information about the poisoning cases reported to Poison Control Centers nationwide. Since its inception the number of reported poisonings has increased each year, from 251,012 in 1983 to 1,837,939 in 1991, as indicated in the most recent annual report of the AAPCC National Data Collection System (1992). Of the exposures reported in 1991, 36,859 were occupational and 25,588 were environmental.

In the 1960s approximately 600 poison control centers existed in the United States, ranging from a telephone in the emergency department answered by available staff to the establishment of a specific program in a health care facility to deal exclusively with the treatment of poisonings, consultation, professional training, and outreach programs. The number of poison control centers has been significantly reduced, and today there are approximately 100 centers.

Of these centers, approximately 38 are designated as regional poison control centers, which have a special certification awarded by the AAPCC. To obtain this certification, poison centers must fulfill a number of requirements, including 2-hour service; have adequate personnel to handle the numbers of telephone calls coming to the center, sufficient information resources and protocols to provide accurate and complete information, a medical director, a managing director, certified poison information specialists (who have passed a certification examination), educational staff to develop outreach programs, a working relationship with regional treatment facilities, participation in regional and national data collection, and association membership.

Poison control centers are being asked to expand their role from dealing with acute drug and consumer poisonings to include hazardous exposures encountered in the occupational and environmental settings. In this regard, only a few poison control centers have been adequately prepared to address these exposures; however, because the public and health care practitioners are increasingly in need of information about these exposures, these centers are actively seeking to expand their expertise in this area. To meet these needs, poison control centers are acquiring resources to provide better information about chemical hazards, becoming trained in occupational and environmental toxicology and linking themselves to appropriate consultants to help health care professionals better serve their patients. These centers are also beginning to participate in acute exposure situations that require emergency response actions. In this regard, the regional poison control centers can act as a valuable resource in providing information about the toxicity and health effects of hazardous exposures involved in these disasters to emergency responders, emergency medical service personnel, or emergency department staff.

AMERICAN ASSOCIATION OF POISON CONTROL CENTERS
Certified Regional Poison Centers, April 1993

ALABAMA

Regional Poison Control Center, The Children's Hospital of Alabama, 1600 7th Ave. South, Birmingham, AL 35233-1711
Emergency Phone: (205) 939-9201, (800) 292-6678 (Alabama only), or (205) 933-4050

ARIZONA

Arizona Poison and Drug Information Center, Arizona Health Sciences Center, Rm. #3204-K, 1501 N. Campbell Ave., Tucson, AZ 85724
Emergency Phone: (800) 362-0101 (Arizona only), (602) 626-6016

Samaritan Regional Poison Center, Good Samaritan Regional Medical Center, 1130 E. McDowell, Suite A-5, Phoenix, AZ 85006
Emergency Phone: (602) 253-3334

CALIFORNIA

Fresno Regional Poison Control Center of Fresno Community Hospital and Medical Center, 2823 Fresno St., Fresno, CA 93721
Emergency Phone: (800) 346-5922 or (209) 445-1222

San Diego Regional Poison Center, UCSD Medical Center; 8925 225 Dickinson St., San Diego, CA 92103-8925
Emergency Phone: (619) 543-6000, (800) 876-4766 (in 619 area code only)

San Francisco Bay Area Regional Poison Control Center, San Francisco General Hospital, 1001 Potrero Ave., Building 80, Room 230, San Francisco, CA 94122
Emergency Phone: (415) 476-6600

Santa Clara Valley Medical Center Regional Poison Center 751 South Bascom Ave., San Jose, CA 95128
Emergency Phone: (408) 299-5112, (800) 662-9886 (California only)

University of California, Davis, Medical Center Regional Poison Control Center, 2315 Stockton Blvd., Sacramento, CA 95817
Emergency Phone: (916) 734-3692, (800) 342-9293 (Northern California only)

COLORADO

Rocky Mountain Poison and Drug Center, 645 Bannock St., Denver, CO 80204
Emergency Phone: (303) 629-1123

DISTRICT OF COLUMBIA

National Capital Poison Center, Georgetown University Hospital, 3800 Reservoir Rd., NW, Washington, DC 20007
Emergency Phone: (202) 625-3333, (202) 784-4660 (TTY)

FLORIDA

The Florida Poison Information Center at Tampa General Hospital, P.O. Box 1289, Tampa, FL 33601
Emergency Phone: (813) 253-4444 (Tampa), (800) 282-3171 (Florida)

GEORGIA

Georgia Poison Center, Grady Memorial Hospital, 80 Butler St. S.E., P.O. Box 26066, Atlanta, GA 30335-3801
Emergency Phone: (800) 282-5846 Georgia only; (404) 589-4400

INDIANA

Indiana Poison Center, Methodist Hospital of Indiana, 1701 N. Senate Blvd., P.O. Box 1367, Indianapolis, IN 46206-1367
Emergency Phone: (800) 382-9097 (Indiana only), (317) 929-2323

MARYLAND

Maryland Poison Center, 20 N. Pine St., Baltimore, MD 21201
Emergency Phone: (410) 528-7701, (800) 492-2414 (Maryland only)

MASSACHUSETTS

Massachusetts Poison Control System, 300 Longwood Ave., Boston, MA 02115
Emergency Phone: (617) 232-2120 or (800) 682-9211

MICHIGAN

Blodgett Regional Poison Center, 1840 Wealthy S.E., Grand Rapids, MI 49506-2968
Emergency Phone: (800) 632-2727 (Michigan only), TTY (800) 356-3232

Poison Control Center, Children's Hospital of Michigan, 3901 Beaubien Blvd., Detroit, MI 48201
Emergency Phone: (313) 745-5711

MINNESOTA

Hennepin Regional Poison Center, Hennepin County Medical Center, 701 Park Ave., Minneapolis, MN 55415
Emergency Phone: (612) 347-3141, Petline: (612) 337-7387, TDD (612) 337-7474

Minnesota Regional Poison Center, St. Paul–Ramsey Medical Center, 640 Jackson St., St. Paul, MN 55101
Emergency Phone: (612) 221-2113

MISSOURI

Cardinal Glennon Children's Hospital Regional Poison Center, 1465 S. Grand Blvd., St. Louis, MO 63104
Emergency Phone: (314) 772-5200 or (800) 366-8888

NEBRASKA

The Poison Center, 8301 Dodge St., Omaha, NE 68114
Emergency Phone: (402) 390-5555 (Omaha), (800) 955-9119 (Nebraska)

NEW JERSEY

New Jersey Poison Information and Education System, 201 Lyons Ave., Newark, NJ 07112
Emergency Phone: (800) 962-1253

NEW MEXICO

New Mexico Poison and Drug Information Center, University of New Mexico, Albuquerque, NM 87131-1076
Emergency Phone: (505) 843-2551, (800) 432-6866 (New Mexico only)

NEW YORK

Hudson Valley Poison Center, Nyack Hospital, 160 N. Midland Ave., Nyack, NY 10960
Emergency Phone: (800) 336-6997 or (914) 353-1000

Long Island Regional Poison Control Center, Winthrop University Hospital, 259 First St., Mineola, NY 11501
Emergency Phone: (516) 542-2323, 2324, 2325, 3813

New York City Poison Control Center, N.Y.C. Department of Health, 455 First Ave., Room 123, New York, NY 10016
Emergency Phone: (212) 340-4494, (212) P-O-I-S-O-N-S, TDD (212) 689-9014

OHIO

Central Ohio Poison Center, 700 Children's Dr., Columbus, OH 43205-2696
Emergency Phone: (614) 228-1323, (800) 682-7625, (614) 228-2272 (TTY), (614) 461-2012

Cincinnati Drug and Poison Information Center and Regional Poison Control System, 231 Bethesda Avenue, M.L. 144, Cincinnati, OH 45267-0144
Emergency Phone: (513) 558-5111, 800-872-5111 (Ohio only)

OREGON

Oregon Poison Center, Oregon Health Sciences University, 3181 S.W., Sam Jackson Park Rd., Portland, OR 97201
Emergency Phone: (503) 494-8968, (800) 452-7165 (Oregon only)

PENNSYLVANIA

Central Pennsylvania Poison Center, University Hospital, Milton S. Hershey Medical Center, Hershey, PA 17033
Emergency Phone: (800) 521-6110

The Poison Control Center serving the greater Philadelphia metropolitan area, One Children's Center, Philadelphia PA 19104-4303
Emergency Phone: (215) 386-2100

Pittsburgh Poison Center, 3705 Fifth Ave. at DeSoto St., Pittsburgh, PA 15213
Emergency Phone: (412) 681-6669

RHODE ISLAND

Rhode Island Poison Center, 593 Eddy St., Providence, RI 02903
Emergency Phone: (401) 277-5727

TEXAS

North Texas Poison Center, 5201 Harry Hines Blvd., P.O. Box 35926, Dallas, TX 75235
Emergency Phone: (214) 590-5000, Texas WATS (800) 441-0040

Texas State Poison Center, The University of Texas Medical Branch, Galveston, TX 77550-2780
Emergency Phone: (409) 765-1420 (Galveston), (713) 654-1702 (Houston)

UTAH

Intermountain Regional Poison Control Center, 50 North Medical Dr., Salt Lake City, UT 84132
Emergency Phone: (801) 581-2151, (800) 456-7707 (Utah only)

VIRGINIA

Blue Ridge Poison Center, Box 67, Blue Ridge Hospital, Charlottesville, VA 22901
Emergency Phone: (804) 924-5543 or (800) 451-1428

WEST VIRGINIA

West Virginia Poison Center, 3110 MacCorkle Ave., S.E., Charleston, WV 25304
Emergency Phone: (800) 642-3625 (West Virginia only), (304) 348-4211

Appendix C

GOOD INFORMATION ABOUT HAZARDOUS SUBSTANCES

Virginia H. Sublet

Printed materials
  Books
  Fact sheets
  Case studies, profiles, and criteria documents
  Newsletters
Electronic data bases
  On-line computer systems
  On-line access
  Microcomputer data bases
  CD-ROM systems
  CD-ROM access
Organizations and groups
Responsibilities of key federal agencies
Summary

Over the last several years legislation such as the Comprehensive Environmental Response, Compensation, and Liability Act of 1980, Superfund Amendment and Reauthorization Act of 1986 (SARA), the Occupational Safety and Health Administration Hazard Communication Standard, and local right-to-know laws have increased public awareness of the hazards associated with exposures in the workplace and the environment. As communities have become more concerned about the significance of these exposures, physicians have begun to receive more inquiries from patients regarding health effects.

Accidental and intentional exposure to natural and man-made poisons is a serious public health problem. In 1991, 1,837,939 poisonings were reported to the American Association of Poison Control Centers (Annual Report, *Emergency Medicine,* September, 1992). This statistic is considered only a minimal estimate of the number of actual poisonings occurring that are unreported. This conclusion is based on the prevalence of drug prescribing, with the danger of side effects and drug interactions; the improper use of consumer and industrial products containing hazardous chemicals that may result in illness and injury; and the significant health effects resulting from chronic or acute exposures to hazardous substances in the workplace or environment that occur in the United States.

Because the public has become increasingly aware of the potential health effects associated with exposure to hazardous chemicals and because the use of chemicals in industry and manufacturing is escalating, health care professionals in private practice, public health, emergency medicine, emergency medical services, and poison control centers are increasingly being faced with situations that require a knowledge of occupational and environmental toxicology.

What constraints affect physicians' treatment of patients exposed to hazardous chemicals? The report from the National Academy of Sciences/Institute of Medicine on the *Role of the Primary Care Physician in Occupational and Environmental Medicine* (1988) states that one of the leading concerns of physicians about treating occupational and environmental exposure cases is the "lack of information support available to the primary care practitioner." Most physicians have used journals, texts, and hard-copy materials to obtain information about unknown areas of expertise. Referrals are also a popular resource for information. Computer data bases have been less used. The leading recommendation from the National Academy of Sciences report to aid the primary care practitioner to function effectively and knowledgeably when faced with a patient whose symptoms suggest an occupational or environmental disease was to have a "single-access point for all necessary clinically pertinent information." Currently, this point is being investigated but is not a reality. Therefore, available resources, including printed materials, computer data bases, and telephone numbers that may be helpful to the health care professional regarding hazardous exposures, are the focus of this appendix. See also Table 65-2 for resources useful to the medical practitioners who respond to chemical emergencies.

PRINTED MATERIALS

A number of factors must be considered in the use of printed information materials. They are less current than electronic data bases. Information is often found in many different references and not compiled in one resource. There is often a lack of information diversity. Finding answers to questions can be frustrating and require significant time. Many printed resources are extremely expensive, costing several hundred dollars. One of the great advantages of use of these materials is that the printed material is available to read at one's leisure without dependence on a computer to retrieve this information. Significant printed materials, including books, factsheets, case studies/profiles/criteria documents, and newsletters, are discussed on the following pages.

The books listed below are helpful in obtaining background information about hazardous chemicals.

Books

Klassen CD, Amdur MO, Doull J, eds: *Cassarett and Doull's toxicology: the basic science of poisoning,* ed 4, New York, 1991, Macmillan.

Target: Toxicologists and physicians

Topics: Groups of chemicals. Text designed to describe toxic responses and mechanisms, not treatment. Useful as a background resource.

Agency for Toxic Substances and Disease Registry: *Chemical emergencies: hospital emergency department guidelines,* Atlanta, 1991.

Target: Emergency medical services (EMS) personnel and physicians

Topics: Information on emergency department response to hazardous material incidents, patient management, planning systems, and the like. Good information for first responders and emergency medical personnel.

Agency for Toxic Substances and Disease Registry: *Chemical emergencies: guidance for the management of chemically contaminated patients in the prehospital setting,* Atlanta, 1991.

Target: Emergency response personnel

Topics: Basic information on hazard recognition, decontamination and assessment of victims, resources available for planning how to handle emergency incidents. Valuable resource.

Proctor NH, Hughes JP, Fischman ML: *Chemical hazards in the workplace,* Philadelphia, 1988, JB Lippincott.

Target: Physicians and toxicologists

Topics covered: Specific chemicals (400)
Very useful medical and toxicology information. Easy to use, contains information on exposure routes, toxicology, diagnosis of poisoning, and treatment. Medical treatment information is useful. Excellent resource; concise; does not give complete medical treatment information.

US Coast Guard, Department of Transportation: *CHRIS (chemical hazards response information system),* Washington, DC, 1985, US Government Printing Office.

Target: Emergency response personnel

Topics: Gives chemical and physical properties, fire hazards, toxicity and symptoms, and first-aid treatment. No medical treatment information.

Gosselin RE, et al: *Clinical toxicology of commercial products,* Baltimore, 1990, Williams & Wilkins.

Target: Physicians and toxicologists

Topics: Commercial chemical products. Very useful toxicology information for poisonings in the home due to commercial products. Very useful textbook.

Sax NI: *Dangerous properties of industrial materials,* New York, 1988, Van Nostrand Reinhold.

Target: Toxicologists

Topics: Information on 19,000 industrial chemicals. A massive handbook.

Bronstein AC, Currance PL: *Emergency care for hazardous materials exposure,* St. Louis, 1988, CV Mosby.

Target: EMS

Topics: Provides 82 guidelines for a variety of chemicals. Provides good initial medical management information. Hospital treatment not addressed. Principal concerns are the lack of secondary contamination information and recommendation of SCBA for response to all hazardous materials.

Department of Transportation: *Emergency response guidebook,* Washington, DC, 1990, US Government Printing Office.

Target: Emergency responders

Topics: Information on commonly transported chemicals. First-aid information; no medical treatment. Essential for emergency response personnel.

Rom W, Editor: *Environmental and occupational medicine,* Boston, 1992, Little, Brown.

Target: Physicians and toxicologists

Topics: This textbook focuses on the mechanisms of occupational disease and injury, target systems, agents, physical environment, personal and general environment, and control measures. A classic in the field of occupational medicine.

National Fire Protection Association: *Fire protection guide on hazardous materials,* ed 9, Quincy, Mass, 1986, The Association.

Target: Firefighters

Topics: Covers a wide variety of chemicals. Life-hazard information is brief. Useful for first responders.

Dreisbach RH: *Handbook of poisoning: prevention, diagnosis and treatment,* ed 12, Norwalk, Conn, 1987, Appleton & Lange.

Target: Physicians and toxicologists

Topics: Covers general classes for chemicals. Inadequate medical information.

Rosenstock L, Cullen MR, eds: Textbook of occupational, and environmental medicine, Philadelphia, 1994, WB Saunders.

Target: Clinicians

Topics: An up-to-date and useful resource focusing on evaluation and treatment as well as the hazards and toxicology, primarily in the occupational setting.

Sittig M: *Handbook of toxic and hazardous chemicals and carcinogens,* ed 2, Park Ridge, NJ, 1985, Noyes.

Target: Physicians and toxicologists

Topics: Medical treatment not included. Contains identification numbers, exposure sources, incompatibilities, routes of entry, medical surveillance procedures, personal protective procedures, and respiratory protection.

Sax NI, Lewis RJ: *Hazardous chemicals desk reference,* New York, 1987, Van Nostrand Reinhold.

Target: Emergency responders, EMS, toxicologists, physicians

Topic: Consists of information on chemicals, including hazard rating, CAS, DOT, physical properties, synonyms, and current standards for exposure limits. Abstracted version of *Dangerous properties of industrial chemicals,* but easier to carry. Good reference.

Stutz DR, Janusz SJ: *Hazardous materials injuries: a handbook for pre-hospital care,* ed 2, Greenbelt, Md, 1988, Bradford Communications.

Target: EMS

Topics: Provides field treatment protocols in the form of guidelines. Covers 300 chemicals. Protective clothing recommendations are excessive. Hospital treatment not addressed.

Borak J, Callan M, Abbott W: *Hazardous materials exposure: emergency response and patient care,* Englewood Cliffs, NJ, 1991, Brady.

Target: EMS and health care providers

Topics: Provides good emergency response information about treatment of victims in the field; recognition of hazardous materials; personal protective clothing, planning the EMS response; injuries to the lungs, eyes, and skin; systemic complications; and so on. A well-written reference book.

Sullivan JB, Kreiger GR, editors: *Hazardous materials toxicology,* ed 1, Baltimore, 1992, Williams & Wilkins.

Target: Physicians and toxicologists

Topics: Provides information on basic scientific principles, regulatory safety, emergency response, industry and sites, and specific toxins. Most of the book is devoted to a discussion of specific toxins. A good reference book.

Ricks RC, Leonard RB: *Hospital emergency department of radiation accidents,* 1984, Emergency Management Institute, National Emergency Training Center.

Target: Physicians

Topic: Covers basic principles of medical care for radiation-accident victims in the hospital emergency department. Represents the Federal Emergency Management Authority recommendations for these incidents.

Ellenhorn M, Barcelaux D: *Medical toxicology: diagnosis and treatment of human poisoning,* New York, 1988, Elsevier.

Target: Toxicologists and physicians

Topics: Covers a wide variety of chemicals. Well written, with good discussions of toxicology and treatment of chemical poisoning. Very good textbook.

Mackison FW: *NIOSH/OSHA occupational health guidelines for chemical hazards,* Washington, DC, 1981, Department of Health and Human Services.

Target: Physicians and toxicologists

Topics: Contains information on symptoms, medical monitoring procedures, and respiratory and personal protective equipment use. Gives first-aid information.

Zenz C, editor: *Occupational medicine,* Chicago, 1993, Year Book.

Target: Physicians and toxicologists

Topics: Covers the clinical, physical, and chemical aspects of occupational disease. Discusses the work categories of concern, psychosocial considerations, epidemiology, reproductive toxicology, investigation of health hazards, occupational considerations for women, and the like. Classic textbook in occupational medicine.

Clayton GD, Clayton FE: *Patty's industrial hygiene and toxicology,* ed 4, New York, 1990, John Wiley & Sons.

Target: Toxicologists and physicians

Topics: A comprehensive four-volume textbook on chemicals. Medical treatment is not major emphasis, but a very good reference for toxicology.

Olsen K: *Poisoning and drug overdose,* San Mateo, Calif, 1990, Appleton and Lange.

Target: Physicians and toxicologists

Topics: Well-written reference on chemical exposures. Good medical treatment information. Valuable resource.

Arena JM, Drew RH, editors: *Poisoning,* ed 5, Springfield, Ill, 1986, Charles C Thomas.

Target: Physicians and toxicologists

Topics: General information about poisonings. Subjects include pesticides, industrial hazards, occupational diseases, environmental hazards, drugs, and consumer products. Excellent information on toxicology. Good textbook.

Hayes AW: *Principles and methods of toxicology,* New York, 1982, Raven Press.

Target: Toxicologists and physicians

Topics: Contains a thorough introduction to toxicology. Current testing procedures, guidelines, and so on are discussed. A valuable resource.

Morgan DP: *Recognition and management of pesticide poisonings,* ed 4, Washington, DC, 1988, US Environmental Protection Agency.

Target: Physicians and toxicologists

Topics: Organized by class of pesticide. Discusses treatment procedures. Good information. Easy-to-use resource.

Goldfrank LR, et al: *Toxicologic emergencies,* ed 3, Norwalk, Conn, 1986, Appleton-Century-Crofts.

Target: Physicians and toxicologists

Topics: Chemicals, pharmaceutical, botanicals, and food poisoning are covered. Good overview of toxicology; discusses treatment alternatives. Very useful textbook.

Fact sheets

Fact sheets provide quick, easy-to-read information about chemicals, which is an advantage to busy physicians. A number of state health departments, such as that in New Jersey, have prepared chemically specific fact sheets that provide information about symptoms and medical management procedures. The Hazard Evaluation System and Information Service, a part of the California State Health Department, also has prepared fact sheets available to physicians and other health care professionals. The Environmental Protection Agency (EPA) has developed fact sheets for a number of extremely hazardous substances. These sheets provide no medical treatment information but supply first-aid directions.

Case studies, profiles, and criteria documents

The Agency for Toxic Substances and Disease Registry (ATSDR) has developed the *Case Studies in Environmental Medicine* and *Toxicological Profiles*. The *Case Studies in Environmental Medicine* are self-instructional documents that provide continuing medical education for physicians. The *Case Studies* discuss the symptoms, diagnosis, treatment, and surveillance of exposure to hazardous substances. Fifteen of these documents have been completed, and 15 more are currently being written. They are available at no cost from ATSDR.

The *Toxicological Profiles* are longer documents that include a public health statement written in nontechnical language. The remainder of the profile contains very detailed information and is meant for toxicologists, physicians, and others needing technical information about health effects, chemical and physical properties, exposure limits, production, releases into the environment, and similar information. More than 100 of these profiles are available through NTIS.

The National Institute for Occupational Safety and Health (NIOSH) and the EPA both have developed comprehensive *Criteria Documents*. These documents review the toxicology research that is the basis of recommended exposure standards and are available from the respective agencies.

Newsletters

Newsletters generally contain new findings and events in a brief journalistic format. A number of state and federal agencies, as well as private industry, offer these information materials. ATSDR publishes *Hazardous Substances and Public Health*, the Agency newsletter, which provides health care professionals a forum for exchanging information about environmental health. Subscriptions are free to primary-care providers and other health professionals.

ELECTRONIC DATA BASES

The development of computerized data bases has revolutionized the retrieval of up-to-date, accurate, and comprehensive information. These resources are valuable to health care professionals, because when treating a patient exposed to hazardous substances the health care provider can obtain information about the health effects and treatment of exposure to these chemical hazards.

Data bases are commonly accessed through on-line retrieval of information, floppy disk, or compact disc–read only memory (CD-ROM). Each of these media is discussed in subsequent sections.

Data bases can provide factual information, providing information similar to a handbook of chemical facts; or bibliographic information, containing the names of journal articles, reports, documents, and so on. Special-purpose bulletin boards also can be a valuable resource because of the large variety of topics included and the meetings listed. In addition, there are whole-text (complete articles from journals); special-purpose (for example, Agricola, which is concerned with food and agriculture); and directory (for example, Directory of Databases) data bases. This section on information resources concentrates on factual, bibliographic, and bulletin-board data bases.

A number of factors influence the use of electronic data bases. Health professionals have not had the opportunity to learn about computer data bases until recently and thus have not been aware of these available toxicology resources and their usefulness. Many electronic data bases have been created without professional or legal precedents to standardize the materials presented. Initial investment in computer equipment can be costly. The advantages of use of electronic media to search for toxicology information include the speed of retrieval of information, the diversity of information available from one source, the ease of searching the user-friendly data bases, and the up-dated quality of material obtained.

On-line computer systems

On-line systems require a computer modem to dial up a mainframe located at an outside location to access the required information. The information obtained from the mainframe is shown on the user's terminal and can be printed. The disadvantages of use of on-line systems are as follows: (1) The strategies necessary to search these data bases have not been user-friendly and in the past required special education. (Many of these data bases are developing menu-driven systems to make searching easier.) (2) The expense involved when inexperienced users search on-line can be very costly. (Charges are made on a per/hour basis.) The advantages of the on-line system are that information obtained is current and this system provides the greatest versatility and comprehensiveness in obtaining different kinds of information because several data bases can be cross-searched.

On-line access

The Toxicology Data Network (TOXNET), developed by the National Library of Medicine (NLM), is a computerized system of files oriented to toxicology and related areas. The following files are currently included in TOXNET.

The Hazardous Substance Data Bank (HSDB), toxicology data base, was developed by NLM and ATSDR. It is a factual, peer-reviewed data base of more than 4200 chemicals. Records have 12 different information categories, including substance identification, manufacturing/use, chemical/physical properties, safety and handling, toxicity, biomedical effects, pharmacology, environmental fate/exposure summary, exposure standards and regulations, monitoring and analysis methods, additional references, and express data. It includes annotated medical treatment information derived from the Poisindex data base. It is currently being revised into a menu-driven, user-friendly resource to increase its utility to a number of different groups in need of comprehensive information that is easy to search. This change will be particularly helpful for physicians.

The Registry of Toxic Effects of Chemical Substances (RTECS), a factual data base, provides information on more than 100,000 potentially toxic chemicals, including toxicity data, chemical identifiers, National Toxicology Program test status, exposure standards, and so on. RTECS is built and maintained by NIOSH.

The Chemical Carcinogenesis Research Information System, a factual resource, provides scientifically evaluated data from carcinogenicity, mutagenecity, tumor-promotion, and tumor-inhibition tests on 2100 substances that have been evaluated according to criteria and protocols widely accepted by experts in carcinogenesis.

The Toxic Release Inventory was created by NLM and the EPA. It is a record of estimated releases to the environment reported by industries of more than 300 toxic chemicals, based on information collected by EPA as mandated by SARA. This data base will have community interest as it becomes known to the public.

The Integrated Risk Information System is an EPA data base that contains chemically specific information on more than 370 chemicals. It contains information on reference doses, carcinogenic information, drinking-water health advisory, risk management, and supplementary data.

The Developmental and Reproductive Toxicology Database (DART) is a bibliographic data base containing citations to literature published on birth defects and other aspects of reproductive and developmental toxicology since 1989. The file currently contains more than 1500 records. Plans call for the addition of approximately 3600 records each year. DART continues the Environmental Teratology Information Center Backfile (ETICBACK) file. DART is funded by the National Institute of Environmental Health and Safety (NIEHS) and the EPA.

The Environmental Mutagen Information Center (EMIC) is a bibliographic data base on chemical, biologic, and physical agents that have been tested for genotoxic activity. It contains citations from literature after 1988. The data base is produced by the Oak Ridge National Laboratory in Oak Ridge Tennessee, and is funded by the federal government.

The Environmental Mutagen Information Center Backfile (EMICBACK) is the backfile for the EMIC data base. EMICBACK is a bibliographic data base on chemical, biologic, and physical agents that have been tested for genotoxic activity. It contains approximately 71,000 citations from literature published from 1950 to 1988, including some references published earlier than 1959. The data base is produced by the Oak Ridge National Laboratory in Oak Ridge, Tennessee, and is funded by the federal government.

The Directory of Biotechnology Information Resources (DBIR) is a multicomponent data bank containing information on a wide range of resources related to biotechnology. The resources include on-line data bases and networks, bulletin boards, publications such as books and compendiums, organizations, and collections. The DBIR file currently contains 1400 records.

ETICBACK is a bibliographic data base containing more than 49,000 citations to publications concerning teratology and developmental toxicology. It covers publications dating from before 1950 through 1988. This data base was produced by Oak Ridge National Laboratory in Oak Ridge, Tennessee. ETICBACK is continued by the DART database.

Genetic Toxicology is a product of the EPA; this data base explores the area of chemicals and genetic toxicology.

Other selected On-Line Computer Databases provide toxicology information.

Toxicology Information On-Line (TOXLINE/TOXLIT), from the NLM, is specifically designed to offer comprehensive bibliographic coverage of toxicology information. It covers the pharmacologic, biochemical, physiologic, environmental, and toxicologic effects of chemicals and drugs. Sixteen subfiles can be searched in this data base, and approximately 2.5 million references are found in it. Subfiles are from *Chemical Abstracts, Biological Abstracts, International Pharmaceutical Abstracts,* and so on. TOXLINE is available through the NLM MEDLARS System.

MEDLINE (NLM) is the most familiar data base used by health care practitioners. It is the on-line version of *Index Medicus.* It is a bibliography that indexes more than 3200 journals published in the United States and abroad. It can easily be accessed through the menu-driven Grateful Med.

Chemical Abstracts provides worldwide information about chemical sciences, literature from more than 12,000 journals, patents, books, conference proceedings, and government research reports.

NIOSHTIC (NIOSH Technical Information Center Database) is a compilation of information about toxicology, epidemiology, industrial hygiene, and other areas of occupational safety and health in abstract form. It is produced by NIOSH.

Hazardline (BRS) provides emergency-response, safety, regulatory, and health information on more than 4000 chemicals.

Material Safety and Data Sheets for hazardous substances at a workplace are made accessible to employees by mandate of the Occupational Safety and Health Administration (OSHA) of the Department of Labor.

National Pesticide Information Retrieval System contains registration information on 45,000 pesticides registered by the EPA. It includes specific information about the chemicals, studies, and related documents submitted to the EPA by companies seeking registration.

Reprotox (Reproductive Toxicology Center) includes information on reproductive toxicology. It is an inexpensive data base, is easy to search, and provides a beginning to do more extensive evaluation of these exposures. It contains information about drugs and chemicals.

Bulletin boards. Bulletin boards provide broad information on various subjects. They are accessed by dialing into a telephone number to an on-line system.

DOT/FEMA Hazmat bulletin board. The Hazardous Materials Information Exchange is operated by the Federal Emergency Management Agency (FEMA) and the Department of Transportation (DOT). It includes calendars of events and conferences, listings of literature references, data bases, instructional materials, events, regulations, organizational resources, and electronic messaging.

Microcomputer data bases

The microcomputer data base operates via floppy disk. This type of data base involves the use of a microcomputer and disk drive for the floppy disk containing the data base information. An example of this kind of data base is discussed herein.

Disadvantages include the possible damage to the floppy disk making the system, the limit in the amount of material that can be stored, and the lack of current information. Because of the development of the CD-ROM technology, this access medium is not greatly used.

The Computer-Aided Management of Emergency Operations (CAMEO) program is a data base that uses a floppy disk as the information medium. This data base is designed primarily for emergency planners and first responders. It contains response information on more than 2500 chemicals; an air-dispersion model to evaluate release scenarios and evaluation options; and a group of easily adaptable data bases that can be used to organize response information. This response information can include facility-specific maps with chemical storage locations; contact lists; special population concentrations, such as school and hospitals; response resources; material safety data sheets; and digitized maps of the planning area, overlaid with plumes calculated by the air model for any of the chemicals in the data base. It does not include medical information.

CD-ROM systems

CD-ROM systems use a compact disc reader and a computer software package to read the information on a compact disk (see Figure 6). The CD-ROM systems store a large amount of material, are generally very easy to use, and require minimal time for instruction. In addition, the CD-ROM systems are a known budget item, and users can search for any length of time without additional cost. Because the CD-ROMs are updated quarterly, the information is not as current as that obtained from on-line searching, which is a disadvantage of use of this system. In addition, the compact disc system does not have the same power in searching other data bases as does the on-line system.

CD-ROM access

The following are a few of the CD-ROM databases available.

Canadian Center of Occupational Health and Safety has developed the Canadian Center Information Disk System (CCINFO). The CCINFO disc series consists of three disks and can be purchased very inexpensively. The main disadvantage of the CCINFO system is that it not as user friendly as some of the other CD-ROM products available. Once search strategies are learned, users can gain access to a number of data bases.

1. Chemical Information Series A1 includes material safety data sheets; Tradenames, a data base with more than 50,000 chemicals; Cheminfo, a database of health and safety information on chemicals; and Videotex information packages.
2. Chemical Information Series A2 includes Chem Source; Cheminfo; Pesticide Management, Research Information System; Chemical Infogram; RIPP–Regulatory Information on Pesticides; 49 CFR; CESARS–Chemical Evaluation Search and Retrieval System; NiPERA; and New Jersey Information Sheets.
3. Chemical Information Series B1 includes OSH-CAN-DATA–Canadian occupational health studies, resources, case law, mining accidents, and so on.
4. Chemical Information Series B2 includes OSH-INTERDATA CIS International Labor Organization (CISILO); International Directory of Occupational Safety and Health Institutions; INRS bibliographic database, organizations; INET-research projects (INRS).
5. Chemical Information Series C1 includes NIOSHTIC.
6. Chemical Information Series C2 includes the NIOSH Registry of Effects of Chemical Substances (RTECS).

Micromedex developed the Poisindex CD-ROM system used in poison control centers, containing toxicology information on drugs and consumer products. The TOMES-Plus (Toxicology, Occupational Medicine and Environmental Series Information System) provides toxicology information about short- and long-term exposure to occupational and environmental chemicals. It is a very easy system to search.

The TOMES-Plus System includes Meditext, which contains detailed information on the evaluation and treatment of individuals exposed to industrial chemicals and OSHA permissible exposure limits information; Hazardtext—information on spills, leaks, and fires that may occur in a hazardous materials incident; Saratext—acute and chronic effects of hazardous substances (assists with SARA Title III medical reporting requirements); Infotext—regulatory listings and general information documents; Reprorisk—reproductive risk data about effects of chemicals and environmental agents; First Medical Response Protocols—emergency response to workplace illness and injury; RTECS from NIOSH—compendium of toxicology data on more than 100,000 chemicals; NIOSH Pocket Guide—critical industrial hygiene data for approximately 400 chemicals, including concentrations, exposure limits, and respiratory recommendations; HSDB from the NLM—extensive reviews of the toxicity and hazards of more than 4000 chemicals; DOT Emergency Response Guides—initial response to fires, explosives, and releases involving hazardous chemicals; the U.S. Coast Guard's Chemical Hazard Response Information System (CHRIS)—provides information about the chemical and physical properties of hazardous substances to assist in dealing with emergency situations; the Oil and Hazardous Materials/Technical Assistance Data System (OHM/TADS), developed by the EPA—contains information on petroleum products; IRIS, from the EPA—health and environmental risk assessments for more than 450 chemicals; and New Jersey Hazardous Substance Fact Sheets from the New Jersey Department of Health—employee-oriented exposure-risk information for more than 700 hazardous substances.

Silverplatter has produced a number of CD-ROM discs that can be helpful to health care professionals needing toxicology information in an emergency response situation. A number of compact discs available from this company are mentioned herein. Silverplatter discs are very user friendly.

1. CHEM-BANK includes RTECS, OHMTADS, CHRIS, and HSDB on one disc.
2. OSH-ROM includes NIOSHTIC; the HSALINE, data base of the United Kingdom's Health and Safety Executive; and CISDOC, from the International Labour Organization. The Major Hazard Incident Data Service provides information on more than 3000 major accidents involving chemicals.
3. PEST-BANK contains information on the U.S.-registered pesticides used in agriculture, industry, and general commerce. The information comes from the National Pesticide Information Retrieval System (NPIRS). It contains information on the synonyms, registration dates and registering companies, composition and formulation, sites, pests affected by the pesticide, and the like.
4. TOXLINE is toxicologic information from the NLM. It includes references to published materials on drugs, food, chemicals, occupational hazards, pesticides toxicologic analysis, and so on.
5. MEDLINE contains bibliographic citations and abstracts of biomedical literature.

TELEPHONE RESOURCES

Agency for Toxic Substances and Disease Registry Emergency Response
 404-639-0615
CHEMTREC—Chemical Manufacturers Association
 24-hr. hotline for chemical spill information 800-424-9300
 Non-emergency number 800-262-8200
National Pesticide Telecommunications Network
 800-858-7378
NIOSH Technical Information Service
 800-35-NIOSH (800-356-4674)
Occupational and Environmental Reproductive Hazards Center
 508-856-6162
OSHA Technical Support
 202-219-7031
Poison Control Centers (see Appendix B)

ORGANIZATIONS AND GROUPS

Developing a network of colleagues can be very helpful for the emergency physician or primary care practitioner. The Association of Occupational/Environmental Clinics is a network of 30 clinics throughout the United States that are dedicated to occupational and environmental medicine. This clinic network will eventually expand to cover all states. These professionals can be helpful as consultants regarding the treatment of patients exposed to hazardous chemicals. The National Association of County Health Officers covers more than 4000 jurisdictions in the United States. It is composed of local and county health professionals who are becoming significantly involved in dealing with situations concerned with environmental health. Many state health departments are developing environmental health programs to educate health care professionals about the hazards of exposure to toxic chemicals. The poison control center system in the United States can provide invaluable help during an emergency response incident. Appendix B discusses the use of these facilities and their locations throughout the country.

RESPONSIBILITIES OF KEY FEDERAL AGENCIES

ATSDR is responsible for preventing or mitigating the adverse human health effects and diminished quality of life resulting from exposure to hazardous substances in the environment. It carries out health assessments and health studies. In addition, it provides information resources and training programs for health professionals to help them become more aware of the symptoms, diagnosis, treatment, and surveillance of patients who may have been exposed to hazardous substances. ATSDR also has an emergency consultation function in case of emergency accidents. It has no regulatory function.

The EPA administers nine comprehensive environmental protection laws (see Appendix A). It carries out Title III reporting requirements. It is responsible for the remediation of hazardous waste sites as designated by Superfund laws. It has regulatory responsibility.

The Department of Transportation (DOT) establishes the nation's transportation policy. It is responsible for issuing standards and regulations relating to the transportation of hazardous materials from state to state nationwide. It has regulatory responsibility.

FEMA is responsible for coordinating all civil emergency planning, management, mitigation, and assistance functions of the federal government. SARA Title III establishes this agency as primarily responsible for planning and related training for hazardous materials emergency management. This authority encompasses accidents at manufacturing, processing, storage, and disposal facilities, as well as hazardous materials in transit by highways, on water, by rail, and by air. FEMA assists the states and local communities regarding emergency planning.

OSHA is charged with enforcing workplace health and

safety standards. OSHA regulates the training of emergency personnel involved in emergency response actions and the training of workers who have potential contact with toxic compounds. OSHA sets standards for worker exposure to hazardous substances.

NIOSH is responsible for conducting research on workplace health and safety. NIOSH is required to provide assistance when imminent hazards are suspected.

SUMMARY

Exposure to hazards in the workplace and the environment are a frequent occurrence. The publication of information such as the Toxic Release Inventory allows citizens to determine what chemicals directly influence the quality of life where they work and live. Knowledge of the name of the chemical, however, does not mean that citizens know what health effects or disease risks are associated with exposure to it. It is known that patients regard their physicians as the most trusted person to advise them. Therefore, it is highly likely that the physician will be queried about such problems. In addition, primary care practitioners are increasingly likely to encounter an acutely exposed patient or one that is suffering from disease due to a chronic exposure. For these reasons, health care professionals must become aware of the resources that can help them diagnose and treat these conditions.

REFERENCES FOR INFORMATION RESOURCES SECTION

Sublet V: *Information resources, hotlines, databases,* American Medical Association Conference, 1989.

Wexler P: *Information resources, hotlines, databases,* New York, 1988, Elsevier.

Deck K, Bonzo S: *Some publicly available sources of computerized information on environmental health and toxicology,* Atlanta, 1990, Centers for Disease Control.

INDEX

A

Aberrant differentiation theory, 80-81
Abortion (spontaneous), reproductive toxins and, 74, 97
Absorption, 15f, 17, 37, 38
 of asbestos, 442
 carcinogens and, 84
 in children vs. adults, 123
 developmental toxicology and, 120-123
 dioxin and, 135
 eye exposure and, 38; see also Eyes/vision
 gastrointestinal, 301
 of lead, 131
 of mercury, 132
 of organic solvents, 133
 percutaneous, 184-186, 263-265
 of pesticides, 134, 135
 photochemical transformation and, 186-187
 promotion of, 70
 toxicology and, 66, 67, 71
Acceptable daily intake (ADI), 44, 498t, 501-502
Accidents, 28; see also Emergency
Acetaminophen, 124, 303
Acetic acid, 422, 178
Acetone, 25, 422
Acetylcholine, 141, 147
Acetylcholine-esterase inhibitor; see Aldicarb
Acetylcholine
 gastrointestinal tract and, 301
 respiratory toxicology and, 172, 172
Acetylcholinesterase, neurotoxicity and, 323-324
N-Acetyltransferase, 358
Acid aerosols, 23, 676
Acid rain/precipitation, 676, 746
Acids, 606
 blindness caused by, 38
 carboxylic, 600, 601
 dermatoses and, 266t
 eyes/vision and, 243-244
 in household products, 401
 outdoor air pollution and, 464, 465, 467
 solid waste management and, 633
Acne, 265t, 266; see also Chloracne
Acquired immune deficiency syndrome (AIDS), 147-149, 278
 ears/hearing and, 255
Acrodynia, 119
Acrolein, 21t, 174-175
 fire and, 472t, 474
 tobacco smoke and, 422
Acrylamide, 130, 191t, 322t, 601
Acrylonitrile, 21t, 503-504, 601
ACTH; see Adrenocortical trophic hormone
Activity level/fitness, 67; see also Exercise, physical
Acute mountain sickness (AMS), 579-580, 581
Acute myeloid leukemia (AML), 211-213
Acute nonlymphatic leukemia (ANLL), 211-212
Acute toxicity, 18
Additivity, 73
Adenine, 209
Adenomatous polyposis, 83t
Adenosine triphosphate, 133
ADH; see Antidiuretic hormone
Adhesives, 233
Adolescents, workplace environment and, 408-415
Adrenocortical trophic hormone (ACTH), 103, 162

Tables are indicated by a t following the page number and figures by an f.

Adriamycin, bleomycin, vinblastine, and dacarbazine (ABVD), 213
Adult respiratory distress syndrome (ARDS), 288-290
Aerosols, 39, 41-42, 135
 children and, 390, 465
 immunotoxicology and, 151
 nickel, immunotoxicology and, 151
 outdoor air pollution and, 465, 467
Aerospace medicine, 6, 576-591
Affective symptoms, 134, 191, 197-198; see also Emotional consequences
Aflatoxins, 90
Age, 14, 15
 cancer and, 91
 DNA and, 73
 heat stress and, 569
 immunosurveillance and, 160
 immunotoxicology and, 148t
 inhalation exposure, 38
 susceptibility and, 359
 toxicology and, 115-128
Agency for Toxic Substances and Disease Registry (ATSDR), 31, 190, 233, 595
 asbestos and, 451
 biomarkers and, 306
 hazardous waste and, 637, 641
 responsibilities of, 761
 risk communication and, 739, 742
Agent Orange, 272, 496
Agents, 3, 12-13; see also Hazards (environmental)
 cancer and, 87, 90, 93
 causative; see Causative agents/causality
 clinical diagnosis and, 229-231
 cluster studies and, 53
 included in early environmental medicine, 6
 interaction between host, environment, and, 14f, 17
 in occupational settings, 6
 presence of inordinate numbers of, 40
 selection of, in exposure assessment, 39-40
 susceptibility and, 355-356
 toxic, classification of, 68; see also Toxicology
 tumors specific to certain, 87, 90
Agglutination, and immunology of cancer, 157
Agriculture, 626
 global aspects of, 684-687
 methane and, 672; see also Methane
AIDS; see Acquired immune deficiency syndrome
Air, 4, 43
 children's intake of, 377
 direct discharge into, 10, 11f
 environmental history and, 233, 234
 exposure assessment and, 38
 preventive medicine and, 6
 toxicology and, 66f, 67
Air cleaners, 468
Air monitoring, 726
Air pollution/contamination, 4, 13f, 15f; see also Breathing zones; Clean Air Act
 approach to problem of, 428-431
 ambient; see Air pollution/contamination, outdoor
 benzene and, 205; see also Benzene
 breathing zones and, 119
 cancer and, 86
 children and, 390-397
 chronic pulmonary disease and, 362-364
 community standards regarding, 43-44
 control procedures for, 431-434
 dermatitis and, 335
 developmental toxicology and, 120f
 environmental science and, 4

 eyes/vision and, 242-243
 exposure assessment and, 38, 40, 41-42
 gases and vapors and, 41; see also Gases; Vapors
 immune system and, 74
 indoor, 25-26, 419-437
  asbestos and, 441-442, 448
  carbon monoxide and, 135
  children and, 391-393
  comprehensive standards regarding, 44
  environmental history and, 233
  examples of, 423-425
  exposure assessment and, 38, 43-44
  gastrointestinal-induced disorders and, 305
  human factors influencing responses to, 425-426
  humidity and, 432
  industrial standards for, 44
  inhalation and, 38; see also Inhalation
  pets and, 424, 425, 432-433
  room air-cleaning devices (RACDs) and, 433-434
  sources of, 420-423
 from meterologic inversion, 166
 modification of, 17
 multiple exposure pathways for, 16f, 17
 outdoor, 22-25, 462-469
  air quality standards for; see National Ambient Air Quality Standards (NAAQS)
  carbon monoxide and, 135, 136
  children and, 393-395
  control strategies for, 467-468
  environmental history and, 233
  eyes/vision and, 243
  inhalation exposure and, 38
  ozone in, 150; see also Ozone
  photochemical, 23
  respiratory toxicology and, 166-181
  soil contamination and, 4, 521
  solvents and, 130
  susceptibility and, 355, 357
  waterborne pollutants and, 4
Air ventilation, 40-41
Airway inflammation/resistance, 282-285, 355
Alar (daninozide), 120, 499
Alcohol, 600-601
 cancer and, 92
 concentration of, in blood, 40
 ears/hearing and, 254t, 260
 improving patients' life-style in regard to, 730
 male reproductive function and, 98
 neurobehavioral testing for toxicity and, 191
 neurotoxicity and, 324
 susceptibility and, 353
 toxicology and, 70
 vestibular disorders and, 260
Aldehydes, 600, 601
 respiratory toxicology and, 173, 174-175
Aldicarb, 149, 379, 381-382; see also Acetylcholine-esterase inhibitor
 in food, 499
 in well water, 480t
Aldicarb sulfoxide (ASO), 499
Aldrin, 21t, 135, 604
 in well water, 480t
Algae, 41
Alimentary tract, autoimmunity and, 343t
Aliphatics, 599-600
Alkaline phosphatase, placental, 158t
Alkalis
 dermatoses and, 266t
 eyes/vision and, 244
 in household products, 401

Alkylating agents
 aplastic anemia and, 204t, 209
 dermatoses and, 274
 leukemia and, 213
 nephrotoxicity and, 314t
Alkyl benzene aromatics, 133
Alkyl sulfonates, 209
Allergens, 12t, 141
 immune system and, 328-348, 335
 immunotoxicology and, 149, 152-153
 indoor, 422t, 424-425
 nickel and, 152
 ozone and, 150
 respiratory toxicology and, 174, 177, 187-188
Allergic alveolitis, 222
Allergic bronchopulmonary aspergillosis (ABPA), 336
Allergic conjunctivitis, 243
Allergic contact dermatitis (ACD), 152, 182, 186-188, 266
 immune system and, 335
Allergic reactions, 12
 immune system and, 328-329
 indoor air pollution and, 421t
 to insects, 425, 433
 to pets, 424, 425, 431-432
 Types I and IV, 152
Allergic rhinitis, 329-330
ALOHA data base, 726
Alpha$_1$-antitrypsin, 172, 174
Alpha-fetoprotein (AFP), 158, 162
Aluminum, 18
 in drinking water, 44t
 as EPA priority chemical, 21t
 food contamination and, 494
Ambient air
 respiratory toxicology and, 174, 233
 quality standards for, 745-747; see also National Air Ambient Quality Standards (NAAQS)
Amides, 601
Amidopyrine, 204t, 208
Amines
 dermal toxicology and, 187
 immune system and, 328
 immunotoxicology and, 141, 146, 147
 man-made fibers and, 458
 respiratory toxicology and, 173
Amino acids, 195
 bone marrow toxicology and, 206
 developmental toxicology and, 120
 liver and, 301-302
δ-Aminolevulinic acid (ALA), 131, 210, 211
Aminopyrine, 204t, 208
Aminotriazone, 605
Amitrol, 605
Ammonia, 401, 606
 from blueprint machines, 422
 as EPA priority chemical, 21t
 eyes/vision and, 244
 respiratory toxicology and, 168
 respiratory tract disorders and, 287t
 solid waste management and, 633
Amniocentesis, 112
Amniotic fluid, 122
Analgesics, 152
 ears/hearing and, 254t
 nephrotoxicity and, 313
Anaphylaxis, 147, 152, 327-328
Anaplasia, 79
Androstenedione, 103
Anemia, 152, 201-212
Aniline dyes, 254t
Animals, 17
 allergens derived from, 152
 bioconcentration by, 13, 15f, 17, 69-70
 bites and stings by, parenteral exposure to, 38
 bone marrow toxicology and, 210, 212
 dander from, 25

763

764 INDEX

Animals—cont'd
  diseases transmitted by, 620
  dose-response curve and inbred laboratory, 72
  epidemiology and, 46
  extrapolation to humans from (risk assessment), 33-34
  in female reproductive studies, 107, 109-111, 112
    endpoints used in, 110, 111, 113
    litter-mate effect in, 111
  immunotoxicology and, 149, 149-153
  in vitro testing vs. testing in, 76
  neurobehavioral testing for toxicity and, 192-193, 198
  neurotoxicants and, 135
  as pets, and indoor air pollution, 424, 425, 431-432
  rights of, 76
  sentinel event strategies and, 20
  soil contamination and, 522
  susceptibility, enhanced, in, 73
  toxicology and, 72, 73, 76
Antagonism, 68, 73
  cancer and, 92
  respiratory toxicology and, 167
Antibiotics
  aplastic anemia and, 206
  ears/hearing and, 254
  factory farming and, 504-505
  immunotoxicology and, 151, 152
  nephrotoxicity and, 313
Antibodies, 51, 74, 75
  autoimmunity and, 151
  clinical diagnosis and, 223
  dermatoses and, 273
  gastrointestinal tract and, 300
  immune system and, 327-348
    cancer and, 157, 159, 162-165
    immunodeficiency disorders and, 344
    in various autoimmune diseases, 343t
  immunotoxicology and, 140t, 141-146
  interactions between antigens and, 146-148, 161
  metals and, 151, 152
  respiratory tract disorders and, 286
  tobacco smoke and, 150
Antibody-dependent cellular cytotoxicity (ADCC), 159-160, 332
Antibody-forming cells (AFCs), 151
Anticancer agents/anticarcinogens, 92, 93
  aplastic anemia and, 204t, 209
  female reproductive function and, 74-75
  leukemia and, 213
  natural, in diet, 512-514
Anticholinesterase insecticides, 133, 134, 189
Antidiuretic hormone (ADH), 103
Antigens, 74, 141, 142, 143
  as allergens, 152-153
  clinical diagnosis and, 222
  cosmetics and, 152
  dermal toxicology and, 187
  dermatoses and, 273
  fetal and placental, 158-159, 162, 163f
  immunology and, 326-348
  interactions between antibodies and, 146-148, 161
  respiratory toxicology and, 177
  respiratory tract disorders and, 286
  tissue, 162
  tumor-associated, 157-159
    evaluation and diagnosis to detect, 161-163
    immunotherapy and, 163-165
Antihistamines, 152
Antimony, 21t
Antineoplastics, 254t
Antioncogenes, 82-83
Antioxidants, 75, 513-514
  diet and, 354
  food preservatives and, 501
  respiratory toxicology and, 170f, 171, 172
Antiproteases, 170f, 172, 175
Antipyretics, ears/hearing and, 254t
Antithyroid drugs, 151, 204t, 209
Aplastic anemia, 201, 203-211
  leukemia and, 212-213

Apoptosis (vs. necrosis), 79f
Apraxias, 195
Aquatic biota, 15f, 24; see also Oceanic life
Aquifiers, 517
Aramid fibers, 459
ARDS; see Adult respiratory distress syndrome
Arginine esterases, 147
Armustine, 204t, 213
Aromatic amine, 84t, 87-88, 173
Aromatic hydrocarbons, 81, 84t
  dermatoses and, 272, 274
Arsenic, 24, 25, 610-611
  dermatoses and, 272
  developmental toxicity and, 118, 120
  in drinking water, 44t
  ears/hearing and, 254t, 260
  environmental history and, 237
  as EPA priority chemical, 21t
  eyes/vision and, 244
  factory farming and, 505
  in food, 495
  neurobehavioral testing for toxicity and, 191
  neurotoxicity and, 130, 322t, 323t
  toxicology of, 132-133
  vestibular disorders and, 260
  in water, 483
Arsine, 611
Arterial gas embolism (AGE), 587
Arthropod vector-borne disease, 619-620
Arthus phenomenon, 147, 333-334
Artificial insemination, 97
Aryl hydrocarbon hydroxylase (AHH), 91, 186
  dioxin and, 135
Aryl hydrocarbon receptor (Ah), 18
Asbestos, 24, 39, 40
  in buildings, 438-454
  cancer and, 87, 92
  children and, 391, 392t, 393
  chronologic history of knowlege about, 440t
  cigarette smoking and, 73, 92
  clinical diagnosis and, 222, 227
  control procedures for, 431
  diseases related to, 443-448
  in drinking water, 44t
  environmental history and, 233, 235, 236
  as EPA priority chemical, 21t
  features of toxicity of, 456-458
  forms of, 439t
  immunotoxicology and, 151
  indoor air pollution and, 421t, 431
  measuring, 442, 443t
  nonoccupational exposure to, 441
  preventing exposure to, 448-451
  respiratory toxicology and, 175-177
  respiratory tract disorders and, 290, 292-294
  in school environment, 119
  secondary exposure to, 442
  working safely with, 449
Asbestos-cement piping (ACP), 442, 484
Asbestos-containing building materials (ACBM), 441, 448-451
Asbestos Hazard Emergency Response Act (AHERA), 449
Asbestosis, 293, 294f, 443-444
Ascorbate, respiratory toxicology and, 171
Asphalt emissions, 191-192
Aspirin, 152
Asthma, 282-285
  acid aerosols and, 465
  children with, 363-364, 390, 394
  gas stoves and, 393
  chronic pulmonary disease and, 362-364
  clinical diagnosis and, 222
  as environmental disease agents causing, 284t
  vs. nonenvironmental, occupational, 177-178, 221
  immune system and, 330
  immunotoxicology and, 152
  indoor air pollution and, 424, 428

occupational vs. nonoccupational (environmental), 177-178
outdoor air pollution and, 22, 24, 465, 466
respiratory toxicology and, 166, 167, 174, 177-178
  bronchorestriction and, 172
  ozone and, 174
  TDI type of, 177-178
Astrocyte function, 195-196
Ataxia telangiectasia, 160
Atmosphere, 15f, 23-25, 577-591
Atomic absorption spectrophotometry, 97
Atomic bomb survivors, 530
Atopic dermatitis, 330-331, 424
Atopy, 22, 358, 363
Atrazine (Atrex), 149, 480t
Atropine, 301, 404
Attention, 197
Auranofin, 204t, 209
Aurothioglucose, 204t, 209
Autoimmunity, 147, 149, 336-344
  antibodies in various disorders involving, 343t
  classification of, 338-342
  environmental agents and, 149, 150-152
  laboratory tests for disorders of, 342
  neoplasia and, 342-343
  systemic lupus erythematosus (SLE) as prototype for disorder of, 339-340
  tissue lesions and, 335
  furans in, 25t
  school environment and, 118
Autonomic nervous system (ANS), gastrointestinal tract and, 301
Aviation environment, 582-589
Azoospermia, 74, 97

B

Bacteria, 12t
  composting and, 654
  dermatoses and, 276
  in food, 506; see also Irradiation (of food)
  factory farming and, 504-505
  food contamination and, 617-618
  gastrointestinal tract and, 301
  immunotoxicology and, 140t, 146, 147
  indoor air pollution and, 25, 421t, 424
  reuse of sludge and, 657-658
  soil contamination and, 618-619
  water pollution and, 485, 616-617, 621
Badges, 42
Barbiturates, 108, 109t
Barium, 21t, 44t
Barotrauma, 260, 584-589
Basal ganglia, 195
Bases, 606
Basophilic leukocytes, 140t, 141
Basophil kallikrein of anaphylaxis (BK-A), 147
Basophils, immune system and, 327-328
Batteries, indoor air pollution from, 24
Bayesian reasoning, 231
B-cells/lymphocytes, 74, 140t, 141-143
  AIDS and, 148
  autoimmunity and, 150-151, 337-344
  dermal toxicology and, 187
  HIV and, 148-149
  immune system and, 147, 337-346
  immunoglobulins and, 144
  and immunology of cancer, 159-160, 162, 163t
  mercury and, 151
  ozone and, 150
  PCBs and, 151
  pesticides and, 149
Behavioral development, 120, 192t; see also Neurobehavioral testing
Behavioral risk reduction, 729-730
Behavioral studies, 70
Behavioral teratology, 198
Belladonna, gastrointestinal tract and, 301
Bends, 587-588
Benomyl, 152, 153

Bentazon, in well water, 480t
Benton Visual Retention Test, 197
Benzene, 18, 25, 118, 133, 134, 597-598
  aplastic anemia and, 204-206
  children and, 392t
  in drinking water, 44t, 150
  environmental history and, 233, 236
  as EPA priority chemical, 21t
  eyes/vision and, 244
  fire and, 473
  immunotoxicology and, 150
  leukemia and, 204, 212-213, 228
  neurotoxicity and, 322t
  vs. other solvents, 210
  tobacco smoke and, 422
Benzene dihydrodiol, 205
Benzene hydrochloride, 134
Benzene oxide, 205
Benzidine, 21t, 236
Benzo(a)anthracene, 21t
Benzocaine, dermatoses and, 266t
Benzo(b)fluoranthene, 21t
2,3-Benzofuran, 21t
Benzo[a]pyrene, 21t, 81, 166, 167, 602-603
  dermal toxicology and, 186
p-Benzoquinone, 205f, 206
o-Benzoquinone, 205f, 206
Berksonian bias, 55
Beryllium, 21t, 24, 25, 611-612
Beryllium disease, 285-286
Beryllium oxide, 152
Beta (type II error), 59
Beta-blockers, 151
Betadine scrub solution, 122
Beta lactim antibiotics, 151
Betanaphthylamine, 87, 88
BHA; see 2,3-Tert-butyl-4-hydroxyanisole
Bhopal disaster, 10, 11f, 166, 723
  compared to Cantara disaster, 722
BHT; see 3,5-Di-tert-butyl-4-hydroxytoluene
Bias, 53-55, 196
Bikini bomb test, 532
Bile, 82, 303
Binding, 66f, 70, 71
  alkylating agents and, 209
  arsenic and, 133
  benzene and, 206, 212
  cancer and, 82-84, 86
  carbon monoxide and, 136
  female reproductive function and, 103
  immune system and, 327-328
  lead and, 131
  neurotoxicity and, 324
  receptors and, 73-74
Bioaccumulation, 18, 70, 134
Bioactivation, 71, 75
Bioamplification, 70
Bioassays, 113
Bioavailability
  acid precipitation and, 676
  soil contamination and, 519-520
  toxicology and, 66, 67, 70
  uptake estimate and, 70
Biochemical effect, 17
  male reproductive function and, 97
  neurobehavioral testing for toxicity and, 195-196
  toxicology and, 66, 70, 73
Bioconcentration, 13f, 15f, 17, 69-70
Biodiversity, 6, 10, 11f
  global aspects of, 688
Biologic agents, 3, 12, 14f, 15f, 615-622
  arthropod vector-borne disease and, 619-620
  dermatoses and, 265t, 275-276
  exposure assessment and, 37, 38
  eyes and, 38; see also Eyes/vision
  indoor air pollution and, 25-26, 421t, 427-428, 433
  infectious diseases and, 615-619
  modification of hazardous agent because of, 17
  respiratory toxicology and, 166, 167
  toxicology and, 68
Biological amplification, 69-70; see also Bioconcentration

Index 765

Biologic markers/biomarkers, 18, 21-22, 32, 698-704; *see also* Markers
  benzene and, 205
  epidemiology studies and, 51
  ethical and legal issues in use of, 703
  exposure assessment and, 40
  female reproductive function and, 110
  gastrointestinal-induced disorders and, 306-307
  liver and, 306-307
  male reproductive function and, 97
  nephrotoxicity and, 313
  neurotoxicity and, 322
  of stress, 359
  susceptibility and, 359
  toxicology and, 74-75
  validation of, 701-702
Biomagnification, 70
Biomedical science, 7
Biomedical waste (BMW), 663; *see also* Medical waste
Biomonitors, 6, 222-223
  cancer and, 89-90
  toxicology and, 70
Biostatistics, 31, 39, 57
Biotechnology
  factory farming and, 505
  global aspects of, 686
Biotransformation, 17
  dermal toxicology and, 182, 186
  susceptibility and, 355
Biphenyls, 18
Birth
  bone marrow and, 201
  environmental history and, 234
  lead and, 117f, 117
  neurobehavioral testing for toxicity and, 198
  reproductive toxins and, 74
  uterus and, 103
Birth defects, 18, 20, 21
Bisbenzylisoquinone alkaloids, 177
Bis(2-chloroethyl)ether, 21t
Bis(chloromethyl)ether, 21t
BK-A; *see* Basophil kallikrein of anaphylaxis
Black lung disease, 292
Block Design subtest, 197
Blocking agents, 512-513; *see also* Anticancer agents
Blood
  bone marrow toxicology and, 201-208
  immune system and, 328, 332-333
  immunotoxicology and, 140, 147
  lead and, 131, 210-211, 608-608
  toxicology and, 66f
Blood/brain barrier, 130, 131
Blood flow
  gastrointestinal tract and, 301
  kidneys and, 312-313
  liver and, 302-303
  neurobehavioral testing for toxicity and, 191
  susceptibility and pulmonary, 355
Blood glucose, 22
Blood-lead concentration, 19
Blood transfusions, 13
Bone marrow, 201-208
  aplastic anemia and, 201, 203-211, 212
  causes of toxicity of, 204t
  confounding factors in studies of toxicity of, 210, 211
  dermal toxicology and, 183
  immunotoxicology and, 140, 141, 146
  leukemia and, 201, 211-213
  solvents and, 210; *see also* Benzene
  structure and function of, 201-203
Boron, 21t
Bovine somatotropin (BST), 509
Bradykinin, 147
Brain; *see* Nervous system
Breast cancer, 83t
  diet and, 92
  environment and, 7
  immunology and, 158, 163, 164
  ionizing radiation and, 530-531
  pesticide residues and, 7
Breath analysis, 40
Breathing zones, 119
Brevetoxins, 172
Bromoform, 21t

Bromomethane, 21t
Bronchial asthma; *see* Asthma
Bronchiolitis obliterans, 288-289
Bronchitis, respiratory toxicology and, 166
Bronchoalveolar lavage (BAL), 173, 174, 177
  clinical diagnosis and, 222
  respiratory tract disorders and, 284
Bronchoconstriction, 282, 283, 362
Bronchogenic carcinoma, 82, 91, 92, 295
Bruton-type agammaglobulinemia, 160
BST; *see* Bovine somatotropin
Building-related illness, 6, 25, 420-437
  asbestos and, 438-454
  children and, 393
Bulletin boards, 760
Burkitt's lymphoma, 158, 160
Burns, cancer and, 85
Busulfan, 204t, 209, 210f, 213
1,3-Butadiene, 18
3-Butadiene, 21t
2-Butanone, 21t

C
Cacosmia, 194
Cadmium, 18, 24, 25, 609
  in composts, 655
  in drinking water, 44t
  female reproductive function and, 107, 108
  in food, 490t
  immune system and, 74
  immunotoxicology and, 151, 153
  nephrotoxicity and, 314-315
  reuse of sludge and, 657
Calcium, 121, 123, 354
  children and, 385
  lead and, 121, 123, 131
Calcium hydroxide, 244
Cancer; *see* Carcinogenesis/cancer
Cancer potency slope, 31, 33-34
"Cancers of affluence," 92
Candidiasis, 148t, 163t
Cantara disaster, 722, 723-724, 725
Capping, 142
Captan, 152
Carbamates, 379, 381
  indoor air pollution and, 421t, 404-405
Carbaryl, 153
Carbimazole, 209
Carbofuran, 379
Carbohydrates, developmental toxicology and, 120
Carbon, 24, 92, 459
Carbon dioxide, 25
  climate changes in world and, 672
  indoor air pollution and, 421t, 422, 431
Carbon disulfide, 130, 133, 191, 192, 607
  as EPA priority chemical, 21t
  eyes/vision and, 244
  neurotoxicity and, 323t
Carbon monoxide (CO), 22-25, 422-431, 606-607
  ambient air quality standards and, 43, 167t
  biologic half-life of, 136
  children and, 392t, 393
  cigarette/tobacco smoke and, 40, 422
  developmental toxicology and, 121
  in drinking water, environmental history and, 233
  ears/hearing and, 254t
  environmental history and, 233, 236
  eyes/vision and, 244
  hazardous waste incinerators and, 24
  indoor air pollution and, 421t, 422-431
  neurobehavioral testing for toxicity and, 191, 192
  neurotoxicity and, 322t
  outdoor air pollution and, 464, 466
  from pyrolysis, 472-473
  respiratory toxicology and, 173
  solid waste management and, 633
  source of, in photochemical air pollution, 23, 24
  sources of toxicity from, 130

susceptibility and, 357
  toxicology of, 135-136
Carbon tetrachloride, 18, 21t, 133
  in drinking water, 44t
  hepatotoxicity and, 303, 313
  nephrotoxicity and, 313
Carboxyhemoglobin (COHb or HbCO), 121, 135, 136, 466-477
Carboxylic acids, 600, 601
Carcinoembryonic antigen (CEA), 158, 162
Carcinogenesis/cancer, 78-94; *see also specific types*; Malignancy; Tumors
  age and, 366
  AIDS and, 148
  air pollution and, children and, 391
  Alar (daninozide) and, 120
  alcohol abuse and, 92
  animal models regarding, 80, 81-82, 88
  asbestos and, 444-445, 447-448
  biomonitoring and, 89-90
  bone marrow toxicology and, 204t, 209, 211-213
  burns and wounds and, 85
  chemically modified membranes and, 164
  chloroform and, 600
  chronic inflammation and, 85, 91, 93
  chrysotile and, 447-448
  cigarette smoking and, 92; *see also* Cigarette smoking
  clinical diagnosis and, 222, 227, 228
  cluster studies and, 50
  cohort studies and, 48
  cytogenetic assays and, 88-89
  defined, 78-79
  dermal toxicology and, 186-187
  dermatoses and, 265, 269-274
  developmental toxicology and, 117, 120, 126
  diet and, 92-93, 120; *see also* Diet; Food
  dose-response assessment and, 31-32
  environmental history and, 234, 236
  as environmental/occupational disease, 7, 86-93, 221
  epidemiology and, 90
  in firefighters, 475
  food and, 354-355; *see also* Diet; Food
  gastrointestinal-induced disorders and, 307-308
  geographic areas and, 87
  hereditary vs. nonhereditary, 84
  human models regarding, 80, 82
  immunology and, 156-155
    evaluation and diagnosis and, 161-163
    immunotherapy and, 163-165
  immunotoxicology and, 147, 148, 153
  initiation of, 75, 80, 82-84
  ionizing radiation and, 530-531
  leukemia resulting from treatment of other types of, 213
  mechanisms of, 80-81
  as multistage process, 80, 84, 85
  mutagens and, 74
  mutation and, 80-82, 85, 88
    age and, 91
    initiation and, 84
    molecular epidemiology and, 90
  neoplasia and, 79, 85
    age and, 91
    natural history of, 81f
  nonionizing radiation and, 551-552
  pesticides and, 381t; *see also* Pesticides
  polycyclic hydrocarbons and, 274
  progression of, 80-81, 82-84
    esophageal cancer and, 87
    types of carcinogens and, 85
  promotion of; *see* Tumor, promotion of
  proportional mortality studies and, 49
  psychosocial factors in, 358-359
  public fears/misunderstandings about, 78, 86
  radiation and, 86
    ionizing, 530-531
    nonionizing, 551-552
  radon and, 537-538

registry for, 52-53
  regulatory aspects of, 82
  remission of, and aplastic anemia, 209
  respiratory toxicology and, 167, 174
  reversibility and, 84
  risk of, 32, 91
  sentinel event strategies and, 20
  susceptibility and, 353, 358-359
  terminology concerning, 79
  threshold and, 73
  tumors and, 79-85; *see also* Tumors
  ultraviolet radiation and, 546-547
  unilateral vs. bilateral, 84
  viruses and, 84, 85-86
  water pollution and, 481-482, 485-486
Carcinogens
  alcohol abuse and, 92
  anti-, 92, 93, 512-514
  bone marrow toxicology and, 211-213
  classification of, 80
  co-, 81, 84, 92
  EPA and, 18
  epigenetic, 84, 85
  genotoxic, 84, 85, 89, 92
  hazardous waste incinerators and, 24
  interactions among, 90, 93
  naturally occurring, 7, 86-87, 92, 512-514
  number of, 12
  occupational, 87-88, 90, 92
  potential, 90
  prevention of, 7; *see also* Patients, improving life-style of
  public impression concerning, 78
  respiratory tract and, 166, 295
  stress proteins and, 18
  threshold and, 73; *see also* Threshold
  types of, 84-86
  "weak," 498
Cardiovascular/heart disease, 23, 54, 92, 730
  carbon monoxide and, 136
  environmental history and, 233, 234
  fire and, 475
  high-altitude disease and, 582
  outdoor air pollution and, 467
  as preexisting illness, 364
  susceptibility and, 364
  tobacco smoke and, 25, 428
Cardiovascular system, space environment and, 590
Carmustine (BCNU), 204t, 209
β-Carotene, 354, 513
Car painting, 129, 130
Carpal tunnel syndrome, 12, 12, 320
Cartograms, 20
Case reports/studies, 226, 237-238
  hazardous waste and, 642-643
  nonionizing radiation and, 551-552
Catalase, 172
Catechol, 205, 206
Catecholamines, 141, 147
  depression and, 359
  gastrointestinal tract and, 301
  susceptibility and, 355
Causal inference, 59-60
Causation/causative agents, 12-13
  aplastic anemia and, 210
  clinical diagnosis and, 222, 223, 226, 227
  correlation vs., 46
  dermatoses and, 278
  environmental history and, 233
  epidemiology, 46, 60-61
  neurobehavioral testing for toxicity and, 191
  respiratory toxicology and, 167
  unknown, and markers and surrogates, 40
Cause-and-effect relationship
  between bone marrow toxicology and chemicals, 201, 207, 209-210
  environmental history and, 234
  epidemiology and, 46, 61
  latency and, 73
  toxicology and, 73
Caustics, 401-402
CEA; *see* Carcinoembryonic antigen
Cellular phones, 551-552
Cellular poisons, 74
Cellular protooncogenes (c-oncs), 82-86, 90, 91

Cellular responses, 14f, 15, 17-18
  airway inflammation and, 282-283
  arsenic and, 133
  bone marrow toxicology and, 201-208, 211-213
  in cancer, 78-79, 82-89
    anticarcinogens and, 93
    male vs. female, 91
  carbon monoxide and, 136
  developmental toxicology and, 125-127
  eyes/vision and, 243
  immune system and, 327-336
    autoimmunity and, 337-344
    cancer and, 157-165
    immunotoxicology and, 139-147
      AIDS and, 148-149
      electromagnetic fields and, 151-152
      pesticides and, 149
    man-made fibers and, 457-458
    neurobehavioral testing for toxicity and, 192, 195-196
    neurotoxicants and, 130-131
    respiratory toxicology and, 168-171, 175-177
    susceptibility and, 355
  female reproductive function and, 104-109
  toxicology and, 66, 67, 73-75
Centers for Disease Control (CDC), 38, 51, 273
  air pollution and children and, 393
  biomarkers and, 306
  international travel and, 621
  lead poisoning in children and, 386
  radon and, 539
Central nervous system (CNS), 322, 324
  autoimmunity and, 341, 343t
Centrifugation, 41
Cephalosporins, 152
Cesium-137, 26
Chediak-Higashi syndrome, 148t
Chelation therapy, 131
CHEM-BANK data base, 761
Chemical Abstracts, 759
Chemical analysis, 70
Chemical burns, to eyes, 243-244
"Chemical conjunctivitis," 242
Chemical Control site fire (Elizabeth, New Jersey), 642
Chemical disaster preparedness, 722-728
  information resources for, 727
Chemical Hazard Response Information System (CHRIS), 761
Chemical hazards, 4, 5, 12; see also Chemicals; Hazards (environmental)
  direct discharge of, 10, 11f
  female reproductive function and, 109-112
  as focus of environmental medicine, 4
  screening for, 113
  sources of, 10-12
Chemical manufacture/plants
  furans from, 25
  multiple exposure pathways from, 16f, 17
  dioxins from, 25
Chemical reactivity, 107-108
Chemicals, 3, 592-614; see also Hazards (environmental)
  toxicology and form of, 67, 68
  as allergens, 152-153
  aplastic anemia induced by; see Anemia
  asthma and, 178
  bone marrow and, 201-208
  breathing zones and, 119
  cancer caused by, 12, 84-85, 93, 211-212; see also Carcinogenesis/cancer
  classification of toxic, 594-595, 594t
  clinical toxicology of, 128t; see also Toxicology
  compounds of
    semivolatile, 421t, 423
    volatile; see Volatile organic compounds (VOCs)
  dermatoses and, 264, 265t, 266t, 272-275
  developmental toxicology and, 119

EPA priority, 21t
exposure assessment and, 37, 38; see also Exposure
eyes/vision and, 38, 240-249
in hazardous waste, 638; see also Hazardous waste
and immunology of cancer, 157-158
in immunotherapy, 164
immunotoxicology and, 149-153
information resources on, 592-594, 755-762
inorganic, 594-595, 606-607
interactions among/mixtures of, 12, 17
  hazardous waste and, 640
  modification of agent and, 17
  toxicology and, 68, 73; see also Toxicology
man-made, dermatoses and, 272
molecular weight of, 38
neurotoxicity and, 319
number of, 68
organic, 117, 597-606
  classification of toxic, 594-595
  in composts, 655
  female reproductive function and, 75
  in food, 495-496
  hazardous waste incinerators and, 25
  kidneys and, 311
  respiratory toxicology and, 171
  volatile; see Volatile organic chemicals (VOCs)
organometallic, 605-606
ototoxic, 254
population explosion and, 10, 11f
with and without potential for secondary combustion, 711t
from pyrolysis, 472-478
respiratory toxicology and, 167, 172
response to low levels of; see Exposure, low-level; Low-level radioactive waste
sensitivity to multiple, 74, 200, 368-376
solubility of, 38
structure and toxicology of, 595-597
synthetic, reproductive function and, 74, 108
threshold limits of toxic, 596t; see also Threshold
top ten, from hazardous waste, 638t
toxic, 67, 68; see also Toxicity; Toxicology
transdermal absorption of, 122
types of, 12t
of unknown toxicity, 12
untested, 113
in water, 15f
Chemiluminescence, 42
Chemotaxis, 143, 146, 147
Chemotherapy
  aplastic anemia and, 209
  immunotherapy and, 164, 165
  leukemia and, 213
CHEMTREC, 725, 727
Chernobyl disaster, 10, 11f, 26
  food irradiation and, 507-508
  global aspects of, 689
  immunotoxicology and, 150
  ionizing radiation and, 532
  pregnant women exposed to, 150
Children; see also Development
  absorption in, 123, 130
  acid aerosols and, 465
  vs. adults, 127
  air pollution and, 390-397, 466-467
  aplastic anemia and, 204, 211
  benzene and, 204
  conditions unique or more common to, 391
  food additives and, 502
  food contamination and, 499, 502
  hazardous waste and, 641, 642
  lead and, 383-389
  neurobehavioral testing for toxicity and, 198
  neurotoxicants and, 130, 132
  pesticides and, 377-382, 497
  radon and, 538
  soil ingestion by, 516, 521
  workplace environment and, 408-415
Chi-square (X^2) test, 58
Chloracne, 265t, 266, 272, 277

Chlorambucil, 204t, 204t, 213, 209
Chloramphenicol, 204t, 206-207, 212
  leukemia and, 213
Chlordane, 18, 135, 751
  as EPA priority chemical, 21t
  immunotoxicology and, 149, 153
  in well water, 480t
Chlordecone, 125, 134, 135, 134
Chloride, 41, 44t, 392t
Chlorinated benzene, 134
Chlorinated cyclodienes, 134
Chlorinated cyclohexane, 134
Chlorinated dioxins, 24
Chlorinated hydrocarbons (HC), 12t, 69
  breast cancer and, 7
  indoor air pollution and, 423
  toxicology of, 135
Chlorinated polyaromatic hydrocarbons, 602
fire and, 474
in soil, 521
Chlorine, 17, 92
  pyrolysis and, 472
  respiratory toxicology and, 168, 178
  respiratory tract disorders and, 287t, 289
Chlorine monoxide monomer, 274
Chlorobenzene, 21t, 24, 599
Chlorodifluoromethane, 422
Chloroethane, 21t
Chlorofluorocarbons (CFCs), 672-673
Chlorofluoromethane, 274
Chloroform, 21t, 133, 600
  in drinking water, 480, 482, 484-486
  hepatotoxicity and, 303
Chlorophenols, 24, 25t
Chlorophenoxy herbicides, 605
Chloroquine, ears/hearing and, 254t
Chloromethane, 21t
Chlorpromazine, 151, 204t, 208-209
Chorionic villus sampling, 112
Chromium, 24, 25, 609-610
  dermal toxicology and, 187
  dermatoses and, 266t, 275
  in drinking water, 44t
  immunotoxicology and, 149, 152, 153
  respiratory clearance and, 170t
  in soil, 520
Chromosomes
  bone marrow toxicology and, 212
  cancer and, 83-84, 88-89
  immunotoxicology and, 153
  ionizing radiation and, 18, 529
  mutagens and, 74
  susceptibility and, 356
Chronic mountain sickness, 581-582
Chronic obstructive pulmonary disease (COPD), 352, 363-364
  outdoor air pollution and, 22, 462, 465-468
Chronic pulmonary disease, 362-364
Chronic toxic encephalopathy (CTE), 133, 260
Chronic toxicity, 18
Chrysene, 21t
Chrysotile, 176, 447-448, 457
Cigarette smoking, 10, 11f; see also Tobacco smoke
  asbestos and, 73, 92, 446
  attributable risk and, 57-58
  benzene and, 204
  cancer and, 81, 82, 86, 91, 92
  chronic pulmonary disease and, 362-363
  as confounding factor, 48, 50, 55
  decline in, 730
  developmental toxicology and, 126
  ears/hearing and, 255
  exposure assessment and, 40
  environmental history and, 233
  female reproductive function and, 109t, 111
  fetus and, 122
  glutathione S-transferase (GST) and, 124
  life-style and, 428
  male reproductive function and, 98t
  passive, 363, 426; see also Secondhand smoke
  physical exercise and, 355
  radon and, 538
  relative risk (RR) and, 55-56

respiratory toxicology and, 170, 172, 178
susceptibility and, 352-353, 355
  genetic factors in, 357-358
  outdoor air pollution and, 466t
synergism and, 92
tar and, 92
Circadian variations, 96
Circulation, toxicology and, 66
Cisplatin, 209
Clara cells, 168, 171
Clay silt, 41
Clean Air Act, 43, 745-747
  incineration and, 665
  NAAQS and, 463, 465
  pesticides and, 751
Clean Air Act amendments, 167, 746
  children and, 393-394
Clean Water Act, 480, 744-745
  mercury and, 493
  pesticides and, 751
Climate (worldwide), 671-676, 689
  agriculture and, 686-687
Clinical effect/diagnosis, 5, 217-231; see also Patients
  asbestosis and, 444
  aviation environment and, 582-584
  barotraumas and, 584-589
  categories for, 228t
  cellular response and, 15
  children and
    lead and, 385-386
    pesticides and, 379, 380
  and clinical experience, 226
  and clinical studies, 226
  data bases and, 225-226
  dermatoses and, 277-278
  ears/hearing and, 255-261
  eyes/vision and, 242-248
  female reproductive function and, 111-112
  gastrointestinal-induced disorders and, 306
  hazardous waste and, 641
  hepatotoxicity and, 305
  high-altitude disorders and, 579-582
  immune system and, 329, 332, 335, 339
    allergic disease and, 329
    immunodeficiency disorders and, 344-346
  lead and, children and, 385-386
  mercury and, 132
  multiple chemical sensitivity and, 368-376
  nephrotoxicity and, 313
  neurobehavioral testing for toxicity and, 190, 193-195, 198
  neurotoxicity and, 319-321, 324
  organic solvents, 132
  pesticides and, children and, 379, 380
Exposure—cont'd
  preexisting illnesses and, 227, 228t
  respiratory tract disorders and, 284-285, 290-291
  reuse of sludge and, 659
  temporal relationships and, 227-228, 277
    in contact dermatitis, 277
    in neurotoxicity, 319
  and third parties' effect on diagnosis, 219-220
  toxicology and, 66
  vestibular disorders and, 259-261
Clinicians; see also Health professionals/practitioners
  developmental toxicology and, 127
  future needs regarding, 8
  improving patients' life-style and, 734-735
  neurobehavioral testing for toxicity and, 190, 193-195
  as risk communicators, 65
  role in toxicology, 70
Clonal expansion, 142, 143
Coal, benzene and, 204; see also Benzene
Coal mining, 290, 292
Coal stoves, indoor air pollution and, 421t, 423
Coal workers' pneumoconiosis (CWP), 291, 292
Cobalt, 21t, 187, 233

Index 767

Cocaine, 191t, 273
Cocarcinogens, 81, 84, 92
Coccidioidomycosis, 285
Cochlear disorders, 252; see also Eyes/hearing; Noise pollution
Cognitive functions, 130, 134, 190-198
Coliform counts, 32
Collagen diseases, autoimmunity and, 343t
Colloidal solids, 41
Colon cancer, 82, 83t, 84, 91
  diet and, 87, 92
  immunology and, 163, 164
  predisposition to, 85
Colony forming unit (CFU), 202, 203
  alkylating agents and, 209
  benzene and, 206
  chloramphenicol and, 206, 207
  leukemia and, 212
  phenothizines and, 208-209
Colony-stimulating factor (CSF), 203
  extrinsic allergic alveolitis and, 336
  immunotoxicology and, 146
Color, in drinking water, 44t
Color blindness, 194
Colostrum, 123
Combustion
  children and, 391-392
  complete vs. incomplete (pyrolysis), 472
  exposure assessment and, 42
  indoor air pollution and, 421t, 423, 431
  outdoor air pollution and, 465
Community assistance panels (CAPs), 739
Community environment, 3, 4, 5, 6, 12
  aplastic anemia and, 204
  asbestos in, 442
  benzene in, 204
  dermal exposure and, 38
  different exposure levels in same, 51
  environmental history and, 235
  exposure assessment and, 43-44
  fire and, 472-477
  hazardous waste and, 635-646
  improving patients' life-style and, 731
  lead in, children and, 386-387
  MSDSs and, 224-225
  outdoor air pollution in, 23, 468
  overlap between workplace and, 5
  recreational
    developmental toxicology and, 120
    environmental history and, 233-234, 237
    noise in, 253t
    repeated, low-level exposures in, 10
    trauma in, 12
  school; see School environment
  toxicology and, 66
  toxic profile of, 12
Community medicine, 4, 5
Comparability, 53-54
Complement-dependent antibody lysis, 331-332
Complement system, 147
  AIDS and, 148
  immune system and, 331-334, 344-346
  and immunology of cancer, 159, 162, 163t
  metals and, 151
Composting, 628, 629, 654-656
Comprehensive Environmental Response, Compensation, and Liability Act (CERCLA), 636-637, 648, 650, 747-748
Computer-Aided Management of Emergency Operations (CAMEO), 760
Computer-assisted sperm analysis (CASA), 96
Concanavalin A, 151, 157, 163t
Concentration (as cognitive function), 196, 197
Concentration, 13f, 14, 15f, 17
  of benzene, 204
  carcinogens and, 78, 84
  cytogenic assays and, 89
  dermatoses and, 263-264
  dose and, 37
  exposure assessment and, 38-41

eyes/vision and, 240, 242
female reproductive function and, 112, 113
in hazardous waste, 639
risk assessment and, 32
solvents and, 324
substance abuse and, 70
threshold and, 42
toxicology and, 66, 71
Concentration gradient, toxicokinetics and, 71
Concentration models, 19
Conception
  exposure before, and developmental toxicology, 116-118
  fallopian tubes and, 102-103
  male reproductive function and, 97
Confidence interval, 58-59, 60, 111
Confounding bias/factors, 48, 50, 55, 196, 210
  analytic control of, 57
  causal inference and, 60, 61
  neurotoxicity and, 320, 324
  outdoor air pollution and, 463
Congeners, 596-597
Congenital Disease Surveillance Project, 21
Conjugation, 66f, 71
Contact dermatitis (CD), 265, 277, 278; see also Allergic contact dermatitis
  immune system and, 335
  from plants, 276-277
  temporal relationships and, 277
  from woods, 277
Contact models, 19
Cooking
  food contamination and, 496-497, 504
  indoor air pollution and, 422
COPD; see Chronic obstructive pulmonary disease
Copper, 25
  bile and, 303
  in drinking water, 44t
  as EPA priority chemical, 21t
  furans and, 25t
  hypersensitivity and, 152
  immunotoxicology and, 149, 151, 152
Coproporphyrin, 210-211
Corneal scarring, 38
Cornpicker's pupil, 38
Corpus luteum, 102, 103-105
Corrosives, 401
Corticosteroids, 104, 185, 335
Cortico-striatal-pallidal-thalamic-cortical loop, 195
Corynebacterium parvum (BCG), immunotherapy and, 163, 164
Cosmetics, 152; see also Food, Drug and Cosmetic Act
Cosmic radiation, 75, 590
Cotton dust, 24, 40, 92
Coulometry, 42
Crafts/hobbies, 233-234, 237
  indoor air pollution and, 422
  neurotoxicity and, 320
Creosols, 21t, 599
Creosote
  dermatoses and, 267
  developmental toxicology and, 120
  environmental history and, 237
  as EPA priority chemical, 21t
CREST syndrome, 341-342
Cristobaline, 39
Crystals, 612; see also Quartz crystal; Silica
Cutaneous malignancy, 265t, 269-270, 272
  DNA and, 274
Cyanates, 25
Cyanide, 21t, 472, 601
Cyclamate, 82, 502
Cyclins, 83-84
Cyclodienes, 135
Cyclohexane, 134
Cyclophosamide, 204t, 213
Cyclophosphamide, 108, 109t, 204t, 209
Cypermethrin, 149
Cytochrome oxidase, 136, 206
Cytochrome P-450, 75, 91, 108
  benzene and, 205
  carbon monoxide and, 136

developmental toxicology and, 124
dioxin and, 135
hepatotoxicity and, 305
respiratory toxicology and, 168, 171
soil contamination and, 513
Cytokines, 144, 146
  aplastic anemia and, 206
  dermal toxicology and, 187
  extrinsic allergic alveolitis and, 336
  leukemia and, 212
  ozone and, 150
  respiratory toxicology and, 175
Cytomegalovirus, 160
Cytosine, 209
Cytotoxicity, 159-165, 331-333, 335
Cytotoxin, 85t

D
2,4-D; see 2,4-Dichlorophenoxyacetic acid
Dacarbazine, 204t, 209
Daninozide (Alar), 120, 499
Data bases, 21, 225-226, 238-239, 758-761
  on chemical agents, 593, 758-761
  for chemical disaster preparedness, 727
Data collection; see also Epidemiology
  comparability and biases involving, 53-55
  female reproductive function and, 109-113
  neurobehavioral testing for toxicity and, 190
Datura stramonium, 38
DDT, 108, 109t, 135, 603-604, 751
Decompression sickness (DCS), 587-588
Defense mechanisms, 14f, 15, 17
  gastrointestinal, 299-301
  pulmonary, 169-178
Deforestation, 686
Dehydration, 571
Dehydrochloramphenicol, 207
Delaney Amendment/Clause, 73, 498, 500
Delayed recall index, 197
Deltamethrin, 153
Demographics, and global aspects of environmental health, 679-683
De Morbis Artificium, 232
Deodorants, 25
Deoxyribonucleic acid (DNA); see also DNA-protein crosslinks; Recombinant-DNA techniques
  anticancer alkylating agents and, 209
  benzene and, 206, 212
  cancer and, 75, 79, 80, 82-83
    biomonitoring and, 89-90
    radiation and, 86
    types of carcinogens and, 84
  chloramphenicol and, 207
  chromium and, 153
  clinical diagnosis and, 229
  cross-linked, dermal toxicology and, 187
  dermatoses and, 272, 274
  developmental toxicology and, 126
  Epstein-Barr virus and, 158
  female reproductive function and, 105, 107t, 108
  food additives and, 501
  genetic engineering and, 508-509
  and immunology of cancer, 157-158
  immunotoxicology and, 153
  ionizing radiation and, 527, 529
  male reproductive function and, 97
  man-made fibers and, 457
  ozone and, 676
  respiratory toxicology and, 171, 175
  soil contamination and, 513
  susceptibility and, 356
  toxicology and, 67, 73
  water pollution and, 481
Deposition, 15f, 17, 66f, 71
Depression, 131, 133
  immune system and, 359
  multiple chemical sensitivity and, 373-374
  ingestion or inhalation vs., 13
Dermal toxicology, 38, 182-188; see also Skin

absorption and, 13, 17, 184-186
allergic contact dermatitis and, 182, 186, 187-188
biotransformation and, 182, 186
cancer and, 88
percutaneous absorption and, 184-186
photochemical transformation and photosensitivity and, 182, 186-187
sweat glands and, 183, 185, 187
testing for, 187-188
Dermatitis, 265-266
  allergic contact; see Allergic contact dermatitis
  atopic, 330-331
  as environmental disease vs. nonenvironmental, 221
  of eyelid, 335
  ICD and ACD, 265-266
  immune system and, 330-331, 335
  nickel and, 274
  photocontact, 335
Dermatophytes, 275
Dermatoses, 263-281
  aggravating factors in, 278
  clinical aspects of, 278
  cutaneous malignancy and, 265t, 269-270, 272, 274
  diagnosis of, 277-278
  DNA and, 274
  hygiene and, 278-279
  infection and, 265t, 269
  NMSC and, 265, 269-272, 274
  latency and, 277
  ozone and, 274
  nonoccupational, 277
  pigmentary changes and, 265t, 267-268
  plants and woods and, 276-277
  prevention and treatment of, 278-279
  scleroderma, 265t, 268-269, 273
  sunlight and, 265, 271-272
  temperature-related, 270-271
  urticaria and, 265t, 268
  water-related, 265
DES; see Diethylstilbesterol
Detection bias, 54
Development
  ears/hearing and, 260
  female reproductive function and, 103, 110
  immunodeficiency disorders and, 344
  immunotoxicology and, 139, 140
  ionizing radiation and, 529-530
  lead and, 260
  susceptibility and, 391
  toxicity and, 18; see also Toxicology, developmental
  vestibular disorders and, 260
Developmental and Reproductive Toxicology Database (DART), 759
Diabetes/diabetic symptoms, 234
  autoimmunity and, 343t
  dermatoses and, 278
  neurotoxicity and, 364
Diagnosis; see Clinical effect/diagnosis
Diarrhea, traveler's, 621
Diazinon, 153, 480t
Dibenzo(a, h)anthracene, 21t
Dibenzofurans, 18, 24
1,2-Dibromethane, 21t
Dibromochloropropane (1,2-Dibromo-3-chloropropane) (DBCP), 21t, 74, 97, 479-480, 482, 605
Di-n-butylphthalate, 21t
1,4-Dichlorobenzene, 21t
Para-Dichlorobenzene, 44t
O-Dichlorobenzene, 44t
3,3-Dichlorobenzidine, 21t
Dichlorodiphenylethane, 134
Dichloro-diphenyl-trichloroethane, 153
1,1-Dichloroethane, 21t
1,2-Dichloroethane, 21t, 44t
1,1-Dichloroethylene, 44t
Dichloromethane, 133, 600
2,4-Dichlorophenol, 21t
1,2-Dichlorophenoxyacetic acid (1,2-D), 480t
2,4-Dichlorophenoxyacetic acid (2,4-D), 152, 153, 490t, 496
1,2-Dichloropropene, 21t
1,3-Dichloropropane, 44t,
Dichlorvos, 153

Dieldrin, 135, 480t, 604
Diesal exhaust, 40
  IgE production and, 329
  respiratory toxicology and, 170t
Diet; see also Food
  cancer and, 7, 86, 87, 90-93
    fiber and, 92, 513
    susceptibility and, 354-355
  cigarette smoking and, 355
  developmental toxicology and, 119-120, 121f
  gastrointestinal tract and, 301
  genetic engineering and American, 508-509
  hazardous waste and, 641-642
  improving patients', 730
  metals and, immunotoxicology and, 149
  physical exercise and, 355
  psychosocial factors in, 358
  sentinel event strategies and, 20
  TCDD in, 150
  toxicology and, 70
Diethylenetriaminepentaacetic acid, 173
Di(2-ethylhexyl)phthalate, 21t
Diethylstilbesterol (DES), environmental history and, 234
Diffuse alveolar damage (DAD), 287-290
Diffusion, 15f, 17
Difolatabm 152
Dihydrodiol, benzene and, 205
Diisopropylfluorophosphate, 134
Dilution, 14f, 15f
Dilution (of waste), 651
Dimethoate, 153
Dinitrochlorobenzene (DNCB), 152, 163t
2,4-Dinitrophenol, 164
2,4-Dinitrotoluene, 21t
2,6-Dinitrotoluene, 21t
Dinoseb, 480t
Dioctyl phthalate, 504
Dioxin(s), 596-597, 602-603
  bioavailability of, 70
  categories of, 24-25
  in composts, 655
  dermatoses and, 269, 272-273
  developmental toxicology and, 120
  estrogen receptors and, 74
  "fingerprint" pattern of, 25
  in food, 490t, 496, 496
  hazardous waste incinerators and, 24-25
  immune system and, 74
  incineration and, 664
  neurotoxicity and, 322t
  in soil, 521
  solid waste management and, 632-633
  sources of, 25, 130
  stress proteins and, 18
  Times Beach incident involving, 10, 12, 219, 643
  toxicology of, 135
1,2-Diphenylhydrazine, 21t
2,3-Diphosphoglycerate, 136
Diquat, 380
Directory of Biotechnology Information Resources (DBIR), 759
Disaster, preparedness for chemical, 722-738; see also specific ones (e.g., Bhopal disaster)
Disease registries, 52-53
Disinfectants, 6, 122
Distillation, 41
Distribution, 66, 68, 71
  of asbestos, 442
  developmental toxicology and, 123
  organic solvents and, 133
3,5-Di-tert-butyl-4-hydroxytoluene (BHT), 501-502
Diuretics, ears/hearing and, 254
DNA; see Deoxynbonucleic acid
DNA-protein crosslinks (DPC), 153
DNCB; see Dinitrochlorobenzene
n-dodecane, 81
Dopamine, 131, 141
Dose, 14
  alkylating agents and, 209
  antibiotics and, 206
  bioconcentration of; see Bioconcentration
  biologic markers and effective, 21-22; see also Biomarkers
  bone marrow toxicology and, 206, 209, 210
  in cancer studies, 88
  chloramphenicol and, 206
  clinical diagnosis and, 218, 225-231
  developmental toxicology and, 124
  duration and, 69
  environmental history and, 224
  estimation of, 70
  explanation of, to patients, 70
  exposure assessment and, 37, 38
  female reproductive function and, 109-111
  hazardous waste and, 639
  internal vs. biologically effective, 37
  ionizing radiation and, 529
  lethal vs. effective, 72
  multiple exposure pathways and, 16f, 17
  personal dosimeters and, 51
  pesticides and, immunotoxicology and, 149
  physical activity and, 355
  reference (RfD), 32, 594, 630, 726
  risk assessment and, 31-32
  route of exposure and, 38
  threshold and, 42, 67; see also Threshold
  toxicology and, 66
  water pollution and, 482
Dose models, 19
Dose-response relationship, 39, 66, 67, 71-72
  asbestos and, 446
  and cancer and radiation, 86
  diagnosis and, 219, 228-231
  female reproductive function and, 109-110
  food contamination and, 498
  immunotoxicology and, 149, 151, 153
  ionizing radiation and, 527-528
  neurobehavioral testing for toxicity and, 198
  neurotoxicity and, 318-319
  potency and, 67
  respiratory tract disorders and, 283, 284
DOT/FEMA Hazmat bulletin board, 760
Dredge spoilage, 626, 629-630
Drinking water, 10, 11f, 26, 479-487; see also Safe Drinking Water Act; Water pollution/contamination
  arsenic in, 483
  asbestos in, 442, 479, 484; see also Asbestos
  benzene in, 150; see also Benzene
  cancer and, 86
  carbon monoxide in, 233; see also Carbon monoxide
  children and, 384, 387
  chloroform in, 480, 482, 484-486
  coliform counts from, 32
  copper in, 151
  exposure assessment and, 38, 44
  global aspects of, 683-688
  hazardous waste incinerators and, 24
  immunotoxicology and, 150, 151, 153
  ingestion exposure and, 38
  landfills and, 10-12
  lead in, 13, 130, 384, 387; see also Lead
  metal extraction and, 27
  national regulations regarding, 44
  nitrates in, 233; see also Nitrates
  pesticides and, 381t, 479-480
  radon in, 483-484
  Santa Clara, California, incident involving, 643
Droplets, inhalation exposure, 38
Drug/substance abuse, 70
  male reproductive function and, 98t
  neurobehavioral testing for toxicity and, 191
Drugs; see also Pharmaceuticals
  as allergens, 152
  bone marrow and, 201; see also Anemia
  cancer susceptibility and, 91
  ears/hearing and, 254
  factory farming and animal, 505
  female reproductive function and, 111
  hepatotoxicity and, 303-304
  immune system and, 328, 335
  immunotoxicology and, 152
  lupus induced by, 340
  nephrotoxicity and, 313
  ototoxic, 254
  susceptibility and, 353-354
  toxicology and, 66
  UV light and, 335
  water-soluble, dermal toxicology and, 187
Dry-cleaned clothing, 25
Dumping, 10, 11f, 26
Duration, 14, 17, 224
  benzene and, 204
  development of disease vs., 54
  diagnosis and, 218
  dose and, 69
  environmental history and, 235
  exposure assessment and, 37, 38
  eyes/vision and, 240
  female reproductive function and, 112
  incidence and, 47
  multiple chemical sensitivity and, 372
  toxicology and, 68, 69, 70
Dust, 13f, 24, 521
  arsenic in, 132
  control procedures for, 431-432
  children and, 387
  cotton, 92
  dermatoses and, 270
  fibrogenic vs. nonfibrogenic inorganic, 290t
  indoor air pollution and, 421t, 424, 431-432
  interplanetary, 590
  lead in, 131, 387
  multiple chemical sensitivity and, 372
  respirable, 39
  respiratory toxicology and, 166
  respiratory tract disorders and, 290-293
  silica; see Silica
  soil-borne contaminants and, 4
Dust mites, indoor air pollution and, 25, 26
Dwarfism, 148t
Dypirone, 204t, 208
Dysentery, 621
"Dysfunctional society," 9
Dysplasia, 79

E
Ears/hearing, 250-262; see also Noise
  anatomy and physiology of, 250-253
  neurobehavioral testing and, 194, 197
  nonenvironmental disease of, 254-255
  nonoccupational disease of, 253-254
  vestibular disorders and, 257-261
E. coli, 618, 621
Ecological risk assessment, 6
Ecology, 3 6
  catastrophes of, 10, 11f
  chemical plants and, 16f, 17
  and EPA categories of environmental hazards, 18
  future and, 8, 9
  population explosion and, 10, 11f
  toxicology and, 66
Effective Dose 50% (ED50), 72
Efficacy, 67, 70, 72, 75
Elastase; see Neutrophil elastase
Elderly, 365-367
Electric apparatus, indoor air pollution and, 24
Electric conductivity, 42
Electrochemical analysis, 42
Electromagnetic fields (EMF), 28, 49, 554-556
  environmental history and, 237
  eyes/vision and, 240, 245-249
  immunotoxicology and, 151-152
  nonionizing radiation and, 543-545, 550-551
  school environment and, 118
Electrophysiologic studies, 195
Elimination, 15f, 17
Elizabeth, New Jersey, fire, 642
Embedded Figures task, 197
Embryo, 74, 80
Emergency
  data base regarding response to, 760
  information resources regarding, 755-762
  medical response to chemical/hazardous waste disaster, 705-727
  organizations regarding, 761
  planning levels of medical response to, 724-725
  poison control centers for; see Poison control centers (PCC)
  and treatment of fire victims, 475-476
Emergency medical technicians (EMTs), 713-714
Emergency Planning and Community Right-to-Know Act (EPCRA), 20, 751
Emissions, 10, 11f
  asphalt, 191-192, 25
  automobile
    environmental legislation about, 746-747
  furans in, 254
  lead in, 384, 385, 394
  school environment and, 118
  solid waste management and, 631-632
  environmental legislation about, 746-747
  Geographic Information System (GSI) and, 20-21, 22f, 23f
  from hazardous waste incinerators, 24
  mapping systems for measuring, 21
  multiple exposure pathways from, 16f, 17
  neurobehavioral testing for toxicity and, 191-192
  sources of toxicity from, 130
Emotional state, 15, 131; see also Affective symptoms; Depression
Emphysema
  cigarette smoking and, 357
  in firefighters, 475
  respiratory toxicology and, 166, 174, 175
Employees; see also Occupation; Workplace environment
  improving life-style and health of, 732-733
  sick building syndrome and, 434-435
Employers, 220
EMTs; see Emergency medical technicians
Encephalopathy, 133, 192, 260, 324
Endocrine system, 74
  autoimmunity and, 343t
  cancer and, male vs. female, 91
  female reproductive function and, 101, 103-109, 112
  male reproductive function and, 96-97
Endoplasmic reticulum, 74
Endosulfan, 21t
Endothall, 480t
Endothelium-derived relaxing factor (EDRF), 314
Endotoxins, 286, 424
Endrine aldehyde, 21t
Energy industry, 9-10, 11f
  global aspects of, 686-687
  phototechnical air pollution and, 24
Entamoeba histolytica, 621
Environment, 3, 4
  aplastic anemia and, 210
  cancer and, 7, 86-93
  catastrophes of, 10, 11f
  community; see Community environment
  developmental toxicology and, 117-119
  and environmental physicians, 6-7
  interaction between host, agent, and, 14f, 17
  male reproductive function and, 97-98
  neurotoxicants and, 129-130
  overlaps between different types of, 4f, 5
  persistence of hazardous substances in, 18, 24
  school; see School environment
  recreational; see Community environment, recreational
  three major types of human, 4, 5, 12
  toxicology and, 67

Environmental crisis, 9-10, 11*f*
Environmental engineers, 39, 225
Environmental health, 3-6; *see also*
    Public safety/health
  defined, 5
  global aspects of, 669-691
  surveillance of, 692-697
Environmental history, 70, 232-239;
    see also Exposure history
  case studies and, 237-238
  clinical diagnosis and, 224
  data bases and, 238-239
  female reproductive function and, 111
  personnel and information resources
    for, 238-239
Environmental hygienists, 32, 39; *see
    also* Industrial hygienists
"Environmental illness," 369; *see also*
    Multiple chemical sensitivity
    (MCS)
Environmental legislation, 219, 743-
    751
Environmental measurements, 51
Environmental medicine, 3-8
  classification of diseases in, 233-234
  clinical approach in, 220-231; *see also*
    Clinical effect/ diagnosis
  defined, 3, 5
  diagnosis in, 217-231; *see also*
    Clinical effect/diagnosis
  environmental health and, 5, 6
  future and, 8
  global aspects of, 669-691
  "key players" of, 14*f*, 17
  organizations concerned with, 239
  physicians' bias in, 220
  practitioners of, guidelines for, 35
  preventive medicine and, 4*f*, 7
  primary care practitioners and, 3, 5,
    221
  risk assessment applied to, 6, 30-36
Environmental Mutagen Information
    Center (EMIC), 759
Environmental Mutagen Information
    Center Backfile (EMICBACK), 759
Environmental physicians, 6-7
Environmental Protection Agency
    (EPA), 360; *see also* U.S.
    Environmental Protection Agency
    (USEPA)
  air pollution and children and, 393
  benzo[*a*]pyrene and, 602
  building products and, 422
  case studies available from, 758
  chemical agents and, 594
  chemical disaster preparedness and,
    723, 726, 727
  composting and, 655
  data bases available from, 19, 759,
    761
  drinking water and, 44, 751
  emissions and, 746
  environmental health practitioners
    and, 35
  environmental history and, 233
  environmental law and, 744
  exposure assessment and, 19, 41
  food contamination and, 498-509
  Geographic Information System of,
    20-21
  hazardous waste and, 635-638, 641
  emergency medical response and,
    705-715
  incineration and, 661, 665
  sites listing and, 26-27
  indoor air quality and, 44
  NAAQS and, 745-747
  National Air Pollution Control
    Administration and, 43
  outdoor air pollution and, 462-463,
    468
  permits and, 744, 746
  prevention of asbestos exposure by,
    448-451
  priority chemicals of, 21*t*
  radon and, 539, 540
  RCRA and, 748-749
  responsibilities of, 761
  reuse of sludge and, 657-658
  risk communication and, 739
  risk management and, 30, 32
  sewage and, 620

solid waste management and, 630
state government and, 744
TEAM study of, 600
toxicology and, 66
Toxic Substances Control Act and,
    750
water pollution and, 480-481, 483
hazardous exposure categories and, 18
Environmental science, 3, 4, 5
Environmental Teratology Information
    Center Backfile (ETICBACK), 759
Environmental tobacco smoke (ETS);
    see also Tobacco smoke
  children and, 391-393
  indoor air pollution and, 426, 428
Environmental toxicity, 18
Environmental toxicology, 69
Enzymes, 74
  AIDS and, 148*t*
  anemia and, 210, 211
  benzene and, 205
  cancer and, 83-84, 91
  chloramphenicol and, 206
  clinical diagnosis and, 223
  depression and, 359
  dermal toxicology and, 185
  developmental toxicology and, 123-
    124
  dioxin and, 135
  eyes/vision and, 244
  female reproductive function and,
    108, 109
  hepatotoxicity and, 305
  immune system and, 328, 334-335
  immunotherapy and, 164
  immunotoxicology and, 141, 143,
    146, 147, 151
  lead and, 131, 210, 211
  microsomal induction of, 75, 91
  respiratory toxicology and, 171, 172
  soil contamination and, 513
  susceptibility and, 359
  zinc and, 151
Eosinophil chemotactic factors of
    anaphylaxis (ECF-A), 147 140*t*,
    141, 147
Eosin Y stain exclusion, 96
EPA; *see* Environmental Protection
    Agency
Epidemiology, 5, 7, 46-61; *see also*
    Population(s)
  aplastic anemia and, 207, 210
  asbestos and, 445-446, 447
  and bone marrow toxicology, 201,
    203-204, 207, 210
  cancer and, 90
  case-control studies in, 47, 49, 53
    Berksonian bias in, 55
    confidence interval and, 59
    power and, 60
    risk measures in, 56-60
    type I and II errors in, 58
  causal inference in, 59-60
  cigarette smoke and, 352; *see also*
    Cigarette smoking
  clinical diagnosis and, 225-226
  cluster studies in, 50, 53
  cohort studies in, 47, 49, 53
    healthy worker effect in, 54
    observation and measurement bias
      in, 54
    power and, 60
    risk estimates in, 55-60
  comparability and bias in, 53-55
  confidence interval and, 59
  controversies regarding controls in, 49
  cross-sectional studies in, 47, 48, 60
  data bases for, 225-226
  data collection in, 50-53
  defined, 46
  disease registries and, 52-53
  dose-response relationships and, 39
  environmental health surveillance and,
    692
  environmental measurements and, 51
  female reproductive function and,
    110-111
  gastrointestinal-induced disorders and,
    306
  gastrointestinal tract and, 298
  geographic information system (GSI)
    and, 21

hazardous waste and, 643-644
immune system and, allergic disease
    and, 329
immunotoxicology and, 149-153
incidence vs. prevalence in, 47, 54;
    see also Incidence; Prevalence
incineration and, 664-665
longitudinal studies in, 47, 48-49
male reproductive function and, 97
medical records and, 51-52, 53
molecular, 90
morbidity data in, 51, 53
mortality data in, 49-52
multiple chemical sensitivity and,
    369-370
neurobehavioral testing for toxicity
    and, 190, 198
neurotoxic agents and, 129, 135
outdoor air pollution and, 463
pesticides and, 604
power, sample size, and significance
    tests in, 60
problems in, 47
proportional incidence ratio (PIR)
    studies in, 49-50
proportional mortality ratio (PMR)
    studies in, 49-50
respiratory toxicology and, 174
respiratory tract disorders and, 284-
    285, 289
risk assessment and, 31-32, 35
sample size and, 60
special surveys or studies in, 53
statistics in, 55-60
tobacco smoke and, 428; *see also*
    Tobacco smoke
Epigenetic carcinogens, 84, 85
Epinephrine, 140*t*, 141
Epoxyhydrolase, 171
Epoxy resins, scleroderma and, 269
Epstein-Barr virus (EBV), 85, 158, 160
  multiple chemical sensitivity and, 373
Erethism, 191
Erythrocytes, 89
Erythromycin, 152
Erythropoiesis, 206, 211
Erythropoietin (EPO), 203
Esophageal cancer, 87, 92*t*
Estradiol, 102, 103-109, 112
Estrogen, 104-109, 111, 112
  alpha-fetoprotein and, 158
  cancer and, 91
  dioxin and, 74
  pesticides and, 108
Estrone, 103, 104
Ethanol, 121, 133
Ethereal sulfate, 205
Ethers, 600, 601
Ethics, and environmental hazards in
    the workplace, 220
Ethyl alcohol, 191*t*
Ethylbenzene, 21*t*, 44 *t*, 133, 599
Ethylenediamine hydrochloride, 335
Ethylene dibromide (EDB), 97, 480*t*,
    502, 508
Ethylene dichloride, in well water, 480*t*
Ethylene-*bis*-dithiocarbamate (EBDC),
    497
Ethylene glycol
  indoor air pollution and, 421*t*, 403-
    404
  nephrotoxicity and, 313
Ethylene oxide, 21*t*, 322*t*, 508
Ethylenethiourea (ETU), 497
Ethylenimines, 209
O-Ethyl-*O*-4-nitrophenyl
    phenylphosphonothioate (EPN),
    134
Evaporation, 15*f*, 17
Excretion, 15*f*, 17
  aplastic anemia and, 207, 211
  developmental toxicology and, 123,
    124
  equilibrium between intake and, 69
  toxicology and, 66, 68, 68, 71
Exercise, physical, 730; *see also*
    Activity/fitness level
  outdoor air pollution and, 464, 467
  susceptibility and, 355
Expiration, 15*f*, 17
Exposure; *see also* Hazards
    (environmental)

acute, chronic, subacute, 17, 38, 68-
    69
age and, 365-367
to asbestos, 441-442
  preventing, 448-451
  secondary, 442
assessment of, 37-45; *see also* Risk
    assessment
  clinical diagnosis and, 225
  community standards and, 43-44
  eyes/vision and, 242, 243
  home audit for, 236-237
  markers and surrogates in, 40
  occupational standards and, 42-43
  oxygen deficiency and, 43
  toxicology and, 65, 70
bioaccumulation and, 18
bone marrow toxicology and, 210
cancer and; *see also* Carcinogenesis/
    cancer
  age and, 91
  animal studies and, 88
cardinal indices of, 224-225
categories of, and environmental
    measurements, 51
characterizing, 224-225
children's
  to air pollution, 390-397
  to lead, 383-389
  to pesticides, 377-382
clinical diagnosis and, 218, 220-231
concentration of, 14; *see also*
    Concentration
confounding factors in, 48, 50; *see
    also* Confounding bias/factors
cumulative, 68, 69
cytogenic assays and, 89
defined, 37
dermatoses and, 277-278
developmental toxicology and, 116-
    120
duration of, 13, 17, 224
economic factors in, 422-423
environmental history and, 233, 234-
    235
epidemiological studies regarding; *see*
    Epidemiology
eyes/vision and, 240, 242-248
to fire products, 470-478
frequency of, 13, 14, 17
generic matrix of, 4, 5*t*
hazardous; *see* Hazards
    (environmental)
to hazardous waste, 638-640, 643,
    645
high-level, 17, 68*f*, 69
human activities and, 422
immune system and, 329
innate capability prior to (premorbid
    ability), 196, 197
interaction between humans and
    hazardous, 13-17
ionizing radiation and, 527, 532
kidneys and, 311
lead and, anemia and, 210-211
limits for safe, 42-44
long-term
  to arsenic, 133
  and low-level, neurotoxicity and, 324
  and low-level, respiratory toxicology
    and, 167
low-level, 5, 10, 11*f*, 17, 68, 69
  eyes/vision and, 242
  kidneys and, 311
  hormesis and, 76
  to lead, 385
multiple chemical sensitivity and,
    369
magnitude of, 14
male reproductive function and, 97-98
misclassification regarding, 53, 55
monitoring; *see* Monitoring
multiple pathways of, 16*f*, 17
neurobehavioral testing for toxicity
    and, 190, 192, 193, 196
neurotoxicity and, 319-320, 324
occupational, and children and
    adolescents, 410-411
outdoor air pollution and, 463
potential vs. actual, 70

Exposure—cont'd
  preexisting illness and, 227, 228t, 363t
  rare cases of, 48, 49, 87
  remote, neurotoxicity and, 319
  removal from, 227, 229t
  repeated, 10, 17, 18
  risk communication and, 738; see also
    Risk communication
  risk of; see Risk assessment
  routes of, 4, 5, 12-13
    for arsenic, 132
    cancer animal studies and, 88
    for chromium, 152
    dermatoses and, 278
    developmental toxicology and, 120-123
    environmental history and, 233
    exposure assessment and, 38, 44
    eyes/vision and, 242-248
    female reproductive function and, d 110
    food and, 488-511
    gastrointestinal tract as major one, 298, 305-306
    for lead, 131
    for organic solvents, 133
    for pesticides, in children, 378
    for radon, 536-537
    soil and, 515-523
    toxicology and, 66, 67
  "safe" vs. "dangerous," 17
  short-term
    fire and, 472
    vs. long-term, 38
    and massive, respiratory toxicology and, 166
  single, to arsenic, 132
  surrogates of, 39, 40
  temporal features of, 68-69
  to tobacco smoke; see Cigarette
    smoking; Tobacco smoke
  "total human," 14, 16f, 17, 516
  toxicology and, 66
  unexpected consequences of, 17
  very high over-, 226-227, 229t
Exposure databases, 19; see also Data
  bases
Exposure history, 15; see also
  Environmental history
  case-control studies and, 56
  clinical diagnosis and, 221
  dermatoses and, 277
  epidemiology studies and, 50, 54-55
  latency and, 17
  multiple chemical sensitivity and, 372-373
  neurotoxicity and, 319-320, 324
  susceptibility and, 355-356
  toxicology and, 67
  work/job history and, 51, 52, 111
Exposure matrix, 13f
  hazardous waste and, 639f
  soil and, 516
Extraction, 41
Extrinsic allergic alveolitis, 336
Eyes/vision, 38, 240-249
  anatomy and physiology of, 240-242
  chemical burns and, 243-244
  dermal toxicology and, 187
  foreign-body sensation and, 243
  ionizing radiation and, 530
  neurobehavioral testing of, 194, 197
  prevention and treatment of injuries to, 248-249
  systemic toxicity and, 38, 244-245

F

Factory farming, 504-505
Fame ionization, 42
Family (of patient), diagnosis and, 219
Federal Emergency Management
  Agency (FEMA), 761-762
Federal Emergency Management
  Agency's Fire Administration
  (FEMA/USFA), 476
Federal government/agencies; see
  Government
Federal Insecticide, Fungicide, and
  Rodenticide Act (FIFRA), 33, 497, 498, 750-751
Federal Water Pollution Control Act, 44

Feed additives, 504-505
Feedback mechanisms, 103, 105, 108
  aplastic anemia and, 211
  negative, 141
FEMA; see Federal Emergency
  Management Agency
Female reproductive function, 101-114
  clinical evaluation and, 111-112
  feedback mechanisms in, 103
  hypothalamus and, 101-109, 112
  infertility and, 102, 105, 106, 110-112
  pituitary and, 101-109, 112
  reproductive toxins and, 74-75
  risk assessment and, 109-111, 113
  subfertility and, 111, 112
  target sites for chemical injury in, 105-107
Ferrochelatase, 206, 211
α_2H-Ferroprotein, 158t
Fertility/infertility
  female, 102, 105, 106, 110-112
  ionizing radiation and, 530
  lead and, 125
  male, 95, 97
Fetal alcohol syndrome, 125
γ-Fetoprotein, 158t
Fetus
  clinical evaluation of, 112
  and immunology of cancer, 157-159, 162
  ionizing radiation and, 531
  mercury and, 492-493
  neurotoxicants and, 130
  outdoor air pollution and, 466
  preconception exposure and, 117
  routes of exposure for, 120-123
  susceptibility and, 359
  transplacental route and, 121
Fiber, dietary, 92, 513
Fiberglass, 24
Fibers, 455-461, 612
  asbestos, 24, 39, 40; see also
    Asbestos
  dermatoses and, 270
  exposure assessment and, 37-39
  features of toxicity of, 456-458
  inhalation and, 38; see also Inhalation
  man-made and natural, 612
  man-made vitreous (MMVF), 455-461
  mineral, 39
  respiratory tract disorders and, 290-293
  types and pathogenesis of, 446-447
Fibronectin, 457
Fibrous glass, 455, 458
Fick's law of diffusion, 184, 185
Filtration, 41, 97
Fire, 12, 23, 24, 470-478; see also
  Combustion; Incineration
  children and, 391-392
  dermatoses and, 270
  in Elizabeth, New Jersey, 642
  environmental history and, 236
  furans from, 25t
  identification of hazards pertaining to, 707f
  indoor air pollution and, 421t, 423
  and unique hazards and exposures of firefighting, 470-472, 475
Firefighters, 470-472, 475, 642
  EPCRA and, 751
  NFPA and, 707, 708, 714
Fish (toxins in), 24, 69, 618, 621
  cancer and, 92
  global aspects of, 687-688
  mercury in, 129
  neurotoxicants in, 129, 135
Fluorides, 41, 21t, 44t
Fluoroacetate, 38
Fluorocarbon polymer fumes, 92
Foaming agents, in drinking water, 44t
Fog, 24
Follicle stimulating hormone (FSH)
  female reproductive function and, 102-109, 112
  male reproductive function and, 96-97
Food, 4, 12, 488-511; see also Diet
  agencies and regulations dealing with, 497-500, 506-507, 509
  animal products for, 504-505
  cancer and, 7, 86-87, 90

children and, 377, 384, 387
dioxins in, 130; see also Dioxins
environmental history and, 233, 234
factory farming and, 504-505
fat and sugar substitutes in, 502
gastrointestinal-induced disorders and, 306
genetic engineering and, 508-509
global aspects of, 683-688
heavy metals in, 490-495
immune system and, 328
irradiation of, 505-508
lead in, 237, 384, 387
naturally occurring anticarcinogens in, 512-514
naturally occurring carcinogens in, 7, 86-87, 92, 512-514
nephrotoxicity and, 313
neurotoxic agents in, 129
nickel in, 274, 275t
"organic," 488, 505
packaging of, 502-504
pesticides in, 497-500; see also
  Pesticides/insecticides
preparation and cooking of, 496-497
preservation of, 92, 501-509
toxicology and, 66f
Food additives, 500-502
  cancer and, 86
  children and, 502
  for color, 501
  irradiation regulated as one, 507
Food chain
  biological amplification and, 69-70
  global aspects of, 689
  inadequate landfills and, 10-12
  insecticides and, 134
  mercury and, 130
  waterborne pollutants and, 4
Food contamination, 4
  airborne pollutants and, 4
  arsenic and, 132; see also Arsenic
  cancer and, 7, 86; see also
    Carcinogenesis/cancer
  developmental toxicology and, 119-120, 121f
  dioxins and, 135, 135
  exposure assessment and, 38, 44
  eye exposure and, 38; see also Eyes/vision
  home gardens and, 13
  ingestion exposure and, 38
  infectious diseases and, 617-618
  lead and, 131
  preventive medicine and, 6
  proximate and ultimate sources of, 489t
  soil contamination and, 13, 522; see
    also Soil contamination
Food and Drug Act, 66
Food and Drug Administration (FDA), 66, 497-509
Food, Drug, and Cosmetic Act, 73, 498-509, 751
Food extracts, 513
Foreign body/substance, 66, 74
  eyes and, 243
  skin and, 182, 186-187, 270
Formaldehyde, 24, 25, 117, 601
  children and, 392t, 393
  dermatoses and, 266t
  environmental history and, 236
  fire and, 473-474
  immunotoxicology and, 152-153
  indoor air pollution and, 421t, 423, 431
  respiratory clearance and, 170t
  respiratory toxicology and, 171, 174-175
Fossil fuel burning, 24
Free radicals, 75, 172-177, 365
  age and, 365
  respiratory toxicology and, 172, 176, 177
French-American-British (FAB)
  Cooperative group, 211
Freon, 422, 481
Frequency, 13, 14, 17, 37, 38
  epidemiology studies and, 47
Friction, dermatoses and, 270
Fructose, 97
FSH; see Follicle stimulating hormone

Fumes
  chronic pulmonary disease and, 362
  fire and, 474
  lead in, 131
  neurobehavioral testing for toxicity and, 194
Fumigants, 152, 153
Fungi, 12t, 25, 26, 84t, 87
  immunotoxicology and, 140t
  indoor air pollution and, 421t
  respiratory tract disorders and, 285
  water pollution and, 485
Fungicides, 33, 152, 153, 273, 378t, 605; see also Federal Fungicide,
  Insecticide, and Rodenticide Act
  (FIFRA); Pesticides/insecticides
  indoor air pollution and, 421t, 423
  neurotoxicity and, 323t, 324
Furadan, 379
Furans, 24, 25, 602-603
  in composts, 655
  solid waste management and, 632-633
Furniture refinishing, 129, 130
Furocoumarins, 187

G

G-CSF; see Granulocyte colony-
  stimulating factor
G6PD; see Glucose-6-phosphate
  deficiency
Gaia Hypothesis, 688
b-Galactosidase, 18
Gamma-aminobutyric acid, 131, 135
Gamma globulins, 74
Garbage, 24, 26; see also Incineration;
  Landfills; Solid waste management
Gardening (home), 13, 129
Gaseous phase, 38
Gases, 38, 130, 191, 606-607
  barotraumas and, 584-589
  chronic pulmonary disease and, 362
  diffuse alveolar damage and, 287-290
  exposure assessment and, 38, 40
  and concentration of, 41
  sampling and, 42
  eyes/vision and, 244
  greenhouse, 672-676
  outdoor air pollution and, 464
  respiratory protective equipment for, 468
  respiratory toxicology and, 168
  respiratory tract disorders and, 287-290
  solid waste management and, 633
Gas-exchange surfaces, 168
Gasoline, 133, 204
  indoor air pollution and, 423
  lead in, 384, 385
Gas stoves, 421t, 423
Gastrointestinal system/tract, 298-310
  allergy and, 330
  asbestos and, 445
  cancer of, 85, 307-308
  defense mechanisms of, 299-301
  developmental toxicology and, 122-123
  dioxin and, 135
  exposure types and sources of illness of, 305-306
  immune system and, 329, 330
  lead and, 131
  mercury and, 132
  nickel and, 274
  organic solvents and, 133
  pesticides and, 134
  sewage and, 621
Gender/sex, 14, 15
  inhalation exposure and, 38
  heat stress and, 569
Genetic engineering, 508-509
Genetic makeup, 6, 15
  aplastic anemia and, 207, 208
  autoimmunity and, 337-338
  cancer and, 75, 79-80, 83-84
    vs. diet, 87
  immunology of, 157
  susceptibility and, 91
  chloramphenicol and, 207
  dermatoses and, 273
  developmental toxicology and, 115, 126
  gastrointestinal tract and, 301

Genetic makeup—cont'd
 immune system and, 157, 329
 immunotoxicology and, 140
 indoor air pollution and, 425-426
 ionizing radiation and, 18, 528-529
 male reproductive function and, 97
 mutagens and, 74
 susceptibility and, 73, 356, 357-358
 toxicology and, 67, 73
 tumors and, 79-80
Genetic Toxicology data base, 759
Genotoxic carcinogens, 84, 85, 89, 92
Geographic Information System (GIS), 20-21
Geographic mapping, 20
Gerontogens, 365
Giardiasis, 616-617
Ginger jake paralysis, 129
Glands, immune system and, 328
Global warming, 10, 11*f*
Glomerular filtration, 124
Glucoroic acid, 205
Glucose, liver and, 301-302
Glucose-6-phosphate deficiency (G6PD), 357
Glucose-6-phosphate dehydrogenase, 211
 AIDS and, 148*t*
Glucuronide, 207
Glue sniffing, 260, 313, 322*t*
Glutamate, 195
Glutathione, 513, 205
Glutathione-dependent peroxidases, 75
Glutathione peroxidase, respiratory toxicology and, 172
Glutathione S-transferase (GST), 124, 171
Glycerylphosphorylcholine (GPC), 97
Glyceryl trinitrate, 186
Glycine, anemia and, 210
Glycol ethers, 97
Glycoproteins, 146
 HIV and, 148-149
 and immunology of cancer, 157
 respiratory toxicology and, 172
Gold, ears/hearing and, 254*t*
Gold salts, 151, 152
Gold sodium thiomalate, 204*t*, 209
Gonadotropin-releasing hormone (GnRH), 103-109, 112
Gonadotropins, 97, 106-109, 112
Gonads, 103
Government, 51-52, 67; *see also specific agencies/acts*
 carcinogens and, 90
 and diagnosis in environmental medicine, 219, 225
 environmental community hazards and, 12
 environmental legislation and, 743-751
 epidemiology studies and, 51-52
 exposure assessment and, 41, 42-44
 MSDSs required by, 239
 responsibilities of key federal agencies of, 761-762
 testing requirements by, 236
 toxicology and, 73
Grab samples, 42
Graft rejection/graft-versus-host reactions, 140*t* 146, 164
Grain handling/milling, 166
Granulocyte colony-stimulating factor (G-CSF), 203
Granulocyte macrophage colony-stimulating factor (GM-CSF), 203, 206
Granuloma formation, 285-287, 335
Granulomatous disease, 148*t*
Granulosa cells, 106-107
Greenhouse gases, 672-676
Green Revolution, 669, 686
Green tea, 513
Griseofulvin, 335
Grooved Pegboard test, 197
Ground water, 4, 479-487
 exposure assessment and, 42
 from wells, 15*f*
 gastrointestinal-induced disorders and, 305
 immunotoxicology and, 150
 persistence of environmental hazards in, 18

soil contamination and, 4, 517-518, 521
 vs. surface, 42
 toluene and benzene in, 150
 treatment of, 650
Growth factors/hormones; *see also* Hormones; Transforming growth factors (TGF)
 bone marrow toxicology and, 201-208
 cancer and, 79, 80, 82-85
 cancer and, microbial and mammalian cell culture assays and, 88
 developmental toxicology and, 125-127
 factory farming and, 505
 female reproductive function and, 102-109, 112
 immunotoxicology and, 146
 leukemia and, 212
 respiratory toxicology and, 175-177
Guanine, 209
Gut, 66*f*; *see also* Intestinal tract
Gut-associated lymphoid tissue (GALT), 300

H
Habitat destruction, 10, 11*f*
Hageman factor pathway enzymes, 146, 147, 328
Hallucinogens, 191*t*
Haloethers, 17
Halogenated aliphatics, 599-600
Halogenated alkanes and alkenes, 133
Halogenated aromatic hydrocarbons (HAH), 135, 150
Halogenated compounds, respiratory toxicology and, 173
Halogenated hydrocarbons, 97, 109*t*
 dermatoses and, 274
 nephrotoxicity and, 311, 313, 314*t*
Halogenated polyaromatic hydrocarbons, 149-150
Halstead-Reitan test battery, 190
Haptens, 74, 152-153, 187
Hardpans, 517
Hassall's corpuscles, 140*t*, 149
Hay fever, 6
Hazardline (BRS) data base, 759
Hazardous Substance Data Bank (HSDB), 758-759, 761
Hazardous waste, 626; *see also* Solid waste management; Waste disposal
 amount of, 12
 asbestos as, 448
 assessment and remediation of, 647-653
 burning of, 24; *see also* Incineration
 case studies of exposure in, 642-643
 characteristics of, 636*t*
 cleanup criteria for, 649
 community exposure to, 635-646
 definition of, 636
 emergency medical response involving, 705-721, 751
 federal regulations for, 636-637, 745-749, 751
 inadequate landfills and, 10-12
 incineration of, 662-663; *see also* Incineration
 infectious diseases and, 620-621
 liquid, 651, 652
 at Love Canal, 10, 219, 642
 prevention of exposure to, 645
 protective equipment for, 714-716
 radioactive, 644-645
 reducing exposure to, 643
 risk communication, 738
 simple aromatics in, 599
 sites of, 26-27, 637-638, 648
 social considerations regarding, 652
 soil contamination and, 518
 types of, 637*f*
Hazard potential, 7
Hazards (environmental), 6, 11*f*-12
 causative agents of, 12-13; *see also* Causation/causative agents
 defined, 12
 elderly and, 365-367
 employers and, 220
 environmental history and, 233; *see also* Environmental history
 EPA categories of, 18

EPCRA and, 751
 female reproductive function and, 109-112
 forced relocation because of, 219
 gastrointestinal tract and, 298
 identification of
  chemical, 724-725
  fire, 707*f*
  risk assessment and, 30, 31
 immunotoxicology and, 149-153
 information about, 755-762
 male reproductive function and, 97-98
 measurement of, 18-19, 39; *see also* Exposure, assessment of
 preexisting illness and, 361-365
 proximity to, 70
 public response to, 7, 10, 11*f*
 recognition of, 7, 18-22
 sources of, 9-29
 susceptibility and, 351-360
 types of, 9-29, 12, 28
HbCO; *see* Carboxyhemoglobin
hCG; *see* Human chorionic gonadotropic
Health departments/agencies, 51-52
Health care professionals/practitioners; *see also* Physicians
 clinical experience of, 226
 environmental crisis and, 10, 11*f*
 environmental medicine and, 3, 5, 35, 217-231
 EPCRA and, 751
 global aspects for consideration by, 689
 guidelines for, 35
 improving patients' life-style and, 729-736
 parenteral exposure and, 38
 primary care, 3, 5, 735
 public health and, 411
 radon and, 540
Health promotion, 733-735
Health status, susceptibility and, 73
Healthy People 2000, 729
Healthy worker effect, 70
Heart disease; *see* Cardiovascular/heart disease
Heart transplants, 333
Heating, ventilation, and air-conditioning system (HVAC), 419, 429-431
 ASHRAE and, 41, 44
Heat shock, 17
Heat stress, 475, 563-575
 acute illnesses of, 569-572
 chronic illnesses of, 572
 prevention of, 572-573
Heavy metals, 12*t*, 17, 24, 607-612; *see also* Metals
 aplastic anemia and, 204*t*, 209
 diagnosis and, 221, 222
Household products—cont'd
 ears/hearing and, 260
 environmental history and, 233, 236, 237
 female reproductive function and, 74
 in food, 490-495
 hazardous waste incinerators and, 24
 male reproductive function and, 97
 nephrotoxicity and, 311, 313
 solid waste management and, 633-634
 vestibular system and, 260
Hematopoiesis, immunotoxicology and, 146
Hemoglobin, 116, 121
 aplastic anemia and, 206, 211
 carbon monoxide and, 135, 136
 chloramphenicol and, 206
 lead and, 211
Hemolysins, 74
Hemolytic anemia, 152
Hepatic disease, 88, 227
Hepatitis virus, 51, 85, 621
Hepatochlor, immunotoxicology and, 149
Hepatotoxicity, 303-305
 respiratory toxicology and, 166
 susceptibility and, 358
Heptachlor, 21*t*, 134, 480*t*
Herbicides, 378*t*, 605; *see also* Pesticides/ insecticides
 children and, 378-379, 380
 chlorophenoxy vs. bipyridyl, 380

genetic engineering and, 508-509
immunotoxicology and, 149, 153
indoor air pollution and, 423
respiratory toxicology and, 168
Herpes virus, 158, 160, 275
Heterocyclic amines, 17
Hexacarbons, neurotoxicity and, 322*t*
Hexachlorobenzene (HCB), dermatoses and, 273-274
Hexachlorocyclohexane, 21*t*
Hexachlorophene, 122, 130
n-Hexane, 130, 190, 191*t*, 599
 neurotoxicity and, 322*t*, 323*t*
2-Hexanone, 21*t*
High-altitude and aerospace medicine, 576-591
High-altitude cerebral edema (HACE), 581
High-altitude pulmonary edema (HAPE), 580-581
Hiroshima, 530, 532
Histamines
 immunotoxicology and, 140*t*, 141, 146, 147
 urticaria and, 331
Histamine-releasing factors (HRFs), 146
Histiocytes, and immunology of cancer, 159-160
Histoplasmosis, 285
History; *see* Environmental history; Exposure history;
HIV; *see* Human immunodeficiency virus
HLA; *see* Human leukocyte antigens
Hodgkin's disease
 AIDS and, 148*t*
 immune system and, 160, 162
Home environment, 3, 4, 5, 6, 12
 aplastic anemia and, 204
 asbestos in, 448
 benzene in, 204
 developmental toxicology and, 117, 119*f*
 diagnosis and, 219; *see also* Clinical effect/diagnosis
 environmental history and, 233, 235, 236-237
 eyes/vision and, 240
 family psychosocial agents in, 12
 hazardous waste and, 641
 indoor air pollution in, 419-437
 nephrotoxicity and, 313
 neurotoxicity and, 320
 noise in, 253*t*
 pesticides and, 377
 radon in, 537-540
 repeated, low-level exposures in, 10
 vs. school, 11*f*
 toxic profile of, 12
 workplace/occupation environment and, 4*f*, 5, 219
 trauma in, 12
Homeostasis, immunotoxicology and, 139
Hormesis, 76
Hormones
 alpha-fetoprotein and, 158
 bone marrow toxicology and, 211
 cancer and, 79, 80, 82, 91
 factory farming and, 504-505
 of female reproductive function, 101-109, 112
 immunotherapy and, 164
 immunotoxicology and, 140*t*, 141
 of male reproductive system, 96-97
 neuroendocrine poisons and, 74
 receptors and, 74
 reproductive toxins and, 74
 stress and, 359
 susceptibility and, 359
Hospital records, 51-52, 53
Host
 defense mechanisms of; *see* Defense mechanisms
 interactions between agent, environment, and, 14*f*, 17
 susceptibility; *see* Susceptibility
House dust, 13; *see also* Dust
Household accidents, 28
Household products, 6, 25, 233, 236-237, 398-407

INDEX

Household products—cont'd
 ears/hearing and, 260
 eyes/vision and, 244
 neurotoxicity and, 320
 nontoxic, 398-399
HSALINE data base, 761
Human chorionic gonadotropic (hCG), 105, 158t, 162
"Human exposure topology," 14
Human immunodeficiency virus (HIV), 13, 91, 148-149
 parenteral exposure and, 38
Human leukocyte antigens (HLA), 142, 164
 immune system and, 332, 333, 338
 autoimmunity and, 340, 341
 SLE and, 340
Human placental lactogen (HPL), 162
Human responses, 14f, 19
 cellular; see Cellular response
 factors in, 13, 14, 17
Humoral response, in immunology of cancer, 157-165
Hydralazine, 151
Hydrazine, nephrotoxicity and, 314t
Hydrocarbons
 ambient air quality standards and, 43
 dermatoses and, 272
 environmental history and, 236
 indoor air pollution and, 421t, 402
 nephrotoxicity and, 313t, 314t, 315-316
 respiratory toxicology and, 173
 in soil, 521
 source of, in photochemical air pollution, 23
Hydrochloric acid, 244
Hydrogen chloride, 606
 hazardous waste incinerators and, 24
 from pyrolysis, 472, 473
 solid waste management and, 633
Hydrogen cyanide, 473
Hydrogen fluoride, solid waste management and, 633
Hydrogen peroxide, hepatotoxicity and, 303
Hydrogen sulfide, 191t, 192, 287t, 289
Hydroquinone, 205, 206
5-Hydroxyindoleacetic acid, 131
Hydroxyl radical, 75, 303
Hydroxymethylbilane, 210
γ-Hydroxyphenylbutazone, 208
Hygiene
 dermatoses and, 278-279
 industrial, 6; see also Industrial hygienists
 sanitation vs., 6
Hyoscyamine, 38
Hyperbilirubinemia, 122
Hypergammaglobulinemia, 148
Hyperplasia, 75, 79, 142
Hyperproliferation, 79
Hyperreactivity of respiratory tract, 282-285, 358
Hypersensitivity, 140, 143
 AIDS and, 148
 chemical mediators of, 146-147
 delayed (DH), 144, 146, 149
 allergic contact dermatitis and, 335
 atopic dermatitis and, 331
 cadmium and, 151
 dermal toxicology and, 187
 dermatoses and, 278
 immune competence tests and, 162, 163
 organ transplantation and, 333
 environmental agents and, 149, 152-153
 immune system and, 328-329
 type I disorders and, 329-331
 type II disorders and, 331-333, 335
 type III disorders and, 333-334
 type IV disorders and, 334-335
 interferons and, 146
 transfer factor and, 144
Hypersensitivity pneumonitis (HP), 286-287, 336
Hypertrophy, 75, 79
Hypogammaglobulinemia, 148t
Hypoosmotic swelling (HOS assay), 96
Hypoplasia, 148t

Hypothalamic-pituitary-ovarian-uterine axis (HPOU-axis), 104, 105, 108, 112
Hypothalamus, 101-109, 112
Hypothyroidism, 122
Hypoxanthine-guanine phosphoribosyltransferase (HPRT), 356

I

"Ice minus" case, 508
IgA, 144, 148t, 327
 gastrointestinal tract and, 300
 HAHs and, 150
 mercury and, 151
 metals and, 151
 PCBs and, 151
 trimellitic anhydride and, 152
IgD, 142, 144
IgE, 144, 146, 327-328
 ABPA and, 336
 atopic dermatitis and, 331
 autoimmunity and, 151
 enhancement of antigen entry and production of, 329t
 eyes/vision and, 243
 hypersensitivity and, 152
 metals and, 152
 penicillin senstivity and, 152
 pesticides and, 152
 trimellitic anhydride and, 152
 urticaria and, 331
IgE antibody, 140t
IgG, 143, 144
 ABPA and, 336
 AIDS and, 148t, 149
 gastrointestinal tract and, 300
 HAHs and, 150
 metals and, 151
 ozone and, 150
 PCBs and, 151
 respiratory toxicology and, 174
 respiratory tract disorders and, 286
 SLE and, 340
 trimellitic anhydride and, 152
 type I immune system reactions and, 327, 331, 336
 type II immune system reactions and, 331-333, 336
 urticaria and, 331
IgM, 142, 143, 144, 327
 AIDS and, 148t
 gastrointestinal tract and, 300
 HAHs and, 150
 herbicide and, 149
 metals and, 151
 respiratory tract disorders and, 286
 SLE and, 340
 trimellitic anhydride and, 152
 type II immune system reactions and, 331-333
IL-2, 149, 150
Immediately dangerous to life or health (IDLH), 42-43
 chemical disaster preparedness and, 726-727
 fire and, 472
Immune complex diseases, 334
Immune enhancement, 149, 150-152
 and immunology of cancer, 161
 immunotherapy and, 163
Immune response (IR) genes, 142
Immune response/immunity, 139, 142-143
 chemical mediators of, 146-147
 to tumor, 159-160
Immune surveillance, 160-161, 163
Immunization, 334, 346
Immunoassay, 89, 112t
Immunoblastic lymphadenopathy, 342-343
Immunocompetence, tests for, 162-163
Immunodeficiency diseases, 147-149, 344-346
 cancer, 160-161
 congenital, 160
 environmental agents and, 149-150
 immunotherapy and, 164
Immunogen, 141, 142
Immunoglobulins, 123, 143-144; see also entries beginning Ig
 AIDS and, 148t, 149

and immunology of cancer, 159, 162, 163t
 ionizing radiation and, 150
 metals and, 149
Immunologic memory, 143
Immunologic tissue injury, 147
Immunologic tolerance, 143
Immunology/immune system, 326-348
 allergic and atopic disorders and, 328-329
 anaphylaxis and, 327-328
 asbestos and, 445
 autoimmunity and, 335, 336-344
 bone marrow toxicology and, 202, 209, 212
 cancer and, 75, 86, 91, 156-165
 evaluation and diagnosis in, 161-163
 immunotherapy and, 163-165
 clinical diagnosis and, 222, 227, 228
 depression and, 359
 dermal toxicology and, 186, 187
 dermatoses and, 265, 278
 eyes/vision and, 243
 gastrointestinal tract and, 300-301
 ionizing radiation and, 529
 mixed reactions of, 336
 multiple chemical sensitivity and, 372
 nephrotoxicity and, 313
 organ transplantation and, 333
 reasons for failure of, 326
 respiratory toxicology and, 167, 170f, 173
 respiratory tract disorders and, 284, 286
 susceptibility and, 358, 359
 toxicology and, 68, 74
 type I reactions of, 327-331
 type II reactions of, 331-333
 type III reactions of, 333-334
 type IV reactions of, 334-335
Immunorestoration, 164
Immunosuppression, 85t, 86, 149-150
 vs. immunoenhancing, 146
 immunotherapy and, 164
 multiple chemical sensitivity and, 372
 organ transplantation and, 160, 333
 renal transplants and, 160
 tobacco smoke and, 150
 tumors and, 153
Immunotherapy, 163-165
Immunotoxicology, 74, 139-155
 of AIDS, 148-149
 environmental agents and, 149-153
 mechanisms of immunologic and related diseases, 147-149
 metals and, 149, 151, 152, 153
 primary immune response and, 142-143
 secondary (anamnestic) response and, 143
 tumors and, 149, 152, 153
 TNF and, 146
 tobacco smoke and, 150
Incidence, 47
 bias for, 54
 in cohort studies, 48
 proportional ratio of (PIR), 49-50
 standardized ratio (SIR) of, 56
 of tumors, 87-88
Incident command system (ICS), 709
Incineration, 12, 20, 24, 628, 630, 660-666; see also Fire
 biomedical, 25t
 furans from, 25
 lead from, 130
 mobile incinerators for, 651
 research needs regarding, 665-666
 treatments for, 651
 types of, 24
Indomethacin, 204t, 209
Indoor air pollution, 464
Industrial hygienists, 6, 32, 39
 asbestos and, 451
 associations for, 709, 726-727
 environmental history and, 235
 epidemiology studies and, 51
 fire and, 472
 respiratory tract disorders and, 286
 threshold limit values set by, 596t
Industrial operations
 arsenic from, 130
 benzene from, 204
 cancer and, 86, 87

 dermal exposure and, 38
 developmental toxicology and, 118
 dioxins from, 130, 135
 environmental history and, 233
 furans from, 25
 immunotoxicology and, 152
 lead from, 130, 384
 mercury from, 130
 soil contamination and, 518
Infection, 4, 12, 13; see also Viruses
 aplastic anemia and, 204
 cancer and, 85-86
 children and, 378
 dermatoses and, 265t, 269, 270, 277
 female reproductive function and, 111
 food contamination and, 617-618
 immune system and, 335
 immunotoxicology and, 139, 148
 chemical mediators and, 147
 tobacco smoke and, 150
 indoor air pollution and, 421t
 inflammatory response to, 139
 international travel and, 621
 male reproductive function and, 98
 ozone and, 150
 reuse of sludge and, 657-658
 soil contamination and, 618-619
 susceptibility to, in children, 391
 T-cells and, 140t, 141
 toxicology and, 68
 water pollution and, 615-617
Infertility, 95
 female reproductive function and, 102, 105, 106, 110-112
 male reproductive function and, 95, 97
Inflammation
 of airway, 282-285
 eyes/vision and, 242
 immune system and, 336
 immunotoxicology and, 139-141, 146, 147
 nervous system and, 320
 respiratory toxicology and, 170f, 172, 173, 175
Infrared analysis, 42
Ingestion, 13, 15f, 17; see also Intake
 of asbestos, 441t
 bioconcentration and, 15f
 of chromium, 152
 exposure assessment and, 38
 inhalation or dermal absorption vs., 13
 insecticides and, children and, 379
 of lead, 387
 of soil, 516, 521
Inhalation, 13, 15f, 17
 of arsenic, 132
 of asbestos, 441t
 of benzene, 204
 cancer and, 88
 of carbon monoxide, 136
 by children, 379
 of chromium, 152
 chronic pulmonary disease and, 363-364
 of dioxin, 135
 exposure assessment and, 38
 ingestion or dermal absorption vs., 13
 insecticides and, in children, 379
 of man-made fibers, 455-461
 of mercury, 132
 outdoor air pollution and, 464
 pesticides and, 135
 rate of, risk assessment and, 33
 respiratory toxicology and, 166, 168, 173-175
 respiratory tract and, 282-297
 of smoke, 474-477
 volatility and, 135
Inhibition, 73, 93
Injury
 inflammatory response to, 139
 occupational, and children and adolescents, 409-410
Insecticides; see Pesticides/insecticides
Insects, 17
 diseases transmitted by, 619-620
 indoor air pollution and, 25
Insulin, 104, 112t
Insurance companies, and diagnosis in environmental medicine, 219

Intake
  of children, 377
  developmental toxicology and, 120f
  equilibrium between excretion and, 69
Integrated Risk Information Service, 31, 759
Intellectual functions, 133, 196-197, 198
Intensity, environmental history and, 235
Interferons, 144, 146
  AIDS and, 148
  PCBs and, 151
Interleukin (IL), 144, 145t, 203, 206
  allergic contact dermatitis and, 266
  organ transplantation and, 333
Interleukin-6, respiratory toxicology and, 174
International Agency for Research on Cancer (IARC), 31, 33, 90, 91, 212
International Classification of Diseases (ICD), 51, 52
International Food Biotechnology Council (IFBC), 498t, 509
International travel, 621; see also Environmental medicine, global aspects of
Interstitial fibrosis, 290-295
Intestinal tract, 67, 207
Intracellular membrane alteration, 67
Intravascular spaces, immunotoxicology and, 140
In vitro testing, vs. animal testing, 76
Iodine, 122
Ionized silanol groups, 175
Ions, 195
Iron
  aplastic anemia and deficiency of, 211
  children and, 385
  dermatoses and, 271
  in drinking water, 44t
Irradiation (of food), 505-508
Irritant contact dermatitis (ICD), 265-266, 277
Isolation, 6
Isomers, 40, 596-597
Isoniazid, 151
Isophorone, 21t
2-Isoproposyphenyl methylcarbamate (Unden), 149
Isotopes, 26

J
Jewelry, 233
Jimson weed, 38
Job's syndrome, 148t

K
Kaposi's sarcoma, 148
Kara Sea dumping, 26
Kepone, 125, 135, 751
Kerosene, 25, 133, 421t, 423
Ketones, 173, 601
Kidneys, 18, 311-317
  anatomy and physiology of, 311-312
  arsenic and, 132
  cancer of, 83t
  developmental toxicology and, 124
  environmental history and, 233
  lead and, 125, 131
  mercury and, 151
  solvents and, 133
  transplants of, 333
Killer (K) cells; see NK (natural killer) cells
Kinase C, 131
Kindling mechanisms, 372
Kinins, 140t, 141, 146, 147

L
Laboratory testing, 222-224, 235-236
  immune system and
    autoimmunity and, 342
    immunodeficiency disorders and, 344
  for lead, in children, 385-386
  multiple chemical sensitivity and, 373
  nervous system and, 320-321, 322
Lack of specificity, 15
Lactate dehydrogenase, respiratory toxicology and, 174
Landfills, 650
  environmental law about, 745

inadequate, 10, 11f
soil contamination and, 518
treatment techniques for, 652
Langerhans' cells, 183, 187, 266
Lasers, 550
Latency, 17
  allergic contact dermatitis and, 266
  asbestos and, 441, 446
  cancer and, viruses and, 86
  children and, 391
  cohort studies and, 48
  environmental history and, 234
  toxicology and, 73, 76
Latex, 119, 335
Law; see Environmental legislation; Government
Lawyers, effect of, on diagnosis, 219-220
LD50; see Lethal Dose 50%
Leachate, 518
Leaching, 10, 11f, 15f, 17
Lead, 13, 25, 607-608
  ambient air quality standards and, 43, 167t
  anemia induced by, 210-211
  as biological marker, 51
  calcium and, 121, 123, 131
  children and, 198, 383-389
  clinical diagnosis and, 223
  in composts, 655
  developmental toxicology and, 117f, 117, 120, 125
    calcium and, 121, 123
    distribution and, 123
  development and, 260
  in drinking water, 44t
  ears/hearing and, 254t, 260
  emotional consequences of poisoning from, 131
  environmental history and, 233, 236, 237
  as EPA priority chemical, 21t
  eyes/vision and, 244
  female reproductive function and, 108
  fertility and, 125
  in food, 237, 490t, 493-495, 504
  hazardous waste incinerators and, 24
  history of toxicity of, 129
  immune system and, 74
  immunotoxicology and, 149
  iron deficiency and, 211
  male reproductive function and, 96, 97
  measuring airborne, 19
  need for further research regarding, 387-388
  nephrotoxicity and, 313-314
  neurobehavioral testing for toxicity and, 189-192, 198
  and neuronal response to injury, 131
  neurotoxicity and, 322t, 323
  occupation and, 125
  outdoor air pollution and, 22, 466
  from paint, 10, 11f, 13, 384
  persistence of, 131
  pregnancy and, 117f, 117, 234
  reproductive toxicity of, 18
  reuse of sludge and, 657
  risk assessment of, 30-31
  in school environment, 117
  in soil, 520
  sources of, 129-130, 383-384
  storage of, in bone, 66, 68, 123, 131
  toxicity of, 131, 132t
  vestibular disorders and, 260
  VOCs and, 25
Lead acetate, 82
Leaf burning, 24
Learning, 130, 133, 191, 193, 197
Legionellosis, 617
Leprosy, 148t, 160
Leptophos, 134
Lethal Dose 50% (LD50), 72
Leukemia, 80
  benzene and, 204, 212-213, 228, 598
  bone marrow toxicology and, 201, 211-213
  EFT and, 237
  EMF exposure and, 49, 50
  immune system and, 162
  immunotherapy and, 163, 164
  immunotoxicology and, 153

ionizing radiation and, 530
RNA viruses and, 158
skin tests for, 163
Leukocytes, 80, 85, 89, 91, 140t
  dermal toxicology and, 187
  respiratory toxicology and, 174
Leukotrienes, 147
Levamisole, 164
Levin's attributable risk, 57
LH; see Luteinizing hormone
Lifestyle/culture, 14, 70, 86, 92-93
  improving patients', 729-736
  male reproductive function and, 98
Li-Fraumeni syndrome, 83t
Ligands, 74
Light bulbs, 24
Lime, 244, 271, 275, 401
Lindane, 153, 480t, 604
Love Canal incident involving, 10, 219, 642
Lipid peroxidation, 74, 75, 303
Lipids, 69
  dermal toxicology and, 184, 187
  dermatoses and, 264
  developmental toxicology and, 120f
  dioxin and, 135
  immune system and, 328
  and immunology of cancer, 157
  immunotoxicology and, 146, 147
  liver and, 301-302
  organic solvents and, 133
  toxicokinetics and, 71
Lipophilic compounds/substances
  developmental toxicology and, 121
  dioxin and, 135
  gastrointestinal tract and, 301
  organic solvents and, 133
  preexisting illness and, 364
Lipopolysaccharide, 151
Lipoprotein saccharide (LPS), 151
15-Lipoxygenase, 171
Liquid hazardous waste, 651, 652
Liquid phase, 38
Lissencephaly, 125
Listeria, 618
Lithium carbonate, 151
Liver, 18, 301-310
  anatomy of, 302-303
  aplastic anemia and, 205, 209
  autoimmunity and, 343t
  biomarkers and, 306-307
  cancer of, 82, 87, 88
  developmental toxicology and, 124
  environmental history and, 233
  immunotoxicology and, 140
  male reproductive function and, 96
  nephrotoxicity and, 131, 313
  respiratory toxicology and, 172
  solvents and, 133
  susceptibility and, 355
Local anesthetics, 152
Logistic regression, 57
Lomustine (CCNU), 204t, 209, 213
Long-acting anticoagulants (LAA), 405
Loop of Henle, 311-312
Love Canal incident, 10, 219, 642
Lowell, Massachusetts, incident, 643
Lowest-observed-adverse-effect level (LOAEL), 32 109-110, 594
Low-level radioactive waste (LLRW), 27-28
Lung cancer
  ACTH and, 162
  asbestos and, 444-445
  clinical diagnosis and, 227
  immunology of, 162, 163, 164
  ionizing radiation and, 530
  radon and, 537-538
  respiratory toxicology and, 166, 167
  tobacco smoke and, 428
Lungs
  acute toxicity and, 18
  age and, 365
  anatomic features of, 168-169
  asbestos and, 442, 445-446, 447
  children and, 390
  chronic toxicity and, 18
  developmental toxicology and, 122, 123t, 125-126
  environmental history and, 233
  exposure assessment and, 39
  hazardous waste incinerators and, 24

mercury and, 131, 132
nickel and, 151
obesity and, 364
ozone and, 363; see also Ozone
pesticides and, 134
respiratory toxicology and, 168
silica and, 34-35, 39
susceptibility and, 355, 390
toxicology and, 66f
trimellitic anhydride and, 152
Lupus, 340, 343t; see also Systemic lupus erythematosus (SLE)
Luteinizing hormone (LH)
  female reproductive function and, 102-109, 112
  male reproductive function and, 96-97
Lye, 244
Lyme disease, 619
Lymphangiectasis, 148t
Lymph nodes
  and immunology of cancer, 159-160
  immunotoxicology and, 140, 141-143
  nickel and, 151
Lymphocytes, 140t, 141, 142
  atopic dermatitis and, 331
  dermal toxicology and, 187
  HIV and, 148-149
  immune system and, 153, 327-328
  and immunology of cancer, 159-160, 162, 163
  immunotoxicology and, pesticides and, 149
  organ transplantation and, 333
  ozone and, 150
  PCBs and, 151
  respiratory toxicology and, 174, 177-178
  susceptibility and, 356
  transfer factor and, 144
Lymphoid tissue, tobacco smoke and, 150
Lymphokines, 142, 144, 163t
  allergic contact dermatitis and, 266
  immune system and, 333, 334-335
  organ transplantation and, 333
Lymphoma, 80
  AIDS and, 148
  autoimmunity and, 342-343
  Burkitt's, 158
  immune system and, 148, 153, 162
  renal transplants and, 160
  Smith Hall, New Jersey, study of, 643
Lymphotoxins (LT), 144, 146
Lysosomal hydrolases, 140t
Lysozyme, 140t

M
Macroglobulinemia, 148t
Macrolide antibiotics, 152
Macromolecules, 71, 74
  hepatotoxicity and, 303
  and immunology of cancer, 157
  immunotoxicology and, 141, 152
  reactive oxygen species and, 75
Macrophages, 140t, 141, 142, 143
  cadmium and, 151
  CSF and, 146
  dermal toxicology and, 187
  hepatotoxicity and, 303
  HIV and, 148-149
  immune system and, 327-328, 335
  and immunology of cancer, 160, 163t-164
  interferons and, 146
  man-made fibers and, 457-458
  outdoor air pollution and, 464
  respiratory toxicology and, 169-177
  respiratory tract disorders and, 283
Magnesium, dermatoses and, 271
Magnetic field, 28; see also Electromagnetic fields (EMF)
Magnetic resonance imaging (MRI), 112t
Magnitude, 14
  dose-response relationship and, 71-72
  exposure assessment and, 37
  female reproductive function and, 111
Major histocompatibility locus (MHC), 333
  autoimmunity and, 337-338
Malaria, 621
Malathion, 152, 153

INDEX

Male reproductive function, 95-100
  azoospermia and, 74, 97
  cyclophosphamide and, 108
  infertility and, 95, 97
  pesticides and, 74, 97, 98t, 605
Malignancy, dermatoses and, 278
Malignant mesothelioma, 294-295
Mammary cancer, immunology and, 87, 91, 158, 161, 163
Manganese, 21t, 44t, 606, 610
  bile and, 303
  ears/hearing and, 260
  neurobehavioral testing for toxicity and, 191
  neurotoxicity and, 323t
Man-made vitreous fibers (MMVF), 455-461
Mapping systems, 21
Markers, 158, 162; see also Biomarkers
Mast cells, 140t, 141, 146, 147
  dermal toxicology and, 187
  eyes/vision and, 243
  immune system and, 327-328
  respiratory tract disorders and, 283
Material safety data sheets (MSDSs), 224-225, 239
  chemicals and, 592-593
  data bases and, 759
  emergency medical response and, 708, 727
Mathematical modeling, 19, 57, 70, 673
Measurement bias, 54
Mechanical injuries
  nervous system and, 320
  skin and, 270
Mechanism of action, 67, 73-75
Mechlorethamine, 204t, 209, 210f, 213
Mechlorethamine Oncovin (vincristine sulfate), procarbazine, and prednisone (MOPP), 213
Medical history, 6, 51-52, 53, 222
  dermatoses and, 277
  female reproductive function and, 111
  multiple chemical sensitivity and, 372-373
  toxicology and, 67, 70
Medical waste, 626, 629, 663
  environmental legislation about, 749
  indoor air pollution and, 24
Medical Waste Tracking Act, 749
Meditext, 760
MEDLARS, 759
MEDLINE, 759, 761
MEDTREC, 727
Melanoma, 163
Membranes, 67, 74
  cancer and, 82-83
  free radicals and, 75
Memory, 130, 133, 189-197
Mepazine, 204t, 208
Meperidine, 191
Mercury, 18, 25, 609
  biological amplification and, 69
  biologic half-times of, 132
  in composts, 655
  developmental toxicology and, 119
  dose-response curve for poisoning from, 72f
  in drinking water, 44t
  ears/hearing and, 254t, 260
  as EPA priority chemical, 21t
  eyes/vision and, 244
  female reproductive function and, 107, 108
  in fish, 129
  in food, 490t, 491-492
  fumes of, 13
  hazardous waste incinerators and, 24
  immunotoxicology and, 151, 152
  nephrotoxicity and, 313, 315
  neurobehavioral testing for toxicity and, 189, 191, 192
  and neuronal response to injury, 130
  neurotoxicity and, 322t, 323t
  replaced by tributyl tin, 606
  in soil, 520
  sources of neurotoxicity from, 130
  toxicology of, 131-132
  vestibular disorders and, 260
Mesothelioma, 294-295
  asbestos and, 445
  in teachers, 233
Metabolic poisons, 17, 67, 74
Metabolism
  age and, 366
  of anticancer alkylating agents, 209
  aplastic anemia and, 205, 207, 209, 211
  of benzene, 205f, 212
  bone marrow toxicology and, 205-212
  carcinogens and, 84
  of chloramphenicol, 207
  dermal toxicology and, 184-185, 186
  developmental toxicology and, 119, 121, 123-124
  dioxin and, 135
  exposure assessment and, 40
  female reproductive function and, 103, 105, 108
  gastrointestinal tract and, 300, 301
  immunotoxicology and 147
  intermediary, 67
  lead poisoning and, iron deficiency and, 211
  leukemia and, 211-212
  male reproductive function and, 96
  neurotoxicants and, 131, 133, 134
  organic solvents and, 133
  pesticides and, 135
  respiratory toxicology and, 167-168, 170f, 171
  toxicology and, 66, 67, 68, 71
    male reproductive function and, 96
    microsomal enzyme induction and, 75, 91
    toxicokinetics and, 71
Metal recovery, 25, 25t
Metals, 131-133; see also Heavy metals
  bile and, 303
  cancer and, 84
  in composts, 655
  dermal toxicology and, 187
  eyes/vision and, 244
  fire and, 474
  food contamination from, 495, 504
  hair and, 187
  immunotoxicology and, 149, 151, 152, 153
  naturally occurring, in soil, 520
  nephrotoxicity and, 313, 314t, 315
  neurobehavioral testing for toxicity and, 191
  neurotoxicity and, 319, 322t, 323t
Metal salts
  aplastic anemia and, 204t, 209
  cancer and, 84, 87
  dermatoses and, 266t
  immune system tumor and, 153
Metam, 722, 723, 481
Metaplasia, 79
Meterologic conditions/weather, 15f, 17, 166; see also Climate
Methane, 599, 672
Methanol
  eyes/vision and, 244
  indoor air pollution and, 421t, 402-403
Methemoglobinemia, 116, 117f, 123
Methimazole, 204t, 209
Methomyl, 379
8-Methoxypsoralen, 186t, 187
N-Methyl-D-aspartate receptors, 195-196
Methyl bromide, neurotoxicity and, 322t
Methyl n-butyl ketone, neurotoxicity and, 322t, 323t
N-Methyl carbamates, 379
Methyl-CCNU; see Semustine
Methyl chloride, water pollution and, 481
Methylchloroform, 133
Methylcholanthrene, 157
Methyldithiocarbamate (metam), 722
Methyldopa, 151
Methylene, children and, 392t
Methylene chloride, 21t, 133, 191t, 600
  environmental history and, 236
  eyes/vision and, 245
Methyl isocyanate, 10, 11f, 166
Methylisothiocyanate (MITC), 481, 722-724
Methyl mercaptan, 21t
Methyl mercury; see Mercury
Methyl methacrylate, 322t
2-Methylnaphthalene, 21t
Methyl parathion, 21t
1-Methyl-4-phenyl-1,2,3,6-tetrahydropyridine (MPTP), 189, 191, 195
Methyl tert-butyl ether, 481, 601
MHC; see Major histocompatibility locus
Microenvironmental samplers, 18-19
β_2-Microglobulines, 149
Microgravity, 589-590
"Micro-mercurialism," 132
Micrometroids, 590
Microsomal enzyme induction, 75, 91
Microwaves, 86, 548-550, 552
Minamata disease, 129, 609
Mineral fibers, 39
Mineral oil hypothesis, 447
Mineral spirits, 133
Mineral wool, 455, 458-459
Mining waste, 27, 626
Minnesota Multiphasic Personality Inventory-2 (MMPI-2), 197-198
Mipafox, 134
Mirex, 134
Miscarriages, 18
Misclassification bias, 53, 55
Mites, 276
Mitochondria, 74
  aplastic anemia and, 206, 210, 211
  benzene and, 206
  carbon monoxide and, 136
  chloramphenicol, 206
  ears/hearing and, 260
  lead and, 131, 210
  respiratory toxicology and, 168
Mitogens, 150, 151, 163t
Mitomycin, 209
Mobilization, 66f
Modification, 14f, 17
Molds, 424
Molecular epidemiology, 90
Molecular level
  airway inflammation and, 283-284
  allergens and, 152
  aplastic anemia and, 210-211
  dermal toxicology and, 186-187
  developmental toxicology and, 121
  female reproductive function and, 108
  immune system and, 327-344
  immunotoxicology and, 139-147
  neurobehavioral testing for toxicity and, 192
  organic solvents and, 133
  respiratory toxicology and, 172, 175-177
  toxicology and, 66, 75
Molinate, 480t
Monitors, 71
  ambient, 32
  aplastic anemia and, 205, 210
  benzene and, 205
  biologic; see Biomarkers
  exposure assessment and, 39
  personal, 19
  risk assessment and, 32
Monochlorobenzene, in drinking water, 44t
Monocyte/macrophage colony-stimulating factor (M-CSF), 203
Monocytes, 140t, 143
  CSF and, 146
  dermal toxicology and, 187
  HIV and, 148-149
  immune system and, 327-328
  ionizing radiation and, 150
  organ transplantation and, 333
Monokines, 140t, 144
Mononucleosis, 158
Monosodium glutamate, 130
"Montreal Accords," 672
Mood alterers/changes, 191t, 197-198
Morbidity rates, 51, 53, 56-57
Mortality rates, 51, 52, 54
  proportional (PMR), 49-50, 56
  standardized (SMR), 55, 56-57
Morula, 105
Mosaic, 678
Motion sickness, 588-589
Motor function; see Psychomotor functions
Mount St. Helens eruption, 243
Mouth, acute toxicity and, 18
MRI; see Magnetic resonance imaging
Muconaldehyde, 206
Muconic acid, 206
Mucosa-associated lymphoid system (MALT), 300
Mucous membranes, 242
  gastrointestinal tract and, 300, 301
  immune system and, 328
  respiratory tract disorders and, 283-285
Mud, 13f
Multifactorial etiology, 14-15
Multiple chemical sensitivity (MCS), 74, 200, 368-379
  psychiatric hypotheses for, 371-372
Multiplicative effect, 73
Mumps, 163t
Mustard gas, 18
Mutagens/mutation, 74
  cancer and, 80-81, 82, 85
  age and, 91
  initiation and, 84
  microbial and mammalian cell culture assays and, 88
  molecular epidemiology and, 90
  ionizing radiation and, 529
  susceptibility and, 355
Mycobacteria, 140t
Myeloma, multiple, 148t, 153
Myeloperoxidase, 140t, 148t
Myopathy, 320

N

Nagasaki, 530, 532
Naleb, 152
Naphtha, 25, 133
Naphthalene, 21t, 480t
β-Napthylamine, 236
Nasopharyngeal carcinoma, 158, 160
National Academy of Sciences (NAS), 30
National Air Pollution Control Administration, 43
National Ambient Air Quality Standards (NAAQS), 23, 43, 167t, 174, 463-466, 745-747
National Cancer Institute (NCI), 52
National Center for Health Statistics (NCHS), 51
National Environmental Policy Act (NEPA), 743-744
National Fire Protection Association (NFPA), hazardous waste and, emergency medical response and, 707, 708, 714
National Institute for Occupational Safety and Health (NIOSH), 7, 31, 95, 96
  benzo[a]pyrene and, 602
  case studies available from, 758
  chemical disaster preparedness and, 727
  children and adolescents and, 409
  data bases and, 759, 760
  exposure assessment and, 41, 42-43, 44
  fire and, 472t
  hazardous waste and, emergency medical response and, 710
  incineration and, 664-665
  man-made fibers and, 456
  neurobehavioral testing for toxicity and, 190, 191
  responsibilities of, 762
National Institute of Environmental Health Sciences (NIEHS), 6
  data bases available from, 759
National Library of Medicine (NLM), 758, 759, 761
National Pesticide Information Retrieval System (NPIRS), 759 761
National Research Council, 37, 39, 40
National Toxicology Program, 90, 212
Natural resources, future and, 10, 11f
Necrosis, 79f
  vs. apoptosis, 79f
  immunotoxicology and, 143
Needle sticks, 13

Negative feedback, immunotoxicology and, 141
Neningioma, 83t
Neomycin, dermatoses and, 266t
Neoplasia, 79, 85
 age and, 91
 autoimmunity and, 342-343
 esophageal cancer and, 87
 and immunology of cancer, 159-161
 leukemia and, 211-212, 213
 natural history of, 81f
Nephrotic syndrome, 148t
Nephrotoxicity, 312-317
Nerve cells, 141
Nervous system, 18, 318-325; see also Central nervous system (CNS)
 anatomy and physiology of, 130
 aplastic anemia and, 211
 arsenic and, 130, 132-133
 developmental toxicology and, 122
 female reproductive function and, 101-103
 gastrointestinal tract and, 301
 lead and, 129-131, 132t, 131
 learning and memory and, 130, 133
 male reproductive function and, 96-97
 mercury and, 129-132
 nephrotoxicity and, 313
 neuroendocrine poisons and, 74, 96-97
 neuropathy and, 320-321; see also Neuropathy
 pathophysiology of, 195-196
 peripheral, 132, 320-321, 324
 and selected neurotoxic agents, 129-136
 solvents and, 133
 target components of, 190-191
 and testing for toxicity, 189-198
Neuraminidase, 164
Neurobehavioral Evaluation System, 190
Neurobehavioral testing, 76, 189-194
 children and, 386-387
 clinical considerations in, 193-195
 confounders in, 196
 and developmental neurobehavior, 197-198
 history of, 190
 intellectual ability and, 196
 language and, 196, 198
 pathophysiology and, 195-196
 psychometric testing and, 195-198
Neuroendocrine system, 74
 immunotoxicology and, 151-152
 male reproductive function and, 95, 96-97
Neuroma, 83t
Neurons, 125, 130
 injury and, 130-131
 neurobehavioral testing for toxicity and, 195, 198
 organic solvents and, 133
Neuropathy, 131f, 132, 320-321; see also Polyneuropathy
 carbon disulfide and, 191
 encephalopathy and, 192
 eyes/vision and, 244, 245
 mono- and focal vs. poly-, 320
 neurobehavioral testing for toxicity and, 190, 192
 organophosphate-induced delayed neurotoxicity and, 134
Neuropathy target esterase (NTE), 324
Neuropsychological toxicology, 129, 136, 195-198
 environmental history and, 233
 multiple chemical sensitivity and, 372-372
Neuroreceptors, 74
Neurotoxicity, 18, 40; see also Neurobehavioral testing; Nervous system; Toxicity, 318-325
 age and, 366
 coasting and, 319
 confounding factors in, 320, 324
 encephalopathy and, 324
 mass hysteria and, 320
 psychoorganic syndrome and, 324
 respiratory toxicology and, 166
 selected disorders due to, 322-324
 temporal relationships and, 319

Neurotransmitters, 74, 130
 female reproductive function and, 108
 gastrointestinal tract and, 301
 lead and, 131
 neurobehavioral testing for toxicity and, 190
Neutralized sulfate salts, 24
Neutrophil elastase, 172
Neutrophilic leukocytes (PMN), 140t
Neutrophil inhibitory factor (NIF), 140t, 141
Neutrophils
 immune system and, 334
 respiratory toxicology and, 174
New source performance standards (NSPS), 746
Nezelof's syndrome, 148t
Nickel, 25, 69, 610
 dermal toxicology and, 187
 dermatoses and, 266t, 274-275
 as EPA priority chemical, 21t
 immune system and, 335
 immunotoxicology and, 151, 152
Nicotine, 40, 153; see also Tobacco smoke
 ears/hearing and, 254t
 gastrointestinal tract and, 301
NIOSH; see National Institute for Occupational Safety and Health
NIOSHTIC, 759, 761
Nitrates, 24, 92
 cyanide from, 472
 developmental toxicology and, 116, 117f, 123
 in drinking water, 44t, 233
 environmental history and, 233
 in food, 501
 water pollution and, 484
Nitrate salts, 24
Nitric acids, 24, 244
Nitriles, 601
Nitrites
 in drinking water, 44t
 in food, 501
 water pollution and, 484
Nitroarene, 84t
Nitrobenzene, 599
Nitrogen dioxide (NO_2), 24, 25
 ambient air quality standards and, 43, 167t
 children and, 392t, 393
 climate changes in world and, 672
 outdoor air pollution and, 464, 465-467
 respiratory tract disorders and, 284, 287, 288
 respiratory toxicology and, 168, 171t, 172, 174
 tobacco smoke and, 422
Nitrogen oxides; see Oxides of nitrogen
Nitrophenol, 21t
Nitrosamine, 84t, 93
Nitrosochloramphenicol, 207
Nitroso compounds, nephrotoxicity and, 314t
N-Nitrosodi-n-propylamine, 21t
N-Nitrosodimethylamine, 21t, 21t, 422
 tobacco smoke and, 422
Nitrosureas, 204t, 209, 213
Nitrous acids, 24
Nitrous oxide, 24, 191t
NK (natural killer) cells, 142, 143, 331-335
 AIDS and, 148
 and immunology of cancer, 160
 PCBs and, 151
 type I immune system reactions and, 331
 type II immune system reactions and, 331-333
Noise, 5, 12, 28, 234
 ears/hearing and, 250, 253-262
 neurotoxicity and, 319
 solid waste management and, 633
 toxicology and, 68
Noise-induced hearing loss (NIHL), 253-257
Noise trauma, 260
Non-Hodgkin's lymphoma (NHL), 148, 153
Nonmedical disciplines, 3, 4f

Nonmelanoma skin cancer (NMSC), 265, 269-272, 274
 latency and, 277
 ozone and, 274
Nonresponse bias, 54
Nonsteroidal anti-inflammatory agents, aplastic anemia and, 204t, 208, 209
No-observed-adverse-effect level (NOAEL), 32, 109-110, 113, 594
 chemical disaster preparedness and, 723-726
 food contamination and, 503
 water pollution and, 481-482
Norepinephrine, 140t, 141
Normal temperature and pressure (NTP), 41
North Carolina incident, 643
Nose
 eyes and, 242
 mucus and, 169-171, 174, 242
 olfaction and, 172-173
 respiratory toxicology and, 168
Nosocomial infections, 38
"No threshold" curve, 72-73
Nuclear power/energy, 26-28; see also Energy
 leak of, 10, 11f
 ionizing radiation and, 531-532
Null hypothesis, 111
Nutrition, 14, 15
 of children, 385
 factory farming and, 504-505
 improving patients', 730
 lead and, 385
 susceptibility and, 354-355
 toxicology and, 67

O

Obesity, 364-365
Occupation; see also Workplace environment
 animal bites and stings and, parenteral exposure and, 38
 asbestos and, immunotoxicology and, 151
 asthma and, 152, 177-178; see also Asthma
 beryllium disease and, 285
 cancer and, 7, 81, 86-92
 dermatoses and, 277
 developmental toxicology and, 119, 126
 dioxins and, 135
 disease registries and, 53
 employer and
  and diagnosis in environmental medicine, 219-220
  MSDSs and, 224-225
 environmental history and, 233
 epidemiology studies and, 48
 exposure assessment and, 38
 exposure from, and children and adolescents, 410-411
 healthy worker effect in epidemiological studies of, 54
 history for, 51, 52
 home environment vs. environment of, 219, 226
 immunotoxicology and, 151, 152, 153
 injury from, and children and adolescents, 409-410
 lead exposure and, 125, 130, 383-384
 male reproductive function and, 95, 97-98
 mortality rates according to, 49, 50
 multiple chemical sensitivity and, 369, 372-373
 nephrotoxicity and, 313
 neurotoxicants and, 129, 324
 organic solvents and, 133
 radon and, 537, 538
 rare types of, 48, 87
 solvents and, 324
 stress and, 359
 susceptibility and, 359
 trauma and, 12
Occupational acroosteolysis, 273
Occupational medicine, 3, 4f
 environmental medicine and, 5-6
 government and, 51
 preventive medicine and, 6

Occupational Safety and Health Administration (OSHA), 360, 749-750
 benzo[a]pyrene and, 602
 children and adolescents and, 408-409
 data bases and, 759, 760
 exposure assessment and, 42, 43-44
 fire and, 472
 hazardous waste and, emergency medical response and, 705-713
 man-made fibers and, 456
 MSDS and, 759
 responsibilities of, 762
 toluenediisocyanate and, 40
Oceanic life, 26; see also Aquatic biota
Odds ratio, 56-57, 59
Odor/odorants, 25, 633
Office of Environmental Health Hazard Assessment (OEHHA), 722-725
Oil and Hazardous Materials/Technical Assistance Data System (OHM/TADS), 761
Oil of chenopodium, ears/hearing and, 254t
Oil spills, 15f, 26
Olfaction, 194
Omethoate, 153
β-Oncofetal antigen, 158t
Oocytes, 106, 107
Optacon, 194
Oral contraceptives, 108, 505
Ores, extraction of, 27
Organelles, 71, 74
Organization for Economic Cooperation and Development (OECD), 109
Organochlorine insecticides, 133, 134-135, 191t, 603-604
 children and, 379, 381
Organomercurials, 605-606
Organometallic compounds, 605-606
Organophosphate-induced delayed neurotoxicity (OPIDN), 134
Organophosphate-induced delayed polyneuropathy (OPIDN), 379
Organophosphate pesticides, 189, 191t, 604-605
 children and, 377-382
 eyes/vision and, 244
 immunotoxicology and, 152, 153
 indoor air pollution and, 421t, 404
 neurotoxicity and, 322t, 323-324
 susceptibility and, 355
Organophosphorous ester, 129, 134
Organotin, 323t, 324
Organs
 autoimmunity specific to, 338-339, 343t
 classification of toxic chemicals by target, 595t
 clinical diagnosis and, 221-222
 environmental history and, 233
 toxicology and, 66f, 73
Organ transplantation, 333
OSHA; see Occupational Safety and Health Administration
Osteosarcoma, 83, 86, 163
Ototoxic agents, 254
Oxepin, 205
Oxidants, 23
 age and, 365
 dermatoses and, 266t
 diet and, 354-355
 man-made fibers and, 457
 respiratory toxicology and, 172
Oxidative stress, 75
Oxides of nitrogen, 23, 24
 children and, 392t
 environmental history and, 236
 indoor air pollution and, 421t, 422
 outdoor air pollution and, 465-466
 from pyrolysis, 473
 respiratory toxicology and, 173, 174
 solid waste management and, 633
Oxides of sulfur, 167, 170, 173, 465
Oxygen
 carbon monoxide and, 136
 deficiency OF, 43
 dermal toxicology and, 183, 186-187
 developmental toxicology and, 119
 man-made fibers and, 457-458
 respiratory toxicology and, 172
 toxicology and, 75

Oxygen free radicals; see Free radicals
Oxyphenylbutazone, 208
Oxytocin, 103
Ozone, 22, 23-24, 150, 606
  ambient air quality standards and, 43, 167t
  children and, 394
  depletion of, 676
  dermatoses and, 274
  environmental law about, 746
  eyes/vision and, 245-246
  hyperreactivity and, 284
  indoor air pollution and, 422
  outdoor air pollution and, 465, 467
  preexisting illness and, 362, 363
  respiratory toxicology and, 170, 172-174
  susceptibility and, 355
  tolerance to, 283
  ultraviolet radiation and, 545

P

Packaging (of food), 502-504
Paint, 129, 130, 152
  children and, 384, 387
  immunotoxicology and, 152, 153
  indoor air pollution of, 24
  lead in, 10, 11f, 13, 384, 387
  waste site of, incident involving, 643
Painters' syndrome, 324
Pancreatic oncofetal antigen, 158t
Paper pulp bleaching, 25, 25t
Para-aminosalicylic acid, immunotoxicology and, 151
Paradichlorobenzene, 25, 236
Paraphenylenediamine, 335
Paraquat, 168, 380, 381
Parasites
  dermatoses and, 276
  immunotoxicology and, 140t
  reuse of sludge and, 659
Parenteral environment, 13, 38
  exposure assessment and, 38
Parkinsonism, 189, 191, 195
Particles
  ambient air quality standards and, 167t
  children and, 392t
  dermatoses and, 270
  radioactive, in food, 508
  respiratory clearance and, 170t
  respiratory protective equipment for, 468
  respiratory toxicology and, 170-172, 173
  tobacco smoke and, 422
Particulates; see also Dust; Fibers
  ambient air quality standards and, 43
  children and, 394-395
  chronic pulmonary disease and, 362-364
  dermatoses and, 270
  developmental toxicology and, 119
  environmental history and, 236
  exposure assessment and, 37, 39
  exposure assessment and, inhalation and, 38
  IgE production and, 329
  indoor air pollution and, 25
  inspirable vs. respirable, 42
  outdoor air pollution and, 22, 24, 464, 465
  respirable, cigarette smoke and, 40
  solid waste management and, 632
Partitioning, 66f, 67, 68, 71, 133
Passive dosimetry, 42
Patch (of land), 677-678
Patch testing, 278, 335
Patients
  fears/concerns of, 6-7, 6-7, 65-66, 218-220
  about cancer/AIDS, 78, 86, 740
  risk communication and, 739-742
  subjective, 221
  improving life-style of, 729-736
  risk communication to, 737-742
PCBs; see Polychlorinated biphenyls
PCP; see Pentachlorophenol
Penicillin, 151, 152
2,3,4,7,8-pentachlorodibezofuran (PeCDF), 150

Pentachlorophenol (PCP), 25t, 237, 603
  as EPA priority chemical, 21t
  in food, 490t, 496
Pentobarbital, ears/hearing and, 254t
Pentose, 211
Peptides
  bone marrow toxicology and, 206
  cancer and, 85, 87, 91
  female reproductive function and, 103
  immune system and, 328
  immunotoxicology and, 146, 147
  respiratory toxicology and, 178
Perchlorethylene (PCE), 25, 236, 133, 191t, 480, 482, 600
Percutaneous route, 120, 121-122
  dioxin and, 135
  for organic solvents, 133
  for pesticides, 135
Perfumes, 25
Perfusion rate, toxicokinetics and, 71
Peripheral nervous system, 125, 320-321, 324
Permeability, toxicokinetics and, 71
Permissable exposure level (PEL), 42, 599
  fire and, 472
  for man-made fibers, 456
  hazardous waste and, emergency medical response and, 709-710
  solid waste management and, 630
  for toluenediisocyanate, 40
Peroxidase, 140t
Perphenazine, 204t, 208
Persistence (of environmental hazards in environment), 18, 24
Personal care/hygiene products, 25, 153, 399, 400t
Personal dosimeters, 51
Personality, neurobehavioral testing for toxicity and, 197-198
Personal monitors, 19
Personal psychosocial agents, 12t
Pesticide residues
  cancer and, 90
  chlorinated hydrocarbons as, breast cancer and, 7
  developmental toxicology and, 117
  environmental health and, 4
  environmental medicine vs. other disciplines in regard to, 5
  factory farming and, 505
  measurement of, 497-498
  surface, vs. that taken up into plant tissue, 69
  toxicology and, 69
Pesticides/insecticides, 4-5, 12t
  as allergens, 152, 152
  anticholinesterase, 133, 134, 133, 134, 189
  arsenic in, 130
  Bhopal disaster and; see Bhopal disaster
  cancer and, 153
  carbamate, 379, 421t, 404-405
  children and, 377-382, 390
  dermatoses and, 264, 272
  developmental toxicology and, 125
  environmental history and, 233, 236
  environmental legislation about, 750-751
  eyes/vision and, 244, 244
  factory farming and, 504-505
  female reproductive function and, 75, 108, 108, 111
  in food, 497-500
  global aspects of, 685-686
  household, 6, 25
  immune system and, 74
  immunotoxicology and, 149, 150-151, 153
  indoor air pollution and, 421t, 404-405, 423
  male reproductive function and, 74, 74, 97, 98t
  National Pesticide Information Retrieval System and, 759, 761
  nephrotoxicity and, 313t
  neurobehavioral testing for toxicity and, 189, 191
  neurotoxicity and, 319, 323-324
  number of, 12
  organic, 25

organochlorine, 133, 134-135, 191t, 603-604
  children and, 379, 381
  preexisting illness and, 364
organophospate; see Organophosphate insecticides
  preexisting illness and, 364
  pyrethrin, 322t, 421t, 404, 405
  pyrethroid, 134, 152, 191t
    indoor air pollution and, 421t, 404, 405
  pyrethrum, 379, 605
  risk assessment and, 33
  sources of toxicity from, 130
  toxicology of, 66, 133-134, 133-134
  triazine, 153
  VOCs and, 25
Petroleum, 133, 192, 521, 647t
  benzene and, 204
  nephrotoxicity and, 313t
pH, in drinking water, 44t
Phagocytosis/phagocytes, 139, 140-142, 147
  AIDS and, 148
  HIV and, 148-149
  immune system and, 332, 344-346
  interferons and, 146
  ionizing radiation and, 150
  respiratory toxicology and, 169, 170-171
  susceptibility and, 355
  zinc and, 151
Pharmaceuticals; see also Drugs
  abuse of, 70
  immunotoxicology and, 151-152
  male reproductive function and, 98
  toxicology and, 66
Pharmacology, 66
Phenol, 205, 599
  as EPA priority chemical, 21t
  fire and, 473
Phenolic disinfectant, 122
Phenothiazines, aplastic anemia and, 204t, 208-209
Phenoxyacetic acids, 153
Phenylbutazone, 204t, 208, 212
p-Phenylenediamine, 38
Phenytoin, 151, 204t, 209
Pheochromocytoma, 83t
Phosgene, 18, 287t, 289, 474
Phosphates, arsenic and, 133
Phosporus 32 labeling, 89
Photoallergic reactions, 265t, 268
Photochemical air pollution, 23, 465
Photochemical pollution, 465
  transformation and, 182, 186-187
Photocontact dermatitis, 335
Photographic products, 153
Photoionization, 42
Photons, 543
Photosensitivity, 182, 186-187
  dermatoses and, 265t, 266-267
Phototoxicity
  dermatoses and, 267
  immune system and, 335
Physical activity, susceptibility and, 355
Physical agents, 3, 12, 14f, 15f, 28
  dermatoses and, 265t, 270-272
  exposure assessment and, 37
  exposure assessment and, eyes and, 38; see also Eyes/vision
  as focus of environmental medicine, 4
  and immunology of cancer, 157-158
  immunotoxicology and, 149-153
  modification of hazardous agent caused by, 17
  neurotoxicity and, 319
  toxicology and form of, 67
Physical examination
  environmental history and, 234
  multiple chemical sensitivity and, 372-373
  neuropathy and, 320
Physicians; see also Health care professionals/practitioners
  bone marrow toxicology and, 210
  clinical experience of, 226
  environmental, 6-7
  environmental crisis and, 10, 11f
  primary care, 3, 5

information resources for, 755-762
  organizations for, 761
  Response to Chemical Emergencies package for, 727
  as risk communicators; see Risk communication
Physiologic capacity, 15
Physiologic effect, toxicology and, 66, 70
Phytophotodermatitis, 276-277
Pigmentary changes, 265t, 267-268
Pituitary, 101-109, 112
Placenta, 121, 158-159, 162
Plague, 619-620
Plankton, 41, 69
Planned Approach to Community Health (PATCH), 731
Plants, 69
  agglutinins of, 157
  allergens derived from, 152
  bioconcentration/bioaccumulation and, 17, 18
  cancer and, 84t, 92
  dermatoses and, 276-277
  hemolysins in, 74
  pollution in, 13, 15f
  uptake by, 520, 522
  waterborne pollutants and, 4
Plaque forming cells (PFC), 149
Plasma, immunotoxicology and, 140t, 142-143
Plasma pyrolysis, 26
Plasminogen activator (PA), 177
Plastics, 152, 204, 503-504
Platelet activating factors (PAF), 140t, 141, 147
Platinum refining, 152
Plumes, 515
Plutonium, 21t
Pneumocytes, respiratory toxicology and, 169
Pneumonia, hypersensitivity and, 152
Point estimate, confidence interval and, 59
Poison control centers (PCC), 711-712, 752-754
  list of, 753-754
  MEDTREC and, 727
  statistics regarding, 755
Poisoning
  acute, 306, 593-594
  common causes of food, 617t
  fish and shellfish food, 618
Poison ivy/oak/sumac, 266, 278, 335
Poisons, metabolic, 17
Pokeweed mitogen, 149, 163t
Poliovirus, 621
Pollen, 25, 421t
Polyaromatic hydrocarbons, 21t, 601-601
Polybrominated biphenyls (PBBs), 108, 109t, 602
  in food, 490t, 496
Polychlorinated aromatic compounds, 18
Polychlorinated biphenyls (PCBs), 24, 25t, 66, 68, 82
  in composts, 655
  in cooking oils, 129, 135
  developmental toxicology and, 116, 120, 121
  discussion of, 596-597, 602
  as EPA priority chemical, 21t
  female reproductive function and, 108, 109t
  fire and, 474
  in food, 490t, 495-496
  immunotoxicology and, 151
  neurotoxicity and, 322t
  North Carolina incident involving, 643
  obesity and, 364
  in soil, 521
  toxicology of, 135
Polychlorinated dibenzo-p-dioxins, 135
Polychlorinated dibenzodioxins (PCDDs), 490t, 496
Polychlorinated dibenzofurans (PCDFs), 135, 496
Polychlorinated dioxins, 24
Polychlorinated quaterphenyls (PCQs), 135

Polycyclic aromatic hydrocarbons (PAH), 18, 24, 25, 81, 91, 108, 109*t*
  in composts, 655
  dermal toxicology and, 186
  dermatoses and, 274
  developmental toxicology and, 121
  environmental history and, 236
  as EPA priority chemical, 21*t*
  respiratory toxicology and, 173
  tobacco smoke and, 422
Polycyclic compounds, indoor air pollution and, 423
Polyhalogenated aromatic compounds, 74
Polymerase chain reaction (PCR), 90
Polymers, fire and, 474
Polymorphisms, 83-84
Polyneuropathy, 131, 132, 135, 320-321, 322*t*
  solvents and, 324
Polypeptide chains, 143-144
Polystyrene, 204, 503
Polyurethane foam, immunotoxicology and, 152
Polyvinyl chloride (PVC), 503
  pyrolysis and, 472
  scleroderma and, 269
Polyvinyl pyridine-*N*-oxide (PVPNO), 457-458
Population(s); *see also* Epidemiology
  cancer registry and, 52-53
  cartograms regarding, 20
  census data on, 50-51
  cluster studies and, 50, 53
  cohort studies of, 48, 49, 53, 54
  cross-sectional studies of, 47-48
  elderly, 365-367, 466
  English language and, 196
  environmental health surveillance and, 695-696
  exposure assessment and, 5, 37, 44
  hazardous waste and, 642
  heat stress and, 568-569
  incidence vs. prevalence in, 47
  longitudinal studies of, 48-49
  male reproductive function studies based on, 96-97
  neurobehavioral testing for toxicity and, 190, 196
  PCBs and, 602
  with preexisting conditions, 361-365
  proportional mortality studies in, 49-50
  radon and, 538
  susceptibility of, 351-360, 361-362
    biomarkers and, 700-701
    outdoor air pollution and, 466-467
Population attributable risk (PAR), 57-58
Population explosion/growth, 9, 10, 11*f*, 680-683
  land-use changes and, 676-677
Porphyria turcica, 273-274
Position sense, 195
Postural/body sway, 194, 195
Potassium
  ears/hearing and, 254*t*
  man-made fibers and, 459
Potassium dichromate, 152
Potency, 67, 75, 67
Potentiation, 73, 167
Power, 59-60, 110
Power lines, 118
Practolol, ears/hearing and, 254*t*
Pralidoxime, 404-405
Preexisting illness, 14, 227, 228*t*, 361-365
Pregnancy, 102, 105
  acetaminophen and, 124
  cadmium and, 151
  environmental history and, 234
  immune system and previous, 333
  immunotoxicology and, 150
  lead and, 117*f*, 117
  outdoor air pollution and, 23
  PCBs and, 116
  prolactin and, 104
  susceptibility and, 357
Premature infants, 117
Premercapturic acid, 205
Premorbid ability, 196, 197

Pressure, dermatoses and, 270
Prevalence, 47-48
  bias for, 54
  type I and II errors and, 60
Preventive medicine, 5, 6
  environmental medicine and, 3, 4, 7
  sentinel event strategies and, 19-20
Primary amebic meningoencephalitis, 617
Printing, 130
Pro-adrenocortical trophic hormone (pro-ACTH), 162
Probability (*p*-value), 58, 59-60
Procainamide, immunotoxicology and, 151
Procarbazine, 204*t*, 213
Processing (in immunotoxicology), 141, 142
Prochlorperzine, 204*t*, 208
Profile of Mood States, 198
Progesterone, 102, 103-109, 112
  factory farming and synthetic, 505
Progressive massive fibrosis (PMF), 291-292
Project Smoky, 532
Prolactin (PRL)
  female reproductive function and, 104
  male reproductive function and, 96-97
Prolactin inhibiting factor (PIF), 104
Promazine, 204*t*, 208
Proportional incidence ratio (PIR), 49-50
Proportional mortality ratio (PMR), 49-50, 56
Proposition 65, 33
Propylthiouracil, 204*t*, 209
Prostaglandins, 141, 147, 172, 174
Prostate, 91, 97
Protein-limiting filtration, 97
Proteins
  allergic contact dermatitis, 335
  bone marrow toxicology and, 206
  dermal toxicology and, 187
  developmental toxicology and, 120
  dioxin and, 135
  female reproductive function and, 108
  fetal, 158-159
  immunotoxicology and, 140*t*
  lead and, 131
  respiratory toxicology and, 171-172, 174
  stress, 17-18
Proteoglycans, 146, 147
Protoporphyrin, 210-211
Protozoans, 616-617
  composting and, 654
  immunotoxicology and, 140*t*, 146
Proximity analysis, 20
Psychiatric/psychologic factors, in multiple chemical sensitivity and, 371-372, 373-374
Psychiatric disease, neurotoxicity and, 324
Psychometric testing, 195-198
Psychomotor functions, 131, 133
  neurobehavioral testing for toxicity and, 193, 195, 197
Psychoorganic syndrome, 324
Psychophysiologic factors, susceptibility and, 353-359
Psychosocial factors, 12, 14*f*, 358
  toxicology and, 68
Public; *see also* Patients
  EPCRA and, 751
  fears/concerns of, 6-7, 65-66
    about cancer, 78, 86
    food irradiation and, 507-508
    risk communication and, 739-742
    response of, to environmental hazards, 7, 10, 11*f*
    risk communication and, 738-742
Public health medicine, 3, 5, 10, 11*f*
  environmental health as part of, 4
  government and, 51-52
  occupational medicine and, 6
Public safety/health
  children and adolescents and, 411
  composting and, 654-656
  environmental legislation and, 743-751
  policy of, and epidemiology, 60
  gastrointestinal tract and, 298

genetic engineering and, 509
hazardous waste and, 643-645
improving patients' life-style and, 730
indoor air pollution and, 426-428
ionizing radiation and, 531-532
lead and, 383
man-made fibers and, 458
outdoor air pollution and, 464-466
radon and, 537-540
solid waste management and, 630-632
water pollution and, 482
Pulmonary defense mechanisms, 169-173
Pulmonary fibrosis, 175-177
  clinical diagnosis and, 222, 228
Pulmonary function tests, 235
Pulmonary overpressure accident, 586-587
p-value; *see* Power
PVC; *see* Polyvinyl chloride
Pyrethrins
  indoor air pollution and, 421*t*, 404, 405
  neurotoxicity and, 322*t*
Pyrethroids, 134, 152, 191*t*
Pyrethrum, 379, 605
Pyrimidine 5'-nucleotidase, 211
Pyrogens, 140*t*
Pyrolysis products, 91, 470-478; *see also* Fire

Q

Quarantine, 6
Quartz, 33, 39, 151, 175, 457, 458; *see also* Silica
Quinacrine, 204*t*, 209
Quinidine, 151, 204*t*, 209
Quinine, ears/hearing and, 254*t*

R

Rabies, 620
Race, 15
  cancer and, 91
  cigarette smoking and, 730
  inhalation exposure and, 38
Radiation
  cancer and, 75, 86
  cosmic, 75, 590
  developmental toxicology and, 125
  electromagnetic; *see* Electromagnetic fields (EFT)
  ears/hearing and, 245-248
  eyes/vision and, 240, 245-249
  female reproductive function and, 111
  fire and, 474
  genetic and chromosomal mutation and, 18
  immunotherapy and, 164
  immunotoxicology and, 150
  ionizing, 12, 28, 524-533, 542-543
    dermatoses and, 272
  leukemia, 204*t*, 213
  male reproductive function and, 98*t*
  nephrotoxicity and, 313*t*
  neurotoxicity and, 319
  nonionizing, 12, 28, 524-533, 542-553
    dermal toxicology and, 186
  infrared, 548
  lasers and, 550
  microwave, 86, 548-550, 552
  radiofrequency, 86, 548-550, 551
  ultraviolet; *see* Ultraviolet radiation (UV)
  space environment and, 590
  spectrum of, 245*t*
  threshold and, 72
  toxicology and, 68
  ultraviolet, 37, 38
    cancer and, 86
    dermal toxicology and, 186, 187
    eyes/vision and, 245-249
Radiation film badges, 51
Radioactive waste, 10, 11*f*, 644-645
  dumping of, 26
  low-level vs. high-level, 27
Radiofrequency radiation, 86, 548-550, 551
Radium, as EPA priority chemical, 21*t*
Radon, 21*t*, 65, 92, 534-541
  children and, 392*t*, 393
  developmental toxicology and, 119
  environmental history and, 233, 236

indoor air pollution and, 421*t*, 431
water pollution and, 483-484
Ragweed, 335
Rail Accident and Immediate Deployment (RAPID) plan, 725-726
Rain, 17
Rape *seed* oil, 273
Reactive airways dysfunction syndrome (RADS), 178, 285, 401
Reactive oxygen species, 75, 93
Recall bias, 55
Receptor enzymes, 18
Recombinant-DNA techniques, 18
Recommended exposure limit (REL), 42, 44
Recreational environment; *see* Community environment, recreational
Rectum, cancer of, 92*t*
Recycling, 627, 629
Reference exposure levels (RELs), 723-724
Refractory ceramic fibers (RCF), 455, 459
Registry of Toxic Effects of Chemical Substances (RTECS), 759, 760, 761
Rejection/graft-vs.-host reactions, 140*t*, 146, 164, 333, 335
Relative risk (RR), 48, 55-56
  confidence interval and, 58-59
  power of study and, 60
  type I and II errors and, 60
Renal transplants, 160
Reproductive toxicology, 18, 74-75, 105-112; *see also* Female reproductive function; Male reproductive function
  critical period for, 111
  environmental history and, 233, 234
Reserpine, 151
Resins, dermatoses and, 272
Resource Conservation and Recovery Act (RCRA), 24, 747-749
  hazardous waste and, 636-638, 650
  incineration and, 662, 665
Respiratory system
  in children, 390-397
  developmental toxicology and, 122-123
  disorders of, 282-297
  eyes/vision and, 242
  in firefighters, 475
  immune system and, 329
  inhalation exposure and, 38; *see also* Inhalation
  lead and, 131
  multiple chemical sensitivity and, 372
  photochemical air pollution and human, 24
  sensitizers in, 74
Respiratory toxicology, 166-181
  age and, 366
  airway epithelium and, 172
  alveolar macrophages and, 173, 175-177
  and anatomic features of respiratory system, 168-169
  biochemical mechanisms and, 171-172
  bronchial asthma and, 177-178
  bronchorestriction and, 172, 175
  cancer and, 166, 167, 174
  clearance mechanisms and, 169-170
  environmental history and, 233
  failure of defense mechanisms and, 175-178
  important airborne pollutants and, 173-175
  mucus flow and, 169-170; *see also* Nose
  olfaction and, 172-173
  pulmonary defense mechanisms and, 169-173
  and unique features of respiratory system, 168
Respiratory tract disorders
  airway inflammation and hyperreactivity as, 282-285
  diffuse alveolar damage (DAD) as, 287-290
  granuloma formation in, 285-287

Respiratory tract disorders—cont'd
  hypersensitivity pneumonitis as, 286-287
  interstitial fibrosis as, 290-295
  malignant mesothelioma as, 294-295
Response bias, 196
Restriction endonucleases, 83-84
Retinoblastoma, 83-84, 86, 91
Reversibility, 73, 74
  bone marrow toxicology and, 206
  in carcinogenesis, 75
  female reproductive function and, 110
  neurobehavioral testing for toxicity and, 191
  of tumor-promoting agents, 84
Rheumatoid arthritis (RA), 340-341, 342, 343t
Ribonucleic acid (RNA)
  benzene and, 206
  female reproductive function and, 108
  and immunology of cancer, 157, 158, 164-165
Risk (environmental)
  "attributable," 48, 57-58
  "relative"; see Relative risk (RR)
Risk assessment, 30-36
  adolescents and, 119
  age and, 359, 365-367
  aplastic anemia and, 204
  benzene and, 204
  biomarkers and, 700
  chemical agents and, 594
  of chemical disaster, 723-724
  data bases for, 225-226
  dermatoses and, 277-278
  female reproductive function and, 109-111, 113
  food contamination and, 498
  hazardous waste and, 638
  steps in, 30, 31f
  susceptibility and, 358
  voluntary vs. involuntary, 8
  water pollution and, 482
  xenobiotics and, 67
Risk communication, 3, 7-11f, 65, 217-218, 737-742
  information resources for, 738
  principles of, 741-742
Risk estimates
  bone marrow toxicology and, 201
  in epidemiological studies, 55-58
  xenobiotics and, 67
Risk management, 724, 725-727
Rivers and Harbors Act, 480
RNA; see Ribonucleic acid
Rocky Mountain spotted fever, 619
Rodenticides, 33, 378t, 605
  indoor air pollution and, 421t, 405-406
Romberg tests, 195
Room air-cleaning devices (RACDs), 433-434
Rubber compounds, immune system and, 152, 335
Runoff, 10, 11f, 15f, 17

S
Saccharin, 82, 502
Safe Drinking Water Act (SDWA), 480, 481, 751
Salicylates, 254t, 260
Salmonellosis, 7, 618, 621
Sampling, 60, 88, 110
  exposure assessment and, 39, 41-42, 44
Sanitation, 4, 6
Santa Clara, California, incident, 643
Sarcoidosis, 148t, 160, 285
School environment, 4, 5, 6
  air pollution in, 390, 393
  developmental toxicology and, 117-119
  vs. home, 117
  improving patients' life-style and, 731-732
  preventive medicine and, 6
  repeated, low-level exposures in, 10
Schwann-cell degeneration, 130, 131
Scleroderma, 151, 265t, 268-269, 273
  autoimmunity and, 341-342, 343t
Scrotal cancer, 126
Seafood, 621; see also Fish; Shellfish
Sea of Japan dumping, 26

Secondary contamination, 710-711
Secondhand smoke, 6; see also Cigarette smoking, passive
  ear infections and, 234
  environmental history and, 233, 234, 236
Sediment, 18, 517
Sedimentation, 15f, 17, 41
Selenium, 21t, 611
  in drinking water, 44t
  in soil, 520-521
Self-contained breathing apparatus (SCBA), 714-715
Semivolatile organic compounds, 421t, 423
Semustine (methyl-CCNU), 204t, 209, 213
Sensitization
  allergic contact dermatitis and, 266
  clinical diagnosis and, 228-229
  immune system and, 327-328, 335
Sensitizers, 74
Sentinel event strategies, 19-20, 21
Serotonin, 131, 140t, 141, 147
Serum cortisol, 359
Serum sickness, 147, 152, 334
Sewage, 519, 626-626
  untreated, 10, 11f
  in composts, 655
  infectious diseases and, 620-621
Shellfish, toxins in, 618
Shigella, 621
Short-chain hydrocarbons, 71
Short-term exposure limits (STELs), 472, 710
Sick building syndrome (SBS), 233, 420, 426-427
  children and, 393
  philosophic approaches to, 434-435
Sickle cell trait, 358
Side effect, 66, 70
Silica, 24, 612
  amorphous or crystalline dust of, 39
  dermatoses and, 273
  exposure assessment and, 39
  nephrotoxicity and, 315
  PVPNO and, 457
  risk assessment example using, 30, 33-35
Silicon, nephrotoxicity and, 313t
Silicon carbide, 459
Silicon dioxide, silicosis and, 291-292
Silicon breast implants, 151, 273
Silicosis, 290, 291-292
  scleroderma and, 269
Silver, 25
  in drinking water, 44t
  as EPA priority chemical, 21t
  furans and, 25t
Simazine, 480t
Simple aromatics, 597-599
SIR; see Standardized incidence ratio
Sjögren's syndrome (SS), 341, 342
Skin; see also Dermal toxicology; Dermatoses
  acute toxicity and, 18
  biologic factors affecting, 265t, 275-276
  chemical factors affecting, 265t, 272-275
  chromium and, 152
  developmental toxicology and, 118, 122
  environmental history and, 233
  environmentally induced disorders of, 265t
  excretion from, 187
  foreign body/substance and, 182, 186-187, 270
  immune system and, 329, 335
  mechanical factors affecting, 270
  organic solvents and, 133
  percutaneous absorption by, 263-265; see also Absorption
  pesticides and, 135
  physical factors affecting, 265t, 270-272
  as route of exposure, 13, 17
  sensitizers in, 74
  soil contamination and, 521
  structure and function of, 182-184
  toxicology and, 66f, 67, 70

Skin cancer, 81; see also Nonmelanoma skin cancer (NMSC)
  dermal toxicology and, 186
  developmental toxicology and, 117
  immunology and, 160, 161
  melanoma and, 269-270
  ultraviolet radiation and, 546-547
Skin tests for cancer, 163
Slag, garbage transformed into, 26
SLE; see Systemic lupus erythematosus
Slow-reacting substance of anaphylaxis (SRS-A), 140t, 141, 47
Sludge, 13f, 518, 625-626, 629
  in composts, 655
  reuse of, 657-659
Smith Hall, New Jersey, study, 643
Smog, 24, 150
Smooth muscle contraction, 147, 172
  asthma and, 283
  immune system and, 328, 342
Snake venom, 74
Soaps and detergents, 399-400
Society
  "dysfunctional," 9
  response to hazards by, 7, 10, 11f
Sodium chlorate, 152
Sodium dichloropropionate, 152
Sodium hydroxide, 244
Soil, 4, 12-13, 515-523
  cadmium or aluminum in, 18
  changes in
    throughout world, 675f
    in United States, 676f
  direct discharge into, 10, 11f
  environmental history and, 233, 234
  land-use changes and, 676-677, 689
  landscape patterns and, 677-678
  lead in, 13
  "night," 621
  persistence of environmental hazards in, 18
  physical and chemical constraints of, 687t
  physical and chemical properties of, 516
  profiles of, 516-517
  sediments in, 517
  siting and, 518-519
  toxicology and, 66f
  types of, 516
Soil contamination/pollution, 4, 10, 11f, 12-13
  airborne pollutants and, 4
  aquifers and, 517
  cancer and, 7
  children and, 384, 393
  composting and, 655
  dermal exposure and, 38
  dilution of, 651
  environmental science and, 4
  evaluating, 522-523
  exposure assessment and, 38, 44
  food-borne contaminants and, 4
  by garbage and solid waste, 26
  gastrointestinal-induced disorders and, 306
  hazardous waste incinerators and, 24
  home gardening and, 13, 384
  infectious diseases and, 618-619
  ingestion exposure and, 38, 44
  measuring, 5
  preventive medicine and, 6
  sewage and, 519
  sources of, 516, 517-523
  types of, 520-521
  waterborne pollutants and, 4
Solar flares, 590
Solid phase, 38
Solids in water, 41
Solid waste management, 26, 623-634; see also Hazardous waste; Waste disposal
  environmental legislation about nonhazardous, 749
  incineration in, 660-666; see also Incineration
  pollution control devices and, 631
  social considerations regarding, 652
  treatment techniques in, 647-643
Solubility, 38, 66f, 68, 70
  organic solvents and, 133
  toxicology and, toxicokinetics and, 71

"Solvent drag," 301
Solvents, 12t, 25, 31, 97, 130, 132t
  biologic half-life of organic, 133
  bone marrow toxicology and, 210; see also Benzene
  dermatoses and, 266t, 269, 272
  ears/hearing and, 260
  encephalopathy from exposure to, 192
  environmental history and, 233
  eyes/vision and, 244, 245
  nephrotoxicity and, 311, 313, 314t, 323t, 324
  neurobehavioral testing for toxicity and, 190, 191, 192
  toxicology of organic, 133
  vestibular system and, 260
Somatic mutation theory, 80
Somatoform disorders, 198
Soot, 24, 126
Sorption, 15f, 17
Space environment, 589-590
Specific macrophase arming factor (SMAF), 160
Sperm morphometry, 96
Spinal cord damage, 18
Spiramycin, 152
Spleen, 140, 143, 151
Spontaneous miscarriage, 234
Sporothrix, 275-276
Stabilization, 651
Standardized incidence ratio (SIR), 56
Standardized mortality rates (SMR), 55, 56-57
Statistical analysis, in female reproductive studies, 111
Statistical significance, 50, 59, 110, 111
  confidence intervals and, 59
  power and, 60
Statistics, in epidemiological studies, 55-60
Sterility, ionizing radiation and, 530
Steroid hormones, 104, 185, 335
  developmental toxicology and, 124
  female reproductive function and, 102-109, 112
  male reproductive function and, 91, 96-97
  factory farming and, 505
Stomach, 87, 92t, 123
Storage (of toxins), 66, 71, 364; see also Depot
Storage mites, 424-425, 431-432
Storage tanks, leaking underground, 644, 650
Stratification, 57
Streptokinase-streptodornase, 163t
Streptomycin, 152
Streptozotocin, 204t, 209
Stress, 17-18
  heat, 475, 563-575
  male reproductive function and, 98t
  oxidative, 75
  susceptibility and, 358, 359
Stroop Color Word test, 197
Structure activity relationship (SAR), 67
Strychnine, 406
Styrene, 133, 191t
  children and, 392t
  in drinking water, 44t
  as EPA priority chemical, 21t
Subacute environmental toxicity, 306
Subcellular poisons, 74
Sublimation, 15f, 17
Substance abuse, 70; see also Drug abuse
Succinyl coenzyme A, 210
Suicide, 28
Sulfa compounds, dermatitis and, 335
Sulfates, 24, 41, 44t
Sulfhydryl groups, 131, 133
Sulfites, 501-502
Sulfoglycoprotein (fetal), 158t
Sulfonic acid, 24
Sulfur dioxide (SO_2), 22, 24, 25
  ambient air quality standards and, 43
  asthma and, 283-285
  indoor air pollution and, 422
  outdoor air pollution and, 464, 465
  respiratory toxicology and, 170t, 172, 174
  respiratory tract disorders and, 283-289

Index 779

Sulfur dioxide—cont'd
  solid waste management and, 633
  susceptibility and, 355
Sulfuric acid, 24, 170t, 244
Sulfuric oxide, 167, 170, 465
Sulphasalazine, 151
Sunlight, 17, 23-24, 90; see also
    Photosensitivity; Ultraviolet light
    (UV)
  dermal toxicology and, 186
  dermatoses and, 265, 271-272
  eyes/vision and, 248
  immune system and, 335
  skin cancer and, 117
Superfund Amendments and
    Reauthorization Act (SARA), 20,
    24, 747-748, 751; see also
    Comprehensive Environmental
    Response, Compensation, and
    Liability Act (CERCLA)
Superoxide dismutase, 75, 172
Surface water
  exposure assessment and, 42
  gastrointestinal-induced disorders and,
    305
  soil contamination and, 4, 521-522
Surveillance, Epidemiology, and End
    Results (SEER) Program, 52
Susceptibility, 14f, 15, 17
  age and, 359, 365-367
  to aplastic anemia, 204-205, 207, 208
  to benzene, 204-205
  biomarkers and, 22, 700-701
  to cancer, 90-93
  of children
    to air pollution, 390-397
    to lead, 385
  to chloramphenicol, 207
  cigarette smoke and, 352-353
  clinical diagnosis and, 226-231
  defined, 67
  developmental toxicology and, 124-127
  dose-response curve and, 72
  elderly and, 365-367
  general principles of, 351-360
  genetic factors influencing, 356, 357-358
  immunotoxicology and, 149, 151
  indoor air pollution and, 426
  intercurrent diseases and, 358
  to neurotoxicants, 130
  outdoor air pollution and, 463, 466-467
  ozone and, 150
  to phenothiazines, 208-209
  preexisting conditions and, 361-365
  psychophysiologic factors and, 358-359
  stress and, 358, 359
  toxicology and, 73
  unexpected interactions between
    hazards and human, 5
  unusual, 6; see also Exposure, low-level
  xenobiotics and, 67
Susceptibility curves, 72f
Suspended solids, 41
Sweat glands, 183, 185, 187
Switzerland incident, 723
Sympathetic (adrenergic) nervous
    system, 301
Symptom Checklist-90, 198
Synergy/syngerism, 68, 73
  cigarette smoking and, 92
  respiratory toxicology and, 167
Synthetics, VOCs and, 25
Systemic lupus erythematosus (SLE),
    339-340
Systemic toxicity
  caustics and, 401
  dermal toxicology and, 184
  eyes/vision and, 38, 244-245
  male reproductive function and, 98
  polyneuropathy and, 320
  respiratory toxicology and, 168

T
2,4,5-T; see Trichloroacetic acid
Taking an Exposure History, 233
Target cells, 66f
Target organ, 66, 70
Tar smarts, 267
Tartrazine, 151
Taste function, 194
1,1,2,2-TCA, 480t
2,3,7,8-TCDD; see 2,3,7,8-
    Tetrachlorodibenzo-p-dioxin
T-cells/lymphocytes, 140t, 141-143
  AIDS and, 148
  autoimmunity and, 150-151
  beryllium and, 285
  HIV and, 148-149
  immune system and, 147, 334-335
  immunodeficiency disorders and,
    344-346
  cancer and, 159-164t
    immunotherapy and, 163-164
  interferons and, 146
  ozone and, 150, 150
  pesticides and, 149
  specifically reactive, 143
Technology, workplace accidents and,
    28
Telone, 480t
Temperature, 12, 577-578
  cellular response to, 17
  climate changes in, 671-676
  dermatoses and, 270-271
  developmental toxicology and, 122
  neurobehavioral testing for toxicity
    and, 190, 194
  toxicology and, 67, 68
Temporal relationships, 227-228, 277
  hazardous waste and, 640-641
  neurotoxicity and, 319
Teratogens, 12, 75
  ETICBACK data base on, 759
Terrestrial biota, 15f, 24
2,3-Tert-butyl-4-hydroxyanisole
    (BHA), 501-502
Testing
  neurobehavioral; see Neurobehavioral
    testing
  laboratory; see Laboratory testing
  patch, 278, 335
  screening for, 236
Testosterone, 96, 103
Tetanus, 618-619
2 3,7,8-Tetrachlorodibenzo-p-dioxin,
    25t, 74, 135; see also Dioxins
  as EPA priority chemical, 21t
  in food, 490t, 496, 504
  immunotoxicology and, 150
2,3,7,8-Tetrachlorodibenzofuran
    (TCDF), 150
1,1,2,2-Tetrachloroethane, 21t
Tetrachloroethylene (PCE), 21t, 133,
    600
  children and, 392t
  in drinking water, 44t
Tetrachloroterephthalate, water
    pollution and, 481
Tetracyclines
  dermatitis and, 335
  factory farming and, 505
Tetraethyl lead, 605
Textiles, VOCs and, 25
Thalassemia, 358
Thallium, 21t, 191
Thecal cells, 106, 107
Theophylline, 124
Thermal oxiders, 651
Thiopthalimides, 152
Thioridazine, 204t, 208
Thiotepa, 209
Thiouracil, 204t, 209
Thiourea, 204t, 209
Thorium, 21t
Three Mile Island incident, 10, 532
Threshold, 72-73, 596t
  cancer and, 82
  clinical diagnosis and, 228
  defined, 42, 67
  developmental toxicology and 116, 117f
  explanation of, to patients, 70
  hazardous waste and, 639-640
  neurobehavioral testing for toxicity
    and, 190
Threshold limit value (TLV), 40, 42-43, 44
  chemical disaster preparedness and,
    709-710, 726-727
  neurotoxicity and, 324
Thyl antigen, 177
Thymic epithelial cells, 140t, 149
Thymine, 209
Thymosin
  AIDS and, 148, 149
  and immunology of cancer, 151, 163
  PCBs and, 151
Thymus gland, 140, 146
  HIV and, 148-149
  immunotherapy and, 164
  nickel and, 151
  ozone and, 150
  TBTO vs. TBTC and, 150
Thyroxine, prolactin and, 104
Ticks, 619
Tight building syndrome, 233, 420; see
    also Sick building syndrome
Tilletia tritrici, 273
Times Beach incident, 10, 12, 219, 643
Tin, 130, 132t, 606
  ears/hearing and, 260
  as EPA priority chemical, 21t
  food contamination and, 494-495, 504
  neurobehavioral testing for toxicity
    and, 191
Tissue antigens, 162
T-lymphocytes, 74
  allergic contact dermatitis and, 266
  dermal toxicology and, 187
  immune system and, 334-335
  autoimmunity and, 337-344
  immunodeficiency diseases and, 344-346
  respiratory tract disorders and, 286
Tobacco smoke, 6; see also Cigarette
    smoking; Environmental tobacco
    smoke (ETS); Nicotine
  carbon monoxide and, 136
  clinical diagnosis and, 227
  environmental history and, 236
  eyes/vision and, 242-243
  immunotoxicology and, 150
  indoor air pollution and, 421t, 422
  as main environmental factor in
    cancer, 7
  secondhand, 6, 233, 234, 236
  toxicology and, 70
  VOCs in, 25
Tolbutamide, 204t, 209
Tolerance, 283, 337
Toluene, 133, 191t, 598-599
  benzene and, 150
  in drinking water, 44t
  ears/hearing and, 260
  as EPA priority chemical, 21t
  eyes/vision and, 244, 245
  neurotoxicity and, 323t
  ozone and, 150
2,4-Toluenediamine, 504
Toluenediisocyanate (TDI), 40, 44,
    152, 177-178
TOMES-Plus data base, 760
Topical antibiotics, 152
"Total human exposure," 14, 16f, 17
Touch, 190, 194
Toxaphene, 21t, 135, 153, 480t
Toxicants
  and agent-host-environment
    interactions, 14f, 17
  defined, 67
  dermal, 186t; see also Dermal
    toxicology
  direct acting, 107-108
  exposure to several, 14; see also
    Multiple chemical sensitivity
    (MCS)
  female reproductive function and,
    105-111
  indirect acting, 108-109
  learning and memory and, 130, 133
  male reproductive function and, 95-98
  nervous system and selected, 129-136,
    129-136
  neuro-, 319; see also Neurotoxicity
  neurobehavioral, 189-194
  stress proteins and, 18
  in water, 483-486
Toxic Chemical Release Inventory
    (TRI), 20, 21
  top-ranking facilities for, 20-21, 22f,
    23f
Toxic effect, 67
"Toxic encephalopathy," 192
Toxicity
  acute, 18
  behavioral impairments from; see
    Neurobehavioral testing
  chemicals of unknown, 12
  chronic, 18
  defined, 67
  developmental, 18
  factors modifying, 67, 71
  fiber, 456-461
  mechanisms of, 67, 73-75
  neuro-; see Neurotoxicity
  opthalmic, 240
  oxygen and, 75
  ratings, for acute chemical exposures,
    593t
  reproductive; see Reproductive
    toxicology
  reversibility of, 73, 74
  selective, 67
  subacute environmental, 306
  substance abuse and, 70
  systemic toxicity; see Systemic
    toxicity
  temporal features of, 68-69
  testing for; see Neurobehavioral
    testing
  vestibular disorders and, 259-261
Toxicodendron, 335
Toxicokinetics, 71
Toxicology, 5, 65-77
  activation vs. detoxification in, 71
  animal welfare/rights and, 76
  bone marrow, 201-208
  confounding factors in studies of,
    210
  National Toxicology Program and,
    212
  classification of chemical agents
    according to, 594, 595-597
  data bases for, 226; see also Data
    bases
  dermal, 182-188; see also Dermal
    toxicology
  developmental, 115-128; see also
    Development
  absorption and, 120-123
  distribution and, 123
  excretion and, 124
  exposure and, 116-120
  metabolism and; see Metabolism
  neurobehavioral testing for toxicity
    and, 198
  physical location and, 117-119
  pregnancy and, 121
  dose-response relationship and, 66,
    71-72
  environmental, 69
  female reproductive function and,
    105-111, 113
  of food irradiation, 506-507
  hormesis and, 76
  immunology and; see
    Immunotoxicology
  latency and, 73, 76
  learning and memory and, 130, 133
  male reproductive function and, 95-98
  microsomal enzyme induction and, 75
  neuropsychological, 129, 136, 195-198
  outdoor air pollution and, 462-469
  oxygen and, 75
  reproductive function and, 74-75
  respiratory, 166-181
  reversibility and, 73, 74
  of selected neurotoxic agents, 129-136
  susceptibility and, 73; see also
    Susceptibility
  taxonomy of, 67
  teratogens and, 75
  toxic significance in, 75-76
"Toxic profile," 12
Toxic Release Inventory, 759
Toxic Substances Control Act, 747,
    750
Toxins
  clinical diagnosis and, 228-231
  defined, 67
  elderly and, 365t
  environmental history and, 236
  eyes/vision and, 244-245

Toxins—cont'd
  food, 618
  red tide (brevetoxins), 172
TOXLINE/TOXLIT, 759, 761
TOXNET, 758
Transfer factor, 144, 164-165
Transforming growth factors (TGF), 146
Transplacental route, 120, 121
Transport, 14f
  toxicology and, toxicokinetics and, 71
  by weather, 15f, 17
Transportation, photochemical air pollution from, 23
Trauma, 12, 14f, 28
  cancer and, 272
  dermatoses and, 270, 272
  ears/hearing and, vestibular disorders, 260-261
  vestibular disorders and, 259-261
Traveler's diarrhea, 621
Triazenines, 209
Triazine herbicides, 149
5,5,5-Tributyl phosphorothioate, 134
Tributyl tin, 606
Tri-n-butyltin chloride (TBTC), 150
Tri-n-butyltin oxide (TBTO), 150
Tricarboxylic acid, 133
2,4,5-Trichloroacetic acid, 25t, 135, 490t, 496
1,1,1-Trichloro-2,2-bis-ethane (DDT), 21t, 108, 109t, 134, 135, 603-604, 751
1,1,1-Trichloroethane, 18, 21t, 44t
1,1,2-Trichloroethane, 21t
Trichloroethylene, 21t, 133, 191t, 600, 643
  dermatoses and, 273
  in drinking water, 44t
  eyes/vision and, 244, 245
  neurotoxicity and, 322t, 323t
2,4,6-Trichlorophenol, 21t
1,2,3-Trichloropropane, as EPA priority chemical, 21t
Trichophytin, 163t
Tridymite, 39
Triethyl tin (TET), 130, 133t, 260
Triflupromazine, 204t, 208
Trihalomethanes, 600
1,2,4-Trihydroxybenzene, 205f, 206
Trimellitic anhydride (TMA)
1,2,4-Trimethylbenzene, 191
Trimethyl benzene, 599
Tri-ortho-cresyl phosphate, 129, 134
Trithiobutyl compounds, 134
Tryptophan, 131, 269, 273
TU; see Turbidity units
Tuberculosis, 292
Tuftsin deficiency, 148t
Tumor, 73, 79-84
  benign vs. malignant, 79-81, 84-85
  defined, 79
  immune response to, 159-160
    tests for, 162-163
  immune surveillance and, 160-161
  immunotherapy and, 163-165
  immunotoxicology and, 149, 150, 152, 153
  markers for, 158, 162
  promotion of, 75, 80-93
    blocking agents against, 512-513
    partial, 85
  respiratory toxicology and, 167
  thresholds and, 82
  tobacco smoke and, 150
  water pollution and, 485
Tumor-associated antigens (TAA), 157
  evaluation and diagnosis to detect, 161-163
  immunotherapy and, 163-165
Tumor-associated phase-specific antigens (TAPSA), 157
Tumor necrosis factor (TNF), 203
  extrinsic allergic alveolitis and, 336
  immunotoxicology and, 146
Tumor-specific antigens (TSA), 157-159, 164
Tumor-specific transplantation antigens (TSTA), 157-158
Tumor-suppressor genes, 82-86, 91
Turbidity units (TU), 41, 42

Tylosin, 152
Type I and II errors, 59-60
Type II cells, respiratory toxicology and, 169

U
Ultrasound, 112
Ultraviolet (UV) radiation, 271-272, 545-548
  cancer and, 86
  dermal toxicology and, 186
  dermatitis and, 335
  exposure assessment and, 37, 38
  eyes and, 38
  halogenated hydrocarbons and, 274
  infrared combined with, 548
  NMSC and, 269-272
  short-term vs. long-term, 271-272
  from VDTs, 551
Ultraviolet visible photometry, 42
United Nations Environmental Program (UNEP), 670
U.S. Department of Agriculture (USDA), 497-509
U.S. Environmental Protection Agency (USEPA), 6
Unsymmetrical 1,1-dimethylhydrazine (UDMH), 499
Upholstery, immunotoxicology and, 152
Upper confidence limit (UCL), 31, 34
Uptake, 15f
  of asbestos, 442
  bioavailability and, 70
  inhalation exposure and, 38
  soil contamination and plant, 520, 522
  toxicology and, 66, 67, 70
Uranium, 26, 92
  children and, 393
  environmental history and, 236
  as EPA priority chemical, 21t
  nephrotoxicity and, 313t
Urinary tract, 313, 314
Uroporphyrin, 210-211
Urticaria, 265t, 268, 331
USDA; see U.S. Department of Agriculture
USEPA; see U.S. Environmental Protection Agency
UV light; see Ultraviolet (UV) radiation

V
Vaccines
  factory farming and, 504-505
  immunotherapy and, 164
  immunotoxicology and, 152
Vacor, 322t
Vanadium, 21t
Vanishing zero, 70-71
Vaporization, 15f, 17
Vapors, 13f
  exposure assessment and, 38, 40-42
  mercury as one, 131, 132
Vector-borne disease, 619-620
Ventilation rates, 427
Vestibular system, 195, 257-261
  space environment and, 589-590
Veterinarians, parenteral exposure and, 38
Vibration, 12, 557-562
  dermatoses and, 270
  neurobehavioral testing for toxicity and, 190, 194-195
Vibratron II, 190, 194
Video display terminals (VDTs), 551
Vinyl acetate, 21t
Vinyl chloride, 25, 87, 600
  dermatoses and, 273
  in drinking water, 44t
  as EPA priority chemical, 21t
  immunotoxicology and, 151
Vinyl chloride monomer (VCM), 503
Viruses, 12t
  aplastic anemia and, 204
  biological markers and, 51
  cancer and, 84, 85-86
  composting and, 654
  dermatoses and, 275
  immune system and, 335
    cancer and, 157-158, 161, 163, 164
  immunotherapy and, 164

immunotoxicology and, 140t, 147, 150
indoor air pollution and, 25, 26, 421t, 424
neoplasms and, 85t
reuse of sludge and, 657-658
sewage and, 620-621
stomach, 621
tobacco smoke and, 150
water pollution and, 616-617
Visual function; see eyes/vision
Visuospatial functions, 133
Vital statistics, preventive medicine and, 6
Vitamins
  as anticarcinogens, 513
  cancer and, 80, 92t
  food preservatives and, 502
  respiratory toxicology and, 172
  susceptibility and, 354-355
  toxicology and, 75
Volatile organic compounds (VOCs), 25, 597-601
  children and, 392t, 393
  composting and, 655
  examples and sources of, 423t
  indoor air pollution and, 421t, 422-423, 426-431
  solid waste management and, 633
  water pollution and, 482
Volatility, 70, 71
  organic solvents and, 133
  pesticides and, 135
Volatilization, 521
Volcanoes, 24

W
Waste disposal, 15f, 17; see also Hazardous waste; Solid waste management
  dioxin from, 130
  leaching and, 10, 11t, 15f, 17
  preventive medicine and, 6
  runoff and; see Runoff
Water, 4, 12, 13
  children's intake of, 377
  color of, 41
  direct discharge into, 10, 11f
  environmental history and, 233, 234
  global aspects of, 683-688
  palatable/potable, 41
  swimming and, 621
  taste and odor of, 41
  toxicology and, 66f
Water pollution/contamination, 4, 13f, 479-487; see also Clean Water Act
  abandoned mines and, 27
  airborne pollutants and, 4
  cancer and, 7; see also Caricinogenesis/cancer
  cooking or washing and, 12
  dermal exposure and, 38
  dermatoses and, 271
  developmental toxicology and, 119, 120t
  of drinking water; see Drinking water
  ears/hearing and, 260
  environmental science and, 4
  exposure assessment and, 38, 41, 42
  food-borne contaminants and, 4
  gastrointestinal-induced disorders and, 305
  of ground water; see Ground water
  infectious diseases and, 615-617
  modification of, 17
  multiple exposure pathways for, 16f, 17, 482
  nitrates and, 116
  noncancer vs. cancer endpoints and, 481-482
  preventive medicine and, 6
  regulatory programs/standards regarding, 480-481
  soil contamination and, 521-522
  of surface water; see Surface water
  swimming and, 38
    environmental history and, 233-234
    gastrointestinal-induced disorders and, 305
  vestibular system and, 260
  volatile organics and, 482

weather and, 15f
in wells; see Well water
Weather; see Meterologic conditions/weather
Wechsler Adult Intelligence Scale (WAIS-R), 190, 196-197
Wechsler Memory Scale-Revised, 197
Weight, inhalation exposure, 38
Well water, 116, 123, 130, 479-487
  immunotoxicology and, 149, 150
  Woburn, Massachusetts incident of contaminated, 642-643
Wetlands, 745
Wheat germ agglutinins, 157
Wildlife, 18
Wilms' tumor of kidney, 83t
Wind, 15f, 17
Wire coating, 152
Wiring, 24
Wisconsin River incident, 723
Wiskott-Aldrich syndrome, 148t, 160
Woburn, Massachusetts, incident, 642-643
Wood preservatives, 25, 421t
Wood stoves/smoke, 25t, 421t, 423
  children and, 391, 392t
  environmental history and, 236
Workplace environment, 3, 4, 5, 12; see also Occupation
  accidents in, 28
  agricultural, 409
  aplastic anemia and, 210
  benzene and, 204, 212
  children and adolescents and, 408-415
  co-worker psychosocial agents in, 12
  different exposure levels in same, 51
  exposure assessment and, 42-44
  eyes/vision and, 240
  improving patients' life-style and, 732-733
  indoor air pollution in, 419-437
  industrial settings and, 44
  inhalation exposure and, 38
  man-made fibers and, 458
  MSDSs and, 224-225, 592-594
  occupational medicine and, 5
  OSHA and, 43-44
  overlap between community and, 5
  overlap between home and, 4f, 5
  preexisting conditions and, 362-365
  repeated, low-level exposures in, 10
  sick building syndrome and, 434-435
  toxic profile of, 12
  trauma in, 12
World Health Organization (WHO), 7, 44
  food contamination and, 498-500
  IARC of, 90
  neurobehavioral testing for toxicity and, 190
Wounds, cancer and, 85, 87

X
Xenobiotics, 66, 67
  activation vs. detoxification and, 71
  age and, 365
  dermal toxicology and, 182
  developmental toxicology and, 117-127
  female reproductive function and, 105-109, 113
  gastrointestinal tract and, 300, 301
  liver and, 302-305
  and mechanisms of toxicity, 73-75
  metabolism and, 66
  microsomal enzyme induction and, 75
  multiple chemical sensitivity and, 372
  respiratory toxicology and, 168, 171
  toxicokinetics and, 71
Xylene, 21t, 133, 191t, 599
  ears/hearing and, 260
  eyes/vision and, 245

Y
YuCheng, 129, 135
Yusho, 116, 129, 135

Z
Zinc, 82, 97, 223
  in drinking water, 44t
  immunotoxicology and, 151